THE SECRETORY IMMUNE SYSTEM

ANNALS OF THE NEW YORK ACADEMY OF SCIENCES
Volume 409

THE SECRETORY IMMUNE SYSTEM

Edited by Jerry R. McGhee and Jiri Mestecky

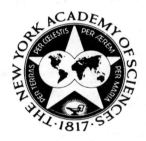

The New York Academy of Sciences
New York, New York
1983

Cover photo: A section of small intestine (rabbit) stained with FITC anti-α. Numerous IgA-plasma cells are apparent in the lamina propria, and transport of pIgA from the basement membrane across the epithelium to the brush border is evident.

Library of Congress Cataloging in Publication Data

Main entry under title:

The Secretory immune system.

(Annals of the New York Academy of Sciences; v. 409)
Proceedings of the Conference on the Secretory
Immune System, held May 4–7, 1982, at the New York
Academy of Sciences.
Bibliography: p.
Includes index.
1. Immune response—Congresses.   2. Immunity—
Congresses.   3. Immunoglobulins—Congresses.   I. McGhee,
Jerry R.   II. Mestecky, Jiri, 1941– .   II. Con-
ference on the Secretory Immune System (1982: New
York Academy of Sciences)   IV. Series.   [DNLM:
1. Allergy and immunology—Congresses.   W1 AN626YL
v. 409/QW   504   S446 1982]
Q11.N5   vol. 409   [QR186]   500s [616.079]
83-12118

SP
Printed in the United States of America
ISBN 0–89766-210-5 (cloth)
ISBN 0–89766-211-3 (paper)

ANNALS OF THE NEW YORK ACADEMY OF SCIENCES
VOLUME 409
June 30, 1983
THE SECRETORY IMMUNE SYSTEM*

Editors and Conference Organizers
JERRY R. MCGHEE AND JIRI MESTECKY

———————◆———————

CONTENTS

*This series of papers is the result of a conference entitled The Secretory Immune System
held May 4–7, 1982 by The New York Academy of Sciences.

Part IV. Transport of IgA and the Role of the Liver

Part V. Secretory and Systemic Immunity and Immune Dysfunctions

Part VIII. Poster Papers

Financial assistance was received from:
- ABBOTT LABORATORIES
- BURROUGHS WELLCOME COMPANY
- FOOD AND DRUG ADMINISTRATION—BUREAU OF BIOLOGICS
  NATIONAL INSTITUTES OF HEALTH
- ICI AMERICAS INC.
- IMPERIAL CHEMICAL INDUSTRIES PLC, PHARMACEUTICALS DIVISION
- McNEIL PHARMACEUTICAL
- MERCK SHARP AND DOHME RESEARCH LABORATORIES
- NATIONAL SCIENCE FOUNDATION
- OFFICE OF NAVAL RESEARCH
- ORTHO PHARMACEUTICAL CORPORATION
- SEARLE RESEARCH AND DEVELOPMENT
- UNITED STATES ARMY MEDICAL RESEARCH AND DEVELOPMENT COMMAND

INTRODUCTORY REMARKS

Jerry R. McGhee

Department of Microbiology
University of Alabama in Birmingham
Birmingham, Alabama 35294

The induction of immune responses to foreign antigens in external secretions comprises many cellular and molecular events that have only been partially elucidated. The expression of IgA in external secretions and serum represents one of the most important forms of immunity to the host. The decade of the 1960s began with the discovery that IgA is the principal immunoglobulin isotype found in external secretions and saw the infancy of mucosal immunity. The 1970s was a period during which the precise composition of secretory IgA was determined and in which it was discovered that IgA-producing plasma cells are present in the highest percentage in mucosal tissues. This decade was also characterized by the realization that a common mucosal immune defense system exists, and that exposure to environmental antigens either by inhalation or ingestion leads to IgA-antibody responses in several mucosal tissues.

IgA research has grown exponentially. Areas now receiving close attention include regulation of the IgA response, characterization of mucosal inductive sites including GALT and BALT, and the basis for the induction of oral tolerance. Other studies examine mechanisms used in the activation of IgA-precursor B-cells and their selective homing to mucosal tissues. Considerable attention is also being given to the precise effector functions of secretory and serum IgA. These important studies include both IgA-immune complexes and polymeric IgA removal by the hepatobiliary route. These and other currently important areas are the topic of this conference on the secretory immune system. It is worthy of note that this represents the first New York Academy of Sciences conference devoted entirely to this subject. The fast pace of research in this area probably now dictates large symposia at closer intervals or smaller workshops.

The first session of this conference deals with environmental influences on the induction of the IgA response. This includes regulation of B-cells for IgA synthesis, expression of IgA genes, and lymphoreticular cell types present in IgA-inductive sites.

The second session focuses on the important observation that oral administration of antigen can simultaneously lead to IgA responses in secretions and systemic unresponsiveness or oral tolerance. These presentations also fully address the subject of homing of sensitized lymphoid cells from GALT and BALT to other lymphoid areas.

The third session focuses more closely on regulatory aspects of cells engaged in the IgA response. These studies include discussion of the IgA-rheumatoid factor and the role of IgE in mucosal immunity. Aging and mucosal immunity also receives emphasis.

The fourth session largely focuses on recent aspects of transport of IgA and IgA-immune complexes by the liver. These studies report immunohistochemical characterizations of transport and the function of the liver in maintenance of IgA homeostasis. Newer aspects of IgA transport into other external secretions are also covered.

The fifth session is devoted entirely to IgA immunity and immune dysfunctions in man. Emphasis is placed on studies of patients with selective IgA deficiency and the cellular and molecular basis for this immune dysfunction. Other subjects addressed are oral immunization for induction of IgA responses to antigens of microbial pathogens and cell-mediated immunity at mucosal surfaces.

The sixth session is devoted entirely to effector functions of IgA. These include studies of mechanisms of IgA inhibition of microbial adherence at mucosae and IgA$_1$ protease produced by mucosal pathogens. A series of papers also addresses specific adjuvants for enhancement of the IgA-immune response.

The last session focuses on practical aspects of induction of IgA responses to current vaccines. Newer approaches to immunization that give attention to antigen form and its delivery to inductive sites for IgA responses are addressed.

Perhaps the most obvious benefit of past symposia on the secretory immune system is that they have allowed young investigators the opportunity to present their findings to others in this field. For this reason, poster papers have been included.

MUCOSAL IMMUNITY*

L. Å. Hanson,†‡ S. Ahlstedt,‡ B. Andersson,‡ B. Carlssoh,‡
M. F. Cole,§ J. R. Cruz,¶ U. Dahlgren,‡ T. H. Ericsson,‖ F. Jalil,#
S. R. Khan,#
L. Mellander,‡ R. Schneerson,** C. Svanborg Edén,‡
T. Söderström,‡ and C. Wadsworth‡

‡Department of Clinical Immunology
Institute of Medical Microbiology
and Department of Pediatrics
University of Göteborg
Göteborg, Sweden
§National Caries Program, National Institute of Dental Research
National Institutes of Health
Bethesda, Maryland 20205
¶Institute of Nutrition of Central America and Panama
Guatemala City, Guatemala
‖Department of Cariology
University of Umeå
Umeå, Sweden
#Department of Pediatrics
King Edward Medical College
Lahore, Pakistan
**Bureau of Biologics
Food and Drug Administration
Bethesda, Maryland 20857

In phylogeny and ontogeny, IgA arises relatively late. Once appearing, this immunoglobulin seems to take on an important role. More than half of all immunoglobulin-producing cells may be synthesizing IgA, and according to Heremans, it is produced at a higher rate than any other immunoglobulin.[1] The high number of mostly IgA-producing cells in the intestinal mucosa, amounting to approximately 10^{10} cells per meter of gut,[2] indicates the importance of the secretory IgA system for the protection of the mucous membranes. For IgA-producing cells to be present in approximately 40 m^2 of intestinal mucosa presupposes tremendous numbers of cells, irrespective of their protective role. The fact that so many individuals deficient in IgA are not having infectious problems[3,4] can be used to question the protective role of IgA. On the other hand, it may only illustrate that secretory IgA (sIgA) is just one of many defense factors

*Keynote address.

This review is based on work supported by grants provided by the Medical Faculty, University of Göteborg, Sweden; the Swedish Medical Research Council (No. 215); the Swedish Agency for Research Cooperation with Developing Countries; the National Swedish Board for Technical Development; the Volkswagen Foundation, West Germany; The Ellen, Walter, and Lennart Hesselman Foundation for Scientific Research, Sweden; and the First of May Flower Campaign Fund, Sweden.

†To whom correspondence should be addressed: Department of Clinical Immunology, Guldhedsgatan 10 A, S 413 46 Göteborg, Sweden.

1

in operation at the mucosal membranes, and that compensatory mechanisms exist.

Mucosal antigenic exposure, for example in the colon, results in local production and secretion of specific sIgA antibodies in the mucosa, as demonstrated by the classical study of Ogra and Karzon, who introduced poliovirus vaccine into the gut by means of colostomies.[5] It is not as obvious why antigenic exposure on mucous membranes results in sIgA antibodies appearing in secretions from, for example, mammary, salivary, and lacrimal glands that are remote from mucous membranes. The local IgA is produced by transferred committed B-lymphoblasts from the gut and bronchial-associated lymphoid tissues (GALT and BALT) to, among others, the mammary glands, as illustrated by animal experiments.[6,7] IgA-producing cells are abundant in the mammary glands of several species, including man.[8,9] The local stimulus to the IgA synthesis in the gland is not known; it has not been ruled out that antigen may reach the gland. Another possibility is an uptake of dimeric serum IgA by means of the glandular epithelial secretory component (SC) with a transfer into the exocrine secretion, as demonstrated in the liver of rats.[10] Halsey et al.[11] have recently demonstrated such a transfer, to account for a major portion of the milk sIgA in mice, at least early in lactation. This happens presumably before the homing to the gland of IgA-producing cells, directed by lactogenic hormones, reaches its peak.[12] It is surprising, however, that Halsey et al. find the level of polymeric IgA in serum to increase during lactation. Either this is the result of a backflow of IgA produced in or taken up by the mammary glands—which would disturb their conclusions—or lactogenic hormones increasing the polymer IgA production in other sites.

Brandtzaeg has demonstrated the same density of IgA-producing cells in the mammary and parotid glands in man, and he has also noted large amounts of sIgA in acinar and tubular cells of the mammary gland.[9] A contribution of IgA, originating from the serum polymer IgA fraction, to the sIgA in human milk has not been excluded. Studies of human milk, by thin-layer chromatography in Sephadex G-200 Superfine, followed by a superimposed antibody-containing agar layer,[13] show obvious changes during the onset of lactation. The sIgA, 11S component dominates the precolostrum, but there is often some 7S IgA. Free SC is also present, as well as fragments thereof.[14] 7S IgA is usually not seen in colostrum; there is only SC in addition to the major sIgA fraction (FIGURE 1). As the milk volume increases during the early phase of lactation, this patterns seems to remain. The significant 7S IgA component, as noted in mouse milk[11] is not seen.

There are other species differences; in the rat we could not show any transfer of thoracic duct lymph IgA antibodies into milk, as was noted in bile.[15] In these studies we noticed that after Ductus thoracicus drainage, the total bile IgA levels decreased rapidly, whereas the levels of specific IgA antibodies induced by immunization of the rats with E. coli O6 remained. Passively administered, IgA anti-O4 antibodies decreased as rapidly as the total IgA levels. Cell cultures suggested a synthesis of the IgA anti-O6 antibodies, in among other places, the spleen. Such an IgA synthesis, followed by transport by means of the serum reaching the liver, might explain the persistence of the bile anti-O6 antibodies; alternatively lymph, carrying IgA produced in the thorax, could be the origin. In

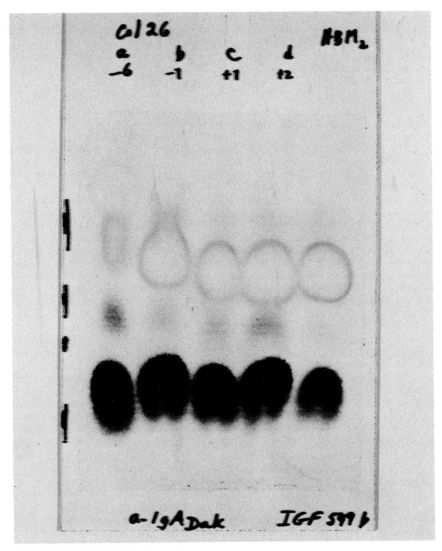

FIGURE 1. Thin-layer gel chromatography in Sephadex G-200 Superfine of milk samples. From left to right: precolostrum, taken 6 and 1 days before parturition (a and b), colostrum taken days 1 and 2 after parturition (c and d), all from the same mother. HBM$_2$ is a milk pool. After the separation step with buffer flow downwards an agar layer containing anti-α and anti-SC antibodies was overlayered. The heavy precipitate, formed with the fastest filtering component, corresponds to 11S secretory IgA; behind that is 7S IgA, followed by SC, which is seen as fragments in the precolostrum samples. In the left margin is indicated in ink the localization of human serum proteins included in the same run, showing as the three main fractions, the 19S, 7s, and albumin components.

the human, Brown et al.[16] did not find any difference in the level of polymeric IgA in thoracic duct lymph, portal vein, or aortic blood. They suggested that this does not support hepatic clearance of serum IgA as a major origin of bile sIgA in the human. They also had some evidence for the existence of IgA-synthesizing cells adjacent to the bile ducts in the liver hilus. Possibly serum IgA does not significantly contribute to the sIgA in secretions in man.

THE INDUCTION OF sIgA ANTIBODIES IN SECRETIONS BY IMMUNIZATION

Since sIgA antibodies can protect against many viral infections, including myxo- and rhinoviruses,[17] as well as against various bacterial infections, such as cholera,[18] many studies have been devoted to finding the most efficient mode of immunization for an sIgA response.[19] In previous studies, we found that parenteral vaccination of lactating women against cholera[20] and polio,[21] boosted the naturally acquired milk and saliva sIgA antibodies. In unexposed individuals no or a limited, short-lasting response was obtained.[20,21] Primary oral immunization in mice against cholera may require repeated doses to be successful,[22] whereas oral exposure to the bacteria, followed by parenteral booster, was most efficient in inducing intestinal antibodies in this species.[23,24] Recently a cholera enterotoxin-in-B-subunit-vaccine was found to give similar intestinal IgA booster responses in naturally exposed humans, whether given perorally or intramuscularly.[25]

By contrast, oral immunization with live poliovirus vaccine in naturally exposed lactating women was often found not to increase but rather to decrease the milk sIgA anti-poliovirus antibody levels.[21,26] A simultaneous parenteral cholera vaccination further decreased the sIgA poliovirus antibody response, although the cholera sIgA antibody response in milk and saliva was undisturbed, suggesting a specific defect of the poliovirus response. In ongoing studies, we confirmed the boosting effect on milk sIgA antibodies to poliovirus by parenterally administered inactivated vaccine. The Swedish inactivated vaccine gave, in most instances, a milk sIgA response which lasted only 2–3 months; whereas preliminary data, with a new more antigen-rich Dutch vaccine kindly provided by Dr. van Wezel, showed a longer-lasting sIgA response (FIGURES 2a and b). With two exceptions the live peroral poliovirus vaccine decreased the sIgA anti-poliovirus titers or had no effect (FIGURE 2c). One of the unvaccinated controls showed a response during follow-up, indicating the presence of the wild virus in Lahore, Pakistan, where the study was performed (FIGURE 2d).

We compared modes of immunization with Escherichia coli O6 in rats, that is perorally (p.o.), intravenously (i.v.), and into the Peyer's patches (PP). Whereas the levels of IgG antibodies in serum, milk, and bile appeared to be similar, the IgM response was lower in milk and bile after the iv injection than after the PP injection. The serum IgM anti-O6 levels were equally high after iv or PP injection (FIGURE 3a). More IgA anti-O6 antibodies were also formed in milk and in bile after the PP injection than after iv administration (FIGURE 3b). Peroral immunization induced no response in milk, whereas the milk IgA and IgM antibodies were high on day 9 after immunization in the PP, but were not demonstrable after 30 days. In contrast, the IgG milk antibodies remained elevated (FIGURE 4).

Recently, Peri et al.[27] showed that peroral and intratracheal, but not iv, immunization of rabbits with respiratory syncytial virus, resulted in milk, bronchial, and intestinal IgA antibodies. Similar administration of bovine serum albumin (BSA) induced only IgG antibodies, illustrating possible species differ-

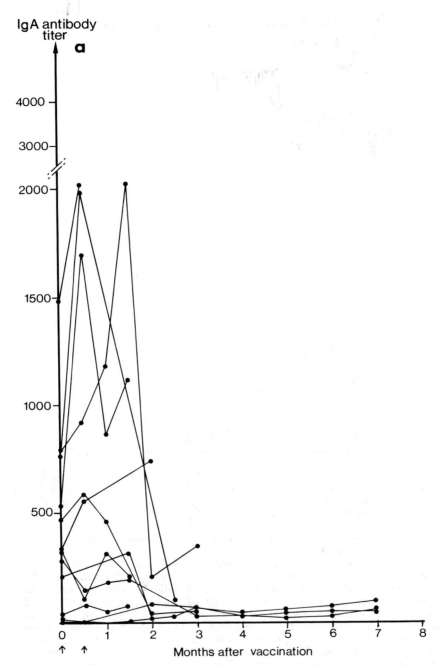

FIGURE 2. Milk sIgA antibodies in lactating Pakistani women against poliovirus type 1 antigen determined with ELISA. Titers given as the highest dilution reciprocal showing an O.D. of 0.2 above background. They were vaccinated about four weeks after parturition. Arrows indicate vaccinations.

Figure 2a) The response after two subcutaneous injections, two weeks apart, of the Swedish commercial inactivated poliovirus vaccine.

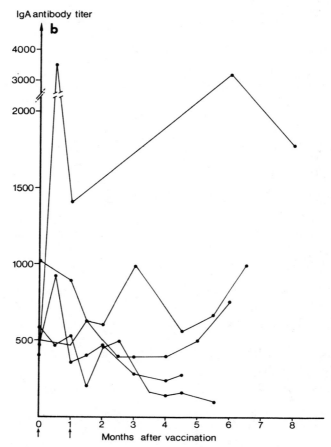

Figure 2b) The response after two subcutaneous injections, one month apart, of a Dutch inactivated poliovirus vaccine kindly provided by Dr. van Wezel, Rijks Institut voor de Volksgezondheid, Bilthoven, the Netherlands.

ences, but also differences in response against various antigens, as noted previously by Ebersole et al.[28,29]

Rats were given p.o. either live or formalin-killed E.coli O6:K13:H1, followed one month later by a K13-BSA conjugate subcutaneously. Utilizing the ELISA technique, IgM and IgG, but no IgA antibodies to the K13 polysaccharide, were detected (TABLE 1). In saliva, however, the best IgA response against the K13 antigen was obtained in the rats who were given the K13 conjugate after peroral exposure to the K13 antigen on either live or killed bacteria. Peroral bacterial exposure or parenteral K13 conjugate administration alone induced lower antibody levels. These studies support our observations in humans that the most efficient sIgA response may be obtained by parenteral booster following mucosal exposure.[20,21]

Many vaccines contain components to which the vaccinee has already been naturally exposed and primed. Vaccine-boosted mucosal responses may play a

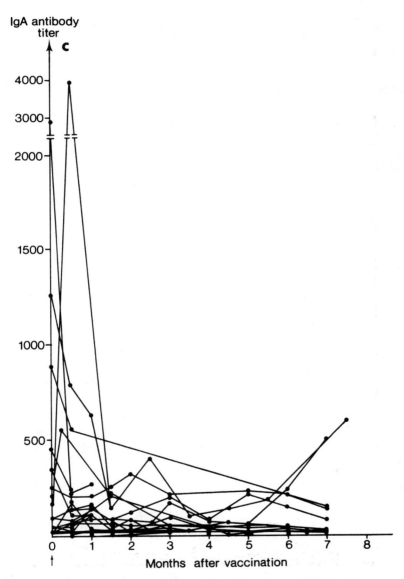

Figure 2c) The response after oral vaccination with a commercial live poliovirus vaccine, kindly provided by Behringwerke AG, Marburg/Lahn, FRG.

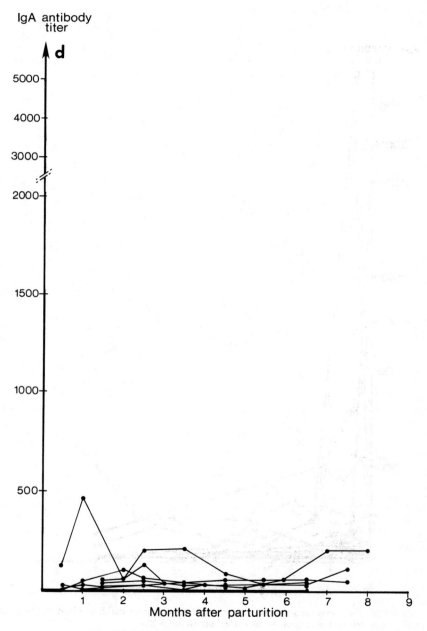

Figure 2d) Antibody levels in unvaccinated women.

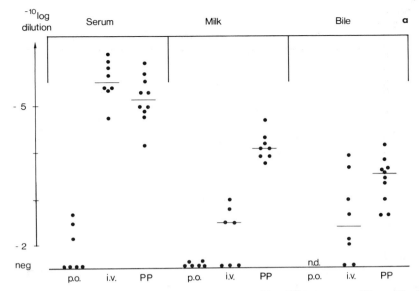

FIGURE 3a. IgM anti-O6 antibodies in rats immunized by different routes. The antibody activity was measured with ELISA and expressed as the dilution giving 0.1 absorbance units (405 nm) above background, at 100 minutes of enzyme/substrate reaction time. Each dot represents one rat, and the bars denote the median. The samples were taken eight days after the last immunization. Neg = no detectable antibodies at 1/100 sample dilution. p.o. = 10^9 live *E. coli* O6:K13 daily for six days by gastric intubation. i.v. = 10^9 formalin-killed *E. coli* O6:K13 intravenously. P.p. = 10^9 formalin-killed *E. coli* O6:K13 in the Peyer's patches.

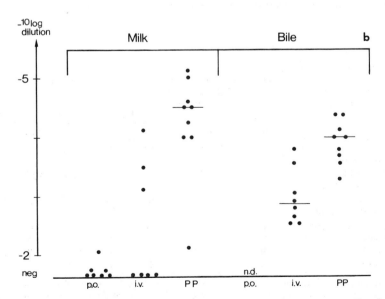

FIGURE 3b. IgA anti-O6 antibodies in rats immunized by various routes. For further information see legend to FIGURE 3a.

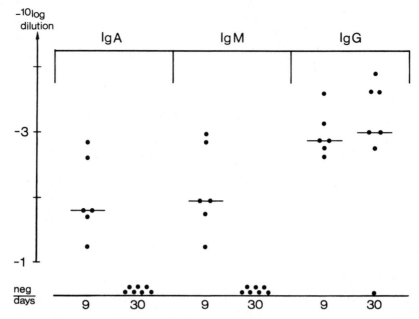

FIGURE 4. *E. coli* anti-O6 antibodies in rat milk 9 and 30 days after immunization. The rats were immunized in the Peyer's patches with 10^9 formalin-killed *E. coli* O6:K13. Milk was collected on day 9 and 30 after parturition. The antibody activity was measured with the ELISA and expressed as the dilution giving 0.1 absorbance units above background at 100 minutes of enzyme/substrate reaction time. Each dot represents one rat and the bars denote the median. Neg = no detectable antibodies at 1/10 sample dilution.

TABLE 1

IMMUNE RESPONSE TO THE K13 POLYSACCHARIDE INDUCED BY LIVE OR FORMALIN-KILLED *ESCHERICHIA COLI* O6:K13:H1 BACTERIA FOLLOWED BY K13 POLYSACCHARIDE-BSA CONJUGATE*

	Number of Animals	Serum Antibodies			Saliva Antibodies		
		IgG	IgM	IgA	IgG	IgM	IgA
Live *E. coli*	8	508	427	<100	612	441	424
Live *E. coli*, K13-BSA	9	234	335	<100	534	408	517
Formalin-killed *E. coli*	8	<100	158	<100	403	385	432
Formalin-killed *E. coli*, K13-BSA	8	496	404	<100	607	426	521
K13-BSA × 1	9	112	210	<100	650	400	372
K13-BSA × 2	9	378	1,374	<100	607	448	404
Unimmunized	5	148	233	<100	282	232	352

*SPF rats, 28 days old, were fed 10^8 live *E. coli* or 10^8 formalin-killed *E. coli* every second day for 39 days and/or injected subcutaneously with 2.5 µg of K13-BSA conjugate once or twice. The antibody levels by ELISA of the pooled sera were expressed as OD readings at 405 nm above background after 100 minutes.

role in the protection attained by some vaccines, often attributed to the serum antibody response alone.

Secretory IgA antibodies against food proteins appear in secretions in humans, including milk. In previous studies sIgA antibodies to cow's milk proteins, black beans, and soy proteins were frequently found in the milk of Guatemalan women.[30,31] It was suggested that sIgA antibodies against these antigens and against *E.coli*, *Salmonella*, and *Shigella* antigens are formed equally efficiently in undernourished and in well-nourished mothers. It is possible that the migration of lymphoid cells to the lactating mammary gland, being directed by the lactogenic hormones, makes the mammary gland an immunologically privileged site. This may be true since the levels of lactogenic hormones are higher in undernourished than in well-nourished lactating mothers.[32] By peroral administration of an uncommon protein from cow peas, to lactating Guatemalan women, we could induce a milk IgA response in women without anti-food protein antibodies. One mother with a high antibody level showed a temporary depression of her response.[33] This mother may illustrate the development of tolerance. It is of interest to determine whether or not such a mechanism is involved also in the deficient sIgA responses against perorally given live poliovirus vaccine.

THE ONTOGENY OF THE sIGA RESPONSE

It is intriguing that the neonate can handle the load of microorganisms that colonize its mucosal membranes after birth, especially the respiratory and gastrointestinal tracts. Various bacteria, including *E.coli*, carry adhesins such as fimbriae or pili, which mediate attachment of the bacteria to various ligands in mucus or on epithelial cells.[34] Other pili exist, some of which are present on pyelonephritogenic *E.coli* and bind to receptors encompassing the Galα1→4Gal moiety of globoseries glycolipids on urinary tract epithelium.[34-36] Little is known about how the mucosal antibody response is developed against these various *E.coli* antigens in the infant.

We investigated the *E.coli* that comprised the major aerobic flora colonizing the throat and gut of 22 neonates during the first week of life. O antigen and the presence of type 1 pili were determined and related to the sIgA in the saliva of infants and children. Most *E.coli* strains carried adhesins, but less than a third had the mannose-sensitive type 1 pili. These were expected to be important for colonization since they may be associated with intestinal mucus.[37] The majority of the strains carried adhesins with the Galα1→4Gal specificity (FIGURE 5). This fact is surprising, since the Galα1→4Gal-containing receptor glycolipids are not found on adult human small-intestinal epithelium.[35] Other, as yet undetected, adhesins pili may also be present with specificities for structures in the intestinal mucus or mucosa.

Whole, unstimulated saliva was collected from infants and children starting on the day of birth. sIgA was quantitated with a modified ELISA,[38] and IgA and sIgA antibodies against *E.coli* O and pili antigens were determined by ELISA. sIgA appeared in saliva during the first few days of life and increased slowly (FIGURE 6). The levels of sIgA anti-O antibodies were low during the major part of the first year and increased thereafter (FIGURE 7). Inhibition experiments supported specificity of the IgA antibodies against *E.coli* O antigens. The infants obviously produced salivary sIgA antibodies early but at low levels. Burgio *et al.*,[39] studying infants older than two months, also found a slow increase of salivary IgA antibodies. Some previous studies suggested that adult levels of salivary IgA were attained during the first few months of life.[40] These differing results may have technical explanations.

Preliminary studies on salivary IgA antibodies against *E.coli* pili in infants showed very low antibody levels against type 1 pili and against the Galα1→4Gal-binding pili. There was a rise in level according to increasing age, but slower than that found for anti-O antibodies (cp TABLE 2 and FIGURE 7).

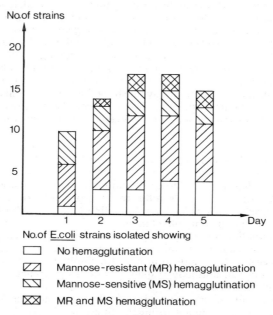

No.of E.coli strains isolated showing

☐	No hemagglutination
▨	Mannose-resistant (MR) hemagglutination
◺	Mannose-sensitive (MS) hemagglutination
▧	MR and MS hemagglutination

FIGURE 5. The dominating *E. coli* strains in the aerobic stool flora from the first five days of life of 22 healthy newborns. The strains were investigated for presence of pili by hemagglutination in the presence and absence of mannose. The type 1 pili were identified by their mannose-sensitivity (MS); the mannose-resistant (MR) ones were further characterized by their specificity for the globoseries glycolipid receptor.

HUMAN MILK AND MUCOSAL DEFENSE

Human milk contains sIgA antibodies against numerous *E.coli* O and K antigens.[41-43] Secretory IgA antibodies against various *E.coli* pili are also found in milk.[44] The milk provides a rich source of sIgA antibodies against virulence factors on the potentially pathogenic *E.coli* colonizing the newborn and infant. With the slow development of the infant's own sIgA response as judged from the saliva studies, the mother's milk antibodies may be important, as is illustrated by the fact that gastrointestinal and upper respiratory infections are less common in breast-fed than nonbreast-fed infants. This protection is most evident for the more heavily exposed infants in developing countries, but it also exists in developed countries, independent of the parents' socioeconomic level.[45-48]

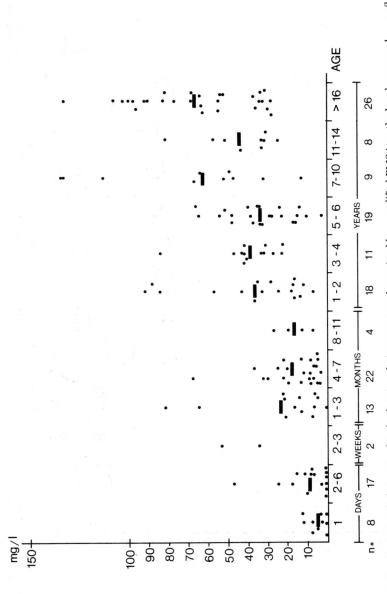

FIGURE 6. Total sIgA in whole unstimulated saliva in relation to age as determined by a modified ELISA method and expressed as mg/l. The numbers of subjects in the age groups are given, and the bars represent the mean values.

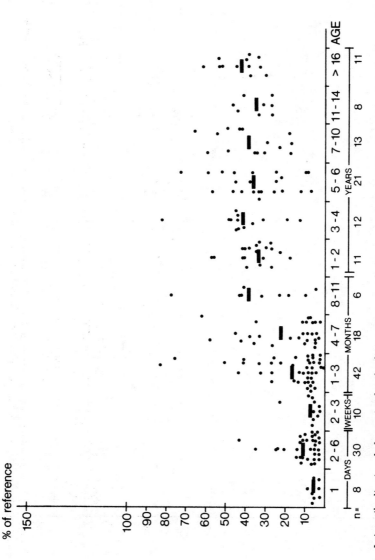

FIGURE 7. sIgA antibodies in whole unstimulated saliva against a pool of ten common *E. coli* O antigens in relation to age as determined by ELISA and expressed in percent of a milk pool reference. The bars represent the means for the age groups. The numbers of subjects in the age groups are given.

It should be noted that the protective effect of milk need not depend on the sIgA antibodies alone, since there are a number of other protective factors in milk.[49] Recently Holmgren et al.[50] showed that hemagglutination of red cells by V. cholerae and E.coli, presumably mediated by adhesins, was inhibited more efficiently by a nonimmunoglobulin-containing milk fraction than by the immunoglobulin-containing one.

Otitis media has been reported to occur at a lower frequency in breast-fed than in formula-fed infants.[45,47,51] The mechanism is unknown but a breast-fed suckling baby is "bathing" its upper respiratory mucosa in milk. We have noticed that pneumococci causing otitis media attach more efficiently to retropharyngeal

TABLE 2

IgA Antibodies in Salivas from Infants and Children (4–6 Pooled Per Age Group) Against Various E. coli Pili Antigens

	Antibody Levels (ELISA)*		
Age	NMS Pilus†	Junior Type 1 Pilus	MR Pili Pool‡
Week			
1	<100	<100	<100
Months			
1	<100	<100	<100
2	<100	<100	<100
3	224	n d§	295
4	315	n d	340
5	132	<100	119
6	106	<100	160
7	122	<100	141
8–9	103	138	201
Years			
1–2	177	<100	nd
2–3	103	<100	322
3–4	102	109	288

*Values given as $E_{405} \times 100$ is ELISA above background. Values below 100 considered negligible.
†NMS pilus = Nonmannose sensitive pilus, similar to the colonization factor I, was, as type 1 pilus, kindly provided by Dr. C. Brinton, Pittsburgh, Pa.
‡MR = Mannose-resistant, urinary tract E. coli pilus pool.
§nd = not done.

cells than do pneumococci of other origin.[52] Human milk was found to efficiently prevent this attachment (TABLE 3). Attachment was also prevented, however, by milk from an IgA deficient mother, and by both a high and a low molecular weight (MW) fraction of pooled normal milk. Decreasing the immunoglobulin content in the high MW fraction to 1/25 with an anti Ig-immunosorbent did not decrease the anti-attachment. Intermediate MW fractions did not inhibit the attachment. Svanborg Edén et al.[36] present results showing that pneumococci bind to the oligosaccharide moiety of neolactoseries glycolipids on retropharyngeal cells. Such oligosaccharides are present in human milk[36] and may prevent attachment of pneumococci to epithelial cells as specifically as antibodies. The presence of such oligosaccharide components in milk, in addition to milk sIgA antibodies against pneumococci, may explain why breast-feeding seems to protect against *otitis media.*

IgG AND IgM ANTIBODIES AND MUCOSAL IMMUNITY

Brandtzaeg has demonstrated large amounts of IgG in the extracellular spaces of the gastrointestinal mucosa.[53] It may well be that the IgG antibodies in this locale, and in the passage into the lumen, can prevent microbial invasion by way of mucous membranes. If so, the maternal IgG antibodies acquired by the human offspring transplacentally can also play a role in mucosal defense.

To study the prevention of bacteremia by parenterally injected antibodies, we used a model of neonatal rats colonized perorally with *E.coli* K_1 strains. It was found that monoclonal IgM anti-K_1 antibodies, when given subcutaneously,

TABLE 3

INHIBITION OF ADHESION OF *S. PNEUMONIAE* TO RETROPHARYNGEAL CELLS
BY HUMAN MILK

	sIgA g/l	Bacteria/epithelial Cell	
		Test	Saline
Milk pool	1.2	1	132
Milk fraction*			
High MW	1.28	0	133
High MW after			
immunoadsorption†	0.054	3	133
Intermediate MW	nd‡	265	234
Low MW	0.0017	12	138
IgA deficient milk	0	8	246

*The milk pool fractions were obtained by Sephacryl S-300 chromatography and designated according to molecular weight (MW) of the components.
†Anti-human Ig conjugated to Sepharose.
‡nd = not done

protected efficiently against invasion from the intestinal tract.[54] In contrast, anti-type 1 pili gave no protection, perhaps because the antibodies were directed only against type 1 pili, weakly recognized by the antibodies. As indicated by Svanborg Edén et al.,[36] antibodies against type 1 pili may protect at the bladder mucosal level against urinary tract infections, although they protect poorly against intraperitoneal *E.coli* infections in mice.[60] It seems that type 1 pili may occur more often on *E.coli* present on mucous membranes, than on *E.coli* infecting tissues.[61] This may explain why protection should only be expected at the mucosal level.

Polysaccharide capsules are obligatory virulence factors for *Hemophilus influenzae, E.coli, Neisseria meningitidis* and pneumococci–all important pathogens for infants and small children. Antibodies against these polysaccharides belong primarily to the IgG_2 class. The B-lymphocytes producing IgG_2, are as slow to appear ontogenetically as are the IgA-producing cells.[52a] At 24 months of age these B-lymphocytes are still few, which may explain the poor response of children under two years of age to polysaccharide vaccines.[55] The prevalence of infections with these encapsulated bacteria in this age group may be similarly explained.

The importance of IgG_2 antibodies for host defense is illustrated by the predominance of upper and lower respiratory tract infections in IgG_2 deficient individuals.[57] Among 39 individuals with IgA deficiency, discovered during workup for various diseases, we found IgG_2 deficiency in nine of the individuals with most infections.[58] Among 22 ataxia-telangiectasia patients, those with severe respiratory tract infections showed decreased levels of IgG_2 rather than IgA deficiency.[59] Whereas IgA deficiency may be compensated for by increased local production of IgM and possibly other factors, IgG_2 deficiency may remain uncompensated.

SUMMARY

Mucosal defense is provided by a number of host factors countering the specific virulence factors of the many microorganisms infecting the mucous membranes. Secretory IgA antibodies presumably play an important role. Increase of the sIgA antibodies may most advantageously be attained by parenteral immunization, following mucosal priming. This was demonstrated in a rat model, where it was also noted that antigen injection into PP induced high milk IgA antibody levels.

In man, parenteral vaccination against polio increased the sIgA antibody levels in the milk of mothers previously exposed naturally to the poliovirus. The response was relatively short-lived. In the previously unexposed, there was little or no response. By contrast peroral immunization with live poliovirus vaccine did not increase, or even decrease, the milk sIgA poliovirus antibody levels.

Although salivary sIgA antibodies against antigens of colonizing *E.coli* appear during the first days of life, they are slow to increase. This deficiency is richly compensated for by all the sIgA antibodies that are provided the baby through the milk.

No transfer of dimeric IgA into the milk could be shown in lactating rats, in contrast to what has been reported in mice. There is no evidence for a contribution to milk sIgA from serum in man. Close to parturition, human milk often contains some 7S IgA and various sizes of free SC, in addition to the dominating 11S sIgA. A few days later there is almost exclusively monomeric SC and 11S sIgA.

IgG antibodies also play a role at the mucosal level. IgG_2 antibodies against the bacterial polysaccharide capsule are as slow to appear as sIgA in ontogeny, possibly explaining the prevalence of infections with encapsulated bacteria and the poor response to polysaccharide vaccines in early childhood.

Other defense factors preventing infections by way of mucous membranes may be important. Thus, oligosaccharides present in human milk seem to specifically prevent pneumococcal attachment to retropharyngeal cells. This anti-attachment capacity, in addition to that provided by milk and salivary IgA antibodies, may explain why breast-fed babies have less *otitis media* than formula-fed ones.

REFERENCES

1. HEREMANS, J. F. 1975. The secretory immune system. A critical reappraisal. *In* The Immune Systems and Infectious Diseases. E. Neter and F. Milgrom, Eds.: 376–385. Karger. Basel, London.
2. HEREMANS, J. F. 1974. Immunoglobulin A. *In* The Antigens. M. Sela, Ed. Vol. II: 365–522. Academic Press. New York.
3. ROCKEY, J. H., L. Å. HANSON, J. F. HEREMANS & H. G. KUNKEL. 1964. Beta 2A-aglobulinemia in two healthy men. J. Lab. Clin. Med. **63:** 205–212.
4. HANSON, L. Å., J. BJÖRKANDER & V. OXELIUS. 1982. Selective IgA deficiency. *In* Immunodeficiency Diseaes. R. K. Chandra, Ed. Churchill Livingstone. Edinburgh. In press.
5. OGRA, P. L. & D. T. KARZON. 1969. Distribution of poliovirus antibody in serum, nasopharynx and alimentary tract following segmental immunisation of lower alimentary tract with poliovaccine. J. Immunol. **102:** 1423–1431.
6. BIENENSTOCK, J., M. MACDERMOTT & D. BEFUS. 1979. A common mucosal immune system. *In* Immunology of Breast Milk. P. L. Ogra & D. H. Dayton, Eds.: 91–98. Raven Press. New York.
7. LAMM, M. E., P. WEISZ-CARRINGTON, M. E. ROUX, M. MCWILLIAMS & J. M. PHILLIPS-QUAGLIATA. 1979. Mode of induction of an IgA response in the breast and other secretory sites by oral antigen. *In* Immunology of Breast Milk. P. L. Ogra & D. Dayton, Eds.: 105–109. Raven Press. New York.
8. PUMPHREY, R. S. H. 1977. A comparative study of plasma cells in the mammary gland in pregnancy and lactation. Symp. Zool. Soc. Lond. **41:** 261–276.
9. BRANDTZAEG, P. 1983. Immunohistochemical characteristics of the secretory immune system of lactating human mammary glands. Ann. N.Y. Acad. Sci. This volume.
10. JACKSON, G. D. F., I. LEMAITRE-COELHO, J. P. VAERMAN, H. BAZIN & A. BECKERS. 1978. Rapid disappearance from serum of intravenously injected rat myeloma. IgA and its secretion into bile. Eur. J. Immunol. **8:** 123–126.
11. HALSEY, J. F., C. MITCHELL, R. MEYER & J. J. CEBRA. 1982. Metabolism of immune globulin A in lactating mice: origins of immunoglobulin A in milk. Eur. J. Immunol. **12:** 107–112.
12. WEISZ-CARRINGTON, P., M. E. ROUX & M. E. LAMM. 1977. Plasma cells and epithelial immunoglobulins in the mouse mammary gland during pregnancy and lactation. J. Immunol. **199:** 1306–1309.
13. HANSON, L. Å., J. HOLMGREN & CH. WADSWORTH. 1971. A radial immuno-gel filtration method for characterization and quantitation of macromolecules. Int. Arch. Allergy. Appl. Immun. **40:** 806–819.
14. BRANDTZAEG, P. 1971. Human secretory immunoglobulins. 3 Immunochemical and physiochemical studies of secretory IgA and free secretory piece. Acta Path. Microbiol. Scand. Section B. **79:** 165–188.
15. DAHLGREN, U., S. AHLSTEDT, L. HEDMAN, CH. WADSWORTH & L. Å. HANSON. 1981. Dimeric IgA in the rat is transferred from serum into bile but not into milk. Scand. J. Immunol. **14:** 95–98.
16. BROWN, W. R., P. D. SMITH, E. LEE, R. T. MCCALMON & H. NAGURA. 1982. A search for an enriched source of polymeric IgA in human thoracic duct lymph, portal vein blood and aortic blood. Clin. Exp. Immunol. **48:** 85–90.
17. PERKINS, J. C., H. L. KNOPF, A. Z. KAPIKIAN & R. M. CHANOCK. 1969. The relative role of serum and nasal secretory neutralizing antibodies in protection against experimental rhinovirus illness. *In* The Secretory Immunologic System. National Institute of Child Health and Human Development. Bethesda, MD.
18. FUBARA, E. S. & R. FRETER. 1973. Protection against enteric bacterial infection by secretory IgA antibodies. J. Immunol. **111:** 395–403.
19. ROWLEY, D. 1982. Immune responses to enterobacteriae presented by various routes. *In* Progress in Allergy. Host Parasite Relationships in Gram-Negative Infections. L. Å. Hanson, P. Kallós and O. Westphal, Eds.: Vol. **33:** 159–174. Karger. Basel.
20. SVENNERHOLM, A.-M., L. Å. HANSON, J. HOLMGREN, B. S. LINDBLAD, B. NILSSON &

F. QURESHI. 1980. Different secretory IgA antibody response to cholera vaccination in Swedish and Pakistani women. Infect. Immun. **30:** 427–430.

21. SVENNERHOLM, A.-M., L. Å. HANSON, J. HOLMGREN, B. S. LINDBLAD, SHAUKAT R. KHAN, A. NILSSON & B. SVENNERHOLM. 1981. Milk antibodies to live and killed polio vaccines in Pakistani and Swedish women. J. Inf. Dis. **143:** 707–711.

22. LANGE, S., H. NYGREN, A.-M. SVENNERHOLM & J. HOLMGREN. 1980. Antitoxic cholera immunity in mice: Influence of antigen deposition on antitoxin-containing cells and protective immunity in different parts of the intestine. Infect. Immun. **28:** 17–23.

23. BLOOM, L. & D. ROWLEY. 1979. Local immune response in mice to *V. cholerae*. Aust. J. Exp. Biol. and Med. Sci. **57:** 313–323.

24. HORSFALL, D. J. & D. ROWLEY. 1979. Intestinal antibody to *V. cholerae* in immunised mice. Aust. J. Exp. Biol. Med. Sci. **57:** 75–85.

25. SVENNERHOLM, A.-M., J. HOLMGREN, D. A. SACK & P. K. BARDHAN. 1982. Intestinal antibody responses after immunisation with cholera B subunit. Lancet **1:** 305–307.

26. HANSON, L. Å., B. CARLSSON, F. JALIL, B. S. LINDBLAD & A.-M. SVENNERHOLM. 1981. Implications for immunization. The milk IgA antibody response to live and inactivated poliovirus vaccines. *In* Immunology of Infant Feeding. A. W. Wilkinson, Ed.: 137–144. Plenum Publ. Corp. New York.

27. PERI, B. A., C. M. THEODORE, G. A. LOSONSKY, J. M. FISHAUT, R. M. ROTHBERG & P. L. OGRA. 1982. Antibody content of rabbit milk and serum following inhalation or ingestion of respiratory syncytial virus and bovine serum albumin. Clin. Exp. Immunol. **48:** 91–101.

28. EBERSOLE, J. L., J. A. MOLINARI & D. PLATT. 1975. Sequential appearance of salivary antibodies after oral immunization of axenic mice. Infect. Immun. **12:** 353–359.

29. EBERSOLE, J. L. & J. A. MOLINARI. 1976. Specificity of secretory antibodies to bacterial immunogens. Infect. Immun. **13:** 53–62.

30. HANSON, L. Å., B. CARLSSON, J. R. CRUZ, B. GARCIA, J. HOLMGREN, SHAUKAT R. KHAN, B. S. LINDBLAD, A.-M. SVENNERHOLM, B. SVENNERHOLM & J. URRUTIA. 1979. Immune response in the mammary gland. *In* Immunology of Breast Milk. P. L. Ogra and D. H. Dayton, Eds.: 145–157. Raven Press. New York.

31. CRUZ, J. R., B. GARCIA, J. J. URRUTIA, B. CARLSSON & L. Å. HANSON. 1981. Food antibodies in human milk from Guatemalan women. J. Pediatr. **99:** 600–602.

32. LUNN, P. G., A. M. PRENTICE, S. AUSTIN & R. G. WHITEHEAD. 1980. Influence of maternal diet on plasma-prolactin levels during lactation. Lancet **1:** 623.

33. CRUZ, J. R. & L. Å. HANSON. Specific immune response in human milk to oral immunization with food proteins. Ann. N. Y. Acad. Sci. This volume.

34. SVANBORG EDÉN C., L. HAGBERG, L. Å. HANSON, T. K. KORHONEN, H. LEFFLER & S. OLLING. 1981. Adhesion of *E.coli* in urinary tract infections. *In* Adhesion and Microorganism Pathogenicity. Ciba Symp. **80:** 161–178. Pittman's Medical. London.

35. LEFFLER, H., & C. SVANBORG EDÉN. 1980. Chemical identification of a glycosphingolipid receptor for *Escherichia coli* attaching to human urinary tract epithelial cells and agglutinating human erythrocytes. FEMS Microbiol. Lett. **8:** 127–134.

36. SVANBORG EDÉN C., L. HAGBERG, L. Å. HANSON, H. LEFFLER, G. MAGNUSSON & T. SÖDERSTRÖM. Receptor analogues and anti-pili antibodies as inhibitors of attachment *in vivo* and *in vitro*. Am. N.Y. Acad. Sci. This volume.

37. ØRSKOV, I., F. ØRSKOV, & A. BIRCH-ANDERSEN. 1980. A fimbria *E.coli* antigen, f7, determining uroepithelial adherence. Comparison with type 1 fimbriae which attach to urinary slime. Infect. Immun. **27:** 657–663.

38. SOHL ÅKERLUND, A., L. Å. HANSON, S. AHLSTEDT & B. CARLSSON. 1977. A sensitive method for specific quantitation of secretory IgA. Scand. J. Immunol. **6:** 1275–1282.

39. BURGIO, G. R., A. LANZAVECCHIA, A. PLEBANI, S. JAYAKAR & A. G. UGAZIO. 1980. Ontogeny of secretory immunity: Levels of secretory IgA and natural antibodies in saliva. Pediatr. Res. **14:** 1111–1114.

40. HAWORTH, J. C. & L. DILLING. 1966. Concentration of γ-globulin in serum, saliva and nasopharyngeal secretions of infants and children. J. Lab. Clin. Med. **67:** 922–933.

41. GINDRAT, J.-J., L. GOTHEFORS, L. Å. HANSON & J. WINBERG. 1972. Antibodies in human milk against *E.coli* of the serogroups most commonly found in neonatal infections. Acta Paediatr. Scand. **61:** 587–590.

42. CARLSSON, B., L. GOTHEFORS, S. AHLSTEDT, L. Å. HANSON & J. WINBERG. 1976. Studies of *Escherichia coli* O antigen specific antibodies in human milk, maternal serum and cord blood. Acta Paediatr. Scand. **65:** 216–224.
43. CARLSSON, B., B. KAIJSER, S. AHLSTEDT, L. GOTHEFORS & L. Å. HANSON. 1982. Antibodies against *Escherichia coli* capsular (K) antigens in human milk and serum—their relation to the *E.coli* gut flora of the mother and neonate. Acta Paediatr. Scand. **71:** 313–318.
44. SVANBORG EDÉN, C., B. CARLSSON, L. Å. HANSON, B. JANN, K. JANN, T. KORHONEN & T. WADSTRÖM. 1979. Anti-pili antibodies in breast milk. Lancet **2:** 1235.
45. CUNNINGHAM, S. S. 1979. Morbidity in breast-fed and artificially fed infants II. J. Pediatr. **95:** 685–689.
46. LARSEN, S. A. & D. R. HOMER. 1978. Relation of breast versus bottle feeding to hospitalization for gastroenteritis in a middle-class US population. J. Pediatr. **92:** 417–418.
47. CHANDRA, R. K. 1979. Prospective studies of the effect of breast feeding on incidence of infection and allergy. Acta Paediatr. Scand. **68:** 691–694.
48. MATA, L. J. & J. J. URRUTIA. 1971. Intestinal colonization of breastfed children in a rural area of low socio-economic level. Ann. N.Y. Acad. Sci. **176:** 93–109.
49. HANSON, L. Å. & J. WINBERG. 1972. Breast milk and defence against infection in the newborn. Arch. Dis. Child. **47:** 845–848.
50. HOLMGREN, J., A.-M. SVENNERHOLM & C. ÅHRÉN. 1981. Nonimmunoglobulin fraction of human milk inhibits bacterial adhesion (hemagglutination) and entero-toxin binding of *Escherichia coli* and *Vibrio cholerae*. Infect. Immun. **33:** 136–141.
51. SAARINEN, U. M. 1982. Prolonged breast feeding as prophylaxis for recurrent otitis media. Acta Paediatr. Scand. **71:** 567–571.
52. ANDERSSON, B., B. ERIKSSON, E. FALSEN, A. FOCH, L. Å. HANSON, O. NYLÉN, H. PETERSON & C. SVANBORG EDÉN. 1981. Adhesion of *Streptococcus pneumoniae* to human pharyngeal epithelial cells *in vitro:* Differences in adhesive capacity among strains isolated from subjects with otitis media, septicemia, or meningitis or from healthy carriers. Infect. Immun. **32:** 311–317.
52a. ANDERSSON, U., A. G. BIRD, S. BRITTON & R. PALACIOS. 1981. Humoral and cellular immunity in humans studied at the cell level from birth to two years of age. Immunological Rev. **57:** 5–38.
53. BRANDTZAEG, P. & K. BAKLIEN. 1980. Immunohistochemical studies of the immuno-globulin-producing cell systems of the human intestinal mucosa. Acta Histochem., Suppl. **XXI:** 105–119.
54. SÖDERSTRÖM, T., C. C. BRINTON JR, S. HOSEA, C. BURCH, H. A. HANSSON, L. Å. HANSON, A. KARPAS, R. SCHNEERSON, K. STEIN, A. SUTTON & W. VANN. 1982. Analysis of *Escherichia coli* K1, K13 and type 1 pilus antigens with monoclonal antibodies. *In* Progress in Allergy. Host Parasite Relationships in Gram-Negative Infections. L. Å. Hanson, P. Kallós and O. Westphal, Eds.: Vol. **33:** 259–274. Karger, Basel.
55. SHIFFMAN, G. 1982. The immune response to pneumococcal polysaccharide antigens: status report. *In* Seminars in Infectious Disease. Bacterial Vaccines. L. Weinstein & B. N. Fields. Eds.: Vol. 4: 294–304.
56. SCHNEERSON, R., O. BARRERA, A. SUTTON & J. B. ROBBINS. 1980. Preparation, characteri-zation and immunogenicity of *Haemophilus influenzae* type b polysaccharide-protein conjugates. J. Exp. Med. **152:** 361–376.
57. OXELIUS, V.-A. 1974. Chronic infections in a family with hereditary deficiency of IgG2 and IgG4. Clin. Exp. Immunol. **17:** 19–27.
58. OXELIUS, V.-A., A.-B. LAURELL, B. LINDQUIST, H. GOLEBLOWSKA, U. AXELSSON, J. BJÖRKANDER & L. Å. HANSON. 1981. IgG subclasses in selective IgA deficiency; Importance of IgG 2-IgA deficiency. N. Engl. J. Med. **304:** 1476–1477.
59. OXELIUS, V.-A., A. I. BERKEL & L. Å. HANSON. 1982. IgG2 deficiency in ataxia-telangiectasia. New. Engl. J. Med. **306:** 515–517.
60. SÖDERSTRÖM, T., C. C. BRINTON JR, P. FUSCO, A. KARPAS, S. AHLSTEDT, K. STEIN, A. SUTTON, S. HOSEA, R. SCHNEERSON & L. Å. HANSON. 1981. Analysis of pilus-mediated pathogenic mechanisms with monoclonal antibodies. Proc. ASM Conference on Bacterial Adhesion in Pathogenesis. Atlanta, GA. In press.

61. SÖDERSTRÖM, T., C. C. BRINTON JR., L. Å. HANSON, P. LARSSON, K. G. ROSÉN, A. SUTTON and R. SCHNEERSON. 1982. Intestinal colonization and the antibody response. Infection 10: 324–326.

PART I. ENVIRONMENTAL ANTIGENS AND THEIR EFFECTS ON SECRETORY AND SYSTEMIC IMMUNITY

THE IMPORTANCE OF IgA IN
NONMUCOSAL IMMUNE RESPONSES

Byron H. Waksman

Director of Research Programs
National Multiple Sclerosis Society
New York, New York 10017

I wish to introduce the first section of this monograph by commenting on the widely held view that IgA represents primarily mucosal (secretory) antibody, and that IgA is the principal immune system operative at mucosal surfaces. Nonmucosal IgA responses are in fact common and important, and may play a significant role in diseases like rheumatoid arthritis and multiple sclerosis. At the same time, IgE or IgG antibody may dominate the mucosal response in some situations, and mucosa-specific T-cell-mediated immunity in others.[1]

The traditional view is expressed in this volume. Fifteen papers on mucosal IgA are presented, while only two are presented on nonmucosal IgA; one is given on mucosal IgE, and five on T-cell-mediated immunity in the mucosae. In a substantial volume published in 1981 on the mucosal immune system[2] only one paper dealt with nonmucosal IgA (in the rheumatoid factor) and one with IgE. The same emphasis can be seen in earlier symposia.[3]

In TABLE 1, published examples of IgA formation in the central nervous system (CNS) compartment are listed. In patients with virus and other infections of the CNS, local specific IgA antibody formation has been repeatedly demonstrated, and such antibody may continue to be formed for years after an acute infection.[13,14] Sindbis virus, in mice, provides a convenient model of this process.[15] Virus replication in the brain is high two days after infection. At three to five days, there is maximal meningeal inflammation and transudation of serum protein into the cerebrospinal fluid (CSF). During the recovery phase, there is a striking local immune response, shown by an increased ratio of CSF immunoglobulin to albumin, as compared with the ratio in serum. Both IgA and IgG antibody are formed: the predominant serum isotype is IgG, while that in the CSF is IgA.

In multiple sclerosis, the local formation of oligoclonal IgG has been emphasized in all literature on the subject. Yet IgA of unknown specificity is formed as well in the CNS compartment, in as many as thirty percent of patients, and IgA-producing lymphoid cells can be demonstrated by plaque-formation techniques in a very high proportion of MS patients' CSF samples (TABLE 1). It is a common speculation that the bulk of the CSF immunoglobulin may be antibody against one or more components of myelin, which serves as the target of the disease process. The production of IgA rheumatoid factor, described elsewhere in this volume, appears to be a similar process.

The importance of mucosal immune responses of IgE isotype has been pointed out elsewhere,[1,16,17] and is emphasized again in the present volume by Dr. Ogra's presentation. Oral immunization gives unusually strong specific IgE responses, and IgE-secreting plasma cells are found in major numbers in the mucosal lamina propria and in draining lymph nodes like the mesenteric node. Whereas much attention has been given to the possibility that IgE-bearing B-lymphocytes arise in mesenteric lymph nodes and elsewhere,[16] Durkin has provided strong evidence,

22

0077-8923/83/0409-0022$1.75/0 © 1983, NYAS

in a recent study of germfree rats, that these cells are generated initially in mucosal lymphoid aggregates such as the Peyer's patches.[18] In fact, half the IgE-bearing cells in germfree Peyer's patches appear to carry IgA as well; thus there may be a more than casual association between the two isotypes in response to mucosal immunization.[18] It must be added that IgG can also serve as the principal mucosal antibody under appropriate conditions of immunization, as

TABLE 1

PRODUCTION OF IgA IN
CENTRAL NERVOUS SYSTEM COMPARTMENT

Year	Authors	Findings*	Remarks	Reference
1966	Lamoureux, Borduas			4
1971	Link, Müller		Also in polyneuropathy	5
1973	Olsson, Link	Relative increase of CSF IgA in multiple sclerosis	Also transferrin, complement components	6
1981	Stendahl-Brodin		Intrathecal synthesis	7
1981	Schuller		Contains antiviral antibodies	8
1981	Laurenzi		Is oligoclonal	9
1967	Cohen, Bannister			10
1974	Sandberg-Wollheim	IgA synthesis by CSF cells in multiple sclerosis		11
1981	Henriksson, et al.		Also by peripheral blood lymphocytes	12
1971	Link, Müller		Mumps, neurosyphilis	5
1980	Esiri	Increased CSF IgA in various CNS infections containing specific antiviral antibodies	Poliomyelitis	13
1981	Vandvik		Mumps, Herpes simplex, varicella-zoster	14
1981	Griffin		Sindbis (in mice)	15

*CSF = cerebrospinal fluid
 CNS = central nervous system

shown recently in studies of rabbits immunized orally or transtracheally with bovine serum albumin.[19] Mucosal cell-mediated responses are adequately discussed elsewhere in the present volume, and need no further emphasis here.

SUMMARY

IgA may be an important component of nonmucosal immune responses, like those occurring in the central nervous system, in certain virus infections, and in multiple sclerosis. Mucosal immune responses, in appropriate, natural, and experimental situations, may be predominantly IgE or IgG, or indeed T-cell mediated.

REFERENCES

1. WAKSMAN, B. H. & H. OZER. 1976. Specialized amplification elements in the immune system. Prog. Allergy **21:** 1–113.
2. OGRA, P. L. & J. BIENENSTOCK, Eds. 1981. The mucosal immune system in health and disease. Proceedings of the 81st Ross Conference on Pediatric Research. Ross Laboratories. Columbus, Ohio.
3. OGRA, P. L. & D. H. DAYTON, Eds. 1979. Immunology of Breast Milk. Raven Press. New York.
4. LAMOUREUX, G. & A. G. BORDUAS. 1966. Immune studies in multiple sclerosis. Clin. Exp. Immunol. **1:** 363–376.
5. LINK, H. & R. MÜLLER. 1971. Immunoglobulins in multiple sclerosis and infections of the nervous system. Arch. Neurol. (Chicago) **25:** 326–344.
6. OLSSON, J.-E. & H. LINK. 1973. Immunoglobulin abnormalities in multiple sclerosis. Relation to clinical parameters: Exacerbations and remissions. Arch. Neurol. (Chicago) **28:** 392–399.
7. STENDAHL-BRODIN, L. 1981. Studies on humoral immunity and HLA antigens in multiple sclerosis, optic neuritis and hereditary optic atrophy. Linköping University Medical Dissertation, No. 112, Linköping.
8. SCHULLER, E. 1981. Les protéines du liquide céphalorachidien et les maladies immunitaires du système nerveux. Institut Behring. J. B. Bailiere.
9. LAURENZI, M. A. 1981. Immunochemical characterization of immunoglobulins and viral antibodies synthesized within the central nervous system in patients with multiple sclerosis and controls. Acta Neurol. Scand. **63** (Suppl. 84).
10. COHEN, S. & R. BANNISTER. 1967. Immunoglobulin synthesis within the central nervous system in multiple sclerosis. Lancet **1:** 366–367.
11. SANDBERG-WOLLHEIM, M. 1974. Immunoglobulin synthesis in vitro by cerebrospinal fluid cells in patients with multiple sclerosis. Scand. J. Immunol. **3:** 717–730.
12. HENRIKSSON, A., S. KAM-HANSEN & R. ANDERSSON. 1981. Immunoglobulin producing cells in CSF and blood from patients with multiple sclerosis and other inflammatory neurological diseases enumerated by protein-A plaque assay. J. Neuroimmunol. **1:** 299–309.
13. ESIRI, M. M. 1980. Poliomyelitis: Immunoglobulin-containing cells in the central nervous system in acute and convalescence phases of the human disease. Clin. Exp. Immunol. **40:** 42–48.
14. VANDVIK, B. 1981. Personal communication.
15. GRIFFIN, D. E. 1981. Immunoglobulins in the cerebrospinal fluid: Changes during acute viral encephalitis in mice. J. Immunol. **126:** 27–31.
16. ISHIZAKA, K. & T. ISHIZAKA. 1978. Mechanisms of reaginic hypersensitivity and IgE antibody response. Immunol. Rev. **41:** 109–148.
17. JARRETT, E. E. 1978. Stimuli for the production and control of IgE in rats. Immunol. Rev. **41:** 52–76.
18. DURKIN, H. G., H. BAZIN & B. H. WAKSMAN. 1981. Origin and fate of IgE-bearing lymphocytes. I. Peyer's patches as differentiation site of cells simultaneously bearing IgA and IgE. J. Exp. Med. **154:** 640–648.
19. PERI, B. A., C. M. THEODORE, G. A. LOSONSKY, J. M. FISHAUT, R. M. ROTHBERG & P. L. OGRA. 1982. Antibody content of rabbit milk and serum following inhalation or ingestion of respiratory syncytial virus and bovine serum albumin. Clin. Exp. Immunol. **48:** 91–101.

IgA COMMITMENT:
MODELS FOR B-CELL DIFFERENTIATION AND POSSIBLE ROLES FOR T-CELLS IN REGULATING B-CELL DEVELOPMENT*

J. J. Cebra, E. R. Cebra, E. R. Clough, J. A. Fuhrman,
J. L. Komisar, P. A. Schweitzer, and R. D. Shahin

Department of Biology
University of Pennsylvania
Philadelphia, Pennsylvania 19104

INTRODUCTION

We propose to analyze those processes that prime for and stimulate a secretory IgA response. We will stress the role of mucosally applied antigen in driving B-cell differentiation to generate IgA-committed cells. We will further emphasize B-cell isotype potential as determining mucosal IgA responsiveness to antigenic challenge. Finally, we will consider possible roles for T-lymphocytes in promoting a secretory IgA response, and mechanisms by which such cells might act.

Mucosal Priming with Antigen Stimulates the Appearance of IgA-Committed Cells in Mucosal Follicles

The isotype potential of a specific B-cell refers both to the membrane isotype(s) being synthesized and expressed, and to the possibilities remaining in its genome for switching to expression of other isotypes over succeeding generations of clonal outgrowth. To assess isotype potential, which changes in a manner correlated with exposure to antigen and cell division,[1,2] we used a limiting dilution assay in which antigen-sensitive cells are stimulated *in vitro* in monofocal splenic fragments.[3] This assay discerns antibody produced over many clonal generations and allows direct inference of the minimal isotype potential of single clonal precursor cells.[4] It should be stressed that the failure of a clone to express detectable quantities of a particular isotype cannot be taken rigorously to exclude that isotype from the repertoire of the clonal precursor cell.

Mucosal B-cell follicles in the intestinal and respiratory tracts have been implicated in the generation of cells enriched in precursors for IgA plasma cells.[5-7] Significant to understanding their generation was the observation that populations of some B-cell specificities, but not others, in Peyer's patches (PP), contained a high proportion of cells apparently committed to exclusive IgA expression.[8] Clonal progeny derived from such cells secreted only IgA. Usually, such IgA-committed cells were most prevalent in PP and decreased in frequency in more distal lymphoid tissue: frequency in PP > MLN > Spl > PLN.[1,8] The antigenic specificities correlated with increased numbers of IgA-committed B-cells included those corresponding to antigenic determinants common in the

*These studies were supported by a grant from the National Institute for Allergy and Infectious Diseases (AI 17997).

25

murine environment,[1,8,9]—for example, phosphocholine (PC), $\beta 2 \rightarrow 1$ fructosyl or inulin (In), and β-galactosyl (β-Gal). TABLE 1 shows an extreme case of the prevalence of IgA-committed cells to the β- galactosyl determinant occurring naturally in healthy mice not deliberately immunized. If mice born of germfree (GF) parents are raised germfree, then frequencies of PC- and In-sensitive cells remain almost as low as in newborn mice, and there are few IgA-committed cells in any lymphoid tissue.[1,9,10] Deliberate conversion of these mice into specific pathogen free animals by colonization with normal commensals or by monoassociation with *Proteus morganii*, stimulates a marked increase in the frequencies of B-cells, with specificities normally dominant in conventionally raised mice.[1] This colonization further establishes a gradient of IgA-committed cells of the PC and In specificities from PP, where they become most prevalent, to more distal lymphoid tissues. These observations suggest that natural intestinal stimulation by antigens leads to increases in frequencies of specific B-cells, and to the prevalence of IgA-committed cells in PP.

TABLE 1

ISOTYPE POTENTIALS OF β-GALACTOSYL SENSITIVE B-CELLS OCCURRING NATURALLY IN BALB/c MICE

	Percent of Clones (No.)			
	Germfree → SPF → Conventionalized		Conventionally Raised	
Isotype(s) Expressed by Clones	Spl	PP + MLN	Spl + PLN	PP + MLN
IgM only	0(0)	0(0)	7(1)	0(0)
Some IgM	0(0)	0(0)	29(4)	0(0)
IgG ± IgA, no IgM	10(1)	15(2)	43(6)	25(2)
Some IgA	90(9)	92(12)	36(5)	75(6)
IgA only	90(9)	85(11)	29(4)	75(6)
Some IgG	10(1)	15(2)	58(8)	25(2)
Some IgG₃	10(1)	0(0)	7(1)	0(0)
Total clones	10	13	14	8

To test these possibilities and to analyze the priming process, we administered cholera toxin (TXN) by intraduodenal injection.[2] TXN is a potent stimulator of a secretory immune response when given orally.[11,12] Normal mice have barely detectable levels of TXN-specific B-cells in any lymphoid tissue ($\sim 1/10^6$ B-cells). Within two weeks after stimulation the frequency of TXN-reactive B-cells increases about 50-fold[2] and, as shown in TABLE 2, up to one half of these cells in PP becomes committed to IgA expression. Similar to the status of colonized, previously GF mice, a focus of IgA-committed cells is established in PP with diminishing prevalence of such cells in more distal lymphoid tissues.[1,2,8] As also shown in TABLE 2, priming with either TXN or toxoid (TXD) by a variety of other routes, including intratracheally, fails to equal intraduodenal priming in generating IgA-committed cells in PP or in any other lymphoid tissue, although such stimulations result in comparable increases in overall frequencies of antigen-sensitive cells in PP and in all other lymphoid tissues tested (Spl, PLN, MLN,

TABLE 2

ISOTYPE PROFILES OF PP-DERIVED ANTI-TOXOID CLONES

Isotype(s) Expressed by Clones	Unprimed	B-cell Donors Primed by Following Routes With:								
		TXN,* id† 2 Wk	TXD, ip 2 Wk	TXN, sc 2 Wk	TXN, id 4 Wk	TXN, it 4 Wk	TXN, id 6 Wk	TXD, sc 6 Wk	TXN, id 12 Wk	TXD, ip 12 Wk
M only	5	0	0	9	0	0	0	0	0	0
Some M	75	4	61	18	11	54	15	62	75	5
G ± A, no M	10	45	28	82	55	44	62	31	8	90
Some A	20	77	50	0	72	63	85	62	100	42
A only	10	50	11	0	33	9	23	8	17	10
No. of clones	20	22	18	11	18	11	13	12	12	19

*TXN = Toxin; TXD = Toxoid
†id = intraduodenal; sc = subcutaneous; ip = intraperitoneal; it = intratracheal

bronchial-associated lymphoreticular tissue [BALT], or peripheral blood [PB]). Since the appearance of a high proportion of IgA-committed cells in the PP after intraduodenal priming correlates with a pronounced appearance of IgA anti-toxin-producing plasma cells, *in vivo* in the gut lamina propria after a secondary intraduodenal challenge,[2] the generation of such cells seems to explain at least partly the greater efficacy of mucosal priming for a secretory response.

TABLE 3 shows that concomitant with the appearance of IgA-committed TXN-sensitive cells in PP after intraduodenal priming, a rise in the frequency of such cells also occurs in PB.[13] Thus, intestinal stimulation not only drives terminal IgA plasmablasts toward secretory tissue,[14,15] but also releases IgA-committed antigen-sensitive B-cells into the circulation. Such cells are competent to generate a clone of IgA-secreting cells upon antigen driven division. The longevity of these circulating B-cells has not been established, nor is it known whether they continue to recirculate, but a pool of such cells could at least partly account for the effectiveness of gut mucosal priming for the expression of secretory IgA at a distant site upon subsequent challenge at this latter location.[16]

TABLE 3

CIRCULATING TXD-SENSITIVE PRECURSORS GENERATED BY INTESTINAL PRIMING*

| | Percent Clones Expressing Product, B-cell Source: | | |
Clonal Product	PBL	PP	BALT/Lungs
IgM	22	0	0
Some IgM	55	4	57
IgG ± IgA, no IgM	22	45	14
Some IgA	66	77	57
IgA only	22	50	14
Some IgE	11	0	14
No. of clones analyzed	9	22	7

*Tissues analyzed two weeks after id priming.

A MODEL FOR B-CELL DIFFERENTIATION LEADING TO IGA COMMITMENT

We postulated that B-cell differentiation with respect to isotype potential was division dependent, based on the PP being the most active site of natural antigen-stimulated B-cell division of any lymphoid tissue, and the coincidence there of a high proportion of IgA-committed cells of many specificities.[17] The mechanism for linking these processes was suggested by the model for plasmacytoma differentiation presented by Kataoka and Honjo.[18] They proposed that a V_h to C_h gene translocational event, with the deletion of intervening DNA, preceded expression of a particular isotype of antibody. Since normal progenitors of cells, expressing any of the IgG, IgE, or IgA isotypes first express IgM,[19] it seems reasonable that at least two V_h to C_h recombinational events can occur in the same B-cell line—V_h to C_μ followed by V_h/C_μ to V_h/C_h switching. We thus suggested a model for linking the extensive B-cell division, occurring in the absence of plasma-cell maturation that is peculiar to PP, with the accumulation of these IgA-committed cells.[8,17,20-22] This model proposes that V_h/C_μ to V_h/C_h isotype switching can occur repeatedly in a single normal B-lymphocyte line, with deletion of intervening C_h genes at each recombinational event. The switching process is taken to be vectorial, occurring in the 5' to 3' order of C_h genes, which is $C_\mu - C_{\gamma 3} - C_{\gamma 1} - C_{\gamma 2b} - C_{\gamma 2a} - C_\epsilon - C_\alpha$ in the murine genome.[23] The successive switching to a downstream (3') gene is random, but may be of unequal probability for each C_h gene, depending on the particular V_h/C_h combination existing before the switch. The consequence of this process is that extensive clonal outgrowth, in the absence of maturation to nondividing plasma cells that would attenuate lines within a clone, should result in the accumulation of B-cells in the terminal, productive V_h/C_α state. These cells, still retaining antigen-sensitivity, would be committed to generating clones exclusively secreting IgA. We believe that this model is consistent with our finding of gradients of IgA-committed B-cells decreasing from PP to distal tissues, following chronic or acute, natural or deliberate, gut mucosal stimulation with antigens.

Having attempted to support our model with diverse observations and tests,[1,20,21,24] our next consideration was the nature of the antigenic stimuli and T-lymphocyte interactions that may naturally influence B-cell differentiation leading to IgA commitment.

An Assessment of the Role of T-Cells, both in the Process Leading to B-Cell Commitment to IgA, and to the Expression of Secreted IgA Antibody

Athymic mice have antigen-sensitive cells of common specificities (PC, In) in all lymphoid tissues, including PP, in frequencies similar to those of euthymic mice.[25] Few of those cells, however, are committed to IgA expression. Rather, these populations of cells include a very high proportion of those cells that generate clones expressing some IgM (80-90%) or exclusively IgM (~40%). Thus, a deficiency in normally functioning T-cells in the presence of environmental antigens seems to curtail that part of natural priming leading to extensive IgA commitment, and results in a steady state of B-cells with fewer differentiated characteristics than seen in euthymic mice. However, TABLE 4 shows that acute, gut mucosal application of the TXN antigen to either euthymic or athymic mice results in similarly elevated frequencies of antigen-sensitive cells in both Spl and PP, and in a lesser but still evident commitment of PP cells to IgA in athymic mice, compared with euthymic mice. The simplest interpretation of these observations is that antigen-driven priming of PP B-cells leading to IgA commitment can proceed in the absence of T-cells, but is more efficient in their presence, in euthymic mice.

Most of our assessments of the isotype potential of B-cells from euthymic and athymic mice utilized unfractionated cellular inocula injected into lethally irradiated, carrier-primed recipients. Since the TXN-sensitive B-cells of athymic mice were analyzed in the absence of accompanying antigen-primed T-cells, we evaluated the effect of removing such cells from the TXN-primed PP B-cells of euthymic mice, to allow a more symmetric comparison of isotype potentials.[13] We found little difference between the frequencies of antigen-sensitive B-cells from untreated PP cells, including TXN-primed T-cells, and the same cells treated with anti-Thy-1 plus complement (37 vs $30/10^6$ B-cells), or in the proportions of these cells generating clones expressing some IgA (70% vs 77%) or exclusively IgA (50% vs 40%).[13] Thus, the expression of some IgA or only IgA by clones seems an inherent property of the precursor B-cell, acting with antigen-specific T_h cells, and does not depend on specialized, viable T-cells that occur in primed PP that somehow favor IgA expression. However, we did observe a quantitative difference between some of the clones developed in the irradiated splenic fragments in the presence of accompanying, primed T-cells and those arising in their absence. This difference involved clones exclusively expressing IgA or making some IgA. When such clones developed from inocula containing accompanying T-cells, their output of antibody was considerably greater than when they arose without nonirradiated T-cells (>25 ng/20 λ vs 5 ng/20 λ for clones exclusively expressing IgA and 20 ng/20 λ vs 8 ng/20 λ for clones making some IgA). Clones that did not express any IgA did not show this distinction.

TABLE 4

INTESTINAL PRIMING WITH CHOLERA TOXIN GENERATES IgA-COMMITTED B-CELLS IN ATHYMIC MICE WITHIN TWO WEEKS

Clonal Product	Percent Anti-toxoid Clones Expressing Product, B-cell Source:			
	BALB/c PP	nu/nu PP	BALB/c Spl	nu/nu Spl
IgM only	0	9	14	19
Some IgM	4	18	38	75
IgG ± IgA, no IgM	45	64	23	12
Some IgG$_3$	0	0	0	0
Some IgG$_1$	36	54	23	31
Some IgG$_2$	36	9	8	0
Some IgA	77	36	62	62
IgA only	50	18	38	12
Some IgE	0	9	0	12
No. of clones analyzed	22	11	13	16
Freq./10^6 B-cells	37	100	30	24

In general, a greater output of antibody product by these clones could be achieved in at least three ways, which would not involve the instructed switching of B-cells to IgA-expression, postulated later in this volume:[26] 1) by increased clone size due to more cell divisions by its members; 2) an increased "burst size," whereby more clonal members matured to secretory plasma cells and contributed antibody; and 3) a greater output per cell by either increased synthesis and secretion, or by the continuation of synthesis and secretion over a longer period. Antigen-primed T-cells could modulate any of these processes in a way that would appear to favor IgA expression, without being specific for the IgA isotype, if terminal IgA-committed cells required somewhat more support for growth, maturation, or survival than less differentiated B-cells, and if all viable, long-lived, dividing clones could eventually generate some members expressing IgA by successive isotype switching. We have not yet analyzed the mode of action of the accompanying T-cells, and only would point out the salient difference between the two sorts of splenic fragment cultures; one contains only irradiated, antigen-primed T-cells, whereas the other includes supplementary, viable, antigen-primed T-cells over the 15 day assay period.

All of these observations suggest that IgA-committed cells can arise in the absence of functional T-cells and T-cells can expand or facilitate IgA commitment and expression. It has long been accepted that IgA responses are T-dependent,[17,27] but athymic mice express IgA antibodies;[28] certain thymus-independent antigens, such as polysaccharides, do stimulate an IgA component as part of the response in euthymic mice.[29,30] We would like to conclude by considering the role of thymus-independent antigens—such as bacterial polysaccharides common in the environment—and the subset of B-cells that respond to them, in the development of IgA responses and of IgA-committed B-cells.

ROLE OF THYMUS-INDEPENDENT ANTIGENS AND THE SUBSET OF B-CELLS THAT RESPOND TO THEM IN THE DEVELOPMENT OF IgA RESPONSES AND IgA-COMMITTED B-CELLS

Recently, we and others succeeded in stimulating clonal outgrowth of single, antigen-sensitive cells in splenic fragments with TI-2 antigens.[31-33] The lethally irradiated recipients used to score these B-cells need not be antigen-primed and the B-cell inocula need not come from deliberately primed donors and need not contain accompanying T-cells. Antigens such as bacterial levan, TNP-Ficoll, and purified C-carbohydrate or heat killed R36A pneumococcal vaccine (PnC) stimulate anti-In, anti-TNP, and anti-PC responses respectively in splenic fragments containing limiting dilutions of B-cells, with the same order of frequencies as their thymus-dependent counterparts In-, TNP-, and PC-conjugated hemocyanin (Hy).[31] Of considerable interest was our own finding that clones stimulated to develop by these TI-2 antigens, underwent isotype switching and expressed all combinations of IgM, IgG, and IgA isotypes (IgE was not tested). The most salient characteristic of these clones is that most express some IgM (70–100%). Otherwise, the different TI-2 antigens each gave clones showing different spectra of isotype patterns: PnC clones frequently expressed some IgG3, TNP-Ficoll clones often made some IgA, and levan clones frequently gave IgA, IgM, and some IgG isotypes. However, all isotypes could be found as products from some clones stimulated by each antigen.

Next, we addressed the extent of overlap, if any, between the populations of antigen-reactive cells responding to these TI-2 antigens, and those reactive with the same determinants in thymus-dependent (TD) form. We analyzed B-cells from spleens of donors that had not been deliberately primed, in order to address this point. Portions of the same B-cell pool were inoculated into many Hy-primed, irradiated, scoring animals, and the resulting splenic fragments were stimulated with either PnC, PC-Hy, or mixtures of the TI-2 and TD form of the PC antigenic determinant. We found that frequencies of B-cells responsive to each form of antigen were similar and that little, if any, additivity of frequencies was evident when mixtures of the two forms of antigenic determinant were used to stimulate specific clonal outgrowth.[31] Thus, it seems that considerable overlap exists between the populations of B-cells responsive to the TI-2 and TD forms of the PC-determinant in the splenic cells of these unprimed mice. A further finding supports this conclusion. The patterns of isotype expression given by clones responding to PnC were different from those shown by clones stimulated by PC-Hy. However, mixtures of PnC and PC-Hy resulted in clones with superimposed characteristics from TI-2 and TD clones. Particularly, clones responsive to PnC frequently expressed IgG3 along with IgM, whereas IgG_1 and IgG_2 were rarely detected. Clones stimulated by PC-Hy seldom expressed IgG_3, but often made IgG_1 and/or IgG_2. The mixture of forms of the PC-determinant resulted most conspicuously in frequent coexpression of IgG_3 with IgG_1 and/or IgG_2.[31]

If the population of unprimed B-cells responsive to TI-2 antigens considerably overlaps the population reactive with TD antigens, and can evidence isotype switching in response to TI-2 antigens, it seems likely that this former population is situated astride a linear pathway of B-cell differentiation that could lead to IgA-committed cells. A corollary of this model for B-cell development is that TI-2 antigens administered to mice should prime (i.e., increase the frequency of

TABLE 5

ISOTYPE AND FREQUENCY ANALYSIS OF ANTI-TNP-PRODUCING CLONES FROM UNIMMUNIZED MICE, AND MICE PREVIOUSLY IMMUNIZED WITH TNP-FICOLL*

Isotype Expressed	TNP-Ficoll Primed	Unprimed
Some IgM	97	100
Some IgA	97	93
IgM + IgA only	41	52
Some IgG_2	32	31
Some IgG_1	26	21
Some IgG_3	9	3
IgA only	3	0
IgM only	3	3
IgG ± IgA, no IgM	3	0
No. of cells analyzed	5×10^7	8.2×10^7
No. of clones analyzed	34	29
Frequency TNP-reactive Cells/10^5 B-cells	5.9	2.3

*Adult male BALB/c mice were immunized with 100 μg TNP_{150}-Ficoll i.p. Unimmunized littermates served as controls. Three weeks following immunizations, splenocytes from each group of mice served as donor inocula for clonal analysis. Splenic fragments were stimulated with a cocktail of TNP-Hy + PC-Hy, each at 5 μg/ml. Culture supernatants were collected on days 6, 9, 12, and 15, and tested for hapten-specific antibodies by RIA.

specific B-cells) for subsequent responses to the same determinants in TD form in the presence of the appropriate T_h cells. Support for this possibility has been obtained by using in vivo secondary responses to the TD version of the determinant as indicative of priming with TI antigens or by testing cell populations in vitro.[34-36] Priming has been quantitated using in vitro clonal assays to show the rise in frequency of B-cells responsive to the TD form of antigen following in vivo stimulation with the TI-2 form.[10,36,37] Thus, bacterial levan and TNP-Ficoll have been shown to prime one to three day old mice for TD responses to In- and TNP-Hy respectively.[10,34] Recently, Speck and Pierce have shown a similar effect of TNP-Ficoll given to either young adult athymic or euthymic mice.[37] TABLE 5 indicates that TNP-Ficoll stimulation results in a 2.5-fold increase in antigen-sensitive cells reactive to TNP-Hy in a TD splenic fragment assay.

Typically, increases of the order of two to fourfold are observed following TI-2 priming.[10,37] TABLE 5 also shows that most (97%) clones responsive to TNP-Hy from cells out of TNP-Ficoll primed donors, express some IgM, and almost all of these also make IgA. IgG isotypes are also coexpressed by a majority of these clones (56%). Such patterns of isotype expression are typical of clones derived from unprimed, young adult mice responding to the In-determinant on levan, a TI-2 antigen, or to the TD form of this determinant, In-Hy.[10] However, if one to three day old mice are primed with levan, resulting in a 3.5-fold rise in In-reactive B-cells, most of the resulting clones stimulated by In-Hy (78%), only express IgM. If extra (0.8×10^6) T-cells, taken from PP of mice, primed intraduodenally with cholera toxin, are added to the levan-primed, neonatal B-cell inocula (40×10^6 splenic B-cells), then the resultant clones stimulated by In-Hy mostly express both IgA (75%) and/or IgG3 (33%) together with (75%) or without (25%) IgM.[38] This is a preliminary observation, but it does seem related to the phenomenon of T-cell dependent enhancement of IgA expression reported in this volume.[26] The implication of our observation is that TXN-primed T-cells, which also would include T-cells freshly primed to a variety of environmental antigens accompanying TXN, can induce clones that would otherwise only express IgM to also make IgA and IgG_3. The mechanism by which this increase in expression of non-IgM isotypes is achieved is yet to be established. Teale and Mandel have pointed out the prevalence of antigen-sensitive cells that generate clones, making IgM plus IgA in inocula from fetal liver and spleen.[39] This apparently preferred isotype switch may simply reflect the higher probability of random V_h/C_μ to V_h/C_α switches, and cells displaying it may be less obscured in perinatal tissue by more differentiated B-cells. The T-cell effect we have noticed might reflect a higher threshold in neonatal cells for T-cell signals, allowing the expression of IgM to IgA and IgM to IgG_3 isotype switches, and hence a continuing requirement for viable T-cells over the 9–15 day lifetime of their clones, which is not met in the irradiated splenic fragment.

CONCLUSIONS

In conclusion, all these observations lead to the concept of a linear pathway for B-cell differentiation, which includes TI-2 responsive cells that can both undergo isotype switching to express IgG and IgA, and can give rise to generations of cells further stimulable by TD forms of antigen in concert with T-cells. The principal distinction between models for branched and linear pathways for differentiation is that, in the former, B-cells undergo asymmetric divisions after acquisition of antigen-sensitivity, leading to separate sets of IgM-bearing clonal precursors (FIGURE 1). One set is predestined to react with TI-2 antigens, and according to some models,[40] to generate progeny expressing IgM or IgG_3. The other set of precursors is responsive to specific T-cell signals, and TD antigens stimulate their clonal outgrowth and the expression of mainly IgG_1 and IgG_2 isotypes (FIGURE 1A). Our observations support a linear pathway for B-cell differentiation, in which cells responsive to TI-2 antigens occur in the same cell line that gives rise to cells stimulable by TD antigens. Some, but not all, of the B-cells responsive to TI-2 and TD antigens may overlap on a generational level (FIGURE 1B). We also favor a linear pathway of B-cell development with respect to isotype expression, wherein B-cells of the same lineage can undergo successive, random, but vectorial $V_h/D/J_h$ to C_h gene switches in the 5' to 3' order of C_h genes. In this model, each isotype switch further restricts the isotype potential of

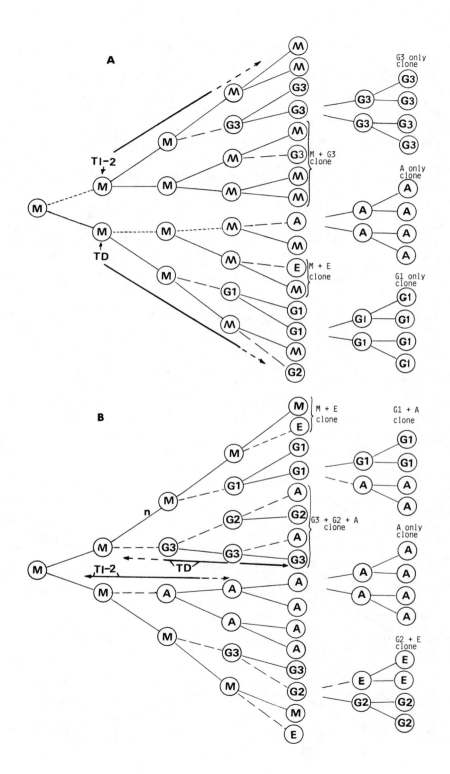

TABLE 6

COEXPRESSION BY CLONES OF IgG$_3$ OR IgE WITH OTHER ISOTYPES

Isotype Expressed	No.	Percent	Isotype Expressed	No.	Percent
Some IgG$_3$	67		Some IgE	90	
IgG$_3$ only	9	13	IgE only	3	3
IgG$_3$ + IgM	5	7	IgE + IgM	8	9
IgG$_3$ + IgA	12	18	IgE + IgA	12	13
IgG$_3$ + IgGX	4	6	IgE + IgGX	24	27
IgG$_3$ + IgM + IgA	7	10	IgE + IgM + IgA	7	8
IgG$_3$ + IgM + IgGX	1	1	IgE + IgM + IgGX	12	13
IgG$_3$ + IgA + IgGX	19	28	IgE + IgA + IgGX	14	15
IgG$_3$ + IgM + IgA + IgGX	10	15	IgE + IgM + IgA + IgGX	10	11

the B-cell line by the deletion of intervening 5′ C$_h$ genes (FIGURE 1B). The alternative model of branched differentiation with respect to isotype potential would involve asymmetric divisions by IgM-bearing cells, leading to separate populations, each predestined to generate clones that express only one particular IgG, IgE, or IgA isotype or to one particular pattern of isotypes (FIGURE 1A). Separate sets of predestined B-cells have been suggested to account for IgG$_3$ and IgE expression.[40,41] Elsewhere in this volume we present an analysis of IgE expression in relationship to IgA, by clones from B-cells, derived from PC-Hy primed, *Ascaris*-infected mice.[42] TABLE 6 presents a summary of isotypes, coexpressed by 67 clones making anti-PC or anti-In IgG$_3$, and by 90 clones making anti-PC IgE, the former from nonprimed donors, and the latter from *Ascaris*-infected mice. The general observation is that both IgG$_3$ and IgE are randomly coexpressed with one or several of all other isotypes. These data do not support the common occurrence of distinct subsets of B-cells predestined to generate clones, making one particular isotype or one pattern of isotypes. Finally, if branched differentiation through asymmetric divisions were common, and only single isotype switches from V$_h$/C$_\mu$ to V$_h$/C$_h$ occurred in any single B-cell line, then one might expect rather balanced frequencies of specific B-cells, that give

FIGURE 1. The schematic drawings attempt to illustrate the subtle differences between asymmetric divisions without isotype switching (dotted lines), occurring in dividing antigen-sensitive cells and resulting in a branched pathway of differentiation (FIGURE 1A), and asymmetric divisions defined by isotype switching (broken lines) giving a linear pathway for differentiation (FIGURE 1B). In the branched scheme, separate B-cells that continue to express membrane IgM become committed to respond to either TI-2 or to TD antigens, or become predestined to give rise to either IgM- plus IgG$_3$- or IgM- plus IgE-, etc., secreting clones by asymmetric divisions. This predestination could also arise in stages and be independent of division, as recently suggested by Honjo and his coworkers.[43] By this mechanism, cells would first make and use polycistronic mRNA that would be processed to allow continued expression of both IgM and some IgG, IgE, or IgA isotype. Such cells would then be committed to generating clones expressing a particular pattern of isotypes. In the model for a linear pathway for differentiation (FIGURE 1B), no B-cell continuing to express IgM is predestined to switch to any other particular isotype (i.e., IgA, IgE, or IgG$_3$). However, once a switch has occurred, it is irreversible. These schemes also illustrate the consequences of B-cells being restricted to making a single isotype switch (IgM → IgX) in the same cell line (here arbitrarily associated with the branched scheme), vs. B-cells being capable of undergoing successive switches within the same B-cell line (here arbitrarily included in the scheme for a linear pathway).

rise to clones exclusively making each of the IgG, IgE, and IgA isotypes, especially if these cells derived from deliberately or environmentally primed donors. Instead, we find the sole expression of any one of the IgG isotypes, or of IgE by clones, to be extremely rare. This phenomenon is so, even when B-cell donors have been intensively primed, deliberately or by monoassociation with particular gut bacteria. Rather, such animals characteristically contain high proportions of cells that generate clones, making mixtures of IgG isotypes with or without IgA in the absence of detectable IgM. Only IgA is found frequently as an exclusive clonal product, and it also occurs as the commonest isotype—other than IgM—in switching clones that express other isotypes. Of 286 clones making anti-PC or anti-In, surveyed from a variety of tissues from mice that had not been deliberately immunized, 38% expressed IgA exclusively (110/286) and 84% expressed some IgA antibody. These observations are consistent with a linear pathway for B-cell development, wherein successive switches occur in the same B-cell line, leading to eventual V_h/C_h to V_h/C_α switching to the 3′ terminal C_α gene and to IgA commitment. Presumably, switching clones undergoing many divisions, eventually yield some progeny, making IgA *in vitro*; this accounts for its being the commonest non-IgM isotype.

Finally, our observations indicate that IgA commitment is an inherent property of a subset of B-cells, but that relevant specific T-cells may potentiate IgA commitment and IgA expression.

REFERENCES

1. CEBRA, J. J., P. J. GEARHART, J. F. HALSEY, J. L. HURWITZ & R. D. SHAHIN. 1980. J. Reticuloendothelial Soc. **28:** 61s–71s.
2. FUHRMAN, J. A. & J. J. CEBRA. 1981. J. Exp. Med. **153:** 534–544.
3. KLINMAN, N. R. 1969. Immunochemistry **6:** 757–759.
4. GEARHART, P. J., N. H. SIGAL & N. R. KLINMAN. 1975. Proc. Nat. Acad. Sci. USA **72:** 1707–1711.
5. CRAIG, S. W. & J. J. CEBRA. 1971. J. Exp. Med. **134:** 188–200.
6. BIENENSTOCK, J., O. RUDZIK, R. CLANCY, R. DAY & D. PEREY. 1974. Fed. Proc. Fed. Am. Soc. Exp. Biol. **33:** 594.
7. CRAIG, S. W. & J. J. CEBRA. 1975. J. Immunol. **114:** 492–502.
8. GEARHART, P. J. & J. J. CEBRA. 1979. J. Exp. Med. **149:** 216–227.
9. CEBRA, J. J., J. A. FUHRMAN, D. J. HORSFALL & R. D. SHAHIN. 1982. *In* Seminars in Infectious Diseases. J. B. Robbins, J. C. Hill and J. C. Sadoff, Eds.: **4:** 6–12. Thieme-Stratton, Inc. New York.
10. SHAHIN, R. D. & J. J. CEBRA. 1981. Infec. Immun. **32:** 211–215.
11. PIERCE, N. F. & J. L. GOWANS. 1975. J. Exp. Med. **142:** 1550–1563.
12. SVENNERHOLM, A-M., S. LANGE & J. HOLMGREN. 1978. Infec. Immun. **21:** 1–6.
13. FUHRMAN, J. A. 1982. Dissertation, The Johns Hopkins University, Baltimore, Md.
14. HUSBAND, A. J. & J. L. GOWANS, 1978. J. Exp. Med. **148:** 1146–1160.
15. McWILLIAMS, M., J. M. PHILLIPS-QUAGLIATA & M. E. LAMM. 1975. J. Immunol: **115:** 54–58.
16. PIERCE, N. F. & W. C. CRAY, JR. 1981. J. Immunol. **127:** 2461–2464.
17. CEBRA, J. J., P. J. GEARHART, R. KAMAT, S. M. ROBERTSON & J. TSENG. 1977. Cold Spring Harbor Symposium on Quantitative Biology **41:** 201–215.
18. HONJO, T. & T. KATAOKA. 1978. Proc. Nat. Acad. Sci. USA **75:** 2140–2144.
19. PIERCE, C. W., S. M. SOLLIDAY & R. ASOFSKY. 1972. J. Exp. Med. **135:** 675–697.
20. GEARHART, P. J., J. L. HURWITZ & J. J. CEBRA. 1980. Proc. Nat. Acad. Sci. USA. **77:** 5424–5428.
21. HURWITZ, J. L., C. COLECLOUGH & J. J. CEBRA. 1980. Cell **22:** 349–359.
22. CEBRA, J. J., J. A. FUHRMAN, P. J. GEARHART, J. L. HURWITZ & R. D. SHAHIN. 1982. *In*

Recent Advances in Mucosal Immunity. W. Strober, L. A. Hanson, and K. W. Sell, Eds.: 151–169. Raven Press, New York.
23. SHIMIZU, A., N. TAKAHASHI, Y. YAOITA & T. HONJO. 1982. Cell **28:** 499–506.
24. GEARHART, P. J. & J. J. CEBRA. 1981. J. Immunol. **127:** 1030–1034.
25. CEBRA, E. R. & J. J. CEBRA. Unpublished observations.
26. STROBER, W. & H. KAWANISHI. 1983. Ann. N.Y. Acad. Sci. This volume.
27. TORRIGIANI, G. 1972. J. Immunol. **108:** 161–164.
28. PIGUET, P.-F. 1980. Scand. J. Immunol. **12:** 233–238.
29. BARTHOLD, D. R., B. PRESCOTT, P. W. STASHAK, D. F. AMSBAUGH & P. J. BAKER. 1974. J. Immunol. **112:** 1042–1050.
30. KAGNOFF, M. F. 1979. J. Immunol. **122:** 866–870.
31. HURWITZ, J. L., V. B. TAGART, P. A. SCHWEITZER & J. J. CEBRA. 1982. Eur. J. Immunol. **12:** 342–348.
32. FUNG, J. & H. KOHLER. 1980. J. Immunol. **125:** 640–646.
33. MONGINI, P. K. A., W. E. PAUL & E. S. METCALF. 1982. J. Exp. Med. **155:** 884–902.
34. MOSIER, D. E. 1978. J. Immunol. **121:** 1453–1459.
35. HOSOKAWA, T. 1979. Immunology **38:** 291–299.
36. PILLAI, P. S., D. W. SCOTT & R. B. CORLEY. 1982. Fed. Proc. Fed. Am. Soc. Exp. Biol. **41:** 425; Abs.# 909.
37. SPECK, N. A. & S. K. PIERCE. 1982. J. Exp. Med. **155:** 574–586.
38. SHAHIN, R. D., P. A. SCHWEITZER & J. J. CEBRA. 1983. Ann. N.Y. Acad. Sci. This volume.
39. TEALE, J. M. & T. E. MANDEL. 1980. J. Exp. Med. **151:** 429–445.
40. SLACK, J., G. P. DER-BALIAN, M. NAHM & J. M. DAVIE. 1980. J. Exp. Med. **151:** 853–862.
41. SHIGEMOTO, S., T. KISHIMOTO & Y. YAMAMURA. 1981. J. Immunol. **127:** 1070–1075.
42. CLOUGH, E. R. & J. J. CEBRA. 1983. Ann. N.Y. Acad. Sci. This volume.
43. YAOITA, Y., Y. KUMAGAI, K. OKUMURA, & T. HONJO. 1982. Nature **297:** 697–699.

———————◆———————

DISCUSSION OF THE PAPER

J. R. McGHEE (*The University of Alabama in Birmingham*): Since you are employing TI-2-antigens, you assume that the switches occur in Lyb-5$^+$, and Lyb-7$^+$ cells. Have you done any work with the CBA/N (*xid*)-defective mice, and examined Lyb-5$^-$ cells in terms of switching to IgA?

J. J. CEBRA (*University of Pennsylvania, Philadelphia, Pa.*): We have looked at defective-*XID* mice for commitment to IgA; Dr. Clough's poster will explain how we did this. It involves PC-hemocyanin-priming followed by *Ascaris* infection, which results in not only about 40% IgA-expressing clones, but also in a time-dependent increase in IgA-committed cells in the Peyer's patches.

W. STROBER (*National Institutes of Health, Bethesda, Md.*): Is it appropriate to speak about thymic-independent antigen in relation to IgA and certain other isotypes? Dr. Mongini at NIH, together with Drs. Paul and Metcalf, have shown that IgG$_2$a-responses to TNP-Ficoll are dependent on the presence of T-cells in the splenic focus assay. This is an example of a thymic-independent antigen that is dependent on the presence of T-cells. Although TI antigens are defined in terms of their ability to induce responses in the absence of T-cells, perhaps in certain isotypes, the concept of thymic-independence is not really valid.

CEBRA: I would suggest, that for all isotypes, thymic-independent antigens should be operationally defined. When the antigen acts in an athymic mouse, it may be acting as a thymic-independent antigen. On the other hand, in a euthymic mouse, several second order T-cells might be involved. Of course, the Paul group at NIH, and our group, have deliberately gone into stimulation of clones in order to detect the T-cell influences that might be more obscure in a potent thymus-dependent assay, like the hemocyanin-primed spleen. The clonal analysis tells what the cells have the potential to do, but the lack of appearance of isotypes does not tell what they cannot do.

R. M. E. PARKHOUSE (*National Institute for Medical Research, London, England*): Since it is absolutely crucial to the interpretation of your data on the clonability of the system, would you briefly summarize for us the evidence that proves that the system is totally clonal?

CEBRA: To some extent we base our observations on a wealth of data that the Klinman laboratory has brought forward. It indicates that approximately 10% of the fragments are positive, that is, less than one in twenty clones could likely have more than one antigen-sensitive cell. In fact, we work at that level of 10% positive splenic fragments. Dr. Gearhart has done careful quantitation of idiotype versus isotype of the total antibody. If one accepts allelic exclusion, she can account for all of the idiotype positive cells as making 100% of the antibody. Dr. Cooper in our group has looked at responses to three antigens administered simultaneously and performed studies on the probability of two specificities of cells in the same fragment. He observed complete random assortment. Limiting dilution assays are a statistical consideration in terms of whether you accept clonability.

SEROLOGIC AND MOLECULAR GENETIC STUDIES OF RABBIT Ig HEAVY CHAINS: EVIDENCE FOR ADDITIONAL C_α AND C_γ GENES

Katherine L. Knight, Karen L. Muth, Christine L. Martens,
Steven J. Currier, James L. Gallarda, and W. Carey Hanly

Department of Microbiology and Immunology
Department of Preventive Medicine and Community Health
University of Illinois at the Medical Center
Chicago, Illinois 60680

INTRODUCTION

Two subclasses of rabbit IgA, IgA-f and IgA-g, have been identified, and genetic variants, allotypes, of each subclass have been characterized.[1] The allotypic specificities f69, f70, f71, f72, and f73 are found on IgA-f subclass molecules and appear to be controlled by allelic genes at the $C\alpha f$ locus; the allotypic specificities g74, g75, g76, and g77 are found on IgA-g subclass molecules and appear to be controlled by allelic genes at the $C\alpha g$ locus.[1] The $C\alpha f$ and $C\alpha g$ loci are closely linked to each other and to the loci controlling synthesis of the variable (V_h) and constant (C_h) regions of immunoglobulin (Ig) heavy chains.[2]

Previous studies with the $C\alpha g$ allotypic specificities have shown that the g-allotypes are complex, that is, each has multiple allotypic determinants, many of which are shared among the IgA-g allotypes.[3] The $C\alpha f$ allotypic specificities also appear to be complex in that the allotypic determinants are found on both the Fc and Fd portions of αf molecules.[4] The complexity of these IgA-f allotypes has been further investigated by quantitative radiobinding studies of each $C\alpha f$ allotype, with several alloanti α-chain antibodies. Through these studies, at least two subsets of IgA-f molecules of each $C\alpha f$ allotype have been identified; as each subset is, presumably, the product of different $C\alpha$ structural genes, we propose that there are at least three $C\alpha$ genes in the rabbit genome, $C\alpha f_1$, $C\alpha f_2$ and $C\alpha g$.

SEROLOGIC CROSS REACTIONS AMONG sIgA-f MOLECULES

Rabbit secretory IgA (sIgA) was isolated from milk of rabbits homozygous for various α-chain allotypes;[5] the sIgA-f subclass molecules, which are resistant to proteolytic digestion, were separated by gel filtration from $Fab_2\alpha$ and $Fc_2\alpha$ fragments, subsequent to papain cleavage of the sIgA-g subclass.[6] These sIgA-f molecules were labeled with ^{125}I, and were reacted with various anti-IgA-f allotype reagents in quantitative radiobinding assays.[5,6] Individual reagents were found to react not only with molecules of the immunogen allotype, but also with molecules of other allotypes. For example, anti-f70 antibody obtained from a rabbit with the f72 allotype reacted not only with all f70 sIgA molecules, but also with all f69 and f71 sIgA molecules, and with nearly all f73 sIgA molecules (FIGURE 1). Similar cross-reactions among the sIgA-f allotypes were observed with approximately 40 additional anti-IgA-f alloreagents (FIGURE 1 and unpublished data). In no case did an antiserum react with sIgA molecules of the same allotype

0077–8923/83/0409–0039$1.75/0 © 1983, NYAS

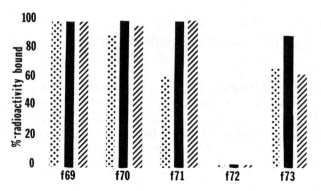

FIGURE 1. Quantitative radiobinding analyses of ^{125}I-labeled f69, f70, f71, f72, and f73 sIgA with three anti-IgA-f alloreagents. ▨ = f72 anti-f69 ■ = f72 anti-f70 ▨ = f72 anti-f71.

as that of the rabbit in which the antiserum was made (e.g., f72 sIgA molecules in FIGURE 1).

IDENTIFICATION OF SUBPOPULATIONS OF sIGA-f MOLECULES

Whereas many of the cross-reactive alloreagents reacted with nearly all sIgA-f molecules of a particular allotype, some reagents reacted with a subset of sIgA-f molecules of one or more of the allotypes. For example, an anti-f71 reagent, which was raised in an f72 rabbit, reacted with 60% of the f73 sIgA molecules (FIGURE 1). These data indicate that f73 sIgA molecules can be separated into at least two subpopulations, one that reacts with anti-f71 and thus apparently shares allodeterminants with f71 molecules, and another that does not react with anti-f71, and thus, does not share allodeterminants with f71 molecules. After adsorption of this anti-f71 antiserum with f73 sIgA molecules—in order to remove antibodies that cross-reacted with f73 sIgA—the antiserum still retained the capacity to react with the f69, f70, and f71 sIgA molecules, but did not react with all of these molecules. The adsorbed antiserum, when used in excess, reacted with 42 to 67% of these molecules (TABLE 1), and thus identified subsets of the f69,

TABLE 1

SUBSETS OF sIGA-f MOLECULES: QUANTITATIVE RADIOBINDING ANALYSIS OF ^{125}I-LABELED sIGA-f MOLECULES WITH ANTI-IGA-f ALLOREAGENTS

	Percent ^{125}I-sIgA-f Bound*				
	f69	f70	f71	f72	f73
f73 adsorbed f72 anti-f71	57	42	67	3	9
f71 anti-f69	67	17	1	57	43
f71 adsorbed f69 anti-f72	ND†	ND	1	44	ND
Goat anti-rabbit Fcα	81	86	82	91	88

*The values reported are the average results of duplicate samples which varied from each other by a maximum of 3%.
†Not done

TABLE 2

Subsets of sIgA-f Molecules: Quantitative Radiobinding Analysis of ^{125}I-Labeled
sIgA-f Molecules with Anti-IgA-f Alloreagents

Antiserum	Percent ^{125}I-sIgA-f Bound*				
	f69	f70	f71	f72	f73
f70 adsorbed f72 anti-f71	52	6	53	1	10
f69 adsorbed f72 anti-f71	1	6	32	2	3
Goat anti-rabbit Fcα	80	86	82	91	88

*The values reported are the average results of duplicate samples which varied from each
other by a maximum of 3%.

f70, and f71 molecules. Subsets of the f72 allotype were identified with two
reagents, an anti-f69 antiserum from an f71 rabbit, and an f71 adsorbed anti-f72
antiserum, made in an f69 rabbit; these reagents reacted with 57% and 44%,
respectively, of the f72 sIgA molecules (TABLE 1).

The specificities of the cross-reactive antibodies of the anti-f71 antiserum
were investigated further by adsorption of the antiserum with f69 and f70 sIgA-f
molecules, and subsequent quantitative radiobinding assays (TABLE 2). The f70
adsorbed antiserum reacted with a subset of f69 and f71 molecules (52 and 53%,
respectively) and not with f70, f72, or f73 molecules; thus, some f69 and f71
molecules share an allodeterminant not found on f70, f72, or f73 molecules.
Adsorption of the anti-f71 antiserum with f69 molecules removed essentially all
of the antibodies that could react with other f-allotype molecules, but left the
antiserum with the capacity to react with a subpopulation of the f71 molecules.

Based on results from the quantitative radiobinding studies, a series of
alloantigenic subspecificities were identified and designated A, B, C, and D.
Subspecificity B, for example, was defined by the reaction of f73 adsorbed
anti-f71 antiserum with subsets of f69, f70, and f71 sIgA molecules. The distribution of the shared subspecificities A, B, and C (and D) among the subsets of each of
the sIgA-f allotypes is shown in a model containing two subsets for each allotype
(FIGURE 2). Unique subspecificities, that is, specificities found only on sIgA
molecules of one allotype, were also found for each IgA-f allotype and are
designated by symbols in FIGURE 2.

In order to study further the relationships of the subpopulations of each of the

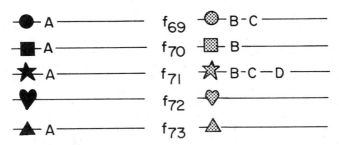

FIGURE 2. Schematic representation of the IgA-f subsets identified by serologic cross-
reactions. Unique allosubspecificities are represented by symbols; cross-reactive allosubspecificities are represented by letters.

sIgA-f allotypes to one another, sIgA-f molecules were tested in sequential radiobinding assays with the various antibodies that identified the subpopulations. Results from these studies indicated that the sIgA-f allotypes are more complex than shown in FIGURE 2. For example, for the f73 sIgA molecules, two preparations of α-chain specific antibodies were used: an f72 anti-f71 antibody preparation that reacted with 43% of f73 sIgA molecules, and an f71 anti-f72 antibody preparation that reacted with 31% of f73 sIgA molecules. After the f73 sIgA molecules that reacted with the f72 anti-71 antibody preparation were removed, an additional 15% of the molecules were found to react with the f71 anti-f72 antibodies (FIGURE 3-1). In the reciprocal experiment, f71 anti-f72 reacted with 31% of f73 sIgA molecules; an additional 26% of the molecules subsequently reacted with the f72 anti-f71 antibodies. These results indicate that the f73 sIgA subpopulations, identified by these two reagents, are not mutually exclusive. This observation was confirmed by a radiobinding assay in which a mixture of the two antibodies bound 55% of the f73 sIgA molecules, rather than the 74% (43% + 31%), which would be expected if the subpopulations were nonoverlapping (FIGURE 3-1). As not all of the f73 sIgA molecules reacted with the f72 anti-f71 and/or the f71 anti-f72 alloreagents, there apparently is another subset of f73 molecules that does not bear the cross-reactive determinants identified by either of these alloreagents. Thus, there may be more than two subsets of f73 sIgA molecules.

Results of sequential radiobinding assays with f71 sIgA molecules also illustrate the complexity of the sIgA-f allotypes. In these studies, however, distinct and nonoverlapping subsets of f71 sIgA were identified (FIGURE 3-2), one by its reactivity with f72 anti-f73 and another by its reactivity with the f73 adsorbed f72 anti-f71. The nonoverlapping nature of the subsets representing 30% and 31% of the f71 molecules, respectively, was confirmed by results of a radiobinding assay in which 58% of the f71 molecules were bound by a mixture of the two alloreagents. Results of sequential radiobinding studies done with each of the other sIgA-f allotypes, f69, f70 and f72, demonstrated that each Cαf allotype appears to be comprised of multiple subsets (data not shown).

GENETIC IMPLICATIONS OF sIgA-f SUBPOPULATIONS

Because the IgA-f allotypic specificities are controlled by genes within the heavy chain chromosomal region, and because the subsets of sIgA-f molecules presumably reflect amino acid differences in the constant region of α-heavy chains, it would appear that there are multiple Cαf genes in the rabbit. This interpretation is dependent on the anti-allotype antisera being specific for the primary structure of α-chains and inactivity for carbohydrate residues or for conformational determinants formed by the association of a given V$_h$a and/or kappa light chain allotype with a particular Cαf allotype. In the studies described, antibodies to such conformational determinants were presumably not involved in identification of subsets, because specific antibodies were prepared by adsorption to, and elution from, immunoadsorbent columns containing sIgA of the immunogen sIgA-f allotype, but of a different V$_h$a and/or kappa light chain allotype.

The IgA-f subsets identified in these studies were presumably not due to carbohydrate moiety differences, as periodate oxidized and non-oxidized sIgA-f molecules[7] reacted nearly identically with the various anti-allotype antisera.

Also, the identification of subsets was not due to structural differences induced by papain hydrolysis of the sIgA molecules, as the subsets were identified in preparations of native sIgA molecules. Thus, we conclude that these subsets must reflect primary structural differences in the α-chains and are presumably encoded by separate genes in the genome. Because we have firmly identified at

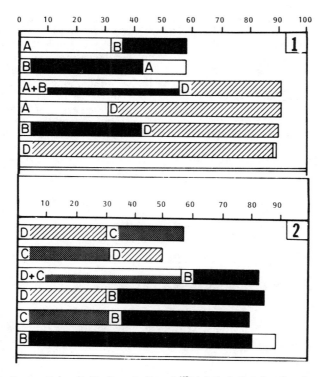

FIGURE 3. Sequential radiobinding studies of ^{125}I-labeled sIgA-f molecules with various alloanti-IgA-f antibodies. ^{125}I-labeled sIgA-f molecules were mixed with the first antibody and the antigen-antibody complexes were removed with *Staphylococcus aureus*; the second antibody was added to the remaining ^{125}I-labeled sIgA and those antigen-antibody complexes were removed with *Staphylococcus aureus*. The percent radioactivity bound by each antibody was determined. Panel 1, subsets of f73 sIgA; Panel 2, subsets of f71 sIgA. Reagent A is f71 anti-f72, B is f72 anti-f71, C is f73 adsorbed f72 anti-f71, and D is f72 anti-f73.

least two subsets of each of the IgA-f allotypes, there must be at least two genes encoding constant regions of α-f molecules, designated $C\alpha f_1$, and $C\alpha f_2$. Results from the sequential radiobinding studies, however, suggest there may be as many as four $C\alpha f$ genes. To determine the precise number and organization of genes encoding rabbit α-chains, we have begun to clone the genes within the heavy chain chromosomal region.

PREPARATION OF cDNA PROBES FOR Cγ AND Cα GENES

Because mammary tissue of lactating animals has been shown to be rich in IgA plasma cells,[8,9] we isolated poly(A)$^+$ RNA from mammary tissue and used this as a template for the preparation of double stranded cDNA encoding α-chains. Similarly, we isolated poly(A)$^+$ RNA from spleen of a rabbit hyperimmunized with *Micrococcus lysodeikticus* and used this as a template for preparation of double stranded cDNA encoding γ-chains.[10,11] The double stranded cDNA was cloned into the *Pst* I site of pBR322. The plasmids were used to transform *E.coli* MC1061, and the resulting cDNA libraries were plated on nitrocellulose filters. Because the C_{h2} domains of rabbit and mouse α-chains are approximately 80% homologous,[3,12] the cDNA library from mammary tissue was screened with a ^{32}P-labeled mouse α-chain cDNA[13] in order to identify one or more plasmids carrying Cα sequences. A cDNA clone with an insert of approximately 500 nucleotides has been isolated by this technique, and has been shown to hybridize specifically to mouse Cα cDNA. Nucleotide sequence studies of this clone are currently in progress in order to confirm that it encodes rabbit Cα. After establishing that this clone encodes rabbit Cα, it will be used as a probe on restriction digests of rabbit germ line DNA in a Southern blot analysis,[14] in order to determine the number of Cα genes in the germ line.

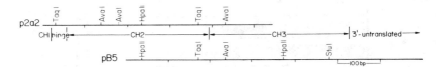

FIGURE 4. Restriction map of two rabbit Cγ cDNA clones, p2a2 and pB5.

From the cDNA library derived from splenic poly(A)$^+$ RNA, several clones were picked, and found to hybridize to a fragment of mouse germ line DNA, encoding the $C\gamma_3$ chain. The nucleotide sequences of two of these clones, p2a2 and pB5 have been totally (p2a2) or partially (pB5) determined and both have been shown to encode rabbit Cγ chains; together, these clones encode the C-terminal eight amino acids of the C_{h1} domain, the entire hinge region and C_{h2} and C_{h3} domains (FIGURE 4). In addition, bases for approximately 150 residues of the 3′ untranslated region were found.

ISOLATION AND CHARACTERIZATION OF TWO Cγ GERM LINE GENES

The Cγ cDNA (p2a2) was used to screen a recombinant phage library made with rabbit liver DNA.[15] Three genomic clones were obtained and, by restriction mapping, appeared to represent two different segments of genomic DNA, each of which hybridized with Cγ cDNA probe, p2a2 (FIGURES 5 and 6). The region of the DNA clone which hybridized with Cγ cDNA was subcloned into pBR322, and comparison of detailed restriction maps of these to each other showed several restriction site differences, both 5′ and 3′ to the regions hybridizing with the Cγ cDNA probe (FIGURE 7). These data further indicate that the two Cγ DNA segments were derived from different regions of the genomic DNA. Partial

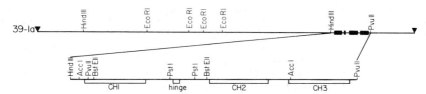

FIGURE 5. Restriction map of recombinant phage clone 39-1a obtained from a library of rabbit liver DNA. A detailed restriction map of the region encoding rabbit Cγ-chains is shown below. The exons encoding the C$_{h1}$ domain, hinge, C$_{h2}$, and C$_{h3}$ domains are indicated.

nucleotide sequence analysis of one of the clones, 39-1a, has established that this segment of DNA encodes rabbit γ-chains in a manner similar to that found for mouse γ-chains; that is, individual gene segments, separated by intervening sequences, encode the C$_{h1}$ domain, the hinge, the C$_{h2}$ domain, and the C$_{h3}$ domain (FIGURE 5). These exons are distributed along approximately 1400 bases of genomic DNA. The nucleotide sequence obtained thus far for these exons is identical to that found for the cDNA, and appears to encode the γ-chain of the IgG molecules present in rabbit serum.

Only a single subclass of rabbit IgG has been well-defined, and thus we did not expect to find two germ line Cγ genes. Nucleotide sequence analysis of the second genomic clone, 20b, revealed that the gene has an unusual structure (FIGURE 7): it encodes approximately 60% of the γ-chain and has an unusual splice site. The gene encodes the entire C$_{h3}$ domain, and all but the N-terminal 23 amino acids of the C$_{h2}$ domain. The nucleotide sequence for these regions is identical to that of the Cγ cDNA, with an intervening sequence of 80 nucleotides between the C$_{h2}$ and C$_{h3}$ domains, and with normal 3' and 5' splice sites at the ends of the intervening sequence. To the 5' side of the nucleotides that encode amino acid 23 of the C$_{h2}$ domain, no sequences were found within 125 bases that would encode the N-terminal 23 amino acids of the C$_{h2}$ domain. Moreover, a consensus RNA splice site is found immediately 5' to the nucleotides encoding amino acid 23. In an effort to locate the C$_{h1}$ domain within this phage clone, a subclone of the DNA encoding the C$_{h1}$ domain in phage clone 39-1a was made and was hybridized to restriction fragments of the entire 20b phage clone. No hybridization of the C$_{h1}$ subclone to the 20b phage clone was detected. Thus, clone 20b does not appear to have sequences that encode the C$_{h1}$ domain. If a genomic sequence encoding the C$_{h1}$ domain is associated with the C$_{h2}$ and C$_{h3}$ domain gene segments

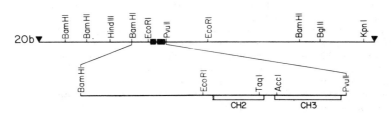

FIGURE 6. Restriction map of recombinant phage clone 20b obtained from a library of rabbit liver DNA. A detailed restriction map of the regions encoding Cγ-chains is shown below; the exons encoding the C$_{h2}$ and C$_{h3}$ domains are indicated.

of clone 20b, it must reside more than four kb upstream. Such a gene structure would be unusual, as no such arrangement has been found for genes encoding mouse heavy chains. If the Cγ gene found in phage clone 20b is expressed as it is found in that clone, that is, without the nucleotides encoding C_{h1} or the N-terminal 23 residues of the C_{h2} domain, then an mRNA smaller than the 16S mRNA that encodes the normal γ-chain should be found. Hybridization of ^{32}P-labeled Cγ cDNA to rabbit splenic poly(A)+ RNA that had been electrophoresed in agarose and blotted onto nitrocellulose,[16] revealed only a single species of RNA, approximately 16S; no hybridization was seen with poly(A)+ RNA smaller than 16S. Thus, if the Cγ gene of clone 20b is expressed as a short γ-chain, this species of γ-chain must be present in minute amounts.

There is no apparent reason why the Cγ-gene in clone 20b cannot be expressed. This Cγ-gene does not appear to be a pseudogene, as there are no stop codons within the coding sequences, and the splice sites at the 5' and 3' ends of the C_{h2}-C_{h3} intervening sequence are normal. The splice site at the 5' end of the C_{h2} coding region also appears to be normal, albeit in an unexpected position.

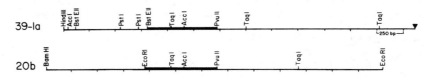

FIGURE 7. Restriction maps of subclones of recombinant phage clones 39-1a and 20b. The regions hybridizing with Cγ cDNA (p2a2) are indicated by heavy lines.

CONCLUSIONS

We have investigated the genes encoding rabbit α- and γ-heavy chains. Serologic analysis of the allotypes of rabbit IgA-f subclass molecules with over 40 alloreagents has revealed that each of the Cαf allotypic specificities is complex; for each allotype, there appear to be multiple allotypic determinants, some of which are shared with one or more of the other Cαf allotypes. Quantitative radiobinding studies with these alloreagents have revealed that molecules of each IgA-f allotype can be separated into at least two subsets. These subsets presumably reflect primary structural differences in the α-chain, as the alloreagents used in these studies were made α-chain specific. Results of sequential radiobinding studies with several alloreagents have confirmed the existence of subsets of the Cαf allotypes and have indicated that each allotype may in fact comprise as many as four subsets. If, indeed, these subsets reflect α-chains that differ in their primary amino acid sequence in the constant regions, then each of these Cα-chains is presumably encoded by separate germ line genes. Thus, we propose there must be at least two germ line genes encoding Cαf molecules, $C\alpha f_1$ and $C\alpha f_2$, as well as a gene encoding α-chains of the IgA-g subclass, Cαg. Characterization of Cα cDNA clones and DNA hybridization studies with these probes and restriction fragments of rabbit DNA should allow us to determine the precise number of α-chain genes in the rabbit genome.

By recombinant DNA technology, we have cloned a cDNA for rabbit γ-chains and have isolated two genomic clones from a recombinant phage library. One of these clones appears to encode the normally expressed γ-chain of rabbit serum

IgG, whereas the other clone encodes a small γ-chain, including the C_{h3} domain and all but the N-terminal 23 amino acids of the C_{h2} domain. At present, we cannot evaluate the physiologic significance of this gene encoding the small γ-chain. It will be important to establish whether this gene is normally expressed, and if so, the nature of the gene product.

REFERENCES

1. CONWAY, T. P., S. DRAY, & E. A. LICHTER. 1969. J. Immun. **102:** 544–554.
2. KNIGHT, K. L. & W. C. HANLY. 1975. *In* Contemporary Topics in Molecular Immunology. F. Inman, and W. Mandy, Eds.: **4:** 55–88. Plenum Publishing Corporation. New York.
3. KNIGHT, K. L., B. FRIEDENSON, W. C. HANLY, T. R. MALEK, & B. E. PETERSON. 1978. *In* Experimental Medicine and Biology. J. McGhee, J. Mestecky, and J. Babb, Eds.: **107:** 513–522. Plenum Publishing Corporation. New York.
4. MALEK, T. R. & K. L. KNIGHT. 1977. Immunochemistry **14:** 493–496.
5. HANLY, W. C., E. A. LICHTER, S. DRAY, & K. L. KNIGHT. 1973. Biochemistry **12:** 733–741.
6. KNIGHT, K. L., E. A. LICHTER, & W. C. HANLY. 1973. Biochemistry **12:** 3197–3203.
7. MATTES, M. J. & L. A. STEINER. 1978. Nature **273:** 761–763.
8. WEISZ-CARRINGTON, P., M. E. ROUX, & M. E. LAMM. 1977. J. Immunol. **119:** 1306–1309.
9. LEE, H., W. C. HANLY, & K. L. KNIGHT. 1977. Fed. Proc. Fed. Am. Soc. Exp. Biol. **38:** abstract # 5515.
10. EFSTRATIADIS, A., T. MANIATIS, F. C. KAFATOS, A. JEFFREY, & J. N. VOURNAKIS. 1975. Cell **4:** 367–378.
11. ROYCHOUDHURY, R., & R. WU. 1980. *In* Methods in Enzymology. L. Grossman and K. Moldave, Eds.: **65:** 43–62. Academic Press. New York.
12. ROBINSON, E. A. & E. APPELLA. 1980. Proc. Natl. Acad. Sci. USA **77:** 4904–4913.
13. EARLY, P. W., M. M. DAVIS, D. B. KABACK, N. DAVIDSON, & L. HOOD. 1979. Proc. Natl. Acad. Sci. USA **76:** 857–861.
14. SOUTHERN, E. M. 1975. J. Mol. Biol. **98:** 503–517.
15. MANIATIS, T., R. C. HARDISON, E. LACY, J. LAUER, C. O'CONNELL, D. QUON, G. K. SIM, & A. EFSTRATIADIS. 1978. Cell **15:** 687–701.
16. THOMAS, P. S. 1980. Proc. Natl. Acad. Sci. USA **77:** 5201–5205.

DISCUSSION OF THE PAPER

W. STROBER (*National Institutes of Health, Bethesda, Md.*): There is a study at NIH on alpha chain genes in man. They have identified, using cDNA probes, two alpha genes in man, as well as two epsilon genes, one of which is a pseudo gene. Could the method that you have described be explained by small differences in the way V-D-J-joining occurs?

K. L. KNIGHT (*University of Illinois at the Medical Center, Chicago, Ill.*): For the alpha chain allotypes, we do not precisely know where they are localized. We know they are only found on IgA. The only information I can give you is that we have done numerous adsorptions of our reagents to remove any activities which might be due to any V-D-J interaction with a particular alpha chain gene. We believe in general that most of these allotypes are recognizing $C\alpha$ determinants.

THE IgA RESPONSE: INDUCTIVE ASPECTS, REGULATORY CELLS, AND EFFECTOR FUNCTIONS*

Suzanne M. Michalek, Jerry R. McGhee, Hiroshi Kiyono,
Dawn E. Colwell, John H. Eldridge, Michael J. Wannemuehler,
and William J. Koopman

*Departments of Microbiology, Pathology, and Medicine
Institute of Dental Research
and
Comprehensive Cancer Center
The University of Alabama in Birmingham
University Station
Birmingham, Alabama 35294*

IINTRODUCTION

Immune defenses against pathogens, allergens, and environmental toxicants, which enter the host by ingestion, utilize a mobilization of cells in gut-associated lymphoreticular tissue (GALT), for example, Peyer's patches (PP). All major cellular immune elements are present in GALT, and these include the two principal accessory cell types [macrophages and dendritic cells], regulatory T-lymphocytes [T-helper (T_h) and T-suppressor (T_s) cells], and precursor IgA B-cells. Following exposure of PP to antigen, necessary cell interactions for initial induction of immune responses occur; however, these interactions do not result in a local immune response in GALT itself. Instead, antigen sensitive cells leave GALT by way of efferent lymphatics and follow a migration pathway, which involves their passage through mesenteric lymph nodes, thoracic duct lymph, and the blood circulation. These migrating cells have a temporary residence in peripheral lymphoid tissue such as spleen, and finally populate the lamina propria regions of the gastrointestinal, upper respiratory, and genitourinary tracts; and interstitium of glands, for example, salivary, lacrimal, and mammary tissues. A large body of evidence has accumulated since the last meeting of mucosal immunologists in Birmingham,[1] that points to the existence of a common mucosal immune defense system for induction of secretory immune responses. In this regard, ingestion or inhalation of antigen results in the sensitization of lymphoid cells in GALT and bronchial-associated lymphoreticular tissues (BALT), respectively, and subsequent migration of precursor IgA B-cells to distant mucosal sites.[2,3] Many aspects of the mucosal immune defense system are still undefined. The precise inductive events, which occur in PP, including regulation of IgA isotype responses and suppressor mechanisms, which may account for lack of local immune responses in GALT and systemic unresponsiveness (oral tolerance) to enterically encountered antigens, are not yet understood. The differentiation of GALT-derived lymphoid cells that occurs during homing and the mechanisms involved in the localization of precursor IgA B-cells in distant secretory tissues have not been determined. Lastly, the signals required for final differentiation of

*This work was supported by United States Public Health Service Grants DE 04217, DE 02670, AI 14807, AM 03555 and CA 13148 and contract DE 02426. SMM is the recipient of Research Career Development Award DE 00092.

0077-8923/83/0409-0048$1.75/0 © 1983, NYAS

precursor IgA cells into plasma cells expressing IgA at mucosal sites are largely unknown.

We have been interested in the cells engaged in the inductive aspects of IgA responses, including antigen presenting macrophages and regulatory cells. To effectively study cell interactions, however, it is also necessary to fully understand how oral antigen encounter results in systemic unresponsiveness.[4] It is now well established that oral administration of antigen,[5-7] and even of simple chemicals,[8] is perhaps the most effective way for induction of tolerance in the host. Numerous studies have shown that oral administration of either particulate antigen,[5,6,9,10] for example, sheep erythrocytes (SRBC), or soluble antigen forms[7] to mice, results in the induction of oral tolerance. Various mechanisms have been proposed for oral tolerance, including induction of T_s-cells,[7,9-11] suppressor factors,[12] immune complexes,[5] and anti-idiotypic antibodies.[6] Compelling evidence exists that oral administration of SRBC or ovalbumin results in the induction of T_s-cells in GALT and that the selective migration of these T_s-cells to peripheral lymphoid tissues, such as spleen, constitutes a major mechanism for oral tolerance.[11] It is also clear that this same oral antigen presentation results in the induction of T_h-cells[13] and precursor IgA B-cells[14] in GALT. Thus, both oral tolerance and secretory IgA responses simultaneously occur following GALT encounters with antigen.[15] Nevertheless, the relationship between oral tolerance and IgA response induction remains a mystery, and thus, we have given this area considerable attention.

ROLE OF GUT BACTERIAL LPS ON ORAL TOLERANCE AND IgA RESPONSES

The demonstration that high IgA responses are induced in LPS-nonresponsive C3H/HeJ mice to orally administered thymic-dependent (TD) antigens,[16,17] suggested that LPS from the indigenous gut microflora profoundly affected these responses. The effect of LPS on GALT was determined by direct comparison of immune responses to gastrically administered SRBC in either C3H/HeJ mice or in syngeneic, LPS-responsive C3H/HeN animals. C3H/HeJ mice, orally primed (SRBC) and subsequently immunized with TNP-SRBC by gastric intubation (GI), exhibited greater T_h-cell induction in GALT and elevated IgA anti-TNP PFC responses when compared with similarly treated C3H/HeN mice. Subsequent studies[17] demonstrated a direct relationship between Lps^d gene expression and elevated IgA responses to orally administered antigen. From these results, we postulated that environmental LPS normally induces precursor T_s-cells in GALT of LPS-responsive mice, and that continued oral exposure to antigen results in mature T_s-cells, which negatively regulate the induction of immune responses. In LPS-nonresponsive mice, orally ingested antigen induces largely a T_h-cell pathway, which results in elevated IgA responses following gastrointestinal exposure to immunogen. If systemic (and perhaps local GALT) unresponsiveness (oral tolerance) is mediated by T_s-cells, then the C3H/HeJ mouse may lack sufficient LPS-induced precursors of this cell type, and thus, offers a model for discriminating between T-cell regulation of IgA immune responses and oral tolerance.

When LPS-responsive and nonresponsive mice were given SRBC daily by GI for 14 consecutive days and subsequently challenged (i.p.) with SRBC, complete unresponsiveness was noted in LPS-responsive mouse strains, while the two LPS-nonresponsive strains tested exhibited full responsiveness to SRBC (FIGURE 1). These results indicated a lack of oral tolerance induction in LPS-nonresponsive mice and indeed, continued oral exposure to SRBC primed these mice for

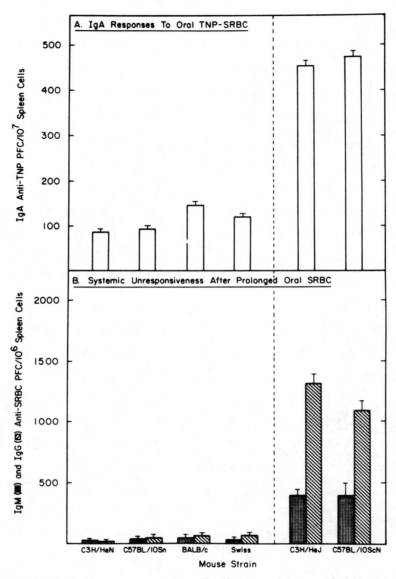

FIGURE 1. Splenic immune response to orally administered antigen of LPS-responsive (C3H/HeN, C57BL/10Sn, BALB/c, and Swiss) and nonresponsive (C3H/HeJ and C57BL/10ScN) mice. A. Groups of mice were given SRBC for two consecutive days by GI, and following GI of TNP-SRBC; the splenic IgA anti-TNP PFC response was assessed. B. Groups of mice were given SRBC daily for 14 days and following i.p. challenge with SRBC, the splenic IgM (▨) and IgG (▧) anti-SRBC PFC responses were assessed. Values are expressed as the mean ± SEM.

secondary responses as evidenced by anti-SRBC PFC responses of the IgG_1, IgG_2, and IgA isotypes.

The cellular basis for oral tolerance in C3H/HeN mice and for heightened responsiveness in C3H/HeJ mice to SRBC was mediated by regulatory T-cells induced in GALT. When both splenic and PP T-cell-enriched fractions from mice given SRBC daily by GI for two weeks were assessed for effector function, C3H/HeJ T-cells showed principally helper activity, while C3H/HeN T-cell fractions exhibited largely T_s-cell activity. Prior treatment of C3H/HeJ T-cells with anti-Lyt-1.1 and rabbit C completely abrogated T-cell help, while treatment of T-cells from spleen or PP of C3H/HeN mice with anti-Lyt-2.1 and C removed suppression.

Evidence that T_s-cells probably originate in PP and mediate oral tolerance in systemic lymphoid tissues such as the spleen was provided by experiments that demonstrated that anti-Lyt-2.1 and C treatment of disassociated PP or spleen cells from C3H/HeN mice, given SRBC by GI for 14 days, completely abrogated

TABLE 1

ANTI-LYT-2 TREATMENT OF SPLEEN OR PP CULTURES ABROGATES SUPPRESSION OF ORALLY TOLERIZED MICE*

Cell Source	Treatment	Anti-SRBC PFC/Culture†		
		IgM	IgG	IgA
Peyer's patch	None	38 ± 11	17 ± 5	6 ± 3
	Anti-Lyt-2 + C	595 ± 37	958 ± 72	2942 ± 65
Spleen	None	42 ± 7	34 ± 17	22 ± 4
	Anti-Lyt-2 + C	352 ± 35	1287 ± 44	1528 ± 42

*Single cell preparations of PP or spleen from C3H/HeN mice given SRBC by GI for two weeks were either untreated or treated with anti-Lyt-2 and C, cultured (5×10^6 cells) with SRBC ($2-3 \times 10^6$) and bioassayed on day 5.
†Values are the mean $\pm$ SEM.

suppression (TABLE 1). It should be noted that good IgA PFC responses occurred in PP cell cultures treated in this manner. Furthermore, both IgG and IgA splenic PFC responses were obtained, clearly suggesting that prolonged oral administration of SRBC primed GALT B-cells for immune responses. Similar results have been obtained with PP and spleen cell preparations from three other LPS-responsive mouse strains.

If endogenous gut LPS induces precursor T_s-cells in GALT, which subsequently become mature antigen-sensitive cells following oral exposure to antigen, mice that have never encountered LPS should exhibit aberrant patterns of oral tolerance induction. Groups of germfree (GF) and conventionally raised (CONV) mice were given SRBC by GI for 14 days and then assessed for systemic unresponsiveness to i.v. administered antigen (FIGURE 2). GF mice were fully responsive to SRBC and manifested largely anamnestic-type responses, whereas similarly treated CONV mice were tolerant. To clearly establish that LPS is

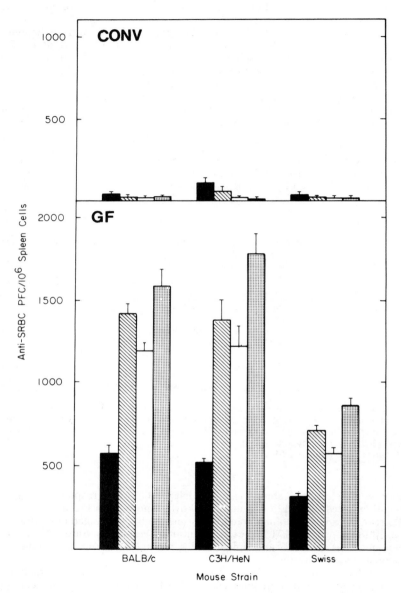

FIGURE 2. Effect of prolonged, daily GI of SRBC to CONV and germfree strains (BALB/c, C3H/HeN, and Swiss) of mice on oral tolerance induction. Groups of mice were given SRBC daily for 14 consecutive days by GI, and following i.v. challenge, with SRBC; the splenic IgM (■), IgG$_1$ (▨), IgG$_2$ (□) and IgA (▥) anti-SRBC PFC responses were assessed. Values are expressed as the mean ± SEM.

responsible for priming to affect oral tolerance induction, GF BALB/c mice were first given LPS orally, prior to prolonged oral administration of SRBC by GI. When these mice were subsequently challenged (i.v.) with SRBC, complete tolerance was observed (FIGURE 3).

In summary, our results provide compelling evidence that oral tolerance to SRBC is mediated by T_s-cells. We further suggest that precursors of T_s in GALT are uniquely sensitive to LPS, and require stimulation by this active substance in order to maintain a regulatory cell population, which is responsible for systemic unresponsiveness. This mechanism would be an obvious host benefit, since common encounters with oral antigens and subsequent migration of cells to the periphery would result in considerable immune regulation.

Thus, in the normal host, LPS from the gut directly influences GALT T-cells,

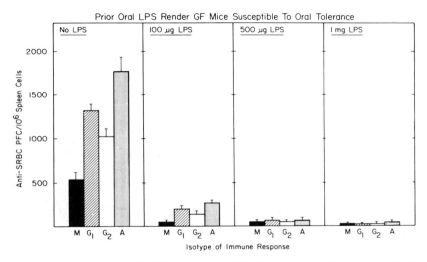

FIGURE 3. Effect of prior GI of LPS to germfree BALB/c mice on oral tolerance induction. Groups of germfree mice were given various doses of LPS by GI prior to daily GI of SRBC for two weeks and following i.v. challenge with SRBC, the splenic IgM (■), IgG₁ (▨), IgG₂ (□), and IgA (▨) anti-SRBC PFC responses were assessed. Values are expressed as the mean ± SEM.

which are important in natural negative homeostasis. We further propose that LPS affects precursors of T_s-cells (Lyt-2^+, I-J$^-$ phenotype). This is an important distinction, since it has been shown that a contrasuppressor circuit, consisting of Lyt-2^+, I-J$^+$ inducer cells, and Lyt-1^+, 2^+, I-J$^+$, Qa-1^+ contrasuppressor cells, occurs in mice.[18] We predict that this circuit is resistant to LPS effects and in the normal host, continued oral exposure to TD antigens results in the induction of Lyt-2^+ T-cells, including those involved in contrasuppression. These interactions are summarized in FIGURE 4. Evidence for the contrasuppressor circuit in GALT has already been provided by Green and associates,[19] who demonstrated that treatment of PP T-cells with anti-I-J and C removed contrasuppressor cells and yielded an Lyt-2^+, I-J$^-$ T-cell population that was highly suppressive. In our model, GF mice (LPS-free) and LPS-nonresponsive C3H/HeJ mice should possess diminished numbers of precursor Lyt-2$^+$, I-J$^-$ T-cells in GALT, and continued oral administration of TD antigens would result in predominantly an Lyt-1$^+$ population of T$_h$-cells that continually promotes IgA responses (FIGURE 4).

CHARACTERIZATION OF LYMPHORETICULAR CELLS IN
MURINE PEYER'S PATCHES

Murine PP contain antigen-sensitive T- and B-cells[20] and accessory cell-types (macrophages and dendritic cells),[14,21] and are covered by an active pinocytotic epithelium of M-cells that readily delivers gut lumenal antigens to underlying

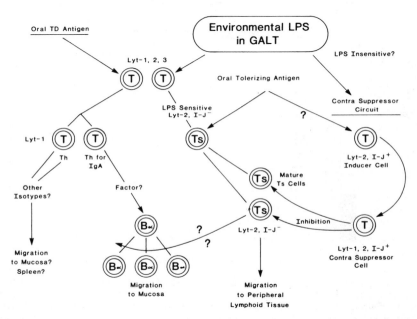

FIGURE 4. Model for T-cell regulation of the inductive events for IgA responses and oral tolerance in GALT.

lymphoreticular cells. Our laboratories have recently developed an enzymatic (Dispase®) method, which releases the total cell population present in the PP. Approximately equal numbers of T- and B-cells are obtained following dissociation (TABLE 2), and a significant percentage of esterase positive cells are obtained. It should be noted that the enzyme dissociation method results in recovery of approximately three-fold more cells than mechanical manipulation, and the latter method largely yields only T- and B-lymphocytes.[22]

When individual immunoglobulin isotype distributions were compared on PP B-cells from either C3H/HeN or C3H/HeJ mice (TABLE 3), the highest percentage of B-cells ($\kappa^+ + \lambda^+$) also stained for IgM. A significant percentage of B-cells bore surface IgA and a small percentage were sIgG.$^+$ Approximately 60 percent of

TABLE 2

DISTRIBUTION OF T- AND B-LYMPHOCYTES AND MACROPHAGES IN MURINE SPLEEN AND PEYER'S PATCHES

Mouse Strain	Peyer's Patch*			Spleen		
	Immunofluorescence			Immunofluorescence		
	Anti-Thy 1.2	Anti-κ + λ	Esterase Positive (M∅)	Anti-Thy 1.2	Anti-κ + λ	Esterase Positive (M∅)
C3H/HeJ	37.3	40.6	6.5	28.9	53.1	10.1
C3H/HeN	37.5	41.2	6.8	31.0	52.2	9.8
C57BL/10ScN	35.2	38.2	6.0	31.4	54.4	9.2
C5BL/10Sn	36.2	40.1	6.4	34.2	52.0	8.3
BALB/c	36.1	41.5	7.7	31.3	53.4	8.9
Swiss/Webster	35.1	38.3	6.7	33.6	54.1	8.6

*PP were enzymatically dissociated (with Dispase®) into single cell suspensions prior to staining.

TABLE 3

SURFACE ANTIGENS PRESENT ON MURINE PP B-LYMPHOCYTES

Mouse Strain	Immunofluorescence (Percent Staining)				
	Anti-κ + λ	Anti-μ	Anti-α	Anti-γ	Anti-I-A$^{\kappa}$
C3H/HeJ	100	91.3	15.3	1.1	99.6
C3H/HeN	100	92.3	12.8	0.9	98.7

sIgA$^+$ B-cells did not bear sIgM (data not shown). Essentially all C3H PP B-cells possessed I-A^k (TABLE 3).

Since differences have been noted in responses to orally administered TD antigens between C3H/HeN and C3H/HeJ mice (reviewed above), which are due largely to regulatory T-cells (T$_h$- and T$_s$-cells), it was of interest to compare surface phenotypes of isolated PP T-cells from these two strains of mice (TABLE 4). As can be seen, greater numbers of T-cells from PP of C3H/HeJ mice bear Fc$_\alpha$ receptors (FcR$_\alpha$). This would suggest a correlation between FcR$_\alpha$ and greater numbers of Lyt-1$^+$-cells, and would perhaps indicate that T$_h$-cells for IgA responses bear Fc$_\alpha$ receptors. In data not shown, we have characterized accessory cell populations present in murine PP. This cell population contains significant numbers of dendritic cells. Furthermore, the accessory cells bear large amounts of surface I-A. A clear demonstration of the ability of PP accessory cells to support *in vitro* immune responses is provided in FIGURE 5. Good *in vitro* immune responses to SRBC were induced in cultures containing irradiated PP accessory cells and purified T- and B-cells from either spleen or PP. Prior treatment of C3H/HeN PP accessory cell populations with anti-I-A$^\epsilon$ and C, completely abrogated *in vitro* immune responses. Thus, the murine PP possesses all of the necessary cellular elements required for immune responses, including cells for IgA isotype responses.

ANALYSIS OF T-HELPER CELL CLONES FROM GALT

The IgA response is T-cell dependent;[23-25] nevertheless, it has been difficult to study T-cell regulation of the IgA response to specific antigens. This was, in part, due to nonuniform methods for isolation of T-cells from GALT, and to low frequencies of antigen-specific T$_h$-cells in the T-lymphocyte population. The availability of methods for continuous proliferation of antigen-specific T-lymphocyte clones in culture has been a recent significant advance in studies directed toward a molecular understanding of T-cell function. In studies reported here, we have adapted the method of Watson[26] to directly isolate and grow T-cells from murine PP. Single T-cell clones have been established, which are antigen-

TABLE 4

SURFACE ANTIGENS PRESENT ON MURINE PP T-LYMPHOCYTES

Mouse Strain	Immunofluorescence (Percent Staining)				Fc Receptor for IgA (Percent Rosettes)
	Anti-Thy 1.2	Anti-Lyt-1	Anti-Lyt-2	Anti-I-A	
C3H/HeJ	100	80	16	<1	9.3
C3H/HeN	100	56	29	<1	2.4

specific and dependent upon T-cell growth factor (TCGF), that is, interleukin 2 (IL 2), for continuous growth. These clones have been maintained for long periods in continuous culture, and a number of these clones exhibit helper activity for IgA responses.

For establishment of PP T-cell clones, C3H/HeJ mice were given SRBC by GI,

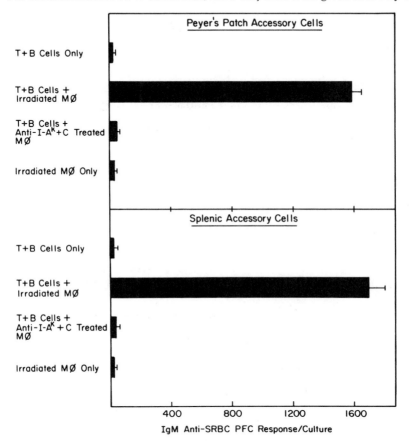

FIGURE 5. Functional capability of Peyer's patch accessory cells for support of *in vitro* immune responses to SRBC. Purified C3H/HeN splenic T- and B-cells (2.5 × 10⁶/culture) were incubated with either irradiated (1500 rads) or anti-I-A^K and C treated Peyer's patch (upper panel); or splenic (lower panel) accessory cells (2.5 × 10⁶ equivalent cells/culture) and SRBC (2–3 × 10⁶). The IgM anti-SRBC PFC response/culture was determined on day 5 of incubation. Values expressed are the mean ± SEM. MØ = macrophages.

and one week later, dissociated PP cells were enriched for T-cells. Purified PP T-cells were cultured in the presence of IL 2, feeder cells, and SRBC, arid wells exhibiting clonal growth were expanded into several wells of macroculture plates (FIGURE 6). Cultures were subcloned by limiting dilution into 96-well microculture plates[26] and subclones were incubated with IL 2 and feeder cells, but without

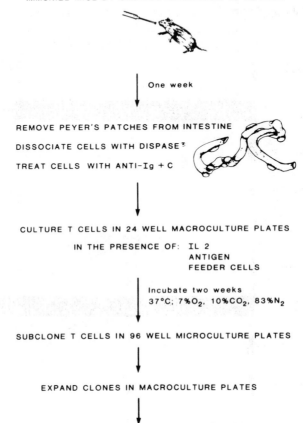

IMMUNIZE MICE BY GASTRIC INTUBATION OF ANTIGEN

One week

REMOVE PEYER'S PATCHES FROM INTESTINE

DISSOCIATE CELLS WITH DISPASE℗

TREAT CELLS WITH ANTI-Ig + C

CULTURE T CELLS IN 24 WELL MACROCULTURE PLATES

IN THE PRESENCE OF: IL 2
                     ANTIGEN
                     FEEDER CELLS

Incubate two weeks
$37°C$; $7\%O_2$, $10\%CO_2$, $83\%N_2$

SUBCLONE T CELLS IN 96 WELL MICROCULTURE PLATES

EXPAND CLONES IN MACROCULTURE PLATES

BIOASSAY CLONES FOR T CELL FUNCTION

FIGURE 6. Experimental procedure employed for the production of murine Peyer's patch T-cell clones.

antigen. A cloning efficiency of approximately 45 to 55% was seen. We have established clones from murine PP from mice orally primed with SRBC, horse erythrocytes (HRBC), or keyhole limpet hemocyanin (KLH). For simplicity, our results with SRBC specific clones are presented here.

Approximately 25% of over 200 clones, established from murine PP exhibit

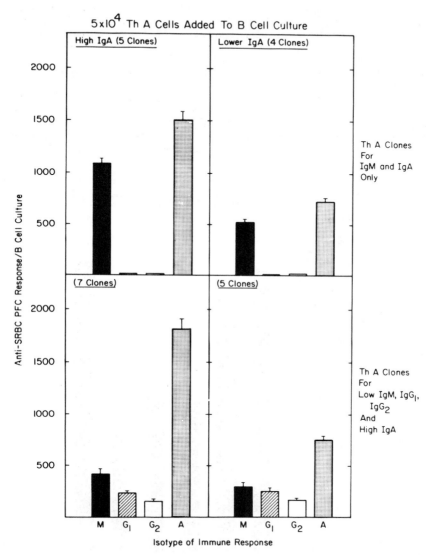

FIGURE 7. Characterization of helper activity of cloned Peyer's patch T_h A-cells for *in vitro* immune responses of splenic B-cell cultures from normal C3H/HeN mice to SRBC. Splenic B-cell cultures (2.5×10^6 cells) were incubated with cloned T_h A-cells (5×10^4/culture) and SRBC ($2-3 \times 10^6$) and assessed on day 5 for IgM (■), IgG$_1$ (▨), IgG$_2$ (□), and IgA (▧) anti-SRBC PFC responses. Values are the mean ± SEM.

T_h-cell activity (63 clones) and of these, 21 exhibit T_h-activity for support of IgA responses (FIGURE 7). Generally, these 21 clones could be divided into two broad groups, that is, those supporting IgM and IgA anti-SRBC PFC responses, and those that supported low IgM, IgG$_1$, and IgG$_2$ and high IgA anti-SRBC PFC responses. The distinction in T_h-cell activity for IgM and IgA on the one hand and for IgM, IgG$_1$, IgG$_2$, and IgA on the other hand was not due to mixed clones, because recloning of T-cells in each category yielded progeny with exactly the same properties as the parent clones. Because these clones largely support IgA isotype responses, they have been designated PP T_h A-clones.

Six PP T_h A-clones (Nos. 1, 5, 7, 9, 11, and 14) were selected for further analysis, because each of these clones supports good IgA anti-SRBC PFC responses. Our past work[14] indicated that although PP lymphoreticular cells from normal mice support *in vitro* immune responses to SRBC, IgA responses were only seen in PP cell cultures from mice orally primed, suggesting that antigen-

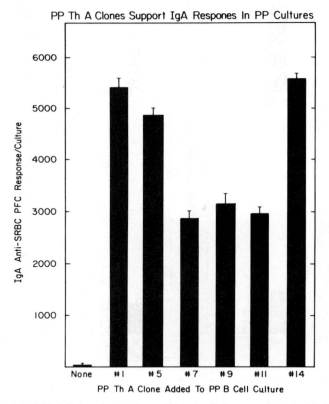

FIGURE 8. Capability of cloned Peyer's patch T_h A-cells to support *in vitro* IgA responses of Peyer's patch B-cell cultures from normal C3H/HeN mice. Peyer's patch B-cell cultures (2.5×10^6 cells) were incubated with cloned T_h A-cells (5×10^4/culture) and SRBC (2–3×10^6) and assessed on day 5 for IgA anti-SRBC PFC responses. Values are the mean ± SEM.

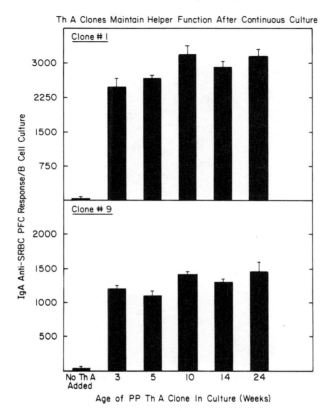

FIGURE 9. Stability of Peyer's patch T_h A-cell clones after continuous culture for support of IgA responses. Splenic B-cell cultures (2.5×10^6 cells) from SRBC orally primed C3H/HeN mice were incubated with cloned T_h A-cells (5×10^4/culture), which had been maintained in culture for various lengths of time, and SRBC ($2-3 \times 10^6$), and assessed on day 5 for IgA anti-SRBC PFC responses. Values are the mean ± SEM.

primed cells were required for IgA responses. When PP T_h A-cells were added to normal PP B-cell cultures (FIGURE 8) that were immunized with SRBC, excellent IgA responses were noted. This clearly suggests that T_h-cells for IgA responses are of central importance for expression of this isotype, and that primed PP B-cells are not a significant prerequisite.

At present, cloned T-cells from murine PP have been maintained in continuous culture for 50 weeks. Clones that exhibit T_h-activity have maintained their ability to support IgA responses (FIGURE 9). It is interesting that cloned T-cells that support either high (clone No. 1) or moderate (clone No. 9) IgA responses have maintained this property for long periods in culture. Similar results were obtained with other clones.

Cloned T_h A-cells are TCGF dependent and antigen independent (after an initial two week incubation with antigen) and exhibit good growth in micro- and macroculture wells (FIGURE 10). Somewhat surprisingly, T_h A-cell clones (T_h A

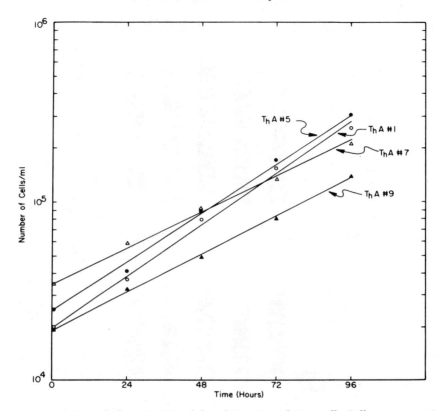

FIGURE 10. Growth characteristics of cloned Peyer's patch T_h A-cells. Cells were grown in microculture wells in complete medium containing TCGF; cells were harvested daily, and viable cells (>95%) enumerated. Individual clones assessed were No. 1 (—O—), No. 5 (—●—), No. 7 (—△—), and No. 9 (—▲—).

Nos. 1 and 5) for only IgM and IgA isotype responses, exhibited higher growth rates than clones supporting low IgM and IgG, and high IgA responses (T_h A Nos. 7 and 9). This has been a consistent finding with all 21 clones tested thus far (data not shown). Addition of excess TCGF to T_h A-clones supporting all three isotype responses did not significantly increase their rate of division (approximately one division every 36 hours).

All PP T_h A-clones tested are antigen-specific and support *in vitro* IgA responses only in the presence of the homologous antigen, SRBC (FIGURE 11). Cloned T_h A-cells do not support *in vitro* immune responses of B-cell cultures immunized with HRBC or chicken erythrocytes (CRBC). Previous studies with cloned T_h-cells suggested a stringent requirement for H-2 compatibility[26] for effective T-cell help. Our experiments also clearly indicate that H-2 compatibility is required for T_h-cell promotion of IgA isotype responses (TABLE 5). T_h A-clones

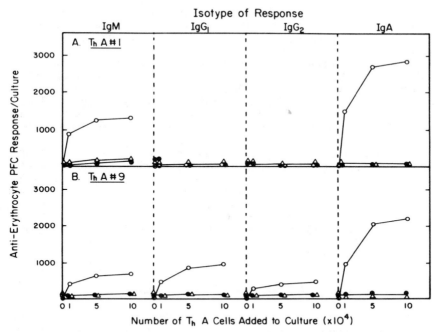

FIGURE 11. Antigen-specificity of helper activity of cloned Peyer's patch T_h A-cells for IgM, IgG_1, IgG_2, and IgA isotype responses. Various numbers of T_h A-cells from clone No. 1 (panel A) or No. 9 (panel B) were added to C3H/HeN splenic B-cell cultures immunized with SRBC (—○—), HRBC (—●—) or CRBC (-△-). The isotype (IgM, IgG_1, IgG_2, or IgA) of anti-erythrocyte PFC responses was determined on day 5 of culture.

TABLE 5

H-2 SPECIFICITY IS REQUIRED FOR T-CELL HELP IN THE IgA RESPONSE*

	IgA Anti-SRBC PFC/Culture† (PP T_h A-clone number)	
	No. 1	No. 2
Source of Spleen Cells		
Nu/nu		
BALB/c	232 ± 17	187 ± 21
C3H/HeN	2487 ± 93	2292 ± 104
B-Cell Culture		
BALB/c	137 ± 7	155 ± 18
C57BL/10Sn	102 ± 8	121 ± 17
C3H/HeN	2662 ± 48	2171 ± 88

*Spleen cells or purified splenic B-cells (2.5×10^6/culture) were incubated with SRBC (2–3×10^6) and cloned T-cells (5×10^4/culture) and bioassayed on day 5.
†Values are the mean ± SEM.

supported good IgA responses in C3H/HeN nude splenic or B-cell cultures, but not in cell cultures derived from H-2 incompatible mice. Thus, complete H-2 compatibility is required for efficient cell interactions involved in the IgA response.

All PP T_h A-cell clones tested thus far are Thy-1.2$^+$ and Lyt-2$^-$ (TABLE 6). In addition, T_h A-cells are Lyt-1$^+$; however, a different pattern of surface staining is seen between cloned T-cells and normal splenic or PP T-cells examined for surface Lyt-1 antigen. Cloned T_h A-cells exhibit a complete halo of dull fluorescence, whereas normal splenic or PP Lyt-1$^+$ T-cells exhibit strong, patchy surface immunofluorescence. None of the clones examined thus far exhibit surface Ig or I-A.

Previous studies have shown that both murine[27] and human[28] T-cell subpopulations form rosettes with IgA-coated erythrocytes, which clearly suggests the presence of T-cell subpopulations with Fc receptors for IgA. We have tested this property with cloned T_h A-cells (FIGURE 12). No IgM or IgG$_{2a}$ rosetting occurred with PP T_h-cell clones; however, the majority of T_h A-cells formed rosettes with IgA-coated erythrocytes. This clearly suggests that PP T_h A-cells bear surface Fc receptors for IgA. In other studies using FITC-labeled MOPC-315 IgA, greater than 99% of T_h A-clones were positive by immunofluorescence or by fluorescence-activated cell-sorter (FACS) analysis.

HIGH FREQUENCY INDUCTION OF IGA HYBRIDOMAS

We have recently developed immunization regimens that have allowed the production of B-cell hybridomas with high frequencies for the IgA isotype. The regimen basically involves either gastric intubation of GF BALB/c mice with appropriate antigens or long-term intravenous injection of CONV mice with killed bacteria. This has allowed us to produce a large number of mouse monoclonal IgA antibodies to major surface determinants of the gram-positive bacterium *Streptococcus mutans* and to somatic determinants of *Salmonella typhimurium* and *Escherichia coli*. Of the hybridomas tested, which produced murine antibodies to surface determinants of *S. mutans*, *S. typhimurium* and *E. coli*, 83%, 48%, and 50%, respectively, were of the IgA isotype. In additional studies, GF Fischer rats were GI with killed *S. mutans* whole cells, and 73% of the subsequent rat-mouse hybridomas secreted rat monoclonal anti-*S. mutans* antibodies of the IgA isotype.

TABLE 6

CHARACTERIZATION OF PP T_h A-CLONES FOR CELL SURFACE ANTIGENS

PP T_h A-Clone No.	Percentage of Cells Bearing Antigen*				
	Thy-1.2	Lyt-1	Lyt-2	I-A$^\kappa$	Ig($\kappa + \lambda$)
1	>99	99.5	0	0	0
5	>99	97.0	0	0	0
7	>99	97.0	0	0	0
9	>99	98.0	0	0	0
11	>99	93.5	0	0	0
14	>99	98.0	0	0	0

*Values are the mean percentage of three separate experiments.

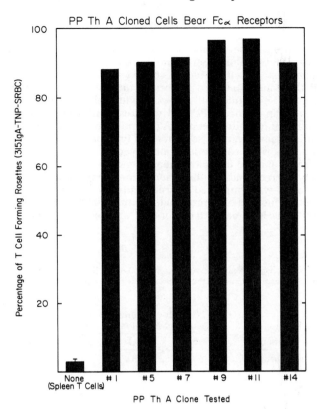

FIGURE 12. Isotype of Fc receptors present on cloned Peyer's patch T_h A-cells. Monoclonal IgM (κ), IgG_{2_a} (κ), or IgA (λ) anti-DNP antibodies were reacted with TNP-SRBC, followed by incubation with cloned T_h A-cells. The number of rosettes were enumerated in 10–15 fields. At least 1500 lymphoid cells were scored for each slide/experiment. Values are the mean percent of T_h A-cells forming rosettes.

The precise specificities of representative hybridoma antibodies were determined by hemagglutination of either *S. typhimurium* or *E. coli* LPS-coated erythrocytes and by ELISA for individual cell surface determinants of *S. mutans* (TABLE 7). Thirty-three percent of the anti-*E. coli* hybridomas and 10% of the anti-*S. typhimurium* hybridomas tested exhibited antibody specificity to the appropriate LPS. Mouse and rat monoclonal antibodies to *S. mutans* were predominantly specific for carbohydrate antigens; however, some monoclonal antibodies were reactive with other cell surface determinants, for example, lipoteichoic acid and cell surface protein.

Our laboratory is currently characterizing the IgA monoclonal antibodies for molecular size, light chain types, and for possible allotype antigen differences. These antibodies will then be used to determine precise effector functions for IgA in host defense against pathogenic bacteria.

DISCUSSION

It is now well established that immune responses to TD antigens are dependent upon the precise interaction of antigen-presenting accessory cells and T- and B-lymphocytes. *In vitro* studies suggest that cell contact, macrophages, T-cells, and their mediators are important for induction of proliferation and differentiation of B-cells into antibody-producing cells. Our studies show that all of these events can occur in PP cell cultures. Furthermore, the presence of T_h-cells is sufficient for induction of IgA isotype specific responses.

The technique employed for separation of lymphoreticular cells from PP is of utmost importance, since early studies employed methods that did not release all cell types present and led to the erroneous conclusion that GALT is deficient in certain cell types required for induction of antibody-forming cells. When the enzyme Dispase® was employed, a true lymphoreticular cell population was obtained, which consisted of approximately equal numbers of T- and B-cells and accessory cell types. Richman and coworkers[29] showed that collagenase treatment

TABLE 7

SPECIFICITY OF MONOCLONAL ANTIBODIES TO S. *MUTANS* CELL WALL COMPONENTS*

Cell Surface Component	Number of Clones Producing Murine Monoclonal Antibody			Number of Clones Producing Rat Monoclonal Antibody†	
	IgA	IgG	IgM	IgA	IgG
Serotype carbohydrate	14	8	6	3	5
Lipoteichoic acid	7	10	14	3	0
Dextran	23	12	18	3	1
Cell surface protein	2	15	10	NT‡	NT

*As determined by ELISA. Analysis of representative clones only.
†Of the 19 hybridomas tested, 13 produced IgA and 6 produced IgG isotype antibodies. Four of the hybridomas produced IgA antibody that reacted with S. *mutans* whole cells but not with serotype carbohydrate, lipoteichoic acid, or dextran.
‡NT: not tested.

of PP yielded a macrophage population capable of presenting antigen to primed T-cells. Our past experience has been that conventional, mechanical disruption of PP yields populations rich in T- and B-cells, but deficient in macrophages.[22] Thus, numerous studies of others, indicating accessory cell requirement for induction of regulatory T-cells, were supported by our own results, and it must be now accepted that antigen presentation to precursor T-cells in GALT can lead to full maturation of T-cells within this tissue.

The unique environment of GALT, including the continued interaction of lymphoreticular cells with gastrointestinal immunostimulants and suppressants, coupled with the propensity of lymphoid cells from this tissue to migrate to other locales, including mucosal sites, provides the host with obvious benefits. Although much remains to be done to elucidate the contribution of nonspecific stimulation of GALT, our work clearly demonstrates that bacterial endotoxin (LPS) is of central importance. The finding that C3H/HeJ mice and GF mice do not become tolerant to orally administered TD antigen, suggests that the pathway for T_s-cell induction is either absent or deficient in these mice. We further suggest that precursors of T_s-cells in GALT are affected by LPS from the indigenous flora or by orally administered LPS in GF mice, and that these cells are induced toward a suppressor pathway. Chronic oral exposure to TD antigens, such as SRBC, would subsequently result in the induction of significant numbers of antigen-specific T_s-cells, which upon migration to peripheral lymphoid tissues, such as spleen, would mediate unresponsiveness to systemically encountered antigen. Thus, LPS in the normal host would represent a central element in maintenance of homeostasis by induction of regulatory T-cells.

The C3H/HeJ mouse also offers us a unique model for studies of T-cell regulation of IgA responses. We have used this unique mouse strain to induce clones of PP T-cells that are able to promote IgA immune responses. Cloned T_h-cells from murine PP have been grown in continuous culture for seven months without affecting their ability to promote IgA responses. Thus far, two broad groups of T_h-cells have been defined; the first promotes IgM and high IgA responses, whereas the second supports low, but significant IgM and IgG subclasses, and elevated IgA responses. Clones of T-cells from both groups are Thy-1.2^+, Lyt-1^+, and Lyt-2^-. It should be noted that T_h A-clones promote even greater IgA PFC responses in GALT B-cell cultures, further corroborating the importance of GALT as a major inductive site for the IgA response. At present, we do not understand why full collaboration for IgA responses fails to occur in the PP itself, but is instead manifested after sensitized cells have migrated to distant mucosal sites. One distinct possibility would be the simultaneous induction of T_s-cells in GALT that would act either on T_h A-cells or IgA precursor B-cells to prevent local immune responses. In this regard, it is well known that T_s-cells can specifically inhibit IgG responses.[30] In some instances, T_s-cells may negatively regulate expression of IgG subclasses.[31] Some evidence for IgA isotype-specific T_s-cells has been derived from studies with IgA deficient subjects.[25] We are currently exploring this possibility by isolation and growth of T_s-cells from murine PP; cloned T_s-cells will be tested for isotype-specific suppression either at the level of T_h A-cells or directly on precursor IgA B-cells.

Summary

In this review, we have emphasized our current studies on the inductive aspects of the IgA immune response and homeostatic mechanisms involved in the induction of oral tolerance. By use of unique inbred mouse strains in restricted microbial environments, we have provided evidence for a central role of LPS in systemic unresponsiveness to orally encountered antigens. We have continued studies on characterization of GALT lymphoreticular cell types, including accessory cells, regulatory T-cells, and precursor IgA B-cells. We have placed recent emphasis on characterization of antigen-specific T_h-cell clones derived from murine PP, which preferentially support IgA isotype responses. Relevant areas for continued research have been emphasized in this review.

References

1. McGHEE, J. R., J. MESTECKY and J. L. BABB. 1978. Secretory Immunity and Infection. **107:** 1–905. Plenum Press. New York.
2. McDERMOTT, M. R. and J. BIENENSTOCK. 1979. Evidence for a common immunologic

immune system. I. Migration of B lymphocytes into intestinal, respiratory and genital tissues. J. Immunol. **122:** 1892–1898.

3. McDermott, M. R., D. A. Clark and J. Bienenstock. 1980. Evidence for a common immunologic immune system. II. Influence of the estrous cycle on B immunoblast migration into genital and intestinal tissues. J. Immunol. **124:** 2536–2539.

4. Tomasi, T. B., Jr. 1980. Oral tolerance. Transplantation **29:** 353–356.

5. André, C., J. F. Heremans. J.-P. Vaerman, and C. L. Cambiaso. 1975. A mechanism for the induction of immunological tolerance by antigen feeding: antigen antibody complexes. J. Exp. Med. **142:** 1509–1519.

6. Kagnoff, M. F. 1978. Effects of antigen-feeding on intestinal and systemic immune responses. III. Antigen-specific serum-mediated suppression of humoral antibody responses after antigen feeding. Cell. Immunol. **40:** 186–203.

7. Richman, L. M., J. M. Chiller, W. R. Brown, D. G. Hanson, and N. M. Vaz. 1978. Enterically induced immunological tolerance. I. Induction of suppressor T lymphocytes by intragastric administration of soluble proteins. J. Immunol. **121:** 2429–2434.

8. Chase, M. W. 1946. Inhibition of experimental drug allergy by prior feeding of the sensitizing agent. Proc. Soc. Exp. Biol. Med. **61:** 257–259.

9. Kiyono, H., J. R. McGhee, M. J. Wannemuehler, and S. M. Michalek. 1982. Lack of oral tolerance in C3H/HeJ mice. J. Exp. Med. **155:** 605–610.

10. Michalek, S. M., H. Kiyono, M. J. Wannemuehler, L. M. Mosteller, and J. R. McGhee. 1982. Lipopolysaccharide (LPS) regulation of the immune response: LPS influence on oral tolerance induction. J. Immunol. **128:** 1992–1998.

11. Richman, L. K., A. S. Graeff, R. Yarchoan, and W. Strober. 1981. Simultaneous induction of antigen-specific IgA helper T cells and IgG suppressor T cells in the murine Peyer's patch after protein feeding. J. Immunol. **126:** 2079–2082.

12. Mattingly, J. A., J. M. Kaplan, and C. A. Janeway, Jr. 1980. Two distinct antigen-specific suppressor factors induced by the oral administration of antigen. J. Exp. Med. **152:** 545–554.

13. Kiyono, H., J. L. Babb, S. M. Michalek, and J. R. McGhee. 1980. Cellular basis for elevated IgA responses in C3H/HeJ mice. J. Immunol. **125:** 732–737.

14. Kiyono, H., J. R. McGhee, M. J. Wannemuehler, M. V. Frangakis, D. M. Spalding, S. M. Michalek, and W. J. Koopman. 1982. In vitro immune responses to a T cell-dependent antigen by cultures of disassociated murine Peyer's patch. Proc. Natl. Acad. Sci. USA. **79:** 596–600.

15. Challacombe, S. J., and T. B. Tomasi, Jr. 1980. Systemic tolerance and secretory immunity after oral immunization. J. Exp. Med. **152:** 1459–1472.

16. Babb, J. L., and J. R. McGhee. 1980. Mice refractory to lipopolysaccharide manifest high immunoglobulin A responses to orally administered antigen. Infect. Immun. **29:** 322–328.

17. Michalek, S. M., H. Kiyono, J. L. Babb and J. R. McGhee. 1980. Inheritance of LPS nonresponsiveness and elevated splenic IgA immune response in mice orally immunized with heterologous erythrocytes. J. Immunol. **125:** 2220–2224.

18. Gershon, R. K., D. D. Eardley, S. Durum, D. R. Green, F.-W. Shen, K. Yamauchi, H. Cantor, and D. B. Murphy. 1981. Contrasuppression. A novel immunoregulatory activity. J. Exp. Med. **153:** 1533–1546.

19. Green, D. R., J. Gold, S. St. Martin. R. Gershon, and R. K. Gershon. 1982. Microenvironmental immunoregulation: possible role of contrasuppressor cells in maintaining immune responses in gut-associated lymphoid tissues. Proc. Natl. Acad. Sci. USA. **79:** 889–892.

20. Kagnoff, M. F., and S. Campbell. 1974. Functional characteristics of Peyer's patch lymphoid cells. I. Induction of humoral antibody and cell-mediated allograft reactions. J. Exp. Med. **139:** 398–406.

21. Faulk, W. P., J. N. McCormick, J. R. Goodman, J. M. Yoffey and H. H. Fudenberg. 1971. Peyer's patches: morphologic studies. Cell. Immunol. **1:** 500–520.

22. Kiyono, H., J. R. McGhee, J. F. Kearney, and S. M. Michalek. 1982. Enhancement of in vitro immune responses of murine Peyer's patch cultures by concanavalin A, muramyl dipeptide and lipopolysaccharide. Scand. J. Immunol. **15:** 329–339.

23. CREWTHER, P. and N. L. WARNER. 1972. Serum immunoglobulins and antibodies in congenitally athymic (nude) mice. Aust. J. Exp. Biol. Med. Sci. **50:** 625–635.
24. CLOUGH, J. D., L. H. MIMS, and W. STROBER. 1971. Deficient IgA antibody responses to arsenilic acid-bovine serum albumin (BSA) in neonatally thymectomized rabbits. J. Immunol. **106:** 1624–1629.
25. WALDMANN, T. A., S. BRODER, R. KRAKAUER, M. DURM, B. MEADE, and C. GOLDMAN. 1976. Defect in IgA secretion and in IgA specific suppressor cells in patients with selective IgA deficiency. Trans. Assoc. Am. Physicians **89:** 215–224.
26. WATSON, J. 1979. Continuous proliferation of murine antigen-specific helper T lymphocytes in culture. J. Exp. Med. **150:** 1510–1519.
27. STROBER, W., N. E. HAGUE, L. G. LUM, and P. A. HENKART. 1978. IgA Fc receptors on mouse lymphoid cells. J. Immunol. **121:** 2440–2445.
28. LUM, L. G., A. V. MUCHMORE, D. KEREN, J. DECKER, I. KOSKI, W. STROBER, and R. M. BLAESE. 1979. A receptor for IgA on human T lymphocytes. J. Immunol. **122:** 65–69.
29. RICHMAN, L. K., A. S. GRAEFF, and W. STROBER. 1981. Antigen presentation by macrophage-enriched cells from the mouse Peyer's patch. Cell. Immunol. **62:** 110–118.
30. HERZENBERG, L. A., K. OKUMURA, H. CANTOR, V. L. SATO, F.-W. SHEN, E. A. BOYSE, and L. A. HERZENBERG. 1976. T-cell regulation of antibody responses: Demonstration of allotype-specific helper T cells and their specific removal by suppressor T cells. J. Exp. Med. **144:** 330–344.
31. LÖWY, I., M. JOSKOWICZ, and J. THEZE. 1982. Characterization of suppressor cells regulating *in vitro* expression of IgG_{2A} and IgG_{2B} antibody responses. J. Immunol. **128:** 768–773.

DISCUSSION OF THE PAPER

D. E. BOCKMAN (*Medical College of Georgia, Augusta, Ga.*): Is it possible that your helper-cell preparations, after enzymatic digestion, would include esterase-positive epithelial cells in addition to macrophages? Have you done anything to rule out this possibility?

S. M. MICHALEK (*The University of Alabama in Birmingham*): We have shown that murine Peyer's patches contain dendritic cells in the accessory cell population. We have not characterized I-A-positive epithelial or epithelioid cells in the enzymatic digests thus far, although we are currently performing experiments of this nature.

M. F. KAGNOFF (*University of California at San Diego, La Jolla*): We have heard about T-cells that may be specific for IgA responses, or T-cells that help IgA responses. Should we envision this T-helper cell as being active in a specific instructional mode, or are we looking at more of a selection stochastic model, such as Dr. Cebra referred to? Does the T-cell that you envision, which is MHC restricted and antigen specific, also have another receptor, presumedly for isotype or something coexpressed with isotype? Do you further envision this cell as delivering a specific instructional signal to an alpha switch site, or do you see this as just enhancing the cell proliferation, such as the sort of model that Dr. Cebra talked about?

MICHALEK: Obviously that is difficult to answer. We have characterized T-cell clones, which help the normal B-cell to respond to antigen, with principally an IgA response.

J. R. MCGHEE (*The University of Alabama in Birmingham*): In response to Dr.

Kagnoff's question, we think we are looking at a specific instructional T-cell. First of all, there were no antibody responses to other types of antigens that were used. These cloned T-cells were put in normal B-cell cultures and largely IgA responses occurred. There was no polyclonal stimulation. In other words, we think these are antigen-specific T-helper cells.

J. J. CEBRA (*University of Pennsylvania, Philadelphia*): I lost your main point in your model that showed all the cell interactions, where you compare the LPS-responding and nonresponding mice. Do you think that the induction of suppressor T-cells is a downstream effect of LPS-responsiveness, or do you think LPS is acting by way of an LPS receptor, by affecting T-cells rather than the B-cells that define responding and nonresponding mice? Maybe if you carefully examine F-1-offspring, you might be able to learn something about a gene-dose effect for LPS receptors? Have you done that experiment?

MICHALEK: We are currently looking at this point and Ms. Gollahon is attempting to isolate the LPS receptor. Preliminary studies indicate that the receptor may be in the cell cytoplasm.

CEBRA: Do you think that LPS is acting to generate helper cells as a downstream effect, or do you think it is a directional action? In other words, what do you think the target of the LPS really is?

MICHALEK: We feel it is acting on a precursor T-cell population.

B. H. WAKSMAN (*National Multiple Sclerosis Society, New York, N.Y.*): I think Dr. Cebra is asking if you think those T-cells have two different receptors, one for LPS and one for antigen, or if those appear in successive stages in the life history of those cells?

MICHALEK: We feel that it acts on a precursor T-suppressor cell, which then, following antigen exposure, results in a more mature T-suppressor cell, that is, the LPS-sensitive cell may be a precursor to the antigen-specific, mature T-suppressor cell.

J. A. MATTINGLY (*Ohio State University, Columbus, Ohio*): Did you take any real precautions to keep your germfree mice LPS-free, since the food given to germfree mice is basically filled with dead bacteria? The water, unless you were using special precautions, contains LPS. Since you already showed that it takes a relatively small amount of LPS to stimulate these responses, how did you control for that?

MICHALEK: Yes, we did extensive autoclaving of food and water (for several hours) to remove pyrogen.

WAKSMAN: I believe many people think LPS is quite resistant to autoclaving. Have you tested for the presence of LPS?

MICHALEK: We have tested the food and water for the presence of LPS by Limulus assay; these were always negative.

G. H. LOWELL (*Walter Reed Army Institute of Research, Washington, D.C.*): Considering the fact that human beings generally are less responsive to LPS for both *in vitro* stimulation as well as in other systems, particularly in polyclonal activation, where murine B-cells are so exquisitely sensitive to LPS, would you speculate that the role of LPS in humans is more akin to that of the C3H/HeJ mouse or the normal mouse?

MICHALEK: This is a difficult and speculative answer; however, although human B-cells are more difficult to trigger with LPS, the human is exquisitely sensitive to LPS or endotoxin effects *in vivo*.

M. D. COOPER (*The University of Alabama in Birmingham*): We have known for about 10 years that there is a switch in the life history of B-cell clones that switch in heavy chain isotype expression, and that T-cells affect terminal differentiation of cells that express various isotypes. There is still a controversy about how the switch occurs and how the T-cells help the B-cells express different isotypes. For example, we have evidence that IgA B-cells come directly from IgM-cells, rather than by successive switches as suggested by Dr. Cebra. I will give some of the reasons why our group thinks that this switch is not driven by antigens or T-cells, and why if the switch occurs very early, the T-cells actually preferentially help these B-cells that are already committed to express a given isotype. One key point has been brought up in this debate, which has been ongoing for a long time: is the Klinman assay, indeed, looking at clones? If they are real clones, and if the cells in each fragment are the immediate progeny of one cell, then the argument is over, or at least there is a clear demonstration of successive switches occurring as a consequence of antigen and T-cell help in that instance. Not everyone is willing to accept that those are true clones. Drs. Stohrer and Kearney have evidence, using phosphorylcholine-driven antibody responses in the Klinman assay, for a very low frequency of responsive cells; they found only four positive fragments per spleen, and they used specific monoclonal anti-idiotype antibodies. A panel of antibodies was used to look at the idiotypic representation in each of these phosphorylcholine-producing fragments. They found multiple patterns among these, which were all too frequent. These results raise the question of whether these are true clones, or whether there is some concentration factor, or helper factors that are involved? Could I ask about these T-helper cell clones, specifically? Have you looked to see if these can help the B-cells respond to antigen by soluble factors? If so, are these IgA specific helper factors in culture supernatants from T-cell clones? Lastly, have you looked at a function for Fc_α receptors? If you add IgA in culture with the T-helper cell clones, does it affect their function?

MICHALEK: In answer to your first question, we are currently performing these studies and we have evidence for a soluble factor which does help the IgA response specifically. It is not IL 2. As far as looking at the function of the Fc receptor, we have not progressed that far yet. These studies are currently being done.

BINDING OF BACTERIAL LIPOPOLYSACCHARIDE
TO MURINE LYMPHOCYTES*

Diane M. Jacobs, Dianna B. Roberts†, John H. Eldridge,‡
and Allen J. Rosenspire§

Department of Microbiology
State University of New York at Buffalo
Buffalo, New York 14214

INTRODUCTION

Lipopolysaccharide (LPS), a component of the outer membrane of gram-negative bacteria, possesses a wide spectrum of biological activities, including activation of cells of the immune system and modulation of the immune response.[1-3] LPS stimulates cell division and immunoglobulin secretion in murine B-cells,[4-8] activates macrophage function and secretion of pharmacologically active materials,[9,10] and appears to have some effect on a small subset of T-cells.[4,12-14] For the past several years, my colleagues and I have sought to understand better the mechanism by which LPS activates cells, by evaluating the nature of the interaction of this bacterial constituent with murine lymphocytes. The selectivity of LPS in activating B- rather than T-lymphocytes would be consistent with a selectivity of interaction with a specific site on the plasma membrane of target cells; yet the hydrophobic nature of lipid A, the structural subunit responsible for most LPS biological activities, might favor a nonselective hydrophobic interaction between the lipid A moiety of LPS with membrane lipids (FIGURE 1). A few investigators[15-17] have demonstrated selective binding of LPS or lipid A to B-cells, whereas others[18-20] have not been able to detect differences in binding between T-cells and B-cells. We have used two approaches to study this question: immunofluorescence microscopy (IF) and radiobinding (RB), and found evidence for "specific" binding, which will be summarized below. In addition, we have examined the cell-bound LPS, and have some evidence that there is selectivity in binding of certain fractions of LPS to different murine cells.

NATURE OF LPS BINDING

TABLE 1 summarizes the major findings of this combined approach.[21-24] In immunofluorescence microscopy, cell-bound LPS is detected using a hapten sandwich technique in which the intermediate layer is antibody directed to the specific O-antigens of the LPS we use: *E. coli* 055:B5. The use of double labeling techniques allows simultaneous detection of other membrane markers to determine the surface phenotype of LPS-binding cells. Radiobinding assays quantify

*This research was supported by PHS Grant AI 16915 and 5T32 AI 07088.

†Present address: Division of Allied Health and Life Sciences, University of Texas at San Antonio, San Antonio, Texas 78285.

‡Present address: Department of Microbiology, University of Alabama in Birmingham, University Station, Birmingham, Alabama 35294.

§Present address: Sloan-Kettering Institute for Cancer Research, 145 Boston Post Road, Rye, New York 10580.

0077–8923/83/0409–0072 $1.75/0 © 1983, NYAS

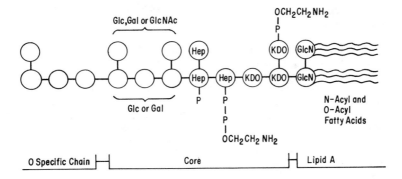

Hep= L-glycero-D-manno-heptose
KDO= 2-keto-3-deoxy-D-manno-octonic acid

FIGURE 1. Schematic representation of LPS. Reproduced from Jacobs.[32] By permission of Raven Press.

the amount of iodinated LPS specifically bound to cell populations, and thus allow some analysis of the characteristics of the binding site.

Binding by either method is saturable with respect both to dose of LPS and time of exposure. In the IF assay, we have observed that the number of LPS⁺ splenic lymphocytes reaches a plateau of 50-60% at 20-30 μg/ml LPS after 30 minutes of incubation at 0° . Radiolabeled LPS reaches equilibrium-binding in 50 minutes at 0° . Temperature dependence was demonstrated in both cases: binding occurred at lower concentrations of LPS at 37° C rather than at 0° C, but the plateau level of LPS⁺ cells remained the same; with RB, more LPS was bound at the higher temperature. As these observations held true, whether or not cells were incubated in the presence of azide, the temperature dependence did not

TABLE 1

CHARACTERISTICS OF LPS BINDING TO MURINE LYMPHOCYTES DETERMINED BY
IMMUNOFLUORESCENCE MICROSCOPY AND RADIOBINDING.*

	Binding Detected by:	
	IF	RB
Saturable: dose and time	Yes	Yes
Temperature dependence	Yes	Yes
Energy independent	Yes	Yes
Inhibitable	Yes	Yes
Correlation between LPS⁺ cells and mitogenic response in lymphoid cells	Yes	ND
Selective for B-cells	Yes	ND
Evidence for nonspecific binding	Yes	Yes
Responder vs nonresponder cells	Same	Same

*LPS used in these experiments was extracted from lyophilized *E. coli* 055:B5 by the phenol-water procedure and purified by enzymatic treatment and chromatography.[25] It did not stimulate mitogenesis in cultures of C3H/HeJ spleen cells.

reflect an energy-dependent binding event, but a temperature-dependent step that modulated the efficiency of binding.

Inhibition experiments were carried out to examine the specificity of binding and to determine the structural component responsible for binding. In RB experiments, unlabeled LPS of the same serotype clearly inhibited 25–45% of the binding of labeled material; this inhibition allowed us to analyze the affinity and number of sites involved in specific binding, which are approximately 3×10^7 M^{-1} and 10^4/cell respectively. As the IF assay used antibody to the 0-specific antigen of *E. coli* 055:B5 to detect cell-bound LPS, a similar approach, examining inhibition by the same serotype could not be used. Nevertheless, we were able to detect inhibition of LPS binding when incubations were carried out with a mixture of 055:B5 and noncrossreactive LPS from *S. typhimurium*. Because the structural determinant common to these two LPS is lipid A, it is likely that this moiety plays a major role in binding to cells, as would be expected from its biological activity.

Double-labeling IF studies have shown that LPS binds selectively to B-cells, predominantly those of the mature subclass with the surface markers $\mu^+Ia^+\delta^+$. A small number of T-cells and null cells are also LPS$^+$. The distribution of LPS$^+$ cells in various lymphoid organs parallels the mitogen response elicited by LPS in cell populations from the same sources. This distribution and the selectivity for B-cells suggest that the binding of LPS we detect is related to the activation of cells by this material, and the characteristics of binding are consistent with the presence of a plasma membrane receptor for this ligand.

Evidence can also be found for nonspecific binding by LPS. After the initial rapid rise to plateau levels of LPS$^+$ cells with increasing doses of LPS, the number of positive cells continues to increase gradually, and at the very high concentration of 2 mg/ml, may be 90% of the total cells. We consider this increase to reflect nonspecific binding. It probably occurs at low doses as well, but is not distinguishable in this assay system. It can, however, be detected using the RB assay, where binding is always measured in the presence and absence of unlabeled LPS. In this case, even at the very low doses of LPS used (usually 0.1 μg/ml), 55–75% of the total LPS bound is not inhibitable by excess cold LPS, and is considered to be bound nonspecifically.

The above results are all consistent with the possibility that LPS selectively binds to lymphocytes by a biologically relevant specific binding site or receptor. With these results in mind, we compared the binding of LPS to lymphocytes of two strains of mice: C3H/St, which responds normally to LPS activation, and C3H/HeJ, which does not "recognize" any activation signals delivered by LPS and is therefore referred to as an LPS nonresponder. We could find no major differences between the strains with respect to the amount of LPS bound, the nature of the binding, or the number and nature of LPS-binding cells. It would therefore appear that the genetic lesion in this strain is not solely a result of altered ligand-binding properties of a cell membrane structure.

CHARACTERIZATION AND FATE OF CELL-BOUND LPS

[125]I-labeled LPS used in radiobinding experiments, described above, was prepared by chloramine T-iodination of LPS that was made reactive by addition of a phenyl group by reaction with p-hydroxy phenylacetic acid (pHPAA) in the presence of carbodiimide.[26] We had previously found that LPS derivatized for iodination had biological activities similar to native material. Therefore, binding

of radiolabeled LPS was assumed to measure the same material as the IF technique, and both were assumed to reflect the starting material. As this assay is more susceptible to misinterpretation when either the cell populations or the ligand are heterogenous or impure, we examined the bound radioactivity to confirm that it was, in fact, LPS and to ascertain whether that LPS that bound to cells was representative of native LPS. We analyzed ^{125}I-labeled LPS and the cell-bound radioactive material, using electrophoretic separation on disc gels of 15% acrylamide containing sodium dodecyl sulfate (SDS), according to the procedure of Laemmli.[27]

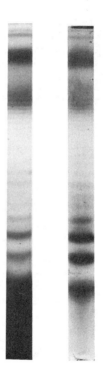

FIGURE 2. Fractionation on LPS of acrylamide gels. The gel on the left was loaded with 0.1 mg LPS and was stained for carbohydrate with Alcian blue. The gel on the right was loaded with 0.25 mg LPS and was stained with Sudan Black B. The dark smear on the bottom of the left-hand gel is an artifact of staining and obscures the band corresponding to that seen on the right-hand gel.

In aqueous solution, LPS exists as aggregates of many subunits of the structure diagrammed in FIGURE 1.[28] In the presence of SDS, the large molecular aggregates are dissociated and will migrate through an SDS acrylamide gel.[29,30] Surprisingly, the subunits are heterogenous as seen in FIGURE 2. The pattern is the same when LPS is stained either with the carbohydrate stain, Alcian blue,[31] or the lipid stain, Sudan Black B. The intensities are different, however, and the top appears to be carbohydrate-rich whereas the bottom bands appear to be lipid-rich. The pattern is similar to that reported by Palva and Makela,[30] and Goldman and Leive.[29] These investigators concluded, on the basis of the mobility of biosynthetically-labeled LPS, that heterogeneity is due to differences in molecular size, based on differences in the number of antigenic side-chain units per subunit. Thus, the number of 0-antigen side-chains in FIGURE 1 varies from none, to over forty.

Iodinated LPS was analyzed quantitatively by identical electrophoretic separation. The gel was sliced, and radioactivity in the fractions was determined in order to give the profile seen in FIGURE 3. The fastest moving peak was coincident with the dye front and had the same mobility as ^{125}I-pHPAA. We see that some amount of this small molecule used for attachment to LPS remains adsorbed but not covalently bound, and it was subsequently iodinated; or else a similar small molecule is a breakdown product of the iodinated derivative of LPS. We have assumed that all counts in this peak are not intact structural subunits of LPS. The remainder of the material in the LPS preparation resolves into several broad overlapping peaks. A peak always exists at $R_f = 0.82$ called peak 1, as well as at $R_f = 0.29$, and sometimes a small peak at $R_f = 0.15$. For purposes of discussion, we have pooled the latter two components and called them peak 3. In different experiments, the radioactive material between these two major peaks may be resolved into a separate peak, or it may be a shoulder to peak 1, or a high plateau.

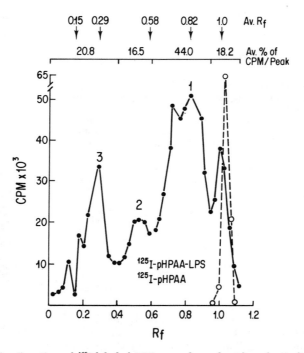

FIGURE 3. Fractionation of ^{125}I-labeled LPS on polyacrylamide gels. Radioiodine was introduced to LPS by chloramine T-iodination of LPS, which first had a reactive phenyl group attached by reaction with p-hydroxy phenylacetic acid (pHPAA) in the presence of carbodiimide. ^{125}I-labeled pHPAA was also prepared. Iodinated materials were treated with SDS and electrophoresed on 15% polyacrylamide gels by the procedure of Laameli.[27] Two mm wide fractions were cut and counted, and the profile of counts are depicted here. R_f values of major peaks of 30 gels were determined and averaged to give the figures above the curve. "Peak 3" refers to all material with an R_f value less than 0.3. The area under each peak was determined, and the fraction of total counts in each peak was calculated. The average value of 11 gels is given.

TABLE 2

PREFERENTIAL BINDING OF DIFFERENT LPS COMPONENTS
BY REACTIVE CELLS AND ANTIBODY

Binding Substrate	Adherent ^{125}I-LPS/Starting ^{125}I-labeled LPS in Peaks			
	3*	2	1	pHPAA
C3H/St splenic lymphocytes	0.60 ± 0.15	0.94 ± 0.51	1.43 ± 0.23	0.77 ± 0.28
C3H/HeJ splenic lymphocytes	0.71	0.98	1.45	0.76
Mouse erythrocytes	0.32	1.34	1.39	0.52
Splenic macrophages	0.75	1.79	1.07	0.47
Glass tubes	0.22	0.46	1.83	0.44
Specific antibody	1.23	1.37	0.94	0.26
Polystyrene tubes (BSA)	0.83	1.24	1.19	0.01

*R_f values of peaks: 3, <0.3; 2, 0.58; 1, 0.82; pHPAA set equal to 1.0. Lymphocytes were the interface cells from a Ficoll-Hypaque separation of spleen cell suspension. Macrophages were the population of cells remaining adherent after a 24 hour incubation of spleen cells in glass tubes. Cells were incubated with ^{125}I-labeled LPS in RPMI-1640 for one hour at 0° C and washed in medium. All cells except for macrophages were transferred to clean glass tubes with fresh medium and centrifuged. The cell pellet or adherent macrophages were lysed in 0.1 ml distilled water. Material adherent to glass tubes after incubation and washing was analyzed in a similar fashion. Polystyrene tubes were coated with the IgG fraction of specific anti-055:B5 as in the solid phase radioimmunoassay for LPS,[26] incubated with iodinated LPS and washed. Control polystyrene tubes were incubated in the same buffer containing BSA before incubating with labeled material. Lysates and adherent material were treated with sample buffer containing SDS and run on 15% acrylamide gels containing SDS. The percentage of total counts of each gel distributed in each major peak was determined. The figures given are the ratios of adherent LPS/starting LPS for each peak. Those underlined are considered to be appreciably different from 1.00.

Counts in this region are called peak 2. The percentage of radioactivity in each peak was measured; the percentage of total counts, migrating in each gel, that falls into each peak is calculated. The average distribution of ^{125}I-LPS in each fraction is also seen in FIGURE 3. About half the LPS is in peak 1 and the remainder is equally divided among peaks 2, 3, and low molecular weight material.

With this approach as a reference point, we carried out similar analyses of ^{125}I-LPS that bound to lymphocytes and other cell types. For each experiment, the distribution of counts in the peaks was determined for cell-bound LPS and the starting material. To determine if any components were preferentially bound, the ratio of adherent material to starting material for each peak was calculated. If a component was bound to the same degree as it was represented in the starting material, it would be expected to have a ratio of 1.0. A preferentially bound component would therefore have a ratio greater than 1.0 and other components would by default have ratios less than 1.0. A summary of these results is outlined in TABLE 2.

Splenic lymphocytes of either C3H/St or C3H/HeJ appear to preferentially bind components in peak 1. In contrast, adherent splenic macrophages preferentially bind peak 2. Erythrocytes, which are known to bind LPS but have no known biological response to it, preferentially bind both peak 1 and peak 2 and have a more pronounced negative preference for peak 3 than any cell type examined. To confirm that these apparent differences in preferential binding are not due solely to LPS binding to tubes, particularly in the case of macrophages, where cells are not transferred before being lysed, we also examined the LPS that bound to glass tubes. This surface appears to have a preference for peak 1, even more pronounced than lymphocytes, and its profile is quite different from that of macrophages.

Because the material we refer to as the carbohydrate-rich peak 3 has more repeating antigenic structures than the lipid-rich components, we also asked if antibody would more easily react with any of the components separated by this method. This point was evaluated by analyzing LPS that was bound to tubes that had been coated previously with the IgG fraction of specific anti-055:B5.[26] In comparison to tubes coated only with bovine serum albumin (BSA), specific antibody preferentially bound peak 3 components, which contain more antigenic side-chains.

Having looked at cell-bound LPS, we continued to analyze the fate of the LPS in/on these cells. The information we have on the rate of loss of cell-bound LPS is summarized in TABLE 3. In these experiments, cells were "loaded" by incubation with ^{125}I-labeled LPS in the cold for one hour, washed, and transferred to clean tubes with fresh medium for incubation at 37°. Samples were taken at subsequent intervals, and the amount of radioactivity remaining on cells was determined. We

TABLE 3

LOSS OF CELL-BOUND LPS FROM MURINE CELLS*

Cell or Surface	Rate of Loss of ^{125}I-labeled LPS $t_{1/2}$ in Hours	
C3H/St splenic lymphocytes	7	220
CeH/HeJ splenic lymphocytes	7	400
Mouse erythrocytes	10	127
Splenic macrophages		164
Glass tubes	36	148

*Cells were incubated with ^{125}I-labeled LPS in RPMI-1640 for one hour at 0° C, washed in medium, transferred to clean glass tubes with fresh medium and incubated for 72 hours at 37° C. Samples were taken at intervals, cells and supernatant fluid were separated by centrifugation, and radioactivity was determined.

saw a loss of lymphocyte-bound label to a level of about 50% of the initial label but little further loss after 24 hours. Macrophages retained the label for longer periods. A detailed analysis indicated that the initial rate of loss from lymphocytes and erythrocytes was fairly rapid. In contrast, macrophages lost label very slowly, possibly because it was internalized when the cells were transferred to 37°.

Differential binding of LPS components to different cell populations provides additional evidence for selectivity of LPS binding. Because not all cells bind each component to the same degree, it is unlikely that the cell surface structure(s) to which LPS binds in each population has identical characteristics. Furthermore, not all cells have a preferential affinity for the most hydrophobic or lipid-rich subunits in peak 1, so binding would not appear to be governed strictly by hydrophobic forces. The results also raise a quite different question about the structure of LPS aggregates in solution. The preferential binding of subunit components could be explained by segregation, such that some aggregates are more homogenous and are composed exclusively or preferentially of the components represented in the individual peaks. If all aggregates were composed of representative proportions of, for example, peaks 1, 2, and 3, regardless of which component interacted with the cell, all components would be part of the adhering aggregate and be detected on analysis. Alternatively, cells could be selectively removing components of certain structure from the large aggregates. Perhaps the most likely explanation for preferential adherence of individual components is that the individual subunits (or dimers or trimers) present in low concentrations in equilibrium with the micellar (aggregate) structures are the active interacting components. While they are being removed from solution by binding to the cell, they may be replaced by futher dissociation of the aggregates if the conditions for such dissociation are met. If this concept can be verified by experiments currently in progress in the laboratory, it will change the way we think about LPS interactions with cells and provide a fruitful analytical approach for examining the molecular nature of LPS interactions with cell surfaces.

CONCLUSION AND SUMMARY

Does LPS activate lymphocytes by binding to a specific cell-surface receptor or by nonspecific hydrophobic interaction with the plasma membrane? We examined this question by detecting cell-bound LPS using immunofluorescence microscopy and radiobinding techniques. LPS binding to splenic lymphocytes from C3H/St mice has characteristics of specific binding: saturability with respect to dose and time, selectivity for a subclass of B-cells, and a correlation between binding and mitogenesis. ^{125}I-labeled LPS bound to cells and analyzed quantitatively by SDS-PAGE separated into 3 major components: peaks 1, 2, and 3 (1 equals the fastest moving). Lymphocytes preferentially bound peak 1, murine RBC peaks 1 and 2, and macrophages peak 2. In contrast, specific antibody preferred peaks 2 and 3. Differential staining of gels suggested that peak 3 is carbohydrate-rich and peak 1 is lipid-rich. LPS was released from these cells at different rates. We conclude that selectivity of LPS binding may be reflected in preferential binding of LPS subunits of different size and/or composition, as well as differential retention of bound LPS.

ACKNOWLEDGMENTS

We thank Patricia Cotter and Swastika Majumdar for technical assistance in many of the experiments discussed here.

REFERENCES

1. MORRISON, D. C. & R. J. ULEVITCH. 1978. Am. J. Pathol. **93:** 527–612.
2. MORRISON, D. C. & J. L. RYAN. 1979. Adv. Immunol. **28:** 293–450.
3. JACOBS, D. M. 1981. J. Immunopharm. **3:** 119–132.
4. GERY, I., J. KRUGER & S. Z. SPIESEL. 1972. J. Immunol. **108:** 1088–1091.
5. ANDERSSON, J., F. MELCHERS, C. GALANOS & O. LÜDERITZ. 1973. J. Exp. Med. **137:** 943–953.
6. ANDERSSON, J., G. MÖLLER, & O. SJÖBERG. 1972. Cell. Immunol. **4:** 381–393.
7. ANDERSSON, J., O. SJÖBERG & G. MÖLLER. 1972. Eur. J. Immunol. **2:** 349–353.
8. ANDERSSON, J., A. COUTINHO & F. MELCHERS. 1977. J. Exp. Med. **145:** 1520–1530.
9. ROSENSTREICH, D. L. & S. N. VOGEL. 1980. *In* Microbiology 1980. D. Schlesinger, Ed.: 11–15. American Society for Microbiology. Washington, D.C.
10. WEINBERG, J. B., H. A. CHAPMAN & J. B. HIBBS. 1978. J. Immunol. **121:** 72–80.

11. SKIDMORE, B. J., J. M. CHILLER & W. O. WEIGLE. 1977. J. Immunol. **118:** 274–281.
12. KONDA, S., Y. NAKAO & R. T. SMITH. 1972. J. Exp. Med. **136:** 1461–1477.
13. GOODMAN, M. G., & W. O. WEIGLE. 1979. J. Immunol. **122:** 2548–2553.
14. NORCROSS, M. A., & R. T. SMITH. 1977. J. Exp. Med. **145:** 1299–1315.
15. GREGORY, S. H., D. H. ZIMMERMAN & M. KERN. 1980. J. Immunol. **125:** 102–107.
16. ZIMMERMAN, D. H., S. GREGORY & M. KERN. 1977. J. Immunol. **119:** 1018–1023.
17. BONA, C., D. JUY, P. TRUFFA-BACHI & G. J. KAPLAN. 1976. J. Microsc. Biol. Cell.
      25: 47–56.
18. KABIR, S., & D. L. ROSENSTREICH. 1977. Infect. Immun. **15:** 156–164.
19. MÖLLER, G., J. ANDERSSON, H. POHLIT & O. SJÖBERG. 1972. Clin. Exp. Immunol.
      13: 89–99.
20. SYMONS, D. B. A. & C. A. CLARKSON. 1979. Immunology **38:** 503–508.
21. ELDRIDGE, J. H., F. J. SWARTZWELDER & D. M. JACOBS. Submitted for publication.
22. JACOBS, D. M. & J. H. ELDRIDGE. Submitted for publication.
23. JACOBS, D. M. & A. J. ROSENSPIRE. 1980. Fed. Proc. Fed. Am. Soc. Exp. Biol. **39:** 917.
24. JACOBS, D. M. & A. J. ROSENSPIRE. 1980. Fourth Int'l. Congress of Immunol., Paris,
      France.
25. MORRISON, D. C. & L. LEIVE. 1975. J. Biol. Chem. **250:** 2911–2919.
26. GUTOWSKI, J. A. & D. M. JACOBS. 1979. Immunol. Commun. **8**(3): 347–364.
27. LAEMMLI, U. 1970. Nature (London) **227:** 680–685.
28. GALANOS, C., O. LÜDERITZ, E. T. RIETSCHEL & O. WESTPHAL. 1977. In International
      Review of Biochemistry: Biochemistry of Lipids II. T. W. Goodwin. Ed.: Vol.
      14: 239–335. University Park Press. Baltimore.
29. GOLDMAN, R. C. & L. LEIVE. 1980. Eur. J. Biochem. **197:** 145–153.
30. PALVA, T. & H. MAKELA. 1980. Eur. J. Biochem. **107:** 137–143.
31. WARDI, A. H. & G. A. MICHOS. 1972. Anal. Biochem. **49:** 607–609.
32. JACOBS, D. M. In Recent Advances in Mucosal Immunity, W. Strober, Ed., Raven Press.
      New York. In press.

DISCUSSION OF THE PAPER

M. BLAKE (*Rockfeller University, New York, N.Y.*): I would like to know the nature of the LPS preparation you are using. Have you ruled out the possibility that cell digestion of LPS is occurring? DeVol and Gilchrist suggested that LPS was being digested by the cell and then released as lower molecular weight forms.

D. M. JACOBS (*State University of New York, Buffalo, N.Y.*): I will answer your second question first. All of the binding studies that I have shown have been done with cells incubated at 0°C in the presence of sodium azide for no more than one hour. Whether or not digestion can take place under these conditions I will leave up to you to decide. The LPS that we use is prepared by a phenol-water extraction of lyophilized *E. coli* 055:B5 that we make ourselves and that we further purify with RNAse, Pronase treatment and column chromatography. Our LPS preparation does not stimulate mitogenic responses in C3H/HeJ spleen cell cultures.

J. R. MCGHEE (*The University of Alabama in Birmingham*): You mentioned experiments regarding LPS binding to B-cells in baby mice, and you looked at relatively immature B-cells versus more mature B-cells with surface IgM and IgD. Have you also looked at LPS binding in CBA/N, X-linked immunodeficient mice?

JACOBS: No. The maturity was based on the surface phenotype; when lymphocytes from newborns were studied, we found no LPS-binding B-cells. We have not looked at any other mouse strains. Of course, other obvious experiments would involve LPS binding to cells from germfree mice.

M. D. COOPER (*The University of Alabama in Birmingham, Ala*): Could you discuss the subclasses of B-cells that bind LPS? For example, the triggering studies would suggest that B-cells have those receptors as soon as they are formed. As soon as they are transformed from pre-B-cells or as soon as you see surface immunoglobulin-positive cells, you find cells that can be triggered to plasma cell differentiation with LPS. Is this lost later on, or, is it just a subset that does not relate to differentiation? Finally, has anyone looked at Peyer's patch B-cells, for example, for their binding of LPS?

JACOBS: We have looked at Peyer's patch cells. This organ has the smallest number of LPS$^+$ cells: approximately 4% of total lymphocytes. We have only 11% μ^+ cells in the Peyer's patches. These cell preparations were not made by enzyme dissociation, but by teasing, so we may have lost cells. LPS will activate B-cells as soon as μ^+ cells appear; but this is at the same time at which δ and Ia begin to appear. If you look at both markers, when the LPS$^+$ cells appear—we have looked at six days—we have a small fraction of δ^+ and Ia-positive cells as well as a larger fraction of μ^+ cells. Comparing neonates of 6 days, which is the time at which the LPS$^+$ B-cells start to appear, as determined by double labeling experiments, we see LPS$^+$ μ^+ cells in the same numbers and at about the same time as LPS$^+$ δ^+ and LPS$^+$ Ia$^+$ cells. The other problem of interpreting the triggering data with the time of appearance of a marker—and I think Melchers and others have also found this—is that if one puts B-cells in culture, two days are required for maturation to LPS-responsiveness. If one puts cells into culture with LPS, one finds responses three days later, and yet the cells may have taken two days to mature in culture.

QUESTION: Have you looked to see whether there is any difference in the fluidity of the membranes after addition of LPS?

JACOBS: No, but others have found a difference in fluidity, depending on whether you use rough LPS, which is predominantly lipid-A, or smooth LPS, which also has carbohydrate. There is a problem with those experiments, however, because most people do not use pure populations of cells and one does not really know what one is looking at if you use a mixture.

QUESTION: How do you interpret your data with the macrophages binding of this LPS? Everyone uses *E. coli* 055 lipopolysaccharide by tradition. The structure however, has been determined recently, and it contains colitose and branched sugars. This structure is a bacterium that is frequently cultured from food. It would be better to use LPS from bacteria that are not normally in contact with the mouse. Your data indicates that peak 2 bound better to the macrophages. Could this binding be due to recognition from the macrophages on the O-polysaccharide side-chain, rather than binding by the lipid-A moiety?

JACOBS: Yes. We have no additional data on the nature of the binding other than that which I presented by the polyacrylamide gel electrophoresis.

COLOSTRUM-DERIVED IMMUNITY
AND MATERNAL-NEONATAL INTERACTION

Pearay L. Ogra,* Genevieve A. Losonsky,
and Mark Fishaut

*Departments of Pediatrics and Microbiology
State University of New York at Buffalo
and
Division of Infectious Diseases
Children's Hospital of Buffalo
Buffalo, New York 14222*

The human neonate is well endowed with precursor immunocompetent tissue for antibody production and possesses adequate effector mechanisms of T-cell-mediated immunity. Nevertheless, the early newborn period is characterized by the lack of any serum or secretory A immunoglobulin activity in the mucosal surfaces. Although antigen-reactive IgA-precursor lymphoid cells are present in the neonatal gut-associated (GALT) and bronchial-associated lymphorecticular tissues (BALT), the synthesis of IgA does not occur in detectable quantities until the activation of such cells takes place through the environmentally-induced microbial and other dietary antigens in the gastrointestinal and respiratory mucosa. Measurable quantities of IgA are generally observed in the mucosal secretions after the first two to three weeks of life.[1]

It has been suggested that transfer of maternal immunologic reactivity through the process of breast-feeding may serve as an effective replacement in the gap of mucosal immunity during the neonatal period, by virtue of the rather unique immunologic characteristics of the products of lactation.[2]

The investigations summarized in this report were designed to examine the nature of specifically induced immunologic and microbiologic reactivity in the mammary glands, relative to its interaction with the suckling neonate. These studies employed rubella virus, respiratory syncytial virus (RSV) and bovine serum albumin (BSA) as investigative model-antigens. Supporting data for other appropriate antigens employed by other investigators are also summarized.

DEVELOPMENT OF IMMUNE RESPONSE
IN THE MAMMARY GLANDS AND THE MILK

The early colostrum and subsequent products of lactation are replete with immunoglobulins, especially secretory IgA, macrophages, T- and B-lymphocytes, and a variety of other soluble and cellular components.[3] It is believed that at least the IgA in milk is directed against the antigens introduced into the exposed mucosal surfaces rather than the antigens ordinarily associated with the breast directly. This opinion is based on the observation that IgA-bearing B-lymphocytes of BALT or GALT origin will preferentially populate the mucosal lamina propria of the bronchial and intestinal mucosa as well as the mammary glands after

*Correspondence to: Pearay L. Ogra, M.D., Division of Infectious Diseases, Children's Hospital, 219 Bryant Street, Buffalo, New York 14222.

0077-8923/83/0409-0082 $1.75/0 © 1983, NYAS

antigen exposure in the mucosal sites.[4-6] Studies carried out in rabbits with a nonreplicating antigen, dinitrophenylated keyhole limpet hemocyanin or pneumococcal antigen, after bronchial or intestinal immunization, have shown the appearance of specific IgA antibodies in the colostrum and milk.[7] The contribution of gut-associated mucosal immunity to the antibody activity in human milk was clearly demonstrated in an elegant series of experiments by Goldblum, *et al.*[8] and Hanson, *et al.*[9,10] To date, specific antibody activity in the milk has been demonstrated against a variety of microorganisms (TABLE 1).

Epidemiologic studies carried out during a community outbreak of infection with respiratory syncytial virus provided a unique opportunity to study the role of bronchial mucosal exposure to a virus on the development of specific immunocompetence in the milk. Groups of nursing mothers were sequentially evaluated for the presence or appearance of RSV-specific antibody in the breast milk at

TABLE 1

SPECIFIC ANTIBODY REACTIVITY IN HUMAN COLOSTRUM AND MILK

Bacteria	Viruses	Fungi	Others
E. coli (O + K antigens and enterotoxin)	Rotavirus	*Candida albicans*	Milk proteins
Salmonella	Poliovirus 1,2,3		Dietary antigens
Shigella	Echovirus 6,9		Other macromolecules
Vibrio cholera	Coxsackievirus A9,B3		
Bacteroides fragilis	Respiratory syncytial virus		
Streptococcus pneumoniae	Cytomegalovirus		
Bordetella pertussis	Influenza A virus		
Clostridium diphtheriae	Herpes simplex virus		
Clostridium tetani	Arboviruses		
Streptotoccus mutans	Semlike Forest		
	Ross River		
	Japanese B		
	Dengue		

different stages of lactation before, during, and towards the end of the RSV epidemic. Antiviral IgM and IgG were observed in the milk only occasionally and in low titers.[12] Nevertheless, RSV-specific IgA activity was observed in 75% of the specimens of colostrum and in 40% and 57% of the specimens of milk obtained three months and six months after the onset of lactation (TABLE 2). The latter increase in the frequency of antibody-containing milk samples appeared to follow the peak of the RSV infection in the community. Of particular importance was the observation that many subjects, documented as having reinfection with RSV during the outbreak, manifested an increase in the preexisting IgA-antibody titers in the milk (FIGURE 1). In view of the fact that the pathogenesis of RSV is characterized by its exquisite restriction of replication to the respiratory tract mucosa, these observations provide strong support to a bronchomammary axis for the occurrence of virus-specific immunologic reactivity in human milk. These

TABLE 2

TEMPORAL PATTERNS OF CLASS-SPECIFIC ANTIBODY ACTIVITY AGAINST RSV IN THE COLOSTRUM AND MILK OF LACTATING WOMEN

Subjects with RSV Antibody Response in Colostrum and Milk

Day Postpartum	Number Tested	IgG		IgA		IgM	
		Number Positive Percent	RSV Antibody Titer [Mean]	Number Positive Percent	RSV Antibody Titer [Mean]	Number Positive Percent	RSV Antibody Titer [Mean]
1–3	24	7 (29.1)	2.5	18 (75.0)	6.5	1 (4.1)	10
8–28	19	0	—	7 (36.8)	3.1	0	—
85–112	15	0	—	6 (40.0)	4.3	0	—
>168*	7	0	—	4 (57.1)	16.8	0	—

*Corresponds to the onset of infection with RSV in the community.

experiments do not, however, rule out the possible activation of intestinal lymphoid tissue with small amounts of RSV antigen swallowed from the nasopharynx.

In order to examine the differential role of bronchial vs. gut-associated lymphoreticular tissue, as well as the role of the nature of the antigen (soluble vs. particulate), groups of pregnant rabbits were immunized with RSV and BSA, administered intratracheally, intravenously, or by intragastric intubation. Following intragastric and intratracheal immunization, RSV IgA appeared regularly in the colostrum and milk but not after intravenous immunization. Antiviral IgG appeared in the colostrum, milk, and serum regardless of the route of immunization. On the other hand, the responses to BSA in the serum, colostrum, and milk were limited to IgG after immunization by all three routes of immunization. No IgA anti-BSA response was observed. The anti-BSA isotype did not exhibit any change by nursing and was not affected by BSA-ingestion before or during

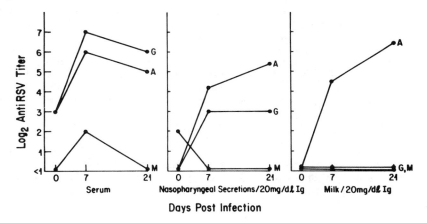

FIGURE 1. Representative data on IgG, IgA, and IgM antibody responses to respiratory syncytial virus (RSV) in three lactating women after RSV infection.

pregnancy, or during nursing.[13] These observations suggest that the appearance of IgA-antibody response in the mammary gland following mucosal immunization is not uniform for different types of antigens. The presence of mammary IgA response to RSV, and its absence to BSA, following respiratory or intestinal immunization, suggests that the physical and chemical nature of the antigens may be important determinants of mammary immune response.

The characteristics of the class of antibody activity observed in the milk may also be influenced by the dissemination of infecting agents from the mucosal sites to the mammary glands by way of the systemic circulation. Unlike RSV, the pathogenesis of rubella virus infection is frequently associated with the development of viremia and involvement of other systemic sites. Of the currently available licensed rubella vaccines, the HPV-77 strain seems to have lost the ability to induce infection in the respiratory tract when administered directly into the respiratory tract. Replication can be consistently demonstrated, however, when administered parenterally. On the other hand, RA27/3 strain of the vaccine can result in mucosal and systemic replication, following intranasal or parenteral inoculation.[14]

The development of immune response to rubella was studied in the milk, serum, and nasopharyngeal secretions in groups of lactating women immunized with the RA27/3 or HPV-77 DE/5 live attenuated rubella vaccines, administered subcutaneously or intranasally. A predictable nasopharyngeal IgA and serum IgG rubella response was observed after intranasal or subcutaneous immunization with RA27/3 vaccine. Little or no nasopharyngeal IgA activity was detected after subcutaneous immunization with HPV-77 vaccine. On the other hand, a rubella-specific IgA response was observed in the milk after subcutaneous immunization with HPV-77 and after subcutaneous or intranasal immunization with RA27/3 vaccine, as shown in FIGURE 2.[15] It should be pointed out that over 69% of the subjects shed rubella virus in the milk after either form of immunization. Virus shedding in the nasopharynx, however, was consistently observed after immunization with RA27/3, but only rarely, and in minimal levels, after immunization with HPV-77 vaccine.[15] The development of IgA response in the milk in the absence of such a response in the nasopharynx in HPV-vaccinated subjects may suggest a direct stimulation by the virus in the mammary gland of the previously uncommitted IgA precursors in the mammary glands. Nevertheless, the bulk of the available evidence would not support this mechanism. Alternately, it is possible that the respiratory mucosa is minimally accessible to the HPV-77 viral antigen when administered parenterally. Such nasopharyngeal availability, although inadequate for nasopharyngeal immune response may activate sufficient numbers of IgA precursors in the respiratory lymphoid tissues that will eventually migrate to the mammary glands.

In view of the frequent detection of rubella virus in the milk, it is proposed that appearance of milk antibody may be partly mediated by the further proliferation of BALT-derived rubella-sensitized IgA cells as a result of local availability of the virus in the breast. This possibility is further supported by the observation that IgA-rubella activity in the milk was highest in subjects who shed measurable amounts of virus in the nasopharynx as well as milk, compared to those who shed the virus only in nasopharynx or milk (FIGURE 3).

EXCRETION OF OTHER MATERNAL PRODUCTS IN THE MILK AND THEIR TRANSFER TO THE INFANT

The investigative effort to date has largely focused on the characterization of the soluble and cellular immunologic components in the mammary gland and milk. Nevertheless, some information is available to suggest that a variety of microorganisms, drugs and antibiotics, dietary proteins, radiopharmaceuticals, and environmental toxins and contaminants are also excreted in milk.[11] Many of the substances are present in the milk in much higher concentration than in the maternal serum, presumably as a result of the well-known bioconcentration phenomenon.[11] A listing of some of these components that have been observed in freshly collected samples of human milk is presented in TABLE 3.

We estimate that a suckling human neonate receives about one gram of IgA and approximately 1/100 of the amount of IgM and IgG every day through breast feeding.[3] Although the fate of the colostral and milk IgG, IgM, and IgA in the neonatal intestinal tract has not been determined with certainty, bulk of the milk immunoglobulins appears to be eliminated in the feces without any systemic absorption. Small amounts of milk IgA, however, appear to be absorbed from the

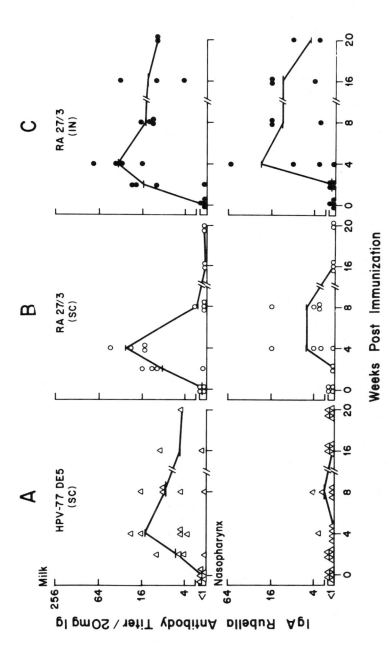

FIGURE 2. Temporal patterns of IgA-rubella antibody response in the milk and nasopharyngeal secretions after subcutaneous (SC) or intranasal (IN) immunization with HPV-77 DE/5 or RA27/3 live attenuated rubella virus vaccines.

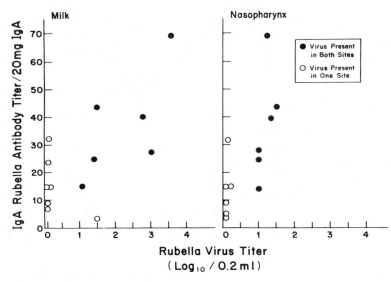

FIGURE 3. Correlation of IgA-rubella antibody titer in the milk to the amount of rubella virus shed in the milk and nasopharynx.

neonatal intestine during the first 24 hours after birth.[16] Other reports have raised the possibility of the transfer of minimal amounts of milk IgA to the nasopharynx during the newborn period.[17] We also have some evidence to suggest the transfer of maternal cellular immune reactivity, through the process of breast-feeding, to the suckling neonate. Human studies have indicated transfer of specific in vitro correlates of cell-mediated immunity against mycobacterium tuberculosis,[16] to the

TABLE 3

TRANSFER OF MATERNAL IMMUNOLOGIC FUNCTIONS, INFECTIOUS MICROORGANISMS, AND OTHER POTENTIAL ANTIGENS TO THE HUMAN INFANT THROUGH BREAST-FEEDING

Components of adoptive immunity	—	In vitro correlates of cellular immunity to Tuberculin*
		IgA antibody to Poliovirus*
Bacteria	—	Mycobacterium tuberculosis
		Pathogenic streptococcus and staphylococcus*
		Enteric pathogens
Viruses	—	Hepatitis B
		Cytomegalovirus*
		Rubella*
		Herpes simplex
Drugs	—	Nicotine
		Cephalosporins
		Organohalides*
Dietary proteins	—	Bovine serum proteins
Radiopharmaceuticals	—	Lead
		Radioisotopes

*With evidence of systemic uptake in the infant.

neonate after prolonged breast-feeding from sensitized mothers. A few studies have raised the possibility of transfer of viral-specific cell-mediated immunity by way of the placenta.[18-20] We do not know whether such reactivity is transferred to infants through breast-feeding as well. Although the transfer of histocompatibile antigens and T-cells has been reported in suckling rats,[21,22] no evidence is available to suggest systemic uptake of intact T-cells in the human neonate. These observations suggest that, in addition to providing a large volume of specific immunologic reactivity in the neonatal intestinal lumen, breast feeding may also provide soluble and possibly cellular immunologic components for systemic uptake in the early neonatal period.

It is apparent that a number of microorganisms are excreted in the milk after naturally acquired or vaccine-induced maternal infections.[11] Fortunately, most published cases have not shown the development of any specific illness in the suckling infant that consumed milk containing such microorganisms.

TABLE 4

MATERNAL-NEONATAL INTERACTION DURING RUBELLA IMMUNIZATION IN
LACTATING FEMALES

	Breast-Feeding	Non-Breast-Feeding
Immunized Mothers		
Number Immunized	16	10
Virus recovery NPS* percent positive	56	50
Peak titers ($\log_{10}/0.2$ml)	0.9	0.7
Virus recovery milk percent positive	68	NA
Peak titers ($\log_{10}/0.2$ml)	1.9	NA
Seroconversion percent subjects	100	100
Nonimmunized Infants		
Number Infants	16	10
Virus recovery NPS percent positive	56	0
Seroconversion in percent of virus positive infants	44	0
Absence of seroconversion in percent of virus positive infants	56	NA

*NPS indicates nasopharynx or throat.

As pointed out earlier, infectious rubella virus was recovered in the milk of 69% of the lactating women immunized with HPV-77 or RA27/3 live rubella vaccine. No differences were observed in the excretion pattern of rubella in the milk between subcutaneously or intranasally immunized subjects. Of particular importance is the observation that rubella virus was recovered in 56% of infants breast-fed by these immunized mothers.[32] None of the non-breast-fed infants were found to shed the virus, in spite of the fact that these mothers were immunized in an identical manner and frequently shed virus in the nasopharynx, as the mothers of breast-fed infants (TABLE 4).

EFFECT OF THE BREAST-FEEDING ON
IMMUNOLOGIC REACTIVITY IN THE NEONATE

Breast-feeding has been strongly implicated in maintaining immunologic homeostasis in the neonatal intestine during the period of functional immaturity of the secretory immune system. Epidemiologic studies carried out in several rural and urban settings have demonstrated a striking resistence of breast-fed infants to mucosal infections with *Escherichia coli*, shigella, *Vibrio cholera* and protozoan infestations, even under field conditions when the risk of natural infection is high.[11] It has also been proposed that breast-feeding favors an environment for establishment of a "normal flora" in the newborn intestine. Conflicting information exists regarding the role of breast-feeding in prevention of rotavirus infection in man.[11] Studies of Banatvala, *et al.* have shown that presence of rotavirus-specific IgA antibody in the milk does not appear to influence the course of rotavirus shedding in feces in naturally infected breast-fed subjects.[10,24] Breast-feeding has been associated with a decrease in the incidence of atopic-allergic disorders, possibly by reducing the uptake of, and increasing the mucosal elimination of foreign antigens and dietary macromolecules. Such immune exclusion may limit the development of systemic and possibly mucosal immune response to allergy-prone antigens.[25,26] Nevertheless, other studies have shown that IgE and specific reaginic antibody activity against egg proteins and bovine milk proteins may be even higher in breast-fed allergic infants than in non-breast-fed infants.[27,28]

Although minimal differences have been observed in the levels of serum immunoglobulin and secretory IgA between breast-fed and non-breast-fed infants, little or no information is available regarding the level of microbial-specific antibody or cell-mediated immune response relative to breast-feeding.[3] Little information is available about the effects on the suckling neonate, of microbial and other antigens excreted in the milk. A few clinical observations have suggested that ingestion of human milk containing hemolytic streptococcus[29,30] and possibly rubella[31] may be associated with the development of clinical disease in the breast-feeding neonate.

Studies carried out in breast-feeding and non-breast-feeding infants after maternal immunization with HPV-77 or RA27/3 live rubella virus vaccine did not evidence any clinical disease in infants who were infected with the vaccine virus.[23] As mentioned earlier, rubella virus was recovered on several occasions from about 56% of breast-fed infants. Significantly, however, only 44% of infants from whom virus was recovered manifested conversion for rubella-specific antibody or cell-mediated reactivity in the serum. The immunologic response appeared to be transient and no reactivity was observed 12 weeks after initiation of breast feeding (FIGURE 4). Such a response is strikingly different from the response observed after naturally acquired or vaccine-induced active infections in infancy and childhood.[14] It is important to appreciate that the remaining 50% of infants excreting rubella virus also failed to manifest any specific seroconversion.

CONCLUSIONS

The information summarized in this report provides strong evidence for the independent contributions of the bronchial-associated lymphoreticular tissue and intestinal lymphoid tissue to the development of viral-specific IgA-antibody activity in the products of lactation. Based on the data with rubella virus immunization, it is suggested that availability of antigen locally in the mammary tissue, as a result of viremia, may potentiate local antibody production by inducing further proliferation of antigen-sensitized IgA-precursor clones, which have migrated from the peripheral mucosal tissues to the stroma of mammary glands. The isotype of breast-milk antibody may be to a major extent determined by the physical-chemical nature of the antigens experienced in the mucosal lumen. This is exemplified by the lack of IgA-specific anti-BSA response in the milk after mucosal immunization in the rabbits, although these animals elicited IgA response to RSV without any difficulty. A small amount of milk-derived IgA antibody appears to be absorbed from the infant intestine during the early neonatal period. In addition, systemic uptake of *in vitro* correlates of cell-mediated immunity also appears to take place as a result of breast-feeding. The implications of such transfer of adoptive immunity remains to be determined especially in the regulation of immune response to specific antigens in the neonate.

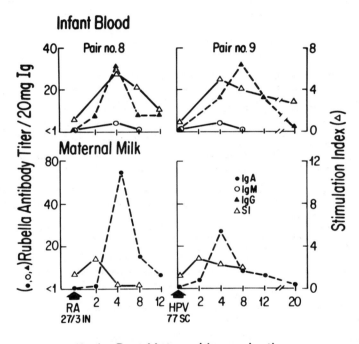

FIGURE 4. Representative data on the outcome of neonatal rubella virus infection acquired in the neonate as a result of virus shedding in the milk after maternal immunization with rubella virus vaccine, administered intranasally (IN) or subcutaneously (SC).

It is clear that a number of infectious microorganisms can be shed in the breast milk after maternal infection. Such infectious agents can induce immunologic and possibly clinical evidence of infection in the neonate. It is also notable that many infants who acquired viral infection through breast-feeding, manifested a transient or no specific immune response despite demonstrable viral shedding. The potential effects of maternally induced sensitization for a virus on the development of immune response and the course of subsequent naturally acquired viral infections or routine immunization with the same virus in such infants remains to be determined. A few animal studies suggest an important role for such sensitization. Administration of ovalbumin to pregnant rats has been shown to result in marked suppression of antigen-specific IgE responses in the suckling offspring after they were immunized with ovalbumin in a similar manner as the mothers.[32] Other studies have suggested that mucosal immunization of pregnant rats, while resulting in high levels of specific antibody response in the mother, induces specific suppression to similar immunization in the neonate.[33] More recently, oral immunization with BSA in pregnant rabbits has been found to induce significant hyporesponsiveness to subsequent immunization in the newborn animals.[34] Based on these observations, the possibility of significant alterations of neonatal immune response to specific antigens introduced postnatally, must be seriously considered in situations of prior exposure to the infectious agent in the neonate through the process of breast-feeding.

REFERENCES

1. OGRA, P. L. 1980. Ontogeny of the local immune system. Pediatrics **64:** 765.
2. OGRA, S. S. & P. L. OGRA. 1979. Components of immunologic reactivity in human colostrum and milk. *In* Immunology of Breast Milk. P. L. Ogra & D. Dayton, Eds.: 185–195. Raven Press. New York.
3. LOSONSKY, G. A. & P. L. OGRA. 1981. Maternal-neonatal interactions and human breast milk. *In* Reproductive Immunology. N. Gleicher, Ed.: 171–182. Alan R. Liss, Inc., New York.
4. BIENENSTOCK, J., M. MCDERMOTT & D. BEFUS. 1979. A common mucosal immune system. *In* Immunology of Breast Milk. P. L. Ogra & D. Dayton, eds.: 91–104. Raven Press. New York.
5. ROUX, M. E., M. MCWILLIAMS, J. M. PHILLIPS-QUAGLIATA, P. WEISZ-CARRINGTON & M. E. LAMM. 1977. Origin of IgA-secreting plasma cells in the mammary gland. J. Exp. Med. **146:** 1311.
6. WEISZ-CARRINGTON, P., M. E. ROUX, M. MCWILLIAMS J. M. PHILLIPS-QUAGLIATA & M. E. LAMM. 1978. Hormonal induction of the secretory immune system in the mammary gland. Proc. Natl. Acad. Sci. USA **75:** 2928.
7. MONTGOMERY, P. C., K. M. CONNELLY, C. COHEN & C. A. SKANDERA. 1978. Remote-site stimulation of secretory IgA antibodies following bronchial and gastric stimulation. Adv. Exp. Med. Biol. **107:** 113.
8. GOLDBLUM, R. M., S. AHLSTEDT, B. CARLSSON, L. A. HANSON, U. JODAL, G. LIDIN-HANSON & A. SOHL-AKERLUND. 1975. Antibody-forming cells in human colostrum after oral immunization. Nature (London) **257:** 797.
9. HANSON, L. A., B. CARLSSON, J. R. CRUZ, B. GARCIA, J. HOLMGREN, S. R. KHAN, B. S. LINDBLAD, A.-M. SVENNERHOLM, B. SVENNERHOLM & J. URRUTIA. 1979. Immune Response in the mammary gland. *In* Immunology of Breast Milk. P. L. Ogra & D. Dayton, Eds.: 145–157. Raven Press. New York.
10. HANSON, L. A., B. CARLSSON, U. DAHLGREN, L. MELLANDER & C. SVANBORG EDEN. 1980. The secretory IgA system in the neonatal period. *In* Perinatal Infections. Ciba Foundation Symposium 77, Excerpta Medica. 187–204. Amsterdam.
11. OGRA, P. L. & H. L. GREENE. 1982. Human milk and breast feeding: An update on the state of the art. Pediat. Res. **16:** 266–271.
12. FISHAUT, M., D. MURPHY, M. NEIFERT, K. MC INTOSH & P. L. OGRA. 1981. Bronchomammary axis in the immune response to respiratory syncytial virus. J. Pediat. **99:** 186–191.
13. PERI, B. A., C. M. THEODORE, G. A. LOSONSKY, J. M. FISHAUT, R. M. ROTHBERG & P. L. OGRA. 1982. Antibody content of rabbit milk and serum following inhalation or ingestion of respiratory syncytial virus and bovine serum albumin. Clin. Exp. Immunol. **48:** 91–101.
14. OGRA, P. L., KERR-GRANT, G. UMANA, J. DZIERBA & D. WEINTRAUB. 1971. Antibody response in serum and nasopharynx after naturally acquired and vaccine induced infection with rubella virus. New Eng. J. Med. **285:** 1333–1339.

15. LOSONSKY, G. A., J. STRUSSENBERG, J. M. FISHAUT & P. L. OGRA. 1982. Effect of immunization against rubella on lactation products. I. Development and characterization of specific immunologic reactivity in breast milk. J. Infect. Dis. **145:** 654–660.
16. OGRA, S. S., D. WEINTRAUB & P. L. OGRA. 1977. Immunologic aspects of human colostrum and milk. III. Fate and absorption of cellular and soluble components in the gastrointestinal tract of the newborn. J. Immunol. **119:** 245–248.
17. ROBERTS, S. A. & D. L. J. FREED. 1977. Neonatal IgA secretion enhanced by breast feeding. Lancet **2:** 1131.
18. GALLAGHER, M. R., R. WELLIVER, T. YAMANAKA, B. EISENBERG, M. SUN & P. L. OGRA. 1981. Cell-mediated immune responsiveness to measles: Its occurrence as a result of naturally acquired or vaccine-induced infection and in infants of immune mothers. Am. J. Dis. Child. **135:** 48–51.
19. SCOTT, R., M. SCOTT & G. L. TOMS. 1981. Cellular and antibody response to respiratory syncytial (RS) virus in human colostrum, maternal blood, and cord blood. J. Med. Virol. **8:** 55–66.
20. SIEBER, O. F., D. L. LUCAS, C. LOHMAN, W. LARTER, H. GILES & T. J. JOHN. 1976. Reactivity of lymphocytes in maternal and cord blood to respiratory syncytial virus. Clin. Res. **24:** 181.
21. BEER, A. E., R. E. BILLINGHAM & J. HEAD. 1974. Proceedings: The immunologic significance of the mammary gland. J. Invest. Dermatol. **63:** 65–74.
22. DUTMERS, B. K. & R. C. PARKS. Altered immunological competence of neonatal mice force fed allogeneic lymphoid cells. Transplantation **26:** 443–445.
23. LOSONSKY, G. A., J. STRUSSENBERG, J. M. FISHAUT & P. L. OGRA. 1982. Effect of immunization against rubella on lactation products. II. Maternal-neonatal interactions. J. Infect. Dis. **145:** 661–666.
24. BANATVALA, J. E., I. L. CHRYSTIE & B. M. TOTTERDELL. 1978. Rotaviral infections in human neonates. J. Am. Vet. Med. Assoc. **173:** 527–530.
25. EASTHAM, E. J. & W. A. WALKER, 1979. Adverse effects of milk formula ingestion on the gastrointestinal tract. An update. Gastroenterology **76:** 365–374.
26. MATTHEW, D. J. & J. SOOTHILL. 1977. Prevention of eczema. Lancet **1:** 321–324.
27. KAPLAN, M. S. & N. J. SOLLI. 1979. Immunoglobulin E to cow's milk protein in breast-fed atopic children. J. Allergy Clin. Immunol. **64:** 122–126.
28. JUTO, P. & B. BJORKSTEIN. 1980. Serum IgE in infants and influence of type of feeding. Clin. Allergy **10:** 593–600.
29. KENNY, J. F. & A. J. ZEDD. 1977. Recurrent group B streptococcal disease in an infant associated with the ingestion of infected mother's milk. J. Pediat. **91:** 158–159.
30. SCHREINER, R. L., T. COATES & P. G. SHACKELFORD. 1977. Possible breast milk transmission of group B streptococcal infection. J. Pediat. **91:** 159.
31. KLEIN, E. B., T. BYRNE & L. Z. COOPER. 1980. Neonatal rubella in a breast fed infant after postpartum maternal infection. J. Pediat. **97:** 774–775.
32. JARRETT, E. & E. HALL. 1979. Selective suppression of IgE antibody responsiveness by maternal influence. Nature (London) **120:** 145.
33. PERI, B. A. & M. WAGNER. 1977. Immune response and dental caries incidence in Streptococcus faecalis-monoassociated Harvard caries resistant and caries susceptible rats. Infect. Immun. **16:** 805.
34. PERI, B. A. & R. M. ROTHBERG. 1981. Specific suppression of antibody production in young rabbit kits after maternal ingestion of bovine serum albumin. J. Immunol. **127:** 2520–2525.

DISCUSSION OF THE PAPER

M. D. COOPER (*The University of Alabama in Birmingham*): I was interested in the implication from your studies that immunization by the tracheal route caused seeding of cells presumably from BALT to lung mucosa and also to the breast, but not to the gut, whereas immunization by way of the oral route also resulted in seeding, but presumably from GALT to intestinal mucosa and into the milk, but not into the lung sphere. Do you think these are separate circuits: the BALT and GALT?

P. L. OGRA (*Children's Hospital, Buffalo, N.Y.*): I think they are distinctly separate circuits, and their contribution to the degree of immunocompetence that one sees in the milk will vary from circumstance to circumstance. This includes different types of antigens, since many antigens completely bypass the respiratory tract, and other antigens completely bypass the gut. As far as syncytial virus is concerned, it is an antigen that does not stimulate the gut, but replicates in fairly large quantities in the respiratory tract. There probably will be distinct patterns of the relative contribution from these two sites on the milk.

J. A. MATTINGLY (*Ohio State University, Columbus, Ohio*): What kind of antibody was produced in the studies using i.v. injection?

OGRA: It is primarily IgG, because, as I first presented, these rabbits do not make detectable quantities of IgA.

MATTINGLY: Could this responsiveness be transferred to the neonate?

OGRA: Yes.

MATTINGLY: Does the feeding of IgG suppress the ability of the neonate to respond to the antigen later?

OGRA: I can not say for sure that this particular response is related to feeding of IgG, because one cannot relate unresponsiveness to the amount of antibody to be assayed in the milk.

MATTINGLY: Dr. Peri and Dr. Rothberg have data that indicates that the rabbit responds differently to an oral challenge and later injection than do other rodents. In rodent systems and in man, an oral introduction of antigen followed by the same antigen i.v. does not yield a very good antibody response: the condition is termed oral tolerance. The rabbit, however, readily responds to systemic antigen. Do you agree with this?

OGRA: All creations are not equal, and I do not think you are going to find similar responses among rabbits, mice, and man. I would urge more studies in man.

R. I. CARR (*National Jewish Hospital, Denver, Colo.*): The appearance of tolerance in the kits after the feeding of the mother raises an interesting point. Do you have any direct evidence, or does Dr. Peri or Dr. Rothberg have any direct evidence to show that this is a passage of cells in milk from mother to kit?

OGRA: I do not think so; but Dr. Rothberg may want to respond.

R. M. ROTHBERG (*The University of Chicago, Chicago, Ill.*): We have no direct evidence that demonstrates a passage of cells from mother to kit.

C. R. WIRA (*Dartmouth Medical School, Hanover, N.H.*): Would you speculate on the possibility that the virus occurs in the milk during lactation, or that viral particles present in milk may actually be shed? Could you explain it by an immune exclusion in which IgA directed against a virus was carried across as an immune complex that could later dissociate?

OGRA: We do not know whether the virus replicates in the breast or simply filters in this organ. There is a well-known bioconcentration phenomenon for removing antigen through the milk. It is well established that immunized subjects, for example, infected women, shed viruses and bacteria in milk, and can infect their suckling neonate. It is also clear that some response occurs in those babies who are sucking this infected milk; there is also a lack of persistence of the response in those babies who do seroconvert after ingesting this infected milk. It will be important to clearly demonstrate significant modulation of the immune response, relative to the shedding of the virus in the milk.

WIRA: There is one report that I am aware of by Yallow that demonstrates the movement of an antigen-bound IgG across the placenta during the latter part of pregnancy. This movement is analogous to what Underdown and others have shown in the bile.

J. BIENENSTOCK (*McMaster University, Hamilton, Ontario, Canada*): I have a comment on the question of separation of the BALT and GALT circuits. I think they are both separate and integrated. I think that the evidence suggests that there is organ specificity for lymphocytes, derived from the lung to go back to the lung. There is also evidence to suggest seeding of other mucosal sites. This raises a question regarding the factors that may be in the milk. Jarret has shown that a factor responsible for apparent IgE suppression is transferred from mother to child. I understand that this factor is an IgG antibody. I wonder if you, or Dr. Rothberg, have any evidence for that activity accounting for this factor?

OGRA: I have no information right now.

J. J. CEBRA (*University of Pennsylvania, Philadelphia*): You suggest that mothers who have high levels of shed virus in milk have higher levels of IgA antibody, and that this situation might indicate that cells primed in the BALT might go to the mammary tissue. Have you ever been able to intercept cells in the peripheral blood that are stimulated either with mitogen or dead viral antigen that in fact will divide and make antibodies?

OGRA: We have attempted to look at this. It is difficult to collect peripheral blood from these babies; however, we have examined this point. In these cultures, we detect anti-rubella, but not anti-varicella-producing cells. We have not succeeded in identifying an isotype-specific, sensitized B-cell, but it may simply be a question of sensitivity of the technique and the number of sensitized cells that are present in the blood at a given time.

T. LEHNER (*Guy's Hospital, London, England*): Cellular immune responses can be transferred from mother to infant. Has your transfer of seropositivity ever been associated with finding fetal cord lymphocytes expressing positivity to the particular virus you were interested in?

OGRA: In this study, we did not examine cord lymphocytes; however, we have looked at other related situations. It is likely that transmission of virus-specific lymphocytes for rubella occur. Dr. Scott at Newcastle in England has provided some evidence for the existence of responses to syncytial virus. In our laboratory, Dr. Tante has suggested, from studies with measles virus, that this response is a distinct possibility.

DEVELOPMENT OF IMMUNOLOGICAL CAPACITY UNDER GERMFREE AND CONVENTIONAL CONDITIONS

H. Tlaskalová-Hogenová, J. Šterzl, R. Štěpánková, V. Dlabač,
V. Větvička, P. Rossmann, L. Mandel, and J. Rejnek

Department of Immunology and Laboratory of Gnotobiology
Institute of Microbiology
Czechoslovakian Academy of Sciences
142 20 Prague 4, Czechoslovakia

INTRODUCTION

The development of immunocompetency in mammals occurs during fetal life.[1-3] The immunological capacity of the newborn organism, however, is not fully mature; the insufficiently adapted organism is delivered into an environment full of microorganisms. At the beginning of life the defence capacity depends to a great extent on a supply of maternal antibodies from placenta, colostrum, and milk. It is the intestinal lymphoid tissues that are exposed to the load of microflora and food antigens. The significance of microbial antigens for a clonal expansion of lymphocytes of certain idiotypes and isotypes was recently critically evaluated.[4,5] The lymphatic tissue of the intestine reacts to antigenic stimuli by a rapid development that is particularly apparent during the first days after birth.[6,7] Signs of activation of an organized lymphatic tissue (Peyer's patches, appendix) can be followed on both morphological and functional levels.[7-10] Later this activation is reflected in a presence of the IgM- and IgA-producing cells in the intestinal mucosa.[11] Cells originating in Peyer's patches and primed by intestinal antigens are supposed to migrate through the mesenteric lymph nodes, the thoracic duct and blood into the gut and other mucosal surfaces, forming the so-called common mucosal system.[12-16] A similar migratory pathway as for IgA-producing cells was described for T-cells originating in the gut.[17] The nature of factors involved in the homing of these cells to distant mucosal surfaces and exocrine glands is still unknown.[15,16]

In our previous studies we compared the immunological capacities of germfree (GF) piglets and rabbits with those of their conventionally raised (CONV) partners and showed that the antigenic stimulation fundamentally affects development of the immunological capacity.[7,18,19] Nevertheless, for some other species, for example mice, the development of the immunological capacity in the GF and CONV individuals was reported to be comparable.[20] We therefore inquired into the development of another available species—rat—and studied factors that affect development and recirculation of lymphocytes.

Because the six-layered placenta of the pig considerably limits transfer of maternal antibodies, the GF piglets seem to be a suitable model for the study of problems concerning the development of immunological capacity, especially in the GALT. In addition, a higher weight of lymphatic organ makes easier some quantitative assays. Our experimental model was therefore used for the study of

0077-8923/83/0409-0096 $1.75/0 © 1983, NYAS

the fate of bacteria present in the intestinal tract, their migration into other tissues, and the development of a protective barrier against bacterial invasion.

MATERIAL AND METHODS

Animals

Inbred Wistar rats were kept in isolators for GF rearing[22,23] or in conventional conditions of animal facilities. Rats on an artificial diet, delivered by hysterectomy, were from the first day of life hand-fed one of the two diets: K50 or LNa 0.5. The K50 diet[22] consisted of natural cow's milk, dried milk, egg yolk, linseed oil, sunflower oil, salts, and vitamins. The LNa diet (an analogue of diet 449C)[24,25] consisted of light cream, natural cow's milk, dried milk, salts, and vitamins. All rats were weaned on the 20th day after birth and fed by a standard pelleted diet with 21% protein.

GF piglets were delivered by a gnotobiotic cesarean section and given a milk-type diet.[26] The GF state was controlled twice a week by cultivation of a rectal swab.

Plaque Method

In cell suspensions prepared from various organs, the number of cells producing hemolytic[18] and bactericidal[7] antibodies was determined. Plaques were checked microscopically for the presence of the central cell.

^{51}Cr Labeling and Evaluation of Cell Distribution

The cells were labeled by a 45-minute incubation with 100 μCi/mL of sodium chromate (^{51}Cr from Radiochemical Center, Amersham) at 37°C under constant agitation. After four washes, cell viability was measured (always greater than 93%). Each recipient was injected through the tail vein with 5×10^7 cells. The animals were killed 20 hours after cell transfer and the radioactivity of different organs was measured on a γ changer (Nuclear-Chicago). In each experiment GF and CONV rats were injected with the same suspension.

Morphology

Ileum with Peyer's patches was examined in two-month-old rats. For light microscopy, paraffin sections of formalin-fixed tissue were stained by hematoxylin and eosin, PAS method, toluidine blue, and methyl green-pyronine. For electron microscopy, 2.5% glutaraldehyde (0.1 M cacodylate buffer) was injected under gentle pressure between two ligatures of an ileal loop harboring a Peyer's patch. The loop was then excised, fixed for 60 minutes (4°C) in the same solution, postfixed with 2% OsO$_4$, and embedded in Vestopal W. Ultrathin sections, contrasted with U-acetate and Pb-citrate, were examined in a Tesla BS 613 microscope at 80 kV.

Colonization of GF Piglets and Rats with
E. coli *and* Salmonella typhimurium

Bacterial strains used for colonization included *E. coli* 086, 083 and S-16, and *Salmonella typhimurium* strain 1591, which is a stable rough His⁻ mutant obtained through the courtesy of Dr. Otto Lüderitz (Freiburg, FRG); the other rough salmonella strains were described earlier.[27]

The bacterial counts in mesenteric nodes and organs were obtained by homogenization of weighed pieces of tissue in PBS and by plating an appropriate dilution on the Endo plates. The antisera used were either from GF animals, colonized for two months or more with the particular strain, or from adult CONV animals immunized with a heat-killed suspension of the same strain. The daily dose per piglet was about 3 and 30 ml, respectively, and 1 ml per day in the case of GF rats.

Peroral Immunization of GF Piglets with Killed Bacteria

For peroral immunization experiments, one batch of *E. coli* 086 was prepared; the bacterial mass was freeze-dried and sterilized by irradiation. Killed bacteria were added to the milk diet in various proportions, and the immunization dose was calculated from the feeding protocol. In different groups of piglets, the medium daily dose per animal was 50, 200, 700, 1500, and 4000 mg of dry weight, respectively. To another group of GF piglets a heat-killed suspension of *Salmonella typhimurium*, strain 1591, was given in a dose of 100 mg/day per animal. After one to eight weeks, piglets were colonized with particular strains, and the degree of penetration was estimated two days later.

Statistics

Student's *t*-test was performed on the results.

RESULTS AND DISCUSSION

*The Role of Microflora Antigens and Nutritional Factors
in the Development of Immunological Capacity*

The occurrence of cells producing natural antibodies to *E. coli* 086 was studied using the bactericidal plaque technique in GF and CONV rats of different ages. We detected the presence of spontaneous bactericidal plaque-forming cells (PFC) in Peyer's patches of CONV rats only; no bactericidal PFC were found in Peyer's patches of GF rats until 12 months of age (FIGURE 1). In spleen and mesenteric lymph nodes the occurrence of background bactericidal PFC was comparable in normal and GF rats (FIGURE 1). In addition, the number of cells producing natural hemolytic antibodies and the capacity to respond to immunization with SRBC in the two-month-old GF and CONV rats was comparable (FIGURE 2).

The finding of antibody-forming cells in Peyer's patches contradicts earlier findings of some other authors,[28] indicating that only in Peyer's patches, does activation take place, without terminal differentiation into antibody-producing cells.[5,16] Our results, which show that organized lymphoid tissue of the gut takes

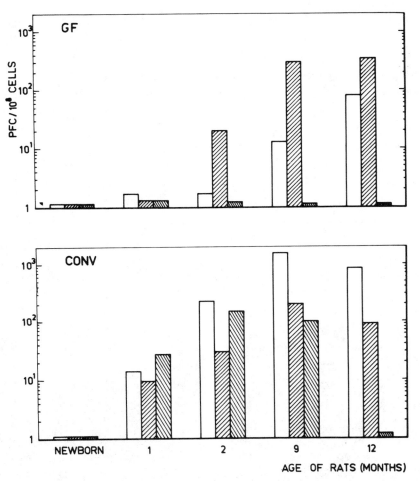

FIGURE 1. Development of natural bactericidal antibody formation in germfree (GF) and conventionally raised (CONV) rats. Number of background PFC against *E. coli* 086 in spleen (□), mesenteric lymph nodes (□), and Peyer's patches (□).

part in antibody formation in rabbits and rats, together with recently published results of other authors,[29] showing that immunoglobulin-producing cells are present in this tissue, suggest that a small number of cells may be activated by antigen and/or by polyclonal B-cell activators in Peyer's patches and differentiate *in situ* directly into antibody-forming cells.

Our morphological studies of intestinal lymphoid tissue confirmed the earlier findings[6,7,9] that the structure of Peyer's patches of GF and CONV animals differs. By light microscopy of rat ileum (PAS staining), we found that in both CONV and GF rats the epithelial layer of mucosal villi was formed by nonvacuolized columnar enterocytes and multiple goblet cells with rare migrating lymphocytes.

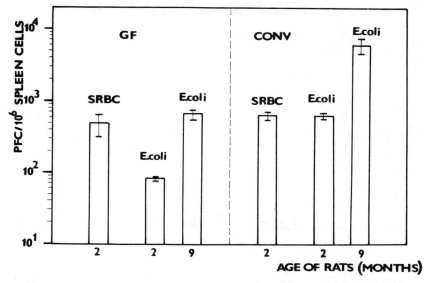

FIGURE 2. Development of hemolytic and bactericidal antibody-forming capacity in GF and CONV rats. Number of PFC in spleen was estimated on day 5 after i.p. immunization of rats with 2×10^9 or heat-inactivated *E. coli* 086 suspension. Arithmetic means ± SD. 4–12 animals per group.

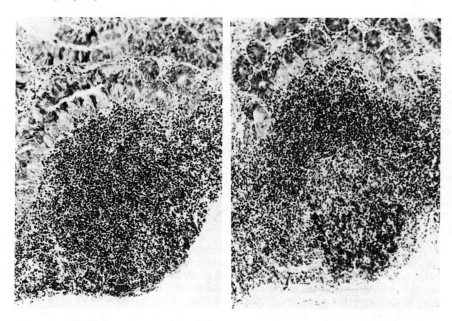

FIGURE 3. (Left): Lymphatic nodule of ileum in GF rat containing small lymphocytes with rudimentary germinal center. (Right): Hyperplastic lymphatic nodule in a CONV rat exhibiting corona and large germinal center with a cluster of basophilic lymphoblasts (bottom). Both parts toluidine blue, (× 115).

The bottom area exhibited many mitoses and scarce granular Paneth's cells. The lamina propria displayed multiple lymphocytes, granular macrophages (shown by PAS staining) and scattered granulocytes. The suprafollicular dome area was covered with enterocytes of the same appearance, and rare but unequivocal goblet cells. Lymphocytic migration was more pronounced in the dome area, especially in the CONV rat. The brush border of dome enterocytes was continuous, without apparent defects of the PAS-staining. The submucosal lymphatic follicles were of distinctly larger volume in the CONV rat (FIGURE 3, right). The well-developed germinal centers were infiltrated by aggregated pyroninophilic

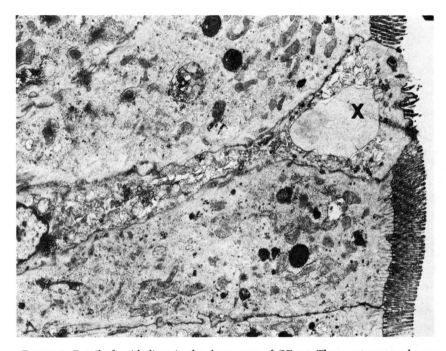

FIGURE 4. Detail of epithelium in the dome area of GF rat. Three enterocytes have a regular microvillous zone, whereas the intercalated M-cell (upper center) displays scarce irregular microvilli. The patch of light cytoplasm (x) probably represents the periphery of an insulated migrating lymphocyte, (× 7200).

lymphoblasts, most densely within the basal portion close to the muscular layer. These centers and the corona were rich in granular macrophages and pyknotic tingible bodies. In the GF rat (FIGURE 3, left), the centers were smaller and hypoplastic, with sporadic lymphoblasts and rare macrophages. Mature plasmacytes were found in both rats within the lamina propria, especially in the base of villi. They were abundant in the CONV rat and less numerous, but still not rare, in the GF animal.

The electron microscopy was used to examine the ultrastructure of the epithelia in the suprafollicular dome area. Most dome enterocytes resembled those of the villi by a regular dense microvillous brush border with an underlying terminal web. Scattered cells, however, exhibited irregular, short and plump villi (FIGURES 4, 5). These intercalated cells were narrow and bottle-shaped with a broader base and had a more dense cytoplasmic matrix than the enterocytes. Their cytoplasm contained multiple mitochondria and well-developed Golgi areas. Characteristically, single or clustered lymphocytes were in close contact with these narrow cells (FIGURE 5). The cytoplasm of the latter formed narrow belts and strands, largely but not fully, insulating the incorporated lymphocytes. There were also close contacts between the base of the intercalated cells and the migrating lymphoid cells. The lymphocytes displayed a broad rim of cytoplasm

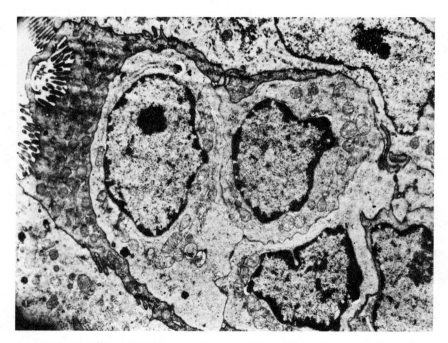

FIGURE 5. M-cell in a CONV rat with short irregular microvilli. Its dense cytoplasm encircles a group of lymphoid cells. Right bottom: nucleus of M-cell; right top: nucleus of enterocyte, (× 7200).

with multiple polyribosomes and some profiles of granular endoplasmic reticula. Mature plasmacytes were not found. The dome goblet cells also had basal nuclei and dense cytoplasm similar to those of intercalated cells, but they showed more copious granular endoplasmic reticula. In the lymphatic follicles of the CONV animal, small and medium lymphocytes prevailed with scattered macrophages with lymphoblasts. Mature plasmacytes were not found within the depth of follicles or in dome epithelia.

This shows that the intestinal lymphatic tissue of CONV and GF rats differed in both the quantitative and qualitative aspects, thus permitting an easy distinction in the blind test. In both animals, the intercalated epithelia, devoid of a well-organized brush border, were readily seen in the dome area. They probably corresponded to the M-cells described in various species[30,31] and had a more cytoplasmic matrix than the adjacent enterocytes. In contrast to our previously unpublished observations in GF piglets and the results of others, for example, in rabbit ileum,[32] the dome epithelium included rare but characteristic goblet cells.

In GF rabbits and piglets, delivered by a cesarean section into isolators for GF rearing, no signs of growth of the immunological potential were found until the third month of life; in CONV individuals this increase in the immunological capacity was substantial.[18,19] Nevertheless, when studying the development of the immunological capacity of mice and rats, different results were obtained: the development in the GF and CONV individuals was comparable. Apart from the species difference, this could be due to a different pattern of feeding: the animals delivered by a cesarean section were kept on an artificial diet, whereas the mice were breast-fed. Therefore we decided to study the effect of the artificial nutrition of rats on the development of their immunological capacity.

Baby rats of the inbred strain, delivered by hysterectomy, were fed with one of the two milk diets: the LNa diet and the K50 diet. Hand-fed and breast-fed rats were weaned on day 20 after birth and fed with a standard pelleted diet. In rats on the LNa diet, the weight gain was lower than in breast-fed or hand-fed rats given the K50 diet (FIGURE 6). In two-month-old animals the inadequate LNa diet brought about histological changes in the endocrine system and other organs.[33]

At the age of 60 days, we compared the immunological capacities of the breast-fed and the artificially fed rats. The animals were immunized intraperitoneally with 2×10^9 SRBC and the antibody response was measured by a hemolytic plaque technique in the spleen 5 days after the immunization. The lowest immune response was in the group of the GF and CONV rats hand-fed with the LNa diet (FIGURE 7).

From the group of nonimmunized rats, the highest number of natural antibody-producing cells (background plaques) was in the breast-fed rats, whereas minimal number of such cells was found in rats reared on the LNa diet (FIGURE 8). It is interesting to note that in the group of CONV rats reared on the K50 diet, the presence of background plaques and the number of plaques after immunization were comparable with those in the breast-fed rats. It is therefore possible that colonization with microflora may, to a certain degree, compensate for deficiencies that appear when the newborn rats do not get maternal milk.

Apart from the antibody response, we studied the effect of nutrition on the cellular immunity by following the growth of the Yoshida sarcoma[34] in the peritoneum of rats. Whereas the breast-fed rats are resistant to 10^3 intraperitoneally injected cells of this sarcoma, the LNa-reared rats were killed by it after 16 to 30 days of life.

Results of this study support the significance of feeding with maternal milk for the development of the immunological capacity. An artificial diet applied after birth may deeply influence the defense capacity of an adult organism.

The Role of Antigen, Present in the Intestine, on the Lymphocyte Migration Pattern

The specific homing mechanism that makes possible preferential localization of lymphoblasts originating in the organized lymphatic intestinal tissue and committed to production of the IgA antibodies on the mucosal surfaces still remains unclear.[14-16] Despite the fact that some findings[35,36] eliminate the role of

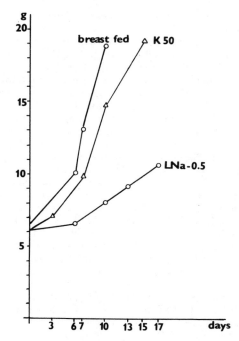

FIGURE 6. Growth curve of breast-fed and hand-fed rats with K50 and LNa 0.5 milk diets for the first days of life.

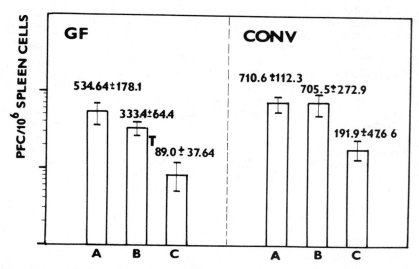

FIGURE 7. Antibody-forming capacity of GF and CONV two-month-old rats. The number of hemolytic PFC in spleen was estimated on day 5 after intraperitoneal immunization of rats with 10^9 SRBC. (A): breast-fed rats; (B): rats fed for the first 20 days of life with K50 diet; (C): rats fed for the first 20 days of life with LNa 0.5 diet.

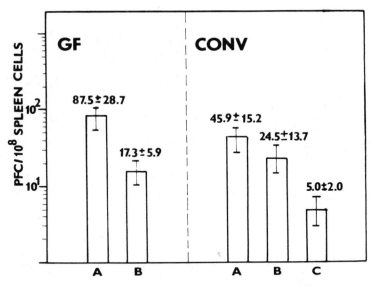

FIGURE 8. Number of background hemolytic PFC in spleen of GF and CONV two-month-old rats. (A): breast-fed rats; (B): rats fed for the first 20 days of life with K50 diet; (C) rats fed for the first 20 days of life with ONa 0.5 diet.

antigen, we, together with other authors,[37] do not take these proofs as fully convincing. We therefore decided to scrutinize again the role of antigen in the migration patterns, by using the opportunity to work with GF and CONV inbred rats. Because it has been proved that there exists in sheep a migration of ^{51}Cr-labeled small lymphocytes from the intestinal lymph into the intestine,[38,39] we used the same label for our assays.

The comparison of homing of the radiolabeled cells isolated from the mesenteric nodes, popliteal lymph nodes and Peyer's patches of CONV rats (TABLES 1, 2 & 3) yielded the following conclusions. (1) The salivary gland and

TABLE 1

LOCALIZATION OF ^{51}Cr-LABELED CELLS
FROM MESENTERIC LYMPH NODES OF CONV RATS
20 HOURS AFTER TRANSFER INTO SYNGENEIC GF OR CONV RATS*

| | Percentage of Injected Radioactivity In | |
Localization In	GF Recipients	CONV Recipients
Popliteal lymph nodes	3.28 ± 0.29	1.11 ± 0.16
Mesenteric lymph nodes	3.59 ± 0.69	3.37 ± 1.00
Small intestine	7.81 ± 1.60	14.26 ± 1.93
Salivary gland	3.42 ± 0.32	2.21 ± 0.30
Spleen	29.88 ± 5.03	19.15 ± 3.19
Liver	22.48 ± 4.11	14.33 ± 2.89
Lung	11.70 ± 1.88	3.40 ± 0.52
Thymus	3.65 ± 0.53	1.66 ± 0.64

*Six animals were used in each group. Arithmetic means ± SD.

TABLE 2

LOCALIZATION OF ^{51}Cr-LABELED CELLS FROM POPLITEAL LYMPH NODES OF CONV RATS 20 HOURS AFTER TRANSFER INTO SYNGENEIC GF OR CONV RATS*

Localization In	Percentage of Injected Radioactivity In	
	GF Recipients	CONV Recipients
Popliteal lymph nodes	1.00 ± 0.11	1.04 ± 0.16
Mesenteric lymph nodes	1.02 ± 0.19	2.00 ± 0.37
Small intestine	2.52 ± 0.67	3.59 ± 0.66
Salivary gland	0.90 ± 0.12	0.87 ± 0.09
Spleen	28.31 ± 5.63	22.27 ± 4.35
Liver	13.21 ± 4.90	12.52 ± 2.12
Lung	3.44 ± 0.58	3.04 ± 0.68
Thymus	1.03 ± 0.39	1.55 ± 0.33

*Six animals were used in each group. Arithmetic means ± SD.

intestine of both the CONV and GF rats were seeded by significantly more cells from mesenteric nodes of CONV rats than by cells from popliteal nodes or Peyer's patches. We thus confirmed in our system the homing mechanism, described about the mesenteric node lymphoblasts by other authors.[14,16,17,35-37,40,41,58] (2) Homing of the mesenteric node cells into the small intestine is significantly higher in CONV recipients than in the GF ones (TABLE 1). Nevertheless because we may assume a higher homing of cells in the intestine of CONV rats in which a massive development of lymphatic tissue takes place, and thus also the blood flow is higher, we tried to exclude the role of an increased blood flow. We also studied the fate of lymphatic cells isolated from mesenteric nodes of GF rats. We found no significant differences in homing of cells obtained from mesenteric nodes of GF rats in the intestine of GF and CONV rats; the homing in the intestine of the GF rats was even higher (TABLE 4). Homing of these cells in the intestine and salivary gland is lower than that of cells obtained from mesenteric nodes of CONV rats (TABLES 1, 4). The homing affinity to the intestine, therefore, seems to be only a property of cells obtained from CONV rats, that is of cells that were in contact with the antigen. A comparison of these cells with those from popliteal nodes of

TABLE 3

LOCALIZATION OF ^{51}Cr-LABELED CELLS FROM PEYER'S PATCHES OF CONV RATS 20 HOURS AFTER TRANSFER INTO SYNGENEIC GF OR CONV RATS*

Localization In	Percentage of Injected Radioactivity In	
	GF Recipients	CONV Recipients
Popliteal lymph nodes	0.15 ± 0.02	0.12 ± 0.02
Mesenteric lymph nodes	0.15 ± 0.07	0.15 ± 0.05
Small intestine	0.34 ± 0.11	0.44 ± 0.20
Salivary gland	0.19 ± 0.04	0.24 ± 0.06
Spleen	9.87 ± 0.68	7.81 ± 1.02
Liver	14.80 ± 2.64	9.30 ± 1.97
Lung	2.02 ± 0.31	1.62 ± 0.28
Thymus	0.38 ± 0.16	0.35 ± 0.17

*Seven animals were used in each group. Arithmetic means ± SD.

GF rats, which is being performed in our laboratory, may bring a solution to this interesting problem.

Our results indicate that antigens of microflora present in the intestine enhance homing of cells from mesenteric nodes that were activated by these antigens. The antigens seem not only to increase proliferation of cells localized in the intestine,[37,59] but due to a direct attraction, increase the number of homed cells. This conclusion is in keeping with findings of Cahill[42] et al., according to which a subpopulation of intestinal lymphocytes that migrates preferentially through the small intestine of adult sheep was not found in the fetus. Our results are not in keeping with the findings in mice.[43] The question is whether in our system the chief role is played by the small lymphocytes, as in sheep, or whether there is a higher binding of the ^{51}Cr label to the population of lymphoblasts.[14] Therefore, at present we are studying the migration streams of cells that incorporate labeled uridine.

Antigens of the external environment seem to affect to a considerable degree the development of the lymphocyte-circulation pattern. We should therefore

TABLE 4

LOCALIZATION OF ^{51}Cr-LABELED CELLS FROM MESENTERIC LYMPH NODES OF GF RATS 20 HOURS AFTER TRANSFER INTO SYNGENEIC GF OR CONV RATS*

| | Percentage of Injected Radioactivity In | |
Localization In	GF Recipients	CONV Recipients
Popliteal lymph nodes	2.24 ± 0.39	2.50 ± 0.43
Mesenteric lymph nodes	2.55 ± 0.56	2.78 ± 1.21
Small intestine	5.87 ± 1.30	4.63 ± 1.03
Salivary gland	1.32 ± 0.20	1.62 ± 0.45
Spleen	23.35 ± 1.35	22.74 ± 4.72
Liver	18.93 ± 5.10	19.42 ± 3.05
Lung	9.85 ± 4.17	7.34 ± 1.75
Thymus	2.06 ± 0.56	2.64 ± 0.86

*Five animals were used in each group. Arithmetic means ± SD.

keep in mind that CONV individuals with natural migratory circuits (found in fetuses and GF individuals) exhibit changes brought about by sensitization with antigens and attraction of lymphocytes into sites where these antigens are localized. This finding holds not only for antigens of the microflora but for food antigens as well.

The Development of Barrier Function of the Intestine after Peroral Colonization of GF Piglets and Rats

It has been repeatedly shown that under conventional conditions the presence of normal microbial flora effectively competes with colonization of the intestine with artificially introduced strains of bacteria, including known enteric pathogens.[44] The colonization of CONV animals with various strains of enteric bacteria is extremely difficult and transitional success was achieved only with very high doses of bacteria (10^9 or more). This so-called colonization resistance,[44] which certainly represents a very important factor of anti-infectious resistance,[45] could be dramatically reduced, if normal flora was suppressed, for example, by suitable antibiotics, and completely eliminated under GF state conditions. Enteric bacteria applied perorally to GF animals readily multiply, with generation time similar to *in vitro* conditions; bacterial counts in the intestine reach a plateau within one or two days, with maximal values in colon and terminal ileum.[46] In many strains of *E. coli* and salmonella species, the colonization is accompanied by septicemia, resulting in death,[47,48] whereas colonization with some *E. coli* and rough strains of *Salmonella typhimurium* does not evoke clinical symptoms of disease, and histological findings show only signs of "physiological inflammation."[7,49] Nevertheless, after peroral infection of GF piglets with such strains, appreciable counts of viable bacteria were detected in mesenteric nodes and eventually in liver and spleen. If the viable counts in various organs were continuously estimated, characteristic curves would be obtained. FIGURE 9 shows a typical pattern obtained after peroral infection of GF piglets with avirulent strain 1591 of *Salmonella typhimurium*. It is apparent that within three to six days after the introduction of bacteria, maximal counts were reached in mesenteric nodes, spleen, and liver, followed by a continuous decrease for several weeks thereafter, with a complete disappearance within about eight weeks. Similar curves were

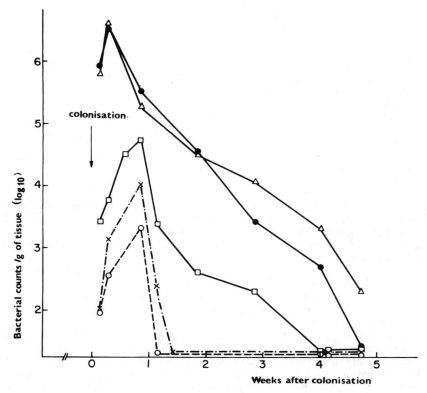

FIGURE 9. Penetration of *Salmonella typhimurium*, strain 1591 to mesenteric nodes of jejunum (□), ileum (△), colon (●), spleen (x), and liver (○) of monoassociated piglets.

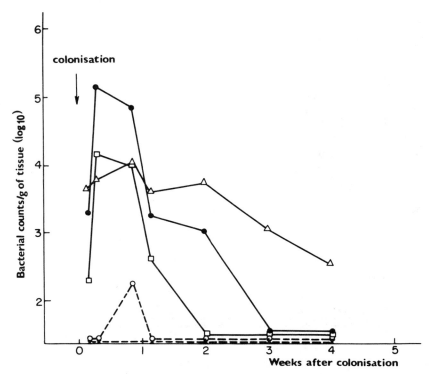

FIGURE 10. Penetration of *E. coli* 086 to mesenteric nodes of jejunum (□———□), ileum (△———△), colon (●———●), spleen (x --- x) and liver (O --- O) of monoassociated piglets.

obtained with other rough strains of the salmonella species and a number of innocuous strains of *E. coli*. In the latter case, however, viable bacteria were only exceptionally found in liver and spleen, and the estimated counts were usually by one or two orders lower in comparison with the estimates in the *Salmonella typhimurium*-infected animals (FIGURE 10). It should be stressed that similar results, using the same strains, were obtained also in GF rats,[50] and additionally, the dynamics of bacterial counts in mesenteric counts of GF piglets, monoassociated with "innocent" *E. coli* strains, were quite comparable with changes of viable counts of "coliforms" in mesenteric nodes of CONV piglets, during the first weeks after birth (FIGURE 11).

This more general and more widely encountered consequence of the first contact with at least some bacterial species seems to have an important immunological background, leading to an extraordinary high degree of protection against the used strain.[44,51]

It seems that in the observed phenomena, specific local immunity plays a role. Despite the pronounced antibody response in groups subjected to a higher dose regimen, we were not able to prevent or modify the degree of penetration of either *E. coli* or *Salmonella typhimurium* by peroral vaccination of GF piglets using different doses of killed bacteria and immunization schedules as outlined

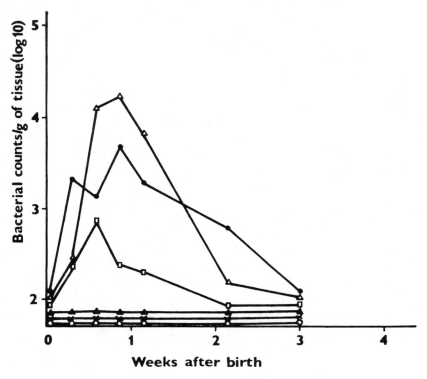

FIGURE 11. Penetration of "coliforms" from the gut of CONV piglets to mesenteric nodes of jejunum (□), ileum (△), colon (●), spleen (x), liver (○), and blood (▲).

above. One such example is shown in FIGURE 12. Some piglets and rats were treated perorally with hyperimmune sera obtained from either immunized adults or from long-term colonized animals. No appreciable effect was observed irrespective of the dose given to any group of monoassociated piglets (FIGURE 12) or rats.[50] If we accept the view that piglets born under CONV conditions are colonized with the mother's own E. coli strains and at the same time suckle colostrum containing antibodies against such strains, then the fairly "normal" course of penetration in the conventionally bred piglets (FIGURE 11) can serve as another argument against the participation of antibodies in the phenomenon presented herein. This observation is somewhat surprising, because peroral immunization with killed bacteria, or drinking of sera or colostrum was shown to be quite successful in prevention of illness, caused by some known enteric pathogens, for example, Vibrio cholerae and enteropathogenic strains of E. coli.[48,52-54] In these cases, however, antibodies against the colonization antigen[53,55] or flagella[56] were found to be effective, mainly by blocking firm adhesion of bacteria to columnar cells. Using the above-mentioned strains, we were not able to demonstrate any significant association with columnar cells in vivo or in vitro,[57] and therefore, different mechanisms may be involved.

Since our efforts with peroral vaccination or application of hyperimmune sera

were quite unsuccessful in both GF piglets and rats, we tried to modify the extent
of penetration of intestinal bacteria by an adoptive transfer of spleen cells from
the long-term colonized inbred rats. For technical reasons only, an avirulent
mutant of *Salmonella typhimurium* was used in most experiments. If 3.3 to 5.1 ×
10^8 spleen cells from the long-term monoassociated rats were injected into the tail
vein of GF rats, simultaneously with peroral infection of the same strain, no viable
bacteria were found two days later in mesenteric nodes and spleen; viable counts
in control animals were 1.1 × 10^7/g and 5.5 × 10^3/g in mesenteric nodes and
spleen, respectively. Our preliminary results suggest that protective cells could be
eliminated by filtration through nylon wool. The presence of living or multiplying
microorganisms in lymphatic tissue represents an antigenic stimulus, which in
comparison to the effect of peroral immunization with killed bacteria, might lead
to a quantitatively or qualitatively different immune response. The elucidation of
effector immunological mechanisms that control the penetration of microorganisms through the intestinal barrier has begun.

CONCLUSIONS

Using *E. coli* and SRBC as antigens in CONV and GF rats, we observed that
the development of immunological capacity (the response to *E. coli* antigens) is
affected by the presence of microflora. Spontaneous bactericidal PFC against *E.*

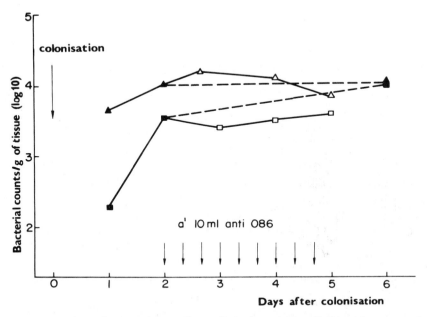

FIGURE 12. The influence of perorally applied pig anti *E. coli* 086 antiserum on the
penetration of *E. coli* 086 to mesenteric nodes of jejunum (□ · ■) and ileum (Δ · ▲). Full
symbols represent estimates in control group; empty symbols represent estimates in monoassociated piglets receiving 10 mL of antiserum three times daily (short arrows).

coli in Peyer's patches were found in CONV rats only. It seems that in the organized lymphoid tissue, antigens or polyclonal B-cell activators of bacterial origin cannot only activate cells, but can also stimulate some of them to terminal differentiation. Morphological studies showed signs of activation in lymphoid tissue of Peyer's patches in CONV rats. In dome epithelia of GF and CONV rats, cells similar to M-cells of other species were found.

Artificial milk diets applied during the first days after birth greatly influenced the development of immune potential: even as adults the artificially fed rats exhibited decreased immunological capacity compared with the breast-fed rats. The nature of the factors from maternal milk that affect the long-term development of immunological capacity is not known and is at present under study.

When following the migratory pattern of lymphocytes, we found that independently of the blood flow, the gut microflora increased the homing of mesenteric node cells into the gut of CONV rats. We also compared trappings of cells, isolated from mesenteric nodes of CONV and GF donors, in the gut and salivary glands of GF and CONV rats. A higher degree of localization in these organs was found when mesenteric node cells from CONV donors were used. This phenomenon indicates that activation of cells by microflora antigens increases their homing affinity for mucosal surfaces.

Colonization of the gastrointestinal tract leads to an immune response against a number of microbial antigens. Such immune response may be critical in the development of a functional barrier controlling the penetration of intestinal microorganisms and/or their antigens.

REFERENCES

1. ŠTERZL, J. & A. M. SILVERSTEIN. 1967. Adv. Immunol. **6:** 337–459.
2. SOLOMON, J. B., Ed. 1971. Foetal and Neonatal Immunology. Elsevier Biomed. Press. Amsterdam.
3. COOPER, M. D. & D. H. DAYTON, Eds. 1977. Development of Host Defences. Raven Press. New York.
4. GEARHART, P. J. & J. J. CEBRA. 1979. J. Exp. Med. **149:** 216–227.
5. CEBRA, J. J., P. J. GEARHART, J. F. HALSEY, J. L. HURWITZ & R. D. SHAHIN. 1980. J. Reticuloendothelial Soc. **28:** 619s–715s.
6. THORBECKE, G. J. 1959. Ann. N.Y. Acad. Sci. **78:** 237–246.
7. TLASKALOVÁ, H., J. ŠTERZL, P. HÁJEK, M. POSPÍŠIL, I. ŘÍHA, H. MARVANOVÁ, V. KAMARÝTOVÁ, L. MANDEL, J. KRUML & F. KOVÁŘŮ. 1970. In Developmental Aspects of Antibody Formation and Structure. J. Šterzl & I. Říha, Eds.: 767–790. Academia. Prague.
8. CARTER, P. B. & F. M. COLLINS. 1975. J. Reticuloendothelial Soc. **17:** 38–46.
9. WAKSMAN, B. H. & H. OZER. 1976. Progr. Allergy **21:** 1–113.
10. TLASKALOVÁ-HOGENOVÁ, H., J. ŠTERZL, M. POSPÍŠIL & J. HOFMAN. 1977. In Developmental Immunobiology. J. B. Solomon & J. D. Horton, Eds.: 355–362. Elsevier/North-Holland. Amsterdam.
11. BRANDTZAEG, P. 1981. Monogr. Allergy **17:** 195–221.
12. McGHEE, J. R., J. MESTECKY & J. L. BABB, Eds. 1978. Secretory Immunity and Infection. Plenum Press. New York.
13. HANSON, L. A., S. AHLSTEDT, B. ANDERSSON, B. CARLSSON, U. DAHLGREN, G. LIDIN-JANSON, I. MATTSBY-BALTZER & C. SVANBORG-EDEN. 1980. J. Reticuloendothelial Soc. **28:** 1s–9s.
14. HALL, J. G. 1980. Monogr. Allergy **16:** 100–111.
15. MESTECKY, J., J. R. McGHEE, S. S. CRAGO, S. JACKSON, M. KILIAN, H. KIYONO, J. L. BABB & S. M. MICHALEK. 1980. J. Reticuloendothelial Soc. **28** (Suppl. 45): 45s–60s.

16. BIENENSTOCK, J. 1981. Monogr. Allergy **17**: 233–249.
17. PAROTT, C. R. & A. FERGUSON. 1974. Immunology **26**: 571–588.
18. ŠTERZL, J., J. VESELÝ, M. JÍLEK & L. MANDEL. 1965. *In* Molecular and Cellular Basis of Antibody Formation. J. Šterzl, Ed.: 463–476, Academia. Prague.
19. TLASKALOVÁ-HOGENOVÁ, H. & R. ŠTĚPÁNKOVÁ. 1980. Folia Biol. **26**: 81–93.
20. BOSMA, M., T. MAKINODAN & H. E. WALBURG. 1967. J. Immunol. **99**: 420–430.
21. TLASKALOVÁ-HOGENOVÁ, H., J. ČERNÁ & L. MANDEL. 1981. Scand. J. Immunol. **13**: 467–472.
22. ŠTĚPÁNKOVÁ, R., J. KLEPALOVÁ & J. KRUML. 1972. Folia Microbiol. **17**: 505–512.
23. ŠTĚPÁNKOVÁ, R. 1979. Folia Microbiol. **24**: 11–15.
24. PLEASANTS, J. R. 1959. Ann. N.Y. Acad. Sci. **78**: 116–126.
25. WOSTMANN, B. S. 1959. Ann. N.Y. Acad. Sci. **78**: 175–182.
26. TRÁVNÍČEK, J., L. MANDEL, A. LANC & R. RŮŽIČKA. 1966. Čs. Fyziol. **15**: 240–246 (In Czech).
27. DLABAČ, V. 1968. Folia Microbiol. **13**: 439–449.
28. BIENENSTOCK, J. & J. DOLEZEL. 1971. J. Immunol. **106**: 938–945.
29. BENNER, R., A. M. RIJNBEEK, R. R. BERNABE, C. MARTINEZ-ALONSO & A. COUTINHO. 1981. Immunobiology **158**: 225–238.
30. OWEN, R. L. & A. L. JONES. 1974. Gastroenterology **66**: 189–203.
31. CHU, M. R., R. D. GLOCK & R. F. ROSS. 1979. Am. J. Vet. Res. **40**: 1720–1728.
32. FAULK, W. P., J. N. CORMICK & J. R. GOODMAN, 1970. Cell. Immunol. **1**: 500–520.
33. ŠTĚPÁNKOVÁ, R., J. ŠTERZL & I. TREBICHAVSKÝ. 1981. Proc. Intern. Symp. on Human Milk Banking. Hradec Králové. Czechoslovakia. In press.
34. YOSHIDA, T. 1952. J. Natl. Cancer Inst. **12**: 947–969.
35. HALSTEAD, T. E. & J. G. HALL. 1972. Tranplantation **14**: 339–346.
36. FERGUSON, A. 1974. Clin. Exp. Immunol. **17**: 691–696.
37. HUSBAND, A. J., H. J. MONIE & J. L. GOWANS. 1977. *In* Immunology of the Gut. P. J. Lochmann, S. Ahlstedt, Eds.: 29–54. Elsevier/North-Holland. Amsterdam.
38. SCOLLARY, R. G., J. HOPKINS & J. G. HALL. 1976. Nature (London) **260**: 528–529.
39. CAHILL, R. N. P., D. C. POSKITT, H. FROST & Z. TRNKA. 1977. J. Exp. Med. **145**: 420–428.
40. WEIZS-CARRINGTON, P., M. E. ROUX, M. McWILLIAMS, J. M. PHILLIPS-QUAGLIATA & M. E. LAMM. 1979. J. Immunol. **123**: 1705–1708.
41. MONTGOMERY, P. C., I. M. LEMAITRE-VOELHO & J. P. VAERMAN. 1980. Immunol. Comm. **9**: 705–713.
42. CAHILL, R. N. P., D. C. POSKITT, I. HERON & Z. TRNKA. 1980. Blood Cells **6**: 35–37.
43. FREITAS, A. A., M. L. ROSE & D. M. V. PARROT. 1977. Nature (London) **270**: 731–733.
44. VAN DER WAAIJ, D., J. M. BERGHUIS DE VRIES & J. E. C. LEKKERKERK-VAN DER WEES. 1972. J. Hyg. **70**: 335–342.
45. FRETER, R. 1981. Proc. VIIth Intern. Symp. Gnotobiol. p. 111.
46. DLABAČ, V., J. KLEPALOVÁ & L. MANDEL. 1971. Folia Microbiol. **16**: 533.
47. DLABAČ, V., I. MILER, J. KRUML, F. KOVÁŘŮ & M. LEON. 1970. *In* Developmental Aspects of Antibody Formation and Structure. J. Šterzl & I. Říha, Eds.: 105–134. Academia. Prague.
48. REJNEK, J., J. TRÁVNÍČEK, J. KOSTKA, J. ŠTERZL & A. LANC. 1968. Folia Microbiol. **13**: 36–42.
49. ABRAMS, G. D., H. BAUER & H. SPRINZ. 1963. Lab. Invest. **12**: 355–364.
50. DLABAČ, V., L. MANDEL, R. ŠTĚPÁNKOVÁ & M. TALAFANTOVÁ. 1981. Proc. VIIth Intern. Symp. Gnotobiol. p. 105.
51. BERG, R. G. & A. W. GARLINGTON. 1979. Infect. Immun. **23**: 403–411.
52. KOHLER, E. M. & E. H. BOHL. 1966. Can. J. Comp. Med. **30**: 233–237.
53. FRETER, R., 1969. Tex. Rep. Exp. Biol. Med. (Suppl. 1) **27**: 299–316.
54. TLASKALOVÁ, H., J. REJNEK, J. TRÁVNÍČEK & A. LANC. 1970. Folia Microbiol. **15**: 372–376.
55. WILSON, M. R. & A. W. HOHMANN. 1974. Infect. Immun. **10**: 776–782.
56. GUENTZEL, M. N. & L. J. BERRY. 1975. Infect. Immun. **11**: 890–897.
57. TALAFANTOVÁ, M. & V. DLABAČ. Unpublished results.
58. OGRA, P. L. & D. DAYTON, Eds. 1979. Immunology of Breast Milk. Raven Press. New York.
59. PIERCE, N. F. & J. L. GOWANS. 1975. J. Exp. Med. **142**: 1550–1563.

HUMORAL ANTIBODY RESPONSES TO THE BACTERIAL POLYSACCHARIDE DEXTRAN B1355*

Martin F. Kagnoff†

Department of Medicine
University of California
San Diego, La Jolla, California 92093

Immune responses to bacterial polysaccharides are important in host-environment interactions at mucosal surfaces, and are clinically relevant when considering immunization programs. Nevertheless the induction and regulation of antibody responses to purified polysaccharides differs in several respects from that of most protein antigens. Antibody responses to bacterial polysaccharides traditionally have been regarded as thymus independent, that is not requiring T-cell help.[1-5] Many bacterial polysaccharides have a limited number of antigenic determinants and elicit an antibody response of restricted heterogeneity[6,7] and with little evidence of immunologic memory.[8] Genes that govern antibody responses to determinants on various polysaccharides have been shown to be linked to genes mapped to the immunoglobulin heavy chain constant region allotype (Igh-C) locus.[9-16] Anti-polysaccharide antibody appears to be largely of the IgM class, or as more recently reported, the IgG_3 subclass in mice[17,18] and the IgG_2 subclass in humans.[19,20] In contrast to proteins, only low level antibody responses to polysaccharide antigens are seen in mice and humans in early life.[21-25] This latter observation has important implications for immunization programs in infants.

We recently reported that BALB/c (H-2^d, Igh^a) mice produce substantial T-cell and age dependent IgAλ_1 antibody responses to α (1,3) glucan determinants on dextran B1355, a capsular polysaccharide derived from *Leuconostoc mesenteroides*.[10,26,27] These findings represent a significant departure from previous observations and may have particular relevance for mucosal immunity. In addition, our observations suggest the need to reevaluate the mechanisms involved in the induction and regulation of anti-polysaccharide antibody responses. This paper summarizes our studies on the induction and regulation of antibody responses to dextran B1355.

Kinetics and Age of Onset of Anti-Dextran B1355 Responses in Vivo

As shown in TABLE 1, IgA anti-dextran splenic plaque-forming cell (PFC) responses after injection of BALB/c mice with dextran B1355 i.p. were optimal on day 5 and followed the same kinetics as the IgM response. IgG anti-dextran responses were seen in 40% of mice, but were less than 15% of the IgA response.

*This work was supported in part by the National Institutes of Arthritis, Diabetes, Digestive, and Kidney Diseases, and the National Foundation for Ileitis and Colitis.

†Address Correspondence to: Martin F. Kagnoff, University of California, San Diego, Department of Medicine, M-023-D, School of Medicine, La Jolla, Calif. 92093.

0077-8923/83/0409-0114 $1.75/0 © 1983, NYAS

TABLE 1

KINETICS OF THE HUMORAL ANTIBODY RESPONSE TO
DEXTRAN B1355*

Days After Injection	PFC/10^6 Spleen Cells†	
	IgA	IgM
0	2 ± 0.8	0 ± 0
2	1 ± 0.1	6 ± 2
4	175 ± 34	402 ± 16
5	508 ± 62	1,058 ± 111
7	56 ± 20	161 ± 16
11	6 ± 2	74 ± 4
14	2 ± 0.8	75 ± 7

*Eight-week old BALB/c mice were injected with 100 μg dextran B1355 i.p. Injection of titrated doses of dextran B1355 between 0.1 μg and 10 mg produced no greater IgA or IgM response.

†Mean ± S.E.M. Six mice/group. IgA and IgM responses were totally inhibited by the incorporation of dextran B1355 but not dextran B512 (95% [1,6]α-D-glucopyranosidic linkages) into the PFC assay.

By radioimmunoassay, over 95% of the IgA antibody to dextran B1355 was of the λ_1 light chain class and directed to α (1,3) determinants. Little to no IgA or IgM memory response was seen in mice reinjected with a second dose of dextran B1355 between 10 and 14 days after the primary immunization.[10]

Unlike the IgM anti-dextran response, the magnitude of the IgA anti-dextran response was age dependent. As shown in TABLE 2, significantly greater splenic IgA anti-α (1,3) glucan responses were obtained in 4–12-week-old mice than in 3-week-old mice. By 24 weeks of age, still greater IgA anti-dextran responses were seen. The ratio of the IgA:IgM response in various experiments ranged from 0.3 to 3.5.

TABLE 2

AGE DEPENDENCE OF THE IgA ANTI-DEXTRAN B1355
RESPONSE IN VIVO*

Age of Mice	PFC/10^6 Spleen Cells†	
	IgA	IgM
Weeks		
3	80 ± 48	1,508 ± 89
4	670 ± 20 ‡	1,560 ± 33
12	575 ± 60 ‡	1,609 ± 228
24	1,665 ± 156‡§	1,553 ± 187

*BALB/c mice were injected with 100 μg dextran B1355 i.p. and assayed on day 5. Six to twelve mice/group.

†Values represent mean ± S.E.M.

‡Value significantly different from 3-week-old mice (p < 0.01).

§Value significantly different from 4 to 12-week-old mice (p < 0.05).

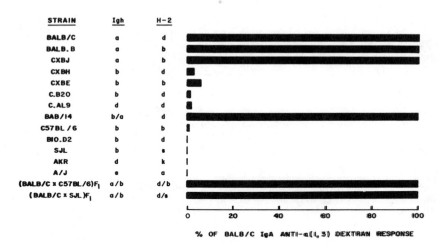

% OF BALB/C IgA ANTI-α(1, 3) DEXTRAN RESPONSE

FIGURE 1. Linkage of the IgA anti-α (1,3) dextran response to the immunoglobulin heavy chain allotype locus. Mice of various strains were injected with 100 μg dextran B1355 i.p. and splenic IgA anti-α (1,3) dextran responses were assayed five days later. Responder mice had the Igh^a haplotype. In crosses between responders and nonresponders, high response was dominant. Data represent results from three or more six to eight-month-old mice per group. CXB mice are recombinant inbred strains between BALB/c and C57BL/6. BALB.B and BALB/c are H-2 congenic strains. C.B20, C.AL9, BAB/14, and BALB/c are allotype congenic strains. The intra-V region recombinant strain BAB/14 has the Igh^b allotype, but some of the immunoglobulin heavy chain variable region (V$_h$) genes of BALB/c.

TABLE 3

T-CELL DEPENDENCE OF THE IgA ANTI-α(1,3) DEXTRAN B1355 RESPONSE IN VIVO*

		PFC/10^6 Spleen Cells†			
	Mice Injected	IgA	p	IgM	p
Experiment 1	BALB/c nude (nu/nu)	0 ± 0		354 ± 59	
			<0.01		<0.01
	BALB/c nude (nu/nu) reconstituted with 5 × 10^7 thymus cells‡	713 ± 141		1,533 ± 333	
Experiment 2	BALB/c nude (nu/nu)	18 ± 14		307 ± 55	
			<0.01		<0.01
	BALB/c nude (nu/nu) reconstituted with 5 × 10^7 thymus cells‡	698 ± 174		1,294 ± 258	

*3–6 month-old mice were injected with 100 μg Dextran B1355 i.p. and responses were assayed on day 5 after injection. Six mice/group.
†Mean ± S.E.M.
‡Thymus cells from littermate heterozygous nude mice (nu/+). Thymus cells from 17–19 day old nu/+ or BALB/c mice also reconstituted the response.

Genes That Determine the IgA Anti-Dextran B1355 Response
Are Linked to the Igh^a Haplotype

As shown in FIGURE 1, the ability of mice to produce an IgA anti-α (1,3) glucan response mapped to the Igh-C locus and not to H-2. Igh^a mice were high responders. In crosses between responders and nonresponders, high response was dominant.

T-Cell Dependence of the IgA Anti-Dextran Response in Vivo

The IgA anti-α (1,3) glucan response was markedly T-cell dependent. As shown in Table 3, spleen cells from BALB/c nude (nu/nu) mice injected with dextran B1355 produced little to no IgA response on day 5. By contrast, BALB/c nude mice reconstituted with thymocytes from heterozygous BALB/c nudes (nu/+) produced significant IgA anti-dextran responses. Although BALB/c nude mice produced low level IgA anti-dextran responses by day 7 after injection, responses never exceeded 25% of that seen in thymus-reconstituted littermates. It is worthwhile noting that nude mice produced significantly lower IgM responses than their matched T-cell-containing controls.

Anti-Dextran B1355 Responses in Vitro

The immune response to purified polysaccharide antigens such as dextran B1355 has been difficult to study in the past, partly due to the lack of suitable culture methods for examining the induction and regulation of immune responses to these antigens *in vitro*. We have successfully applied Mishell-Dutton lymphoid cell culture methods[28] to the study of the antigen-specific induction of antibody responses to purified dextran B1355. Optimal antigen-stimulated responses were obtained after stimulation of 2.5×10^6 lymphoid cells in 0.5 ml cultures with 0.2 – 2.0 ng dextran B1355 per culture.[26,27] As shown in FIGURE 2, mesenteric lymph node (MLN) cultures produced substantial IgA anti-α (1,3) dextran responses, but only when MLN were obtained from older mice. IgA anti-α (1,3) dextran responses in spleen cultures often were lower than in MLN cultures (TABLE 4), but also depended on the age of the mice from which the spleen cells were obtained. Like IgA, the IgM anti-α (1,3) glucan response in MLN cultures was age-dependent, but the age-dependence was not as marked for IgM splenic anti-α (1,3) dextran responses.

The inability to stimulate significant IgA anti-α (1,3) dextran responses in cultures from young mice was not due to cell-mediated suppression. Thus, spleen or MLN cells from young mice did not suppress the response of spleen or MLN cells from old mice when the two were mixed together in culture.[26] In addition, studies using admixtures of B- and T-cells from young and old mice revealed that T-cells from young and old mice were equally effective in supporting the induction of an IgA anti-α (1,3) dextran response in B-cell cultures from old mice. By contrast, B-cells from young mice did not produce significant IgA anti-α (1,3) glucan responses regardless of the age of the mice from which the T-cells were obtained (data not shown).

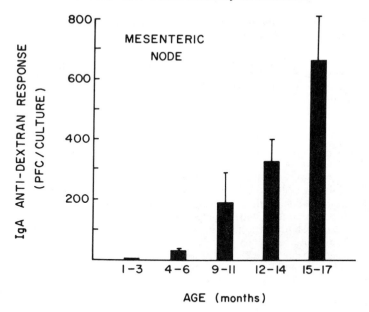

FIGURE 2. Age dependence of the IgA anti-α (1,3) dextran B1355 response in MLN cultures. Cultures containing 2.5×10^6 MLN cells from BALB/c mice of various ages were stimulated in culture with 0.2 ng dextran B1355, and IgA anti-α (1,3) responses were determined on day 5 after culture. Results represent mean ± S.E.M. of 5-9 repeated experiments.

Serum Anti-Dextran B1355 Antibody in Normal BALB/c Mice

We examined by radioimmunoassay age and sex-matched cohorts of BALB/c mice over a period of 12 months for the development of naturally occurring class and subclass-specific serum anti-α (1,3) dextran antibody. As shown in FIGURE 3, IgA anti-α (1,3) dextran antibody increased progressively in the serum of

TABLE 4

AGE DEPENDENCE OF THE ANTI-α (1,3) DEXTRAN B1355 RESPONSE
IN MESENTERIC LYMPH NODE AND SPLEEN CULTURES

	PFC/Culture*			
	MLN		Spleen	
Age of Mice	IgA	IgM	IgA	IgM
1–3 months	0	0	38 ± 28	70 ± 13
4–6 months	30 ± 8	38 ± 8	48 ± 18	100 ± 28
9–11 months	188 ± 90	73 ± 20	50 ± 13	128 ± 38
12–14 months	325 ± 88	98 ± 30	128 ± 53	110 ± 28
15–17 months	668 ± 175	148 ± 25	143 ± 60	153 ± 53

*2.5×10^6 cells/culture. PFC assay on day 5 after culture. Values represent means ± S.E.M. of results obtained in 5–12 repeated experiments.

unimmunized mice between three and six months of age, reaching a plateau at 30–40 μg/ml IgA. IgM anti-α (1,3) glucan antibody levels increased to a peak of 5 μg/ml at four months and decreased thereafter. Levels of "naturally" occurring IgG$_3$ anti-α (1,3) anti-body did not exceed 1 μg/ml over the 12-month period in this cohort, although in other studies, we have noted background IgG$_3$ anti-α (1,3)

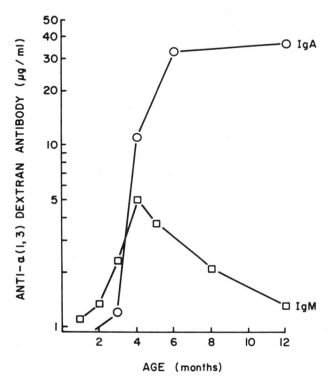

FIGURE 3. Serum anti-α (1,3) dextran antibody in unimmunized BALB/c mice. A cohort of 20 BALB/c mice (10 males and 10 females) were bled monthly between 1 and 12 months of age. IgA, IgM, and IgG subclass anti-α (1,3) dextran antibody was determined on serum pools by RIA. Not shown: levels of IgG$_3$ anti-α (1,3) dextran antibody did not exceed 1 μg/ml in this cohort and significant levels of IgG$_1$, IgG$_{2a}$, IgG$_{2b}$, and IgE anti-α (1,3) dextran antibody were not detected at any age. In other experiments, IgG$_3$ anti-α (1,3) dextran levels have ranged as high as 10 μg/ml in unimmunized individual BALB/c mice. Specificity for α (1,3) determinants was assessed by inhibition with dextran B1355 and dextran B512.

glucan levels as high as 10 μg/ml in individual BALB/c mice. Significant levels of IgG$_1$, IgG$_{2a}$, IgG$_{2b}$, and IgE anti-α (1,3) dextran antibody were not detected.

T-Cell Regulation of the IgA Anti-a (1,3) Dextran Response in Vitro

The IgA anti-α (1,3) dextran response *in vitro*, like the response *in vivo*,[10] was markedly T-cell dependent.[26] Thus, the removal of T-cells from spleen or MLN

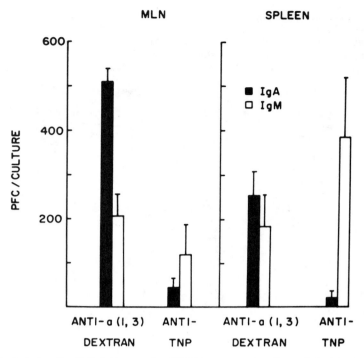

FIGURE 4. IgA anti-α (1,3) dextran and anti-TNP responses in culture. Cultures containing 2.5 × 10⁶ MLN or spleen cells from 15–17-month-old TNP-ovalbumin or TNP-KLH-primed BALB/c mice were stimulated with TNP-dextran B1355. Cultures were assayed five days later for IgA and IgM anti-α (1,3) dextran and anti-TNP responses. Data represent mean ± S.E.M. of three experiments using MLN and three experiments using spleen. Control cultures from TNP-protein-primed mice stimulated with TNP on the homologous carrier yielded > 1000 IgA anti-TNP PFC/culture. Similar results were obtained also with spleen and MLN cells from unprimed mice.

populations eliminated the IgA anti-α (1,3) response, and such responses were restored by the addition of T-cells.[26] Nevertheless T-cell help did not appear to depend on carrier-specific or MHC-restricted T-helper cells. As shown in FIGURE 4, stimulation of spleen or MLN cultures from TNP-protein-primed mice with TNP-dextran resulted in an IgA and IgM anti-α (1,3) dextran response and an IgM anti-TNP response. Such cultures, however, did not produce significant IgA anti-TNP responses. IgA anti-TNP responses were seen in parallel control cultures stimulated with TNP-protein. Finally, as shown in FIGURE 5, non-MHC restricted supernatants from concanavalin A (Con A) activated spleen cells, or a Con A-activated T-cell hybridoma (AOFS 21.10) could substitute for T-cells in our culture system. Similar results were also seen using supernatants from Con A-activated Peyer's patches cells. Such supernatants supported the production of IgA anti-α (1,3) glucan responses in MLN cultures (FIGURE 5) or spleen cultures (data not shown) that had been severely T-cell depleted.

DISCUSSION

These studies demonstrate significant T-cell and age-dependent IgA antibody responses to α (1,3) glucan determinants on the bacterial capsular polysaccharide dextran B1355. IgA anti-α (1,3) dextran responses far exceeded responses in the IgG subclasses including IgG$_3$, and in older mice the IgA response equaled or exceeded the IgM response. Previously, murine antipolysaccharide responses were thought to belong predominantly to the IgM and relatively minor IgG$_3$ subclass.[17,18] IgG$_3$ and IgG$_{2a}$ anti-α (1,3) dextran antibody responses have been reported in dextran B1355 immunized BALB/c mice, but substantial responses were obtained only when the mice were subsequently injected with *E. coli* B, an antigen thought to have determinants that cross-react with dextran B1355.[29]Unlike the IgA response seen in our studies, murine IgG responses to polysaccharides are thought to be thymus-independent.[30-33] T-cells recently, however, have been shown to influence IgG subclass expression to a haptenated polysaccharide, DNP-Ficoll[34,35] and anti-polysaccharide responses can be rendered T-cell-dependent when the polysaccharide is coupled to a carrier protein.[36,37] IgG anti-polysaccharide responses in humans are largely of the relatively minor IgG$_2$

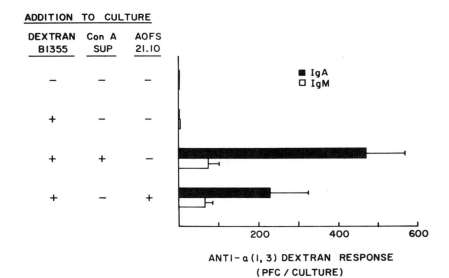

FIGURE 5. Anti-dextran response in T-cell depleted cultures. T-cell depleted MLN from BALB/c mice were cultured at 5×10^5 cells in 0.2 ml. Cultures were stimulated with 0.1 ng dextran B1355 or no antigen as indicated. Additional cultures were supplemented with either a) supernatant from Con A-activated spleen cells (Con A Sup.) or b) supernatant from a Con A-activated T-cell hybridoma (AOFS 21.10). These Con A supernatants did not stimulate significant IgA anti-α (1,3) dextran responses in the absence of added antigen. Similar results were obtained using a supernatant from Con A-activated Peyer's patch cells (data not shown). For T-cell depletion, BALB/c mice were treated on day 3 and day 1 before sacrifice with antithymocyte serum. MLN cells from these mice were treated with anti-Thy 1.2 and anti-Lyt 2.2 and complement and passed over a Sephadex G-10 column.

subclass.[19,20] IgA constituted, however, a substantial quantity of the human antibody response to pneumococcal and *H. influenza* type b-polyribose phosphate polysaccharide antigens.[25] Our studies clearly indicate the need to reexamine isotype expression and regulation in response to various polysaccharide antigens and to determine the functional importance of different isotypes, including IgA, in the host interaction with polysaccharide antigens. Such investigations are particularly relevant for mucosal immunity.

The age dependence of the IgA anti-α (1,3) glucan response in mice may have relevance to the clinical situation. Thus, humans respond poorly to polysaccharide antigens and vaccines (e.g., pneumococcal vaccine, *H. influenza* type b-polyribose phosphate) before two years of age[23-25,38] and the inability to produce such antibody responses has impeded immunization programs. In human studies with bacterial capsular polysaccharide antigens, preimmunization antibody levels have correlated with the magnitude of the antigen-stimulated antibody response.[25,39,40] With increasing age, we noted an increase in the level of naturally occurring IgA anti-α (1,3) dextran antibody in serum, which correlated with the ability to stimulate an IgA anti-α (1,3) response *in vivo*. Although mice were not intentionally immunized with dextran B1355, aging mice are not antigenically naive since bacterial polyglucans are ubiquitous antigens in the mammalian intestine.[41-44] Thus, we favor the notion that the development of increasing levels of naturally occurring serum anti-α (1,3) antibody with age reflects the activation of B-cells following exposure to cross-reacting antigens and/or mitogens (e.g., bacterial lipopolysaccharide) at gut mucosal surfaces. In support of this notion, the relative frequency of B-cell precursors[45] and antibody to certain polysaccharide determinants was significantly lower in germfree than in conventionally raised mice and increased when germfree mice were conventionalized.[46] With additional information regarding B-cell activation by polysaccharide antigens, it may be possible to define ways to manipulate the onset, character, and repertoire of such responses at an early age.

The relative age dependence of the IgA anti-α (1,3) dextran response *in vitro* compared to the intact animal warrants comment. The age at which substantial IgA anti-α (1,3) dextran responses could be stimulated *in vitro*, particularly in MLN, was delayed for months, and splenic responses *in vitro* also appeared to be delayed. Such findings, although not absolute, may be an artifact of the culture system, reflecting differences in the microenvironment or the relative lack of efficiency of a large carbohydrate antigen ($\sim 4 \times 10^7$ daltons) in stimulating an *in vitro* immune response. In addition, our data suggest that the age delay both *in vitro* and *in vivo* reflects a relative deficiency of appropriate precursor B-cells and/or mature accessory cells required for the induction of the IgA anti-α (1,3) dextran response. By contrast, we found *in vivo* and *in vitro* that T-cells capable of helping the IgA anti-α (1,3) dextran response are present in young (i.e., 17-19-day-old) and in old mice.

Antibody responses to bacterial polysaccharide antigens traditionally are regarded as T-cell independent,[1-5] that is, not requiring T-cell help. Our studies demonstrate that the IgA antibody response to α (1,3) determinants on dextran B1355 is markedly T-cell dependent. The finding that cooperative events in the presence of TNP-dextran were sufficient to induce an IgA anti-α (1,3) glucan response, but not an IgA anti-TNP response, suggested that T-cell help for the IgA anti-α (1,3) dextran response was not mediated by carrier-specific T-helper cells. It may be that T-cell help for the IgA anti-α (1,3) dextran response is mediated by anti-idiotypic T-helper cells[47-51] (i.e., T-helper cells directed to anti-α (1,3) dextran antibody on the B-cell surface). Alternatively, our finding with TNP-dextran may reflect differences in the state of activation, and thus the requirements for triggering, of an IgA anti-TNP compared with an IgA anti-α (1,3) dextran B-cell, or differences in the presentation and binding of TNP to the B-cell, when associated with dextran in our culture system rather than a protein carrier. The IgA anti-α

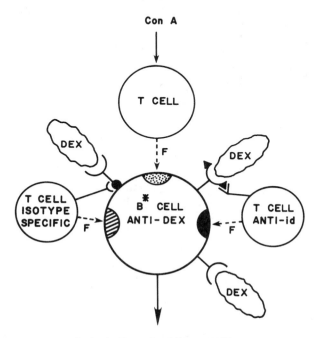

IgA ANTI-α (1, 3) DEXTRAN

FIGURE 6. T-cell help for the IgA anti-α (1,3) dextran response. Specificity of the response is determined by B-cell recognition of α (1,3) determinants on dextran B1355 (DEX). T-cell help is delivered by one or more T-cell-derived B-cell growth or differentiation factors (F). In this model, such factors (F) are depicted as deriving from a) Con A-activated T-cells (e.g., spleen, Peyer's patch or hybridoma T-cells), b) autoantiidiotypic T-cells (T-cell anti-id) that recognize idiotypic determinants on anti-α (1,3) dextran antibody on the B-cell surface, or c) isotype-specific T-cells that recognize determinants specific for, or coexpressed with, an immunoglobulin isotype on the cell surface (e.g., IgA). B-cells responding to such signals are already likely in an "activated" state and are depicted as B* as a result of prior exposure to cross-reacting environmental antigens and/or mitogens (e.g., bacterial lipopolysaccharide). It is not known if the B*-cell induced to secrete IgA anti-α (1,3) dextran antibody is committed to IgA before exposure to the T-cell-derived helper factor or if theT-cell-derived factor plays a role in isotype switching into the IgA class.

(1,3) response was not stimulated by polyclonal B-cell activating properties of dextran as shown by the high degree of antigen specificity of the response.

Recently, we have noted that non-MHC restricted, nonantigen-specific factors produced by concanavalin A (Con A) activated spleen[52] or Peyer's patches cells or supernatants of a Con A-activated T-cell hybridoma known to contain among other factors, high levels of interleukin 2,[53] can substitute for T-cell help in the IgA anti-α (1,3) glucan response *in vitro*. Thus, regardless of the cognitive interactions involved in T-cell help for the IgA anti-α (1,3) dextran response, one or more T-cell derived B-cell growth or differentiation factors appear to be involved as part of the mechanism activating the IgA response (FIGURE 6). Although we favor the notion that such factors expand a preexisting population of anti-α (1,3) dextran B-cells committed already to the IgA isotype, we cannot exclude the possibility that such factors enhance isotype switching of anti-α (1,3) dextran precursor B-cells into the IgA class. We are currently examining this possibility.

ACKNOWLEDGMENTS

I am grateful to Ms. Leslie Arner, Ms. E. Hom, and Mr. Raleigh Austin, whose technical expertise has been extremely valuable to these studies. I thank Dr. A. Jeanes and Dr. M. E. Slodki for generously supplying the dextran B1355 and dextran B512 used in these studies. Dr. M. Cohn, Dr. S. Swain, Dr. D. Rivier, and Dr. P. Trefts are acknowledged for their contributions to various aspects of these studies. Finally, I thank Dr. R. Langman for his helpful comments on the manuscript and Ms. Debby Glazer for typing the manuscript.

REFERENCES

1. HOWARD, J. G. & B. M. COURTENAY. 1975. Influence of molecular structure on the tolerogenicity of bacterial dextrans. II. The α1-3-linked epitope of dextran B1355. Immunology. **29:** 599–610.
2. VICARI, G. & B. M. COURTENAY. 1977. Restricted avidity of the IgM antibody response to dextran B512 in mice: studies on inhibition of specific plaque forming cells by oligosaccharides. Immunochemistry. **14:** 253–258.
3. FERNANDEZ, C. & G. MOLLER. 1977. Immune response against two epitopes on the same thymus-independent polysaccharide carrier. 1. Role of epitope density in carrier-dependent immunity and tolerance. Immunology. **33:** 59–68.
4. HOWARD, J. G., G. VICARI & B. M. COURTENAY. 1975. Influence of molecular structure on the tolerogenicity of bacterial dextrans. I. The α1-6-linked epitope of dextran B512. Immunology. **29:** 585–597.
5. HOWARD, J. G., G. H. CHRISTIE, B. M. COURTENAY, E. LEUCHARS & A. J. S. DAVIES. 1971. Studies on immunological paralysis. VI. Thymic-independence of tolerance and immunity to type III Pneumococcal polysaccharide. Cell. Immunol. **2:** 614–626.
6. BRAUN, D. G. & J. C. JATON. 1974. Homogeneous antibodies: induction and value as probe for the antibody problem. Curr. Top. Microbiol. Immunol. **66:** 29–76.
7. HANSBURG, D., B. CLEVINGER, R. M. PERLMUTTER, R. GRIFFITH, D. E. BRILES & J. M. DAVIES. 1979. Analysis of the diversity of murine antibodies to α(1 → 3) dextran. *In:* Cells of Immunoglobulin Synthesis. B. Pernis and H. J. Vogel, Eds.:295–308. Academic Press. New York.
8. BASTEN, A. & J. G. HOWARD. 1973. Thymus independence. Contemp. Top. Immunobiol. **2:** 265–291.
9. FERNANDEZ, C., R. LIEBERMAN & G. MOLLER. 1979. The immune response to the alpha 1-6 epitope of dextran is determined by a gene linked to the Ig CH locus. Scand. J. Immunol. **10:** 77–80.
10. KAGNOFF, M. F. 1979. IgA anti-dextran B1355 responses. J. Immunol. **122:** 866–870.
11. BLOMBERG, B., W. R. GECKELER & M. WEIGERT. 1972. Genetics of the antibody response to dextran in mice. Science. **177:** 178–180.
12. RIBLET, R., B. BLOMBERG, M. WEIGERT, R. LIEBERMAN, B. A. TAYLOR & M. POTTER. 1975.

Genetics of mouse antibodies. I. Linkage of the dextran response locus, V_H DEX, to allotype. Eur. J. Immunol. 5: 775–777.

13. GECKELER, W., B. BLOMBERG, C. DE PREVOL & M. COHN. 1977. On the genetic dissection of a specific humoral immune response to α(1,3) dextran. Cold Spring Harbor Symposia on Quantitative Biology. XLI: 743–748.

14. LIEBERMAN, R., M. POTTER, E. B. MUSHINSKI, W. HUMPHREY, JR. & S. RUDIKOFF. 1974. Genetics of a new IgV_H (T15 idiotype) marker in the mouse regulating natural antibody to phosphorylcholine. J. Exp. Med. 139: 983–1001.

15. EICHMANN, K. 1972. Idiotypic identity of antibodies to streptococcal carbohydrate in inbred mice. Europ. J. Immunol. 2: 301–307.

16. LIEBERMAN, R. 1978. Genetics of IgCH (Allotype) locus in the mouse. Springer Seminars in Immunopathology 1: 7–30.

17. PERLMUTTER, R. M., D. HANSBURG, D. E. BRILES, R. A. NICOLOTTI & J. M. DAVIE. 1978. Subclass restriction of murine anti-carbohydrate antibodies J. Immunol. 121: 566–572.

18. DER BALIAN, G. P., J. SLACK, B. L. CLEVINGER, H. BAZIN & J. M. DAVIE. 1980. Subclass restriction of murine antibodies. III. Antigens that stimulate IgG_3 mice stimulate IgG_{2c} in rats J. Exp. Med. 152: 209–218.

19. YOUNT, W. J., M. M. DORNER, H. G. KUNKEL & E. A. KABAT. 1968. Studies on human antibodies. VI. Selective variations in subgroup composition and genetic markers. J. Exp. Med. 127: 633–616.

20. RIESEN, W. F., F. SKVARIL & D. G. BRAUN. 1968. Natural infection of man with Group A Streptococci. Levels, restriction in class, subclass, and type; and clonal appearance of polysaccharide-group-specific antibodies. Scand. J. Immunol. 5: 383–390.

21. BONA, C., J. J. MUND, K. E. STEIN, S. HOUSE, R. LIEBERMAN & W. E. PAUL. 1979. Immune response to levan. III. The capacity to produce anti-inulin antibodies and cross-reactive idiotypes appears late in ontogeny. J. Immunol. 123: 1484–1490.

22. FERNANDEZ, C. & G. MOLLER. 1978. Immunological unresponsiveness to native dextran B512 in young animals of dextran high responder strains is due to lack of Ig receptor expression. Evidence for a nonrandom expression of V-genes. J. Exp. Med. 147: 645–655.

23. GOLD, R., M. L. LEPOW, I. GOLDSCHNEIDER, T. L. DRAPER & E. C. GOTSCHLICH. 1975. Clinical evaluation of Group A and Group C meningococcal polysaccharide vaccines in infants. J. Clin. Invest. 56: 1536–1547.

24. ROBBINS, J. B., R. SCHNEERSON, M. ARGAMAN & Z. T. HANDZEL. 1973. Haemophilus influenzae type b: disease and immunmity in humans. Ann. Intern. Med. 78: 259–269.

25. SIBER, G. R., P. H. SCHUR, A. C. AISENBERG, S. A. WEITZMAN & G. SCHIFFMANN. 1980. Correlation between serum IgG-2 concentrations and the antibody response to bacterial polysaccharide antigens. N. Engl. J. Med. 303: 178–182.

26. TREFTS, P. E., D. A. RIVIER & M. F. KAGNOFF. 1981. T cell-dependent IgA anti-polysaccharide response in vitro. Nature. (London) 292: 163–165.

27. RIVIER, D. A., P. E. TREFTS & M. F. KAGNOFF. 1983. Age-dependence of the IgA anti-α (1 $\rightarrow$ 3) dextran B1355 response in vitro. Scand. J. Immunol. In press.

28. MISHELL, R. I. & R. W. DUTTON. 1967. Immunization of dissociated spleen cell cultures from normal mice. J. Exp. Med. 126: 423–442.

29. HANSBURG, D., R. M. PERLMUTTER, D. E. BRILES & J. M. DAVIE. 1978. Analysis of the diversity of murine antibodies to dextran B1355. III. Idiotypic and spectrotypic correlations. Eur. J. Immunol. 8: 352–359.

30. AUGUSTIN, A. A. & A. COUTINHO. 1980. Specific T helper cells that activate B cells polyclonally. In vitro enrichment and cooperative function. J. Exp. Med. 151: 587–601.

31. FERNANDEZ, B. & G. MOLLER. 1979. A thymus-independent IgG response against dextran B512 can be induced in C57BL but not in CBA mice, even though both strains possess $V_H$dex gene. Scand. J. Immunol. 10: 465–472.

32. SHARON, R., P. R. B. MCMASTER, A. M. KASK, J. D. OWENS & W. E. PAUL. 1975. DNP-Lys-Ficoll: A T-independent antigen which elicits both IgM and IgG anti-DNP antibody-secreting cells. J. Immunol. 114: 1585–1589.

33. MARTINEZ-ALONSO, C., A. COUTINHO & A. A. AUGUSTIN. 1980. Immunoglobulin C-gene expression. I. The commitment of IgG subclass of secretory cells is determined by the quality of the nonsepcific stimuli. Eur. J. Immunol. **10:** 698–702.

34. MONGINI, P. K. A., K. E. STEIN & W. E. PAUL. 1981. T cell regulation of IgG subclass antibody production in response to T-independent antigens. J. Exp. Med. **153:** 1–12.

35. MONGINI, P. K., W. E. PAUL & E. S. METCALF. 1982. T cell regulation of immunoglobulin class expression in the antibody response to trinitrophenyl-Ficoll. Evidence for T cell enhancement of the immunoglobulin class switch. J. Exp. Med. **155:** 884–902.

36. WARD, R. & H. KOHLER. 1981. Regulation of clones responding to dextran B1355. II. Response of T-dependent and T-independent precursors. J. Immunol. **126:** 146–149.

37. SCHNEERSON, R., O. BARRERA, A. SUTTON & J. B. ROBBINS. 1980. Preparation, characterization, and immunogenicity of haemophilus influenzae type b polysaccharide-protein conjugates. J. Exp. Med. **152:** 361–376.

38. SELL, S. H., G. SCHIFFMAN, W. K. VAUGHN & P. F. WRIGHT. 1978. Clinical trial of octavalent pneumococcal polysaccharide vaccine in infants—a preliminary report. *In:* Eighteenth Interscience Conference on Antimicrobial Agents and Chemotherapy. Sponsored by the American Society for Microbiology. Atlanta, Georgia.

39. AMMANN, A. J., G. SCHIFFMAN & R. AUSTRIAN. 1980. The antibody responses to pneumococcal capsular polysaccharides in aged individuals. Proc. Soc. Exp. Biol. Med. **164:** 312–316.

40. BAKER, C. J., D. L. KASPER, M. S. EDWARDS & G. SCHIFFMAN. 1980. Influence of preimmunization antibody levels on the specificity of the immune response to related polysaccharide antigens. N. Engl. J. Med. **303:** 173–182.

41. POTTER, M. 1971. Antigen-binding myeloma proteins in mice. Ann. N.Y. Acad. Sci. **190:** 306–321.

42. LIEBERMAN, R., M. POTTER, W. HUMPHREY & C. C. CHEN. 1976. Idiotypes of inulin-binding antibodies and myeloma proteins controlled by genes linked to the allotype locus of the mouse. J. Immunol. **117:** 2105–2111.

43. HANSBURG, D., D. E. BRILES, & J. M. DAVIE. 1976. Analysis of the diversity of murine antibodies to dextran B1355. I. Generation of a large, pauciclonal response by a bacterial vaccine. J. Immunol. **117:** 569–575.

44. TAUBMAN, M. A. 1982. *In:* Workshop on Mechanisms on Mucosal Immunity. Raven Press. In press.

45. CEBRA, J. J., C. A. CRANDALL, P. J. GEARHART, S. M. ROBERTSON, J. TSENG & P. M. WATSON. 1979. Cellular events concerned with the initiation, expression, and control of the mucosal immune response. *In:* Immunology of Breast Milk. P. L. Ogra & D. H. Dayton, Eds.:1–18. Raven Press. New York.

46. LIEBERMAN, R., M. POTTER, E. B. MUSHINSKI, W. HUMPHREY, JR. & S. RUDIKOFF. 1974. Genetics of a new IgV_H (T15 idiotype) marker in the mouse regulating natural natibody to phosphorylcholine. J. Exp. Med. **139:** 983–1001.

47. BOTTOMLY, K. & D. E. MOSIER. 1979. Mice whose B cells cannot produce the T15 idiotype also lack an antigen-specific helper T cell required for T15 expression. J. Exp. Med. **150:** 1399–1409.

48. WOODLAND, R. & H. CANTOR. 1978. Idiotype-specific T-helper cells are required to induce idiotype positive B memory cells to secrete antibody. Eur. J. Immunol. **8:** 600–606.

49. HETZELBERGER, D. & K. EICHMANN. 1978. Recognition of idiotypes in lymphocyte interactions. I. Idiotypic selectivity in cooperation between T and B lymphocytes. Eur. J. Immunol. **8:** 846–852.

50. ADORINI, L., M. HARVEY & E. E. SERCARZ. 1979. The fine specificityof regulatory T cells. IV. Idiotypic complementarity and antigen-bridging interactions in the anti-lysozyme response. Eur. J. Immunol. **9:** 906–909.

51. BOTTOMLY, K. & D. E. MOSIER. 1981. Antigen-specific helper T cells required for dominant idiotype expression are not H-2 restricted. J. Exp. Med. **154:** 411–421.

52. ANDERSSON, J., O. SJOBERG & G. MOLLER. 1972. Mitogens as probes for immunocyte activation and cellular cooperation. Transplant. Rev. **11:** 131–177.

53. HARWELL, L., B. SKIDMORE, P. MARRACK & J. KAPPLER. 1980. Concanavalin A-inducible, interleukin-2-producing T cell hybridoma. J. Exp. Med. **152:** 893–904.

B. H. WAKSMAN (*National Multiple Sclerosis Society, New York, N.Y.*): The phrase T-dependence or T-independence has always meant, for me, two quite different things. The first is that there are cells that make antibodies without any T-cell help. The other is the classic phenomenon where T-cells clearly are helping the response, because in the absence of T-cells the response does not occur. Would you care to comment about this?

M. F. KAGNOFF (*University of California at San Diego, La Jolla*): T-cell dependence is relative. Our experiments, and those of others, have shown that there are different types of T-cell help. There are clearly MHC restricted, carrier-specific, T-helper cells that are required in the induction of responses to T-dependent antigen. There are a variety of other T-helper cells that may or may not have all those particular characteristics and that may act by different means. To some extent, I believe that the response to all antigens, including the IgM response, is T-dependent.

C. G. Bell. (*University of Illinois, Chicago, Ill.*): You observed an IgM response that is slightly lower in the nude than in the conventionally raised mouse; however, did you perform the T-cell reconstitution study in parallel? This method is important, because the amount of dextran on the sheep cells will determine the magnitude of the response. Do you have an idiotypic analysis on the IgA, the IgM anti-dextran PFC, and the serum antibody levels? This analysis is important because of low levels (5–10 micrograms) of IgM anti-dextran responses at 12 months of age and 40 micrograms of anti-dextran specific IgA at 12 months of age. If these are naturally occurring antibodies, are they of a specific idiotype?

KAGNOFF: The data I have presented refer to anti-α (1,3) antibody that has the J558 and MOPC 104E cross-reacting idiotype.

BELL: Have you measured anti-dextran antibodies that are not of the J558 idiotype?

KAGNOFF: We have not detected large amounts of idiotype negative antibody.

J. R. McGHEE (*The University of Alabama in Birmingham*): Is dextran 1355 a polyclonal B-cell activator?

KAGNOFF: Not in our hands.

McGHEE: In your studies of factors for B-cell responses, does the material contain TCGF or IL 2 and TRF?

KAGNOFF: The AOFS 21.10 supernatant is rich in IL 2, but does not have TRF activity. In one assay system, this material also was shown to have weak BCGF activity. The Con A supernatant has both IL 2 and TRF activity.

M. ZAUDERER (*Columbia University, New York, N.Y.*): You have taken advantage of the age-dependence of the IgA response, and you show that IgA-producing cells represent a different B-cell set that is not simply due to development of IgA-specific T-helper cells. I am surprised that you should invoke isotype or idiotype-specific T-helper cells, because you can account for all of your own data, simply in terms of different T-cell functions required for activation of different B-cell sets. What you call B* is a B-cell that can apparently be activated by a soluble factor, which may be produced by some T-cells and not by others. In your system, such a T-cell would give the appearance of isotype specificity without any real need to be isotype specific. I think that the results presented by the McGhee group this morning lend themselves to a similar interpretation.

KAGNOFF: I largely agree and would propose that factors that can activate the IgA response, appropriate differentiation factors, can be produced by T-cells other than the MHC restricted, carrier-specific helpers.

J. J. CEBRA (University of Pennsylvania, Philadelphia): The previous questioner asked a question similar to my own. What do you think sets the clock in the age-dependent IgA responsiveness in the young maturing mice? Is it idiotype specific T-cells or maturation of the B-cell compartment? We know that in the young adult, the B-cell compartment, with respect to specificity to polysaccharide determinants, is much different than the B-cell compartment with respect to TNP specificity.

KAGNOFF: I believe maturation of the B-cell compartment is responsible, with the proviso that there also may be involved some dependence on maturation of accessory cell lines as well.

H. GREGORY (I.C.I.P.L.C. Pharmaceuticals Division, Mereside, Macclesfield, Cheshire, England): Have you separated dextran into the fraction L and fraction S? If so, have you noticed any differences?

KAGNOFF: I have not used L. This research was done with S.

THE ROLE OF EPITHELIAL CELLS IN
GUT-ASSOCIATED IMMUNE REACTIVITY*

Dale E. Bockman, William R. Boydston, and Donald H. Beezhold

Department of Anatomy
Medical College of Georgia
Augusta, Georgia 30912

INTRODUCTION

One feature that distinguishes the immune reactivity of the gastrointestinal tract from systemic responses involving primarily spleen and lymph nodes is the participation of epithelial cells. The acronym GALT, in its fullest usage, refers to gut-associated lymphoepithelial tissue. Epithelial cells and their products are essential participants in both initial and final stages of reactivity to foreign materials in the gut lumen. Their participation is not passive and isolated, but rather involves active cooperation with lymphoid cells.

It will be the purpose of this paper to focus on the role of epithelial cells in immune reactivity in the gastrointestinal tract, although it is assumed that the principles apply also to interactions at other mucosal surfaces. Specifically, we will review information that is pertinent to the participation, by epithelial cells, in the following facets of gut-associated immune reactivity of the adult: antigen exclusion, transport of antigens from the lumen, bidirectional transport, degradation of antigens, and antigen presentation. A role of epithelium in each of these areas is supported by present data or is subject to experimental testing by methods that are currently available.

ANTIGEN EXCLUSION

Most potential antigens in the gut lumen never interact with lymphoid tissue. A multilayered barrier is provided by an epithelial layer joined by tight junctions, an underlying basal lamina that is a component of the basement membrane and is capable of molecular selection, and a surface mucous layer formed primarily by epithelial-cell secretions.

Most potential food antigens are broken down before absorption. In fact, most potential antigens in the gut lumen never interact with the cell membrane (or surface glycocalyx) of epithelial cells. The physical arrangement of intestinal elements provides a mechanism by which the bulk of luminal concepts flow through the center, touching only the mucous coat at the periphery. Thus a proportionately small, but antigenically significant, quantity of antigens initiate immune reactivity. It is the handling of these antigens, and the augmentation of nonspecific exclusion by specific immune products that will be addressed below and in other papers in this volume.

*This work was supported in part by National Institutes of Health Grant AI14222.

0077–8923/83/0409–0129 $1.75/0 © 1983, NYAS

TRANSPORT OF ANTIGENS FROM THE LUMEN

Transport by Columnar Absorptive Cells

A number of experiments in the earlier parts of the century indicated that antigenically intact foreign proteins were transmitted from the gut lumen to blood and lymph (reviewed by Bazin[1]). The development of electron microscopic tracer techniques made it possible to elucidate the mechanism by which this transport occurs. Bockman and Winborn[2] first demonstrated directly in 1966 that intact macromolecules were transported by pinocytosis, from the intestinal lumen of adult animals, through columnar absorptive cells into capillaries and the lamina propria, where they were available to lymphoid cells. Ferritin from horse spleen was traced to hamster small intestines. Cornell et al.[3] confirmed this finding in 1971 by following the transport of horseradish peroxidase (HRP) through columnar absorptive cells of rat small intestine. Transmitted HRP could be detected in the intestinal lymph and portal blood.[4]

Transport by Follicle-Associated Epithelium (FAE)

The efficiency with which epithelial cells could transmit material from the lumen did not prove to be uniform throughout the gastrointestinal tract. Gut-associated lymphoepithelial tissue demonstrated an affinity for this activity. Joel et al.[5] administered India ink to adult mice by a stomach tube and observed greater uptake of carbon particles by epithelium covering Peyer's patches than by epithelium of intestinal villi. The carbon particles accumulated in macrophages in the Peyer's patches and remained there for at least a week. Hanaoka et al.[6] found carbon particles in the lamina propria and blood vessels after intraluminal administration of India ink in rabbit appendix. Carbon particles were again concentrated in macrophages.

Bockman and Cooper[7,8] studied the fine structure and pinocytotic capabilities of epithelium overlying lymphoid follicles in the appendix, the bursa of Fabricius, and Peyer's patches. In all three examples of GALT were found morphologically similar cells, characterized by short, irregular microvilli and by numerous tubules, vesicles, and vacuoles in the apical cytoplasm. FIGURES 1 & 2 demonstrate the similarity between the cells in mouse Peyer's patch and chick bursa of Fabricius. In all three locations, these specialized cells were shown to be efficient in transporting ferritin and carbon particles from the lumen to underlying lymphoid cells, as compared with nearby cells lacking those characteristic features. These cells were referred to collectively as FAE and were named and referred to as FAE cells. It was suggested that they were specialized to sample intestinal contents to induce lymphoid differentiation along plasma-cell lines.[7] The presence of morphologically similar cells in human GALT was described later in Peyer's patches by Owen and Jones[9] and in appendix by Bockman and Cooper.[10] The greater efficiency of FAE in transporting tracer from the lumen was confirmed when HRP uptake was studied in adult mice.[11]

Terminology of GALT Epithelium

Some confusion exists in the literature concerning the appropriate designation for the epithelial cells of GALT. Follicle-associated epithelium cells have also

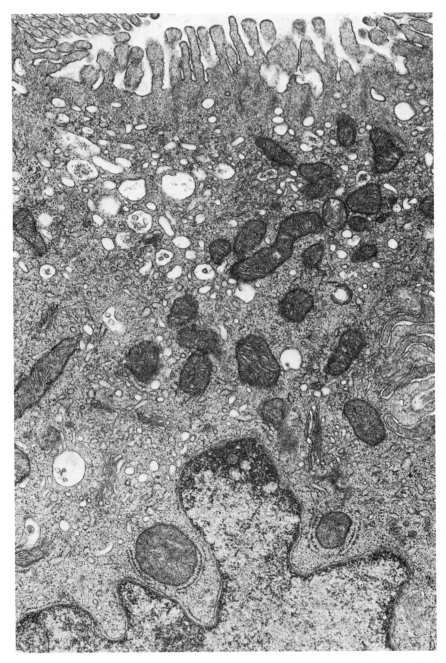

FIGURE 1. Follicle-associated epithelial cell from mouse Peyer's patch. Note the short, irregular microvilli bordering on the lumen (top) and the numerous apical vesicles and vacuoles. (D. E. Bockman & M. D. Cooper.[8] With permission from the *American Journal of Anatomy*).

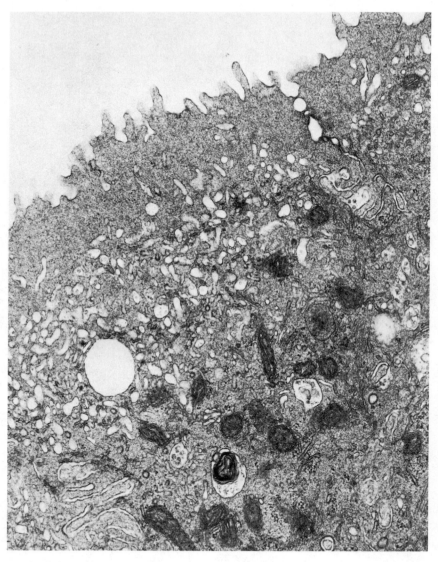

FIGURE 2. Apical portion of FAE cell from bursa of Fabricius. The ultrastructural features are quite similar to FAE in Peyer's patch (FIGURE 1). (D. E. Bockman & M. D. Cooper.[8] With permission from the *American Journal of Anatomy*).

been referred to as M-cells. The designation M for these cells was originally used by Owen and Jones[9] because it was thought that they were characterized by "microfolds" on their luminal surface. This hypothesis has not proven to be correct. The "microfolds" may have been on the surface of goblet cells. When questioned about the continued usage of M, Owen responded that a change had been made so that M stands for membrane, because the cells ". . . are thin and function similar to a membrane restricting uncontrolled entry of luminal material into the lamina propria and loss of lymphocytes into the fecal stream."[12]

We strongly recommend that the cells in question be designated FAE for the following reasons. These cells were first described and named FAE by Bockman and Cooper in 1971.[7] They were called M by Owen and Jones in 1974.[9] Follicle-associated epithelium cells are characterized by their association with lymphoid follicles, not by microfolds. Although these cells may sometimes separate lymphoid cells from the lumen by a thin extent of their cytoplasm, they often do not so separate. The reference to membranes, therefore, seems less than compelling as a reason to retain the M designation.

The epithelium covering the surface of follicles in the appendix, Peyer's patches, and solitary follicles of the intestine[13] consists only in part of FAE cells. Columnar absorptive cells and a few goblet cells also are present. This epithelium covers a domelike projection of lymphoid tissue, and should continue to be referred to, as a whole, as dome epithelium.[14]

Significance of Epithelial Transport

The continuing transport by columnar absorptive cells, efficient transport by FAE, and the association of FAE with lymphoid follicles leads to the assumption that epithelium is directly involved with early interactions between foreign materials and cells from the lymphoid system, and initiation of an immune response to molecular antigens and microorganisms.

Follicle-associated epithelium can transport inert particulate material such as carbon particles[8,13,15] and latex spheres[15,16] over 1 μm in diameter, as well as antigenic tracers like ferritin[7,8] and horseradish peroxidase.[12]

Follicle-associated epithelium also appears to be efficient in transmitting microorganisms to reactive lymphoid cells. Wolf *et al.*[17] inoculated Reovirus type 1 into the ileum of young mice and observed a preferential adherence of the viral particles to the surface of FAE-cells. Within one hour virus particles had been transported through the FAE-cells to intercellular spaces containing lymphoid cells. Oral administration of poliovirus to chimpanzees resulted in early accumulation in relatively high concentration in only tonsils and Peyer's patches.[18]

Transport of bacteria through the epithelium covering the domes of lymphoid follicles of rabbit appendix is well recognized,[14,19] because the bacteria are so abundant and apparently cause no adverse effects. It has recently been shown that it is FAE-cells that transport bacteria in rabbit appendix.[20]

Bacterial transport with striking morphological similarity to FAE transport in rabbit appendix has been observed in human nasopharyngeal epithelial cells (D. S. Stephens, Z. McGee, and L. Hoffman, Vanderbilt University, Nashville, Tenn., USA, unpublished). Epithelial cells with short irregular microvilli, overlying adenoidal lymphoid tissue, were shown by scanning electron microscopy to interact with piliated group B meningococci. By transmission electron microscopy, the bacteria were shown to be taken up into cytoplasmic vacuoles. In their studies on the route of infection by *Salmonella enteritidis* in mice, Carter and

Collins[21] observed that Peyer's patches seemed to be intimately involved in the establishment of the primary infection focus. Gaines et al.[22] recognized the involvement of Peyer's patches in orally induced infections of chimpanzees by S. typhi, but thought that they were probably preferential sites of multiplication rather than invasion; typhoid bacilli were thought probably to penetrate the intestinal mucosal lining in random fashion. The latter workers pointed out that their data did not exclude the possibility that the aggregate intestinal follicles were preferential sites of invasion.

There can be little doubt that FAE cells serve as a preferential route for the passage of many kinds of foreign materials, including pathogenic microorganisms. Upon transport through FAE, the materials may interact with macrophages and lymphocytes locally, and/or be transmitted to mesenteric lymph nodes for reaction there.

Processing by Macrophages

Macrophages are numerous in GALT, even attaining an intraepithelial location.[23-27] Thus some antigens are immediately available to macrophages upon completion of transport by the follicle-associated epithelium. The intraepithelial macrophages are phagocytic when formaldehyde-killed Salmonella typhi is administered orally to rabbits previously sensitized intravenously, as shown by Kimura.[24] Intraepithelial macrophages have also been shown to be capable of pinocytosing intraluminally administered ferritin in nonimmunized rats.[27] Phagocytosis of lymphocytes and plasma cells by intraepithelial macrophages has been demonstrated in Peyer's patches[25,27] and appendix.[20] Phagocytosis of Giardia muris has been described to occur through the extensions of pseudopods into the epithelium by macrophages lying beneath the basal lamina.[28] The bacteria indigenous to the lumen of rabbit appendix are engulfed by intraepithelial macrophages after they are transported by FAE[20] and are numerous in macrophages throughout the follicle.

Macrophages are quite numerous throughout the dome area of GALT, and in germinal centers. In these locations there frequently is ample evidence of phagocytosis and breakdown by the cells. Numerous engulfed and degenerating lymphocytes are characteristic for many of the macrophages in germinal centers, forming the so-called tingible body macrophages.

Joel and coworkers[13] carried out a long-term study of the uptake and distribution of carbon particles administered to mice by gavage or ingestion in drinking water. After uptake through Peyer's patch epithelium, the carbon particles were at first visible in macrophages in the subepithelial area. After extended periods, carbon-laden macrophages were present in all areas of Peyer's patches and mesenteric lymph nodes. Mobility of macrophages was thought to play a role in this distribution. Carbon was evident in Peyer's patches and lymph nodes four months after cessation of carbon ingestion. Approximately eight days elapsed between gavage and finding carbon-laden macrophages in germinal centers. A significant observation in this study was that isolated follicles along the intestine handled the carbon in a manner similar to the follicles aggregated into Peyer's patches. Keren et al.[29] have also emphasized the histological similarity of isolated follicles with follicles of Peyer's patches.

Despite the presence of numerous macrophages that are capable of phagocytosis, degradation, and migration within GALT, a question has been raised about their competence to participate in the induction of humoral immune responses.

Kagnoff and Campbell[30] demonstrated the inability of Peyer's patch cells to respond *in vitro* to sheep red blood cells without the addition of adherent peritoneal exudate cells or 2-mercaptoethanol. The capability for an initial response to antigen by Peyer's patch cells may be deduced from the failure of germinal centers to develop in Peyer's patches in germfree situations, and from the disappearance of germinal centers in rabbit appendix when its continuity with the gut lumen is interrupted (discussed by Parrott[31]). Richman *et al.*[32] have recently shown that macrophages from Peyer's patches are capable of antigen presentation if they are isolated in the presence of collagenase. They further theorize that 2-mercaptoethanol may preserve the innate ability of Peyer's patch macrophages to present antigen by preventing the oxidation of glutathione. As will be discussed below, plasma cells are present within and beneath the dome epithelium of GALT. Therefore, some terminal differentiation of B-cells probably does occur locally.

BIDIRECTIONAL TRANSPORT

The capability of GALT to respond to luminal antigens and organisms would include the capability to transmit the end products of immune reaction into the gut lumen. Bockman and Stevens[33] demonstrated that FAE could participate in the efficient transport of materials from the underlying lamina propria into the lumen. Horseradish peroxidase was introduced into the bloodstream and followed through mouse Peyer's patches, rabbit appendix, and chicken bursa of Fabricius. Reaction product for HRP activity was localized in much greater quantities in FAE-cells than in non-FAE. Saline washings from appendiceal and bursal lumina 15 minutes after administration showed peroxidase activity, indicating transport into the lumen.

The conclusions from this study were questioned by Lupetti and Dolfi,[34] on the basis that HRP in the lumen and FAE might have arrived by a route other than the one suggested. These workers injected HRP intravenously and found the development of peroxidase activity, within 15 minutes, in chick urine and the bile of mice and rabbits. This discovery suggested that HRP might be gaining access to the bursal lumen through the cloaca, and to mouse Peyer's patch and rabbit appendix by way of the bile duct and intestinal lumen.

Beezhold and Bockman (unpublished observations) subsequently ligated the bursal duct before i.v. administration of HRP in chicks. Similarly, the proximal jejunum was doubly ligated before i.v. administration of HRP in mice. Transport into and through FAE was again observed. FIGURE 3 shows transport of HRP through FAE in chick bursa, including the reaction product on the luminal surface.

Follicle-associated epithelium, therefore, seems capable of transporting macromolecules both from and to the lumen. It seems possible that this capability might include the transport of immunoglobulins into the lumen. Keren *et al.*[29] have pointed out that IgG can be detected in fluids from most isolated loops of intestines. In fact, although the data presented by Chodirker and Tomasi[35] indicated a decreased ratio of IgG to IgA in intestinal fluid as compared with serum, IgG still was present at twice the concentration of IgA. In addition to IgG, and other immunoglobulins, one could also suggest that antigen-antibody complexes, cell break-down products, and viruses might be transported into the intestinal lumen by follicle-associated epithelium.

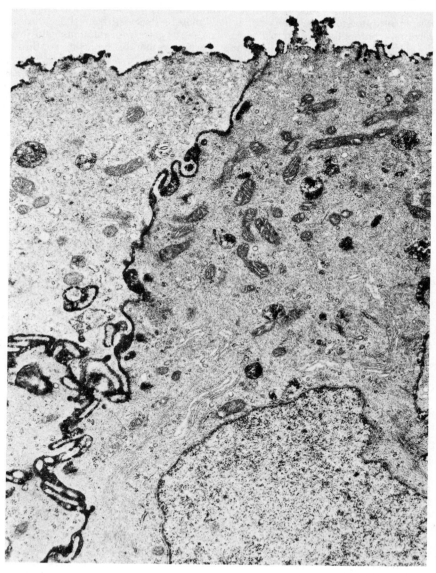

FIGURE 3. FAE from bursa of Fabricius after intravenous administration of horseradish peroxidase. Dense peroxidase reaction product is prominent intercellularly, within vesicles and vacuoles intracellularly, and along the luminal surface (top).

Plasma Cells Associated with Epithelium in GALT

Although plasma cells are not prominent in follicles of GALT, they are present in close association with the dome epithelium of Peyer's patches of rabbits,[24] mice,[25] and rats[26,27] and of rabbit appendix.[20] The failure of previous attempts[36] to locate antibody-forming cells in GALT after immunization may have been due to the restricted distribution of plasma cells in these organs. Plasma cells are located within and immediately beneath the dome epithelium (FIGURES 4 & 5). It should be realized, however, that because of the interruption in basal lamina, which is characteristic for dome epithelium, and is particularly marked in appendix,[19,20] the molecular selection exerted by the basal lamina is deficient, and subepithelial plasma cells are effectively intraepithelial, so far as transport of their secretions is concerned.

It seems likely that the secretions of the plasma cells in this location would react with appropriate antigen immediately upon its arrival, and that it would be transported into the intestinal lumen through FAE cells. In this situation the secretions would be able to modulate uptake of specific antigen. These secretions could be joined by secretions brought to the base of the FAE cells by the capillary plexus, which underlies the dome epithelium.[26,37]

Alteration of Absorption after Immunization

It has been demonstrated quite convincingly that immunization alters the absorption of that antigen. After oral[38,39] or parenteral[40] immunization, transport of antigen through the gut wall *in vitro*,[38,40] or into mesenteric blood *in vivo*,[39] is reduced as compared with nonimmunized controls (see paper by Walker in this volume, for a complete discussion). Brandtzaeg and Tolo[41] demonstrated that transport of albumin through lingual mucous membranes was reduced in rabbits immunized to albumin, but that there was a concomitant enhancement in transport of another protein (transferrin) to which the animals were not immunized. Thus, the possibility of nonspecific alteration in mucosal permeability due to antigen-antibody reaction was raised.

There have been some findings that raise the possibility of enhanced uptake of antigen after immunization. Bockman and Winborn,[2] in a nonquantitative electron microscopic study of ferritin uptake in hamster small intestine, observed apparently increased uptake of antigen by columnar epithelial cells in parenterally immunized animals. Kimura[24] could observe uptake of orally administered killed bacteria in the epithelium of Peyer's patches, and in macrophages within and immediately beneath the epithelium, only in those animals that had been previously immunized intravenously. The i.v. immunized and orally challenged animals also exhibited increased numbers of macrophages in the epithelial cell layer.

Decreased transmission of antigens into blood and lymph is not necessarily inconsistent with increased uptake by epithelium and epithelium-associated macrophages after immunization. Increased epithelial uptake after parenteral immunization might signal participation of epithelial cells in the reactivity to luminal antigens in the presence of circulating antibodies by increased antigen degradation and decreased transmittal into blood and lymph.

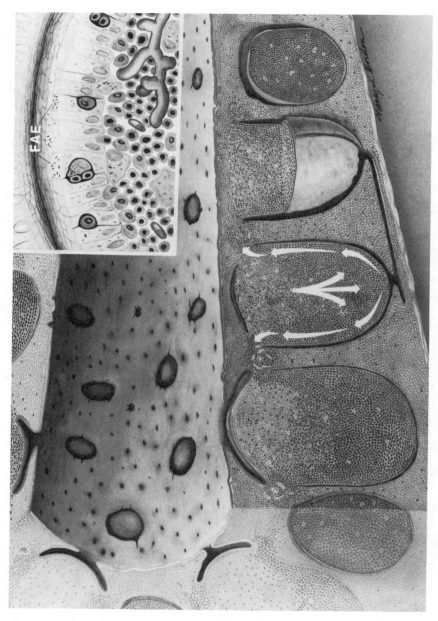

FIGURE 4. Pictorial representation of rabbit appendix. The dome epithelium of each follicle is recessed beneath the general luminal surface. The lumen is continuous, through an ostium, with the space bordering on the dome epithelium. Bacteria are numerous in this space. Bacteria are transmitted through the FAE cells of the dome epithelium and are engulfed by macrophages, which become scattered throughout each follicle. Lymphocyte reactivity is represented by the arrows in one follicle, representing the flow in antigen recognition, DNA synthesis at the base, mitosis laterally, and migration of lymphocytes into lymphatic sinuses surrounding each follicle.

ANTIGEN DEGRADATION

Intracellular degradation of macromolecules by epithelial cells is a well-demonstrated phenomenon. The uptake of ferritin into phagolysosomes within columnar epithelial cells was evident in the previously described studies,[2] particularly in immunized animals. Presumably, degradation within the epithelial cells prevents most of the macromolecules from being transported to the lamina propria antigenically intact. Schaffner *et al.*[15] introduced *E. coli* and *S. albus* into the bursal lumen and looked for transmission into bursal follicles. Intact organisms were not transmitted into the follicles, but some stainable microorganisms could be detected in FAE cells and increasing numbers of periodic acid-Schiff (PAS) positive, myelinlike cytoplasmic inclusions were demonstrated. These workers suggested that, considering the marked enzymatic activities in the epithelial cells covering the follicles, it seemed a reasonable assumption that particulate material of microbial origin would be degraded rapidly and efficiently by these cells.

The possibility of interaction between antigen being transported from the lumen and antibody being transported to the lumen, with enhanced antigen degradation, seems a reasonable possibility that is experimentally approachable.

ANTIGEN PRESENTATION

Just as epithelial cells share with macrophages the capability for antigen degradation, they may also share the capability for the presentation of antigens to

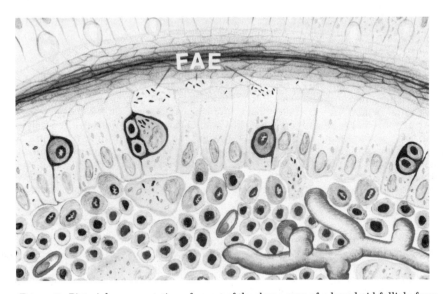

FIGURE 5. Pictorial representation of a part of the dome area of a lymphoid follicle from rabbit appendix, as depicted in FIGURE 4. Some of the epithelial cells of the dome are FAE. Macrophages and plasma cells, as well as lymphocytes, are located within the epithelium. Plasma cells are located immediately beneath the epithelium, with little or no basal lamina intervening.

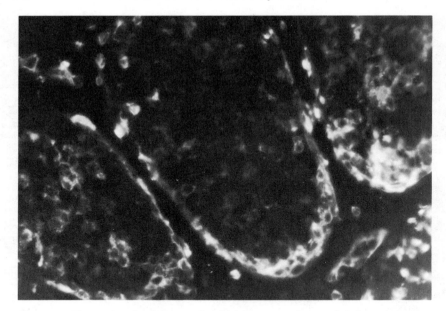

FIGURE 6. Fluorescent localization of Ia-like antigen in bursa of Fabricius. A mouse monoclonal IgM antibody to chick Ia-like antigen was followed by rhodamine-coupled anti-mouse IgM. Prominent localization on the epithelial cells forming the peripheral limit of the medulla of each follicle is evident.

reactive lymphocytes. Ia antigens are membrane-bound glycoproteins, coded for by genes of the major histocompatibility complex, which are present on macrophages and are thought to be involved in antigen recognition and initiation of response by the immune system. Ia-like antigens are also present on intestinal epithelial cells.[42] Mason et al.[43] observed increased expression of Ia antigens, on rat gut epithelial cells, induced by graft-versus-host disease and suggested that the expression of Ia is an indication that, during antigen recognition, the epithelial cells of the gut take on an antigen-presenting or processing function. Similarly, Natali et al.[44] used a monoclonal antibody to localize Ia-like antigens on human epithelial cells of small intestine and colon, as well as other epithelia. These workers suggested that Ia-like antigens may play a role in recognition processes between lymphoid cells and epithelial cells that come in contact with environmental pathogens and carcinogens.

Ia antigens are present on the epithelial cells of mouse thymus,[45,46] but are missing in thymus of nude mice.[46] FIGURE 6 shows the localization of Ia-like antigens on epithelial cells of developing chick bursa (Max Cooper, University of Alabama, Birmingham Ala., USA, unpublished observations). Both thymus and bursa represent microenvironments where appropriate interaction of epithelial cells with developing lymphocytes is necessary for the development of appropriate immune reactivity.

Interaction, in the bursa of Fabricius, between epithelium and lymphoid cells, seems necessary for the normal differentiation of both.[8,47,48] Perhaps this interaction involves Ia-like antigens. Induction of antibody response by the bursa requires the presence of epithelial cells.[49] Perhaps FAE in the bursa and mammalian GALT, as well as columnar absorptive cells of the intestine, can present antigen to lymphocytes.

SUMMARY

Epithelial cells and their products are essential participants in both initial and final stages of reactivity to foreign materials in the gut lumen. Follicle-associated epithelial cells, called "M"-cells by others, more efficiently transport antigens from the lumen than do columnar absorptive cells. Epithelial cells degrade antigens intracellularly. The presence of Ia-like antigens on epithelial cells of the gastrointestinal tract and thymus suggests a role in antigen presentation. Actively phagocytic macrophages are present within the epithelium of Peyer's patches and appendix, providing antigen degradation and presentation. Follicle-associated epithelial cells transport materials from lamina propria into intestinal lumen. Therefore, FAE cells are capable of bidirectional transport. Plasma cells are located within and immediately beneath the epithelium of Peyer's patches and appendix, where defects in the basal lamina indicate diminished capability for molecular selection. Transmission of antibodies into the lumen would modulate further antigen uptake and provide for interaction with organisms.

ACKNOWLEDGMENT

We thank Mrs. Pat O'Meara for typing the manuscript.

REFERENCES

1. BAZIN, H. 1976. The secretory antibody system. *In* Immunological Aspects of the Liver and Gastrointestinal Tract. A. Ferguson and R. N. M. MacSween, Eds.: 33–82. University Park Press. Baltimore, Md.
2. BOCKMAN, D. E. & W. B. WINBORN. 1966. Light and electron microscopy of intestinal ferritin absorption. Observations in sensitized and non-sensitized hamsters (*Mesocricetus auratus*). Anat. Rec. **155**: 603–622.
3. CORNELL, R., W. A. WALKER & K. J. ISSELBACHER. 1971. Small intestinal absorption of horseradish peroxidase. A cytochemical study. Lab. Invest. **25**: 42–48.
4. WARSHAW, A. L., W. A. WALKER, R. CORNELL, & K. J. ISSELBACHER. 1971. Small intestinal permeability to macromolecules. Transmission of horseradish peroxidase into mesenteric lymph and portal blood. Lab. Invest. **25**: 675–684.
5. JOEL, D. D., B. SORDAT, M. W. HESS & H. COTTIER. 1970. Uptake and retention of particles from the intestine by Peyer's patches in mice. Experientia **26**: 694.
6. HANAOKA, M., R. M. WILLIAMS & B. H. WAKSMAN. 1971. Appendix and γM antibody formation. III. Uptake and distribution of soluble or alum-precipitated bovine γ-globulin injected into the rabbit appendix. Lab. Invest. **24**: 31–37.
7. BOCKMAN, D. E. & M. D. COOPER. 1971. Fine structural analysis of pinocytosis in lymphoid follicle-associated epithelium in chick bursa and rabbit appendix. Fed. Proc. Fed. Am. Soc. Exp. Biol. **30**: 511.
8. BOCKMAN, D. E. & M. D. COOPER. 1973. Pinocytosis by epithelium associated with lymphoid follicles in the bursa of Fabricius, appendix, and Peyer's patches. An electron microscopic study. Am. J. Anat. **136**: 455–478.
9. R. L. OWEN & A. L. JONES. 1974. Epithelial cell specialization within human Peyer's

patches: an ultrastructural study of intestinal lymphoid follicles. Gastroenterology **66:** 189–203.

10. BOCKMAN, D. E. & M. D. COOPER. 1975. Early lymphoepithelial relationships in human appendix. A combined light- and electron-microscopic study. Gastroenterology **68:** 1160–1168.

11. OWEN, R. L. 1977. Sequential uptake of horseradish peroxidase by lymphoid follicle epithelium of Peyer's patches in the normal unobstructed mouse intestine: an ultrastructural study. Gastroenterology **72:** 440–451.

12. OWEN, R. L. & P. NEMANIC. 1978. Antigen processing structures of the mammalian intestinal tract: an SEM study of lymphoepithelial organs. Scanning Electron Microsc. **2:** 367–377.

13. JOEL, D. D., J. A. LAISSUE & M. E. LEFEVRE. 1978. Distribution and fate of ingested carbon particles in mice. J. Reticuloendothelial Soc. **24:** 477–487.

14. WAKSMAN, B. H., H. OZER & H. E. BLYTHMAN. 1973. Appendix and γM-antibody formation. VI. The functional anatomy of the rabbit appendix. Lab. Invest. **28:** 614–626.

15. SCHAFFNER, T., J. MUELLER, M. W. HESS, H. COTTIER, B. SORDAT & C. ROPKE. 1974. The bursa of Fabricius: a central organ providing for contact between the lymphoid system and intestinal content. Cell. Immunol. **13:** 304–312.

16. LEFEVRE, M. E., R. OLIVO, J. W. VANDERHOFF & D. D. JOEL. 1978. Accumulation of latex in Peyer's patches and its subsequent appearance in villi and mesenteric lymph nodes. Proc. Soc. Exp. Biol. Med. **159:** 298–302.

17. WOLF, J. L., D. H. RUBIN, R. FINBERG, R. S. KAUFFMAN, A. H. SHARPE, J. S. TRIER & B. N. FIELDS. 1981. Intestinal M cells: a pathway for entry of reovirus into the host. Science **212:** 471–472.

18. BODIAN, D. 1955. Emerging concept of poliomyelitis infection. Science **122:** 105–108.

19. SHIMIZU, Y. & W. ANDREW. 1967. Studies on the Rabbit Appendix. I. Lymphocyte-epithelial relations and the transport of bacteria from lumen to lymphoid nodule. J. Morphol. **123:** 231–250.

20. BOCKMAN, D. E. & W. R. BOYDSTON. 1983. Participation of follicle associated epithelium (FAE), macrophages, and plasma cells in the function of appendix. Scanning Electron Microsc. In press.

21. CARTER, P. B. & F. M. COLLINS. 1974. The route of enteric infection in normal mice. J. Exp. Med. **139:** 1189–1203.

22. GINES, S., H. SPRINZ, J. G. TULLY & W. D. TIGERTT. 1968. Studies on infection and immunity in experimental typhoid fever. J. Infect. Dis. **118:** 293–306.

23. CRABB, E. D. & M. A. KELSALL. 1940. Organization of the mucosa and lymphatic structures in the rabbit appendix. J. Morphol. **67:** 351–367.

24. KIMURA, A. 1977. The epithelial-macrophagic relationship in Peyer's patches; an immunopathological study. Bull. Osaka Med. Sch. **23:** 67–91.

25. ABE, K. & T. ITO. 1978. Fine structure of the dome in Peyer's patches of mice. Arch. Histol. Jpn. (Niigata Jpn.) **41:** 195–204.

26. BOCKMAN, D. E. 1981. Range of function of gut-associated lymphoepithelial tissue. In Aspects of Developmental and Comparative Immunology. J. B. Solomon, Ed.: 273–277. Pergamon Press. Oxford.

27. LAUSE, D. B. & D. E. BOCKMAN. 1981. Heterogeneity, position, and functional capability of the macrophages in Peyer's patches. Cell Tissue Res. **218:** 557–566.

28. OWEN, R. L., C. L. ALLEN & D. P. STEVENS. 1981. Phagocytosis of Giardia muris by macrophages in Peyer's patch epithelium in mice. Infect. Immun. **33:** 591–601.

29. KEREN, D. F., P. S. HOLT, H. H. COLLINS, P. GEMSKI & S. B. FORMAL. 1978. The role of Peyer's patches in the local immune response of rabbit ileum to live bacteria. J. Immunol. **120:** 1892–1896.

30. KAGNOFF, M. F. & S. CAMPBELL. 1974. Functional characteristics of Peyer's patch lymphoid cells. J. Exp. Med. **139:** 398–406.

31. PARROTT, D. M. V. 1976. The gut-associated lymphoid tissues and gastrointestinal immunity. In Immunological Aspects of the Liver and Gastrointestinal Tract. A. Ferguson & R. N. M. MacSween, Eds.: 1–32. University Park Press. Baltimore, Md.

32. RICHMAN, L. K., A. S. GRAEFF & W. STROBER. 1981. Antigen presentation by macro-phage-enriched cells from the mouse Peyer's patch. Cell. Immunol. **62:** 110–118.
33. BOCKMAN, D. E. & W. STEVENS. 1977. Gut-associated lymphopeithelial tissue: Bidirectional transport of tracer by specialized epithelial cells associated with lymphoid follicles. J. Reticuloendothelial Soc. **21:** 243–252.
34. LUPETTI, M. & A. DOLFI. 1980. Concerning bidirectional transport by the lymphoid follicle-associated epithelial cells. Cell. Mol. Biol. **26:** 609–613.
35. CHODIRKER, W. B. & T. B. TOMASI, JR. 1963. Gamma-globulins: Quantitative relationships in human serum and nonvascular fluids. Science **142:** 1080–1081.
36. BIENENSTOCK, J. & J. DOLEZEL. 1971. Peyer's patches: Lack of specific antibody-containing cells after oral and parenteral immunization. J Immunol. **106:** 938–945.
37. BHALLA, D. K., T. MURAKAMI & R. L. OWEN. 1981. Microcirculation of intestinal lymphoid follicles in rat Peyer's patches. Gastroenterology **81:** 481–491.
38. WALKER, W. A., K. J. ISSELBACHER & K. J. BLOCK. 1972. Intestinal uptake of macromolecules: Effect of oral immunization. Science **177:** 608–610.
39. ANDRE, C., R. LAMBERT, H. BAZIN & J. F. HEREMANS. 1974. Interference of oral immunization with the intestinal absorption of heterologous albumin. Eur. J. Immunol. **4:** 701–704.
40. WALKER, W. A., K. J. ISSELBACHER & K. J. BLOCH. 1973. Intestinal uptake of macromolecules. II. Effect of parenteral immunization. J. Immunol. **111:** 221–226.
41. BRANDTZAEG, P. & K. TOLO. 1977. Mucosal penetrability enhanced by serum-derived antibodies. Nature (London) **266:** 262–263.
42. WIMAN, K., B. CURMAN, U. FORSUM, L. KLARESKOG, U. MALMNAS-TJERNLUND, L. RASK, L. TRAGARDH & P. A. PETERSON. 1978. Occurrence of Ia antigens on tissues of non-lymphoid origin. Nature (London) **276:** 711–713.
43. MASON, D. W., M. DALLMAN & A. N. BARCLAY. 1981. Graft-versus-host disease induces expression of Ia antigen in rat epidermal cells and gut epithelium. Nature (London) **293:** 150–151.
44. NATALI, P. G., C. DE MARTINO, V. QUARANTA, M. R. NICOTRA, F. FREZZA, M. A. PELLEGRINO & S. FERRONE. 1981. Expression of Ia-like antigens in normal human nonlymphoid tissues. Transplantation **31:** 75–78.
45. ROUSE, R. V., W. VAN EWIJK, P. P. JONES & I. L. WEISSMAN. 1979. Expression of MHC antigens by mouse thymic dendritic cells. J. Immunol. **122:** 2508–2515.
46. JENKINSON, E. J., W. VAN EWIJK & J. J. T. OWEN. 1981. Major histocompatibility complex antigen expression on the epithelium of the developing thymus in normal and nude mice. J. Exp. Med. **153:** 280–292.
47. BEEZHOLD, D. H., H. G. SACHS & P. J. VAN ALTEN. 1982. The influence of embryonic testosterone treatment on bursal epithelial pinocytotic activity. Dev. Compr. Immunol. **6:** 121–130.
48. BEEZHOLD, D. H., H. G. SACHS & P. J. VAN ALTEN. 1982. The development of transport ability by embryonic follicle-associated epithelium. Submitted for publication.
49. WALTENBAUGH, C. R., H. G. SACHS & P. J. VAN ALTEN. 1977. Antibody production in organ culture by bursae of mature chickens and the development of immunological competence. Dev. Compr. Immunol. **1:** 353–362.

DISCUSSION OF THE PAPER

A. G. PLAUT (*Tufts-New England Medical Center, Boston, Mass.*): In clinical gastroenterology, there is a disease, nodular lymphoid hyperplasia, that involves proliferation of the follicles. Do you know whether there is a follicle-associated epithelium (FAE) over all of those new follicles in these patients?

D. E. BOCKMAN (*Medical College of Georgia, Augusta, Ga.*): We have not looked at those specific follicles. We assume that over all of the normally occurring follicles, not only over the GALT, but over the many individual follicles that are located throughout the G.I. tract, there appears to be an FAE-type of epithelium.

PLAUT: Do these cells have exactly the same origin in the crypt as do columnar absorptive epithelial cells?

BOCKMAN: These cells originate in the crypt, migrate onto the dome, and differentiate there.

PLAUT: Do they contain digestive enzymes?

BOCKMAN: They have some digestive enzymes that appear to be lower in concentration than the non-FAE epithelium.

ORAL TOLERANCE AND ACCESSORY-CELL FUNCTION
OF PEYER'S PATCHES

T. B. Tomasi, W. G. Barr, S. J. Challacombe, and G. Curran

*Cancer Research Center
and
Department of Cell Biology
University of New Mexico
Albuquerque, New Mexico 87131*

The ingestion of a single large dose (1 to 20 mg) of a soluble protein such as human gamma globulin (HGG) or ovalbumin (OVA) in mice results in unresponsiveness to the subsequent systemic administration of the same antigen.[1-4] Tolerance has been observed in the IgM, IgG, and IgE antibody classes; tolerance is antigen specific and lasts for long periods (2–4 months).[5] T-cells are also tolerized as shown by suppression of antigen-induced T-cell proliferation,[6] and by the observation that feeding of a specific carrier such as OVA produces tolerance to dinitrophenylated (DNP)-OVA but not to DNP-keyhole-limpet hemocyanin (KLH).[1]

Several studies have shown that suppressor cells appear early after oral immunization in gut-associated lymphoreticular tissue.[3,7-13] It has been suggested that antigen-specific IgA T-helper cells (T_h) and IgG specific T-suppressor cells (T_s) are induced simultaneously in Peyer's patches (PP), and that T_s migrates to the spleen and peripheral lymphoid tissues and produces systemic tolerance.[10] This notion is consistent with our previous work,[6] showing that secretory immunity and systemic tolerance may occur concomitantly after oral immunization with soluble proteins. An active role for suppressor cells in the induction of oral tolerance, however, has not been established, especially in view of the observations that tolerance to parenterally administered deaggregated HGG (DHGG) may be induced in the apparent absence of suppressor cells.[12-14]

Oral or systemic immunization with soluble antigens does not appear to lead to the production of antibody-secreting cells or an effective T-cell proliferative response in the PP themselves,[6,15,16] although irregular responses have been reported in the rabbit[17] and with particular antigens such as killed *Streptococcus mutans*.[6] Kagnoff and Campbell[18] reported the failure of PP cells to support the induction of a primary humoral response to sheep red blood cells or the development of cytotoxicity to allogeneic cells *in vitro*. Both of these functions were restored by the addition of adherent peritoneal exudate cells (APEC) to the cultures. This discovery suggested that the immunological shortcomings of PP cells might exist secondarily to a decrease in the number of functional capacity of accessory cells. The apparent deficiency of accessory cell function is of particular interest in relationship to the development of suppressor cells, because in other systems it has been shown that deficient antigen presentation and the failure to generate a large number of proliferating T-helper cells is related to the apparent ease with which suppressor cells develop.[19] Thus, the apparent deficiency of accessory cell function of PP could be related to the development of T_s and oral tolerance. This study was undertaken to further explore the parameters of the

145

accessory cell function within PP and to further elucidate the role of suppressor cells in the development of oral tolerance.

MATERIALS AND METHODS

Animals

Inbred mice CBA/J, C3H/HeJ, B6AF1, B10.BR, BALB/c, and SJL/J female mice were purchased from Jackson Laboratories, Bar Harbor, Maine; C3H/AnF female mice were obtained from Cumberland View Farm, Clinton, Tennessee, and C3H/Cr female mice from Charles River Laboratories, Wilmington, Massachusetts. B10.S5 (12R) and A-TFR-1 mice were kindly provided by Dr. Chella David.

Lymph Node Cell (LNC) Proliferative Assay

Methods of immunization and the *in vitro* culture techniques employed were essentially those described by Alkan.[20] Human gamma globulin (Fraction II), human serum albumin (HSA, gamma globulin free), and bovine serum albumin (BSA) (all purchased from Sigma Chemical Co., St. Louis, Missouri) and ragweed antigen E were used as antigens. All determinations were done in triplicate and data are expressed as stimulation index or CPM ± standard error (SE).

Presentation of Antigen to Sensitized Lymph Node Cells (SLNC)

Method I: Cell preparations were incubated in triplicate in flat-bottomed tissue culture trays (Falcon 3042, Falcon Co., Oxnard, Calif.) at six different concentrations calculated to give 0.1 to 3.2×10^5 adherent cells per well. After incubation for 60 minutes at 37°C, nonadherent cells were removed by washing the cells ($\times$ 3) in cold RPMI-2.5 (RPMI 1640 + 2.5% FCS). For pulsing, 200 μg of antigen in 200 μl of medium was added to each well; the trays were then incubated for a further two hours or in some experiments 24 hours. After washing ($\times$ 3) with warm media, 4×10^5 SLNC were added to each well; the trays were incubated for four days with no further addition of antigen. One μCi of tritiated thymidine was added to each well 16 hours before cultures were harvested. As controls, SLNC were added to duplicate cultures of nonpulsed adherent cells or pulsed adherent cells were incubated alone.

Method II: In a separate series of experiments, cells were adhered to 6 cm plastic petri dishes as outlined above. The cells were pulsed with antigen for two hours and then thoroughly washed in RPMI-2.5. Adherent cells were removed with .02% ethylenediaminetetracetate (EDTA) and added to 4×10^5 SLNC in concentrations ranging from 0.1×10^5 to 1.6×10^5 (viable cells) in a total volume of 200 μl and then incubated for four days at 37°C. Results in both methods were expressed as the difference in counts between pulsed adherent cells plus SLNC, and nonpulsed adherent cells plus SLNC.

Enrichment for Low Density Populations

Populations of spleen and PP cells were enriched for low density cells by equilibrium density centrifugation on dense bovine plasma albumin (BPA) solutions. Single cell suspensions were spun at 10,000 g in an SW39 swinging bucket rotor for 20 minutes at 4°C. Two cell fractions (pellicle and pellet) were then harvested with Pasteur pipettes and washed in RPMI prior to suspension in the final media for counting. Bovine plasma albumin solutions were prepared from BPA powder (fraction V, Reheis Chemical Co., Phoenix, Ariz.). The pH and density were adjusted if necessary to give a final solution with a pH 7.35–7.45 and a density of 1.080–1.082. The solution was subjected to Millipore filtration and kept at 4°C prior to use.

Morphologic Examination for Dendritic Cells

Examination by phase-contrast microscopy was performed on specimens fixed for five minutes at room temperature in 2.5% glutaraldehyde buffered with phosphate-buffered saline (PBS) pH 7.40 following adherence to glass coverslips for two hours at 37°C. Nonadherent cells were bound to coverslips previously coated with poly-l-lysine (Type VII, Sigma Chemical) (25 μg/ml in PBS). The cells were allowed to adhere for 20 minutes, fixed with glutaraldehyde and examined for the morphological feature of dendritic cells as described by Steinman and Cohn.[21]

Preparation of T-Cells

Cloned T-cells specific for poly l-Glu^{60}:l-Ala^{30}:l-Tyr^{10} (GAT) were kindly donated by Drs. M. Kimoto and C.F. Fathman and were prepared as previously described.[22] Alloreactive long-term T-cell cultures were the result of long-term repetitive mixed lymphocyte reactions (MLR) with initially unfractionated responder cell populations. 3–6 × 10^6 cells (responder cells from PP or spleen) were maintained in 20 ml of RPMI supplemented with 25 mM HEPES, 100 U/ml penicillin, 100 μg/ml of streptomycin, 2 mM glutamine, Garamycin (400 μg/ml), and fungizone (3 μg/ml) with 5% fetal calf serum (FCS) and 2-mercaptoethanol (2-ME, 5 × 10^{-5}M) in 75 cm tissue culture flasks (Corning, Corning Glass Works, Corning, N.Y.). Every 10–14 days these cells were pulsed with 50–60 × 10^6 irradiated (3300 rads) spleen cells. T-cells recognizing B6AF1 determinants were derived from CBA/J Peyer's patch cells stimulated with irradiated B6AF1 spleen cells. T-cell lines recognizing CBA/J determinants were derived from B10 spleen cells stimulated by irradiated CBA/J spleen cells.

Mixed Lymphocyte Reactions

Variable numbers of irradiated (3300 rads) spleen or Peyer's patch cells served as stimulators and 10^5 alloreactive T-cells as responder cells. Cells were cultured in round bottom tissue culture plates (Linbro, Flow Laboratories, Hamden, Conn.) and stimulation was measured by uptake of tritiated thymidine in a two day proliferative assay. Primary MLR were performed as described by Murgita and Tomasi.[23]

Presentation of GAT to Cloned T-Cells

10^4 cloned GAT T-reactive cells were mixed with 40 μg of GAT and variable numbers of irradiated cells from the spleen or PP of B6AF1 in a total volume of 200 μl. Cells were cultured in flat bottom (Falcon 3042) tissue culture plates for three days, and stimulation was measured by uptake of tritiated thymidine.

Intragastric and Intraperitoneal Immunization

Antigens were centrifuged at 150,000 g for three hours at 4°C and the upper third of this solution was collected and used as the deaggregated tolerogen. Mice were tolerized with 1.0 to 10.0 mg in a volume of 0.5 ml, either intragastrically (IG) (animals were anesthetized with ether and a 21-gauge needle with a hollow steel ball of 2 mm diameter soldered onto the blunted end was inserted into the stomach) or intraperitoneally (IP). Seven days later, IG and IP tolerized and normal control (ID) (immunized but not tolerized) mice were given 100 μg of the antigen in adjuvant subcutaneously at the base of the tail.[20]

Elimination of ^{125}I-Labeled Antigen

Mice were passively immunized as previously stated by subcutaneous challenge with antigen. Seven days later IG, IP, ID as well as nonimmunized control mice were injected IP with 10 μg of ^{125}I-labeled antigen. Whole body counts were monitored at time 0 and 24 hours later, as determined in a NaI crystal scintillation counter, and results were expressed as the percent of total injected protein-bound radioactivity eliminated at 24 hours.[24]

Solid-Phase Radioimmunoassay

Micro-enzyme-linked immunosorbent assay (ELISA) removable strips (Cat. No. 1-223-35, Dynatech Laboratories, Alexandria, Va.) were used as the solid-phase. HGG, BSA, or HSA were coupled to the solid-phase with 100 μg of antigen added to each well in a total volume of 300 μl. These strips were incubated at 4°C overnight to complete the initial coupling step. Each well was then thoroughly washed and blocked with 5% normal rabbit serum diluted in phosphate-buffered saline. Serial dilutions of control and experimental serums were added (total volume in each well was equal to 300 μl) and then incubated for three hours at room temperature. After washing, ^{125}I-labeled rabbit anti-mouse Ig (with κ and IgG Fc specificity) was added to each well and incubation was continued for an additional three hours. The wells were then washed three times with 0.05% PBS-Tween 20, and the strips were counted in a Packard Auto-Gamma Scintillation Spectrometer.

RESULTS

Antigen Presentation to Sensitized Lymph Node Cells

Adherent spleen cells (ASC) pulsed with antigen (Method I—MATERIAL AND METHODS) were most efficient in presenting antigen to SLNC. Significant stimulation of SLNC was found with 2.5% ASC, and the proliferative response increased in proportion to the number of cells added to a maximum at 40% ASC (FIGURE 1). Pulsed APEC also stimulated SLNC to a maximum at 10–20% APEC; greater

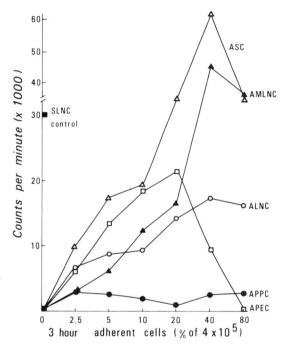

FIGURE 1. Presentation of ovalbumin to sensitized lymph node cells (SLNC) by adherent Peyer's patches cells (APPC = ●), spleen (ASC = △), mesenteric lymph nodes (AMLNC = ▲), lymph nodes (ALNC = O) and peritoneal exudate (APEC = □). Adherent cells pulsed with 200 μg ovalbumin for two hours, washed and SLNC added at 4×10^5 per well and cultured for four days. ■ = SLNC control, 100 μg ovalbumin added to 4×10^5 SLNC. Mean of three experiments. Control values (nonpulsed adherent cells plus SLNC) have been subtracted.

concentrations causing a progressive decrease in the response. Presentation of antigen by adherent lymph node cells (ALNC) appeared to be less effective than with ASC or APEC. At concentrations of 40% or greater, pulsed adherent mesenteric lymph node cells showed significantly greater counts than ALNC ($p < 0.05$), although the gross cellular characteristics of mesenteric and peripheral

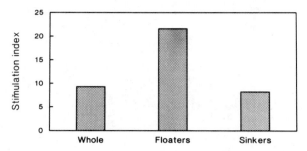

FIGURE 2. Antigen presentation by irradiated (3300 rads) syngeneic Peyer's patch cells to B6AF₁ cloned GAT specific T-cells. 200 μg/ml of GAT added and [³H]thymidine incorporation measured after two days of culture. CPM on whole Peyer's patches = 2309 ± 155, floaters = 3321 ± 82, sinkers = 1517 ± 109. Floaters and sinkers separated on BPA (1.080 density).

lymph nodes are very similar. Data very similar to that shown in FIGURE 1 with OVA as antigen was also obtained with HGG and purified protein derivative (derived from mycobacterium tuberculosis) (PPD). As shown in FIGURE 1, pulsed adherent Peyer's patch cells (APPC) did not elicit stimulation of SLNC at any of the concentrations tested (between 2.5 and 80% of the number of SLNC). Lengthening the period of antigen pulsing to 24 hours did not improve presentation. Antigen pulsed APPC were also unable to present HGG or PPD to SLNC. Ten percent APPC added to APEC or ASC did not significantly affect their ability to present antigen, suggesting that suppressor cells were not responsible for the deficient presentation by APPC.

When adherent cells were pulsed in petri dishes, removed with EDTA and transferred to trays (Method II—MATERIALS AND METHODS), similar results were obtained. Viabilities of the adherent cells for each of the cell preparations were similar.

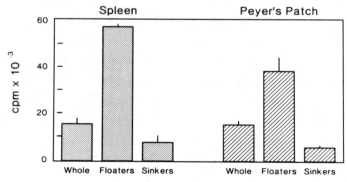

FIGURE 3. Mixed lymphocyte reactions comparing irradiated (3300 rads) stimulators from CBA spleen and Peyer's patch populations separated on BPA gradients. Responding cells were obtained from long-term T-cell cultures (see MATERIALS AND METHODS). Whole spleen SI = 41; spleen floaters SI = 158; Spleen sinkers SI = 26; whole PP SI = 49; PP floaters SI = 113; PP sinkers SI = 15.

The lack of presentation by APPC did not appear to be restricted to CBA/J mice because identical results were found with mice of the A.TFR-1 and B10.S (12R) strains (data not shown).

Antigen Presentation to Cloned T-Cells

Both unfractionated PP and spleen cells from B6AF$_1$ mice were shown to be capable of presenting antigen to cloned GAT reactive T-cells. Density centrifugation on BPA (p = 1.080) separates spleen and PP cells into two fractions: a low density population ("floaters") and a high density fraction ("sinkers"). The antigen-presenting cell in the spleen was significantly enriched in the floaters (containing 5–15% of total cell population). Similar findings were found with PP cells (see FIGURE 2) where low density cells made up 10–30% of the total. Repeated experiments showed PP floaters to be less efficient in presenting antigen to the cloned cells than spleen cells at the same cell concentrations.

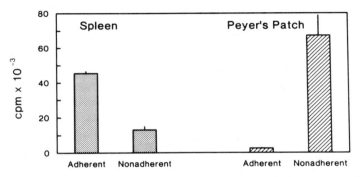

FIGURE 4. Mixed lymphocyte reactions with irradiated (3300 rads) low density spleen and Peyer's patch cells comparing the stimulating capacity of their adherent and nonadherent fractions. Responders were long-term alloreactive T-cell cultures. Spleen adherent SI = 228; spleen nonadherent SI = 65; PP adherent SI = 6; PP nonadherent SI = 174.

Mixed Lymphocyte Reaction Stimulation by Peyer's Patch Cells

Whole Peyer's patch cells provide good stimulation in the allogeneic MLR, approaching, although usually inferior to, spleen cells. The stimulating capacity of the nonadherent population was similar to that of the whole Peyer's patches. Long-term T-cell cultures enriched for alloreactive cells by repetitive MLR were used as responder cells. Stimulation of 10^5 of these T-cells by as few as 2×10^4 irradiated spleen or PP cells provided an excellent response when two-day MLR were assessed. Separation of spleen and PP cells into high and low density cells resulted in enrichment for the stimulating cell in the low density fraction (FIGURE 3). In repeated experiments, PP floaters provided good stimulation, though consistently less than spleen cells.

PP and spleen cells differed when low density cells were separated into adherent and nonadherent fractions. In spleen cell populations the MLR stimulating cell was present primarily in the adherent fraction, whereas in the PP it was recovered only in the nonadherent population (FIGURE 4). Experiments using a T-cell line derived from B10.BR mice recognizing CBA/J determinants yielded results similar to those outlined above.

Dendritic Cells in Peyer's Patches

Phase contrast examination of low density adherent cells (LODAC) from PP revealed significant differences when compared to the spleen. Spleen LODAC preparations were consistently characterized by 40% or more cells with typical morphological features of dendritic cells (DC) as described by Steinman and Cohn.[21] Peyer's patch LODAC populations did not contain, or at best showed small numbers (<5%) of cells resembling splenic dendritic cells. The nonadherent low density cells from PP were attached to glass coverslips previously treated with poly-l-lysine. These cells, however, did not demonstrate the typical morphology exhibited by splenic DC after similar treatment. Furthermore, observation of the nonadherent PP population in culture for up to five days did not reveal the development of dendritic cells.

Oral Tolerance to HGG Measured by T-Cell Proliferation and Humoral Responses

The IP and IG administration of DHGG produces systemic tolerance to a subsequent injection of aggregated HGG in Freund's adjuvant (FIGURE 5). A

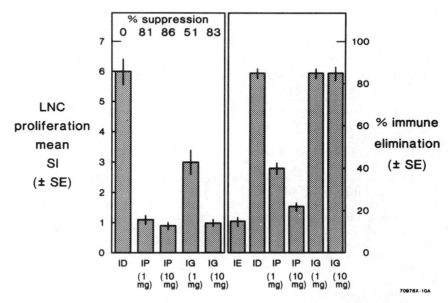

FIGURE 5. IP and IG administration DHGG (1 and 10 mg) produces systemic tolerance as measured by the T-cell proliferative assay. Only IP DHGG tolerizes for humoral response as measured by percent elimination of [125I]HGG administered IP. Five mice per group.

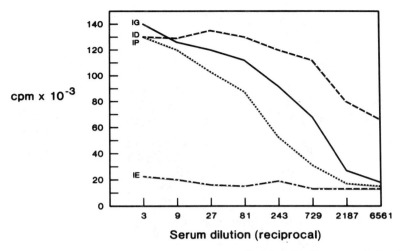

FIGURE 6. Solid phase radioimmunoassay using ^{125}I-labeled affinity purified rabbit anti-mouse Ig. Effect of 10 mg of DHGG IG and IP on systemic antibody response. Illustrates suppression of serum titers by IP > IG.

consistent feature illustrated in FIGURE 5 is the greater efficiency of the IP route in inducing tolerance to DHGG compared to the IG route. It is also noted that T-cell tolerance is more readily induced and more complete than humoral tolerance. In fact, as shown in FIGURE 5 using the immune elimination assay that we initially employed, tolerance induction by the IG route was not observed even at 10 mg intragastrically. As shown in FIGURE 6, however, employing a more sensitive radioimmunoassay to detect serum antibodies specific for HGG, partial tolerization of the humoral response by prior feeding is evident.

Effect of Colchicine and Cyclophosphamide on Systemic and Oral Tolerance

FIGURE 7 demonstrates that colchicine at 20 µg per mouse administered two hours prior to the tolerizing dose does not affect the development of tolerance as measured by either the T-cell or humoral responses. The effects of colchicine and Cytoxan are compared in TABLE 1. Colchicine and Cytoxan, at the doses regularly employed, enhanced T-cell proliferation in the control cultures, suggesting that suppressor cells sensitive to these agents have a regulating effect on the lymph node proliferative response. Our previous studies of oral tolerance demonstrated T-suppressor cells by passive transfer.[6] In additional experiments we demonstrated that the doses of colchicine and Cytoxan employed inhibited adoptive transfer of tolerance to syngeneic recipients (data not shown).

Genetic Control of Oral Tolerance

It has been reported[25] that both H-2 and non-H-2 genes control systemic tolerance. To determine whether similar genetic influences were also operative

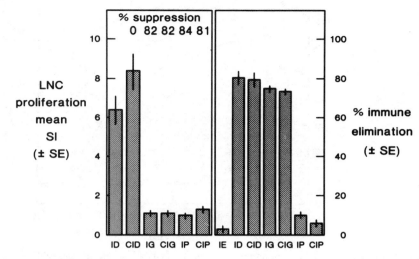

FIGURE 7. Lack of effect of colchicine (20 μgm/animal) on tolerance as measured by the T-cell proliferative assay. Colchicine enhances T-cell proliferation in control culture, but does not affect the development of tolerance after 10 mg of DHGG IP or IG. Colchicine does not inhibit induction of tolerance at the humoral level (as measured by immune elimination of [^{125}I]HGG) after 10 mg IP DHGG. IG DHGG does not induce tolerance as measured by immune elimination. Five mice per group.

TABLE 1

EFFECT OF COLCHICINE AND CYTOXAN ON THE INDUCTION OF ORAL TOLERANCE*

	CPM ± SE		
Treatment	Media	OVA	SI
Saline IV Saline IG OVA SC	3,535 ± 253	27,364 ± 2,079	7.7
Saline IV OVA IG OVA SC	1,794 ± 185	2,675 ± 310	1.5
Colchicine IV Saline IG OVA SC	4,223 ± 306	39,177 ± 1,112	9.3
Colchicine IV OVA IG OVA SC	1,700 ± 106	2,402 ± 202	1.4
Cytoxan IV OVA IG OVA SC	3,226 ± 293	6,271 ± 264	1.9

*Eight CBA/J mice per group. Colchicine IV (20 μg) given 2½ hours and Cytoxan (280 μg) two days prior to intragastric (IG) saline or OVA (10 mg). Seven days later OVA (100 μg) given SC in tail in H37 Ra adjuvant. Eight days later regional (para-aortic and inguinal) nodes removed and cultured in media or media plus OVA (250 μg/ml). Incorporation of [^{3}H]thymidine determined after four days.

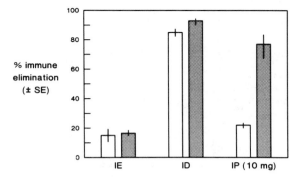

FIGURE 8. Ease of tolerance induction (measured by serum antibody levels) in CBA/J (H.2^k) (open bar) mice compared to resistance of B10.BR (H.2^k) (stippled bar). Five mice per group. Antibody levels quantitated by elimination of [^{125}I]HGG administered IP.

in oral tolerance, the experiments illustrated in FIGURE 8 and TABLES 2 and 3 were performed. Tolerance was easily induced in the CBA/J mice compared to the resistant B10.BR (FIGURE 8). TABLE 2 summarizes the data obtained with five different mouse strains of the H-2^k haplotype and illustrates significant differences in the ease of tolerance induction between these strains. The SJL/J (H-2^s) mice are as difficult to tolerize by the oral route as they are systemically. The BALB/c strain has been shown to be resistant to systemically produced tolerance, whereas DBA/2 are much more sensitive. As shown in TABLE 3, however, the ease of induction of oral tolerance in DBA/2 versus BALB/c is reversed compared with systemically induced suppression.

Tolerance to Human Versus Bovine Serum Albumin

FIGURE 9 demonstrates data obtained following IP or IG tolerization with human serum albumin and bovine serum albumin. One or 10 mg of HSA readily tolerized CBA/J mice in both the T-cell (FIGURE 9) and humoral responses (data not shown). As noted in FIGURE 10, however, BSA produces little suppression and is not statistically significant (compared with controls).

TABLE 2

EFFECT OF GENETIC BACKGROUND ON TOLERANCE INDUCTION IN
MICE OF THE H-2^k HAPLOTYPE*

Strain	H-2 Type	T-Cell Proliferative Response Percent Suppression	
		IP	IG
CBA/J	k	81	51
C3H/HeJ	k	72	35
C3H/Anf	k	78	40
C3H/Cr	k	73	0
SJL/J	s	40	9

*Tolerance induced by 1 mg of DHGG given IG or IP.

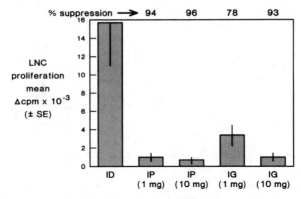

FIGURE 9. Systemic tolerance as measured by the proliferative response to HSA after IP or IG administration of 1 or 10 mg of deaggregated HSA.

DISCUSSION

Adherent cells from PP are deficient in their ability to present soluble antigens (OVA, HGG, PPD) to sensitized lymph node cells when compared to adherent cells from peripheral lymph nodes, spleens, or peritoneal exudate. The number of adherent cells in PP is significantly less than spleen or lymph nodes, although we cannot be sure this discrepancy is not attributable to technical problems, such as the manner in which the patches are collected. Perhaps macrophages are concentrated close to the intestinal lumen. In this regard we have not been able to

TABLE 3

STRAIN DIFFERENCES IN ORAL TOLERANCE

		LNC Proliferative Assay Stimulation Index	
Strain		HGG	PPD
CBA/J	Saline	9.3	14.3
BALB/c	Saline	6.4	14.8
DBA/2	Saline	13.7	12.3
CBA/J	1 mg DHGG	1.4	25.2
BALB/c	1 mg DHGG	10.6	18.8
DBA/2	1 mg DHGG	7.5	14.6
CBA/J	5 mg DHGG	1.2	22.1
BALB/c	5 mg DHGG	6.4	13.0
DBA/2	5 mg DHGG	9.1	12.1
CBA/J	10 mg DHGG	1.4	31.7
BALB/c	10 mg DHGG	2.6	18.4
DBA/2	10 mg DHGG	5.6	18.9
CBA/J	20 mg DHGG	1.2	37.9
BALB/c	20 mg DHGG	2.2	18.7
DBA/2	20 mg DHGG	5.6	11.8

improve yields of adherent cells by using collagenase (type 2) or trypsin plus collagenase, nor did we find significant differences with the manner with which the patches are obtained (deep cuts versus more superficial). Defective antigen presentation cannot, however, be attributed to cell numbers alone, because equivalent numbers of adherent cells were used from each source. It also seems unlikely that APPC contained a population of suppressor cells. The addition of APPC to SLNC did not suppress the response, and mixing APPC with APEC or ASC did not alter their ability to present antigen.

Our data demonstrate that whereas whole Peyer's patches present antigen, they do so less efficiently than equivalent numbers of spleen cells; this phenomenon is not a result of the suppression by adherent cells. Nonadherent PP cells and reconstituted mixtures of adherent and nonadherent PP cells are equal in presentation of antigen to unfractionated PP populations. It has not been excluded that the deficiency of APPC to present antigen may apply only to certain antigens. This possibility is raised by the observation that T-cell proliferative

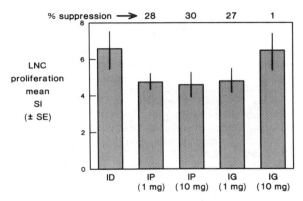

FIGURE 10. The *in vitro* proliferation to BSA after IP or IG administration of 1 or 10 mg of deaggregated BSA. Note that the degree of suppression is considerably less than with HSA (see FIGURE 9) and is not statistically significant (p > .05).

responses of PP following intragastric administration of soluble (tolerogenic) protein antigens such as OVA is negligible, whereas significant stimulation occurs after the administration of a particulate antigen such as *Streptococcus mutans*.[1,6]

The response of cloned T-cell lines to a synthetic polymer such as GAT depends on the presence of a supporting population of antigen-presenting cells. We have found that flotation of whole spleen or PP cells on BPA (density 1.080) produces a heterogeneous low density population as first reported by Steinman and Cohn,[21] and that this population is enriched in antigen presenting cells. Repeated experiments, however, have shown that equivalent numbers of low density cells from PP are less efficient in their ability to present antigen to cloned T-cells than those derived from spleen.

The initial work of Steinman and Cohn[21] has directed attention to a novel mononuclear lymphoid cell with distinctive morphological characteristics; the lymphoid dendritic cell. Dendritic cells have been reported to be critical for a variety of accessory cell functions including antigen presentation,[26] oxidative mitogenesis,[27] and the development of cytotoxic T-cells.[28] In addition, they appear to act as potent stimulators of both the allogeneic and syngeneic mixed lymphocyte reactions.[29,30] In this study, whole PP act as good stimulators of the primary and secondary mixed lymphocyte reaction. In both the spleen and PP, the MLR-stimulating cell was found predominantly within the low density population. Whereas adherent floaters from the spleen were potent stimulators of the MLR, this activity was found exclusively in the nonadherent low density population of Peyer's patches. Also, unlike spleen, the low density nonadherent population of PP does not contain cells with typical morphological characteristics of dendritic cells. It is possible that dendritic cells are present within PP, but have different morphological characteristics than those within the spleen. Alternatively, a different type of cell or cells in PP may be responsible for antigen presentation and/or stimulation in the allogeneic mixed lymphocytic reaction. Recently B-cell tumors and LPS-induced normal lymphoblasts have been reported[31] to have antigen presenting capacity, and we are currently investigating whether PP B-cells may present antigen.

The comparative lack of antigen presentation by APPC is in agreement with a previous report[18] that PP lack the accessory cells needed for a primary in vitro antibody response and fail to produce antibody after oral or parenteral immunization.[15,16] It has been suggested that deficient antigen presentation may facilitate the development of suppressor cells.[19] As mentioned in the introduction, this development is pertinent in regard to oral tolerance because suppressor cells formed in the PP migrate to peripheral lymphoid tissues, and T_s have been implicated in the systemic tolerance that follows the oral administration of certain antigens. It should be emphasized, however, that antigen sensitization must occur in Peyer's patches because cells from this origin are the precursors of antibody-producing cells found in the lamina propria of the gut and other mucosal sites.[32] Moreover, the defect in antigen presentation is only partial, because whole and nonadherent PP do present antigens in the in vitro T-cell proliferative assay, although less efficiently than do spleen cells. Speculative antigen presentation in the gut may occur by unique mechanisms that generate T_h for IgA and T_s for IgG and IgM.[10] The possibility that the presenting cell in gut lymphoid tissues such as PP may have some degree of antigen and/or isotype specificity in their cell interactions as previously suggested[5] should be further explored.

A major unresolved question concerning oral tolerance is whether it is a unique form of tolerance or simply another route of administration of antigen. Perhaps small amounts of monomer or fragments of antigen that are highly tolerogenic are absorbed from the gut, and systemic tolerance results from the same mechanisms as parenteral tolerance. The occurrence of suppressor cells early in the immune response in the gut and later in the spleen, and their specificity for suppression of IgG and IgM classes,[10] suggest that unique mechanisms may be responsible for the systemic suppression that follows the feeding of antigens. This possibility is also suggested by reports that serum factors,[33,34] possibly IgA antibody-antigen complexes, are responsible for oral tolerance. In the present studies, we failed to show an effect on the development of tolerance by pretreatment with Cytoxan or colchicine prior to tolerization. These results are similar to those reported for systemically induced tolerance.[35] Thus, although suppressor cells are present during certain periods in the development of tolerance, they do not appear to be required for its induction. Although we did not test the effect of these drugs on the maintenance of tolerance, the work of Richman,[11] showing that suppressor cells disappear from the spleen and thymus after 30 days even though the animals remained tolerant for several months, suggests that T_s may not be necessary for the maintenance of the tolerant state.

Thus, in this parameter, characteristic oral and parenteral tolerance behave similarly. Suppressive factors, however, have been found in extracts of spleens taken from HGG tolerized animals,[36] and it has not been excluded that only low levels of suppressor activity are necessary to maintain T-cell unresponsiveness late in tolerance and that the cells responsible are undetectable by the relatively crude adoptive transfer experiments employed.

Differences among mice strains and their susceptibility to tolerance induction have been ascribed to the relative efficiency of their macrophages in processing and presenting antigens.[37-39] Cowing et al.[39] in their studies of systemic tolerance noted that the tolerance resistant BALB/c and tolerance susceptible DBA/2 mice differed in the ease with which tolerance could be induced to IgG_3 but not to IgG_1 or IgG_2 subclasses. BALB/c macrophages have receptors for IgG_3, whereas DBA/2 do not. The hypothesis suggested by these workers is that the tolerogenic inducing material in HGG preparations is IgG_3, and that the strain differences result from the manner in which the IgG_3 subclass is handled. BALB/c macrophages would bind IgG_3 and induce cells toward immunity rather than a tolerogenic signal. As mentioned below, however, this explanation would not hold for oral tolerance because DBA/2 are more resistant than BALB/c.

Tolerance induced by the systemic administration of antigen has been shown to be under genetic control by Ranges and Azar.[25] These authors suggested that both H-2 and non-H-2 genes influence tolerance induction to deaggregated human gamma globulin. Our results indicate that within the H-2^k haplotype, there are significant differences in the ease of induction of oral tolerance, suggesting that non-H-2 linked genes are important in oral tolerance. Interestingly, however, differences are seen between oral and parenteral tolerance when the BALB/c and DBA/2 strains are compared. In parenterally induced tolerance, DBA/2 mice are much more susceptible than BALB/c mice, whereas the reverse is true in oral tolerance. This difference has been repeatedly observed using various preparations of HGG and different groups of mice. These results, if confirmed and extended to other strains, would suggest differences in the mechanisms of tolerance induction by the oral and parenteral route. These results, in turn, could be related to the types of macrophages (including their Fc receptors) present in gut versus peripheral lymphoid tissues.

Finally, studies were reported showing that tolerance to HSA could be easily induced by the oral route. When we attempted, however, to tolerize with BSA, which has a similar half life to HSA in the mouse, we were unable to produce tolerance even at the T-cell level. This finding is in striking contrast to all other soluble proteins we have so far examined (OVA, KLH, HGG, and HSA). One feasible explanation is the presence of significant amounts of BSA in the chow that is normally fed to mice in our animal facility. These results are similar to those of Carr et al.,[40] showing that the administration of bovine casein intragastrically failed to induce tolerance to a subsequent immune response to parenteral casein. Casein was a constituent of the normal mouse chow and when mice were bred and raised on a casein-free diet, oral tolerance could be readily induced. These data demonstrate the need, in studies on the tolerogenicity of proteins, to consider the dietary status of the animal.

SUMMARY

Whole and nonadherent Peyer's patch cells were shown to present antigen to cloned antigen specific T-cells, albeit less efficiently than spleen cells. Unlike spleen cells, adherent PP cells did not present antigen, and PP lacked cells with classical dendritic morphology. The antigen presenting and MLR-stimulating cell in both spleen and PP were concentrated in the low density (BPA floaters) population. Soluble antigens (OVA, HGG, HSA, and KLH) are poorly presented by PP and do not elicit a T-cell proliferative response in PP when fed orally. These antigens induce oral tolerance and T_s cells in PP, MLN, and spleen. As with systemic tolerance, however, T_s (as measured by adoptive transfer) are not necessary for the induction of tolerance and can be eliminated by colchicine and Cytoxan without a significant effect on the initiation of tolerance.

Evidence from studies in various inbred strains of mice suggests that oral tolerance is dependent on genetic factors, but the susceptibility of the strain is different from that induced by the systemic injection of the same antigen. Data are also presented that suggest that in studies of oral tolerance to various antigens, care must be exercised in excluding the effect of diet.

REFERENCES

1. CHILLER, J. M., R. G. TITUS & H. M. ETLINGER. 1979. In Immunological Tolerance and Macrophage Function. T. Baram, J. R. Battista and C. S. Pierce, Eds.: 195. Elsevier/North-Holland Publishing Co. Amsterdam.
2. VAZ, N. M., L. C. S. MAIA, D. G. HANSON & J. J. LYNCH. 1977. Inhibition of Homocytotropic Antibody Responses in Adult Inbred Mice by Previous Feeding of the Specific Antigen. J. Allergy Clin. Immunol. 60: 110.
3. RICHMAN, L. K., J. M. CHILLER, W. R. BROWN, D. G. HANSON & N. M. VAZ. 1978. Enterically Induced Immunologic Tolerance. I. Induction of Suppressor T Lymphocytes by Intragastric Administration of Soluble Proteins. J. Immunol. 121: 2429.
4. STOKES, C. & E. T. SWARBRICK. 1977. Induction of Tolerance After Oral Feeding of Soluble Protein Antigen. Biochem. Soc. Trans. 5: 1573.
5. TOMASI, T. B. 1980. Oral Tolerance (overview). Transplantation 29: 353.
6. CHALLACOMBE, S. J. and T. B. TOMASI. 1980. Systemic Tolerance and Secretory Immunity After Oral Immunization. J. Exp. Med. 152: 1459.
7. MATTINGLY, J. A. & B. H. WAKSMAN. 1978. Immunologic Suppression After Oral Administration of Antigen I. Specific Suppressor Cells Formed in Rat Peyer's Patches After Oral Administration of Sheep Erythrocytes and Their Systemic Migration. J. Immunol. 121: 1878.
8. NGAN, J. & L. S. KIND. 1978. Suppressor T Cells for IgE and IgG in Peyer's Patches of Mice Made Tolerant by the Oral Administration of Ovalbumin. J. Immunol. 120: 861.
9. ASHERSON, G. L., L. M. ZEMBALA, M. A. C. C. PERERA, B. MAYHEW & W. R. THOMAS. 1977. Production of Immunity and Unresponsiveness in the Mouse by Feeding Contact Sensitizing Agents and the Role of Suppressor Cells in Peyer's Patches, Mesenteric Lymph Nodes and Other Lymphoid Tissues. Cell. Immunol. 33: 145.
10. RICHMAN, L. K., A. S. GRAEFF, R. YARCHOAN & W. STROBER. 1981. Simultaneous Induction of Antigen-Specific IgA Helper T Cells as IgG Suppressor T Cells in the Murine Peyer's Patch After Protein Feeding. J. Immunol. 126: 2079.
11. RICHMAN, L. K. 1979. Immunological Unresponsiveness after Enteric Administration of Protein Antigens. In Immunology of Breast Milk. P. L. Ogra and D. H. Dayton, Eds.: 49 Raven Press. New York.
12. PARKS, D. E., M. V. DOYLE & W. O. WEIGLE. 1978. Induction and Mode of Action of Suppressor Cells Generated Against Normal Gamma Globulin. I. An Immunologic Unresponsive State Devoid of Demonstrable Suppressor Cells. J. Exp. Med. 148: 625.
13. WATERS, C. A., L. M. PILARSKI, T. G. WEGMAN & E. DIENER. 1979. Tolerance Induction During Ontogeny. I. Presence of Active Suppression in Mice Rendered Tolerant to Human γ-globulin In Utero Correlates with the Breakdown of the Tolerant State. J. Exp. Med. 149: 1134.

14. MILLER, S. D., M. S. SY & H. N. CLAMAN. 1977. The Induction of Hapten-Specific T Cell Tolerance Using Hapten-Modified Lymphoid Membranes. II. Relative Roles of Suppressor T Cells and Clone Inhibition in the Tolerant State. Eur. J. Immunol. **7:** 165.

15. BIENENSTOCK, J. & J. DOLEZEL. 1971. Peyer's Patches: Lack of Specific Antibody Containing Cells After Oral and Parenteral Immunization. J. Immunol. **106:** 938.

16. HENRY, C., W. P. FAULK, Z. KUHN, J. M. YOFFEY & H. H. FUDENBERG. 1970. Peyer's Patches: Immunologic Studies. J. Exp. Med. **131:** 1200.

17. CLANCY, R. & A. PUCCI. 1978. Sensitization of Gut-Associated Lymphoid Tissue During Oral Immunization. AJEBAK **56:** 337–340.

18. KAGNOFF, M. F. & S. CAMPBELL. 1974. Functional Characteristics of Peyer's Patch Lymphoid Cells. I. Induction of Humoral Antibody and Cell-Mediated Allograft Reactions. J. Exp. Med. **139:** 398.

19. PIERRES, M. & R. N. GERMAIN. 1978. Antigen-Specific T Cell-Mediated Suppression. IV. Role of Macrophages in Generation of L-glutamic acid^{60}-L-alanine^{30}-L-tyrosine^{10} (GAT)-Specific Suppressor T Cells in Responder Mouse Strains. J. Immunol. **121:** 1306.

20. ALKAN, S. S. 1978. Antigen-Induced Proliferation Assay for Mouse T Lymphocytes Response to a Monovalent Antigen. Eur. J. Immunol. **8:** 112.

21. STEINMAN, R. M. & Z. A. COHN. 1973. Identity of a novel cell type in peripheral lymphoid organs of mice. I. Morphology, quantitation and tissue distribution. J. Exp. Med. **137:** 1142.

22. KIMOTO, M. & C. G. FATHMAN. 1980. Antigen-reactive T cell clones. I. Transcomplementing hybrid I-A region gene products functions effectively in antigen presentation. J. Exp. Med. **152:** 759.

23. MURGITA, R. A. & T. B. TOMASI. 1975. Suppression of the immune response by α-fetoprotein. II. The effect of mouse α-fetoprotein on mixed lymphocyte transformation. J. Exp. Med. **141:** 440.

24. AZAR, M. M., G. E. RANGES, E. J. YUNIS & C. CLARK. 1978. Genetic Control of Tolerance Induction to Human γ-Globulin in Mice. J. Immunol. **121:** 1251.

25. RANGES, G. E. & M. M. AZAR. 1979. Inheritance of Tolerance Susceptibility to Human γ-Globulin in Congenic Mice. J. Immunol. **123:** 1151.

26. SUNSHINE, G. H., D. R. KATZ & M. FELDMAN. 1980. Dendritic Cells Induce T-Cell Proliferation to Synthetic Antigens Under IR Gene Control. J. Exp. Med. **152:** 1817.

27. KLINKERT, W. E., J. H. LaBADIE, J. P. O'BRIEN, C. F. BEYER & W. E. BOWERS. 1980. Rat Dendritic Cells Function as Accessory Cells and Control the Production of a Soluble Factor Required for Mitogenic Responses of T Lymphocytes. Proc. Nat. Acad. Sci. USA **77:** 5414.

28. NUSSENZWEIG, M. C., R. M. STEINMAN, B. AUTCHINOV & Z. A. COHN. 1980. Dendritic Cells are Accessory Cells for the Development of Anti-Trinitrophenyl Cytotoxic T Lymphocytes. J. Exp. Med. **152:** 1070.

29. STEINMAN, R. M. & M. D. WITMER. 1978. Lymphoid Dendritic Cells are Potent Stimulators of the Primary MLR in mice. Proc. Nat. Acad. Sci. USA **75:** 5132.

30. NUSSENZWEIG, M. C. & R. M. STEINMAN. 1980. Contribution of Dendritic Cells to Stimulation of the Murine Syngeneic MLR. J. Exp. Med. **151:** 1196.

31. CHESNUT, R. W., S. M. COLON & H. M. GREY. 1982. Antigen Presentation by Normal B Cells, B Cell Tumors and Macrophages: Functional and Biochemical Comparison. J. Immunol. **128:** 1764.

32. CRAIG, S. W. & J. J. CEBRA. 1971. Peyer's Patches: An Enriched Source of Precursors for IgA-Producing Immunocytes in the Rabbit. J. Exp. Med. **134:** 188.

33. ANDRÉ, C., J. F. HEREMANS, J. P. VAERMAN & C. L. CAMBIASO. 1975. A Mechanism for the Induction of Immunological Tolerance by Antigen Feeding: Antigen-Antibody Complexes. J. Exp. Med. **142:** 1509.

34. KAGNOFF, M. F. 1978. Effects of Antigen-Feeding on Intestinal and Systemic Immune Responses. III. Antigen-Specific Serum-Mediated Suppression of Humoral Antibody Responses After Antigen Feeding. Cell. Immunol. **40:** 186.

35. PARKS, D. E., D. A. SHALLER & W. O. WEIGLE. 1979. Induction and Mode of Action of

Suppressor Cells Generated Against Human Gamma Globulin. II. Effects of Colchicine. J. Exp. Med. **149:** 1168.

36. TANIGUCHI, M. & J. F. A. P. MILLER. 1978. Specific Suppression of the Immune Response by a Factor Obtained from Spleen Cells of Mice Tolerant to Human γ-Globulin. J. Immunol. **120:** 21.

37. LUKIC, M. L., H. H. WORTIS & S. LESKOWITZ. 1975. A Gene Locus Affecting Tolerance to BGG in Mice. Cell. Immunol. **15:** 457.

38. FUJIWARA, M. & B. CINADER. 1974. Cellular Aspects of Tolerance. VII. Inheritance of the Resistance to Tolerance Induction. Cell. Immunol. **12:** 214.

39. COWING, C., C. GARABEDIAN & S. LESKOWITZ. 1979. Strain Differences in Tolerance Induction to Human γ-Globulin Subclasses: Dependence on Macrophages. Cell. Immunol. **47:** 407.

40. CARR, R. Personal Communication.

DISCUSSION OF THE PAPER

D. F. KEREN (*University of Michigan, Ann Arbor, Mich.*): Can you suppress a previously existing systemic IgG-immune response by oral administration of the same antigen?

T. B. TOMASI (*University of New Mexico, Albuquerque, N. Mex.*): Yes, but it is difficult to do. If the animal has had prior contact with the antigen and the antigen is then given orally, one usually sees a boost. If small doses of antigen are given over a long period of time, the animals progressively become tolerant. This question has distinct implications in terms of any kind of oral therapy, for example, in individuals that are already sensitized.

M. ZAUDERER (*Columbia University, New York, N.Y.*(: As I understand your experiment, the observation that encouraged you to believe that you have induced a switch from IgM to IgA is that when you give both activating signals, that is, both LPS and T-cell help, you get a large increase in IgA responses and IgA plaques, whereas, IgM plaques, that would otherwise predominate, do not occur. Have you checked for an alternative interpretation, other than an IgA-negative feedback, that prevents the activation of the IgM cells when you have that response going on at the same time?

TOMASI: Would you clarify your point, because we have performed some experiments in this regard; I want to make sure I fully understand your question.

ZAUDERER: An alternative interpretation to your observation is that when you activate IgA-secreting cells, IgA feeds back on potential IgM-producing cells to prevent them from being activated; therefore, they disappear. Thus, it is not a switch in the same cell, but rather, different cells being activated under different circumstances.

TOMASI: We have added IgA to cultures and then treated them with LPS or with alloreactive cells separately. Under these circumstances IgM plaques mainly occur.

QUESTION: How long did you culture the Peyer's patch cells before concluding that they did not have dendritic cell-type morphology?

TOMASI: You are probably referring to the fact that rat cells cultured require five days for dendritic cells to develop. We cultured Peyer's patch cells for up to five days, and cells with dendritic morphology did not increase significantly over the five days in culture.

J. R. McGHEE (*University of Alabama in Birmingham*): I would like to inquire how you have characterized these cells as dendritic. Have you used monoclonal antibodies to the dendritic cell, or anti-Mac and IA?

TOMASI: We really have not characterized them. We have recently obtained from Dr. Ralph Steinman, dendritic-specific monoclonal antibody, and we will try to characterize them. There are Mac 3 positive cells in Peyer's patches and we are currently studying the relative distribution of serological markers by fluorescence-activated cell-sorting (FACS) in collaboration with Carleton Steward at Los Alamos National Laboratory.

THE MUCOSAL IMMUNOLOGICAL NETWORK: COMPARTMENTALIZATION OF LYMPHOCYTES, NATURAL KILLER CELLS, AND MAST CELLS*

John Bienenstock, A. Dean Befus, Mark McDermott,
Shelagh Mirski, Ken Rosenthal, and Aldo Tagliabue†

Host Resistance Program
Department of Pathology
McMaster University
Hamilton, Ontario, Canada

LYMPHOBLAST LOCALIZATION

B-cells

It was first shown by Gowans[1] and subsequently elucidated by Hall and coworkers[2] that blast cells from the mesenteric lymph node and thoracic duct lymph had a tendency to localize selectively in the intestinal mucosa. Subsequently, Cebra and coworkers[3] showed that cells from the Peyer's patches had a repopulation potential that exceeded those derived from other lymphoid sources insofar as IgA was concerned. Our group established that cells from both the Peyer's patches and the bronchial-associated lymphoid tissue had an equal propensity to repopulate mucosal tissues with IgA-producing cells. These observations have led to the hypothesis that there is a common mucosal immune system for IgA in which cells sensitized in one mucosa have the capacity to selectively seed distant mucosal sites.[4] This hypothesis received substantiation especially from the work of Lamm, Phillips-Quagliata, and coworkers who showed a selective tendency for IgA B-cells from the mesenteric lymph nodes to localize in lactating mammary gland tissue.[5] This group subsequently gave specificity and biologic significance to this observation by showing that following oral feeding with ferritin, specific antibody-producing IgA cells were found in the respiratory tract, salivary glands, and mammary glands.[6] We found that mesenteric lymph node blast cells selectively repopulated the female cervix and that this localization was under female sex hormonal control,[4] as had been shown for similar experiments with the mammary gland. More recently, Montgomery[7] has shown that mesenteric lymph node blasts that synthesize IgA localize in the salivary glands. Thus the integration of mucosal sites through the migration of IgA cells has been described.

The factors that are responsible for this cellular localization in the mucosal immunological network are not well described, but include blood flow, surface characteristics such as IgA expression, the presence of specific antigens to which the B-cells are committed, the organ derivation of these cells, and the possible local presence of T-helper cells specific for IgA class.[4] In this respect we have shown that lymphoblasts derived from the lung have a tendency to return to that

*This work was supported by the Medical Research Council of Canada, the Canadian Foundation for Ileitis and Colitis, and Fisons Pharmaceuticals.

†Present address: Istituto Steroterapico e Vaccinogeno Toscano Sclavo, Siena, Italy

0077-8923/83/0409-0164 $1.75/0 © 1983, NYAS

organ, whereas those from the gut have a tendency to return to the intenstine. More recently, Pierce[8] has shown a similar tendency for cells sensitized in the colon to return to that organ.

It is less well known and appreciated that there may be a tendency for cells committed to the synthesis of other immunoglobulin isotypes to traffic within the mucosal network. We have shown that bronchial lymph node blasts, which have a tendency to return to their organ of origin, have a selectivity also for the IgG isotype.[9] Thus twelvefold more B-cells making IgG are found in the lung 24 hours after transfer of lymphoblasts from the bronchial lymph node, than are seen after transfer of an equivalent number of blast cells from the mesenteric node. The converse is also true, indicating that there is a selectivity involved in the appearance of mucosally derived IgG-producing cells in mucosal tissues when compared to cells derived from peripheral lymph nodes.

The factors that control the numbers of cells of one or other isotype and their appearance in a mucosal tissue are incompletely understood but must include soluble factors derived from isotype-specific T-cells such as have been described by Elson et al.[10] and more recently by Strober.[11] At present the role of these factors in influencing an isotype switch in B-cells can only be postulated. The factors responsible for mucosal localization of cells appear, however, to be expressed on the cell surface as originally predicted by Gesner and Woodruff.[12] In this regard, our recent study on the role of nutritional factors in selective localization has shown that mesenteric lymph node blasts from vitamin A deficient donors localized inefficiently in recipient animals of various nutritional states.[13] Similarly, donor cells from pair-fed controls localized poorly in the intestine of normal or vitamin A deficient recipients, although slightly better than blast cells from vitamin A deficient donors. It was the characteristic of the donor population that determined the numbers of cells localizing in mucosal tissues, and not the vasculature or other tissue-specific components of the recipients.

In some of the experiments described above, we, as well as many others before us, initially relied upon levels of radioactivity in the recipient tissues for evidence of cell localization. It is clear, however, that the levels of radioactivity localized in mucosal tissues do not correspond well to the actual numbers of cells counted when using autoradiography (TABLE I). A recent series of experiments looking at the effects of gender of the donor versus the recipient on cell localization clearly confirms this finding.[14] Although no differences were established by radiocounting, autoradiography showed that male cells have a tendency to be found in larger numbers in male or female recipient intestine when compared to those from female donor cells of the same species. This phenomenon led us to look at the recipient tissues by autoradiography and then to perform grain counts on the labeled cells in the recipient intestine. Relative to the donor population that is all heavily labeled (grain counts more than 40 per cell) in the recipient tissue 24 hours later, 79% of the cells divided at least once. These studies raise a number of questions, including where and when these cells divided. A kinetic analysis of grain count distribution in lymphoblasts localized in the intestine may provide some clues. Transferred cells may enter the mucosa before they divide, and under the influence of mitogens such as antigen may divide one or more times and then migrate to other mucosal tissues. Alternatively, the dogma that blast cells once localized in mucosal tissues will remain there must be questioned. Indeed, Howard[15] and Smith et al.[16] showed that up to 16% of blasts entering intestinal tissues could be recovered in efferent lymph. Where these cells go and what they do remain to be established.

T-cells

The other advantages of autoradiography over radiocounting became apparent when we looked at the anatomic distribution of B- and T-cell mesenteric lymph node blasts. We have shown that at 24 hours after transfer, about two-thirds of cells localize in the basal lamina propria and are equally T- and B-cells. By contrast, in the villus, T-cells predominated (approximately 70%). In the epithelium, we have evidence for exclusively T-blast localization. The factors that control the differential migration of T-blasts into the gut villus and epithelium, whether they involve a question of time, motility, or chemotactic factors remain to be resolved by future experiments.

Intraepithelial Lymphocytes

Characteristics

In situ, epithelial lymphocytes carry phenotypic markers characteristic of T-cells; up to 40% appear to have granules that vary in number between 5 and 20.

TABLE 1

LACK OF CORRELATION BETWEEN CELL LOCALIZATION AS DETERMINED BY
AUTORADIOGRAPHY AND RADIOCOUNTING*

Recipient Tissue	Donor Cells†	No. Labeled Cells/10^3 HPF	Homing Index‡	Percent Injected Radioactivity
Small Intestine	MLN	93 ± 6	10.3	13.4
	PLN	9 ± 2	1.0	5.8
	BLN	5 ± 1	0.6	5.9
	MLN	39 ± 4	3.0	1.2
Lungs	PLN	13 ± 1	1.0	1.6
	BLN	127 ± 24	9.8	—

*Data derived from McDermott and Bienenstock[9] and unpublished data.
†MLN = mesenteric lymphnode; PLN = peripheral lymphnode; BLN = bronchial lymphnode
‡MLN or BLN/PLN

They appear to contain sulfated mucopolysaccharides, are metachromatic, and may contain small amounts of histamine.[17-19] We have shown recently that these cells can be isolated. In situ they are mostly of the killer/suppressor phenotype, whereas in vitro following isolation these cells express natural killer (NK) activity. The NK activity is more sensitive to anti-Thy-1 antibodies than splenic NK activity, but like the spleen is insensitive to either anti-Lyt-1 or anti-Lyt-2 antibodies.[20] Our results suggest that the granulated cells from the epithelium are responsible for the local NK activity as has also been shown for large granulated lymphocytes from mouse blood and spleen. Thus up to 40% of the cells in the epithelium may be lacking the Lyt-1,2 phenotype. In our hands, this epithelial NK-cell population corresponds to the NK-cell subset described by Bloom and associates as NK_T.[21]

TABLE 2

PHENOTYPE AND LOCALIZATION CHARACTERISTICS OF CLONED NATURAL KILLER CELLS

	NKB61A2 (NK$_I$ or NK$_M$)*	AD-9 (NK$_T$)	H-Y (TK)
Phenotype			
Thy-1	−	+	+
Lyt-1	−	−	−
Lyt-2	−	−	+
Localization			
G.I. Tract	+ +	NT	+ + +
Lungs	+ + + +	NT	+
Skin	+ +	NT	+ + + +

*According to Minato et al.[21]

Localization potential

NK clones   We have examined the migratory properties of three NK clones, which phenotypically are analogous to three of the four NK subsets.[21] Each of these clones has a different selective localization pattern (TABLE 2). The surprising thing that emerged from this study was that some of the clones appear to have a tendency to go into the gut and others into the bronchial epithelium. This localization does not correlate with phenotype, at least as far as Lyt and Thy-1 markers are concerned.

T-cell clones   With Dr. T. Braciale we have recently examined the localization patterns of his two influenza-specific T-cell clones (TABLE 3). These cells showed a propensity to localize in the lung but not in the intestine. Impressive numbers localized in normal uninfected and infected respiratory epithelium. Striking increases in numbers of cells were seen in the lung parenchyma of infected animals, but only the H-2-restricted cytotoxic T-cell line, and not with the clone displaying the helper phenotype. By contrast, recent work from

TABLE 3

LOCALIZATION OF INFLUENZA-SPECIFIC
T-CELL CLONES IN THE LUNGS 22–24 HOURS
AFTER ADOPTIVE TRANSFER INTO SYNGENEIC MICE

Phenotype and Function	Recipient Infected*	Labeled cells/10^3 HPF ± S.E.M.		Parenchyma
		Mucosal		
		Lamina Propria	Epithelium	
Thy-1.2$^+$ Lyt-1$^+$, 2$^+$ H-2 Restricted Cytotoxic	No	31 ± 5	4.4 + 2.4	418 ± 121
	Yes	16 ± 3	1.6 ± 0.6	1423 ± 252
Thy-1.2$^+$ Lyt-1$^+$, 2$^-$ Helper (?)	No	85 ± 10	17.6 ± 6.0	2175 ± 225
	Yes	109 ± 13	10.5 ± 3.3	1922 ± 169

*Mice infected intranasally three days before with A/JAP/57.

deSousa's laboratory[22] has shown that other T-cell clones with cytotoxic phenotype localize in the intestine, especially in the epithelium.

The conclusions that we may reach at present are that the localization of these
cells is not on the basis of the phenotypic characteristics so far examined, but that
when cells from a single clone are examined, they have specific localization
characteristics.

MUCOSAL MAST CELLS

Much work in this area of study has developed from the studies by Enerback
in the 1960's on the atypical nature of mucosal mast cells (MMC).[23] These cells
appear to be smaller, possess granules with lower sulfation or mucopolysacchar-
ide and little or no heparin, and with a lower histamine and serotonin content
than mast cells in other sites. They have a lifespan of less than 40 days, as
compared to one much greater for connective tissue mast cells, and are totally
unresponsive to the secretagogue, compound 48/80. Perhaps the most surprising
thing from a histochemical point of view is that their granules are soluble in
formalin. This discovery has led to much controversy about the existence of MMC
and their abundance.

The proliferation of MMC appears to be dependent on the thymus, despite the
bone marrow derivation of these cells. We have been interested in this cell type
for some time and have shown that it will grow from the mesenteric[24] and
bronchial lymph nodes of appropriately stimulated rats. Adoptive transfer of
intestinal mast cell proliferation can be accomplished by immune mesenteric and
bronchial lymph node cells as well as with serum from similar animals.[25] Miller
and coworkers have similarly shown that the cell responsible for this transfer is in
the thoracic duct and is surface immunoglobulin negative.[26] Subsequent work in
tissue culture has suggested that factors released from T-cells may be necessary
for MMC differentiation and proliferation. It is difficult to discriminate between
the alternatives: transfer of inducer cells or increased numbers of precursors.[27]

Regardless of this situation, the MMC derived from culture as well as from
single cell suspensions from the intestine of *Nippostrongylus* infected animals
have a different profile of responsiveness to a variety of secretagogues than their
connective tissue counterparts.[28] Furthermore, the ability of anti-allergic compounds to inhibit antigen-induced histamine release by MMC is strikingly
different from peritoneal mast cells from the same animals.[29] For example,
disodium cromoglycate has no effect on inhibition of histamine release from
sensitized mucosal mast cells, whereas it is completely active on cells derived
from the peritoneum. On the other hand, doxantrazole, an orally active anti-
allergic that prevents degranulation of peritoneal mast cells, is almost as effective
on both types of cells. Thus, the MMC is functionally different from its connective
tissue counterpart. Whether MMC precursors are derived from Peyer's patches
and have a tendency to circulate to other mucosal tissues as do B- and T-cells is
currently under investigation.

The relationship between the MMC and the NK cell, especially found in the
epithelium, is one that bears closer examination, because the granulated lymphocyte in the epithelium has some of the characteristics associated with mast cells,
such as a low histamine content and granules that are metachromatic. Granulated
lymphocytes also contain mucopolysaccharides.[20] This relationship is strengthened even more by the recent observation that a NK clone has IgE receptors of the
same affinity as mast cells.[30] Our observations of the selectivity of localization in

different mucosal epithelia of different clones of NK cells may also shed some light on the putative relationship between NK cells and mast cells. The continuing study of these various populations, their derivation, distribution, and function may begin to clarify not only their relationships but also the factors that are responsible for their compartmentalization in these various tissues.

CONCLUSION

The concept of a common mucosal immunological system,[4] which was established by studies of the IgA system, must now be explored more fully, given evidence of the mucosal localization of B-cells of other isotypes and of T-cells. Recent evidence that NK cells and MMC in the intestine have unique characteristics dictate that these cell types be considered as candidates in the mucosal immunological networks.

REFERENCES

1. GOWANS, G. L. & E. J. KNIGHT. 1964. Proc. R. Soc. London Ser. B. **159:** 257–282.
2. HALL, J. 1979. Blood Cells **5:** 479–492.
3. CEBRA, J. J., P. J. GEARHART, J. F. HALSEY, J. L. HURWITZ & R. D. SHAHIN. 1980. J. Reticuloendothelial Soc. **28**(Suppl.): 61–71.
4. BIENENSTOCK, J. & A. D. BEFUS. 1980. Immunology **41:** 249–270.
5. ROUX, M. E., M. MCWILLIAMS, J. M. PHILLIPS-QUAGLIATA, P. WEISZ-CARRINGTON & M. E. LAMM. 1977. J. Exp. Med. **146:** 1311–1322.
6. WEISZ-CARRINGTON, P., M. E. ROUX, M. MCWILLIAMS, J. M. PHILLIPS-QUAGLIATA & M. E. LAMM. 1979. J. Immunol. **123:** 1705–1708.
7. JACKSON, D. E., E. T. LALLY, M. C. NAKAMURA & P. C. MONTGOMERY. 1981. Cell. Immunol. **63:** 203–209.
8. PIERCE, N. F. & W. C. CRAY JR. 1982. J. Immunol. **128:** 1311–1315.
9. MCDERMOTT, M. R. & J. BIENENSTOCK. 1979. J. Immunol. **122:** 1892–1898.
10. ELSON, C. O., J. A. HECK & W. STROBER. 1979. J. Exp. Med. **149:** 632–643.
11. KAWANISHI, H., L. E. SALTZMAN & W. STROBER. 1982. Fed. Proc. Fed. Am. Soc. Exp. Biol. **41**(3): 366.
12. GESNER, B. M., J. J. WOODRUFF & R. T. MCCLUSKEY. 1969. Am. J. Pathol. **57:** 215–230.
13. MCDERMOTT, M. R., D. A. MARK, A. D. BEFUS, B. S. BALIGA, R. M. SUSKIND & J. BIENENSTOCK. 1982. Immunology **45:** 1–5.
14. MIRSKI, S., A. D. BEFUS & J. BIENENSTOCK. 1982. Ann. N. Y. Acad. Sci. This volume.
15. HOWARD, J. C. 1972. J. Exp. Med. **135:** 185–199.
16. SMITH, M. E., A. F. MARTIN & W. L. FORD. 1980. Monogr. Allergy **16:** 203–232.
17. RUDZIK, O. & J. BIENENSTOCK. 1974. Lab. Invest. **30:** 260–266.
18. BEFUS, A. D. & J. BIENENSTOCK. 1982. Prog. Allergy **31:** 76–177.
19. GUY-GRAND, D., C. GRISCELLI & P. VASSALLI. 1978. J. Exp. Med. **148:** 1661–1677.
20. TAGLIABUE, A., A. D. BEFUS, D. A. CLARK & J. BIENENSTOCK. 1982. J Exp. Med. **155:** 1785–1796.
21. MINATO, N., L. REID & B. R. BLOOM. 1981. J. Exp. Med. **154:** 750–762.
22. CARROLL, A. M., M. A. PALLADINO, H. F. OETTGEN & M. deSOUSA. 1982. Fed. Proc. Fed. Am. Soc. Exp. Biol. **41:** 303.
23. ENERBACK, L. 1981. Monogr. Allergy **17:** 222–232.
24. DENBURG, J. A., A. D. BEFUS & J. BIENENSTOCK. 1980. Immunology **41:** 195–202.
25. BEFUS, A. D. & J. BIENENSTOCK. 1979. Immunology **38:**95–101.
26. MILLER, H. R. P., Y. NAWA & C. R. PARISH. 1979. Int. Arch. Allergy Appl. Immunol. **59:** 281–285.

27. BIENENSTOCK, J., A. D. BEFUS, F. PEARCE, J. DENBURG & R. GOODACRE. 1982. J. Allergy Clin. Immunol. **70:** 407–412.
28. BEFUS, A. D., F. L. PEARCE, J. GAULDIE, P. HORSEWOOD & J. BIENENSTOCK. 1982. J. Immunol. **128:** 2475–2480.
29. PEARCE, F. L., A. D. BEFUS, J. GAULDIE & J. BIENENSTOCK. 1982. J. Immunol. **128:** 2481–2486.
30. GALLI, S. J., A. M. DVORAK, T. ISHIZAKA, G. NABEL, H. DERSIMONIAN, H. CANTOR & H. F. DVORAK. 1982. Nature (London) **298:** 288–290.

DISCUSSION OF THE PAPER

M. PARMELEY (*University of Kansas Medical Center, Kansas City, Kans.*): In the studies that you have done on transferring mesenteric lymph nodes and looking at grain counts in the intestine, can you estimate the number of cell divisions that occur in either T- or B-cell populations?

J. BIENENSTOCK (*McMaster University, Hamilton, Ontario, Canada*): We have not determined the distribution of grain counts in T- and B-cells. We also have not yet made the calculations, but assuming equal distribution between T- and B-cells, these cells have divided many times. If we assume roughly eight hours for one cell division, then certainly three divisions have occurred in this tissue.

PARMELEY: You indicated that grain counts in the inoculum were greater than 40, so the cell is almost confluent with grains. Do you have any idea about cell repopulation and division at other mucosal sites?

BIENENSTOCK: We have studied the anatomical distribution from the duodenum downwards, but we do not yet have the final numbers. We are looking at it with time, with distribution up and down the G. I. tract, and also in terms of anatomic location within the villus.

PARMELEY: Have you looked at the distribution in salivary or mammary glands?

BIENENSTOCK: No.

W. STROBER (*National Institutes of Health, Bethesda, Md.*): Is there any relationship between the various NK-cell lines? Do they represent different stages of NK-cell differentiation?. This explanation could account for different distributions.

BIENENSTOCK: When some of these lines are cloned, they clearly shift in character, and this shift is a problem with clones in general. At present, however, the assumption has to be made that stages of differentiation ranging from NKI to TK form a continuum, and that we are simply picking out clones from this continuum. Because these cells are derived primarily from spleen, we will probably find more and more heterogeneity among these cells. Their capacity to localize to particular sites will depend upon surface characteristics, or characteristics of the donor population. The factors however, that are responsible for this situation are still unknown. Dr. Sousa has some information in regard to this phenomenon. When she gives interleukin 2 to an animal, together with cloned cytotoxic T-cells, a shift in the distribution of the cell type is observed. Our interest is in the biological significance, the factors that affect this shift, and the fact that some cells will go into the epithelium and that some cells will not.

T. B. TOMASI (*University of New Mexico, Albuquerque, N. Mex.*): Is there any difference in the Lyt phenotype depending on the NK target?

BEINENSTOCK: No, I do not think so.

IgA-IMMUNE COMPLEX RENAL DISEASE INDUCED BY MUCOSAL IMMUNIZATION*

Steven N. Emancipator† and Gloria R. Gallo

Department of Pathology
New York University Medical Center
New York, New York 10016

Michael E. Lamm‡

Case Western Reserve University
University Hospitals of Cleveland
Cleveland, Ohio 44106

INTRODUCTION

In 1969, Berger called attention to a type of glomerulonephritis in which deposition of immunoglobulin A (IgA) was prominent.[1] In the ensuing years, researchers have recognized IgA nephropathy as accounting for about 15% of cases of glomerulonephritis, whose common denominator is mesangial IgA as the predominant, though not necessarily the only, immunoglobulin class deposited.[2] Other features often associated include hematuria, proteinuria, circulating immune complexes containing IgA, and a clinical syndrome suggestive of an acute infectious episode, possibly viral in nature.

The association of a viral-type syndrome with deposition of IgA in the kidney has suggested that IgA nephropathy in general could result from a mucosal immune response to antigens present within the mucosa itself. Whereas such antigens could be derived from infectious agents or absorbed inert molecules, a replicating microorganism would provide an ongoing source of stimulation in which antigen continues to be produced after the initiation of the antibody response. In this view, which is by no means the only possibility, IgA nephropathy would be a variant of classical serum sickness, with IgA largely replacing IgG as the offending antibody, because of a mucosal rather than a systemic antigenic stimulus. Indeed, passively administered IgA-immune complexes have been shown to be capable of lodging in the kidney.[3]

With the above considerations in mind we sought to establish a model for human IgA nephropathy by prolonged oral immunization of mice to an inert protein antigen.

MATERIALS AND METHODS

Young adult BALB/c mice (Charles River Breeding Laboratories) were immunized to bovine gamma globulin (BGG) (Sigma Chemical Co.) by including it in

*This work was supported by NIH Grants AI-19073 and CA-32582 and a Grant-in-Aid from the Kidney Foundation of New York, Inc.

†Research Fellow of the Kidney Disease Institute, New York State Department of Health. Present address: Case Western Reserve University, Cleveland, Ohio.

‡To whom correspondence should be addressed.

171

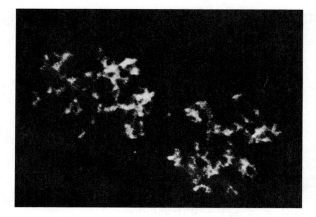

FIGURE 1. Glomerular mesangial deposits of IgA in a mouse orally immunized with BGG antigen, demonstrated by immunofluorescence using fluorescein conjugated anti-mouse IgA. (320×)

the drinking water at 1 mg per ml for 14 weeks, after which the animals were sacrificed.

Immunofluorescence was done on frozen tissue sections. Portions of kidney were fixed in glutaraldehyde, postfixed in osmium tetroxide, embedded in Epon, and stained with uranyl acetate and lead citrate for electron microscopy. All morphological evaluations were done on coded specimens.

Circulating antibody was measured by enzyme (peroxidase)-linked immunosorbent assay (ELISA)[4] of sera taken at sacrifice.

RESULTS AND DISCUSSION

By two criteria, the orally immunized mice generated a mucosal immune response. First of all, by double immunofluorescence, IgA-producing plasma cells capable of binding BGG were readily observable in the intestinal lamina propria and were distinctly more numerous than BGG-binding cells that make other classes of antibody or than BGG-binding cells in control, nonimmunized mice. Second, IgA antibody to BGG was present in the sera of immunized mice to a 16–32 fold greater extent than in controls ($p < 0.001$) (data not shown) as measured by ELISA. By contrast, there was no evidence of an IgG or IgM (systemic) antibody response in the serum.

By morphological evaluation, the kidneys were markedly different in orally

TABLE 1

GLOMERULAR IgA DETECTED BY IMMUNOFLUORESCENCE*

	No. Positive	No. Negative
Orally immunized mice	10	1
Controls	2	10

*$p < 0.01$.

immunized versus control mice. Thus, IgA was readily detected by immunofluorescence in the mesangial regions of the glomeruli in immunized animals, but not in control animals (FIGURE 1 and TABLE 1). On the other hand, there were no differences in glomerular IgM or IgG content between the two groups of mice. As would be expected, if the deposited IgA was part of an immune complex, BGG antigen was also detectable in the mesangial areas of the immunized group (TABLE 2). The data in TABLE 2 were obtained by indirect immunofluorescence in which the sections were incubated for 120 minutes with the first antiserum, that is, unconjugated anti-BGG. When the first incubation was carried out for only 30 minutes, fluorescence for BGG was faint, a result that afforded a means of investigating the specificity of the glomerular IgA. Thus, sections of kidney were initially incubated with 0.1 mg/ml BGG solution, washed, and then evaluated for glomerular BGG as above with a 30 minute incubation of the antiserum to BGG. In this case, fluorescence for BGG was bright in immunized mice but not in control mice, indicating that the glomerular IgA had specificity for BGG. The fact that mouse IgA was much more easily demonstrable than the BGG antigen in sections not treated with exogenous BGG suggests that the glomerular immune complexes were in antibody excess by the time of sacrifice. Mouse C3 was not observed in association with the immune complexes.

Electron dense mesangial deposits were observed in the majority of the orally immunized, but not at all in nonimmunized mice (FIGURE 2 and TABLE 3).

TABLE 2

GLOMERULAR ANTIGEN (BGG) DETECTED BY IMMUNOFLUORESCENCE*

	No. Positive	No. Negative
Orally immunized mice	9	2
Controls	3	9

*$p < 0.05$.

The overall results are most consistent with a mucosal, and hence predominantly IgA response to the ingested BGG antigen maintained in the drinking water throughout the 14 week period. In the initial stage of antibody formation it is likely that immune complexes were formed in the intestinal mucosa by locally produced IgA antibody and some absorbed, intact, or relatively intact, antigen, and that the complexes were in antigen excess and soluble. Once complexes in antigen excess reach the general circulation, they are prone to deposit in the kidney.[5] With the passage of time and a more vigorous immune response to the continuing antigenic stimulation, it may be hypothesized that increasing amounts of specific secretory IgA antibodies in the intestinal lumen would be able to diminish the absorption of antigen, which would be consistent with the failure to detect circulating BGG at the end of the experiment. At the same time the mucosal IgA-antibody response would continue to contribute to the pool of serum IgA, which in turn could bind to BGG antigen previously deposited in the kidney. If this were the case, deposits that had initially been in antigen excess, the kind most likely to be trapped in the kidney from the circulation, could be converted to antibody excess, which would be consistent with the observation that mouse IgA was much more easily demonstrated in the kidney than BGG.

Although the experimental model developed in this work resembles human

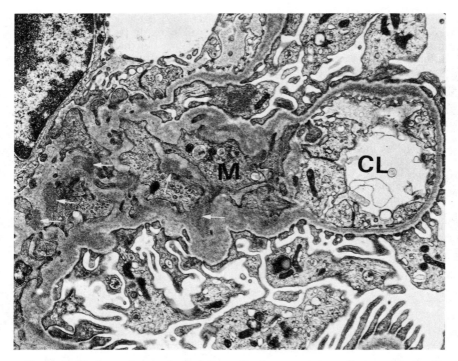

FIGURE 2. Electron micrograph of a glomerulus from a mouse orally immunized with BGG antigen depicting a capillary loop (CL) and mesangium (M) with electron dense deposits (arrows) in the mesangial matrix. (25,000×)

IgA nephropathy in its major features, namely a mesangial localization of mainly IgA immunoglobulin, it differs in one respect: complement (C3) is usually associated with the human disease, but is absent in the mouse model. A number of possibilities could explain this difference. First, in the experimental model, exogenous antigen is being absorbed into the body, whereas in the human disease, antigen may actually be produced within the mucosa, leading to a much greater amount and more acute deposition of immune complexes. Second, mouse IgA-immune complexes are not efficient activators of the alternative complement pathway; they do not bind C3, and activation appears to be incomplete and limited to the fluid phase.[6] Human IgA antibodies could conceivably be more effective activators of complement. Finally, in human IgA nephropathy, IgG

TABLE 3

MESANGIAL DEPOSITS DETECTED BY ELECTRON MICROSCOPY*

	No. Positive	No. Negative
Orally immunized mice	7	4
Controls	0	10

*$p < 0.01$.

antibodies, which are often also present, perhaps contribute to a greater utilization of complement by activating the classical pathway.

The normal function of secretory IgA is to combine with antigens "outside" the body, creating an immunological barrier to the absorption of foreign substances.[7] When, however, antigen in bulk is able to penetrate a mucosal surface or when an infection occurs there, an IgA response would lead to the formation of immune complexes within body tissues. Such complexes could then enter the circulation and reach the kidney. In this view IgA nephropathy would be an inappropriate result of the mucosal immune system responding appropriately to local stimulation.

REFERENCES

1. BERGER, J. 1969. Transplant. Proc. **1:** 939.
2. EMANCIPATOR, S.N., G.R. GALLO & M.E. LAMM. 1981. Surg. Pathol. Q. Index. **3:** 179.
3. RIFAI, A., P.A. SMALL JR., P.O. TEAGUE & E.M. AYOUB. 1979. J. Exp. Med. **150:** 1161.
4. ENGVALL, E. 1980. Methods Enzymol. **70:** 419.
5. COCHRANE, C.G. & D. KOFFLER. 1973. Adv. Immunol. **16:** 186.
6. PFAFFENBACH, G., M.E. LAMM & I. GIGLI. 1982. J. Exp. Med. **155:** 231.
7. LAMM, M.E. 1976. Adv. Immunol. **22:** 223.

DISCUSSION OF THE PAPER

D.F. KEREN (*University of Michigan, Ann Arbor, Mich.*): I was surprised that you had many negative mice in your negative group, because normally in the gut lumen, there are large amounts of different proteins and other complex antigens that must be stimulating some IgA response. If this is the case, why would you not expect to see IgA complexes in virtually all animals unless there was something peculiar about the antigen you employed?

M.E. LAMM (*Case Western Reserve University, Cleveland, Ohio*): It is improbable that there was something peculiar about the antigen used, compared to those generally encountered in the mouse diet. I would estimate that the dose of antigen employed (1 mg/ml) results in a relatively larger amount of antigen absorption than what is normally derived from their diet. For reasons you state, all observations were made double blind to make sure that we would not be misled by background levels.

J. MESTECKY (*University of Alabama in Birmingham*): Do you have any information about the size of the immune complexes in the bile compared to that found in the circulation? Is there a difference?

LAMM: At the time of sacrifice, which is 14 weeks, we do not find any evidence of circulating immune complexes containing antigen. What we are doing now is looking for immune complexes earlier in the course of events. We suspect that early in the course of the experiments, there are circulating immune complexes that are relatively small. If our assumption is correct, then as the IgA immune response becomes greater, we would diminish further absorption of the antigen. Perhaps this would explain the lack of circulating immune complexes at the end of the experiment.

MESTECKY: Did you detect secretory antibodies in saliva or in milk?

LAMM: We have not examined saliva or milk.

MESTECKY: This experiment is important because I would expect that the antigen would be less absorbed.

T.B. TOMASI (*University of N. Mexico, Albuquerque, N. Mex.*): Have you looked at the skin? In dermatitis herpetiformis, there are deposits that are pretty specific for IgA and it has recently been demonstrated that if you feed patients with dermatitis herpetiformis material containing gluten, that almost 100% will have IgA, specifically IgA complexes to this antigen, which is then deposited in the skin. In that case, you can show by elution, which is another technique that you could use in your kidney studies, that the antigen is deposited there. It is sometimes hard to show this fact by immunofluorescence for the reasons you have already described.

LAMM: I agree; in fact, we are doing that now and we should have the answer in a couple of weeks. We were not thinking along those lines initially, and then we found that we could readily find the IgA-immune complexes in the kidney; we agreed that we should look at the skin also.

SALIVARY ANTIBODIES AND SYSTEMIC TOLERANCE IN MICE AFTER ORAL IMMUNIZATION WITH BACTERIAL ANTIGENS*

S. J. Challacombe

Department of Oral Immunology and Microbiology
Guy's Hospital Medical and Dental Schools
London, SE1 9RT England

INTRODUCTION

For many years immunologists have known that oral immunization may lead to the production of systemic tolerance when the animal is challenged.[1,2] It is now generally accepted that under appropriate conditions, systemic tolerance can be induced by oral or intragastric immunization with protein antigens.[3-5] This observation has been made in a number of animal species with a variety of different antigens.

An alternative response resulting from oral immunization is the production of antibodies in secretions. Intragastric immunization may give rise to antibodies in the gastrointestinal (GI) tract,[6] but may also give rise to antibodies in distant sites such as the mammary glands,[7] lacrimal glands,[8] or salivary glands.[9] This discovery has led to the concept of a common enteromucosal secretory antibody system,[10] in which oral immunization leads to the release of antibody precursor cells from the Peyer's patches (PP) that migrate to a variety of mucosal sites.

Previous work has shown that deposition of antigen in the upper GI tract can give rise to secretory antibodies and systemic tolerance at the same time,[11] or to enhanced antigen exclusion from the GI tract (presumably a function of secretory antibodies) at the same time as systemic tolerance.[12] In this study we show that oral immunization with bacteria may give rise not only to salivary antibodies, but also may result in systemic priming rather than tolerance. An attempt is also made to characterize the antibody response in saliva after oral immunization with whole bacteria, and this response is shown to be dose dependent, age dependent and of short duration. Salivary antibodies can be induced in the presence of systemic tolerance or priming.

METHODS

Animals

CBA/CA or BALB/c mice (OLAC Ltd., Bicester, England) were used throughout. In all experiments groups of six or more mice were used. Except in age-related experiments, the mice were aged between 8 and 12 weeks at the beginning of the experiments.

*This work was performed with a grant from the Medical Research Council.

0077-8923/83/0409-0177 $1.75/0 © 1983, NYAS

Bacteria

Whole cells of *Streptococcus mutans* or *Actinomyces viscosus* were prepared as previously described.[11] Antigen I/II is a protein antigen of *S. mutans* of 185,000 molecular weight, and was purified by methods described in detail elsewhere.[13,14] Ovalbumin was obtained from Sigma Chemical Company (Poole, Dorset, England).

Preparation of Cell Suspensions

Cell suspensions from mesenteric lymph nodes (MLN), PP or spleens were prepared as described.[15] For cell transfer experiments, cells were suspended at 2×10^8 per ml in RPMI-1640 medium (Grand Island Biological Co., Grand Island, N.Y.)

Samples

Serum was collected from clotted blood obtained from the tail, and saliva was obtained by injecting 1mg/kg pilocarpine intraperitoneally and allowing the animals to salivate into glass tubes. Saliva was centrifuged at 4,000 rpm for 10 minutes to remove debris.

Antibody Assays

Serum and salivary antibodies to whole cells of *S. mutans*, antigen I/II, or to ovalbumin were assayed by a solid phase radioimmunoassay.[16] Briefly, whole cells of *S. mutans* were bound to the polystyrene wells with methylglyoxal, and the wells were blocked with 0.5% bovine serum albumin overnight at room temperature. Samples of serum (1:100), or saliva (1:50) were then incubated with the bound bacteria for 90 minutes at 37°C. After washing, rabbit antimouse IgG, IgA, or IgM was added in order to obtain isotype specificity and incubated for 90 minute at 37°C. After further washing, radiolabeled sheep anti-rabbit was added and incubated for one hour. After washing, the wells were counted individually. All assays were performed in duplicate. For antibodies to ovalbumin and antigen I/II, the same method was used except that the antigens were bound directly to the polystyrene by overnight incubation in phosphate-buffered saline.

Isotype specificity of the assay was confirmed by titration of the antisera against purified myeloma IgG, IgA, and IgM, kindly supplied by Dr. D. McKean, Mayo Clinic, Rochester, Minn. Antibodies to dinitrophenol (DNP) were assayed by coating wells with dinitrophenylated ovalbumin when the animals were immunized with dinitrophenylated *S. mutans* and vice versa. Less than nanogram amounts of antibody were detectable. Antibodies to trinitrophenol (TNP) were assayed by passive hemagglutination.

Intragastric Immunization

Animals were anesthetized with ether and immunized intragastrically as described.[11] Antigens were given in a volume of 0.5ml (in saline), and controls given saline alone.[11]

Plaque-Forming Cell (PFC) Assay

PFC were assayed using a modification[17] of the method of Cunningham.[18] Chambers were incubated for one hour at 37°C for direct PFC and for two hours for IgG and IgA plaques.

Cell Transfer Experiments

MLN, PP, or spleens were taken four days after intragastric immunization. Into syngeneic recipients 40 × 10⁶ cells were transferred intravenously, and the mice were challenged with the antigen in complete adjuvant (H37 Ra) one day and two weeks after transfer. With S. mutans, 10⁸ organisms were given in 100 μl, and with ovalbumin 100μg was given.

In vitro antibody production. Antibody produced by spleen cell cultures of immunized mice was assayed by a modification of the method of Yarchoan et al.[19] as described in detail elsewhere.[20] Briefly, 5 × 10⁶ spleen cells were cultured in triplicate in the presence of antigen bound to the solid phase, for 4 or 24 hours at 37°C. After washing in EDTA buffer, antibodies were assayed by radioassay as described above.

RESULTS

Salivary Antibody Responses

Single Dose Immunizations

Mice were immunized intragastrically with a single dose of nonviable S. mutans in concentrations from 10⁸ to 10¹⁰ organisms, or with ovalbumin at 1, 5, 10, or 20mg. Single intragastric immunizations did not lead to a reproducible IgA antibody response in saliva. Antibodies could be detected in some experiments, but not on every occasion.

If these same animals, however, were given a second single intragastric dose of antigen eight weeks later, a significant salivary IgA response was detected (FIGURE 1). This was detectable in 7 days and reached maximal levels between days 14 and 21. The response was of short duration and had fallen to preimmune levels by day 35. The response appeared to be highly dose-dependent, and the lower concentration of bacteria given (10⁸) gave a greater response than the higher (10¹⁰) concentration. No serum antibodies of any isotype were detectable.

Weekly Immunizations

When animals were immunized intragastrically weekly with doses of S. mutans from 10⁸–10¹⁰ organisms, or ovalbumin from 1–20mg, and saliva samples assayed weekly, a variable response was found that was on some occasions significantly greater than in the animals immunized with saline. Nevertheless, no consistent pattern of antibody was detected, and a prolonged response was not found.

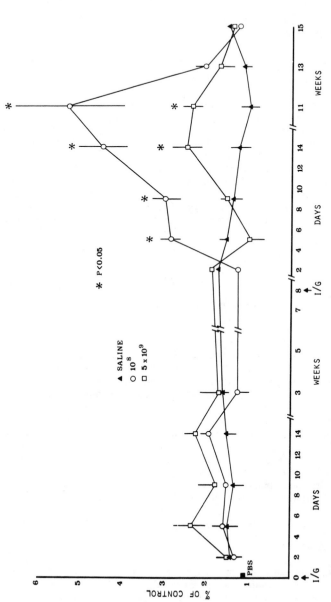

FIGURE 1. Salivary antibody response after intragastric (I/G) immunization with *S. mutans*. Groups of six CBA mice were given a single intragastric challenge at weeks 0 and 8, indicated by arrows. IgA antibodies assayed by radioassay. Mean + − SE antibody units (% of control).

Triple Intragastric Immunization

By contrast to single intragastric immunizations, three consecutive daily intragastric immunizations were able to induce a definite, though small, salivary IgA response. With *S. mutans*, salivary antibodies were detectable after 12 days, and with dinitrophenylated *S. mutans*, antibodies to both *S. mutans* and DNP was detectable at this time (TABLE 1A).

Similarly intragastric immunization with ovalbumin-DNP resulted in detectable salivary IgA antibodies to both hapten and carrier protein in 12 days (TABLE 1B), and immunization with ovalbumin alone resulted only in antibodies to

TABLE 1

SALIVARY ANTIBODIES AFTER TRIPLE INTRAGASTRIC IMMUNIZATION OF CBA/CA MICE*

A. *Streptococcus mutans*

Group	Antibodies to:	
	Streptococcus mutans	DNP
Saline	2.2 ± 0.4	2.02 ± 0.5
S. mutans	3.9 ± 0.5‡	3.65 ± 1.8
S. mutans treated with DNP	3.7 ± 0.6‡	6.29 ± 1.2‡

B. Ovalbumin

Group	Antibodies to:		
	OVA	DNP	TNP
Saline	2.07 ± 0.3	2.49 ± 0.6	0.3 ± 0.2
OVA	4.46 ± 0.8†	2.38 ± 0.7	0.2 ± 0.2
OVA treated with DNP	2.36 ± 0.4	3.48 ± 0.2†	2.3 ± 0.7†

*Mice immunized intragastrically with A.) *S. mutans* or *S. mutans* treated with DNP (4×10^9) and B.) Ovalbumin or ovalbumin treated with DNP (5mg). Saliva taken 12 days later, and antibodies assayed by radioassay or passive hamagglutination (trinitrophenol; TNP) (see Methods). Antibodies expressed as mean ± SE of antibody units (% of standard), or mean Log_2 titer ± SE (starting dilution 1:5) five to six animals/group.
†p < 0.02
‡p < 0.01

ovalbumin. Antibodies to DNP assayed by radioassay correlated with those detected to cross-reactive TNP by passive hamagglutination (TABLE 1B). No serum antibodies were detectable in any group.

Duration of Salivary Response

Triple intragastric immunization with bacterial cells at 10^8, 10^9, and 10^{10} was examined. A significant salivary IgA antibody response was detectable with the 10^8 dose (TABLE 2). This response was maximal between 14 and 21 days after intragastric immunization, but by 28 days had fallen to preimmune levels. The kinetics of the response were similar to those seen after a second single intragastric immunization (FIGURE 1). With the highest dose examined (10^{10}), an apparent initial response at 7 days was not maintained. The 10^9 dose resulted in an intermediate response between that of 10^8 and 10^{10}.

TABLE 2

DURATION OF SALIVARY ANTIBODY RESPONSE TO STREPTOCOCCUS MUTANS AFTER
INTRAGASTRIC IMMUNIZATION*

Group	Week				
	0	1	2	3	4
Saline	2.1 ± 0.6	1.7 ± 1.2	3.0 ± 1.2	3.1 ± 0.7	2.9 ± 1.1
10^8	1.8 ± 0.8	2.5 ± 0.6	6.7 ± 1.2†	5.9 ± 0.2‡	4.2 ± 1.3
10^9	2.0 ± 1.2	3.7 ± 2.1	4.3 ± 1.6	2.7 ± 0.5	4.3 ± 1.4
10^{10}	2.3 ± 0.9	3.8 ± 0.6	2.3 ± 1.3	1.7 ± 1.4	3.9 ± 0.8

*Mice given triple intragastric immunization of Streptococcus mutans. Results expressed as mean ± SE antibody units (% of standard immune serum at 10^4 dilution). Each group contained six mice.
†$p < 0.05$
‡$p < 0.01$ compared with control group

Effect of Age

The effect of age on the salivary response to intragastric immunization was examined by giving 10^{10} S. mutans to groups of CBA mice aged 5, 11, or 17 weeks and comparing the salivary antibody titers with mice given saline intragastrically. In young mice (5 weeks old) some nonspecific uptake was found in the control

TABLE 3

THE EFFECT OF AGE ON THE INDUCTION OF SALIVARY ANTIBODIES BY
INTRAGASTRIC IMMUNIZATION‡

Streptococcus mutans* Age		Day 7	Day 14
5 Weeks	Control	3.1 ± 0.7	2.4 ± 0.3
	Immunized	1.4 ± 0.5	0.5 ± 0.2
11 Weeks	Control	1.3 ± 0.7	0.6 ± 0.5
	Immunized	2.6 ± 0.9	2.8 ± 0.3†
17 Weeks	Control	1.5 ± 0.5	1.3 ± 0.5
	Immunized	5.6 ± 0.6*	5.7 ± 0.5†
Ovalbumin† Age		Day 7	Day 14
5 Weeks	Control	0.8 ± 0.5	0.8 ± 0.7
	Immunized	1.5 ± 0.9	3.2 ± 0.7
11 Weeks	Control	0.8 ± 0.7	1.2 ± 1.4
	Immunized	1.2 ± 0.5	1.6 ± 0.5
17 Weeks	Control	0.9 ± 0.5	2.8 ± 1.0
	Immunized	6.0 ± 1.0*	7.9 ± 0.9†

*CBA/CA mice given 10^{10} Streptococcus mutans intragastrically on three consecutive days. Saliva assayed 7 and 14 days later. Results expressed as antibody units (% standard) ± SE of groups of six mice.
†CBA/CA mice given 20 mg ovalbumin intragastrically on three consecutive days. Results expressed as antibody units (% of standard) ± SE of groups of six mice.
‡$p < 0.01$

animals (TABLE 3). In saliva samples taken 7 days after intragastric immunization, a significant response was found only in the older animals aged 17 weeks ($p < 0.01$, TABLE 3). A similar pattern of results was found in saliva taken after 14 days, when a significant response was found in older animals, but not in young animals. At this time, the response in 11 week old animals also reached statistical significance ($p < 0.05$).

When the experiment was repeated using ovalbumin (20 mg intragastrically), essentially identical results were obtained, except that nonspecific uptake was not found in young animals. Animals aged 17 weeks showed a mean antibody response, in saliva samples taken at 7 days, of 6.0 ± 1.0 (SE) antibody units, compared with 0.9 ± 0.5 in controls ($p < 0.001$), whereas no significant response was detectable in animals aged 5 or 11 weeks (TABLE 3).

Systemic Response to Intragastric Immunization

Ovalbumin

Systemic challenge of animals given ovalbumin by intragastric immunization routinely resulted in a suppression of the subsequent development of serum antibodies. An example is shown in TABLE 4, where single intragastric doses of 1, 5, or 20 mg ovalbumin were followed by intraperitoneal challenge of 100 μg of ovalbumin in adjuvant, one and three weeks later. A dose-dependent suppression of the serum antibody response was apparent in the IgG, IgA, and IgM classes (TABLE 4). With an intragastric dose of 20 mg ovalbumin, suppression of the IgG response by 60%, IgA by 50%, and IgM by 52% was found.

S. mutans

Groups of CBA or BALB/c mice were given triple intragastric doses of bacteria, followed by intraperitoneal challenge of 10^8 bacteria in adjuvant, one and three weeks later. A dose-dependent enhancement of the subsequent serum antibody response was seen (TABLE 5). Serum taken one week after the second intraperitoneal injection showed a significant enhancement of antibodies of the IgG, IgA, and IgM classes ($p < 0.001$). With the highest concentration of bacteria, enhancement of the IgG response was greater than threefold, and with IgA and IgM, was greater than twofold (TABLE 5).

Animals given a single intragastric dose of 10^{10} S. mutans showed a similar enhancement of the subsequent antibody response of greater than twofold for each of the three isotypes. (data not shown)

The enhancement was apparently specific in that intragastric immunization with Actinomyces viscosus cells did not result in an increased systemic response to S. mutans (TABLE 6). In addition, this enhancement was probably due to the induction of T-helper cells because in a hapten carrier system, intragastric immunization with S. mutans resulted in an enhanced systemic response to DNP after intraperitoneal challenge with dinitrophenylated S. mutans as assayed by PFC. This enhancement was proportional to the number of intragastric doses of S. mutans (TABLE 6). The direct PFC assay was unaffected by prior intragastric immunization.

TABLE 4

SERUM ANTIBODIES AFTER LOCAL [INTRAGASTRIC] AND SYSTEMIC [INTRAPERITONEAL] IMMUNIZATION WITH OVALBUMIN*

Intragastric Group	IgG	Percentage Decrease	IgM	Percentage Decrease	IgA	Percentage Decrease
Saline	7,280 + 630		4,880 + 320		2,800 + 180	
1 mg	8,640 + 720	(+18)	3,820 + 190	(22)	2,170 + 130	(23)
5 mg	4,960 + 360	(32)†	3,440 + 230	(30)†	1,980 + 210	(29)†
20 mg	2,880 + 210	(61)‡	2,350 + 160	(52)‡	1,400 + 190	(50)‡

*Results as mean cpm + SE; background values deducted. Mice given single intragastric immunization followed by intraperitoneal immunization one and three weeks later. Serum antibodies assayed at nine weeks.
†p < 0.02
‡p < 0.001

TABLE 5

SERUM ANTIBODIES AFTER LOCAL [INTRAGASTRIC] AND SYSTEMIC [INTRAPERITONEAL] IMMUNIZATION WITH *STREPTOCOCCUS MUTANS**

| Intragastric | Antibodies to Streptococcus mutans [Mean CPM ± SE] Isotype | | | | | |
	IgG	Percentage Increase	IgM	Percentage Increase	IgA	Percentage Increase
Saline	2,137 ± 308		782 ± 76		315 ± 50	
10^8	6,075 ± 1,114	[184]‡	820 ± 131	(4)	343 ± 101	(8)
10^9	7,640 ± 1,131	[257]§	1,427 ± 193	[82]†	583 ± 196	(85)
10^{10}	11,601 ± 2,127	[443]§	1,926 ± 400	[146]†	662 ± 218	[110]†

*CBA mice given 3 intragastric immunizations followed by 2 intraperitoneal immunizations one and three weeks later. Serum antibodies assayed one week after last injection.

†p < 0.02
‡p < 0.01
§p < 0.001

Antigen I/II

Antigen I/II is a surface antigen of S. *mutans*. Intragastric immunization with S. *mutans* followed by intraperitoneal challenge with S. *mutans* led to a similar enhancement of the serum antibody response to antigen I/II (FIGURE 2) as seen for whole cells (TABLE 5). A significant enhancement was found with IgG ($p < 0.01$) and IgA ($p < 0.02$) antibodies at the higher doses of S. *mutans*, but the IgA and IgM responses were low and the enhancement with serum IgM did not reach statistical significance.

By contrast, intragastric immunization with 1, 10, and 50 μg of soluble antigen I/II followed by intraperitoneal challenge of 2 μg of I/II in adjuvant resulted in a suppression of the subsequent systemic response as assayed by PFC (FIGURE 3).

TABLE 6

SPECIFICITY OF ENHANCEMENT OF SYSTEMIC RESPONSE BY INTRAGASTRIC IMMUNIZATION WITH *STREPTOCOCCUS MUTANS**

Intragastric Group	Intraperitoneal	Anti-DNP Plaque-Forming Cells/10^7 Spleen Cells		Percentage Increase
		Direct	IgG	
Saline × 3	Streptococcus mutans-DNP	5,923 ± 849	4,747 ± 607	
Streptococcus mutans × 1	Streptococcus mutans-DNP	5,787 ± 732	6,903 ± 1,798	45%
Streptococcus mutans × 2	Streptococcus mutans-DNP	5,149 ± 807	8,077 ± 1,022	70%†
Streptococcus mutans × 3	Streptococcus mutans-DNP	5,350 ± 699	11,202 ± 2,506	136%†
Actinomyces viscosus	Streptococcus mutans-DNP	4,727 ± 762	5,325 ± 1,017	12%

*CBA mice given 1, 2, or 3 doses of 10^{10} Streptococcus *mutans* or 3 doses of 10^{10} Actinomyces *viscosus* intragastrically followed by intraperitoneal challenge with 10^8 dinitrophenylated Streptococcus *mutans* in adjuvant one and three weeks later. PFC assayed five days after second intraperitoneal injection.
†p < 0.02

Intragastric doses of 10 or 50 μg of antigen I/II lead to significantly depressed PFC responses measured by the direct (IgM) or indirect (IgA and IgG) techniques.

Adoptive Transfer

CBA mice were immunized (×3) intragastrically with S. *mutans*. Four days later, serum and cells from PP, MLN, and spleen were collected. Syngeneic recipients were given 40 × 10^6 cells or 0.2 ml serum intravenously and were then challenged intraperitoneally with S. *mutans* one and fourteen days later. One week after the second intraperioneal injection, spleen cells were collected and assayed for *in vitro* antibody production. Transfer of MLN cells resulted in a small, but statistically significant enhancement of the IgG and IgA responses (TABLE 7). No enhancement was seen after transfer of PP, spleen, or serum.

In a similar experiment with ovalbumin in BALB/c mice, transfer of MLN

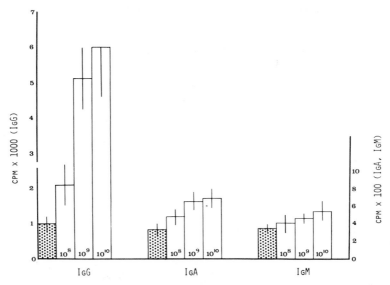

FIGURE 2. Serum antibodies to antigen I/II after intragastric and intraperitoneal immunization with *S. mutans*. CBA mice given three intragastric immunizations followed by two intraperitoneal challenges one and three weeks later. Antibodies assayed at week four.

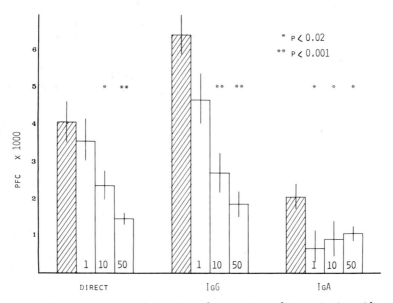

FIGURE 3. PFC response after intragastric and intraperitoneal immunization with antigen I/II. Balb/c mice given three intragastric immunizations with I/II, followed by two intraperitoneal immunizations of 2µg I/II in adjuvant, one and three weeks later.

TABLE 7

ANTIBODY PRODUCTION *IN VITRO* AFTER PASSIVE TRANSFER OF CELLS
OR SERUM FROM MICE GIVEN *STREPTOCOCCUS MUTANS* INTRAGASTRICALLY*

Cells Transferred	IgG	IgA	IgM
None	27.9 ± 0.6	5.7 ± 0.5	2.4 ± 0.4
Peyer's Patches	27.9 ± 0.3	4.7 ± 0.8	2.4 ± 0.6
Mesenteric Lymph Node	31.1 ± 1.2†	7.5 ± 0.4‡	2.2 ± 0.4
Spleen	28.2 ± 1.4	5.6 ± 0.6	1.9 ± 0.5
Serum	28.0 ± 1.7	4.7 ± 0.3	2.3 ± 0.3

*Results expressed as mean ± S.E. antibody units (approx. 1 ng) per culture of 5×10^6 spleen cells. Six mice per group.
†$p < 0.05$
‡$p < 0.02$

cells resulted in a significant inhibition of the IgG responses in the recipients (TABLE 8), whereas transfer of PP and spleen cells did not result in significant suppression. The IgA and IgM responses were not significantly lower than controls. Passive transfer of serum also resulted in significant suppression of the IgG ($p < 0.01$) and IgA ($p < 0.02$) responses in the recipients (TABLE 8).

DISCUSSION

Intragastric immunization may lead to the simultaneous induction of secretory antibodies and systemic suppression;[11] this raises intriguing questions as to the relationship of the two systems. In this paper it has been shown that intragastric immunization with soluble proteins may lead to the induction of salivary antibodies and systemic tolerance, but also that intragastric immunization with bacterial cells may lead to the simultaneous induction of salivary antibodies and systemic priming. This phenomenon suggests that the nature of the antigen may determine whether priming or tolerance results from intragastric immunization.

After intraperitoneal challenge, a marked contrast was found in the serum antibody response between mice that had been intragastrically given ovalbumin

TABLE 8

ANTIBODY PRODUCTION *IN VITRO* AFTER PASSIVE TRANSFER OF CELLS
OR SERUM FROM MICE GIVEN OVALBUMIN INTRAGASTRICALLY*

Cells Transferred	IgG	IgA	IgM
None	22.9 ± 2.8	5.4 ± 0.7	2.2 ± 0.3
Peyer's Patches	17.2 ± 1.5	3.9 ± 0.5	2.9 ± 0.2
Mesenteric Lymph Node	13.3 ± 1.7†	4.9 ± 0.8	1.9 ± 0.1
Spleen	17.1 ± 1.2	4.2 ± 0.2	2.4 ± 0.1
Serum	11.4 ± 1.9‡	3.9 ± 0.4†	1.9 ± 0.2

*Results expressed as mean ± SE antibody units (approx. 1 ng) per culture of 5×10^6 spleen cells. Six mice per group.
†$p < 0.02$
‡$p < 0.01$

and *S. mutans*. In ovalbumin animals, a suppression of all three isotypes was found, including IgA. This suppression is of interest because studies have shown that PP are a source of IgA-specific T-helper cells as well as IgG-specific suppressor cells.[32] A dichotomy between serum IgG and IgA was not apparent in the studies reported here.

With *S. mutans*, intragastric immunization resulted in priming rather than tolerance. Enhancement of the serum antibody response was apparent with all three isotypes (TABLE 5), and was dose-dependent. Enhancement was found with a single intragastric dose even when no salivary antibodies could be detected.

When antibodies to an isolated surface protein antigen of *S. mutans* were assayed in animals given whole cells intragastrically and intraperitoneally, a similar enhancement was found. It has been reported that the systemic response to surface antigens of bacteria after oral immunization may differ, and that it is possible to have tolerance to one antigen and enhancement to another.[34] If antigen I/II was used for intragastric and intraperitoneal immunization, then tolerance was seen (FIGURE 3). Doses of 10 μg, given three times intragastrically, were sufficient to cause significant suppression of PFC of all three isotypes.

These observations suggest that the form of the antigen may determine the type of the systemic response. Soluble proteins lead in most instances to tolerance, whereas particulate antigens such as bacteria may result in an enhanced systemic response. This may be due to differential handling of antigens in PP.[35]

Several different mechanisms have been implicated in the induction and maintenance of oral tolerance. In this study two mechanisms may be operative because both MLN cells and serum were able to transfer tolerance to ovalbumin. An immunosuppressive effect of IgG has been shown *in vitro*,[36] but other factors may be responsible for tolerance *in vivo*.[37,38] The relative importance of cellular and humoral mechanisms is not clear.

The salivary glands can be accepted as part of the enteromucosal system, because salivary antibodies have been induced after intragastric immunization in several species,[8,9,11,21,22] and in addition, IgA-bearing lymphocytes have been shown to migrate from MLN to the salivary glands.[23]

The characteristics of a secretory response after oral immunization have been ill-defined, and it has not been clear whether an anamnestic response can be achieved. Peyer's patches appear to be the source of the antigen-sensitive cells found in the secretory system after oral immunization,[24,25] and possibly such cells reside for a time in the MLN before migrating to salivary glands.[23] Repeated oral immunization may therefore be expected to increase the total number of antigen-sensitive cells arriving at secretory tissue, whereas local antigenic stimulus may increase proliferation and recruitment.[25] Certainly most studies that have successfully induced a salivary response by oral immunization have used long-term feeding of antigen or nonviable bacteria.[21,26]

In this study a single intragastric immunization did not consistently result in a significant salivary response, whereas a more reproducible response was found after three daily intragastric challenges. The failure to consistently detect antibodies after a single intragastric dose may have been due to the detection method used. The values obtained in positive salivas (approx. 5-6% of standard) were equivalent to less than 10 ng of antibody/ml of saliva. These values, however, are calculated on affinity-purified antibody; nonantibody factors in saliva are able to inhibit the detection of antibodies in a radioassay.[26] It is worth noting that Lake *et al.*[28] have shown that deposition of antigen in the gut may lead to goblet-cell mucus release. Although this release has not been shown for saliva, it is possible that any increase in the mucus content could interfere with the detection of antibody.

A repeat immunization of animals who had been given a single intragastric dose of S. mutans resulted in a more consistent response in saliva. This observation clearly suggested an anamnestic response, though the lower (10^8) dose of S. mutans induced a greater salivary response than the 10^{10} one (FIGURE 1). This dose-dependence was also a feature of the salivary response after triple intragastric immunization (TABLE 2) and is consistent with the findings of Michalek et al.[26] in the rat. Because no serum antibodies were detected in any of these experiments, these observations suggest that it is possible to induce a state of hyporesponsiveness to large antigen doses in secretory tissue, as well as in the systemic system. This hyporesponsiveness to large antigen doses may be altered by systemic challenge intraperitoneally.[27]

The salivary antibody response was short-lived (FIGURE 1). This finding is consistent with studies in mice,[29] man,[8] and monkeys,[9] and suggests that after migration of antigen-sensitive cells from PP to salivary glands, cells do not continue to secrete antibodies in the absence of any local challenge.

The salivary response appeared to be age-dependent (TABLE 3) with the greatest salivary responses to either S. mutans or ovalbumin in animals of 17 weeks of age. This phenomenon may indicate that maturation of the secretory response is delayed in comparison with the systemic immune system, although the reverse is thought to be true in man.[30] Mice of all ages were capable of mounting a PFC response, and significant suppression of the PFC response after intragastric application of ovalbumin was found in all ages. (data not shown) It is also possible that priming by cross-reactive antigens in the environment occurred, but the diet did not contain ovalbumin, and S. mutans was not part of the normal murine flora. It is notable that Trefts et al.[31] have found that the IgA antipolysaccharide response in vitro of MLN and spleen cells was highly age-dependent, with significant responses being found only in older mice. Systemic tolerance after oral immunization has been found in mice only two weeks old.[33]

This study shows that deposition of antigen in the GI tract in mice may lead to modulation of the secretory and systemic immune systems. Either system may be stimulated or may become hyporesponsive, and these events can apparently occur independently of one another.

CONCLUSIONS

Secretory and systemic antibody responses were examined after intragastric immunization in mice with bacteria or soluble proteins.

Neither single nor weekly intragastric immunizations gave a reproducible salivary antibody response. A repeated immunization of animals eight weeks later with S. mutans resulted in an IgA salivary antibody response of short duration.

Three daily intragastric challenges with S. mutans or ovalbumin gave a salivary response of short duration and was dose-dependent with apparent hyporesponsiveness with higher antigen doses.

Salivary responses were age-dependent with the greatest responses in mice of 17 weeks of age or older.

Systemic challenge in animals given soluble proteins intragastrically, led to tolerance of antibodies of each of the major isotypes.

Systemic challenge of animals given whole bacteria intragastrically, led to enhancement of antibodies of each isotype.

Tolerance and enhancement could be transferred to syngeneic recipients with MLN cells.

ACKNOWLEDGMENT

I wish to thank Mrs. A. S. Rees for valuable assistance.

REFERENCES

1. WELLS H. G. 1911. Studies on the chemistry of anaphylaxis. III. Experiments with isolated proteins, especially those of the hens egg. J. Infect. Dis. **9:** 147–171.
2. CHASE, M. W. 1946. Inhibition of experimental drug allergy by prior feeding of the sensitizing agent. Proc. Soc. Exp. Biol. Med. **61:** 257–259.
3. THOMAS, H. C. & D. M. V. PARROTT. 1974. The induction of tolerance to soluble protein antigens by oral administration. Immunology **27:** 631–639.
4. VAZ, N. M., L. C. S. MAIA, D. G. HANSON & J. M. LYNCH. 1977. Inhibition of homocytotropic antibody response in adult inbred mice by previous feeding of the specific antigen. J. Allergy Clin. Immunol. **60:** 110–116.
5. RICHMAN, L. K., J. M. CHILLER, W. R. BROWN, D. G. HANSON & N. M. VAZ. 1978. Enterically induced immunologic tolerance. I. Induction of suppressor T. lymphocytes by intragastric administration of soluble proteins. J. Immunol. **121:** 2429–2434.
6. PIERCE, N. F. & R. B. SACK. 1977. Immune response of the intestinal mucosa to cholera toxoid. J. Infect. Dis. **136:** 5113–5117.
7. GOLDBLUM, R. M., S. AHLSTEDT, B. CARLSSON, L. A. HANSON, U. JODAL, G. LIDIN-JANSON, & A. SOHL. 1975. Antibody forming cells in human colostrum after oral immunization. Nature (London) **257:** 797–799.
8. MESTECKY, J., J. R. MCGHEE, R. R. ARNOLD, S. M. MICHALEK, S. M. PRINCE & J. C. BABB. 1978. Selective induction of an immune response in human external secretions by ingestion of bacterial antigen. J. Clin. Invest. **61:** 731–737.
9. CHALLACOMBE, S. J. & T. LEHNER. 1980. Salivary antibody responses in rhesus monkeys immunized with Streptococcus mutans by the oral, submucosal or subcutaneous routes. Arch. Oral Biol. **24:** 917–925.
10. BIENENSTOCK, J., M. MCDERMOTT & A. D. BEFUS. 1979. A common mucosal immune system. *In* Immunology of breast milk P. L. Oga and D. Dayton, Ed.: 91–111. Review Press. New York.
11. CHALLACOMBE, S. J. & T. B. TOMASI. 1980. Systemic tolerance and secretory immunity after oral immunisation. J. Exp. Med. **152:** 1459–1472.
12. SWARBRICK, E. T., C. R. STOKES & J. F. SOOTHILL. 1979. Absorption of antigens after oral immunisation and the simultaneous induction of specific systemic tolerance. Gut **20:** 121–125.
13. RUSSELL, M. W. & T. LEHNER. 1978. Characterisation of antigens extracted from cells and culture fluids of Streptococcus mutans serotype c. Arch. Oral Biol. **23:** 7–15.
14. RUSSELL, M. W. 1978. Purification and properties of a protein surface antigen of Streptococcus mutans. Microbios **25:** 7–18.
15. KRCO, C. J., S. J. CHALLACOMBE, W. P. LAFUSE, C. S. DAVID & T. B. TOMASI, JR. 1981. Expression of Ia antigens by mouse Peyer's patch cells. Cell. Immunol. **57:** 420–426.
16. CZERKINSKY, C., A. S. REES, L. A. BERGMEIER & S. J. CHALLACOMBE. 1983. The detection and specificity of class specific antibodies to whole bacteria using a solid phase radioimmunoassay. Submitted for publication.
17. KONTIAINEN, S. & M. FELDMAN. 1975. Conditions for inducing T. helper cells *in vitro*. Scand. J. Immunol. **4:** 121–128.

18. CUNNINGHAM, A. & A. SZENBERG. 1968. Further improvement in plaque techniques for detecting single antibody forming cells. Immunology **14:** 599–600.

19. YARCHOAN, R., B. R. MURPHY, W. STROBER, H. S. SCHNEIDER & D. L. NELSON. 1981. Specific anti-influenza virus antibody production *in vitro* by human peripheral blood mononuclear cells. J. Immunol. **127:** 2588–2594.

20. CHALLACOMBE, S. J., C. CZERKINSKY & A. S. REES. 1982. Secondary isotype specific antibody responses *in vitro* assayed by a solid phase radioassay. Submitted for publication.

21. MICHALEK, S. M., J. R. MCGHEE, J. MESTECKY, R. R. ARNOLD & L. BOZZO. 1976. Ingestion of Streptococcus mutans induces secretory IgA and caries immunity. Science **192:** 1238–1240.

22. MONTGOMERY, P. C., K. M. CONNELLY, J. COHN & C. A. SKANDERA. 1978. Remote site stimulation of secretory IgA antibodies following bronchial and gastric stimulation. Adv. Exp. Med. Biol. **107:** 113–122.

23. JACKSON, D. E., E. T. LALLY, M. C. NAKAMURA & P. C. MONTGOMERY. 1981. Migration of IgA-bearing lymphocytes into salivary glands. Cell. Immunol. **63:** 203–209.

24. CRAIG, S. W. & J. J. CEBRA. 1971. Peyer's patches: an enriched source of precursors for IgA producing immunocytes in the rabbit. J. Exp. Med. **134:** 188–200.

25. HUSBAND, A. M. & J. L. GOWANS. 1978. The origin and antigen-dependent distribution of IgA-containing cells in the intestine. J. Exp. Med. **148:** 1146–1160.

26. MICHALEK, S. M., J. R. MCGHEE & J. L. BABB. 1978. Effective immunity to dental caries: Dose-dependent studies of secretory immunity by oral administration of *Streptococcus mutans* to rats. Infect. Immun. **19:** 217–223.

27. CHALLACOMBE, S. J. The induction of salivary antibodies by intragastric immunisation in mice (in preparation).

28. LAKE, A. M., K. J. BLOCH, M. R. NEUTRA & W. A. WALKER. 1979. Intestinal goblet cell mucus release. II. *In vivo* stimulation by antigen in the immunized rat. J. Immunol. **122:** 834–837.

29. EBERSOLE, J. L. & J. A. MOLINARI. 1978. The induction of salivary antibodies by topical sensitization with particulate and soluble bacterial immunogens. Immunology **34:** 969–979.

30. SELNER, S. C., D. A. MERRILL & H. W. CLAMAN. 1968. Salivary immunoglobulin and albumin: Development during the newborn period. J Pediatr. **72:** 685–689.

31. TREFTS, P. E., D. A. RIVIER & M. F. KAGNOFF. 1981. T cell-dependent IgA anti-polysaccharide response *in vitro*. Nature (London) **292:** 163–165.

32. RICHMAN, L. K., A. S. GRAEFF, R. YARCHOAN & W. STROBER. 1981. Simultaneous induction of antigen-specific IgA helper T cells and IgG suppressor T cells in the murine Peyer's patch after protein feeding. J. Immunol. **126:** 2079–2083.

33. HANSON, D. G. 1981. Ontogeny of orally induced tolerance to soluble proteins in mice. I. Priming and tolerance in newborns. J. Immunol. **127:** 1518–1524.

34. STOKES, C. R., T. J. NEWBY, J. H. HUNTLEY, D. PATEL & F. J. BOURNE. 1979. The immune response of mice to bacterial antigens given by mouth. Immunology **38:** 497–502.

35. JOEL, D. D., J. A. LAISSUE & M. E. LEFEVRE. 1978. Distribution and fate of ingested carbon particles in mice. J. Reticuloendothelial Soc. **24:** 477–482.

36. CHALON, M.-P., R. W. MILNE & J.-P. VAERMAN. 1979. *In vitro* immunosuppressive effect of serum from orally immunized mice. Eur. J. Immunol. **9:** 747–751.

37. HANSON, D. G., N. M. VAZ, L. C. S. MAIA & J. M. LYNCH. 1979. Inhibition of specific immune responses by feeding protein antigens. III. Evidence against maintenance of tolerance to ovalbumin by orally induced antibodies. J. Immunol. **123:** 2337–2343.

38. MATTINGLY, J. A. & B. H. WAKSMAN. 1980. Immunologic suppression after oral administration of antigen. II. Antigen-specific helper and suppressor factors produced by spleen cells of rats fed sheep erythrocytes. J. Immunol. **125:** 1044–1047.

J. R. MCGHEE (*The University of Alabama in Birmingham*): Do you know the nature of the suppressor or the helper cells transferred from MLN cells? Are they T-cells?

S. J. CHALLACOMBE (*Guy's Hospital, London, England*): They are T-cells in terms of their purification from a nylon wool column; however, we have not yet done deletion experiments.

D. R. GREEN (*Yale University, New Haven, Conn.*): Have you ever mixed the cells that produce the enhancement with the cells that produce the suppression to look for the dominant effect?

CHALLACOMBE: That is an interesting concept; however, we have not done that.

GREEN: Part of the reason I ask is that it seems like quite a paradox that you can produce both effects, that is, immunity and tolerance, in the same animal. Was the inability to transfer enhancement due to the fact that enhancement is actually seen in the presence of suppression, which is the overriding effect?

CHALLACOMBE: That is a possibility. Of course, *Streptococcus mutans* may not be the ideal antigen. There are a number of surface determinants; with a complex antigen, you may have other effects operating concurrently. We would like to attach the soluble protein to some carrier and then look at the nature of the response.

T. B. TOMASI (*University of New Mexico, Albuquerque, N. Mex.*): During the period where there was maximum suppression—tolerance if you will—in animals receiving large doses of *Streptococcus mutans*, were you ever able to transfer suppression to syngeneic animals?

CHALLACOMBE: In these experiments, we have not transferred suppression. Of course, in previous experiments, we were able to transfer tolerance with MLN cells, although we were not able to show that tolerance was due to the T-cell.

TOMASI: The reason I ask is because we have subsequently looked at several particulate antigens, including killed bacteria, and a variety of soluble proteins, that is KLH, ovalbumin, and ragweed pollen. The soluble proteins that induce a long lasting tolerance after a single administration of 1 to 5 milligrams results in a negative T-cell response in the Peyer's patches; however, one does observe suppressor cells. With particulate antigens, such as *Streptococcus mutans*, at doses of 10^9 you find very short lived suppression, that is, in the order of 14 days. You really can not demonstrate suppressor cells; however, a proliferative response occurs in the patches at around 6 to 10 days. Therefore, oral tolerance-producing soluble antigens are quite different from the particulate antigens.

CHALLACOMBE: I agree. We heard this distinction made earlier in Dr. Bockman's work. In fact, Dr. Joel and his group have shown that at least in terms of carbon particles—and one assumes in terms of bacteria—that the antigen can be present in the patches for months, whereas one assumes that the soluble antigen disappears quite quickly. Therefore, the handling and the subsequent responses to these two antigen forms would be different.

MIGRATION AND REGULATION OF B-CELLS IN THE MUCOSAL IMMUNE SYSTEM*

Julia M. Phillips-Quagliata, Maria E. Roux,†
Margaret Arny, Patricia Kelly-Hatfield,
Michael McWilliams, and Michael E. Lamm‡

Department of Pathology
New York University Medical Center
New York, New York 10016

INTRODUCTION

The preponderant immunoglobulin of intestinal secretions is IgA, and its prevalence is reflected in the high proportion of plasma cells producing IgA versus other isotypes in the intestinal lamina propria.[1] The precursors of the IgA-plasma cells are first recognizable as bone marrow-derived (B) cells in the Peyer's patches (PP),[2-5] where they apparently encounter antigens entering from the gut by way of specialized epithelial cells.[6] The precursors may initiate DNA synthesis in the PP, but at some stage leave by way of lymphatics draining into the mesenteric lymph node (MLN), where they proliferate further and eventually mature into IgA-containing blast cells, capable of leaving the MLN and migrating to the small intestine.[7-9] These blasts are transported from the MLN by the efferent and thoracic duct lymph[7,10-13] into the bloodstream from which they emerge at mucosal sites. The whole process by which B-cells originating in PP arrive back in the lamina propria of the small intestine as IgA-containing plasmablasts has been termed the IgA-cell cycle.[1]

THE IgA-CELL CYCLE

That the ability to migrate into intestinal mucosa is largely restricted to lymphoid cells, particularly lymphoblasts, originating in the gut-associated lymphoreticular tissue (GALT) has given rise to the idea that there may be either a unique interaction between GALT-derived lymphoid cells and intestinal endothelial cells or a chemotactic factor that induces the lymphoid cells to leave the circulation at this site. The alternative possibility, that all circulating lymphoblasts can leave the bloodstream in the lamina propria, but that those of GALT origin are preferentially retained, is rendered less likely by the observation that selective migration to the small intestine by MLN, versus peripheral node (PN) blasts, can be observed as early as 30 minutes after intravenous injection (TABLE 1).

The greater ability of MLN blasts than of PN blasts to seek the small intestine

*This work was supported by NIH grants CA 20045, AI 19073, and CA 32582. Dr. Roux was a Fellow of the Arthritis Foundation. Dr. Arny was supported by the Cancer Research Training Program CA 09161.

†Current address: Academia Nacional de Medicina, Instituto de Investigaciones Hematologicas, Departamento de Medicina Nuclear, Buenos Aires, Argentina.

‡Current address: Department of Pathology, Case Western Reserve University School of Medicine, Cleveland, Ohio 44106.

194

TABLE 1

PERCENT INJECTED LABEL RECOVERED 30 MINUTES AND 20 HOURS AFTER INTRAVENOUS INJECTION
OF [^{125}I] IODODEOXYURIDINE PERIPHERAL NODE (PN), MESENTERIC LYMPH NODE (MLN), AND PEYER'S PATCH (PP) CELLS*

Cells Injected	Time of Sacrifice	Recipient Organ					
		PN (Percent per gram)	MLN (Percent per gram)	PP (Percent per gram)	PN/MLN	PN/PP	Small Intestine (Percent per organ)
PN	30 minutes	3.83 ± 0.44	4.00 ± 0.50	2.31 ± 0.17	0.97 ± 0.17	1.67 ± 0.33	1.84 ± 0.11
	20 hours	21.33 ± 3.36	17.16 ± 1.87	6.36 ± 0.77	1.27 ± 0.31	3.42 ± 0.87	2.51 ± 0.23
MLN	30 minutes	1.66 ± 0.48	2.51 ± 0.25	3.70 ± 1.96	0.67 ± 0.23	0.58 ± 0.42	2.47 ± 0.39
	20 hours	4.51 ± 0.22	9.83 ± 0.44	9.93 ± 1.90	0.46 ± 0.03	0.47 ± 0.10	5.69 ± 0.18
PP	30 minutes	1.16 ± 0.48	1.60 ± 0.61	1.74 ± 0.30	0.72 ± 0.06	0.66 ± 0.24	1.54 ± 0.16
	20 hours	0.99 ± 0.37	1.26 ± 0.30	1.87 ± 0.14	0.87 ± 0.46	0.53 ± 0.20	2.10 ± 0.30

*[^{125}I] Iododeoxyuridine was used to label DNA-synthetic [blast] cells in PN, MLN, and PP cell populations of CAF$_1$ mice, and the radiolabeled cells were injected intravenously into groups of three normal, syngeneic recipients. The recipients were sacrificed 30 minutes and 20 hours after injection, and their organs were weighed and counted in a Nuclear-Chicago gamma counter.

in the face of their somewhat diminished ability to seek PN and MLN is revealed by the greater percentage of injected label found in the small intestine at both time points. Only a small proportion of PP blasts ever enters lymph nodes, PP or small intestine, in short-term experiments. That the PN/PP ratios are considerable greater for PN blasts than for either MLN or PP blasts confirms the observations of others, made with an isotopic marker capable of labeling all the cells in the population,[14] that PN cells preferentially seek PN over PP. At both time points, PP blasts and MLN blasts seek the intestine better than PN blasts (relative to their ability to extravasate in lymph nodes), but the percentage accumulation of MLN blasts in small intestine is considerably higher than that of PP blasts. The MLN blasts are clearly a better source of IgA-containing radiolabeled cells accumulated in the small intestine 24 hours after injection.[15] By combined immunofluorescence and radioautography, it is possible to show that 53% of MLN-derived blasts in the lamina propria are IgA-positive versus 22% of PN blasts and only 11% of PP blasts. We have previously shown[8,9] that the majority of MLN blasts that seek the small intestine after intravenous transfer bear surface IgA and can be eliminated with anti-α-chain antiserum plus complement. Once they have arrived in the lamina propria. MLN-derived IgA-bearing blasts rapidly assume the appearance of plasmablasts and may proliferate further in this location.[16-19]

MATURATION OF THE PP PRECURSORS OF INTESTINAL IgA-PLASMA CELLS

Although PP cells show a rather limited potential to seek the small intestine in short-term homing experiments, and only a small proportion of those arriving there make IgA, the PP are clearly the richest source of precursors of the IgA-plasma cells that arrive in and populate the small intestine of irradiated recipients about one week after cell transfer.[2-5,20] In the interim, experiments conducted in irradiated, allotype congenic mice[20] have shown that the majority of the PP precursors mature in the spleen.

We have developed a different system for studying the development of PP-derived IgA-plasma cell precursors.[15] It involves transfer of radiolabeled PP cells into normal (unirradiated), syngeneic recipients, followed, 24 hours later, by a second transfer of the MLN and PN cells of these primary recipients into secondary syngeneic recipients. The tissues of these secondary recipients are then examined by combined immunofluorescence and radioautography. By means of this technique we have demonstrated the existence in PP of a population of IgA-bearing blast cells that seek the MLN in preference to PN of primary recipients and that, 24 hours after transfer of MLN cells of primary recipients, can be identified as radiolabeled IgA-containing cells in the lamina propria of the small intestine of secondary recipients (TABLE 2). It is not yet clear whether this population that takes only 48 hours to arrive in the lamina propria is different from the population that takes five days or more to mature in the spleen of an irradiated recipient.[20] Perhaps maturation of PP-derived IgA-plasma cell precursors simply takes longer in the irradiated spleen due to a relative deficiency of T-cell help and/or enteric antigen. Alternatively, our population may be more mature.

We were intrigued by the ability of these PP-precursors to seek the MLN versus the PN and explored the possibility that this phenomenon was due to recognition of high endothelial venules in the MLN. When, however, we examined by immunofluorescence and autoradiography sections of MLN taken

30 minutes after intravenous injection of ³HT-labeled PP-cells, we found that 41% of the radiolabeled IgA-containing cells in the sections were in the subcapsular sinus, not the paracortex. To reach this location, the cells must have extravasated from blood (to lymph) in the small intestine.

We next examined sections of small intestine taken 30 minutes after intravenous injection of ³HT-labeled PP cells. The transverse sections were cut in such a way that approximately 50% of each section was occupied by Peyer's patch and 50% by the rest of the intestine. In marked contrast to the behavior of IgA-containing MLN-derived blasts, 74% of which extravasated in the lamina propria of the villi and crypts, the vast majority, 93%, of IgA-containing PP-derived blasts in any section were to be found in the Peyer's patches. Because some PP-derived IgA containing cells do extravasate in lamina propria and because throughout the small intestine there is much more lamina propria than PP, we are unable to determine whether the PP-derived IgA-containing cells that reach the MLN are those that extravasated in the PP, or those that extravasated in the lamina propria

TABLE 2

[³H]Thy-Labeled PP Precursors of Intestinal IgA-Containing Cells Preferentially Accumulate in MLN Versus PN 24 Hours after Intravenous Injection*

Injected Label Recovered in Primary Recipients	Cells Transferred	Small Intestine of Secondary Recipients	
		Donor Cells Counted (AR)	Percent IgA Positive Donor Cells (IF)
PN 2.8 ± 0.8 %/g	PN	70	8
MLN 2.7 ± 0.4 %/g	MLN	127	41

*Tritiated thymidine [³H]Thy-labeled PP-cells were injected intravenously into normal syngeneic recipients. The PN and MLN of some of these recipients were harvested 24 hours later, weighed, and counted. Single cell suspensions of the pooled PN and MLN of the remaining mice were injected in equal number into secondary recipients. The small intestine of these secondary recipients was sectioned and examined by combined and autoradiography (AR) and immunofluorescence (IF).

or both. It is remarkable that PP-derived IgA-containing blasts and MLN-derived IgA-containing blasts should behave so differently vis-à-vis extravasation at the two sites. It may reflect either an earlier maturation state of the PP IgA-containing blast or, conceivably, a difference in commitment to becoming a memory cell rather than a plasma cell.

GENESIS AND MAINTENANCE OF THE IGA-CELL CYCLE

We have been considering two major hypotheses for the genesis and maintenance of the IgA-cell cycle. Both are based on the idea that commitment to IgA production does not, per se, control migration of the B-cells to the mucosa. This idea is supported by the fact that T-blasts home as well as B-blasts,[7,21-23] homing is not inhibited by either monomeric or dimeric IgA or by antiserum to secretory component injected intravenously,[8] and the lamina propria of IgA-deficient individuals is populated by plasma cells that make other isotypes.[24] Both hypotheses assume that mucosal homing is antigen-independent,[7,13,21] and both include the possibility that there are T-cells peculiarly capable of helping IgA responses.[25-27]

According to the first hypothesis, the cycle is controlled mainly by instructive mechanisms (FIGURE 1). B-cells of the circulating pool that arrive in the PP either by chance or selection at the level of PP high endothelial venules receive one or both of two kinds of instruction. One instruction, which could come from a T-cell, regulates the switch from IgM to IgA. The other instruction, which might come from the PP stroma, initiates a differentiation sequence such that by the time the PP-cell becomes a plasmablast, it will be capable of extravasation in lamina propria.

According to the second hypothesis the cycle is controlled mainly by selective mechanisms (FIGURE 2). Subsets of B-cells in the bone marrow (or fetal liver) are already committed to extravasation in the lamina propria of the small intestine. On arrival in the intestine by way of the blood they extravasate in the lamina propria rather than the PP and immediately enter the lymph that drains into the MLN. Here they are primed by antigen arriving in the lymph from the Peyer's patches. Antigen and T-cell driven expansion of clones of cells committed to extravasation in lamina propria takes place. The cells leaving the MLN include a mixed population of plasmablasts and memory blasts. On reaching lamina propria, the plasmablasts extravasate and eventually become trapped as their migratory ability declines with maturation into the fully developed plasma cells. The memory cells recirculate through various lymphoid tissues, but are more

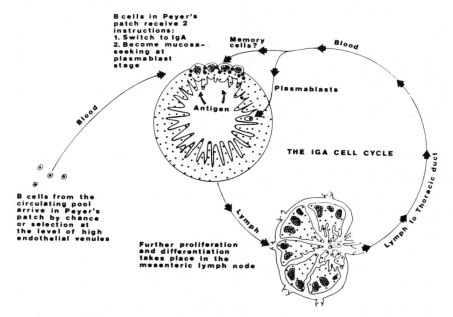

FIGURE 1. Hypothetical scheme for control of mucosal migration by instructive mechanisms.

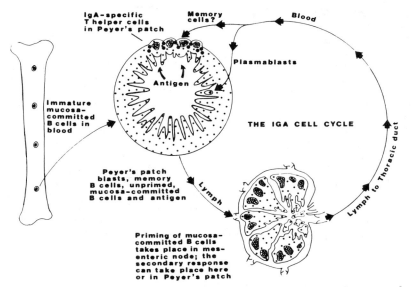

Immature mucosa-committed B cells in blood

IgA-specific T helper cells in Peyer's patch

Memory cells?

Blood

Antigen

Plasmablasts

THE IGA CELL CYCLE

Lymph

Lymph to Thoracic duct

Peyer's patch blasts, memory B cells, unprimed, mucosa-committed B cells and antigen

Priming of mucosa-committed B cells takes place in mesenteric node; the secondary response can take place here or in Peyer's patch

FIGURE 2. Hypothetical scheme for control of mucosal migration by selective mechanisms.

likely to encounter the antigen for which they are specific in GALT, that is, Peyer's patches and mesenteric lymph nodes. Further antigen-driven expansion, perhaps coupled with IgA-specific selective T-cell help results in the predominance in GALT of clones that are both committed to IgA production and have the ability to seek mucosa. Obviously, the two hypotheses could be combined in various ways. For example, an instructive mechanism for controlling the switch to IgA could be coupled with a selective mechanism for expansion of mucosa-seeking B-cell populations.

We tried the following two approaches in our investigation of the selective hypothesis. According to the selective hypothesis, it should be possible to find in bone marrow subsets of B-cells that are able to extravasate in lamina propria and reach the mesenteric lymph nodes. We therefore transformed mouse bone marrow cells *in vitro* with Abelson virus, injected the cells intravenously into syngeneic irradiated recipients and then harvested the MLN or PN cells of the recipients in an effort to select for Abelson transformed cells with the capacity to arrive in the MLN in preference to peripheral nodes. The cells were then expanded in culture and cloned. A total of 54 MLN-passed clones and 12 PN-passed clones were compared in short-term (90 minute) homing experiments. None of the MLN clones showed the kind of selective ability to home to the small intestine or MLN we would have predicted for a clone with a true ability to extravasate in lamina propria.

Although this experiment to some extent argues against the selective hypothesis, it is possible that the pre-B-cells transformed by Abelson virus are simply too immature to show the kind of homing ability predicted or are too large to reach the mesenteric lymph nodes. We are currently growing Abelson-transformed bone-marrow cells, prepared from lamina propria of recipients 24 hours after intravenous injection, in the hope that these might show the ability to return to lamina propria.

In our second approach, we tried to determine whether carrier-primed T-helper cells from GALT, that is, PP and MLN were more capable of helping IgA responses by hapten-primed splenic B-cells than PN T-cells. GALT T-cells were primed by intraduodenal injection and PN T-cells by subcutaneous injection of antigen. Nylon wool nonadherent T-cell preparations were depleted of suppressors with anti-Lyt-2.2 plus complement. The T-cells were then titrated into cultures of T-depleted splenic B-cells plus macrophages from donors primed with 2, 4-Dinitrophenyl-keyhole limpet hemocyanin (DNP-KLH). After four days of culture, IgM, IgG, and IgA anti-TNP plaques were enumerated.

When the T-cells had been primed with sheep erythrocytes (SRBC) and trinitrophenylated-SRBC (TNP-SRBC) was the antigen added to the cultures, T-cell populations from PP, MLN, and PN were all successfully primed and there was no evidence to favor the hypothesis that more help for IgA responses was provided by GALT-derived T-cells (TABLE 3). Initial attempts to prime GALT T-cells with KLH were unsuccessful, but PN T-cells were successfully primed.

TABLE 3

ABILITY OF SRBC-PRIMED PN, MLN, AND PP LYT-2⁻ T-CELLS TO SUPPORT GENERATION OF IgM, IgG, AND IgA PLAQUE-FORMING CELL RESPONSES BY DNP-KLH-PRIMED B-CELLS*

	Source of T-cells	Anti-TNP PFC/culture		
		IgM	IgA	IgG
Experiment 1	PP	5,000	945	2,110
	MLN	5,000	940	2,370
Experiment 2	PN	5,000	2,510	3,160
	MLN	5,000	1,090	2,130

*T-cells were titrated into B-cell cultures. The data shown were taken from titration curves at the same IgM plaque-forming cell (PFC) numbers for ease of comparison.

It became apparent that SRBC-primed T-cells in the presence of TNP-SRBC and KLH-primed T-cells in the presence of DNP-KLH or TNP-KLH could elicit quite different ratios of IgA to IgM and IgG plaque-forming cells from a given DNP-KLH primed B-cell preparation. For example, in one experiment, SRBC-primed T-cell doses supporting 1000 IgM plaque-forming cells in the TNP-SRBC cultures helped 400 IgA plaque-forming cells, whereas KLH-primed T-cells supporting 1000 IgM plaque-forming cells in DNP-KLH cultures helped only 130 IgA plaque-forming cells. T-cell help for IgA (as for IgM and IgG) in TNP-SRBC cultures could be replaced by noncognate help in the form of KLH-primed T-cells plus KLH or supernatants of Concanavalin A (Con A) stimulated spleen cells. By contrast, cognate help was required for IgM and IgA responses in the DNP-KLH cultures, and addition of nonspecific factors generated in Con A splenic supernatants had no augmenting effect.

Our results are compatible with the idea that primed splenic IgA plasma-cell precursors are derived from two pools, one responsive in the presence of TNP-SRBC to the assemblage of nonspecific factors known as T-cell replacing factors, the other requiring cognate help.[28] Such pools have been previously described for IgM and IgG precursors.[29] As yet we have no clear-cut evidence for the existence of IgA-specific T-helper cells, but feel that they are best sought in the cognate rather than the noncognate system where they may be obscured by nonspecific factors.

In considering what would be expected of T-cells capable of promoting IgA responses, it is worth noting that T-cells capable of instructing the switch would not require receptors for IgA, whereas those capable of selecting populations of IgA-bearing B-cells and promoting either their proliferation or differentiation to secretion would require receptors for IgA either alone or combined with antigen and/or Ia determinants. Our experiments to date have indicated that at the start of the cultures, splenic B-cells capable of giving rise to IgA plaque-forming cells four days later in either cognate or noncognate systems are insusceptible to anti-α-chain antiserum plus complement, which suggests that they do not bear surface IgA at this time. This observation limits the time over which a selector T-cell could act to less than four days. Depletion of the T-helper cells on IgA-coated plates also had no effect, which may indicate that they lack receptors for IgA. It may prove necessary, however, to deplete them by the rosette technique.[27]

The high frequency of clones producing only IgA, derived from PP precursor B-cells,[30] could result from instructive or selective T-cell help, or could merely reflect the probability of deletion of C_h genes 5' C_α[31] during proliferation in response to repeated exposure to antigenic and mitogenic stimuli in the Peyer's patches. The idea that the majority of PP precursors of clones producing only IgA are secondary B-cells[30] is based on their ability to respond in an allogeneic environment, which implies that responsiveness to help is unrestricted by the major histocompatibility complex. Because major histocompatibility complex unrestricted help may be equivalent to noncognate help, it is conceivable that the propensity of PP B-cells to make IgA responses reflects the presence of a high proportion of B-cells capable of responses to noncognate help rather than selective or instructive IgA-specific T-cell help.

REFERENCES

1. LAMM, M. E. 1976. Adv. Immunol. **22:** 223–290.
2. CRAIG, S. W. & J. J. CEBRA. 1971. J. Exp. Med. **134:** 188–200.
3. CRAIG, S. W. & J. J. CEBRA. 1975. J. Immunol. **114:** 492–502.
4. RUDZIK, O., D. Y. E. PEREY & J. BIENENSTOCK. 1975. J. Immunol. **114:** 40–44.
5. RUDZIK, O., R. CLANCY, D. Y. E. PEREY, R. P. DAY & J. BIENENSTOCK. 1975. J. Immunol. **114:** 1599–1604.
6. OWEN, R. L. 1977. Gastroenterology **72:** 440–451.
7. GUY-GRAND, D., C. GRISCELLI & P. VASSALLI. 1974. Eur. J. Immunol. **4:** 435–443.
8. McWILLIAMS, M., J. M. PHILLIPS-QUAGLIATA & M. E. LAMM. 1975. J. Immunol. **115:** 54–58.
9. McWILLIAMS, M., J. M. PHILLIPS-QUAGLIATA & M. E. LAMM. 1977. J. Exp. Med. **145:** 866–875.
10. GOWANS, J. L. & E. J. KNIGHT. 1964. Proc. R. Soc. London Ser. B.**159:** 257–282.
11. HALL, J. G., D. M. PARRY & M. E. SMITH. 1972. Cell Tissue Kinet. **5:** 269–281.
12. PIERCE, N. F. & J. L. GOWANS. 1975. J. Exp. Med. **142:** 1550–1563.
13. HALL, J. G., J. HOPKINS & E. ORLANS. 1977. Eur. J. Immunol. **7:** 30–37.
14. BUTCHER, E. C., R. G. SCOLLAY & I. L. WEISSMAN. 1980. Eur. J. Immunol. **10:** 556–561.
15. ROUX, M. E., M. McWILLIAMS, J. M. PHILLIPS-QUAGLIATA & M. E. LAMM. 1981. Cell. Immunol. **61:** 141–153.

16. HUSBAND, A. J. & J. L. GOWANS. 1978. J. Exp. Med. **148:** 1146–1160.
17. MAYRHOFER, G. & FISHER, R. 1979. Eur. J. Immunol. **9:** 85–91.
18. HUSBAND, A. J. 1982. J. Immunol. **128:** 1355–1359.
19. PIERCE, N. F. & W. C. CRAY. 1982. J. Immunol. **128:** 1311–1315.
20. TSENG, J. 1982. J. Immunol. **127:** 2039–2043.
21. PARROTT, D. M. V. & A. FERGUSON. 1974. Immunology **26:** 571–588.
22. SPRENT, J. 1976. Cell. Immunol. **21:** 278–302.
23. GUY-GRAND, D., C. GRISCELLI & P. VASSALLI. 1978. J. Exp. Med. **148:** 1661–1677.
24. BRANDTZAEG, P. J., S. T. GERULDSEN, F. KORSRUD, K. BAKLIEN, P. BERDAL & J. EK. 1979. J. Immunol. **122:** 503–510.
25. ELSON, C. O., J. A. HECK & W. STROBER. 1979. J. Exp. Med. **149:** 632–643.
26. RICHMAN, L. K., A. S. GRAEFF, R. YARCHDAN, & W. STROBER. 1981. J. Immunol. **126:** 2079–2083.
27. ENDOH, M., H. SAKAI, Y. NOMOTO, Y. TOMINO & H. KANESHIGE. 1981. J. Immunol. **127:** 2612–2613.
28. KELLER, D. M., J. E. SWIERKOSZ, P. MARRACK, & J. W. KAPPLER. 1980. J. Immunol. **124:** 1350–1359.
29. ASANO, Y., A. SINGER & R. J. HODES. 1981. J. Exp. Med. **154:** 1100–1115.
30. GEARHART, P. J. & J. J. CEBRA. 1979. J. Exp. Med. **149:** 216–227.
31. HONJO, T. & T. KATAOKA. 1978. Proc. Nat. Acad. Sci. USA **75:** 2140–2144.

DISCUSSION OF THE PAPER

J. J. CEBRA (*University of Pennsylvania, Philadelphia, Pa.*): Because you are using tritiated thymidine-labeled blasts to look for selective homing, you are also looking in a very narrow window. Do you not think it is possible that the blast cells that you get from the Peyer's patches represent younger IgA-bearing cells, whereas those in the mesenteric lymph node would be further along in differentiation, behaving differently. Have you looked for other surface markers on these two cell types to see whether you may be dealing with two distinct lineages, or with cells at different stages of differentiation?

J. M. PHILLIPS-QUAGLIATA (*New York University Medical Center, New York, N.Y.*): We have not looked at tritiated adenosine-labeled PP cells, that contain a somewhat higher proportion of IgA precursors that pass through the peripheral nodes. These could be small lymphocytes that might be part of the recirculating pool. They would enter the peripheral node through the high endothelial venules instead of the route I described. We have not looked at any other surface markers.

With regard to the response to T-cell replacing factor (TRF), however, I was struck by the fact that Dr. Gearhart and you, some years ago, hypothesized that the majority of Peyer's patch B-cells were, in fact, secondary B-cells. This hypothesis was partly based on their ability to respond in noncognate interaction or at least to non-major histocompatibility complex (MHC) restricted T-cell help. I wonder whether, in fact, you have any evidence that Peyer's patch B-cells are more frequently Lyb 5+ than B-cells elsewhere?

CEBRA: We suggested that the IgA-committed cells that produced clones, exclusively making IgA, acted more like secondary cells, but they actually make up a minority of the total Peyer's patch population. I am not sure how many of those would have been labeled in your type of experiment.

PHILLIPS-QUAGLIATA: I was mainly talking about the B-cell response to TRF.

M. F. KAGNOFF (*University of California at San Diego, La Jolla*): We are using similar terminology, but in a somewhat different way. When we talk about instruction, the question is, Is there a T-cell that delivers a signal to a B-cell, which through some intracellular mechanism specifically activates the alpha switch site? One could ask the same question for IgE or for IgG. When I talk about selection, it is a somewhat more complicated issue; there we could talk about organ selection. On the other hand, what I think we are discussing is a stochaistic switching model rather than a specifically instructional switching model. I think we are talking about things at a slightly different level.

PHILLIPS-QUAGLIATA: When I talk about selection, I am suggesting a possible mechanism whereby T-cells selectively work by recognition of IgA on the surface of the B-cell. They promote either proliferation or secretion, or both by that B-cell and its progeny in much the same way as, it is thought, idiotype-specific T-cells function. If one were to have such a selective T-cell, one would more or less expect it to recognize Fd of IgA, rather than Fc.

KAGNOFF: I think that is another issue. What I am calling instruction, you are calling selection, I suppose.

T. B. TOMASI (*University of N. Mexico, Albuquerque, N. Mex.*): One possibility that might be considered is that the alpha message in the Peyer's patches, is almost entirely in the membrane form and not in the secreted form, as it is in the mesenteric lymph nodes. What you really need, in order to get these localization phenomena, is maturation from the membrane to the secreted form. That does not occur in Peyer's patches; therefore, Peyer's patch cells do not home. It does not occur in Peyer's patches either, because the cell leaves rapidly to the mesenteric lymph node, where it matures, or because of some environmental signal perhaps provided by a T-cell, travels from the membrane to the secreted form. You need that signal before you can get these homing properties.

W. STROBER (*National Institutes of Health, Bethesda, Md.*): I would like to make just one comment on this topic. In your studies where you use T-cells from different organs to see whether the different organs have special qualities that help IgA, one concept you have to keep in mind is the concept of preswitch and postswitch B-cells. Because you use B-cells from spleen, that is, what I would consider as cells that had not been switched to membrane IgA-positive cells, you are not really in a position to look for T-cell help. The B-cells were not appropriately prepared. In fact, Dr. Kawanishi and I have some data indicating that if you preexpose B-cells to Peyer's patch cloned T-cells, you will find that the cells can make IgA. This switched B-cell can now respond to a variety of T-cell TRF influences.

PHILLIPS-QUAGLIATA: I want to point out that our B-cells are making IgA. They are not making IgA at the very beginning of the culture, or at least they do not possess IgA at the very beginning, because they can not be depleted with anti-alpha plus complement. They are, however, making IgA by the time the culture is finished. The question is proportion of IgA to other isotypes. I do not deny, for an instant, that there may very well be an IgA specific T-helper cell. I am skeptical about the idea of looking at, for example, a Peyer's patch B-cell in association with the Peyer's patch T-cell, because the controls have to be very rigorous. For example, there may be in GALT idiotype-specific help that functions in relation to idiotypes that are IgA associated.

CELLULAR CIRCUITRY INVOLVED IN ORALLY INDUCED SYSTEMIC TOLERANCE AND LOCAL ANTIBODY PRODUCTION

Jerome A. Mattingly

The Ohio State University
Department of Medical Microbiology and Immunology
Columbus, Ohio 43210

INTRODUCTION

Oral administration of antigen can lead to both help and suppression of the antibody response to that antigen.[1-4] This phenomenon is not unusual, however, because these two modalities of the immune response occur after almost all types of antigen administration. What does appear to be unusual in the oral administration of antigen is that the antibody response that occurs is at the local level, whereas the suppression that occurs is at the systemic level, and the two apparently do not affect each other.

In several different experimental systems where help and suppression were studied simultaneously, one of them appeared to be dependent upon the other; that is, an immunological circuit or network was present.[5-9] It has been shown that these dependencies are due to direct feedback of antibody to cause suppression,[5] by induction of T-suppressor cells (T_s), by T-helper cells (T_h),[6] and by inactivation of T_s by a "helper-like" contrasuppressor cell.[7] Most of these circuits also appear to function through soluble mediators. No such circuits have been reported in the gut-associated lymphoreticular tissue (GALT) immune responses, although the same cell types and mediators appear to function.

The purpose of this study is to define whether the inductions of both help and suppression are connected in a circuitous fashion, or whether each occurs independently of the other. It is reported in this paper that each can take place without the need for the other, that they are two completely independent events, that two different cell types are involved leading to each, that each may have an internal network independent of the other, and that "class-specific" help and suppression may be the end result of various interactions, and not due to "class-specific" T-helper or T-suppressor cells.

MATERIALS AND METHODS

Red Blood Cells

Sheep erythrocytes (SRBC) were obtained (Colorado Serum Co., Denver, Colo.) in sterile Alsevers solution. Before use, they were washed three times in cold RPMI 1640 (Microbiological Associates, Walkersville, Md.) and suspended to the desired concentration. Horse erythrocytes (HRBC) (Colorado Serum Co.) were similarly prepared.

0077-8923/83/0409-0204 $1.75/0 © 1983, NYAS

Mice

Male C57BL/6 (Jackson Laboratory, Bar Harbor, Maine) were used throughout this study. They were shipped at six to eight weeks of age, and were used between one to three weeks of shipping.

Feeding of SRBC

The mice were ether anesthetized and given 0.3 ml of a 50% SRBC suspension through a stomach tube. After a single feeding, the mice were killed either one day or eight days later. In some cases, the mice were injected intraperitoneally (IP) with 200 mg/kg of cyclophosphamide (Cytoxan, Mead-Johnson, Evansville, Ind.) 48 hours before the feeding of sheep erythrocytes.

Cell Separation

Single-cell preparations from Peyer's patches (PP) were made by gentle rubbing between two sterile glass slides. The medium consisted of RPMI 1640 with 100 μg/ml gentamicin (Schering Corp., Kenilworth, N.J.). These cells were washed three times and passed through small nylon-wool columns.[10] The nonadherent cells were used as a source of T-cells (>90% showed positive fluorescence with anti-Thy-1.2 serum). The same process was followed for spleen cells. Approximately 25% of total cells were recovered, and viability was greater than 95 percent. These cells could make no plaque-forming cell (PFC) responses, but they responded well to phytohemagglutinin (PHA, DIFCO).

Cell Culture

One ml of a spleen cell suspension from normal mice that contained 10^7 cells was placed in each well of a tissue culture plate (3008; Falcon Plastics). A modification of the Mishell and Dutton culture system[11] was used. All cultures contained 0.025 ml of 1% SRBC or HRBC. Some cultures contained an additional 10^6 PP or spleen T-cells from either SRBC-fed or normal mice added in 0.1 ml. In other studies, PP T-cells were separated by their ability to bind to peanut lectin (PNA) (see below), and these cells, either PNA$^+$ or PNA$^-$ PP T-cells, were added to the culture at the ratio of 10^6 PP cells to 10^7 spleen cells. The cultures were incubated for five days at 37°C in a 5% CO_2 atmosphere and 100% humidity.

In some cases, the normal spleen cells were treated before culture with monoclonal anti-Lyt-2.2 serum (Becton-Dickinson) plus rabbit complement. This treatment resulted in a spleen cell population that showed only 5–10% positive fluorescence with anti-Lyt-2.2 serum.

Quadruplicate cultures were assayed for indirect PFC[12] using antisera against the heavy chains of IgA and IgG (Miles Laboratories, Elkart, Ind.). Sheep erythrocytes specific PFC were expressed as total plaques minus the direct PFC performed under identical conditions. Results were reported as the geometric mean ($\overset{\times}{\div}$ SD) of each group. Statistics were performed using the Student's t-test for nonpaired data.

Cell Transfer

For in vivo adoptive cell transfer, nylon passed cells from either spleen or PP were suspended to a concentration of 2×10^7/ml in phosphate buffered saline (PBS). One half ml was transferred to recipient mice IV. Sheep erythrocytes (4×10^8) were injected IP 24 hours later, and splenic PFC analysis was done after an additional four days. Results were reported as described under *Cell culture.*

Peanut-lectin (PNA) Binding

PNA (Sigma Chemical Co., St. Louis, Mo) was stored in PBS at 1.0 mg/ml. A modification of the procedure of Reisner et al.[13] was used to separate cells that bind to PNA from the cells that do not bind to PNA in the nylon-wool purified PP T-cells. Equal volumes of PP T-cells (10^7/ml) from SRBC-fed mice (fed 3×10^9 SRBC 24 hours previously), and PNA were incubated for 30 minutes at room temperature in the presence of 1% rabbit erythrocytes (RBC) (RBC are PNA$^+$).[14] These cells were then layered onto a 5% bovine serum albumin column in a 15 ml conical glass tube. After 15 minutes at room temperature, the agglutinated cells sedimented, whereas the unagglutinated cells remained at the top of the bovine serum albumin. The bottom and top layers were removed separately from Pasteur pipets and transferred to different 15 ml conical tubes. The cells were then incubated for 15 minutes at room temperature in the presence of 0.5 M D-galactose in phosphate-buffered saline. The cells were washed two times in the galactose-PBS solution. The RBC were lysed by mixing the suspensions in an RBC lysing buffer (155 mM NH$_4$Cl, 10 mM KHCO$_3$, 0.01 mM EDTA in water). The cells were washed three times in PBS and counted using trypan blue. Approximately 25–30% of the PP T-cells agglutinated in this fashion, and viability was above 85% in both populations.

The ability of cells to bind to PNA after 48 hours in culture was determined by reacting the cells to fluorescein-labeled PNA (Sigma Chemical Co., St. Louis, Mo.) for 30 minutes at 37°C. After thorough washing, the cells were suspended in PBS and examined under fluorescence optics. Freshly isolated PP cells and

TABLE 1

LACK OF EFFECT OF ADDITION OF T-CELLS FROM NORMAL MICE
UPON PFC IN CELL CULTURE

			PFC/Culture§	
Donor Pretreatment*	Day of Transfer†	T-cell Source‡	IgG	IgA
—	—	None	2,760 (1.26)	135 (1.86)
Saline	1	PP	2,840 (1.78)	148 (1.90)
Saline	1	Spleen	3,000 (1.32)	130 (1.58)
Saline	8	PP	3,260 (1.86)	150 (1.46)
Saline	8	Spleen	2,520 (1.05)	164 (1.82)

*Mice were orally given 0.3 ml of saline through a stomach tube.
†Number of days following this saline administration.
‡Organ from which nylon-wool column-passed cells were obtained; 10^6 cells were added to a spleen cell culture of 10^7 cells.
§In vitro PFC reported as PFC/culture $\overset{\times}{\div}$ S.E.M. of triplicate or quadruplicate cultures.

Table 2
LACK OF EFFECT OF ADOPTIVE TRANSFER OF T-CELLS FROM NORMAL MICE
UPON SPLENIC PFC FORMATION *In Vivo*

Donor Pretreatment*	Day of Transfer†	T-cell Source‡	PFC/10^6 Spleen Cells§	
			IgG	IgA
—	—	None	2,788 (1.20)	15.2 (1.68)
Saline	1	PP	2,265 (1.23)	14.1 (1.71)
Saline	1	Spleen	1,886 (1.73)	20.0 (1.58)
Saline	8	PP	2,547 (1.12)	17.6 (1.27)
Saline	8	Spleen	2,500 (1.61)	13.3 (1.82)

*†See footnotes in TABLE 1.
‡10^7 PP or spleen T-cells were injected i.v. into recipient mice.
§*In vivo* PFC reported as PFC/10^6 spleen cells $\overset{\times}{\div}$ S.D. of the responses of five mice.

thymocytes were used as positive controls. Peanut lectin-binding thymocytes remained unchanged after a 48 hour culture.

RESULTS

There are two basic protocols that were followed throughout this study. One consisted of the addition of T-cells from different organs of SRBC-fed mice to the spleen cells of normal syngeneic mice in tissue culture, and the other consisted of the addition of T-cells from the SRBC fed mice to other mice in an *in vivo* syngeneic adoptive transfer. After this transfer, the recipients (either culture or mice) were challenged with SRBC, and PFC analyses were performed after a given time period. TABLE 1 shows that the addition of nylon-wool-passed cells from saline fed mice did not significantly alter the normal PFC response of the *in vitro* system, and TABLE 2 shows that the addition of similar cells had no effect on the *in vivo* PFC response. Also, no effect was found when these recipients were challenged with HRBC and tested for PFC against HRBC (data not shown).

In order to show the dual enhancing and suppressing mechanisms following the feeding of antigens, mice were fed 3×10^9 SRBC by stomach intubation on day zero. On either day 1 or day 8, T-cells from the PP or spleen of these mice were transferred to *in vitro* cultures (10^6 T-cells added to cultures of 10^7 spleen cells). After incubation with either SRBC or HRBC for five days, the cultures were analyzed for PFC against the corresponding antigen. TABLE 3 shows an increase in IgA PFC using PP T-cells, whereas there is a decreased IgG PFC against SRBC when spleen cells were used from mice fed eight days earlier. No effect was seen on the HRBC response (data not shown). The same phenomena are seen *in vivo*, with the increase in IgA being more dramatic (TABLE 4). As can be readily seen from each of these tables, both T-helper cells (T_h) and T-suppressor cells (T_s) for SRBC are found in PP only one day after oral antigen administration. It is also seen that T_s are found in the spleen and T_h are found in the PP eight days following feeding, but not vice versa, and also that the T_h can help both IgG and IgA, when the T_s are not present (day 8 PP cells). Because the results of the experiments indicated that the *in vitro* model correlated very well with the *in vivo* adoptive transfer system, the remaining protocols concentrated solely on the *in vitro* system.

TABLE 3

EFFECT OF ADDITION OF T-CELLS FROM SRBC-FED MICE
UPON PFC IN CELL CULTURE

			PFC/Culture‖	
Donor Pretreatment‡	Day of Transfer§	T-cell Source¶	IgG	IgA
Saline	1	PP	2,840 (1.78)	148 (1.90)
SRBC	1	PP	840 (1.15)*	340 (1.31)†
Saline	1	Spleen	3,000 (1.32)	130 (1.58)
SRBC	1	Spleen	2,780 (1.11)	142 (1.42)
Saline	8	PP	3,260 (1.86)	150 (1.46)
SRBC	8	PP	7,220 (1.46)*	600 (1.50)*
Saline	8	Spleen	2,520 (1.05)	164 (1.82)
SRBC	8	Spleen	1,060 (1.21)*	185 (1.48)

*$p = < 0.01$
†$p = < 0.05$
‡Mice were orally given saline (0.3 ml) or SRBC (0.3 ml of 50% SRBC) through a stomach tube.
§Number of days following administration of saline or SRBC.
¶Organ from which T-cells were removed and added to a spleen cell culture.
‖See footnote in TABLE 1.

To determine if SRBC-specific T_s could be induced by feeding without the induction of the SRBC specific T_h, mice were injected with cyclophosphamide (200 mg/kg) 48 hours before the oral introduction of sheep erythrocytes. Peyer's patch cells removed from these mice 24 hours later were then passed over nylon wool columns and added to cultures as before. The same was done with spleen cells removed after eight days. Results in TABLE 5 indicate that the formation of T_h cells was eliminated from both the PP and the spleen by this procedure but that T_s for IgG were still formed in both lymphoid organs. Again, no effect was seen on the HRBC response (data not shown).

In order to find whether the T_s that are formed in the PP after the oral

TABLE 4

EFFECT OF ADOPTIVE TRANSFER OF T-CELLS FROM SRBC-FED MICE
UPON SPLENIC PFC FORMATION *In Vivo*

			PFC/10^6 Spleen Cells¶	
Donor Pretreatment†	Day of Transfer‡	T-cell Source§	IgG	IgA
Saline	1	PP	2,265 (1.23)	14.1 (1.71)
SRBC	1	PP	960 (1.34)*	65.2 (1.60)*
Saline	1	Spleen	1,886 (1.73)	20.0 (1.58)
SRBC	1	Spleen	2,318 (1.40)	20.4 (1.12)
Saline	8	PP	2,547 (1.12)	17.6 (1.27)
SRBC	8	PP	5,867 (1.41)	66.3 (1.32)
Saline	8	Spleen	2,500 (1.61)	13.3 (1.82)
SRBC	8	Spleen	440 (1.55)	17.4 (1.36)

*$p = < 0.01$.
†‡See footnote in TABLE 3.
§10^7 PP or spleen T-cells were injected i.v. into recipient mice.
¶See footnote in TABLE 2.

TABLE 5

EFFECT OF CYCLOPHOSPHAMIDE ON THE INDUCTION OF T_h
AFTER THE ORAL INTRODUCTION OF SRBC

Donor Pretreatment		Day of Transfer	T-cell Source	PFC/culture	
Day 2 Injection*	Day 0 Feeding†			IgG	IgA
—	Saline	1	PP	2,380 (1.41)	126 (1.16)
Cy	Saline	1	PP	2,640 (1.06)	88 (1.30)
—	SRBC	1	PP	680 (1.68)	442 (1.41)
Cy	SRBC	1	PP	800 (1.31)	110 (1.10)*
—	Saline	8	Spleen	2,940 (1.14)	98 (1.08)
Cy	Saline	8	Spleen	2,433 (1.33)	114 (1.33)
—	SRBC	8	Spleen	860 (1.60)	520 (1.41)
Cy	SRBC	8	Spleen	466 (1.46)	146 (1.22)*

*Mice were injected with Cytoxan i.p. at 200 mg/kg, 48 hours prior to the feeding of SRBC. Controls received the same volume of saline.

†Mice were orally give saline (0.3 ml) or SRBC (0.3 ml of 50% SRBC).

introduction of antigen are T_s inducers or T_s effectors, the spleen cells population to which they were added was depleted of Lyt-2^+ cells by treatment with monoclonal anti-Lyt-2 plus complement. The nylon-wool-passed PP cells were then added to this splenic population of B-cells and Lyt-1^+2^- T-cells. The results of the experiment are shown in TABLE 6, and indicate that the T_s that are formed in the PP are inducers, not effectors, of suppression, as no suppression is seen unless splenic Lyt^{2+} cells are present. Also seen is that the T_h that are formed in the PP within 24 hours of antigen administration can still help in IgA responses, indicating that these are T_h-effector cells, and not inducers, as they obviously do not require the presence of Lyt-123^+ T-cells.

Using the binding of PNA as a marker of immature cells,[13,15] PP cells were tested for their ability to bind PNA. After reacting nylon-passed PP cells from mice fed SRBC 24 hours earlier with PNA, the agglutinated cells (approx.

TABLE 6

EFFECT OF ELIMINATION OF Lyt-2^+ CELLS FROM THE RECIPIENT POPULATION
UPON PFC IN CELL CULTURE

Donor Pretreatment†	T-cell Source	Recipient Pretreatment‡	PFC/Culture	
			IgG	IgA
—	—	—	2,433 (1.21)	88 (1.05)
—	—	Lyt-2 + C	2,840 (1.14)	105 (1.11)
Saline	PP	—	2,680 (1.23)	114 (1.43)
Saline	PP	Lyt-2 + C	2,220 (1.08)	116 (1.61)
SRBC	PP	—	666 (1.31)	520 (1.42)
SRBC	PP	Lyt-2 + C	2,540 (1.17)*	636 (1.66)

*$p = < 0.01$

†Mice were fed saline or SRBC 24 hours before removal of PP.

‡For each culture, 10^7 spleen cells were treated with 1 μg monoclonal anti-Lyt-2.2 for 30 minutes at 4°C, followed by 0.5 ml of a 1:10 dilution of rabbit C for 30 minutes at 4°C. The resulting cell population was used as the Lyt-2 depleted spleen cells.

TABLE 7

EFFECT OF PNA⁺ AND PNA⁻ PP T-CELLS FROM SRBC-FED MICE
ON THE PFC RESPONSE OF NORMAL SPLEEN CELLS

PP T-cells†	PFC/Culture	
	IgG	IgA
—	2,518 (1.10)	126 (1.22)
10^6 PNA⁻	320 (1.41)*	114 (1.06)
10^6 PNA⁺	3,210 (1.33)	540 (1.33)*

*$p = < 0.01$

†Nylon-wool-passed PP cells were separated by their ability to form rosettes in the presence of PNA (see MATERIALS AND METHODS). The PNA was removed from these cells before adding to culture.

25–30% were dissociated with galactose (PNA binds to terminal nonreducing galactose residues). These cells were then transferred to the culture system. As is readily seen in TABLE 7, the PNA binding cells in PP had the ability to help in the antibody responses (most notable to IgA), but had no detectable suppressor activity. When the cells not binding to PNA were used, suppression of IgG was seen, but not of IgA. No helper activity was found in this population.

When the PNA binding T-cells of the PP were allowed to incubate in culture for 48 hours, the ability to agglutinate in the presence of PNA was lost. The results in TABLE 8 also show that the ability to help in IgA production was also lost, but the ability to help in IgG was maintained and even enhanced. Still no suppression was seen in this cell population. Suppressor activity was maintained in the PNA⁻ population of PP T-cells, even after the 48 hours *in vitro* incubation.

DISCUSSION

The present study shows that following the oral administration of an antigen, simultaneous induction of IgA and suppression of IgG occur. These inductions occur independently of one another, and are not affected by one another in any

TABLE 8

EFFECT OF 48 HOUR INCUBATION OF PNA⁺ PP T-CELLS
ON THEIR ABILITY TO BIND PNA AND THEIR FUNCTION

Addition of PP T-cells†	Ability to Bind PNA After Culture‡	PFC/Culture	
		IgG	IgA
—	—	1,930 (1.08)	88 (1.21)
10^6 PNA⁻	No	640 (1.23)	100 (1.16)
10^6 PNA⁺	No	4,160 (1.42)*	126 (1.06)

*$p = < 0.01$

†See footnote in TABLE 7.

‡After removal of the PNA from the PNA binding PP T-cells, the cells were allowed to incubate *in vitro* for 48 hours. They were again tested for their ability to bind PNA using fluorescent labeled PNA (see MATERIALS AND METHODS). These cells were then added to a spleen cell culture and incubated as previously described.

measurable way. One will occur in the complete absence of the other. In addition, the study also shows that the systemic suppression that occurs after the oral ingestion of antigen begins in the GALT with T_s-inducer cells that are not sensitive to high levels of cyclophosphamide, but that the actual T_s-effector cell in this response resides in the spleen. The T_h that is induced in the GALT appears to be the actual T_h-effector and can help IgG, as well as IgA-synthesizing cells.

This study also shows that the induction of T_h in GALT after enteric antigen administration is inhibitable by the administration of cyclophosphamide 48 hours before exposure. We had previously shown that this treatment had no effect upon the T_s formation,[16] but had not studied its effect upon T-helper cells. This approach appears to be a good method for obtaining antigen-specific T_s without the interference of T-helper cells.

This study also showed that the T_h that is induced in the PP after the feeding of antigen is PNA$^+$, and as such, may be an immature T-cell.[13] When the T_h loses its ability to bind PNA, it loses its ability to help in IgA responses, but gains the ability to help in IgG responses. The suppressor cell that is formed in the PP is PNA$^-$, and as such, may be a more mature T-cell.

Rather than supporting the notion that there are distinct classes of T_h that will support the production of only one antibody isotype, these data support an hypothesis that there are different steps in T-cell maturation whereby the T_h can help different isotypic B-cells of the same idiotype. This subtle yet distinct difference is the simplest way to explain the findings and still will account for other seemingly unrelated findings. It also eliminated the need for several different lineages of T-cells, which have not been found, and it allows full advantage for utilizing the entire B-cell repertoire toward a given antigen.

According to this T-cell maturational theory, the cell able to help IgA would be the most immature of the T-helper cells. This hypothesis would support the seemingly unrelated reports concerning lack of memory responses associated with IgA (memory being the property of a mature, long-lived T-cell), and the seemingly loose T-cell control of IgA (greater than 80% of mouse myelomas are IgA).[17] Because control is generally thought to be at the level of the T-cell, this hypothesis would indicate an immature T-cell. To date, no one has found a distinct suppressor cell or suppressor molecule for IgA in a normal situation, but those for IgM, IgG, and IgE have been easily identified.[1,2,18,19] Suppressor cells for IgA have been reported in IgA deficiencies,[20,21] which would explain the deficiency.

The findings presented in this report also show that the T_h-effector cell for IgA has already been formed after initial contact with antigen. There appears to be no need for an inducer for this cell (a more mature step) or for extreme amounts of amplification, as seen in some immune networks. A common maturation and/or amplification step among T-cells shows the Lyt-1 $\rightarrow$ Lyt-123 $\rightarrow$ Lyt-1 effector maturation/amplification scheme that was first advanced by Tada, et al.[8] The T-inducer cell in this scheme is the inducer for IgG help; it does not appear to pertain to IgA synthesis.

In IgA synthesis, the T_h would not need an amplification-maturation step, and the T_h induced by contact with antigen would be the T_h-effector, albeit an immature T-helper cell. It would also have no T_s to control it. The entire control of IgA synthesis would rest upon the internal control mechanisms of the IgA-producing cell itself, and special clearance mechanisms specific for IgA.[22-24] This theory is conceivable, as the IgA-plasma cell is the most mature of the B-cell line, and the only cell that cannot switch isotype class, because its other H-chain genes have been excised. FIGURE 1 shows the maturational scheme of both the T_h and the regulating (T_s) cell that is being proposed.

As can be envisaged in FIGURE 1, the more immature the T_h, the more mature the T_s that controls it, and the more mature the B-cell is upon which it acts. If maturation of the lymphocytes also relates to a more mature controlling mechanism, then this maturation allows for good control of all antibody classes, but especially those of which are potentially dangerous to the host; that is, IgE, IgG, and T-cell dependent IgM. T-cell independent IgM appears to be synthesized by a specific B-cell subset[25] that is not necessarily an immature B-cell and does appear to be under some kind of T-cell control.[26]

Since Ngan and Kind,[27] and Vaz and et al.[28] have shown that the feeding of antigen also suppresses antigen-specific IgE formation, (and others have shown IgE suppression by T_s in other systems),[29,30] IgE appears to be under the same type of control as does IgG. Of all the antibody molecules, IgE probably has the potential to do the most damage to the host, and therefore should be under the strictest control. For this reason, and for where the IgE-producing cell lies on the B-cell maturational schema, one would predict it to be under control of the most mature of the T-suppressor cells. This theory is proposed as part of this hypothesis.

It is readily apparent that FIGURE 1 shows no T_s for IgA; this omission is

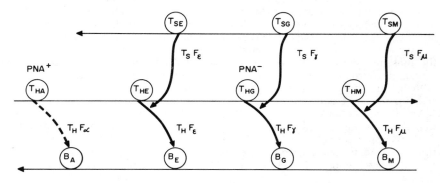

FIGURE 1. Maturation scheme of lymphocytes

justified, as very few studies have ever demonstrated the antigen-specific isotypic suppression of IgA. This study did not demonstrate this IgA specific suppression, although it was examined. IgA-specific suppressor cells have only been shown in cases of specific or generalized immunosuppression,[20,21] which would fit this model, allowing for a defect in either the T_s maturation or the B-cell receptors for suppressor molecules for other isotypes on IgA-producing B-cells.

What makes IgA so special that it needs no T-suppressor cells? First, it is the least dangerous of any of the immunoglobulin classes to the host; that is, it does not fix complement, nor does it cause allergic reactions. It also has a relatively short half-life, and thanks to several recent elegant studies,[22-24] we know that it is actively cleared from the system differently than the other immunoglobulin classes through a bile transport system. Therefore, unlike the other classes, any excess IgA could get cleared before any damage could occur, whatever that damage could possibly be.

It is proposed from these studies, therefore, that there are maturational stages of both T_s and T_h, just as there are with B-cells. The maturational stage of the T-cells is directly related to the ability to control an immunoglobulin response, and the maturational stage of the T_s is directly proportional to the maturational stage of the B-cell that it is to control. The maturational stage of the T_h is inversely related to the maturational stage of the B-cell that it affects.

REFERENCES

1. MATTINGLY, J. A. & B. H. WAKSMAN. 1980. J. Immunol. **125:** 1044.
2. MATTINGLY, J. A., J. M. KAPLAN, & C. A. JANEWAY, JR. 1980. J. Exp. Med. **152:** 545.
3. CRABBE, P., D. R. NASH, H. BAZIN, H. EYSSEN, & J. F. HEREMANS. 1969. J. Exp. Med. **130:** 723.
4. ELSON, C. O., J. A. HECK, & W. STROBER. 1979. J. Exp. Med. **149:** 632.
5. ISHIZAKA, K., & H. OKUDAIRA. 1972. J. Immunol. **109:** 84.
6. EARDLEY, D. D., J. HUGENBERGER, L. McVAY-BOUDREAU, F. W. SHEN, R. K. GERSHON, & H. CANTOR. 1978. J. Exp. Med. **147:** 1106.
7. GERSHON, R. K., D. D. EARDLEY, S. DURUM, D. R. GREEN, F. W. SHEN, K. YAMAUCHI, H. CANTOR, & D. B. MURPHY. 1981. J. Exp. Med. **153:** 1533.
8. TADA, T., T. TAKEMORI, K. OKUMURA, M. NONAKA, & T. TOKUHISA. 1978. J. Exp. Med. **147:** 446.
9. ANDRÉ, C., J. F. HEREMANS, J. P. VAERMAN, & C. L. CAMBIASO. 1975. J. Exp. Med. **142:** 1509.
10. JULIUS, M. H., E. SIMPSON, & L. A. HERZENBERG. 1973. Eur. J. Immunol. **3:** 645.
11. MISHELL, R. I., & R. W. DUTTON. 1967. J. Exp. Med. **126:** 423.
12. CUNNINGHAM, A., & A. SZENBERG. 1968. Immunology **14:** 599.
13. REISNER, Y., L. ITZICOVITCH, A. MESHORER, & N. SHARON. 1978. Proc. Natl. Acad. Sci. USA **75:** 2933.
14. REISNER, Y., G. GACHELIN, P. DUBOIS, J. F. NICHOLAS, N. SHARON, & F. JACOB. 1977. Dev. Biol. **61:** 20.
15. LONDON, J., S. BERRIH, & J. F. BACH. 1978. J. Immunol. **212:** 438.
16. MATTINGLY, J. A., & B. H. WAKSMAN. 1978. J. Immunol. **121:** 1878.
17. POTTER, M. 1971. N. Engl. J. Med. **284:** 831.
18. SY, M-S., M. H. DIETZ, R. N. GERMAIN, B. BENACERRAF, & M. I. GREENE. 1980. J. Exp. Med. **151:** 1183.
19. LEE, W. Y., & A. H. SEHON. 1978. Immunol. Rev. **41:** 200.
20. ATWATER, J. S., & T. B. TOMASI. 1978. Clin. Immunol. Immunopathol. **9:** 379.
21. WALDMANN, T. A., S. BRODER, R. KRAKAUER, M. DURM, B. DEADE, & C. GOLDMAN. 1976. Trans. Assoc. Am. Physicians. **89:** 215.
22. HALSEY, J. F., B. H. JOHNSON, & J. J. CEBRA. 1980. J. Exp. Med. **151:** 767.
23. LEMAITRE-COELHO I., G. D. F. JACKSON, & J. P. VAERMAN. 1978. J. Exp. Med. **147:** 934.
24. ORLANS, E., J. PEPPARD, J. REYNOLDS, & J. HALL. 1978. J. Exp. Med. **147:** 588.
25. ANDERSSON, J. O. SJÖBERG, & G. MÖLLER. 1972. Eur. J. Immunol. **2:** 349.
26. PRIMI, D., L. HAMMORSTROM, & C. I. E. SMITH. 1979. Cell. Immunol. **42:** 90.
27. NGAN, J., & L. S. KIND. 1978. J. Immunol. **120:** 861.
28. VAZ, N. M., L. C. S. MAIA, D. G. HANSON, & J. M. LYNCH. 1977. J. Allergy Clin. Immunol. **60:** 110.
29. FOX, P. C., & R. P. SIRAGANIAN. 1981. Immunology **43:** 227.
30. TAKATSU, K., & K. ISHIZAKA. 1976. J. Immunol. **117:** 1211.

DISCUSSION OF THE PAPER

N. F. PIERCE (*Johns Hopkins University, Baltimore, Md.*): Because you speculate that there are no suppressor cells for the IgA response and that IgA is so carefully and rapidly secreted, what is it that keeps the response from running away with itself?

J. A. MATTINGLY (*The Ohio State University, Columbus, Ohio*): IgA is cleared from the serum much more efficiently than the other immunoglobulins. Even when we do have an abundance of IgA production, we can clear it quite rapidly.

J. BIENENSTOCK (*McMaster University, Hamilton, Ontario, Canada*): I want to ask you a question about your PNA experiments. PNA also reacts, as Dr. Rose has shown, with splenic germinal center cells and also the germinal center cells of the Peyer's patches, which themselves bear IgA. Therefore, would not the following be a reasonable explanation? You are leaving behind the population of cells capable of expressing and then going on to synthesis of IgA.

MATTINGLY: I do not think so, because the Peyer's patch cells that were treated with PNA were purified for T-cells. They had been nylon-wool-passed and then tested for their ability to bind with anti-Thy. About 85% of the cells were positive.

HETEROGENEITY OF B-CELLS

R. M. E. Parkhouse, Elizabeth M. Andrew, Ann Chayen,
and S. Marshall-Clarke

National Institute for Medical Research
Mill Hill
London, NW7 1AA England

INTRODUCTION

The characterization of functionally distinct subclasses of lymphocytes using cell-surface markers has advanced rapidly in recent years. Most success has been achieved in the T-cell area, despite ample evidence for B-cell heterogeneity, for example in differential reactivity to mitogens, T-dependent and T-independent antigens. Other characters, such as size, charge adhesiveness, and recirculation habits, point to heterogeneity of B-cells. A whole set of studies with a variety of cell-surface markers also leads to the same conclusion,[1,2] but without good functional correlates. With all of this in mind, we have used the monoclonal antibody technique to look for antibodies differentially expressed on B-lymphocytes. Here we describe two such antibodies that are by definition differentiation antigens of the B-cell series, in that they are expressed to a greater or lesser extent at different phases of B-cell development. One, NIM-R2, is particularly interesting, in that its complementary determinant changes in density at four discrete stages of cell differentiation.

In addition, a study of the distribution of several well-characterized cell-surface markers and major glycoproteins has been conducted on lymphocytes from different lymphoid tissues.

MATERIALS AND METHODS

Animals

CBA × BALB/c and CBA/N × BALB/c mice, raised under specific pathogen-free conditions were used at 12–20 weeks of age and as stated in the text.

Depletion of T-cells

Spleen cells were depleted of T-cells by treatment with monoclonal rat anti-mouse Thy-1 antibody, NIM-R1,[3] and guinea pig complement. After this treatment the cell suspensions contained <3% Thy-1 positive and 90–95% sIg-positive cells.

Fluorescent Staining of Lymphocytes

Cell suspensions of the various lymphoid organs were prepared by teasing the tissue into PBA, a phosphate-buffered saline (PBS) (130 mM NaCl, 4 mM KCl, 10

215

0077-8923/83/0409-0215 $1.75/0 © 1983 NYAS

mM sodium phosphate, pH 7.4) containing bovine serum albumin (BSA) (1 mg/ml) and NaN_3 (1 mg/ml). Cells were centrifuged and resuspended in 0.83% (wt./vol.) NH_4Cl for five minutes at room temperature (to remove red blood cells (RBC)). For staining, cells were incubated in PBA for 20 minutes on ice with antibody at 0.1–0.3 mg/ml. The washed cell suspension was then similarly treated, when appropriate, with another antibody, and was assessed for fluorescence in the Becton-Dickinson FACS II fluorescence-activated cell-sorter or microscopically with a Leitz instrument.

Cell Lines

The 70Z/3 cell line[4] was provided by Dr. C. Paige (Basel Institute for Immunology, Switzerland) and maintained in RPMI-1640, 10% fetal calf serum (FCS), 2 mM glutamine, 100 U/ml penicillin, 100 μg/ml streptomycin, $5 \times 10^{-5}M$ β-mercaptoethanol, and 2 μg/ml Fungizone. For induction, cells were cultured for 18–24 hours at $5–6 \times 10^5$ cells/ml with lipopolysaccharide (LPS) at 20 μg/ml.

Activation of B-cells with Lipopolysaccharide

Spleen cells from adult CBA × BALB/c strain mice were prepared in the same medium as given above, except that the serum concentration was reduced to five percent. The suspension was depleted of T-cells by treatment with NIM-R1[3] and guinea pig complement. Cultures were dispensed with cells at 2×10^5 per ml, and LPS at 20 μg/ml.

Immunization for Monoclonal Activity NIM-R2

CBA strain spleen cell plasma membranes were prepared[5] and Lou rats were given one mg (as protein) in Freund's complete adjuvant at five sites, distributed over each leg and the nape of the neck. The animals were boosted three months later with 10^8 CBA strain spleen cells (treated with 0.83% (wt./vol.) NH_4Cl to remove RBC), injected intravenously, and sacrificed for fusion after 90 hours.

Immunization for Monoclonal Antibody NIM-R3

The immunization was as above except that the cells used for the booster were CBA spleen cells depleted of T-cells and clearly NIM-R2-positive cells. Depletion of T-cells was achieved by treatment of spleen cells with monoclonal anti-Thy-1, NIM-R1,[3] and guinea pig complement. The cells surviving this procedure were depleted of NIM-R2-positive cells by an indirect version of the panning procedure.[6] The cells were first treated with Ars-NIM-R2 (0.2 mg/ml 20 minutes on ice), washed twice with PBA, and resuspended at 10^7 cells/ml in PBA; 3 ml aliquots were transferred to 90 mm Sterilin single vent (No. 51001.101) Petri dishes. The Petri dishes had previously been coated with affinity purified goat anti-Ars (10 μg/ml in 50 mM TRIS, pH 8.3, 45 minutes room temperature). After 60 minutes at 4° C, with one gentle swirl at 30 minutes, the nonadherent cells were collected and by staining with fluorescein isothiocyanate (FITC)-Goat anti-MIg, the number of B-cells was found to be reduced to 47%. For the booster, 10^8 cells were administered intravenously.

Fusion, Screening, Cloning, and Propagation

Spleen cells (10^8) freed of RBC by treatment with 0.83% (wt./vol.) NH_4Cl, were fused with rat myeloma cells 210RCY3-Ag123,[7] using polyethylene glycol M.W. 4,000 as previously described.[1,3]

Measurement of Immune Responses

Generation of primary immune responses *in vitro*, as well as the assessment of memory cell potential *in vivo* by cell transfer, was done as previously described.[8]

Antibodies

Antibodies were purified and derivatized with haptens and fluorochromes as previously described.[1,3] For the analytical survey of cells in different lymphoid tissues, the following systems were employed: for sIg, a FITC derivative of affinity-purified rat anti-mouse Ig; for I-A^k, a FITC derivative of the monoclonal IgG_2b anti-I-A^{k9} purified on protein A-Sepharose; for Fc receptor (FcR), indirect fluorescence, using as a first layer, tissue culture supernatant from the rat monoclonal antibody 2.4G2,[10] followed by a mixture of FITC-OX12 (a monoclonal mouse IgG_2 anti-rat Kappa chain, purified on protein A-Sepharose, and given to us by Dr. A.F. Williams, Oxford University, England) and affinity purified FITC-Goat anti-rat Ig (absorbed on a column of normal mouse Ig until unreactive with murine B-cells); for NIM-R2 and NIM-R3, staining was similarly indirect, using a 1/100 dilution of ascitic fluid as the first layer and the anti-rat Ig FITC reagents given above; for Lyt-1 and Lyt-2, staining was again indirect, using tissue culture supernatants from the rat cell lines making rat monoclonal antibodies 53-73 (anti-Lyt-1) and 53 6.7 (anti-Lyt-2)[11] in conjunction with the same two FITC-conjugated anti-rat Ig antibodies; for Thy-1, monoclonal antibody NIM-R1 was purified, FITC-coupled and used directly.[3] Controls were normal rat serum or tissue culture fluid followed by the mixed FITC rat anti-Ig (for indirect staining) or affinity purified goat anti-rabbit IgG (for direct staining).

Two-dimensional gel electrophoresis was conducted as previously described,[12] and glycoproteins were subsequently revealed by immersing the gel in ^{125}I-labeled Concanavalin A,[13] washing and autoradiography. The cell lysates for the electrophoresis were mouse lymphoid tissue cell-suspensions depleted of T-cells and RBC, as indicated above, and consisting of >95% sIg-positive cells. The cells were resuspended at 5×10^8/ml in PBS including as protease inhibitors 1 mM phenylmethylsulfonylfluoride, 25 μg/ml N-p-tosyl-L-lysinechloromethyl, L-1-tosylamide-2-phenylethylchloromethylketone, and 1 mM EDTA. The cells were lysed by the addition of Nonidet P40 to 0.5% (vol./vol.), and the mixture was held at 0° C for 10 minutes, and then centrifuged for 20 minutes at 11,000 g. The lysate was stored at $-70°$ C until required, at which stage the other components of O'Farrell's lysis buffer[12] were added.

RESULTS

Tissue Distribution of Monoclonal Antibodies NIM-R2 and NIM-R3

The tissue distribution of cells reactive with monoclonal antibodies NIM-R2 and NIM-R3 is presented in TABLE 1.

In peripheral lymphoid tissue, both NIM-R2 and NIM-R3 stain only B-cells and do so in a reciprocal manner. Thus, although NIM-R2 stains most splenic B-cells, there is a fluorescence intensity distribution ranging from weak or negative to strong, and it is those B-cells that stain, at best, weakly with NIM-R2, that stain with NIM-R3, and vice versa. The reciprocal nature of the two antibodies is most clear when the bone marrow is examined. Here, both antibodies brightly stain nonoverlapping cell populations and additively account for 90–95% of bone marrow cells (TABLE 1). The fact that both antibodies clearly stain more bone marrow cells than are accounted for by the total number within the B-cell lineage is worthy of emphasis, indicating as it does that cell-surface markers are rarely expressed solely within the cells that comprise one defined developmental series, in this case B-cells and their progenitors. This point is further emphasized by the finding of NIM-R2 binding by RBC, thymocytes, and presumably hemopoietic cells in neonatal spleen (TABLE 1). The antibody NIM-R3, on the other hand, recognizes determinants that appear later in development than NIM-R2, both in spleen and bone marrow, and is also absent on thymocytes

TABLE 1

TISSUE DISTRIBUTION OF MONOCLONAL ANTIBODIES NIM-R2 AND NIM-R3

	Percent of Cells Fluorescent in Tissue						
Marker	Newborn Spleen	Adult Spleen	Thymus	Newborn Bone Marrow	Adult Bone Marrow	RBC	CNS
sIg	8	55	0	9	12	−	−
Thy-1	7	43	97	11	7	−	+
NIM-R2	43	46	35	51	62	+	−
NIM-R3	0	20	0	1	28	−	−

*Cell suspensions from 12 CBA × BALB/c mice were stained with affinity-purified FITC-Goat anti-mouse Fab, purified FITC-NIM-R1 (anti-Thy-1), NIM-R2, and NIM-R3. The latter two were ascitic fluids, diluted 1/100 followed by FITC-OX12 (a mouse monoclonal IgG_2a anti-rat kappa chain). The percentages of positive cells were obtained by analysis using the FACS II.

and RBC. This distribution in ontogeny indicates that NIM-R3 does not recognize either pre-B or immature B-cells, but does recognize a differentiation antigen expressed by more mature B-lymphocytes. The antibody NIM-R2, however, binds to all cells within the B-cell series, but to a variable extent, as will become evident below.

Distribution of Selected Cell-Surface Markers and Major Glycoproteins on Lymphocytes of Different Lymphoid Tissue

In this part of the work we looked for differential expression of selected cell-surface antigens and major glycoproteins by B-cells from different lymphoid organs: spleen, peripheral lymph nodes, mesenteric lymph nodes, and Peyer's patches. The marker analysis was done by fluorescent staining, and assessed by the fluorescence-activated cell-sorter. To study major glycoproteins, Nonidet P40-soluble extracts of B-cells were resolved by two-dimensional gel electrophoresis, and then the glycoproteins were selectively revealed by treating the gel with an overlay of ^{125}I-labeled Concanavalin A. The surface marker survey was carried out on B-cells from normal (CBA × BALB/c male) and B-cell defective (CBA/N × BALB/c male) mice,[14] with the hope of detecting differences between the two strains.

The results of the surface marker analysis are presented in TABLE 2, and the main conclusion to be drawn is that B-cells from all organs studied, whether normal CBA or deficient CBA/N, similarly express sIg, I-A^k, and FcR. The same may be said for the monoclonal markers NIM-R2 and NIM-R3, with the possible exception of the slightly lower representation of NIM-R3 by Peyer's patches than other lymphoid organs. Similarly, the expression of T-cell markers, Thy-1, Lyt-1, and Lyt-2 was much the same in all tissues, again with the possible exception of Peyer's patch cells, where the suppressor phenotype Lyt-2 was perhaps less well represented, relative to Lyt-1, than in other tissues.

As with the surface marker study reported above, two-dimensional gel analysis of major glycoproteins expressed by B-cells from different tissues also failed to reveal any major differences (FIGURE 1).

These data raise the possibility that B-cells located in different lymphoid organs, are not distinguished in any major way. Further work is required to establish whether this is the case.

Changes in the Density of a Cell-Surface Determinant During the Differentiation of B-Cells.

In this section, we show how the density of the determinant recognized by NIM-R2 (and in one situation NIM-R3), varies at four defined stages of B-cell differentiation.

Conversion of Pre-B-Cells to B-Cells

The 70Z/3 cell line[4] is a model for the late pre-B-cell stage of differentiation, its only Ig component expressed being cytoplasmic μ-chain. Upon activation with LPS, light-chain synthesis is initiated, and 7S IgM-subunits are assembled and inserted into the plasma membrane. The LPS-driven system, therefore, provides a model for the conversion of a late pre-B-cell to an immature B-cell.

The cells were therefore induced with LPS as described in the MATERIALS AND METHODS, and cell surface expression of NIM-R2 and IgM was evaluated before and after induction. As can be seen (FIGURE 2, bottom), there was a major increase in staining with anti-μ-chain, the percentage of sIg-bearing cells increasing from 4% to 45% upon induction. At the same time (FIGURE 2, top), the density of NIM-R2 binding decreased from 55% positive in the control to 14% in the LPS-induced culture.

Thus, in a model for the conversion of pre-B to immature B-cell, the density of the determinant detected by NIM-R2 decreases.

As might be expected from its distribution, absent in both the spleen and bone marrow of neonatal life, NIM-R3 fails to stain 70Z/3 cells.

Activation of B-cells

Spleen cells from CBA × BALB/c mice were depleted of T-cells using NIM-R1 and guinea pig complement, and activated with lipopolysaccharide.

TABLE 2

DISTRIBUTION OF SURFACE MARKERS IN VARIOUS LYMPHOID TISSUES*

Percentage of Cells Fluorescent in Tissue

Marker	Spleen		Peripheral Lymph Nodes		Mesenteric Lymph Nodes		Peyer's Patches	
	CBA × BALB/c	CBA/N × BALB/c	CBA × BALB/c	CBA/N × BALB/c	CBA × BALB/c	CBA/N × BALB/c	CBA × BALB/c	CBA/N × BALB/c
Lyt-1	42	40	89	91	78	83	31	54
Lyt-2	18	17	32	33	28	29	8	14
Thy-1	43	42	88	92	77	87	33	51
sIg	55	30	14	8	16	11	56	39
I-A^k	49	27	13	9	18	13	56	38
FcR	50	25	14	5	22	11	52	33
NIM-R2	46	32	12	7	19	13	45	32
NIM-R3	20	16	6	4	13	8	9	8

*Cell suspensions from 12 adult mice were stained as indicated in the MATERIALS AND METHODS, and then the percentages of positively stained cells were obtained by analysis using the FACS II. The NIM-R2 and NIM-R3 staining was developed here by the application of two FITC-derivatized antibodies, OX-12, and goat-anti-rat Ig (absorbed on mouse Ig). These two together yield brighter fluorescence than OX-12 alone.

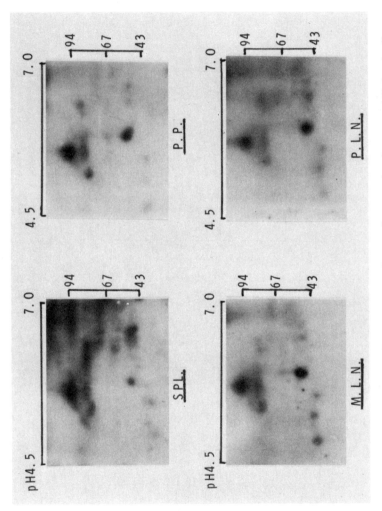

FIGURE 1. Major glycoproteins of lymphoid B-cells. CBA × BALB/c mice, three months of age, were killed and cell suspensions from their lymphoid organs were depleted of T-cells with NIM-R1 and guinea pig complement. They were then lysed in Nonidet-P40, and submitted to two-dimensional "O'Farrell" gel separation. Glycoproteins were revealed by [¹²⁵I]Concanavalin A overlay, washing, and autoradiography. Organs examined in this way were: spleen (SPL), Peyer's patches (P.P.), mesenteric lymph nodes (M.L.N.), and peripheral lymph nodes (P.L.N.). The direction of the pH gradient in the first electrophoretic dimension and the position of molecular weight markers corun in the second, SDS-PAGE, dimension are indicated. Details in MATERIALS AND METHODS. Note the similarity in the profiles.

Cells were removed on various days and stained with NIM-R2 and NIM-R3. Using the cell-sorter, it was possible to assess blastogenesis by counting the total number of blast cells by scattering analysis. Then, the fraction of blast cells staining with NIM-R2, NIM-R3, and anti-Ig was measured, also by sorter-analysis. The results, presented in FIGURE 3, indicate that the number of blast cells

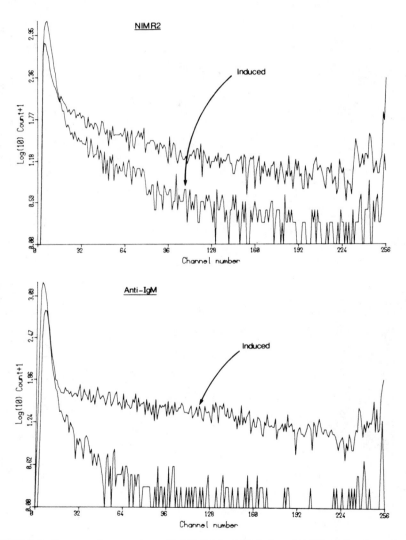

FIGURE 2. Decreased expression of NIM-R2 by LPS-induced 70Z/3 cells. Control and LPS-induced 70Z/3 cells were stained with affinity purified FITC-Goat anti-mouse μ-chain (top) or with NIM-R2 ascites diluted 1/100 followed by FITC-OX12 (a mouse IgG_2a monoclonal anti-rat kappa chain) (bottom) and analysed in the FACS II. The profile given by the induced cells is indicated. Details in MATERIALS AND METHODS.

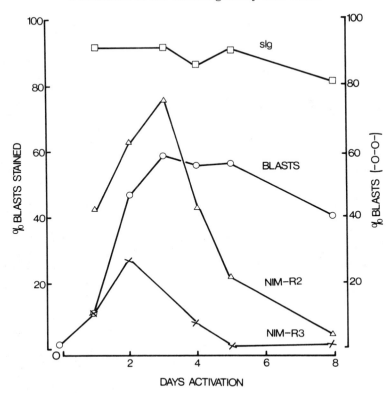

FIGURE 3. Induction of NIM-R2 and NIM-R3 reactivity on splenic B-cells by LPS. Splenic B-cells from CBA × BALB/c were activated by LPS *in vitro* and periodically examined in the FACS II after staining with affinity-purified FITC-Goat anti-mouse Fab, NIM-R2, and NIM-R3. The latter two reagents were ascitic fluid diluted 1/100 and were developed with FITC-OX12. Scatter analysis yielded the number of blast cells, as distinct from lymphocytes. Fluorescence analysis was confined to only the blast cells. Details in MATERIALS AND METHODS.

reactive with both NIM-R2 and NIM-R3 increased to a maximum at two days of culture, and then decreased with further culture. Over the same time period, essentially all of the blasts were positive for sIg.

Thus, during the activation and differentiation processes stimulated by LPS, the density of determinants defined by NIM-R2 and NIM-R3 fluctuated, rising at first and then declining.

Difference in NIM-R2 Expression Between Virgin and Memory-B-Cells

The data described in this section have been reported in detail[8] and will therefore be summarized. When splenic B-cells are stained with NIM-R2, the intensity profile obtained on the FACS ranges from negative, or weak, to very intense (FIGURE 4). The profit was arbitrarily sorted into four numerically equal

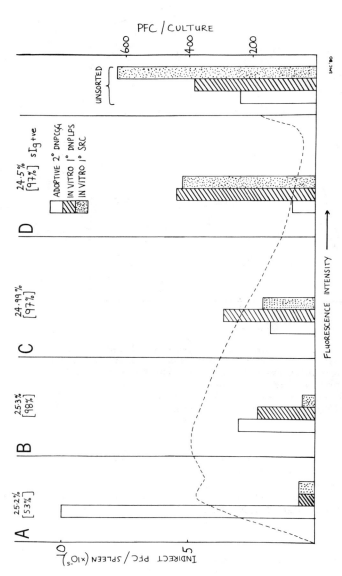

FIGURE 4. Primary and secondary immune responses of B-cells separated on the basis of their staining intensity with NIM-R2. CBA × BALB/c mice, normal or DNP-primed, were depleted of T-cells by treatment with NIM-R1 and guinea pig complement and were incubated (10⁸ cells/ml) with Ars-NIM-R2 (300 μg/ml) followed by affinity purified FITC-Goat anti-Ars (200 μg/ml). The fluorescence profile is indicated (------) and shows a gradation in intensity. For sorting, the profile was divided into four numerically equal-sized fractions from weak (A) through to strong (D), as indicated by the vertical bars on the FIGURE. The number of B-cells in each fraction was obtained by counterstaining the separated cells with affinity-purified TRITC-Goat anti-mouse Fab, absorbed on rat Ig, and the values obtained are the numbers in the square brackets included on the FIGURE. All fractions except A, the weakest stained, which contained 53% of sIg-positive cells, consisted almost entirely of sIg-positive cells. The other numbers included on the figure are the accurate percentages of cells sorted into the four fractions. Primary responses *in vitro* were measured against a T-independent antigen, DNP-LPS (▨), and a T-dependent antigen sheep red blood cell, SRC (▨). The secondary response to DNP was assessed by a transfer of sorted B-cells, antigen, and helper-primed T-cells to X-irradiated recipient mice (□). Further details will be found in reference 8.

fractions, from A, the weakest, through B and C to D, the strongest fluorescence. The fluorescence profile did not change during the period of the sort. Cells collected in each of the four fractions were assessed for the ability to mount a primary response *in vitro*. The results, summarized in FIGURE 4 indicate that the majority of the precursors for both T-dependent (anti-sheep RBC) and T-independent (anti-dinitrophenylated (DNP)-LPS) responses are found among cells with a relatively high degree of fluorescence. Of the recovered direct plaque-forming cells, 76–94% were in fractions C and D. The converse was true when a secondary response was considered. Secondary responses were measured using a secondary adoptive transfer system. Sublethally irradiated mice were given an excess of spleen cells primed with chicken gamma globulin (CGG), and DNP-primed cells, which had been sorted into one of the four populations, A–D. The mice were then challenged with DNP-CGG. The anti-DNP response of the adoptive host was a measure of the ability of the sorted cells to give rise to a secondary response. From the results summarized in FIGURE 4, it was apparent that most of the memory B-cells were located among the least intensely stained cells. Cells in fractions A and B were responsible for generating 83% of the indirect PFC recovered.

In summary, cells that stain weakly with NIM-R2 are enriched for memory B-cells, whereas those that stain strongly are enriched for virgin B-cells. Once again, then, the density of the determinant recognized by NIM-R2 is seen to change as the B-cell undergoes its presumed differentiation from primary to memory cell. These observations also indicate a cell-surface difference between virgin and memory B-cells. Thus memory B-cells must differentiate from virgin B-cells, and are not simply an expanded population, identical to the virgin cells that arise as a result of contact with antigen.

Reactivity of Antibody-Secreting Cells with NIM-R2

Spleen cells from CBA × BALB/c mice on day 7 of a primary or secondary response to a T-dependent antigen were stained with NIM-R2 and separated on the FACS; the positive and negative cells were examined for the presence of antibody-secreting cells (PFC) by the plaque assay.[8]

The results show (TABLE 3), perhaps not surprisingly, that most primary PFC are NIM-R2-negative, although there certainly does exist a significant fraction of NIM-R2-positive plaque-forming cells. More surprising was the finding that secondary PFC, generated, we must assume, from NIM-R2 weak lymphocytes, were almost all NIM-R2-positive. Once again, reactivity with NIM-R2 changes as virgin or memory cells differentiate into their antibody-secreting progeny.

DISCUSSION

There are many indications that B-cells are heterogenous, such as markers defined by allo-antisera,[15–17] responsiveness to T-dependent and T-independent antigens,[18] physical characteristics,[19–20] and surface isotype.[21] More recently, some monoclonal antibodies, reactive with all B-lineage cells, have also been described.[22–24] Using the monoclonal antibody technique, the identification of further cell-surface markers, selectively expressed at different stages of B-cell development, or on independent subpopulations of B-cells, can be anticipated. Such reagents should greatly increase our understanding of the differentiation, triggering, and complexity of cells within the B-cell series.

In this paper, we describe two monoclonal antibodies, NIM-R2 and NIM-R3, that only recognize B-cells in secondary lymphoid organs. Both show differential reactivity in that they react most strongly with nonoverlapping subpopulations of B-cells. They also react differentially with some cells of the primary lymphoid tissue. Thus NIM-R2 and NIM-R3 account for 90–95% of bone marrow cells, but recognize nonoverlapping populations, with NIM-R2 identifying approximately twice the number of cells as NIM-R3. This result merits comment because NIM-R2 was used to bias the fusion that produced NIM-R3, and that fusion was precisely designed to yield an antibody reactive with NIM-R2-negative cells (see MATERIALS AND METHODS). The antibody NIM-R2, but not NIM-R3, also reacted with thymocytes and red blood cells. It is worth emphasizing that the rule, rather than the exception, is to find sharing of cell-surface antigens among widely different cell types. The exact functional significance of this is obscure, but may relate to shared functions or receptor-ligand systems. Whatever the final explanation, the practical importance is that cell-surface markers cannot be used to trace the ontogeny of a given cell type if, as seems to be so frequent, cell-surface determinants are shared among cell types that belong to different cell lineages.

TABLE 3

STAINING OF PRIMARY AND SECONDARY ANTIBODY-SECRETING CELLS WITH NIM-R2§

| | Cells | | | |
Response	Unstained	Unsorted‡	NIM-R2-positive‡	NIM-R2-negative‡
Primary*	1134	1104	500	1342
Secondary†	546	562	992	60

*Spleens from adult CBA × BALB/c mice immunized seven days previously with alum precipitated DNP-human IgG (0.3 mg, intraperitoneally).

†Spleens from mice primed with alum precipitated DNP-KLH (0.1 mg) and boosted with DNP-KLH in saline (0.02 mg) seven days prior to use.

‡Cells were stained with NIM-R2 ascites at 1/100 and FITC-OX12 into positive (the brightest 30%) and negative (the dullest 65%) fractions.

§Results are indirect PFC/10^6 cells and represent the mean of three determinations of DNP-PFC on samples of 2.5–5.0 × 10^5 cells.

The antibody NIM-R2 was of particular interest, because it appeared to recognize a structure that fluctuated at four defined stages of B-cell development. Thus, if the 70Z/3 cell is acceptable as a model for the pre-B cell, the density of the NIM-R2 determinant decreases upon conversion of the pre-B to the immature B-cell. Conversely, when mature B-cells are activated (by LPS), the NIM-R2 (and NIM-R3) determinant rises to a maximum density two to three days post activation and then subsequently declines to a low level over the next four to five days. Most interesting of all was the differential reactivity of NIM-R2 with virgin and memory B-cells. Those cells that stained strongly with the antibody gave excellent primary responses, but were unable to transfer secondary responses, whereas weakly stained B-cells transferred memory, but could not generate primary antibody responses in vitro. From these experiments it appears that NIM-R2 recognizes a cell-surface determinant that is decreased in density as primary B-cells differentiate to memory B-cells. This observation therefore clearly demonstrates a structural membrane difference between virgin and memory cells, and indicates that the generation of memory cells involves changes resulting from differentiation process as well as the presumed expansion due to division. It will be of some interest to examine the density of the NIM-R2 reactive determinant on those memory cells generated soon after antigen contact. The general tendency towards an overall reduction in the NIM-R2 reactive determinant is also seen in the analysis of PFC generated in a primary response, where the majority are relatively weakly stained with NIM-R2 and are, of course, derived from the more highly NIM-R2 reactive population of B-cells. The pattern is, however, disrupted by the finding that the majority of secondary PFC were clearly NIM-R2 positive, although derived from the weakly stained fraction of B-cells.

What may be concluded from this variable up and down fluctuation of reactivity with NIM-R2 during B-cell development? To us, the most appealing speculation, and it is a speculation, is that the structure recognized by NIM-R2 is involved in some sort of recognition system, and fluctuates as it does in order to control the level of communication. Time and appropriate experimentation will indicate whether this is the case.

The structural difference between primary and memory B-cells reported here may reflect previously reported qualitative differences such as half life,[25] ability to recirculate,[26] and physical characteristics.[27,28] The monoclonal antibody NIM-R2, by allowing their separation, should provide a direct approach to determining the physical, physiological, and biochemical properties of virgin and memory B-cells.

Finally, in an attempt to determine gross differences in B-cells located in the different secondary lymphoid organs, an analysis was made of the distribution of sIg, I-A, Fc receptors, and major glycoproteins. No significant differences were detected, and so if there is any preferential location for B-cell subpopulations in these different compartments, then the responsible structural basis will have to be sought outside the molecules studied in this work.

SUMMARY

Two rat monoclonal antibodies, NIM-R2 and NIM-R3, were prepared that only recognize B-cells in murine secondary lymphoid tissues. Both showed differential reactivity in that they reacted most strongly with nonoverlapping populations of B-cells. They also reacted differentially with some cells of the primary lymphoid tissue, recognizing 90–95% of bone marrow cells, again in a nonoverlapping manner and with NIM-R2 accounting for twice as many cells as NIM-R3. The antibody NIM-R2, but not NIM-R3, also recognized thymocytes and red blood cells.

The determinant recognized by NIM-R2 is of interest because it fluctuates at four defined stages of B-cell development: pre-B to immature B, activation of mature B, differentiation of memory cells, and differentiation of antibody-secreting cells. Particularly noteworthy was the differential reactivity of NIM-R2 with virgin and memory B-cells. Those cells that stained strongly with the antibody gave excellent primary responses, but were unable to transfer secondary responses, whereas weakly stained B-cells transferred memory, but could not generate primary antibody responses *in vitro*. Thus NIM-R2 recognized a cell-surface determinant that presumably decreases in density as primary B-cells differentiate into memory B-cells.

A survey of sIg, I-A, Fc receptors, and major glycoproteins of B-cells from spleen, Peyer's patches, mesenteric lymph nodes, and peripheral lymph nodes failed to reveal any major differences between the cells from these different lymphoid organs.

ACKNOWLEDGMENTS

We thank Keith Keeler for operating the FACS II and Graham Preece and N.W.T. Clark for technical assistance. Rachel Woodward operated the word processor.

[NOTE ADDED IN PROOF: Since the submission of this paper, we have noted a great variation in the number of cells reactive with NIM-R3, particularly weakly stained cells measured with the FACS. By binding studies we have shown that the antibodies NIM-R3 also react with granulocytes, and assume that this reactivity is a cause of variability, since the number of non-B, non-T cells in spleens is widely disparate depending upon the biological history of the mouse. At the same time, cells positively selected by NIM-R3 have been shown to transfer antibody responses, and so the reactivity of NIM-R3 with cells of the B-lineage is confirmed, although the number of such cells is normally a low percentage of spleens from mice kept under specific pathogen-free conditions.]

REFERENCES

1. CHAYEN, A. & R. M. E. PARKHOUSE. 1982. Eur. J. Immunol. In press.
2. KINCADE, P. W. 1981. Adv. Immunol. **31:** 177–245.
3. CHAYEN, A. & R. M. E. PARKHOUSE. 1982. J. Immunol. Methods **49:** 17–23.
4. PAIGE, C. J., P. W. KINCADE & P. RALPH. 1978. J. Immunol. **121:** 641–647.
5. SNARY, D., F. R. WOODS & M. J. CRUMPTON. 1976. Anal. Biochem. **74:** 457–465.
6. MAGE, M. G., L. L. MCHUGH & T. L. ROTHSTEIN. 1977. J. Immunol. Methods **15:** 47–56.
7. GALFRÈ, G., C. MILSTEIN & B. WRIGHT. 1979. Nature (London) **277:** 131–133.
8. MARSHALL-CARKE, S., A. CHAYEN & R. M. E. PARKHOUSE. 1982. Eur. J. Immunol. In press.
9. OI, V. T., P. P. JONES, J. W. GODING, & L. A. HERZENBERG. 1978. Curr. Top. Microbiol. Immunol. **81:** 115–129.
10. UNKLESS, J. C. 1980. J. Reticuloendothelial Soc. **28:** 11_s–17_s.
11. LEDBETTER, J. A. & L. A. HERZENBERG. 1979. Immunol. Rev. **47:** 63–90.
12. O'FARRELL, P. H. 1974. J. Biol. Chem. **250:** 4007–4021.
13. BURRIDGE, K. 1978. Methods in Enzymol. **50:** 54–56.
14. PAUL, W. E., B. SUBBARAO, J. J. MOND, D. G. SIECKMANN, I. ZITRON, A. AHMED, D. E. MOSIER & I. SCHER. 1979. *In* Cells of Immunoglobulin Synthesis. B. Pernis & H. J. Vogel, Eds.: 383–396. Academic Press. New York.
15. AHMED, A., I. SCHER, S. O. SHARROW, A. H. SMITH, W. E. PAUL, D. H. SACHS & K. WE. SELL. 1977. J. Exp. Med. **145:** 101–110.
16. HUBER, B., R. K. GERSHON & H. CANTOR. 1977. J. Exp. Med. **145:** 10–20.
17. ZEICHER, M., E. MOZES, Y. REISNER & P. LONAI. 1979. **9:** 119–124.
18. MARSHALL-CLARKE, S. & J. H. L. PLAYFAIR. 1979. Immunol. Rev. **43:** 109–142.
19. SHORTMAN, K. & M. HOWARD. 1979. *In* B lymphocytes in the immune response. M. Cooper, D. E. Mosier, I. Scher and E. S. Vitetta, Eds.: 97–106. Elsevier. North Holland.
20. SCHEGEL, R. A., H. VON BOEHMER & K. SHORTMAN. 1975. Cell. Immunol. **16:** 203–217.
21. PARKHOUSE, R. M. E. & M. D. COOPER. 1977. Immunol. Rev. **37:** 105–126.
22. COFFMAN, R. L. & I. L. WEISSMAN. 1981. J. Exp. Med. **153:** 269–279.
23. DESSNER, D. S. & M. R. LOKEN. 1981. Eur. J. Immunol. **11:** 282–285.
24. PAIGE, C. J., P. W. KINCADE, L. A. SHINEFELD & V. L. SATO. 1981. J. Exp. Med. **153:** 154–165.
25. ELSON, C. J., K. F. JABLONSKA & R. B. TAYLOR. 1976. Eur. J. Immunol. **6:** 634–638.
26. STROBER, S. 1972. J. Exp. Med. **136:** 851–871.
27. SCHRADER, J. W. 1974. Cell Immunol. **10:** 380–393.
28. FIDLER, J. M., M. HOWARD, R. A. SCHLEGEL, M. VADAS & K. SHORTMAN. 1977. J. Immunol. **118:** 1076–1082.

DISCUSSION OF THE PAPER

M. D. COOPER (*University of Alabama in Birmingham*): Why do you think the anti-delta does not affect the thymus-dependent response, that has both delta-positive and negative cells, when anti-μ will? Is that because the IgD gives a different signal, when cross-linked on the cell surface, than the IgM antibodies?

R. M. E. PARKHOUSE (*National Institute for Medical Research, London, England*): I think that is a possible interpretation of it. There is also a relatively trivial explanation for it, which is that most T-independent immune responses are generated by antigens with repeating epitopes. Thus, in this case, IgM alone with antigen may allow cross-linkage in the absence of IgD.

G. T. THORBECKE (*New York University Medical Center, New York, N.Y.*): If you find such shifts in this antigen, for instance when you induce blast formation with LPS, then should you not look every day at the plaque-forming cell-response with your virgin B-cells and with your memory B-cells and really go through it day by day to see how the positivity of the PFC response changes? On which days did you look?

PARKHOUSE: Actually, we only looked on those days; but you are quite right. We do intend to do that experiment.

M. ZAUDERER (*Columbia University, New York, N.Y.*): Am I right in thinking that because of the heterogeneity of surface immunoglobulin, you would not have picked up differences in surface isotype expression on B-cells in different tissues in your gel analysis?

PARKHOUSE: There is an extensive list of different Ig-positive isotypes published by Abney *et al*, (J. Immunol. **120**: 2041, 1978) that looks at all the lymphoid tissues. The IgM and the IgD, which are the major isotypes, are found on most B-cells and are present at the 90% level, whereas the other isotypes are much lower.

ZAUDERER: What is your definition of "memory" in these experiments?

PARKHOUSE: "Memory" in these experiments is defined as the Mitchison three mouse system. You inject mouse one with hapten on a given carrier and then sometime later you challenge in an *in vivo* transfer system. The adoptively transferred cells are challenged with the same hapten on another carrier, and because it is on another carrier, you also provide carrier primed T-cells to the adoptive host. There is an interval of between three to six months from initial priming and the actual execution of the experiment. You noticed in the experiment that approximately 50% of the B-cells did not respond in this system. We are currently determining if B-cell responses shift through that period of short-term priming; it appears that they do.

T-HELPER CELL ACTIVITY IN INTESTINAL LAMINA PROPRIA*

C. O. Elson,† D. B. Weiserbs, W. Ealding, and E. Machelski

Department of Medicine
Medical College of Virginia
Virginia Commonwealth University
Richmond, Virginia 23298

INTRODUCTION

The current concept of the IgA-cell cycle envisions that intestinal antigens stimulate IgA B-cell precursors within the Peyer's patches. These cells, destined to secrete IgA, leave the Peyer's patches and preferentially localize in the intestinal lamina propria as well as other mucosal sites.[1] Although IgA is known to be very T-cell dependent, the role of regulatory T-cells in the IgA-cell cycle is largely unknown. Recent work indicates that regulatory T-cells are also stimulated after antigen exposure in the Peyer's patches. For example, feeding of protein antigens to rodents generates T-suppressor cells in the Peyer's patches, which appear then to migrate to other sites.[2,3] It is known that T-cell blasts obtained from mesenteric lymph nodes preferentially localize in the intestinal lamina propria, just as B-cell blasts do,[4] but the functional properties of these T-cells that "home" to the intestinal lamina propria is unknown. One possibility is that these T-cells regulate the final expression of IgA synthesis toward the eliciting antigen. If so, these regulatory T-cells might well be IgA-isotype specific, considering that previous work has shown that such T-cells are unequally distributed among different tissues.[5] Because of technical difficulties involved in recovering them, lamina propria lymphocytes (LPL) have received little attention. In this study we have recovered LPL from mouse and man and tested their helper function for immunoglobulin synthesis using a pokeweed mitogen system.

MATERIALS AND METHODS

Mitogens

Pokeweed mitogen (PWM) and phytohemagglutinin (PHA-P) were obtained from Difco, Detroit, Michigan. Concanavalin A was obtained from Miles Biochemical, Elkhart, Indiana.

*This work was supported in part by Grant 1 R01 AM28623 from the National Institute of Arthritis, Diabetes, Digestive, and Kidney Diseases and in part by a grant from the National Foundation for Ileitis and Colitis.

†Recipient of Research Career Development Award 5 K04 AM00992 from the National Institute of Arthritis, Diabetes, Digestive, and Kidney Diseases.

0077-8923/83/0409-0230 $1.75/0 © 1983, NYAS

Cell Separations

C3H/He murine lymphoid cells were separated into T-cell and B-cell fractions using the panning technique of Wysoki and Sato.[6] Human lymphoid cells were separated into T-cell and B-cell fractions using rabbit-anti-human Fab_2 affinity columns as previously described.[7]

Isolation of Lamina Propria Lymphocytes

Murine small intestinal LPL were isolated using the method of Davies and Parrott.[8] Human small intestinal LPL were isolated using the method of Bull and Bookman[9] with minor modifications.

Cell Cultures

Cells were cultured in medium containing RPMI 1640, 25 mM N-2-hydroxy-ethyl piperazine-N'-2-ethane sulfonic acid (HEPES), 10% fetal calf serum, 2 mM glutamine, 100 units/ml penicillin, 100 μg/ml streptomycin, 50 μg/ml gentamicin, 2.5 μg/ml Fungizone, and 0.05 mM 2-mercaptomethanol. Cells were cultured in 24-well Costar plates for one week at 37°C in 5% CO_2 and humid air. Supernatants were then collected for assay.

Cell Proliferation Studies

Cells from various tissues were added to individual wells of a 96-well flat bottom microtiter tray (CoStar, Cambridge, Mass.) at a cell concentration of 3 × 10^5 cells/well or 5 × 10^4 cells/well. Various mitogens were added to triplicate wells except for one triplicate set of wells that served as the nonstimulated baseline control. Interleukin 2 was obtained by incubating LBRM 33 1A5 murine lymphoma cells (a gift of Dr. S. Mizel) with diluted macrophage supernatants as a source of interleukin 1, followed by stimulation with phytohemagglutinin.[10] The PHA-P was absorbed out on thyroglobulin-Sepharose 4B.[11] Cells were cultured for 42 hours at 37°C in 5% CO_2 and humid air, then pulsed with tritiated thymidine 0.25 μCi per well. After an additional six hours incubation they were harvested on a mini-MASH (M.A. Bioproducts, Walkersville, Md.) unit, and the degree of incorporation of the tritiated thymidine was assessed using a β scintillation counter.

Measurement of Immunoglobulin Synthesis

The immunoglobulin synthesized in the pokeweed mitogen-stimulated cultures of both mouse and human cells was measured using a sandwich enzyme-linked immunosorbent assay (ELISA) technique. Affinity-purified isotype-specific antisera were purchased from Tago (Burlington, Calif.) and verified before use. A standard curve was generated during each assay using quantitated serums (Miles Biochemicals, Elkart, Ind.). The amount of immunoglobulin in culture supernatants was interpolated from the standard curve using the four parameter logistic model of Rodbard[12] on an Apple II Plus computer.

TABLE 1

PROLIFERATIVE RESPONSE OF MOUSE LYMPHOID CELLS TO MITOGENS

Cells*	None	PHA 0.08 Percent		Con A 2 μg/ml		PWM 1:100	
	CPM	ΔCPM†	SI‡	ΔCPM	SI	ΔCPM	SI
Spleen	2474 ± 213	43968 ± 3559	18.7	52507 ± 21207	22.0	5093 ± 5444	3.0
Peyer's patches	6277 ± 170	21608 ± 5781	4.4	45190 ± 3981	8.2	7280 ± 668	2.2
Lamina propria	149 ± 143	1166 ± 1159	8.8	2100 ± 279	15	831 ± 37	6.6

*Cells were cultured at 3×10^5/ml.

†ΔCPM represents the CPM of stimulated cultures minus the CPM of unstimulated cultures.

‡SI = stimulation index, which represents the CPM of stimulated cultures divided by the CPM of unstimulated cultures.

Proliferation of Murine Lamina Propria Lymphocytes to Mitogens

In initial studies the capability of murine LPL to respond to various T-cell mitogens such as PHA-P, Con A, and pokeweed mitogen was determined and compared to similar capabilities of spleen and Peyer's patch cells (TABLE 1). The spontaneous proliferation of murine LPL was considerably lower than that seen in either spleen or Peyer's patches. When the results are expressed as a stimulation index, the proliferation seen in the lamina propria cells is within the range of that seen in spleen or Peyer's patches. When the results, however, are expressed as the actual number of counts per minute in the presence of mitogen minus the counts per minute without mitogen, the lamina propria cells show considerably lower values than either spleen or Peyer's patches.

Response of Lamina Propria Lymphocytes to Interleukin 2

One explanation of the above results is that the procedure used to isolate the LPL was affecting their ability to respond to mitogens. A second explanation is

TABLE 2

PROLIFERATIVE RESPONSE OF MOUSE LAMINA PROPRIA CELLS TO INTERLEUKIN 2

Lymphocytes Cultured (5×10^4/ml)	Stimulant Added			
	None	PHA 0.08%	IL-2 1:16	IL-2 1:32
Lamina propria	110 ± 81	823 ± 554	431 ± 269	378 ± 229
Mesenteric lymph node	503 ± 70	25984 ± 1600	2764 ± 284	3329 ± 540
Spleen	215 ± 86	13273 ± 906	2120 ± 1299	1588 ± 150
Peyer's patches	162 ± 127	14668 ± 1076	1900 ± 326	1920 ± 558
Peripheral blood	62 ± 16	ND	480 ± 67	338 ± 55

that the lamina propria T-cells might already be activated and thus unable to respond very well to T-cell mitogens. If the latter is correct, LPL should have a heightened response to T-cell growth factor or interleukin 2. In order to address these questions, cells from various mouse lymphoid tissues were obtained, and all the cells were exposed to the same ethylene diamine tetra acetic acid (EDTA) and collagenase isolation procedures that the LPL undergo. The response of these cells to PHA-P and to interleukin 2 was then assessed. The isolation treatment did not appear to have any major effect on the ability to respond to these stimuli. Once again, LPL have a very low rate of spontaneous proliferation and responded to PHA-P with a much lower response than that seen with other lymphoid cells (TABLE 2). Lamina propria cells did respond to interleukin 2, but again the response was quantitatively less than that seen with cells from other tissues. These results suggest that the small intestine lamina propria T-cells are a long-lived, slowly renewed population, rather than a population of recently transformed T-cell blasts.

Immunoglobulin Synthesis by Murine Lamina Propria Lymphocytes

Murine LPL were cultured *in vitro* for one week with and without pokeweed mitogen. The amount of IgA and IgG synthesized by such cultures was then measured. Cultures of LPL spontaneously synthesized substantial amounts of IgA, but not IgG, as compared to spleen cell cultures (TABLE 3). Addition of pokeweed mitogen to lamina propria cell cultures did not stimulate further IgA secretion but appeared to inhibit it.

T-Helper Cell Activity in Mouse Lamina Propria Lymphocytes

B-cells were obtained from a suspension of Peyer's patch cells using a panning technique in which goat anti-mouse immunoglobulin was coated onto plastic petri dishes. Cells that adhered were used as B-cells. T-cells from various mouse tissues were obtained by depleting the B-cells on goat-anti-mouse immunoglobulin-coated plastic dishes. The nonadherent fractions were then coated with a rat anti-Ly2 hybridoma antibody, washed, and layered over a second anti-immuno-

TABLE 3

SYNTHESIS OF IgA AND IgG IN CULTURES OF MOUSE LAMINA PROPRIA AND SPLEEN CELLS

		Experiment 1		Experiment 2	
Culture	PWM	IgA (ng/ml)	IgG (ng/ml)	IgA (ng/ml)	IgG (ng/ml)
Spleen	−	30	<8	35	61
	+	66	118	122	184
Lamina propria	−	218	<8	587	<8
	+	182	<8	214	10

globulin plate. Cells nonadherent to the second immunoglobulin plate, now depleted of both B-cells and Ly2 positive T-cells, were used as the T-cell source for the cultures. B-cells and T-cells were mixed together in a 1:2 ratio and cultured *in vitro* in the presence of pokeweed mitogen for one week. Each fraction was also cultured separately. Supernatants of these cultures were then assayed for the presence of IgA and IgG. As the data in TABLE 4 shows, T-helper cell activity was present in the intestinal lamina propria cells and was similar to that seen in spleen and Peyer's patches, in that help was provided both for IgA and IgG synthesis.

T-Helper Cell Activity in Human Lamina Propria Lymphocytes

Samples of surgically resected human small intestine were obtained and the LPL were isolated. On the same day peripheral blood lymphocytes were obtained from two normal individuals. Each of the cell populations was separated into B-cell and T-cell fractions on anti-human Fab$_2$ affinity columns. Purified normal peripheral blood B-cells were then mixed with T-cells obtained from either

TABLE 4

T-HELPER CELL ACTIVITY IN MOUSE LAMINA PROPRIA, PEYER'S PATHCES, AND SPLEEN LYMPHOCYTES

Culture*		Isotype Secreted†	
B-Cells	T-Cells	IgA	IgG
+	—	66	29
+	Spleen	252	>600
−	Spleen	8	37
+	Peyer's patches	242	>600
−	Peyer's patches	70	94
+	Lamina propria	347	104
−	Lamina propria	77	8

*PWM 1:100 in each
†ng/culture

lamina propria or from the second peripheral blood lymphocyte donor at a 5:1 T-cell to B-cell ratio, and the mixtures were then cultured for one week in the presence of pokeweed mitogen. Each of the cell populations was also cultured alone. Representative data is shown in TABLE 5. Human lamina propria T-cells, similar to murine lamina propria T-cells, were able to provide help for IgA, IgG, and IgM synthesis.

DISCUSSION

In these studies, isolated murine LPL were found to respond to various T-cell mitogens, but less so on an absolute basis than T-cells from other tissues. The LPL, somewhat surprisingly, had a lower rate of spontaneous proliferation than was seen in either spleen or Peyer's patches. When lamina propria cells were cultured *in vitro* they were found to spontaneously synthesize good amounts of IgA, but little or no IgG; stimulation with pokeweed mitogen inhibited the IgA synthesis. In studies on T-helper cell activity using purified populations of B-cells and T-cells in a pokeweed mitogen system, functional T-helper cell activity was demon-

TABLE 5

T-HELPER CELL ACTIVITY OF HUMAN LAMINA PROPRIA LYMPHOCYTES

Culture*		Isotype Secreted†		
B-Cells	T-Cells‡	IgA	IgG	IgM
+	None	<0.5	23	<2
−	LP	17	95	<2
+	LP	2684	1384	>5000
−	PB	2.7	130	<2
+	PB	>5000	809	>5000

*PWM 1:100 in each
†ng/culture
‡LP = lamina propria; PB = peripheral blood

strated in the intestinal lamina propria of both mouse and man. This T-helper cell activity was not restricted to particular isotypes, as help was seen for IgA, IgG, and IgM.

The spontaneous synthesis of IgA by LPL is consistent with the known predominance of this isotype in mucosal tissues. Thus it might appear puzzling that the T-helper cell activity that was demonstrated provided help for all the isotypes. One might have expected the T-cell help in the lamina propria to have been restricted to IgA responses that predominate there. In order to put these results in some perspective, it is helpful to review the hypothesis advanced by Janeway in regard to T-cells that control the quality of antibody produced to a given stimulus.[13] He has postulated that two types of T-helper and suppressor cells exist, one type that recognizes only antigen, and the second type that recognizes both antigen and immunoglobulin determinants. The first type of T-helper cell, denoted T_{h1}, recognizes carrier determinants and provides help to B-cells specific for haptenic determinants when an antigen bridge forms between them. This interaction affects the quantity but not the quality of Ig produced. The second type of T-helper cell, T_{h2}, both requires and synergizes with T_{h1}. T_{h2} recognizes both antigen and Ig determinants, such as idiotype, isotype, or allotype, and thus determines the qualitative composition of the Ig produced. This hypothesis provides as well for a corresponding set of suppressor cells, T_{s1} and T_{s2}. From these considerations, it follows that the assay system used to look for isotype specific help or suppression will be an important variable. It is entirely possible, and in fact likely, that the assay system used in these studies is not particularly well suited to demonstrating anything but T_{h1}-type activity. It is also possible that the IgA predominance in the intestinal mucosa may depend on isotype specific suppression of immunoglobulin classes other than IgA.

The results obtained in the proliferative studies provide some indirect evidence that small intestinal lamina propria T-cells in the mouse may be a slowly turning over population of long-lived cells. If this is true, such T-helper cells, sitting in the mucosa for long periods of time, would be available to direct the expansion of a set of antigen-specific B-cells entering the mucosa in response to a second antigenic challenge, that is, they may be involved in "memory" responses in the intestinal mucosa. In a related manner, these cells may be responsible for the antigen-induced regionalization of mucosal IgA responses that have recently been shown by Pierce, et al., who injected cholera toxin into different regions of the rat intestine. One might speculate that this regionalization might happen in the following fashion. T-cells stimulated by antigen in the Peyer's patches randomly seed to the lamina propria. The T-cells in locations where more antigen is encountered will proliferate in the mucosa and become long-lived cells, remaining there to focus the response to a subsequent antigenic encounter.

It remains to be shown whether antigen-specific T-helper cells appear in the lamina propria after antigen feeding, that is, whether they are among the T-cell blasts that can be shown to preferentially localize in the mucosa.[4] Such studies are currently underway. The existence of these lamina propria T-helper cells, however, represents a new factor to be considered in relation to the understanding of mucosal immunity in general, and more specifically, in relation to the complexity of regulatory signals that an IgA B-cell, leaving the Peyer's patches and dispersing throughout the body, encounters in various tissues. The reaction of these B-cells with such regulatory signals is probably crucial in the final expression of IgA synthesis and in mucosal immunity.

REFERENCES

1. CEBRA, J. J., C. A. CRANDALL, P. J. GEARHART, S. M. ROBERTSON, J. TSENG, & P. M. WATSON. 1979. *In* Immunology of Breast Milk. P. L. Ogra and D. Dayton, Eds.: 1–16. Raven Press, New York.
2. RICHMAN, L. K., A. S. GRAEFF, R. YARCHOAN, & W. STROBER. 1981. J. Immunol. **126:** 2079–2083.
3. MATTINGLY, J. A. & B. H. WAKSMAN. 1978. J. Immunol. **121:** 1878.
4. GUY-GRAND, D., C. GRISCELLI, & P. VASALLI. 1974. Eur. J. Immunol. **4:** 435–443.
5. ELSON, C. O., J. A. HECK, & W. STROBER. 1979. J. Exp. Med. **149:** 632–638.
6. WYSOCKI & SATO. 1978. Proc. Natl. Acad. Sci. USA **75:** 2844–2848.
7. ELSON, C. O., A. S. GRAEFF, S. P. JAMES & W. STROBER. 1981. Gastroenterology **80:** 1513–1521.
8. DAVIES, M. D. J. & D. M. V. PARROTT. 1981. Gut **22:** 481–488.
9. BULL, D. M. & M. A. BOOKMAN. 1977. J. Clin. Invest. **59:** 966–974.
10. GILLIS, S. & S. B. MIZEL. 1981. Proc. Natl. Acad. Sci. USA **78:** 1133–1137.
11. FAGNANI, R. & J. R. BRAATZ. 1980. J. Immunol. Methods **33:** 313–322.
12. RODBARD, D. & D. M. HUTT. 1974. Proceedings, Symposium on radioimmunoassay and related procedures in clinical medicine. International Atomic Energy, Vienna. 165–192. Unipub. New York.
13. JANEWAY, C. A. 1980. *In* Strategies of Immune Regulation. E. E. Sercarz and A. J. Cunningham, Eds.: 179–198. Academic Press. New York.

IgA SPECIFIC T-CELL FACTOR PRODUCED BY A HUMAN T-T HYBRIDOMA*

Lloyd Mayer, Shu Man Fu†, and Henry G. Kunkel

The Rockefeller University
New York, New York 10021

INTRODUCTION

Differentiation of cells of the B-cell lineage is accompanied by immunoglobulin class switching. T-cell requirement for this event has been documented. In the case of IgA, Elson et al. have demonstrated a population of T-helper cells specific for its production in the murine system.[1] Certain evidence has also been obtained to suggest that similar T-helper cells exist in man.[2]

T-T hybridomas with functional supernatants have been obtained in mice and man. These hybridomas have proven to be informative in studies of T-cell functions. Recently, a series of human T-T hybridomas was established in our laboratory. Evidence will be presented to demonstrate that one of these hybridomas is capable of secreting a factor specific for IgA production by isolated human B-cells.

METHODS

Establishment of an Hypoxanthine Guanine Phosphoribosyl Transferase (HGPRT)-Deficient Human T-Cell Line for Fusion

The mutagen ethylmethane sulfonate was added to Jurkat, a human T-cell lymphoma line, at a concentration of 200 μg/ml, according to the method of Epstein et al.[3] Cells were allowed to recover after more than 80% died from this treatment. HGPRT-deficient variants were selected in 6-thioguanine medium and cloned on soft agar with human 6-thioguanine resistant fibroblasts (Gm 1362) as a feeder layer. Resultant clones were tested for aminopterin sensitivity with dose ranges from 10^{-7} to 10^{-9}M. Clones were selected on the basis of their cloning efficiency and presence of a clear-cut level of sensitivity to aminopterin.

Separation and Culture Conditions of Lymphocytes

Leukocyte Concentrate packs obtained from the New York Blood Center were used as a source of peripheral blood mononuclear cells (MNC). Tonsillar tissue was obtained from routine tonsillectomy specimens, and cell suspensions were prepared as previously described.[4] Mononuclear cells were obtained after centrifugation on Ficoll-Hypaque gradients. T- and B-cell separation was performed by a rosetting technique using neuraminidase-treated sheep red blood cells and a Ficoll-Hypaque gradient. Interface cells were rerosetted prior to use.

*This work was supported by National Institutes of Health Grant CA 24338 and American Cancer Society Grant IM-255.

†Present address: Oklahoma Medical Research Foundation, Oklahoma City, Oklahoma 73104.

238

The resultant population of non-T-cells was less than 1% OKT3+ (pan T-cell marker, Ortho, Raritan, N.J.). The isolated T-cells were used in culture. For cell fusion the T-cells were subjected to a further rosetting procedure to enrich for OKT4+ cells (helper/inducer T-cell marker, Ortho, Raritan, N.J.). An indirect rosetting technique was used[5] with some minor modifications. Forty million T-cells were incubated with 0.2 cc of a 1/40 dilution of OKT8 (suppressor/cytotoxic T-cell marker, Ortho, Raritan, N.J.) antibody for one-half hour at 22° C. These cells were washed three times in culture medium and diluted to 0.5 cc in RPMI 1640 (M.A. Bioproducts, Walkersville, Md.) with 10% fetal calf serum (FCS) (Reheis, Phoenix, Ariz.), 1% penicillin, streptomycin (Gibco, Grand Island, N.Y.), and 2mM glutamine (Gibco, Grand Island, N.Y.). Goat anti-mouse Ig-coated ox red blood cells were obtained using a chromium chloride technique.[6] The resulting interface was 90–95% OKT4+ and less than 1% OKT8+ by indirect immunofluorescence. The OKT4+ cells were incubated with Con A (Sigma, St. Louis, Mo.) 10 μg/ml for 72 hours at a concentration of $1-2 \times 10^6$/ml. These stimulated cells were washed three times in serum-free medium prior to use in cell fusions.

Cell Fusion

All fusions were performed with polyethylene glycol (PEG) 1000 (Merck, St. Louis, Mo.). Jurkat 3, an HGPRT-deficient mutant, was fused with Con A-stimulated OKT4+ blasts in PEG for 8 minutes at a ratio of 1:2 (10^7 Jurkat cells:2 × 10^7 OKT4+ cells). Cells were washed free of PEG and cultured in a 96 well microwell plate (Linbro, Hamden, Conn.) using RPMI 1640, 20% FCS, 1% penicillin, streptomycin, and 2mM glutamine. Additionally, hypoxanthine 10^{-4}M and thymidine, 1.6×10^{-5}M were added. After 24 hours, at 37°C 5% CO_2, 95% room air, aminopterin (3×10^{-8}M) was added. After 14-17 days in culture, with feeding every third day, all nonfused control cultures were nonviable. Growth-positive wells were transferred out of aminopterin and into 24 well macrowell cultures (Linbro, Hamden, Conn.). After sufficient numbers of cells were obtained, cell-free supernatants were obtained and tested for functional capabilities.

Functional Assay Systems

Supernatants of documented hybrids, by human leukocyte antigen (HLA)-typing, were tested for their ability to cause B-cell proliferation or B-cell maturation and Ig-production. Assay for B-cell proliferation utilized purified B-cells, tonsillar or peripheral blood (PB) non-T, at a concentration of 1×10^6/ml in RPMI 1640, 10% FCS, 1% penicillin, streptomycin, and 2mM glutamine with 30% supernatant. Triplicate 0.1 ml cultures were incubated at 37° C in 5% CO_2. On days 2-5, 2μCi of aqueous methyl[^{3}H]thymidine (Schwartz-Mann, Division of Becton Dickinson Co., Orangeberg, N.Y.) was added, and after 12 hours the cells were harvested and processed for scintillation counting.

A reverse hemolytic plaque assay was used to evaluate for Ig-isotype production.[7] One milliliter cultures of 1×10^6 B-cells were incubated as above with 30% hybrid supernatant. The cells were washed in RPMI 1640 and assayed for plaque-forming cells on day 6 of culture.

Fusion and Hybrid Characterization

In a representative fusion, 31 wells out of a total of 90 showed positive growth. HLA-typing of selected clones revealed that the hybrids expressed HLA-A, B, or C determinants of both the parental cells. One specific hybrid, J1 and its clone J1.3, are the subject of this paper. The parental line, Jurkat 3, was typed to be HLA-A2, A4, B7, and CW4, and the activated normal T-cells expressed HLA-A1, A30, B35, B17, and CW4. The hybrid J1.3 expressed HLA-A1, A2, B7, B17, and CW4. These results support the conclusion that J1.3 was a fusion product between the two parental cells. This hybrid, as well as the parental line Jurkat 3, was OKT3, 4+, OKT8⁻, and Ia⁻. Both the hybrid and parental line did not have Fc-receptors for IgA or IgG; however, the hybrid was positive for $Fc\mu$, whereas Jurkat 3 was negative.

Functional Characteristics of the Supernatant

Supernatant from hybrid clone J1.3 was added to a purified population of tonsil B-cells to determine its ability to induce B-cell differentiation. In the control cultures, with media alone, 100 IgM plaques/10^6 cells were seen (TABLE 1). With the addition of supernatant from J1.3, 700 IgA-specific plaques were seen. The addition of T-cells, without supernatant, resulted in only 100 IgA-specific plaques and a different isotypic pattern. A repeat experiment with another tonsil B-cell preparation gave similar results with an eight fold increase in IgA-specific plaque-forming cells. Incubation of PB non-T-cells with the supernatant also resulted in an increase in IgA-specific plaques, approaching that seen with the addition of T-cells and pokeweed mitogen (PWM). In general, the addition of supernatant enhanced IgA-secretion to 40–80% of that seen with T-cells and PWM. The addition of unseparated peripheral blood MNC, as well as the addition of isolated autologous T-cells, caused no significant change in the supernatant's ability to promote IgA production. The presence of hybrid supernatant in peripheral blood MNC cultures, stimulated with PWM, did not alter the isotypic patterns of plaque-forming cells. Pokeweed mitogen (1/100) or Con A (10 μg/ml), added to hybrid-cell cultures, failed to generate a more potent superna-

TABLE 1

INDUCTION OF IgA PFC FROM ISOLATED HUMAN B-CELLS BY SUPERNATANT FROM T-T HYBRIDOMA J1.3

Cells	Media Control			Hybrid J1.3 SUP			+T Cells		
	G	A	M*	G	A	M	G	A	M
TONSIL B	0	0	100	200	700	0	0	100	800
TONSIL B	0	300	0	0	2400	0	—		
							+ T Cells + PWM		
PB Non-T	0	0	0	100	700	0	3420	880	1220
PB Non-T	20	50	0	10	420	0			
PB MNC	0	0	0	0	500	0			

*PFC/10^6 cells by reverse hemolytic plaque assay

TABLE 2

EFFECT OF DILUTION OF SUPERNATANT J1.3 ON ABILITY TO ENHANCE IGA PRODUCTION
BY PERIPHERAL BLOOD NON-T-CELLS

Supernatant Dilution	PFC/10^6 Cells*		
	G	A	M
Media control	20	0	0
Undiluted	0	0	0
1:2	90	600	20
1:10	30	310	0
1:50	10	420	0
1.100	10	260	0

*1×10^6 PB non-T-cells were cultured for six days in the presence of supernatant from the hybrid J1.3. On day 6 a reverse hemolytic plaque assay was performed.

tant. The factor could be diluted to 1/50 without loss of activity (TABLE 2). Occasionally, small increases in IgG or IgM PFC accompanying the IgA PFC induction were seen (TABLE 1 AND 2), but this was always much less than the increase in IgA production. The supernatant induced a moderate degree of B-cell proliferation. The incorporation of [^{3}H]thymidine was highest at day 2 (stimulation index 13.99) and fell off thereafter to background levels.

DISCUSSION

We have shown that our T-T hybridoma J1.3 constitutively produces a factor that enhances IgA production and secretion. This extends observations made in mice[2] and man.[1] Elson *et al.* described an IgA-class-specific T-helper cell in murine Payer's patches, capable of enhancing IgA production, while IgG and IgM production was suppressed.[1] Endoh *et al.* showed the presence of such regulatory cells in peripheral blood of humans and enriched for IgA production by isolation of Fcα + T-cells.[2] The addition of these cells to isolated B-cells and PWM resulted in increased IgA production. In this case, some IgG and IgM-plasma cells were seen as well. Atwater and Tomasi, in a study of patients with selective IgA deficiency,[8] described one patient who exhibited lack of T-cell-help in the peripheral blood. Other classes of Ig have been shown to be under specific T-cell control, that is, IgE and IgG, and factors responsible for their control have been demonstrated.[9-11] Relevant to this discussion is the recent report by Isakson *et al.*, that a factor secreted by a T-T hybrid would induce IgG production selectively.[11]

The supernatant from J1.3 hybridoma appears to promote differentiation of isolated B-cells preferentially to IgA plaque-forming cells. This contrasts with other hybrids isolated in our laboratory that induced polyclonal Ig increases. The latter hybrids are similar to those reported by Irigoyen *et al.*[12] in the human system. The accumulated evidence indicates that the J1.3 hybridoma supernatant appears to exert its influence on B-cells directly, although the role played by a small percentage (<1%) of contaminating T-cells in the non-T-cell population cannot be ruled out. Whether the factor mediates its effect on B-cells by inducing a class switch or whether it stimulates B-cells already committed to IgA production is not answered by the present data. Studies of isolated populations of surface IgG, IgA, and IgM-bearing cells are being undertaken to evaluate this question.

SUMMARY

A human T-T hybridoma was produced, which was a fusion product between an HGPRT-deficient T-cell line, Jurkat 3, and an OKT4+ activated peripheral blood T-cell. The hybrid expressed a receptor for IgM Fc and was negative for IgA Fc. It was shown to produce a factor capable of specifically enhancing IgA production and secretion by isolated human B-cells. The factor exerts its effect directly on B-cells and appears to be different from T-cell-replacing factors previously described.

REFERENCES

1. ELSON, C. O., J. A. HECK, & W. STROBER, 1979. J. Exp. Med. **149:** 632.
2. ENDOH, M.H., H. SAKAI, Y. NOMOTO, Y. TOMINO, & H. KANESHIGE, 1981. J. Immunol. **127:** 2612.
3. EPSTEIN, J., A. LEVYA, W. N. KELLEY, & J. W. LITTLEFIELD, 1977. Somatic Cell Genet. **3:** 135.
4. CHIORAZZI, N., S. M. FU, & H. G. KUNKEL, 1980. Clin. Immunol. Immunopathol. **15:** 301.
5. STOCKER, J. W. G. GIAROTTA, B. HAUSMANN, M. TUCCO, & R. CEPELLINI, 1979. Tissue Antigens **13:** 212.
6. GOTTLEIB, A. B., S. M. FU, D. T. Y. YU, C. Y. WANG, J. P. HALPER, & H. G. KUNKEL, 1979. J. Immunol. **123:** 1497.
7. GRONOWICZ, E., A. COUTINHO, & F. MELCHERS, 1976. Eur. J. Immunol. **6:** 588.
8. ATWATER, J. S. & T. B. TOMASI, 1978. Clin. Immunol. Immunopath. **9:** 379.
9. ISHIZAKA, K. & T. ADACHI, 1976. J. Immunol. **117:** 40.
10. HIRASHIMA, J., J. YODOI, & K. ISHIZAKA, 1981. J. Immunol. **127:** 1804.
11. ISAKSON, P. C., E. PURE, E. S. VITETTA, & P. H. KRAMMER, 1982. J. Exp. Med. **155:** 734.
12. IRIGOYEN, O., P. V. RIZZOLO, Y. THOMAS, L. ROGOZINSKI, & L. CHESS, 1981. J. Exp. Med. **154:** 1827.

DISCUSSION OF THE PAPER

J. R. McGHEE (*University of Alabama in Birmingham*): Have you characterized the secreted factor at all, for example, molecular weight, by isoelectric focusing?

L. MAYER (*The Rockefeller University, New York, N.Y.*): We have started growing the hybridoma in serum-free medium to start the isolation procedure of the protein.

REGULATORY T-CELLS IN MURINE PEYER'S PATCHES DIRECTING IgA-SPECIFIC ISOTYPE SWITCHING

Hidenori Kawanishi and Warren Strober

Immunophysiology Section
Metabolism Branch
National Cancer Institute
National Institutes of Health
Bethesda, Maryland 20205

INTRODUCTION

One of the major problems of mucosal immunity relates to the question of why Peyer's patches (PP) act as a source of IgA B-cells.[1,2] One possible answer to this question is based on recent data concerning the molecular biology of B-cell differentiation. It is now known that such differentiation involves successive DNA deletions and rearrangements that result in the coupling of DNA segments coding for the variable region of the Ig molecule with DNA segments coding for the constant region of the Ig molecule.[3-5] Separate DNA segments exist for each Ig class (or subclass), and these occur at more or less regular intervals along the DNA strand. Particular constant region DNA segments are brought into transcription position (next to variable region DNA) during successive cell divisions, and the isotype of the B-cell is determined by the constant region DNA segment linked to the variable region segment at the time the cell moves toward terminal differentiation. Some investigators speculate that the process of DNA deletion and rearrangement occurs in a stepwise fashion along the DNA strand until the most 3' constant region DNA, the region coding for the IgA constant region, is reached; on this basis they propose that the reason PP are the source of IgA B-cells is that they are the repositories of B-cells that have undergone multiple divisions and have therefore reached the ultimate or IgA stage of development.[6,7]

A second possible answer to the question of why IgA B-cells are generated in PP is that PP contain IgA class-specific T-cells that preferentially induce IgA B-cell development. This concept is based chiefly on recent evidence that murine PP T-cell populations contain T-cells that preferentially augment IgA synthesis as compared to T-cells in spleen and peripheral lymph nodes.[8] Whereas it was thought that such class-specific T-cells selectively expand B-cell populations that they already reached the stage of IgA development, such cells could conceivably act at any step in the differentiation process.

MATERIALS AND METHODS

Animals

Normal BALB/c female mice (8 to 16 weeks of age) were used in these studies.

0077-8923/83/0409-0243 $ 1.75/0 © 1983, NYAS

Mitogens and Other Reagents

Lipopolysaccharide (LPS) *S. typhimurium*, concanavalin A (Con A), and L-phytohemagglutinin (PHA) were obtained from commercial sources. Interleukin 2 (IL 2) was generated by stimulation of Sprague-Dawley rat spleen cells with Con A, according to a modification of the method of Gillis et al.[9]

Preparation of Cell Suspensions

Single cell suspensions from spleen, thymus, and mesenteric lymph nodes were made using previously described techniques.[10] Cell suspensions obtained from small intestine were prepared using a modification of a method described by Richman et al.[11]

Long-Term T-Cell Cultures and Cloning

Prior to cloning, unseparated cells (2×10^6/ml) or T-cell enriched fractions (1×10^6/ml) from BALB/c PP and spleens were cultured with Con A (4 μg/ml) in complete culture medium in 75 cm^2 plastic culture flasks (No. 25110, Corning Glass Works, Corning, N.Y.) at 37°C in an atmosphere of 5% CO_2 and 95% air for four days. The nonadherent cells were harvested, and the dead cells were eliminated on Ficoll-Hypaque gradients. The viable Con A-activated lymphocytes were then placed in each well of 24-well plates (No. 3524, Costar, Cambridge, Mass.) at a concentration of 2×10^4 cells per well in complete culture medium supplemented with IL 2 (25%) and additional Con A (0.5 μg/ml) (conditioned medium) under the above culture conditions. Thereafter, half of the culture medium of each well was replaced with fresh conditioned medium every three or four days. When the bottoms of the wells were about two-thirds occupied by cells, the cells were subcultured. After nearly two months of *in vitro* maintenance, the Con A-induced cells were cloned, using a limiting dilution technique.[12] Briefly, cells were diluted into 96-well flat-bottomed microwells at estimated final concentrations of 3, 1, and 0.3 cells per well. Each well contained 0.2 ml of complete medium containing the appropriate number of cells and irradiated syngeneic filler spleen cells (2×10^5 cells/well). The plates were incubated at 37°C in 5% CO_2 and inspected periodically for growth of cells. Cultures were supplemented every four or five days by replacing 0.1 ml of old conditioned culture medium with 0.1 ml of the fresh medium until harvesting. The filler cells were added at every other change of medium. The probability that cells in a given well originated from a single cell was calculated using the Poisson probability distribution.[13]

Recloning

At some point during the above clonal expansion period (three to four weeks after the original cloning), selected cloned cells were recloned using the same method as described above.

Fractionation of T- and B-Cells from Lymphocyte Suspensions

To obtain purified T-cells and B-cells, lymphocytes were first incubated in plastic Petri dishes coated with goat anti-mouse Fab IgG according to the method of Mage et al.[14] The cells not adherent to the plates were passed over nylon wool columns to obtain purified T-cells, according to the method of Julius et al.[15] The cells adherent to the plates were treated with a monoclonal rat anti-mouse Thy-1.2 (New England Nuclear Corp., Boston, Mass.) and complement (C)[11] to obtain purified B-cells. In some experiments the B-cell populations were further purified with the use of an anti-mouse Lyt-1.2 alloserum (Cedarlane Laboratories Limited, Hornby, Ontario, Canada),[16] as described below. Less than 0.5% of the T-cells bore surface Ig as demonstrated by fluoresceinated rabbit anti-mouse polyclonal Ig and anti-mouse $\kappa + \lambda$ antiserum; contamination by nonspecific esterase-positive cells was less than 0.1 percent. More than 99% of the B-cells stained for surface Ig; less than 0.3% of cells in the B-cell population stained with nonspecific esterase.

Cell Cultures for Ig Biosynthesis

Fractionated or unfractionated cells were suspended in RPMI 1640 (GIBCO) supplemented with 10% fetal calf serum (FCS) (GIBCO), 0.3% L-glutamine (GIBCO), 1 mM sodium pyruvate (M. A. Bioproducts, Walkersville, Md.), 0.1 mM nonessential amino acids (M. A. Bioproducts), 5×10^{-5} M 2-mercaptoethanol (Sigma), 25 mM N-2-hydroxyethyl piperazine-N'-2-ethane sulfonic acid (HEPES) buffer and antibiotics (complete culture medium). The cells were then cultured in small vials at 37°C in 5% CO_2 in 95% air humid atmosphere for seven days. To eliminate exogenous Ig in the single cell suspensions, the latter were washed four times through FCS before culture. In some cases, cells received a dose of 1,500 R from a cesium source (Gammator M, Isomedix, Inc., Parsippany, N.J.) prior to culture.

Radioimmunoassays Used for Detection of Ig in Cell Cultures

A double-antibody radioimmunoassay (RIA) employing ^{125}I-labeled purified IgM, IgG, and IgA was used. The details of this technique have been described previously, and the reagents used in these assays are listed in a previous publication.[8]

Anti-Immunoglobulin Antibodies Used in the Enumeration of Surface Ig-Bearing and Cytoplasmic (cIg)-Containing Cells

In studies using direct immunofluorescence, fluorescein isothiocyanate (FITC)-conjugated monospecific (chromatographically purified) goat (G) or rabbit (R) anti-mouse antibodies directed against major Ig heavy chains (μ, γ, α) (Cappel Laboratories, Kirkegaard & Perry Laboratories, Inc., Gaithersburg, Md., and Litton Bionetics) were used. In studies using indirect immunofluorescence FITC-conjugated G anti-R polyvalent antisera against mouse-γ-globulin (Cappel) were used in conjunction with unconjugated antibodies (obtained from the same sources). The specificity of the antiserum or antibodies was confirmed by soft agar precipitin reactions and with blocking studies using chromatographically purified monospecific mouse Ig (Cappel Laboratories, and Kirkegaard and Perry Laboratories). In addition, to rule out nonspecific binding of antibodies by way of the Fc receptor, studies with fluoresceinated Fab$_2'$ fragments of each heavy-chain, monospecific antibodies were employed in representative cases.

Preparation of PP B-Cell Populations with Defined Isotypes

Peyer's patch B-cell populations obtained by the methods described above were, in some studies, further purified into populations bearing only IgM, IgG, or IgA. This purification was accomplished by first adhering cells to an anti-Ig coated plastic dish according to the method of Mage et al.,[14] and then subjecting the adherent cells to anti-Ig + C treatment. To obtain IgM-bearing B-cells, B-cells adherent to anti-IgM plates were subsequently exposed to anti-IgG and anti-IgA; in a similar manner, IgG-bearing B-cells were obtained by adherence to anti-IgG plates followed by exposure to anti-IgM and anti-IgA, and IgA-bearing B-cells were obtained by adherence to anti-IgA plates followed by exposure to anti-IgM and anti-IgG. The resultant B-cell populations were ≥99% homogeneous for the various Ig isotypes.

Detection of Class-Specific Surface Ig and cIg-Bearing PP B-Cells Cocultured with or without Cloned T-Cells

Highly purified PP B-cells (5 × 10^5/2 ml/culture) were cultured in LPS (20 μg/ml) containing complete medium in the presence or absence of PP or spleen cloned T-cells (B/T ratio, 1/4). The cultures were kept in 5% CO$_2$ at 37°C for five days. At harvest, the cultured cells were treated with anti-Thy-1.2 and C, and then overlaid on and spun through Ficoll-Hypaque to deplete them of cocultured cloned T-cells. Finally, to dissociate the cell-bound exogenous Ig present on the cell surface, the cells were treated at 0.05 M acetate buffer (pH 4.0), containing 0.085 M NaCl, 0.005 M KCl, and 0.03% human serum albumin,[17] or incubated at 37°C for one hour, and then washed three times with RPMI-1640. The PP B-cells cultured in this manner were then stained with FITC-conjugated antibodies to determine the number of surface Ig and cIg positive cells present. For this purpose, viable cells (5 × 10^4) were incubated with appropriate dilutions of antibodies and/or FITC-conjugated antibodies for 30 minutes on ice and then washed two times with cold RPMI-1640 containing 0.08% NaN$_3$. To stain cIg, the cell suspensions (5 × 10^4) were layered on a glass slide by using a Shandon cytocentrifuge, air-dried, and fixed with 95% ethyl alcohol plus 5% acetic acid. At this point the spot of cells were overlayed with antibodies, incubated for 30 minutes in a humidified chamber at room temperature, and then mounted in Tris-buffer glycerol (pH 7.0). In each cell suspension (surface Ig) or smear (cIg) examined for immunofluorescence, 300 to 1000 cells were examined in both tungsten and ultraviolet light on a Leitz Ortholux microscope (E. Leitz, Inc., Rockleigh, N.J.) with 100X oil immersion objective and BG 38 and KP 490 excitation filters, coupled with a K530 barrier filter.

TABLE 1

CHARACTERISTICS OF SURFACE PHENOTYPIC MARKERS ON CON A-INDUCED CLONED T-CELLS

T-Cells Tested	Origin of Strain	T-Cell Surface Markers			Ia Antigens				H-2 Antigens	
		Thy-1.2	Lyt-1	Lyt-2	I-A^d	I-E^d	I-A^b	I-E^b	H-2^d(K/D)	H-2^b(K/D)
K-14 (PP)† clone	BALB/c (H-2^d)	+*	+	−	+	+	−	−	+	−
K-24 (PP) clone	BALB/c (H-2^d)	+	+	−	+	+	−	−	+	−
K-8 (Spn)‡ clone	BALB/c (H-2^d)	+	+	−	+	+	−	−	+	−
K-17 (Spn) clone	BALB/c (H-2^d)	+	+	−	+	+	−	−	+	−

* + ≥ 97%, − ≤ 3% in three experiments determined by complement-mediated cytotoxicity.
†PP = Peyer's patches.
‡Spn = spleen.

RESULTS

Clones of Con A-Induced T-Cells

Peyer's patch and spleen T-cells were activated with Con A and adapted to continuous culture according to procedures described above (see METHODS). Two PP (K-14 and K-24) and two spleen (K-8 and K-17) clones were derived from these T-cells by the limiting dilution technique. These cloned T-cell lines were subsequently used in the functional studies described below. Finally, two subcloned T-cell lines were obtained from each original T-cell line and also tested in functional studies.

The characteristics of the cloned T-cells are shown in TABLE 1. All four cloned

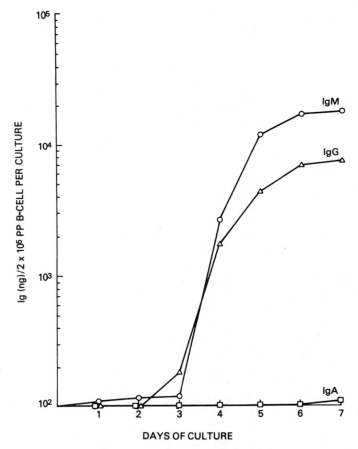

FIGURE 1. Time kinetics of isotype-specific Ig biosynthesis *in vitro* by Peyer's patch (PP), highly purified B-cells (2 × 10⁵ cells per culture) in the presence of LPS (20 μg/ml). Each point expresses the mean of two experiments. O = IgM; Δ = IgG; □ = IgA.

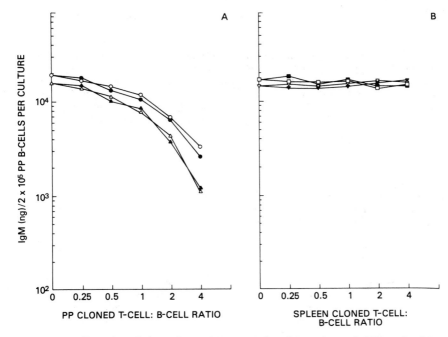

FIGURE 2. Effect of graded numbers of Con A-induced Peyer's patch (PP) and spleen T-cell clones on IgM biosynthesis in fresh PP B-cell-indicator cultures. All cultures contained 2×10^5 PP B-cells and were treated with LPS (20 μg/ml). Each point shows the mean of duplicate experiments. A) Addition of PP T-cell clones to the indicator cultures. K-14 clone, nonirradiated O and irradiated (1,500 R) ●, K-24 clone, nonirradiated △ and irradiated ▲. B) Addition of splenic T-cell clones to the indicator cultures. K-8 clone, nonirradiated □ and irradiated ■; K-17 clone, nonirradiated ▽ and irradiated ▼.

lines expressed Thy-1.2, Lyt-1 antigens, but were devoid of surface and cytoplasmic Ig determinants (including both κ and λ light-chain determinants). In addition, all lines bore Ia and H-2 antigens corresponding to the antigen phenotype of the mouse strain from which they were derived. In studies not shown, it was found that the subcloned T-cell lines exhibited identical properties.

Regulatory Function of Con A-Induced Cloned T-Cells

LPS-Induced Ig Synthesis by Purified PP B-Cells in the Absence of Cloned T-Cells

As shown in FIGURE 1, PP B-cells stimulated by LPS produced IgM and IgG beginning on day 3 of culture. By contrast, little or no IgA was produced under these conditions. In the absence of LPS or with B-cell irradiation (1500 R), essentially no Ig was produced.

LPS-Induced Ig Synthesis by Purified PP B-Cells in the Presence of Cloned T-Cells; IgM Synthesis

As seen in FIGURE 2A, each of the two PP cloned T-cell lines (K-14 and K-24) profoundly suppressed LPS-induced IgM synthesis. Such suppression was proportional to the number of T-cells added (at a 4:1 T/B cell ratio, there was approximately 88% inhibition) and was radiation resistant (1500 R). As seen in FIGURE 2B, a different picture was obtained for the spleen cloned T-cells; in this case, there was neither enhancement nor suppression of IgM synthesis.

IgG Synthesis

As shown in FIGURE 3, both the PP and spleen cloned T-cells suppressed LPS-induced IgG synthesis. Again, the suppression was dose dependent and radiation resistant.

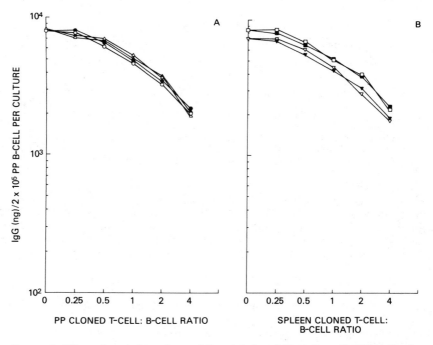

FIGURE 3. Effect of graded numbers of Con A-induced Peyer's patch (PP) and spleen T-cell clones on IgG biosynthesis in fresh PP B-cell-indicator cultures. All cultures were treated with LPS (20 μg/ml) and contained 2×10^5 PP B-cells. Each point shows the mean of duplicate experiments. A) Peyer's patch T-cell clones (K-14 and K-24); B) spleen T-cell clones (K-8 and K-17). All indices are identical to FIGURE 4.

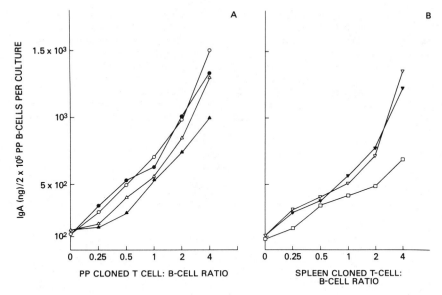

FIGURE 4. Effect of graded numbers of Con A-induced Peyer's patch (PP) and spleen T-cell clones on IgA biosynthesis in fresh PP B-cell-indicator cultures. All cultures were treated with LPS (20 μg/ml) containing 2 × 10⁵ PP B-cells. Each point indicates the mean of duplicate experiments. A) Addition of PP T-cell clones to the indicator cultures. K-14 clone, nonirradiated O and irradiated (1,500 R) ●; K-24 clone, nonirradiated △ and irradiated ▲. B) Addition of spleen T-cell clones to the indicator cultures. K-8 clone, nonirradiated □; K-17 clone, nonirradiated ▽ and irradiated ▼.

IgA Synthesis

As shown in FIGURE 4, the cloned T-cells (from either PP or spleen) augmented IgA synthesis. This augmentation, however, was quantitatively unimpressive and could easily have resulted from IL 2 release by cloned T-cells with subsequent activation of residual T-cells in the purified B-cell populations.

Regulatory Function of Sub-Cloned T-Cells

The above studies were repeated using subcloned T-cell lines derived from the original PP and spleen cloned T-cells. Entirely similar results were obtained (data not shown).

Surface Ig Changes During LPS-Driven PP B-Cell Proliferation and Differentiation in the Presence and Absence of Cloned T-Cells

The effect of cloned T-cells on the nature of surface Ig (as well as cIg) on B-cells cultured in the presence and absence of LPS was then determined. A representative study using a mixed population of PP B-cells (containing IgM, IgG, and IgA-bearing cells initially) is shown in TABLE 2. B-cells cultured in the absence of either LPS or cloned T-cells did not proliferate and contained mostly surface IgM-bearing (77.9%) cells as well as some surface IgG-bearing (4.8%) and surface IgA-bearing (13.5%) cells; few, if any, cells contained cIg (data not shown). Inclusion of LPS into the culture medium led, approximately, to a threefold increase in cell number, a fall in the percentage of cells bearing surface IgM and surface IgA, and the appearance of cells containing cIgM and cIgG.

The addition of cloned T-cells derived from PP (K-14) as well as LPS cultures

TABLE 2

EFFECT OF PEYER'S PATCH (K-14) AND SPLEEN (K-17) CLONED T-CELLS ON SEQUENTIAL SWITCHING OF EACH HEAVY CHAIN OF IMMUNOGLOBULIN (IG) ON/IN HIGHLY PURIFIED PP B-CELLS IN THE PRESENCE OF LPS STIMULATION *IN VITRO* (FIVE DAY CULTURE)*

| | Cultured Conditions of PP B-Cells | | |
| | | PP B-Cells + Cloned T-Cells (B/T:1/4) + LPS | |
	PP B-Cells + LPS	Cloned K-14	Cloned K-17
Total Cell Numbers† ($\times 10^5/2$ ml/culture)	13.70	11.23	12.46
Cell Number and Percent of Each Isotype-Specific surface Ig- or cIg-Bearing Cell Population ($\times 10^5/2$ ml/culture)			
surface IgM	4.329 (31.6%)	3.517 (31.4%)	3.713 (29.8%)
surface IgG	2.190 (16.0%)	1.310 (11.7%)	3.377 (27.1%)
surface IgA	0.615 (4.5%)	4.883 (43.6%)	0.763 (5.4%)
cIgM	3.822 (27.9%)	0.488 (4.0%)	3.339 (26.8%)
cIgG	2.233 (16.3%)	0.157 (1.4%)	0.523 (4.2%)
cIgA	0 (0%)	0.314 (2.8%)	0.162 (1.3%)

*Representative data shown here.
†Initial total cell number for each experiment was 5×10^5 of PP B-cells/2 ml/culture.

led to a marked decrease (as compared to B-cell cultures containing only LPS) in the cells containing cIgM and cIgG, which was accompanied by an eightfold increase in the number of cells bearing surface IgA (but only a modest increase in the number of cells containing cIgA). By contrast, the addition of cloned T-cells derived from spleen (K-17) led to an increase in surface IgG cells and a decrease in cIgG cells; effects on IgA cells were minimal.

Additional studies using B-cell populations containing only surface IgM, surface IgG, or surface IgA-bearing cells were also carried out. In these studies (data now shown) the effect of the addition of cloned PP T-cells to cultures of surface IgM-bearing cells was to greatly augment the occurrence of cells bearing surface IgA-bearing cells (nearly 40% of a total cell number), while decreasing to a moderate extent the occurrence of cells bearing surface IgM and surface IgG. By contrast, the addition of cloned PP T-cells to cultures of surface IgG-bearing B-cells or surface IgA-bearing B-cells had very little effect, if any, on these B-cell populations; in particular, the surface IgG-bearing B-cell cultures did not contain surface IgA or cIgA cells at the end of the culture period; additionally, surface IgA-bearing B-cells did not proliferate, switch, or differentiate into surface IgG, cIgG, or even cIgA B-cells during culture with PP cloned T-cells.

DISCUSSION

In these studies, we describe the immunoregulatory capacity of lines of cloned and subcloned T-cells derived from either Con A-induced spleen or PP cells. These T-cell lines were radioresistant, Ia antigen-positive cells that expressed the surface phenotype of helper or inducer cells (Lyt-1$^+$ 2$^-$).[18] Nevertheless, we found that the addition of cloned or subcloned PP T-cells to LPS-stimulated B-cells profoundly suppressed IgM and IgG synthesis, whereas cloned or subcloned spleen T-cells did not suppress IgM synthesis, but did suppress IgG synthesis. Finally, we found that culture of PP cloned T-cells, but not spleen cloned T-cells with purified PP B-cells (in the presence of LPS) resulted in the appearance of surface IgA-bearing B-cells and that this latter effect was not accompanied by IgA B-cell proliferation or differentiation into plasma cells.

One interpretation of these observations is that the cloned and subcloned T-cells were acting as suppressor cells that were capable of shutting off terminal differentiation of IgM and IgG B-cells. This possibility, however, is unlikely in view of the fact that the cloned and subcloned cells were radioresistant and exclusively of the Lyt-1$^+$ 2$^-$ phenotype; in addition, the cloned cells were capable of producing IL 2 when activated by T-cell mitogens (Kawanishi, Saltzman, and Strober, unpublished observation) and, as a result, slightly augment Ig synthesis by PP B-cells in the absence of LPS stimulation. These properties are characteristic of cells belonging to a helper/inducer subset. A second interpretation is that the cloned cells were acting as inducers of T-suppressor cells; however, because the cloned T-cells were the only T-cells present in the cultures, this possibility is also unlikely.

Yet another interpretation, and one that is strongly supported by the finding that the decrease in IgM- and IgG-bearing and -secreting cells in the presence of cloned PP T-cells is accompanied by a marked increase in IgA-bearing B-cells, is that the apparent suppression of Ig synthesis brought about by the cloned T-cells is actually due to a T-cell effect on B-cell switching. In this view, the cloned T-cells influence B-cells to move rapidly through the differentiation pathway so that cells bypass the intermediate (IgG) stages of differentiation to arrive at a more terminal (IgA) stage of differentiation. The discrepancy between PP and spleen T-cloned cells, as far as their effects on IgM synthesis are concerned, can be explained by assuming that these two types of cells possess the ability to influence switch at different levels of B-cell maturation: the PP T-cell clones, which suppress IgM production, exert their switch function at the $VC_{h\mu}$ to $VC_{h\alpha}$ switch step with the subsequent inhibition of both IgM and IgG plasma-cell development (FIGURE 5); by contrast, the spleen T-cell clones, which do not affect IgM production, exert switch function at the $VC_{h\mu(\delta)}$ to $VC_{h\gamma}$ switch step without significant inhibition of IgM terminal differentiation; alternatively, the spleen T-cell clone mediates some $VC_{h\gamma}$ intersubclass switch. Finally, the fact that IgA synthesis was not greatly augmented by the presence of the cloned T-cells in these experiments can be explained if one assumes that other cells, such as an additional type of T-helper cell, are necessary for terminal IgA B-cell differentiation into IgA-secreting plasma cells (FIGURE 5). In this connection, we have recently shown (H. Kawanishi and W. Strober, unpublished results) that surface IgA-bearing B-cells resulting from prior incubation with cloned PP T-cells ("post-switch B-cells") can differentiate into IgA plasma cells in the presence of uncloned T-cells or T-cell factors and the T-cell-dependent mitogen, staphylococcal protein A.

That the cloned PP T-cells described here are, in fact, operating by causing class-specific effects on B-cell DNA switching events as indicated above is

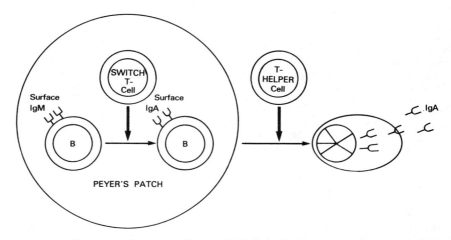

FIGURE 5. Proposed schematic pathway of class-specific immunoglobulin-heavy chain switching and terminal differentiation of PP B-cells. Surface IgM-bearing B-cells switch to surface IgA-bearing B-cells in the presence of IgA class-specific switch T-cells; the post-switch B-cells then differentiate into IgA-secreting plasma cells in the presence of another type of a regulatory cell, such as a T-helper cell.

supported by evidence that 1) the cloned PP T-cells are not simply providing relatively nonspecific proliferative signals to the PP B-cells and thereby driving them, in a stepwise fashion, to ever more 3′ DNA rearrangements; if this were the case, then the surface IgG-bearing B-cells would have yielded surface IgA-bearing B-cells; and 2) the cloned PP T-cells are not merely inducing proliferation and terminal differentiation of surface IgA-bearing B-cells already formed; if this were the case, then the surface IgA-bearing B-cells would have proliferated and begun to secrete IgA when cocultured with the cloned T-cells.

To conclude, the present study provides evidence for the existence of a IgA class-specific "switch T-cell" that directs the early differentiation of B-cells toward IgA B-cell development. Indications are that these "switch T-cells" are preferentially localized in PP, thus accounting for the fact that PP contain IgA precursors. It is of interest that these "switch T-cells" do not result in terminal

B-cell differentiation, a fact that fits well with the observation that PP do not normally contain a large complement of IgA-plasma cells. Recent evidence suggests that such terminal differentiation requires the presence of other T-cells (T-helper cells) that operate on postswitch IgA B-cells and that may or may not be class-specific (H. Kawanishi and W. Strober, unpublished observations). The nature of the switch signal emitted by PP cloned T-cells and resulting in IgA B-cell differentiation is presently unknown. Inasmuch as isotype switching at the DNA level may require switching enzymes that bring together DNA segments coded for variable region and constant regions of the Ig molecule, it is possible (but unproven) that the switch signal could involve induction or activation of Ig class-specific enzymes active in DNA switching mechanisms.

REFERENCES

1. CRAIG, S. W. & J. J. CEBRA. 1971. Peyer's patches: an enriched source of precursors for IgA-producing immunocytes in the rabbit. J. Exp. Med. **134:** 188.
2. HUSBAND, A. J. & J. L. GOWANS. 1978. The origin and antigen-dependent distribution of IgA-containing cells in the intestine. J. Exp. Med. **148:** 1146.
3. HONJO, T. & T. KATAOKA. 1978. Organization of immunoglobulin heavy chain genes and allelic deletion model. Proc. Natl. Acad. Sci. USA **75:** 2140.
4. DAVIS, M. M., S. K. KIM & L. E. HOOD. 1980. DNA sequences mediating class switching in alpha immunoglobulin genes. Science **209:** 1360.
5. SHIMIZU, T., N. TAKAHASHI, Y. YAMAIJAKI-KATAOKA, Y. NISHIDA, T. KATAOKA & T. HONJO. 1981. Ordering of mouse immunoglobulin heavy chain genes by molecular cloning. Nature (London) **289:** 149.
6. GEARHART, P. J. & J. J. CEBRA. 1979. Differentiated B lymphocytes: potential to express particular antibody variable and constant regions depends on site of lymphoid tissue and antigen load. J. Exp. Med. **149:** 216.
7. GEARHART, P. J., J. L. HURWITZ & J. J. CEBRA. 1980. Successive switching of antibody isotypes expressed within the lines of a B cell clone. Proc. Natl. Acad. Sci USA **77:** 5424.
8. ELSON, C. O., J. A. HECK & W. STROBER. 1979. T-cell regulation of murine IgA synthesis. J. Exp. Med. **149:** 632.
9. GILLIS, S., M. M. FERM, W. OU & K. A. SMITH. 1978. T-cell growth factor: parameters of production and a quantitative microassay for activity. J. Immunol. **120:** 2027.
10. CHILLER, J. M. & W. O. WEIGLE. 1973. Restoration of immunocompetency in tolerant lymphoid cell populations by cellular supplementation. J. Immunol. **110:** 1051.
11. RICHMAN, L. K., A. S. GRAEFF, R. YARCHOAN & W. STROBER. 1981. Simultaneous induction of antigen-specific IgA helper T cells and IgG suppressor T cells in the murine Peyer's patch after protein feeding. J. Immunol. **128:** 2079.
12. ROSENBERG, S. A., P. J. SPIESS & S. SCHWARZ. 1980. In vitro growth of murine T cells. IV. Use of T-cell growth factor to clone lymphoid cells. Cell. Immunol. **54:** 293.
13. LEFKOVITS, I. & H. WALDMAN. 1979. Limiting dilution analysis of cells in the immune system, Cambridge University Press. Cambridge, London.
14. MAGE, M. G., L. L. McHUGH & T. L. ROTHSTEIN. 1977. Mouse lymphocytes with and without surface immunoglobulin: preparative scale separation in polystyrene tissue culture dishes coated with specifically purified antiimmunoglobulin. J. Immunol. Methods **15:** 47.
15. JULIUS, M. E., E. SIMPSON & L. A. HERZENBERG. 1974. A rapid method for the isolation of functional thymus-derived murine lymphocytes. Eur. J. Immunol. **3:** 645.
16. OKUMURA, K., K. HAYAKAWA & T. TADA. 1981. Immunoglobulin (Ig) gene restricted augmentation of in vitro secondary antibody response by novel lymphocyte (Thy-1⁻, Ly-1⁺). J. Supramol. Cell. Biochem. Supplement **5:** 73 (Abstract).
17. ABO, T., T. YAMAGUCHI, F. SHIMIZU & K. KUMAGAI. 1976. Studies of surface immunoglobulins on human B lymphocytes. II. Characterization of a population of lymphocytes

lacking surface immunoglobulins but carrying Fc receptor (sIg$^-$Fc$^+$ cell). J. Immunol. **117:** 1781.

18. CANTOR, H. & E. A. BOYSE. 1977. Regulation of cellular and humoral immune responses by T-cell subclasses. Cold Spring Harbor Symp. Quant. Biol. **41:** 23.

DISCUSSION OF THE PAPER

J. J. CEBRA (*University of Pennsylvania, Philadelphia, Pa.*): IgM-bearing cells are the ones that account for clones that switch to give multiple isotype expression in splenic fragments, all the IgG sublasses, and IgA. This has been by cell sorting. The Kearney, Lawton, and Cooper experiments demonstrated that the IgM-bearing cells are the ones that LPS stimulates to divide and switch to IgG cells and IgG-secreting cells, although it is difficult to get these cells to express or secrete IgA. I do not understand why the T-cells that you use can not also act on IgA-bearing cells, because you can expand cells by growth factors to reach the point of IgA expression. Nevertheless, the two populations are quite different. The IgA-bearing cells that account for IgA memory and for generating mucosal immunity are inert to LPS stimulation. You do not have them, as Dutton would say, in the activated form. The cells that have been generated by division from IgM-bearing cells in the process of switching could easily be the target of all kinds of T-cell growth factors. Further division and expansion follows, and ordinarily can not be obtained with LPS, and hence differentiation to IgA expression. How do you get around that problem?

W. STROBER (*National Institutes of Health, Bethesda, Md.*): We have also used appropriate controls. In this regard, we added other kinds of spleen T-cell clones that presumably also provide the nonspecific T-cell factors, and these cells did not act to produce IgA-producing cells. Conversely, when you use the spleen clones, they indeed induce differentiation, probably IgG switching, but not in the IgA direction. Therefore, I think that either LPS alone or other kinds of inductive influences can lead to cell differentiation, but one needs special kinds of T-cells obtained from Peyer's patches to get that IgA switch.

M. D. COOPER (*University of Alabama in Birmingham*): I regard your work as the first good evidence that T-cells can actually cause a switch. My question is, Have you looked at the kinetics of this switch to see when expression of IgA for the first time on those IgM cells occurs, and whether or not it requires division? I ask, because Pernis and Kearney showed that one can induce B-cells that express IgM to express a second isotype that occurs within a matter of six hours or less. It is not blocked by inhibitors of DNA synthesis, but is blocked by inhibitors of RNA and protein synthesis.

STROBER: We have not done the kinetic study. We have simply one time point: a five-day culture of our cloned cells with the B-cells. We do feel that division is necessary, and although the addition of cloned T-cells to the LPS-stimulated cultures does not result in more cells than with LPS alone, you need LPS, which we think is an inductive proliferative influence. We think that it probably requires proliferation, but we have not really looked into this matter.

COOPER: It is an important issue in order to determine whether or not you are influencing already committed cells or, indeed, inducing the switch.

STROBER: I again emphasize that we are starting with IgM cells and, if you expose those IgM cells to other kinds of influences, either LPS alone or other spleen T-cell clones, you do not get the switch; the Peyer's patch T-cells are required for the switch.

M. F. KAGNOFF (*University of California at San Diego, La Jolla*): My question concerns the potential problem of purity of the B-cell population. Because the T-cell clones are producing IL 2, this production might reexpand any residual T-cells present in the B-cell preparation. Are you convinced that the population of IgM-bearing cells is a pure B-cell population?

STROBER: Dr. Kawanishi has obtained populations that are greater than 99% pure.

KAGNOFF: The next question is, Have you looked at whether LPS alone is inducing any DNA gene rearrangement with expression of some alpha message?

STROBER: I think that is a good question, but I would hasten to add that there is IgA on the cell surface and there had to be gene rearrangement. We would like to now think in terms of gene rearrangements, because we know that as soon as you go from a cell that bears one immunoglobulin isotype to another, there has to be, in fact, some gene rearrangement.

M. E. CONLEY (*University of Pennsylvania, Philadelphia, Pa.*): Can you tell me what techniques you have used to rule out the possibility that IgM-bearing cells have very small amounts of IgA on their surface, because we know that immature IgA B-cells can express IgM and small amounts of IgA?

STROBER: I can not exclude that there might be tiny amounts of IgA, but it is important to keep in mind that there was a vast difference in IgA expression, depending upon whether cloned T-cells were added. Therefore, even if you are talking about quantitative differences in IgA, there is still a very large difference.

CONLEY: What I am addressing is the difference between T-cell expansion of a B-cell population that has already isotype switched from that which you favor: the T-cell inducing the switch.

STROBER: All right, let me tell you how we did this experiment. We first panned the cells on anti-IgM plates and then we killed the cells that we took from panning with anti-IgA anti-IgG, and C to get rid of doublet or triplets of IgM cells that express other isotypes.

IgA RHEUMATOID FACTOR: EVIDENCE FOR INDEPENDENT EXPRESSION AT LOCAL SITES OF TISSUE INFLAMMATION*

William J. Koopman,†‡ Randel K. Miller,‡ Sylvia S. Crago,§
Jiri Mestecky,§ and Ralph E. Schrohenloher‡

‡Department of Medicine
Division of Clinical Immunology and Rheumatology
University of Alabama School of Medicine
University of Alabama in Birmingham
and
§Department of Microbiology
University of Alabama School of Medicine
University of Alabama in Birmingham
Birmingham, Alabama 35294

INTRODUCTION

The occurrence of rheumatoid factors (RF) in the sera and synovial fluids of most patients with rheumatoid arthritis (RA) is well recognized. Considerable evidence suggests that RF may contribute to tissue injury in rheumatoid arthritis. This conclusion is based on several lines of evidence, largely derived from studies of IgM and IgG rheumatoid factors in RA, including the demonstration of RF in immune complexes present in sera,[1] synovial fluids,[2] and synovial fluid polymorphonuclear leukocytes[3] of patients with RA; local synthesis of RF by rheumatoid synovial tissue;[4] the capacity of both IgM RF and IgG RF to fix complement under certain conditions;[5,6] evidence of local consumption of complement in the joint space of patients with RA;[7] and correlation of C4 consumption with RF levels in RA.[8]

Considerably less attention has been directed toward examining the properties of IgA rheumatoid factors. Initially detected by Heimer and Levin[9] over 15 years ago, IgA RF has subsequently been repeatedly demonstrated in the sera and synovial fluids of a significant fraction of patients with rheumatoid arthritis.[10-13] Recently, we have developed a sensitive quantitative solid phase radioimmunoassay for IgA RF[14] and have shown IgA RF to be present in the sera and synovial fluids of virtually all seropositive RA patients. Furthermore, striking variability (approximately 50-fold) in the ratio of IgM RF to IgA RF concentrations was observed in RA sera, raising the possibility that expression of IgM RF and IgA RF was governed by distinct regulatory pathways. In order to approach this question at a cellular level, we have initiated studies directed toward investigating patterns of *in vitro* production of IgA RF and IgM RF by peripheral blood mononuclear leukocytes (MNL) and dissociated synovial cells obtained from patients with rheumatoid arthritis. Our results support the hypothesis that distinct regulatory influences modulate expression of IgM RF and IgA RF both in peripheral blood and at local sites of tissue inflammation in rheumatoid arthritis.

*This work was supported by United States Public Health Service Grants AM 03555, AI 14807, AI 18745, and AI 10854.
†To whom correspondence should be addressed.

258

MATERIALS AND METHODS

Study Subjects

Peripheral blood was obtained by venipuncture from 37 patients with definite/classical rheumatoid arthritis.[15] All patients were seropositive as defined by a serum latex fixation titer[16] of at least 1:320. The mean age of the patients was 58 years (range: 38 to 77).

Eighteen healthy adults without personal or family history of RA served as controls (mean age 38 years).

Rheumatoid synovial tissue (knee, hip, or wrist) was obtained at surgery (synovectomy or joint replacement) from 16 patients with seropositive rheumatoid arthritis.

Preparation and Culture of Peripheral Blood Mononulcear Leukocytes

Mononuclear leukocytes were prepared from peripheral blood by density centrifugation using the method of Böyum[17] as previously described.[18] Cells were cultured in plastic tubes at a density of 1×10^6 cells/ml in RPMI 1640 containing 10% fetal calf serum (Microbiological Associates, Walkersville, Md.), 2 mM glutamine, and 20 μg/ml gentamicin. The cells were cultured for seven days at 37° C in a 5% CO_2 and air atmosphere. Pokeweed mitogen (PWM) (Grand Island Biological Co., Grand Island, N.Y.) was added (10 μg/ml) to one-half of the cultures (at least quadruplicates). At the end of seven days, the culture tubes were centrifuged and culture supernatants harvested and frozen at $-20°$ C until assayed for total IgA, IgA RF, total IgM, and IgM RF.

Preparation and Culture of Dissociated Rheumatoid Synovial Cells

Dissociated rheumatoid synovial cells were prepared utilizing a modification of an enzymatic method recently described for preparation of functionally intact Peyer's patch cells.[19] Briefly, surgically removed synovial tissue was immediately transported to the laboratory in chilled saline. The tissue was washed extensively in chilled minimal essential medium and synovial tissue was then separated from capsular tissue using fine dissecting scissors. The synovial tissue was then cut into small fragments (approximately 1-2 mm³), and the resultant fragments were washed extensively with minimal essential medium. The wet weight of the fragments was then recorded, and the tissue then placed into Joklik modified minimal essential medium containing Dispase® (1 mg/ml, grade II, Boehringer Mannheim Biochemicals, Indianapolis, Inc.) at 37° C in a beaker with constant, gentle stirring (generally 50 ml enzyme solution per 10 grams of tissue). At the end of 30 minutes, the medium containing dissociated cells was removed by aspiration and placed into an equivalent volume of RPMI 1640 containing 5% fetal calf serum. Fresh prewarmed enzyme solution was immediately added to the synovial fragments, and the extraction procedure was repeated until cell counts indicated insignificant further cell yields from residual synovial tissue (generally four to five extractions). Dissociated synovial cells were washed five times in RPMI 1640 containing 5% fetal calf serum and two times in complete medium (RPMI 1640 containing 10% fetal calf serum, 2 m M glutamine, and 20 μg/ml gentamycin). Cell viability (trypan blue exclusion) always exceeded 90%, and cell yields varied from 0.5 × 10⁶ cells to 21 × 10⁶ cells/gm tissue (mean = 9.3 × 10⁶ cells/gm). Dissociated synovial cells were cultured at a density of 1 × 10⁶/ml in complete medium for seven days at 37° C in a 5% CO_2 and air atmosphere. Culture supernatants were harvested by centrifugation at the termination of culture and stored at −20° C until assayed for total IgA, IgA RF, total IgM, and IgM RF.

Immunofluorescence Studies

Fixed cytocentrifuge preparations of human synovial cell preparations were examined for the presence of cytoplasmic immunoglobulins, IgA, IgA₁ and IgA₂ subclasses, IgM, and RF (staining with heat-aggregated human IgG).

In initial experiments, slides were incubated with fluorescein isothiocyanate (FITC)-labeled polyvalent anti-human immunoglobulins heavy and light chain specificities) (Behring Diagnostics, Calbiochem, Davis, Calif.) for 45 minutes at room temperature and washed for two hours in phosphate buffered saline (PBS) at 4° C. Preparations containing immunoglobulin-positive cells were then stained to determine the presence of IgA and the distribution of IgA₁ and IgA₂ subclasses. Slides were incubated with unlabeled monoclonal anti-human IgA₁ (Bethesda Research Laboratories, Inc., Gaithersburg, Md.) or monoclonal anti-IgA₂ (Beckton Dickinson, Sunnyvale, Calif.) followed by tetramethylrhodamine isothiocyanate (TRITC)-labeled, affinity-purified goat anti-mouse IgG (Kirkegaard and Perry Laboratories, Inc., Gaithersburg, Md.). After washing, slides were incubated with FITC-labeled polyvalent rabbit anti-human IgA (heavy chain specific). To determine the presence of cytoplasmic RF, preparations were incubated with TRITC-labeled heat-aggregated normal human IgG.[20] Preparations containing cells that bound TRITC-labeled, heat-aggregated human IgG were then examined to determine the isotype of the RF by costaining with FITC-labeled polyvalent goat anti-human IgA or IgM (heavy chain specific). The subclass distribution of IgA RF was determined by costaining with TRITC-labeled heat-aggregated IgG and unlabeled monoclonal anti-IgA₁ or IgA₂ followed by FITC-labeled goat anti-mouse IgG.

Specificity Controls

Preparation of immunoglobulins, antisera, fluorochrome-labeling techniques, and specificity controls for polyclonal reagents have been previously described.[21] TRITC-labeled heat-aggregated IgG did not bind to normal human MNL, that is, MNL stimulated with PWM or synovial cell preparations that did not contain immunoglobulin-positive cells. TRITC-labeled anti-mouse IgG did not stain synovial cells as indicated by the failure to observe staining without first preincubating the cells with monoclonal anti-IgA₁ or IgA₂ reagents. Specificity of monoclonal reagents was determined by their capacity to block the immunoprecipitation of radiolabeled myeloma proteins of relevant and nonrelevant subclass specificity.

Radioimmunoassay (RIA) of IgA Rheumatoid Factors

The procedure used in these studies has previously been reported in detail.[14] Briefly, triplicate aliquots of an isolated monoclonal IgA RF (dose range 0.25–25 ng per well) or unknown samples were placed into polystyrene microtiter wells coated with human IgG and wells coated with bovine serum albumin (BSA) as a control for nonspecific binding. After 18–20 hours incubation at room temperature, the wells were then aspirated, washed three times with veronal buffered saline containing 1% BSA (VBS-BSA) and incubated with 0.25 ml VBS-BSA containing 10 ng of ^{125}I-labeled affinity purified anti-IgA. Standard curves were constructed for each experiment by plotting mean counts per minute (CPM) of ^{125}I-labeled anti-IgA bound per IgG-coated well (minus BSA control) for each input of IgA rheumatoid factor. Quantitative values for unknowns were calculated by determining the mean CPM of ^{125}I-labeled anti-IgA bound (IgG well mean minus BSA tube mean) for each dilution of unknown and then referring to the standard curve. All assays were performed in duplicate or triplicate. The assay has a coefficient of variation of between 5.4% and 5.6% depending on the concentration of IgA RF in the sample.

Radioimmunoassay of IgM Rheumatoid Factor

The procedure used for quantitation of IgM RF has also been described.[22] The assay is essentially identical to that described above for IgA RF except that a purified monoclonal IgM RF is used as a standard. The assay has a coefficient of variation of between 8.2% and 18.6% depending on the concentration of IgM RF in the sample.

Radioimmunoassay of IgM and IgA

Total IgM and IgA in culture supernatants were quantitated by solid phase radioimmunoassay.[23] Microtiter wells were precoated with either the IgG fraction of specific goat anti-human IgM (1 μg/well) or murine ascites fluid containing monoclonal anti-human IgA (1:500 dilution, a kind gift of Dr. Mary Ellen Conley and Dr. John Kearney). Standards for each assay consisted of isolated monoclonal paraproteins of the appropriate isotope and a reference normal human serum containing 1.22 ± 25 mg/dl IgM and 1.78 ± 43 mg/dl IgA as determined by a fluorometric immunoassay (FIAX®, International Diagnostic Technology, Santa Clara, Calif.). Unknowns and standards were incubated overnight at room temperature in microtiter wells coated with anti-human IgM or IgA, and the wells were then washed three times with VBS-BSA. After the final wash, 10 ng of ^{125}I-labeled affinity purified goat anti-human IgA or IgM was added to each well and incubated overnight at room temperature. The wells were then washed three times with VBS-BSA. Individual wells were placed in counting vials and counted in a Beckman 4000 gamma counter (Beckman Instruments Co., Palo Alto, Calif.). Standards were assayed in triplicate and unknowns in duplicate at two different dilutions. Background binding was always less than 3% of the radiolabeled antibody added. Standard curves were constructed for each experiment by plotting CPM of ^{125}I-labeled anti-IgM or IgA bound versus input of reference serum IgM or IgA. Values for unknowns were calculated from the standard curve. Specificity controls performed for each RIA consisted of testing excess quantities (up to 1 μg/well) of unrelated isotypes (e.g. IgA and IgG in the IgM assay) for interference in the radioimmunoassay. No interference was observed, confirming the specificity of the techniques used.

Column Chromatography

Selected synovial cell culture supernatants were fractionated by molecular gel filtration on a column (1 × 106 cm) of Ultragel AcA 22 (LKB Instruments, Inc., Rockville Md.) equilibrated in 0.02 M sodium phosphate buffered normal saline, pH 7.2 (PBS) and calibrated with polymeric IgM, polymeric IgA, and monomeric IgA and IgG. For chromatography in dissociative buffer,[24] samples were dialyzed against 0.05 M NaCl, 0.1 M acetate buffer, pH 4.1 and applied to a Sephacryl S-300 column (1 × 117 cm) equilibrated in the same buffer. Fractions were collected in sufficient saturated Tris to adjust the pH to 7.0–7.5.

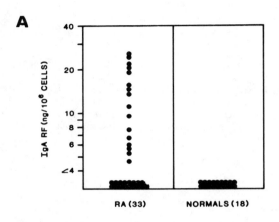

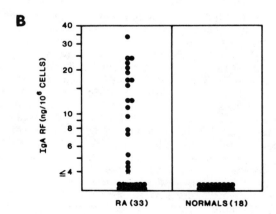

FIGURE 1. Production of IgA RF by MNL from RA patients and normal adult controls. Peripheral blood MNL from RA patients and controls were cultured in the presence (panel B) or absence (panel A) of PWM and culture supernatants were assayed for IgA RF by radioimmunoassay.

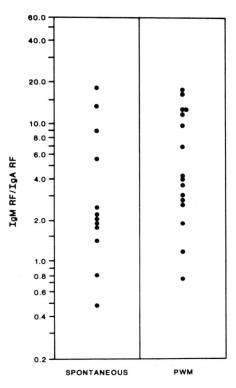

FIGURE 2. Ratio of IgM RF to IgA RF present in supernatants of MNL from RA patients cultured in the presence or absence (spontaneous) of PWM. Results are depicted for supernatants in which both IgA RF and IgM RF were detected.

RESULTS

Synthesis of IgA Rheumatoid Factor by Blood Mononuclear Leukocytes

Peripheral blood MNL from 18 healthy adult controls and 33 patients with seropositive RA were cultured for seven days in the presence and absence of pokeweed mitogen. Culture supernatants were then assayed for IgA RF by solid phase radioimmunoassay. As shown in FIGURE 1, IgA RF synthesis was not observed with unstimulated (panel A) or PWM-stimulated (panel B) MNL from healthy adults. In agreement with previous studies,[18,25] MNL from a significant fraction (9/18) of these healthy adults did elaborate IgM RF *in vitro* (mean ± 1 S.D. = 17.1 ± 9 ng/10^6 cells) when stimulated with pokeweed mitogen.

The pattern of IgA RF production exhibited by MNL from RA patients differed strikingly from control mononuclear leukocytes. Spontaneous production of IgA RF was observed with MNL from 16/33 RA patients (8.4 ± 6.8 ng/10^6 cells). Stimulation of RA MNL with PWM resulted in only a minimal increase in IgA RF production (19/33 patients, 9.9 ± 8.0 ng/10^6 cells). The dependence of IgA RF production (both spontaneous and PWM-induced) on *de novo* protein synthesis was established by demonstrating that cycloheximide (10^{-3} M) consistently blocked expression of IgA RF by RA MNL (>90% inhibition, data not shown).

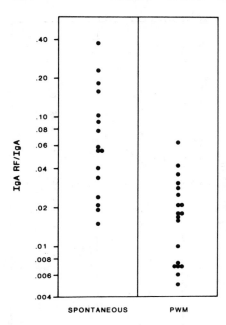

FIGURE 3. Ratio of IgA RF to total IgA present in supernatants of MNL from RA patients cultured in the presence or absence (spontaneous) of PWM. Results are depicted for supernatants in which IgA RF was detected.

Whereas IgA RF synthesis was not observed in the absence of concomitant production of IgM RF, the pattern of IgA RF expression by RA MNL differed from IgM RF in several regards. Unlike IgM RF,[25] PWM stimulation of RA MNL induced negligible overall increases in IgA RF production from that observed with unstimulated mononuclear leukocytes. Furthermore, ratios of IgM RF/IgA RF synthesized by RA MNL (in the presence or absence of PWM) varied markedly (FIGURE 2), a finding in agreement with our previous observations reported for RA sera.[14] As shown in FIGURE 3, IgA RF constituted a significant fraction of the IgA elaborated by unstimulated RA MNL (8.8 ± 9.8%) and a smaller proportion of the IgA elaborated by PWM-stimulated MNL (2.3 ± 1.8%).

We have previously observed that RA MNL synthesize significantly lower quantities of IgM in response to PWM than control mononuclear leukocytes.[25] It was therefore of interest to compare levels of spontaneous and PWM-induced total IgA production by RA MNL with control mononuclear leukocytes. Neither spontaneous (181 ± 142 ng/10^6 cells) nor PWM-induced IgA production (804 ± 622 ng/10^6 cells) by RA MNL differed significantly from control MNL values (spontaneous: 174 ± 170 ng/10^6 cells; PWM-induced: 1082 ± 1142 ng/10^6 cells).

Synthesis of IgA Rheumatoid Factor by Dissociated Synovial Cells

In view of the previously described studies indicating that blood MNL from a significant fraction of RA patients elaborated IgA RF *in vitro*, it was of interest to determine whether production of IgA RF could be demonstrated at local sites of tissue inflammation in RA (e.g. in the synovium). Synovial tissue (17 samples) was therefore obtained from 16 seropositive RA patients undergoing synovectomy or joint reconstruction, and dissociated synovial cells were then prepared by mild enzymatic treatment (Dispase® 1 mg/ml) of the tissue. Synovial cells were cultured for seven days in an identical manner to that described for MNL, and resultant culture supernatants were assayed for IgA RF, total IgA, IgM RF, and total IgM. Synovial cells from 9 out of 16 patients (10 out of 17 samples) elaborated IgA RF (91 ± 221 ng/10^6 cells); this elaboration represented a significant fraction of the total IgA synthesized (10.5 ± 7%). Production of IgM RF occurred with 15 out of 17 synovial cell preparations (1053 ± 2151 ng/10^6 cells); this production represented a substantial portion of the total IgM produced in these cultures (38 ± 29%). The relationship between levels of IgA RF and IgM RF production by synovial cells is depicted in FIGURE 4. Whereas IgA RF production was not observed in the absence of IgM RF synthesis, there was only a weak correlation between levels of the two RF isotypes expressed by synovial cells (r = 0.38).

Immunofluorescence studies of dissociated synovial cells confirmed the

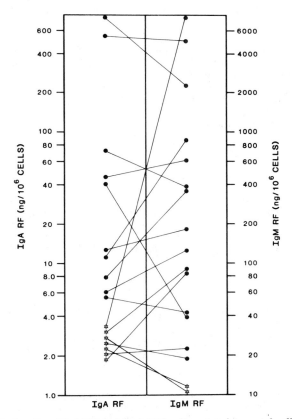

FIGURE 4. Production of IgA RF and IgM RF by dissociated synovial cells from patients with seropositive rheumatoid arthritis. Lines connect points obtained for the same synovial cell preparation. Asterisks (*) depict values that fell beneath the level of detection of the assay for IgA RF or IgM RF.

TABLE 1

IDENTIFICATION OF IgA RHEUMATOID FACTOR PLASMA CELLS IN DISSOCIATED
SYNOVIAL-CELL PREPARATIONS BY IMMUNOFLUORESCENCE

Patient	Cells Staining With aIg* (Percent)	Cells Binding Aggregated IgG† (Percent)	Aggregated IgG-Binding Cells		
			Percent IgA‡	Percent IgA$_1$§	Percent IgA$_2$§
AC	23.0	3.6	41.7	21.5	0.0
ET	18.0	1.9	27.3	—	—
SL	5.2	4.3	13.6	7.7	2.8
RL	3.7	1.7	19.8	11.4	5.7

*Cells exhibiting cytoplasmic staining with FITC polyvalent anti-human Ig.
†Cells exhibiting cytoplasmic staining with TRITC heat-aggregated human IgG.
‡Percentage of cells staining with TRITC heat-aggregated human IgG that also stain with
FITC anti-human IgA.
§Percentage of cells staining with TRITC heat-aggregated human IgG that also stain with
FITC anti-mouse Ig (after preincubation of cells with monoclonal anti-IgA$_1$ or anti-IgA$_2$).

presence of plasma cells containing IgA RF in four of seven preparations
examined. Synthesis of IgA RF *in vitro* occurred with each of the four synovial
cell preparations in which IgA RF staining plasma cells were detected, whereas
in vitro IgA RF production did not occur with synovial cells in which immunofluorescence for IgA RF cells was negative. As shown in TABLE 1, IgA$_1$
represented the predominant subclass of IgA RF staining plasma cells observed
in these synovial cell preparations.

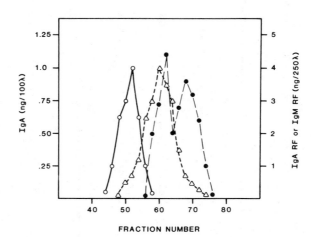

FIGURE 5. Fractionation of concentrated synovial cell culture supernatant from patient
EA. Synovial cell culture supernatant was concentrated tenfold (Amicon C-25 ultrafiltration
membrane cone) and 0.5 ml applied to a 1 × 106 cm column of AcA 22 equilibrated in
phosphate buffered saline. Fractions (0.85 ml) were collected and assayed simultaneously
for IgM RF (O——O) at a 1:3 dilution, IgA RF (△——△) undiluted, and IgA (●——●) at a 1:10
dilution. Results are depicted as raw values and are not corrected for dilution in order to
simplify presentation.

Characterization of IgA Rheumatoid Factor Synthesized by Synovial Cells

Selected synovial-cell supernatants in which significant IgA RF was detected were concentrated and chromatographed at neutral pH on an AcA 22 column as previously described.[26] A typical chromatogram, depicted in FIGURE 5, demonstrates that IgA RF eluted between IgM RF and monomeric IgA, compatible with the IgA RF being complexed or predominantly polymeric. In order to distinguish between these two possibilities, supernatants were chromatographed in acidic buffer on a Sephacryl S-300 column. As shown in FIGURE 6, under these dissociative conditions, IgA RF eluted with the same apparent molecular size. Further studies, including J-chain analysis and secretory piece binding, are currently in progress to establish this point more definitively.

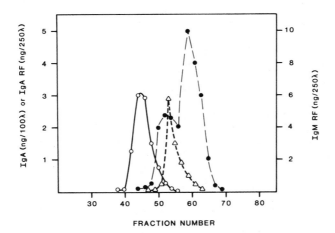

FIGURE 6. Fractionation of synovial-cell culture supernatant from patient AC. Synovial-cell culture supernatant was dialyzed against dissociative buffer (0.05 NaCl, 0.1 *M* sodium acetate buffer, pH 4.1), and 0.5 ml was then applied to a 1 × 117 cm Sephacryl S-300 column equilibrated in the same buffer. Fractions were assayed simultaneously for IgM RF (O——O) at a 1:10 dilution, IgA RF (△——△) undiluted, and IgA (●——●) at a 1:10 dilution. Results are depicted as raw values and are not corrected for dilution in order to simplify presentation.

Comparison of Patterns of IgA Rheumatoid Factor and IgM Rheumatoid Factor Production Exhibited by Paired Blood Mononuclear Leukocytes and Dissociated Synovial Cells

In order to determine the relationship between IgA RF synthesis by synovial cells and blood MNL, we obtained paired samples of synovium and blood from 12 RA patients. Supernatants from cultured blood MNL and dissociated synovial cells were then assayed for IgA RF, total IgA, IgM RF, and total IgM. As shown in TABLE 2, levels of IgA RF and IgM RF production were significantly higher with synovial cells than with paired blood mononuclear leukocytes. Moreover, the ratios of IgA RF/IgA and IgM RF/IgM were significantly higher with synovial cells than with blood MNL, indicating preferential expression of these two RF

TABLE 2

COMPARISON OF IgA RHEUMATOID FACTOR AND IgM RHEUMATOID FACTOR PRODUCTION BY PAIRED BLOOD MNL AND DISSOCIATED SYNOVIAL-CELL CULTURES

Cell Origin	Number	IgA RF*	IgA*	IgA RF/IgA	IgM RF*	IgM*	IgM RF/IgM
Blood MNL	12	4.4 ± 6.2†	314 ± 312‡	0.04 ± 0.04§	17 ± 17§	337 ± 584‡	0.11 ± 0.11§
Synovial Cells	12	82 ± 224†	706 ± 2,022‡	0.12 ± 0.07§	1,019 ± 2,241§	4,350 ± 8,815‡	0.36 ± 0.28§

*ng/10^6 cells ± S.D.
†p < 0.05 (Wilcoxen paired sample test)
‡Not significant
§p < 0.01

isotypes in synovium in comparison to circulating mononuclear leukocytes. A more graphic illustration of this point is provided in FIGURE 7 in which it is evident that expression of IgA RF and IgM RF by synovial cells from individual patients was not related to patterns of IgA RF and IgM RF production exhibited by paired blood mononuclear leukocytes.

DISCUSSION

Despite the well-documented existence of IgA RF in sera and synovial fluids of patients with seropositive RA, details concerning the physical characteristics of IgA RF, source of production and regulation of expression have not been

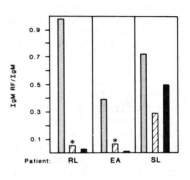

FIGURE 7. Comparison of ratios of IgM RF/total IgM (upper panel) and IgA RF/total IgA (lower panel) synthesized by dissociated synovial cells (stippled bars) and paired peripheral blood MNL cultured alone (striped bars) or in the presence of PWM (solid bars) from three patients with seropositive rheumatoid arthritis. Asterisks above bars indicate that RF was not detected, and the depicted bar represents the maximal possible ratio of RF to total isotype synthesized (obtained by assuming a value at the lower limit of detection for the particular assay).

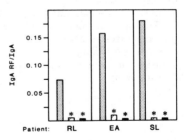

established. Our studies demonstrate that peripheral blood MNL from approximately 50% of seropositive RA patients spontaneously elaborate IgA RF *in vitro*. In marked contrast to IgM RF, stimulation of RA MNL with PWM resulted in insignificant increases in IgA RF production. Moreover, ratios of IgA RF/IgM RF varied widely, a finding that is in agreement with previously reported observations for RA sera.[14] These differences in expression of IgM RF and IgA RF suggest the existence of distinct regulatory influences governing IgA RF and IgM RF expression. In this regard, van Snick and colleagues[27,28] have demonstrated that separate genes influence expression of IgA RF and IgM RF in the mouse. Further studies are clearly necessary in order to determine the basis for variable expression of IgA RF and IgM RF in rheumatoid arthritis.

Previous studies have established that IgM RF[4,20] and IgG RF[20] plasma cells occur in the synovium of seropositive RA patients; however, firm evidence for production of IgA RF has not previously been reported. In our study, synovial cells from a significant fraction (9 out of 16) of RA patients elaborated IgA RF *in vitro*. Moreover, IgA RF staining plasma cells were detectable in those synovial cell preparations in which production of IgA RF was observed. Recent studies of serum IgA RF in Sjögren's syndrome by Elkon et al.,[29,30] have indicated that IgA RF in this disease is predominantly polymeric. These researchers suggested that mucosal involvement in this disease might explain the polymeric nature of the serum IgA RF in these patients. Our results indicating that IgA RF synthesized by synovial cells is predominantly large molecular weight and not dissociated under acid pH conditions raise the possibility that IgA RF exists predominantly as a polymer regardless of tissue of origin. It should be stressed that we cannot exclude, on the basis of our data, either the possibility that monomeric IgA RF is not detected with our assay system or that large molecular weight IgA RF actually represents a tightly complexed IgA RF monomer. We are currently exploring both of these possibilities.

Of particular interest was the clear dissociation between levels of production of IgA RF and IgM RF exhibited by paired synovial cells and blood mononuclear leukocytes. In this regard, ratios of IgA RF/IgA and IgM RF/IgM were significantly higher with synovial cells than with blood MNL, indicating preferential expression of these two RF isotypes at local sites of inflammation in rheumatoid arthritis. These observations are compatible with the view that lymphoid elements localized at sites of inflammation in RA function autonomously and suggest that *in vitro* function of circulating MNL in RA patients bears little relationship to immune processes occurring at local sites of tissue injury in this disease. Recent studies indicating that synovial fluid and synovial tissue MNL, obtained from inflamed joints of patients with RA, consist of markedly different distributions of lymphocyte populations than occur in the circulation of these patients,[31-34] further support this concept.

The precise role(s) of IgA RF in tissue injury associated with RA is unclear. Recent studies establishing that serum polymeric IgA facilitates antigen clearance through the biliary tract[35] raise the possibility that IgA RF may influence the handling of IgG-containing immune complexes in RA, a possibility under current investigation.

ACKNOWLEDGMENTS

The authors are very appreciative of the technical help of Ms. Rose Kulhavy, Ms. Shirley Prince, and Ms. Cindy Moore and are grateful for the assistance of Ms. Joyce Cook in preparing the manuscript.

REFERENCES

1. FRANKLIN, E. C., H. HOLMAN, H. J. MULLER-EBERHARD & H. G. KUNKEL. 1957. J. Exp. Med. **105:** 425–438.
2. WINCHESTER, R. J., V. AGNELLO & H. G. KUNKEL. 1970. Clin. Exp. Immunol. **6:** 689–706.
3. VAUGHAN, J. H., R. F. JACOX & P. NOELL. 1968. Arthritis Rheum. **11:** 135–141.
4. SMILEY, J. D., C. SACHS & M. ZIFF. 1968. J. Clin. Invest. **47:** 624–632.
5. TANIMOTO, K., N. R. COOPER, J. S. JOHNSON & J. H. VAUGHAN. 1975. J. Clin. Invest. **55:** 437–445.

6. BIANCO, N. E., L. W. DOBKIN & P. SCHUR. 1974. Clin. Exp. Immunol. **17:** 91–101.
7. RUDDY, S. & K. F. AUSTEN. 1970. Arthritis Rheum. **13:** 713–723.
8. KAPLAN, R. A., J. G. CURD, D. H. DEHEER, D. A. CARSON, M. K. PANGBURN, H. J. MULLER-EBERHARD & J. H. VAUGHAN. 1980. Arthritis Rheum. **23:** 911–920.
9. HEIMER, R. & F. M. LEVIN. 1966. Immunochemistry **3:** 1–10.
10. TORRIGIANI, G. & I. M. ROITT. 1967. Ann. Rheum. Dis. **23:** 334–339.
11. PANUSH, R. S., N. E. BIANCO & P. H. SCHUR. 1971. Arthritis Rheum. **14:** 737–747.
12. STANKAITIENÉ, D. J., A. A. MATULIS, H. GUOBYS & J. P. JUSENAITE. 1978. Arthritis Rheum. **21:** 120–128.
13. DUNNE, J. V., D. A. CARSON, H. L. SPIEGELBERG, M. D. ASPAUGH & J. H. VAUGHAN. 1979. Ann. Rheum. Dis. **38:** 161–170.
14. KOOPMAN, W. J., R. E. SCHROHENLOHER & A. SOLOMON. 1982. J. Immunol. Methods. **50:** 89–96.
15. A Committee of the American Rheumatism Association. 1958. Arthritis Rheum. **2:** 16–20.
16. SINGER, J. M. & C. M. PLOTZ. 1956. Am. J. Med. **21:** 888–892.
17. BÖYUM, A. 1968. Scand. J. Clin. Lab. Invest. Suppl. **97:** 77–82.
18. KOOPMAN, W. J. & R. E. SCHROHENLOHER. 1980. J. Immunol. **125:** 934–939.
19. FRANGAKIS, M. V., W. J. KOOPMAN, H. KIYONO, S. M. MICHALEK & J. R. MCGHEE. 1982. J. Immunol. Meth. **48:** 33–44.
20. MUNTHE, E. & J. B. NATVIG. 1972. Clin. Exp. Immunol. **12:** 55–70.
21. CRAGO, S. & J. MESTECKY. 1979. J. Immunol. **122:** 906–911.
22. KOOPMAN, W. J. & R. E. SCHROHENLOHER. 1980. Arthritis Rheum. **23:** 302–308.
23. TORII, M., J. R. MCGHEE, W. J. KOOPMAN, S. HAMADA & S. M. MICHALEK. 1981. J. Immunol. **127:** 2106–2111.
24. SCHROHENLOHER, R. E., H. G. KUNKEL & T. B. TOMASI. 1964. J. Exp. Med. **120:** 1215–1229.
25. KOOPMAN, W. J. & R. E. SCHROHENLOHER. 1980. Arthritis Rheum. **23:** 985–992.
26. KUTTEH, W. H., W. J. KOOPMAN, M. E. CONLEY, M. L. EGAN & J. MESTECKY. 1980. J. Exp. Med. **152:** 1424–1429.
27. VAN SNICK, J. L. & P. L. MASSON. 1980. J. Exp. Med. **151:** 45–52.
28. VAN SNICK, J. L. 1981. J. Exp. Med. **153:** 738–742.
29. ELKON, K. B., F. CAEIRO, A. E. GHARAVI, B. M. PATEL, P. P. FERJENCIK & G. R. V. HUGHES. 1981. Clin. Exp. Immunol. **46:** 547–552.
30. ELKON, K. B., D. L. DELACROIX, A. E. GHARAVI, J.-P. VAERMAN & G. R. V. HUGHES. 1982. J. Immunol. **129:** 576–581.
31. GALLILI, U., L. ROSENTHAL, N. GALLILI & E. KLEIN. 1979. J. Immunol. **122:** 878–883.
32. BURMESTER, G. R., D. T. Y. YU, A.-M. IRANI, H. G. KUNKEL & R. J. WINCHESTER. 1981. Arthritis Rheum. **24:** 1370–1376.
33. FOX, R. I., S. FONG, N. SABHARWAL, S. A. CARSTENS, P. C. KUNG & J. H. VAUGHAN. 1982. J. Immunol. **128:** 351–354.
34. SILVER, R. M., D. REDELMAN, N. J. ZVAIFLER & S. NAIDES. 1982. J. Immunol. **128:** 1758–1763.
35. RUSSELL, M. W., T. A. BROWN & J. MESTECKY. 1981. J. Exp. Med. **153:** 968–973.

DISCUSSION OF THE PAPER

K. B. ELKON (*Hospital for Special Surgery, New York, N.Y.*): Because Vaerman in our group has shown that polymeric immunoglobulins can fix IgG, why did you not include this data? Additionally, in our patients with Sjögren's syndrome, we have shown quite clearly that the IgA rheumatoid factor is polymeric, with the presence of J-chain.

W. J. KOOPMAN (*University of Alabama in Birmingham*): Yes, I am aware of your data with Sjögren's patients. You reported that you did not find much IgA rheumatoid factor in sera from patients with rheumatoid arthritis; this may be the result of a difference in the level of sensitivity of the IgA RF assays utilized. Although you suggest that the difference in substrate, for example, rabbit IgG may account for differences, we have also used rabbit IgG, and our results are comparable with this substrate. With regard to your first question, we do not find uptake of radiolabeled goat anti-IgA by IgA rheumatoid factor bound to the side of plates. We have conducted these experiments many times. Goat serum with the second antibody does not alter the results. I think that the rheumatoid factor binds monomeric IgG very poorly, as seen in the assay we employ. We can use 1000-fold excess of monomeric IgG and not block the binding of the rheumatoid factor to solid phase IgG. So, we do not find significant inhibition by monomeric IgG of the IgA-rheumatoid factor assay.

REGULATION OF THE IMMUNE RESPONSES TO A STREPTOCOCCAL ANTIGEN BY HELPER AND SUPPRESSOR FUNCTIONS IN MAN*

Thomas Lehner

Department of Oral Immunology and Microbiology
Medical and Dental Schools
Guy's Hospital
London, SE1 9RT, England

Natural sensitization occurs to a variety of microorganisms residing in the human mouth or gastrointestinal tract. The immune responses have been studied to *Streptococcus mutans*, which is commonly found in the mouth and is one of the most important organisms responsible for dental caries.[1] Serum IgG antibodies to *S. mutans* can be found in the blood of infants and in their mothers.[2] IgG, IgM, and IgA antibodies to this organisms have been found in children from the age of two and one-half years[3] and are also found in adults.[4] Secretory IgA antibodies to *S. mutans* have been reported in colostrum[5] and in saliva.[6]

The presence of serum and secretory antibodies to *S. mutans* has been associated with a variety of cellular immune responses. Lymphoproliferative responses and leukocyte migration inhibition to *S. mutans* have been recorded,[7] and the indices of both these responses increase significantly by the natural effect of dental plaque accumulation. The cellular immune responses in man and subhuman primates have been interpreted in terms of helper function of T-lymphocytes.[8,9] More recently, both helper and suppressor functions have been demonstrated in man and monkeys,[10,11] using a streptococcal protein antigen with a molecular weight of 185,000.[12,13] The streptococcal antigen (SA) stimulates lymphocytes *in vitro* or *in vivo* to generate T-helper or T-suppressor cells that release corresponding helper or suppressor factors after further stimulation with the antigen. Putative T-helper or suppressor cells, however, generated by natural sensitization in man, can be detected by modifying the method, so as to stimulate these cells to release the helper (HF) or suppressor factor (SF). Indeed, this finding revealed that 1 ng of SA will release HF predominantly from lymphocytes with HLA-DRw6, whereas 1000 ng of SA is required to release a corresponding HF activity from HLA-DR4 and other lymphocytes.[8] Suppressor activity showed a reciprocal relationship to helper activity, so that if help is elicited with 1 ng, suppression is elicited with 10 ng or larger amounts of streptococcal antigen.[10]

The aim of this paper is to review the relationship between helper and suppressor activities to the SA with special reference to the HLA-DR antigens. The effect of depletion of the helper population with the monoclonal T4 antiserum,[14] and that of the suppressor population with the T8 antiserum,[15] are then studied in relation to both the helper and suppressor functions.

*This investigation was carried out under a project grant from the Medical Research Council.

0077-8923/83/0409-0273 $1.75/0 © 1983, NYAS

MATERIALS AND METHODS

Subjects and Separation of Mononuclear Cells

Twelve subjects (19–26 years of age) were selected for the HLA-DR antigen that was determined as described before.[8,16] The lymphocytes of six subjects had DRw6 with or without other DR antigens and those of six other subjects had DR4 with or without other DR antigens.

Preparation of Antigens

Streptococcal antigen I/II was prepared from *S. mutans* (serotype *c*, Guy's strain) grown in a semidefined medium as described previously.[12,13] Briefly, the culture supernatant was precipitated by ammonium sulphate and chromatographed on DEAE-cellulose, followed by gel-filtration on Sepharose 6B (Pharmacia, Uppsala, Sweden). The resultant protein showed a single band on polyacrylamide gel electrophoresis and had a molecular weight of about 185,000.[13] Keyhole limpet hemocyanin (KLH) was kindly donated by Dr. M. Ritterberg of Portland, Oregon. Dinitrophenylated-SA was prepared using dinitrofluorobenzene as described before[11] and had five groups of DNP per 100,000 daltons; Trinitrophenylated-KLH was prepared with eight groups of TNP per 100,000 daltons.

Preparation of Helper and Suppressor Factors

In order to induce HF *in vitro* from putative HF *in vivo*, 5×10^6 viable Ficoll-Isopaque separated cells were cultured in 1 ml of tissue culture medium with 0, 1, 10^1–10^5 ng of SA in Marbrook-Diener flasks for 24 hours, as described previously.[8] Any HF released into the supernatant was assayed for antibody-forming cells (AFC). Briefly, a previously determined optimum concentration of 10^{-3} ml of HF per culture was added to 10×10^6 unprimed B10.BR spleen cells and 100 ng/ml of DNA-SA in Costar plates (Cambridge, Mass.). The anti-DNP AFC were assayed on day 4, using the modified Cunningham assay with DNP-Fab-coated sheep red blood cells (SRBC) and uncoated sheep red blood cells. DNP-specific plaques were the difference between the two. All cultures were carried out in triplicate and assayed separately.

Suppressor factor was prepared from putative suppressor cells, assumed to be induced *in vivo*, in the same way as for helper factor. The cells were cultured in the presence of 1–10^5 ng SA for 24 hours, and the supernatants were then assayed for their ability to suppress helper cells.[11] Helper cells were induced from B10.BR mouse spleen cells by culturing these *in vitro* with 100 ng of SA for four days. The SF was then cultured in the presence of 3×10^5 helper cells (HC), 10×10^6 unprimed B10.BR spleen cells, and 100 ng of DNP-SA. Antibody-forming cells were assayed on day 4 as for helper factor. For comparative purposes of HF and SF activity the assays were performed on the same preparation of lymphocytes and were expressed as a percentage of mouse B10.BR helper cells using the following formulas:

$$\text{Helper activity } (\%) = \frac{\text{AFC of HF with SA} - \text{AFC of SA}}{\text{AFC of HC with SA} - \text{AFC of SA}} \times 100$$

$$\text{Suppressor activity } (\%) = 100 - \frac{\text{AFC of SF with SA} - \text{AFC of SA}}{\text{AFC of HC with SA} - \text{AFC of SA}} \times 100$$

Antigen specificity of the HF and SF to SA were demonstrated elsewhere by negative responses to keyhole limpet hemocyanin.[10] Affinity chromatography also showed that SA, unlike KLH bound the HF or SF activity.[10]

Preparation of Helper or Suppressor-Cell-Depleted Lymphocytes

Helper or suppressor-cell-depleted mononuclear cell populations were prepared from the Ficoll-Isopaque separated cells. Samples of 5×10^6 cells, suspended in 1 ml of N-2-hydroxyethyl piperazine-N'-2-ethane sulfonic acid

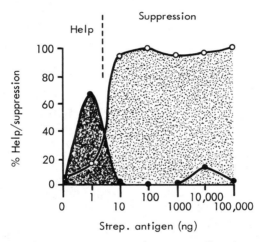

FIGURE 1. Helper and suppressor activities of HLA-DRw6 lymphocytes to streptococcal antigen.

(HEPES)-buffered minimal essential medium (MEM) and 5% fetal calf serum (FCS) were mixed with 25 μl of T4 or T8 antiserum (Ortho Laboratories) for 30 minutes at room temperature. These monoclonal antisera are of the IgG$_2$ subclass and fix complement.[15] The cells were washed twice in the HEPES-buffered MEM and 5% FCS, resuspended in 2 ml of the medium and then rotated with 3.0 ml of reconstituted rabbit complement (Buxted Rabbit Co. Ltd., Sussex) on a blood mixer for 60 minutes at room temperature. The cells were then washed two times in the same medium and 5×10^6 viable cell suspensions were used in the helper and suppressor-cell assays as described above. The proportion of T4 and T8 cells, before and after depletion of the corresponding populations, was assayed by the indirect immunofluorescence test. One $\times 10^6$ cells were incubated with 5 μl of T4 or T8 antiserum for 30 minutes at 4° C and washed. Then 50 μl of FITC-conjugated goat anti-mouse IgG (Fc) (Miles Laboratories) was added and kept for 30 minutes at 4° C. The cells were washed, mounted on microscope slides, and viewed with a Leitz Orthoplan fluorescence microscope. Membrane fluorescence was recorded by counting over 200 cells.

RESULTS

Comparative Assay of Helper and Suppressor Factors

A parallel assay of HF and SF showed two basic patterns (FIGURES 1, 2): DRw6 lymphocytes released HF activity with 1 ng of SA and SF activity with all the other doses (FIGURE 1), whereas DR4 lymphocytes released HF with 1000 ng of SA and SF with all the other doses (FIGURE 2). An analysis of 12 subsets, 6 with DRw6 and 6 with DR4 typed lymphocytes (TABLE 1), showed that in 5 of 6 DRw6 typed subsets, helper activity was restricted to 1 (or 10) ng of SA, but lymphocytes from

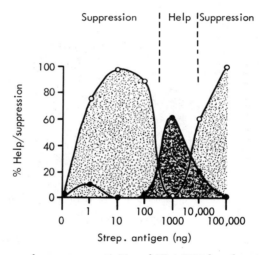

FIGURE 2. Helper and suppressor activities of HLA-DR4 lymphocytes to streptococcal antigen.

the sixth subject responded only to 1000 ng streptococcal antigen. There was negligible SF activity at the corresponding doses of maximum helper activity. Suppressor factor activity between 83% and 100% was elicited by SA at the dose levels of $10-10^5$ ng of SA, except for subject, number four, who yielded HF with 10 ng of SA, and lymphocytes from subject six that released HF with 1000 ng SA (TABLE 1).

Similar parallel assays of lymphocytes from six HLA-DR4 subjects released HF at a dose of 1000 ng of SA, and SF activity at 1–100 ng and at 10^4 ng SA (TABLE 1). In order to exclude the possibility that the antigen alone might be responsible for suppression, SA was added alone to the cooperative culture, in the presence of helper cells. Up to a dose of 1000 ng, there was negligible suppression, a mean of 6.7 ($\pm$5.2)% at 1000 nanograms. Suppression rose to 23 ($\pm$4.2)% with 10^4 ng and to 43.3 ($\pm$8.9)% with 10^5 ng streptococcal antigen. Suppression cannot, therefore, be

TABLE 1

PERCENT OF HELPER AND SUPPRESSOR FUNCTIONS IN 12 SELECTED SUBJECTS, 6 OF WHOM HAD HLA-DRw6 AND 6 OF WHOM HAD HLA DR4-TYPED LYMPHOCYTES*

Subjects	HLA-DR	AFC/Culture Mean (±SE) SA	AFC/Culture Mean (±SE) SA/HC†	Helper Function (Percentage) ng of Streptococcal Antigen 0	1	10	100	1,000	10,000	Suppressor Function Percentage 0	1	10	100	1,000	10,000
1	6,5	13(9)	157[3]	0	67	3	0	0	14	7	17	95	100	95	97
2	6,7	20(12)	197[33]	4	56	13	4	4	4	42	17	83	89	100	100
3	6,5	17(10)	140[12]	0	2	80	0	0	0		ND‡				
4	6	16(12)	120[6]	4	9	97	16	14	1	10	62	16	93	100	87
5	6	30(6)	157[7]	0	97	2	13	0	0	8	19	100	87	0	100
6	6	27(12)	143[15]	0	0	0	5	100	9	5	100	100	100	0	98
7	4,1	30(6)	223[19]	2	0	0	9	100	10	3	90	100	100	21	91
8	4,1	30(6)	280[10]	3	0	4	0	73	13	32	100	93	93	40	76
9	4,2	23(7)	180[15]	0	0	4	2	96	24	20	89	100	100	4	100
10	4,3	23(3)	110[6]	0	0	ND	0	34	100	0	88	100	100	23	100
11	4,3	40(10)	250[17]	0	0	ND	ND	88	ND	29	100	97	100	14	100
12	4,6	20(6)	120[10]	0	0	3	0	100	3	0	83	87	73	23	90

*The results are expressed as a percentage of helper activity, that is, antibody-forming cells (AFC) induced by 100 ng of streptoccal antigen (SA) in mouse B10.BR spleen cells.

†HC = Mouse Helper Cells

‡ND = Not done.

TABLE 2

Effect of Killing HLA-DRw6 Lymphocytes, by T4 or T8 Antibodies and Complement, on Helper and Suppressor Factor Activities to Streptococcal Antigen (SA)

Percentage	Untreated SA(ng)						T4 + C' SA(ng)						Untreated SA(ng)						T8 + C' SA(ng)					
	0	1	10	100	1,000	10,000	0	1	10	100	1,000	10,000	0	1	10	100	1,000	10,000	0	1	10	100	1,000	10,000
Help	5	72	5	5	0		22	11	0	17	0	83	0	97	2	13.4	0	0	0	92	71	89	89	100
Suppression	33	33	100	100	100		37	100	100	100	100	19	19	19	100	87	100	83	2	3	0	29	31	65
Helper Cells	38.5						0						39.2						49.6					
Suppressor Cells	29.5						51						18.1						0					

accounted for by antigen alone, up to a dose of 10^4 ng, because SF induced 90 to 100% suppression, whereas antigen alone induced up to 23% suppression.

Effect of Depletion of Helper or Suppressor-Cells on the Corresponding Functional Activities

Depletion of the T8-positive cells (T-suppressor cells), from 29.5% to 0% with the T8 antiserum and complement, resulted in a decrease in suppression from 87–100% to 0–31%, in the DRw6 lymphocytes (TABLE 2). In addition, however, HF activity could be detected across the whole range of doses of streptococcal antigen. The DRw6 encoded lymphocytes now released HF not only with 1 ng, but also with 10–10^4 ng of streptococcal antigen. A comparable series of T-helper-cell-depletion experiments with T4 antisera and complement showed that untreated DRw6 lymphocytes, with 38.5% of T4-positive cells and 72% HF activity, were decreased to 0% of T4-positive cells and 0–17% HF activity after treatment with T4 antisera (TABLE 2). Suppression was then extended, however, to the entire range of doses of streptococcal antigen. The DR4 lymphocytes showed very similar responses to the DRw6 lymphocytes, after T4 or T8 cell-depletion (TABLE 3). Comparable results were found with four other subjects.

DISCUSSION

Helper and suppressor activities were detected in lymphocytes from all the subjects in this series, suggesting that most normal subjects are sensitized to the SA derived from *Streptococcus mutans*. The latter is commonly found in the human oral cavity. An inverse relationship, however, was observed between the HF and SF activities. The DR4 lymphocytes released HF with 1000 ng of SA and SF with both lower and higher doses of antigen (FIGURE 2). This phenomenon resulted in what seems to be best described for antibodies as low-zone and high-zone tolerance, with an intermediate zone of immunity.[17] The same interpretation is applicable to the DRw6 lymphocytes, except that there is a 1000 ng shift in the dose of antigen (FIGURE 1). Thus, lymphocytes that release HF with 1 ng SA, also release SF, with 10 ng or higher doses of SA.

The HLA-DR-dependent shifts in the dose responses of both helper and suppressor activities were then studied by depleting the lymphocytes of helper or suppressor populations. This depletion was carried out by killing lymphocytes with monoclonal anti-helper (T4) or anti-suppressor (T8) antisera, and rabbit complement. These populations were depleted of most of the helper or suppressor cells, retaining 0–4% of those cells and losing 85% of their helper activity and 69–100% of their suppressor activity (TABLES 2, 3).

The less predictable results, however, were the loss of dose-dependent specificities of the depleted cell populations. Thus, DR4 typed lymphocytes, depleted of suppressor cells, responded with helper activity not only with a dose of 1000 ng, but, also with all other doses used. Similarly, DRw6 lymphocytes responded, in addition to one ng, to the other doses of streptococcal antigen. In the same way, helper-cell-depleted populations showed a broadening of their suppressor activity to all other doses of antigen used. These experiments suggest that the net result of helper or suppressor activity is dependent on the interactions of these cells and factors. As the dose dependency of helper cells is eliminated by killing the suppressor cells, the latter seems to affect all but one antigen dose of

TABLE 3

EFFECT OF KILLING HLA-DR4 LYMPHOCYTES, BY T4 OR T8 ANTIBODIES AND COMPLEMENT, ON HELPER AND SUPPRESSOR FACTOR ACTIVITIES TO STREPTOCOCCAL ANTIGEN (SA)

Percentage	Untreated SA[ng]						T4 ± C' SA[ng]						Untreated SA[ng]						T8 ± C' SA[ng]					
	0	1	10	100	1,000	10,000	0	1	10	100	1,000	10,000	0	1	10	100	1,000	10,000	0	1	10	100	1,000	10,000
Help	0	1	4	2	96	24	0	0	87	91	13	0	0	6.5	0	13	76	6.5	0	31	78	63	54	100
Suppression	20	89	100	100	4	76	17	94	94	96	2	100	8.5	100	100	100	5	90	18	41	26	37	20	31
Helper Cells	46.8						4						45.5						44.3					
Suppressor Cells	20.5						40						31.8						0.3					

the helper response. Alternatively, a subset of suppressor cells might inhibit the suppressor functions, allowing helper activity—described in mice as contrasuppression[18] or abrosuppression.[19] The discrete antigen dose response of helper activity, which seems to be DR dependent, might be related to a subset of antigen-binding suppressor cells that are presently being investigated.[10]

The DR-associated dose shift of 1000 ng of SA is a particularly interesting feature of this investigation and might be an expression of Ir gene control. A monoclonal anti-DRw6,1,2 antiserum (Genox 353) adsorbed both HF and SF from DRw6, but not from DR4 typed lymphocytes.[8] Although this selection suggests a high degree of specificity, it should be noted that DRw6 is a rather ill-defined antigen[20] that is now being split into a number of components. It also appears that the monoclonal anti-DRw6,1,2 (Genox 353) might react with the B-cell alloantigen MT1 (DC1), linked with DRw6,1,2 antigen.[21] Ia antigen has been reported in human HF[22] and in SF.[23] A full characterization of HF and SF by affinity chromatography has been reported elsewhere.[24]

The use of a natural streptococcal antigen, commonly found in the mouth of man,[25,26] to investigate the helper and suppressor activities of human lymphocytes may have some biological significance. It seems that lymphocytes from caries-prone subjects are stimulated by 1–10 ng to induce suppressor activity, whereas this dose of antigen stimulates helper activity from lymphocytes of most caries-resistant subjects. Indeed, there is a 1000-fold difference in the dose of SA required to stimulate a comparable helper activity from lymphocytes of caries-prone and resistant subjects.[8] These findings offer a basis for interpreting the overwhelming incidence of dental caries in developed countries. Whereas sugar encourages the overgrowth of S. mutans, repeated transient bacteremia of S. mutans, which occurs with many oral microorganisms, is likely to induce low-zone or ultra low-zone tolerance, under the immunogenetic control of HLA-DR antigens, and lead to a failure to mount an effective immune response to S. mutans. The SA has been used for immunization of rhesus monkeys and resulted in protection against caries, serum IgG antibodies to the SA, and low-dose helper function.[27]

SUMMARY

Natural sensitization of human lymphocytes to a SA, isolated from *Streptococcus mutans*, has been investigated by stimulating T-lymphocytes *in vitro* with the streptococcal antigen. Helper or suppressor activity released by the lymphocytes was then tested for anti-DNP antibody-forming cells. A differential dose-response of about 1000 ng of SA was found between the specific helper function of HLA DRw6 and DR4 lymphocytes. Specific suppressor activity showed a reciprocal relationship to helper activity. Depletion of suppressor cells, by killing these with the monoclonal T8 antiserum and complement, resulted in loss of suppressor, but increased dose response in helper function. Conversely, helper-cell-depleted cultures showed a loss of helper and increased dose response in suppressor function. The results suggest a reciprocal controlling function of helper and suppressor cells. The HLA-DR linked antigens might be related to significant shifts in the dose response of helper cells.

ACKNOWLEDGMENT

I wish to thank Miss Janet Avery for her excellent technical assistance.

REFERENCES

1. HAMADA, S. & H. D. SLADE. 1980. Biology, immunology, and cariogenicity of Streptococcus mutans. Microbiology Rev. **44**: 331–384.
2. IVANYI, L. & T. LEHNER. 1978. The relationship between caries index and stimulation of lymphocytes by Streptococcus mutans in mothers and their neonates. Arch. Oral Biol. **23**: 851–856.
3. LEHNER, T., J. J. MURRAY, G. B. WINTER & J. CALDWELL. 1978. Antibodies to Streptococcus mutans and immunoglobulin levels in children with dental caries. Arch. Oral Biol. **23**: 1061–1067.
4. CHALLACOMBE, S. J. & T. LEHNER. 1976. Serum and salivary antibodies to cariogenic bacteria in man. J. Dent. Res. **55**: C139–C148.
5. ARNOLD, R. R., J. MESTECKY, & J. R. McGHEE. 1976. Naturally occurring secretory immunoglobulin A antibodies to Streptococcus mutans in human colostrum and saliva. Infect. Immun. **14**: 355–362.
6. CHALLACOMBE, S. J. 1980. Serum and salivary antibodies to streptococcus mutans in relation to the development and treatment of human dental caries. Arch. Oral. Biol. **25**: 495–502.
7. LEHNER, T., S. J. CHALLACOMBE, J. M. A. WILTON & L. IVANYI. 1976. Immunopotentiation by dental microbial plaque and its relationship to oral disease in man. Arch. Oral Biol. **21**: 749–753.
8. LEHNER, T., J. R. LAMB, K. I. WELSH & J. R. BATCHELOR. 1981. Association between HLA-DR antigens and helper cell activity in the control of dental caries. Nature (London) **292**: 770–772.
9. LAMB, J. R., S. KONTIAINEN & T. LEHNER. 1980. A comparative investigation of the generation of specific T cell helper function induced by Streptococcus mutans in monkeys and mice. J. Immunol. **124**: 2384–2389.
10. LEHNER, T. 1982. Human helper and suppressor factors to a Streptococcal antigen. J. Immunol. **129**: 1936–1940.
11. LAMB, J. R., S. KONTIAINEN & T. LEHNER. 1979. The generation of specific T cell suppressor function induced by Streptococcus mutans in monkeys and mice. Infect. Immun. **26**: 903–909.
12. RUSSELL, M. W. & T. LEHNER. 1978. Characterisation of antigens extracted from cells and culture fluids of Streptococcus mutans serotype c. Arch. Oral. Biol. **23**: 7–15.
13. RUSSELL, M. W., L. A. BERGMEIER, E. D. ZANDERS & T. LEHNER. 1980. Protein antigens of Streptococcus mutans purification and properties of a double antigen and its protease-resistant component. Infect. Immun. **28**: 486–492.
14. REINHERZ, E. L., P. C. KUNG, J. M. BREAD, G. GOLDSTEIN & S. F. SCHLOSSMAN. 1980. T cell requirements for generation of helper factor(s) in man: analysis of the subsets involved. J. Immunol. **124**: 1883.
15. MORIMOTO, C., E. L. REINHERZ & S. F. SCHLOSSMAN. 1981. Regulation of in vitro primary anti-DNP antibody production by functional subsets of T lymphocytes in man. J. Immunol. **127**: 69.
16. WELSH, K. I. & J. R. BATCHELOR. 1978. In Handbook of Experimental Immunology. D. M. Weir, Ed.: 35.1–35.20. Blackwell. Oxford.
17. MITCHISON, N. A. 1964. Induction of immunological paralysis in two zones of dosage. Proc. Roy. Soc. London, Ser. B. **161**: 275.
18. GERSHON, R. K., D. D. EARDLEY, S. S. DURUM, D. R. GREEN, F. W. SHEN, K. YAMAUCHI, H. CANTOR & D. B. MURPHY. 1981. Contrasuppression—A novel immunoregulatory activity. J Exp. Med. **153**: 1533.
19. DEKRUYFF, R. H., B. G. SIMONSON & G. W. SISKIND. 1981. Cellular interactions in immune regulation. J. Exp. Med. **154**: 1188.
20. BODMER, J. G. 1978. Ia antigens definition of the HLA-DRw specificities. Br. Med. Bull. **34**: 233.
21. SHACKELFORD, D. A., D. L. MAN, J. J. VAN ROOD, G. B. FERRARA & J. L. STROMINGER. 1981. Human B-cell alloantigens DC1, MT1 and LB12 are identical to each other but distinct from the HLA-DR antigen. Proc. Natl. Acad. Sci. USA **78**: 4566.

22. MUDAWWAR, F. B., E. F. YUNIS & R. S. GEHA. 1978. Antigen-specific helper factor in man. J. Exp. Med. **148:** 1032.
23. KONTIAINEN, S., J. N. WOODY, A. REES & M. FELDMANN. 1981. Induction of human antigen-specific suppressor factors in vitro. Clin. Exp. Immunol. **43:** 517.
24. LEHNER, T. 1983. Characterisation of human helper and suppressor factors with special reference to HLA-DR determinants. Immunology. **48:** 695.
25. KRASSE, B., H. V. JORDAN, S. EDWARDSSON, T. SVENSSEON & L. TRELL. 1968. The occurrence of certain "caries-inducing" streptococci in human dental plaque material, with special reference to frequency and activity of caries. Arch. Oral. Biol. **13:** 911.
26. LOESCHE, W. J., J. ROWAN, L. H. STRAFFON & P. J. LOOS. 1975. Association of Streptococcus mutans with human dental decay. Infect. Immun. **11:** 1252.
27. LEHNER, T., M. W. RUSSELL, J. CALDWELL, & J. R. SMITH. 1981. Immunization with purified protein antigens from Streptococcus mutans against dental caries in rhesus monkeys. Infect. Immun. **34:** 407–415.

DISCUSSION OF THE PAPER

J. A. MATTINGLY (*Ohio State University, Columbus, Ohio*): Your present work stemmed from your earlier studies with C57BL/10 mice. Gershon has published papers concluding that this mouse lacks the contrasuppressor cell. Nevertheless, your findings with the suppressor cell in the human were based upon studies in mice that lack this cell type. Would you care to comment on this situation?

T. LEHNER (*Guy's Hospital, London, England*): In fact, the mouse that we use is the B10BR or CBA. I would not like you to leave with the idea that we are suggesting that these are necessarily contra-suppressor-cells. We have not been able to purify them, because they represent a small percentage of the cells present. The point I am trying to make is that the data are consistent with the concept of contrasuppression.

D. R. GREEN (*Yale University, New Haven, Conn.*): Several groups are interpreting our paper on the B10s as having said that B10s do not contain any contrasuppressor cells. That really is not our observation and applies to a specific suppressor factor system that involves sheep red blood cells. We really do not know what their status is involving *S. mutans*, especially crossing the species barrier.

SUPPRESSION AND CONTRASUPPRESSION IN THE REGULATION OF GUT-ASSOCIATED IMMUNE RESPONSES*

Douglas R. Green and Susan St. Martin

Department of Pathology
Yale University School of Medicine
New Haven, Connecticut

INTRODUCTION

Contrasuppression is an immunoregulatory T-cell activity that renders T-helper cells (and other targets of T-suppressor cells) resistant to suppressor-cell signals. The induction and activity of T-contrasuppressor cells has now been demonstrated in a number of systems, *in vitro* and *in vivo*. In this brief discussion, the possible involvement of contrasuppression in the regulation of gut-associated immune responses will be considered. In addition, a broader perspective will be presented of how contrasuppressor cells may regulate microenvironmentally localized immune responses, perhaps a major role for this regulatory T-cell circuit.

THE STRUCTURE OF THE CONTRASUPPRESSOR CIRCUIT

Three T-cell subpopulations have been identified that interact to produce contrasuppression. These have been analyzed in terms of characteristic arrays of cell surface antigenic markers or "surface phenotypes" by the use of a variety of antisera and lectins. The correlation of a unique surface phenotype with a particular function serves to define a particular cell subset.

The contrasuppressor-inducer cell is an I-J$^+$/Ly-2 T-cell (a T-cell that is Ly-1$^-$ and Ly-2$^+$).[1] This cell produces a cell-free factor (TcsiF) that bears a product of the I-J subregion and binds antigen.[2] In the presence of the contrasuppressor-transducer cell the TcsiF induces contrasuppression that interferes with the activity of Ly-2 T-suppressor cells or their cell-free products.[1,2] The contrasuppressor-transducer cell is an I-J$^+$/Ly-1,2 T-cell (a T-cell that is Ly-1$^+$ and Ly-2$^+$).

The effector of the contrasuppressor circuit is an I-J$^+$/Ly-1 T-cell (a T-cell that is Ly-1$^+$ and Ly-2$^-$).[3] It is dependent upon Ly-2$^+$ cells (the inducer and transducer cells) for its generation. In addition, the contrasuppressor-effector cell can be positively selected on the basis of its adherence to plastic dishes coated with the *Vicia villosa* lectin.[3,4] The contrasuppressor-effector cell functions to render T-helper cells resistant to subsequent suppressor-cell signals;[3,5] it has not been found to inhibit suppressor-cell activity directly.[6]

The contrasuppressor circuit is shown schematically in FIGURE 1. It is suspected that other cells may be involved in this activity, perhaps at a stage preceeding the appearance of the contrasuppressor-inducer cell. The possible existence of such contrasuppressor-initiator cells will be discussed in the following section.

*This work was supported in part by National Institutes of Health Training Grant AI-07019.

0077-8923/83/0409-0284 $1.75/0 © 1983, NYAS

Factors Influencing the Activation of the Contrasuppressor Circuit

There are several variables that determine whether contrasuppressor cells are activated when antigen perturbs the homeostasis of the immune system. So far we have identified roles for antigen presenting cells, B-cells, antigen dose, and antigenic determinants. Each will be considered in turn.

The type of cell that initially presents antigen to the system can be determined by the route of antigen administration or by the use of adjuvants. When hapten is conjugated to certain cell types and injected intravenously, contrasuppression for contact sensitivity is produced. These cells include dendritic cells from the spleen, Langerhans cells from the skin, and peritoneal exudate cells induced by complete (but not incomplete) Freund's adjuvant.[7,8] The amount of helper-cell activity produced, however, is no greater than when antigen is presented on other cell types.

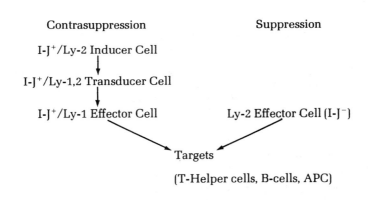

FIGURE 1.

In some cases, contrasuppressor cells seem to be dependent for their activation upon B-cells and/or their products. Mice treated from birth with anti-IgM antiserum fail to produce normal B-cells. These animals also fail to generate contrasuppressor cells in vitro.[9] Hamaoka, et al.,[10] described an immunization protocol involving presentation of antigen coupled to immunoglobulin to produce suppression-resistant immunity. Ptak and colleagues have used this protocol to produce a potent contrasuppressive factor with activity in vitro (personal communication). Another line of investigation implicating B-cells in contrasuppression includes injecting animals that lack late-maturing T-cells with polyclonal B-cell activators to produce autoimmunity. The T-cells in these animals show a preferential generation of contrasuppression.[11]

Antigen dose also has an important role in the activation of contrasuppression. Suppressor cells can be activated at sub- or supraoptimal doses of antigen, whereas optimal doses of antigen allow the activation of dominant contrasuppressor-cell activity (For examples, see the DISCUSSION of this paper and the article by T. Lehner in this volume).

Different regulatory T-cells recognize different features of an antigen. Helper and suppressor cells, for example, recognize distinct determinants of the lysozyme molecule.[12] Contrasuppressor cells have a preference for suppressor determinants on a molecule,[13] an observation that is compatible with the notion of an antigen bridge between the helper-cell target and either of these regulatory-effector cells.

Whereas both suppressor and contrasuppressor cells seem to "see" the same antigenic determinants, it is likely that recognition is achieved by the use of different receptors. Factors from Ly-2 suppressor-effector cells (TsF) specific for sheep red blood cells (SRBC) can be absorbed with SRBC but not horse red blood cells (HRBC). Ly-2 T-cell factor for induction of contrasuppression (TcsiF), however, can be absorbed on either SRBC or HRBC (but not other red blood cells).[2] The wider pattern of cross-reactivity of contrasuppressor cells versus suppressor cells might explain the phenomenon whereby tolerance to specific antigens (including self antigens) can be broken by immunization with a cross-reactive antigen.

EVIDENCE FOR CONTRASUPPRESSOR ACTIVITY IN GUT-ASSOCIATED
LYMPHORETICULAR TISSUE (GALT)

T-cells from the Peyer's patches of most strains of mice have no effect upon the ability of spleen cells to mount an *in vitro* plaque-forming cell (PFC) response to sheep red blood cells. By manipulating either population, however, potent suppressor-cell activity can be revealed.[14]

TABLE 1*

Peyer's Patch T-Cells (Treatment)	PFC Response of Spleen Cells (Treatment)			Comments
	(None)	(Anti-Ly-2 + C')	(Anti-I-J + C')	
No cells	+ +†	+ +	+ +	Control
Cells added (C' alone)	+ +	−	−	Removal of Ly-2$^+$/I-J$^-$ cells from the assay spleen cells allows appearance of suppression.
Cells added (anti-Ly-1 + C')	+ +	−	−	Peyer's patch suppressor cells are Ly-1$^-$.
Cells added (anti-Ly-2 + C')	+ +	+ +	not done	Peyer's patch suppressor cells are Ly-2$^+$.
Cells added (anti-Ly-1 + anti-I-J + C')	−	not done	not done	Removal of Ly-1$^-$/I-J$^+$ cells from Peyer's patch population reveals suppression on unfractionated spleen (compare with group c).

*After Green, et al.[14]

†"+ +" indicates positive response greater than 1000 PFC/culture. "−" indicates suppression to less than 50% of control values.

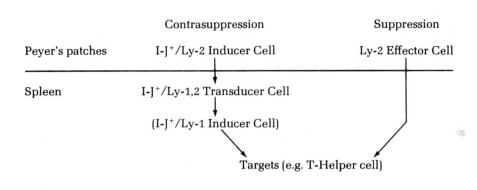

FIGURE 2.

In TABLE 1, the nature and effects of these manipulations is shown schematically. Reading across group B, it can be seen that whereas untreated Peyer's patch T-cells have no effect upon the response of untreated spleen cells, they are capable of suppressing spleen cells treated with either anti-Ly-2 plus complement or anti-I-J plus complement. Groups C and D show that the suppressor cells so revealed in the Peyer's patch T-cells is Ly-1⁻ (group C) and Ly-2⁺ (group D).

Alternatively, this suppression can also be revealed by removing an I-J⁺ cell from the Peyer's patch T-population, such that suppression is then observed when added to the untreated spleen cells (group E).

A tenable explanation for these effects, which is compatible with the independently determined contrasuppressor circuit described above is outlined in FIGURE 2. The Peyer's patch T-cells contain an Ly-2 suppressor-effector cell population (TABLE 1, group D), which is I-J⁻. The effects of this population are masked by the interaction of an Ly-1⁻ I-J⁺ contrasuppressor-inducer cell population in the Peyer's patches (group E) with an Ly-2⁺/I-J⁺ contrasuppressor-transducer cell population in the spleen (group B). It is postulated that this interaction results in activation of contrasuppressor effector cells in the assay that act to render targets of the suppressor cells resistant to the suppressive signals, based upon results from other systems.[3,5] This explanation is the simplest discussion of the data that does not propose hitherto undescribed cell interactions and phenomena.

A role for contrasuppression in the localization of immune responses is suggested by the presence of both contrasuppressor-inducer cells and suppressor-effector cells in Peyer's patches. Suppressor cells, generated by antigens entering through the portals of the gut, might subsequently migrate to the spleen.[15] These cells would suppress any systemic response to nonpathogenic proteins entering the system through the gut, which might otherwise have resulted in immune complex or allergic reactions. Meanwhile, the contrasuppressor cells remaining in the GALT would maintain immunity at the intestine to protect against potential invaders.

The presence of suppressor cells for *in vitro* anti-SRBC responses in naive Peyer's patches may be the result of cross-reacting antigens (perhaps Forsman type) that activate the GALT and can be seen when used in the relatively high ratios and conditions produced *in vitro*. We suggest that the suppression observed *in vitro* is not of sufficient intensity to produce the postulated systemic suppression *in vivo* that was outlined above (SRBC are good systemic immunogens). It has been shown, however, that continued feedings with SRBC can elevate this systemic suppression,[16,17] while allowing localized responses.[17]

AMPLIFICATION OF SUPPRESSION TO OVERCOME CONTRASUPPRESSION IN THE GUT-ASSOCIATED LYMPHORETICULAR TISSUE

The serendipitous contrasuppressive interactions induced by Peyer's patch Ly-2 T-cells described above are not seen in mice that possess the d allele at the D locus of the H-2.[14] Peyer's patch T-cells from animals with the D^d gene suppress unfractionated spleen cells (TABLE 2).

TABLE 2*

Strain: BALB/ByJ (H-2^d)		Assay Spleen Cells		
Peyer's patch T-Cells		PFC/Culture (Percent Suppression)		
	No. Added		Spleen Cells	
	to Assay	Unfractionated	Treated with	
Treatment	Culture	Spleen Cells	Anti-Ly-2 + C'	Comments
—	none	2073	1180	Control
C'	1×10^5	1333 (36%)	2067 (0%)	H-2D^d Peyer's patch T-
	2×10^5	867 (58%)	1387 (0%)	cells suppress only in
	3×10^5	667 (68%)	1447 (0%)	the presence of Ly-2$^+$
				cells in the assay.
Anti-Ly-2 + C'	1×10^5	2440 (0%)	1720 (0%)	H-2D^d Peyer's patch sup-
	2×10^5	2653 (0%)	1800 (0%)	pressor T-cells are Ly-
	3×10^5	2533 (0%)	1400 (0%)	2$^+$.

*Peyer's patch T-cells, prepared as previously described[14] were added to 5×10^6 spleen cells (or the equivalent number of treated spleen cells) under conditions for *in vitro* PFC response to sheep red blood cells.

Peyer's patch T-cells from BALB/ByJ animals added to unfractionated spleen cells produce significant suppression (group B, first column), whereas the same cells have no effect upon spleen cells treated with anti-Ly-2 plus complement (group B, second column). The suppressive effect of the Peyer's patch cells resides in a population also sensitive to treatment with anti-Ly-2 plus complement (group C). Thus Ly-2$^+$ T-cells from the Peyer's patches had interacted with Ly-2$^+$ T-cells in the splenic population to produce suppression. This phenomenon is in contrast to the suppressor-cell effect revealed upon removal of contrasuppression in non-H-2D^d animals (as in TABLE 1). The latter suppressor cells were observed to work effectively in the absence of Ly-2$^+$ splenic T-cells (see TABLE 1, group B, second column).

The interaction of an Ly-2$^+$ T-cell with another Ly-2$^+$ T-population to produce suppression (as in the case shown in TABLE 2) is reminiscent of the "suppressor amplification" circuit described by Tada and others,[18] in which an Ly-2 T-cell interacts by way of an Ly-1,2 T-cell to result in I-J$^+$/Ly-2 suppressor-effector cells.

We have postulated that suppressor amplification or "level two suppression" allows an override of the contrasuppressor circuit.[19] Thus, activation of "level two suppression" might produce a form of tolerance that precludes even gut-associated contrasuppressed responses. Recent advances in characterization of the "level two suppressor circuit" will allow an in depth investigation of this possibility.

CONCLUSION

Using an *in vitro* primary response to SRBC, we have demonstrated that cells involved in contrasuppression and two types of suppression can reside in the Peyer's patch T-cell population. Such observations suggest that responses localized to the GALT might proceed upon an "island" of contrasuppression in an otherwise suppressive "sea". Thus, oral immunization might produce the simultaneous appearance of systemic tolerance and gut immunity.

The results reviewed in this brief discussion generally involved IgM responses *in vitro*. We suggest, however, that similar control and localization of other responses, such as IgA, may proceed by analogous means. In support of this notion, contrasuppressor cells have recently been demonstrated in the regulation of clone growth and secretion of the MOPC 315 myeloma (an IgA producer) *in vivo* (J. Rohrer and J. Kemp, personal communication).

Localized immune responses are not limited to the GALT, and contrasuppression has been implicated in other regions of immunologic importance, such as the thymus[20] and the bone marrow,[21] where they may have a role in the regulation of stem-cell activity. In addition, contrasuppression plays an important role in contact sensitivity,[4,22] which, like the response of the GALT, is another example of immunity proceeding in the face of an otherwise tolerogenic stimulus.[23]

Contrasuppression may be an invaluable concept in the analysis of gut-associated immune responses and in "the paradox that orally encountered antigen can induce protective immunity and systemic tolerance".[24] In turn, a greater understanding of GALT immunity will give us important insights into the regulation of the immune response in general.

ACKNOWLEDGMENTS

The authors wish to thank Dr. Richard K. Gershon for providing the scientific environment that produced the work described herein.

REFERENCES

1. GERSHON, R. K., D. D. EARDLEY, S. DURUM, D. R. GREEN, F. W. SHEN, K. YAMAUCHI, H. CANTOR & D. B. MURPHY. 1981. Contrasuppression: An novel immunoregulatory activity. J. Exp. Med. **153:** 1533–1546.
2. YAMAUCHI, K., D. R. GREEN, D. D. EARDLEY, D. B. MURPHY & R. K. GERSHON. 1981. Immunoregulatory circuits that modulate responsiveness to suppressor cell signals: The failure of B10 mice to respond to suppressor factors can be overcome by quenching the contrasuppressor circuit. J. Exp. Med. **153:** 1547–1561.
3. GREEN, D. R., D. D. EARDLEY, A. KIMURA, D. B. MURPHY, K. YAMAUCHI & R. K. GERSHON. 1981. Immunoregulatory circuits which modulate responsiveness to suppressor cell signals: Characterization of an effector cell in the contrasuppressor circuit. Eur. J. Immunol. **11:** 973–979.

4. PTAK, W., D. R. GREEN, S. K. DURUM, A. KIMURA, D. B. MURPHY & R. K. GERSHON. 1981. Immunoregulatory circuits which modulate responsiveness to suppressor cell signals: Contrasuppressor cells can convert an *in vivo* tolerogenic signal into an immunogenic one. Eur. J. Immunol. **11**: 980–983.
5. GREEN, D. R. & R. K. GERSHON. 1982. Hyperimmunity and the decision to be intolerant. Ann. N.Y. Acad. Sci. **392**: 318–328.
6. GREEN, D. R. 1981. Contrasuppression: An immunoregulatory T cell activity. Doctoral Thesis. Yale University. New Haven, Conn.
7. PTAK, W., D. ROZYCKA, P. W. ASKENASE & R. K. GERSHON. 1980. Role of antigen-presenting cells in the development and persistence of contact hypersensitivity. J. Exp. Med. **151**: 362–375.
8. BRITZ, J. S., P. W. ASKENASE, W. PTAK, R. M. STEINMAN & R. K. GERSHON. 1982. Specialized antigen-presenting cells. Splenic dendritic cells and peritoneal-exudate cells induced by mycobacteria activate effector T cells that are resistant to suppression. J. Exp. Med. **155**: 1344–1356.
9. JANEWAY, C. A., B. BROUGHTON, E. DZIERZAK, B. JONES, D. D. EARDLEY, S. DURUM, K. YAMAUCHI, D. R. GREEN & R. K. GERSHON. 1981. Studies of T lymphocyte function in B cell deprived mice. *In* Immunoglobulin Idiotypes and Their Expression. ICN-UCLA Symposia on Molecular and Cellular Biology. C. A. Janeway, E. E. Sercarz, H. Wigzell, and C. F. Fox, Eds.: Vol. 20: 661–671. Academic Press. New York.
10. HAMAOKA, T., M. YOSHIZAWA, H. YAMAMOTO, M. KUROKI & M. KITAGAWA. 1977. Regulatory functions of hapten-reactive helper and suppressor T lymphocytes. II. Selective inactivation of hapten-reactive suppressor T cells by hapten-nonimmunogenic copolymers of D-amino acids and its application to the study of suppressor T-cell effect on helper T-cell development. J. Exp. Med. **146**: 91–106.
11. SMITH, H. R., D. R. GREEN, E. S. RAVECHE, P. A. SMATHERS, R. K. GERSHON & A. D. STEINBERG. 1983. Induction of autoimmunity in normal mice by thymectomy and administration of polyclonal B cell activators: Association with contrasuppressor function. Clin. Exp. Immunol. In press.
12. ADORINI, L., M. A. HARVEY, D. ROZYCKA-JACKSON, A. MILLER & E. E. SERCARZ. 1980. Different major histocompatibility complex-related activation of idiotypic suppressor T cells. J. Exp. Med. **152**: 521–531.
13. GREEN, D. R. and R. K. GERSHON. 1983. A view from the bridge: Antigenic determinants in immunoregulation. *In* Protein Conformation as an Immunological Signal. F. Celada, V. Schumacher, and E. Sercarz Eds.: Plenum Press. In Press.
14. GREEN, D. R., J. GOLD, S. ST. MARTIN, R. GERSHON & R. K. GERSHON. 1982. Microenvironmental immunoregulation: Possible role of contrasuppressor cells in maintaining immune responses in gut-associated lymphoid tissues. Proc. Natl. Acad. Sci. USA **79**: 889–892.
15. MATTINGLY, J. A. & B. H. WAKSMAN. 1978. Immunologic suppression after oral administration of antigen. I. Specific suppressor cells formed in rat Peyer's patches after oral administration of sheep erythrocytes and their systemic migration. J. Immunol. **121**: 1878–1883.
16. ANDREA, C., J. F. HEREMANS, J. P. VAERMAN & C. I. CAMBIASO. 1975. A mechanism for the induction of immunological tolerance by antigen feeding: Antigen-antibody complexes. J. Exp. Med. **142**: 1509–1519.
17. CHALLACOMBE, S. J. & T. B. TOMASI. 1980. Systemic tolerance and secretory immunity after oral immunization. J. Exp. Med. **152**: 1459–1472.
18. TADA, T. & K. OKUMARA. 1979. The role of antigen-specific T cell factors in the immune response. Adv. Immunol. **28**: 1–40.
19. GREEN, D. R., B. CHUE & R. K. GERSHON. 1983. Two types of suppressor T-cell discriminated by cell surface phenotype as well as function: Regulation of the contrasuppressor circuit. J. Cell. Molec. Immunol. In Press.
20. BRITZ, J. & R. K. GERSHON. Manuscript in preparation.
21. MICHAELSON, J. D. 1982. The characterization and functional analysis of immunoregulatory cells in murine bone marrow. Medical School Thesis. Yale University School of Medicine. New Haven, Conn.
22. IVERSON, G. M., W. PTAK, D. R. GREEN & R. K. GERSHON. 1983. The role of contrasuppression in the adoptive transfer of immunity. Submitted for publication.

23. MACHER, E. & M. W. CHASE. 1969. Studies on the sensitization of animals with simple chemical compounds. XII. The influence of excision of allergenic depots on onset of delayed hypersensitivity and tolerance. J. Exp. Med. **129:** 81–102.
24. Editorial. 1981. Lancet. **1:** 702.

DISCUSSION OF THE PAPER

C. O. ELSON (*Medical College of Virginia, Richmond, Va.*): Was the data that you published in the Proceedings of the National Academy of Sciences USA for IgM responses?

D. R. GREEN (*Yale University School of Medicine, New Haven, Conn.*): Yes, all direct plaque-forming cell (PFC) responses.

ELSON: The dissociation between tolerance and immunity in the lamina propria of the gut is IgA versus IgG. Would you comment on how you would get the notion of contrasuppressors into isotype variations in different areas?

GREEN: As Dr. Mattingly has pointed out, people do not find suppressor cells for IgA responses. We know that you can suppress the IgA response. At least Dr. Lynch has done it in the MOPC 315 system, and other people have shown that Con A supernatants can suppress an IgA response. The question might be, When one does not find suppressor cells for IgA, is it due to either isotype specific contrasuppressors or a failure to produce isotype specific suppressors? I do not know the answer to that. In some cases one sees tolerance to IgA and circulating IgM antibodies. The most intriguing question, however, is, Why is there an IgG, IgA split?

ELSON: I want to point out that in human peripheral blood cultures, one can suppress IgA-isotype responses. We have also provided data in mice for suppression of IgA responses.

GREEN: Again, the question might be, How does one produce one suppressor cell and not another?

J. R. McGHEE (*University of Alabama in Birmingham*): Yes, you can suppress IgA. We have suppressor clones that seem only to suppress IgA.

T. LEHNER (*Guy's Hospital, London, England*): The one point that I found that is HLA-DR (see T. Lehner's paper, this volume) associated is discreet dose response. There is the adage of Mitchison that there is a sea of suppression with an island of immunity. We may be discussing this response. In man, we have found a very discreet dose-related contrasuppressive activity. Do you find this activity in mice?

GREEN: Yes. In the dose response to glycophorin, for example, you cannot prime helper cells to glycophorin and obtain responses in a Mishell and Dutton system. What you can get, however, are suppressor cells and contrasuppressor cells, and the dose response is exactly as you showed. This work by Dr. Schiff, at Yale, has been submitted for publication. There is a dose of glycophorin at which suppressor cells are readily generated, then go away and finally return. At an appropriate dose, we can show the presence of a potent contrasuppressor activity induced *in vitro* in cultures educated to the glycophorin molecule. The delayed-type hypersensitivity (DTH) response has that island of immunity as well, for example, the DTH to sheep red blood cells as Dr. Askenase has shown.

FUNCTION AND BIOSYNTHESIS OF POLYMERIC IgA*

Jiri Mestecky, William H. Kutteh, Thomas A. Brown,
Michael W. Russell, John O. Phillips, Zina Moldoveanu,
Itaru Moro, and Sylvia S. Crago

*Department of Microbiology and Institute of Dental Research
University of Alabama in Birmingham
Birmingham, Alabama 35294*

INTRODUCTION

In lower vertebrates, including fish, reptiles, and amphibians, polymeric IgM in tetrameric and pentameric configurations represents the predominant immunoglobulin isotype in serum as well as external secretions such as skin mucus and bile.[1,2] Predominantly polymeric IgA first appears in birds and mammals,[3] and secretory IgM is replaced by polymeric secretory IgA (sIgA). In man, where IgA appears to be the immunoglobulin isotype produced in largest quantities, further diversification of molecular forms occurs. Thus, IgA$_1$ and IgA$_2$ subclasses, and monomeric and polymeric IgA forms are detectable with a distinctive distribution of subclasses and polymeric/monomeric forms in tissues and body fluids.[3] With the appearance of various isotypes, antibody effector mechanisms became diversified. In contrast to IgM and IgG, IgA does not employ the complement system or phagocytic cells as principal effector mechanisms. This phenomenon is understandable in the case of sIgA, which functions in an environment that is usually deficient in complement components and, with the exception of milk, in significant numbers of intact phagocytic cells. Instead of using products (complement system) and cells (phagocytes) of mesodermal origin, IgA and IgA cells appear to have a closer relationship to cells and products of ectodermal and endodermal origin. Thus, polymeric IgA, which contains the phylogenetically ancient polypeptide J-chain (also found in IgM), interacts specifically with epithelial cells by means of the membrane glycoprotein secretory component (SC), which acts as a receptor and mediates its selective transport into secretions.[4-8] Recent experiments performed in rodent models indicate that the interaction of IgA with SC is involved not only in the selective transport of IgA[7,8] but also as a mechanism for effective antigen disposal. Rodent hepatocytes that express SC on their sinusoidal surfaces[9-11] transport free IgA and thus enrich the intestinal lumen for IgA. They also participate as effector cells in the removal of polymeric IgA-antigen complexes.[12-14]

MECHANISMS OF HEPATOBILIARY DISPOSAL OF IgA IMMUNE COMPLEXES IN MICE

In our experiments, we investigated the fate of immune complexes (IC) composed of radiolabeled dinitrophenylated (DNP) human serum albumin (HSA), mouse myeloma IgA (M315), and hybridoma IgM and IgG with anti-DNP activity.[12] Mice were injected intravenously with DNP-HSA and corresponding

*This work was supported by research grants AI-10854, DE-02670, AM-28537, and AI-18745 from the US Public Health Service.

0077-8923/83/0409-292$1.75/0 © 1983, NYAS

antibodies of IgM, IgG, or IgA isotypes, or with separated immune complexes. Blood and bile were collected one and three hours after the injection and the radioactivity was measured. It is obvious from FIGURE 1 that after one hour (and three hours) radioactive antigen appears in significant quantities in the bile of mice injected with ascitic fluid that contains M315 protein, or with affinity purified M315; IgG and IgM are not effective; purified IC were efficiently transported; and specific antigen-antibody interactions are necessary because unhaptenated HSA, or IgA with antibody specificity other than for DNP, did not result in the appearance of radiolabeled antigen in bile.

Sucrose density gradient centrifugation of the radioactive material found in the bile revealed that approximately 70% of the radioactivity was associated with high molecular weight material, including IgA-immune complexes and free DNP-HSA, and that 60% of the radioactive material was precipitable with anti-HSA and 50% with anti-IgA. By contrast, radioactivity present in the bile of animals injected with radioactive DNP-HSA and IgG was entirely associated with low molecular weight material.

In addition to HSA conjugated with DNP, we have examined the ability of the murine IgA-myeloma protein J558 to transport radiolabeled monoclonal syngeneic anti-idiotypic antibodies of IgG and IgM classes.[15] In these experiments, IgA-IgG complexes were transported into the bile, whereas IgA-IgM complexes were not. Analyses of the radioactivity in the bile by sucrose gradient centrifugation indicated that the IgA-IgG complexes were recovered as high-molecular weight material, whereas the radioactivity in bile of mice receiving IgM, IgG, or IgA-IgM complexes consisted only of low molecular weight fragments. Therefore, it appears that in the case of an IgA-IgG complex, IgA plays the decisive role as to the fate of the mixed immune complex. IgA-IgM complexes may not be transported due to their high molecular weight and the limited ability of the liver to process such large complexes through the hepatocyte pathway.[16]

IgA-mediated hepatobiliary transport was also effective when bacterial antigens such as pneumococcal type III capsular polysaccharide and C carbohydrate were injected with corresponding myeloma or hybridoma antibodies of IgA, but not IgG or IgM isotypes.[17] The transport process involves polymeric but not monomeric IgA; a large excess of IgA of different specificity can inhibit the transport of IgA-IC; blockade of the mononuclear phagocytic system with colloidal carbon greatly decreases the processing of IgG-IC but not the transport of IgA-IC; depletion of C3 by cobra venom factor did not influence the transport of IgA-IC into the bile.[18] These results indicate that the hepatobiliary processing of IgA-IC does not use complement or phagocytic cells as described for IgG and IgM-IC.

The participation of hepatocytes as effector cells raises the possibility that in addition to SC, glycoprotein receptors (e.g. those for mannose and galactose) might be involved in the recognition and transport of IgA. That this is not the case became apparent from the failure to inhibit transport of IgA-IC by previous injections of large quantities of asialo-fetuin (galactose terminal) or yeast mannan (mannose terminal).[18]

Futhermore, comparison of the appearance of intravenously injected IgA-IC in saliva, milk, urine, and bronchial and intestinal washings relative to bile revealed the unique efficiency of the liver in transporting complexed or uncomplexed IgA in contrast to other secretory glands and tissues (FIGURE 2). Radioactivity seen in external secretions other than bile, irrespective of the presence of IgA, was probably due to low molecluar-weight fragments of degraded antigen, and even the passage of intact free antigen.[19]

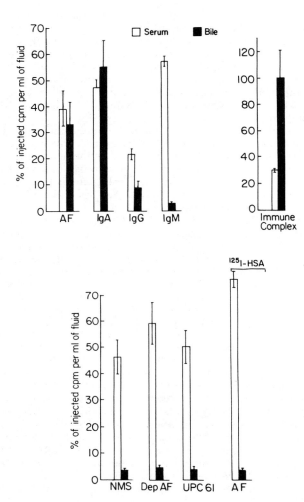

FIGURE 1. Transport of ^{125}I-labeled DNP-HSA into bile by DNP-specific IgA (MOPC 315). Bars represent mean ± S.D. (N = 4).

Top left: Relative serum (open bars) and bile (closed bars) radioactivity one hour after i.v. injection of radiolabeled antigen with MOPC 315 ascites fluid (AF); MOPC 315 IgA purified by affinity chromatography on DNP-Sepharose (IgA); IgG or IgM hybridoma anti-DNP antibody-containing ascites fluids (IgG, IgM).

Top right: Relative serum and bile radioactivity one hour after i.v. injection of MOPC 315/^{125}I-labeled DNP-HSA immune complex partially purified on Sephadex G-200.

Bottom: Controls, showing relative serum and bile radioactivity one hour after i.v. injection of radiolabeled antigen with normal mouse serum (NMS); MOPC 315 ascites fluid depleted of anti-DNP activity by passage over DNP-Sepharose (Dep AF); anti-levan IgA-containing ascites fluid (UPC 61); or ^{125}I-labeled HSA injected with MOPC 315 ascites fluid (AF).

As indicated above, the selective transport of IgA-IC from the circulation into the bile in rodents appears to depend upon polymeric IgA. To investigate whether a similar transport system for IgA occurs in humans, we have studied the cells that produce polymeric IgA in various tissues, and the properties of serum and biliary IgA in normal individuals and in patients with liver diseases.

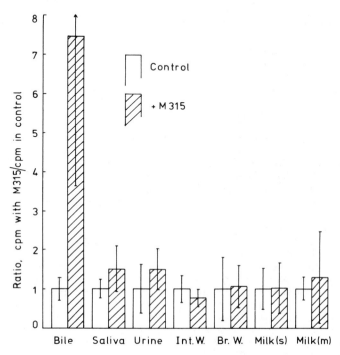

FIGURE 2. Transport of IgA-^{125}I-labeled DNP-HSA immune complexes into secretions. Bars represent mean ± S.D. Samples of bile, saliva, urine, intestinal wash (Int. W.), and bronchial wash (Br. W.) were taken one hour after an injection of radiolabeled antigen alone (open bars) or antigen plus MOPC 315 (hatched bars). Intestinal washes were taken distal to a ligature that was placed around the upper intestine before the beginning of the experiment. Milk samples were taken five hours after injection, either by allowing six pups to suckle for one hour, after which their stomach contents were counted (Milk (s)), or by mechanical milking (Milk (m)). Radioactivity in control samples for each fluid is taken as one, for comparison.

PRODUCTION OF POLYMERIC AND MONOMERIC IgA IN VARIOUS HUMAN TISSUES

Serum IgA consists predominantly of monomer and smaller amounts of polymer (including trace amounts of sIgA). Polymer is estimated to constitute, depending on the analytical method used, up to 15% of the total serum IgA.[3] The cellular origins of polymeric and monomeric IgA have been investigated by indirect methods based on the ability of SC to bind to polymeric IgA, and on the production of J-chain.[20-22] Secretory component followed by labeled anti-SC when applied to cells from various sources, are presumed to bind only to cells that produce polymeric IgA. Because only a small fraction of intracellular IgA occurs as polymers,[23] and because J-chain has been detected in immunocytes producing monomeric immunoglobulins of IgG and IgD classes,[24-26] we have examined the production of IgA in cultures of cells obtained from various human tissues. Lymphoid cell suspensions from tonsils, bone marrow, mediastinal and axillary lymph nodes, gut mucosa, spleen, and peripheral blood were purified and characterized as to the number of Ig and IgA positive cells as described.[23] The amount and the characteristics of the intracellular IgA were determined by radioimmunoassay (RIA) in cell sonicates, and in fractions obtained therefrom by gel-filtration on a standardized Ultrogel AcA 22 column.[23] With the exception of gut mucosa, where polymeric IgA was predominant, cell lysates from all other tissues contained mainly monomeric IgA. The polymeric IgA found in lysates of gut mucosal cells, however, was partially derived from contaminating epithelial cells that contained sIgA: apprpoximately half of the polymeric IgA could be precipitated with an anti-SC reagent.[23]

The amount and characteristics of the secreted IgA were then determined in supernatants of seven day cultures (FIGURE 3). Bone marrow cells released mostly monomeric IgA in quantities exceeding those of any other tissue. Spleen cells also produced monomeric IgA, whereas the lymph nodes and tonsil cells released polymeric and monomeric IgA in approximately equal amounts. Supernatants from the cultures of gut mucosal cells contained predominantly polymeric IgA. Unstimulated peripheral blood (PBL) mononuclear cells released only small amounts of IgA with comparable proportions of polymers and monomers.

We have demonstrated in our previous studies that PBL stimulated with pokeweed mitogen (PWM), lipopolysaccharides or Epstein-Barr virus produce large quantities of predominantly polymeric IgA.[27] Therefore, we examined the effect of PWM on the production of IgA in various human tissues (FIGURE 3. TABLE 1). Pokeweed mitogen-stimulated bone marrow cells produced less than half the amount of IgA compared with unstimulated cells, but there was no significant shift toward polymer production. In the presence of PWM, cells from tonsils and axillary lymph nodes doubled their IgA production, but cells from mediastinal lymph nodes, gut mucosa, and spleen did not respond to PWM stimulation by either increased or decreased IgA production. There appeared to be more polymer produced by PWM-stimulated cells from tonsils and peripheral blood lymphocytes compared to unstimulated cells (TABLE 2). These results suggest that the lymphoid cells in various human tissues are at different stages of maturation and vary in their sensitivity to PWM stimulation.

In addition to various tissues and peripheral blood, we have also investigated the properties of IgA-containing cells from human colostrum and milk. These fluids contain elements that form indirect hemolytic plaques against sheep red blood cells coated with lipopolysaccharide isolated from several species of Gram-negative intestinal bacteria.[28-30] By means of immunofluorescence and histochemistry, we have demonstrated that IgA, IgM, SC, and milk proteins occurred inside colostral macrophages, polymorphonuclear leukocytes, and milk globules probably of epithelial cell origin.[30,31] Such elements costained with fluorochrome-labeled reagents specific for different Ig isotypes, L-chain types, both IgA subclasses, and other milk proteins. Furthermore, cell lysates contained almost exclusively polymeric, SC-associated IgA.[30] This phenomenon was in contrast to the intracellular IgA in PWM-stimulated PBL, which contained mostly monomeric IgA that did not react with anti-SC reagents despite the secretion of predominantly polymeric IgA.[30] Examination of IgA-containing elements in human colostrum by immunoelectron microscopy, using peroxidase-labeled Fab'

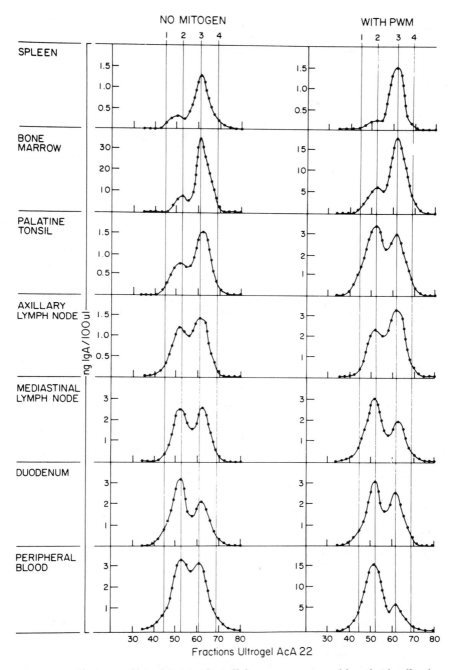

FIGURE 3. Elution profiles of IgA in the cell-free supernatants of lymphoid cells after culture without and with pokeweed mitogen (PWM). Isolated cells were cultured for seven days; culture supernatants were fractionated over an Ultrogel AcA 22 column, and individual fractions were assayed for IgA by radioimmunoassay. Small numbers at the top of the vertical lines represent ^{125}I-labeled marker proteins used to standardize the Ultrogel AcA 22 column: 1: polymeric IgM; 2: polymeric IgA; 3: monomeric IgA; and 4: IgG. Note that scales of IgA concentrations are different for various samples.

TABLE 1

AMOUNTS OF IgA IN CELL-FREE SUPERNATANTS OF CULTURED LYMPHOID CELLS*

Source of Cells†	−PWM	+PWM
Tonsil [3]	47.8	79.0
	(22.4–62.0)	(48.1–94.6)
Bone marrow [3]	1044	420
	(712–1300)	(369–470)
Mediastinal lymph node [3]	41.5	46.0
	(28.5–70.8)	(22.0–82.5)
Axillary lymph node [3]	32.7	61.1
	(29.5–36.5)	(18.2–95.0)
Gut mucosa [3]	126	113
	(87.0–152)	(67.5–140)
Spleen [3]	25.7	26.7
	(20.0–34.8)	(21.6–34.6)
Peripheral blood [5]	48.8	635
	(33.3–106)	(168–1050)

*Numbers represent the mean (range) ng of IgA produced/ml by 10^6 lymphoid cells cultured for seven days in the absence or presence of $8\mu l$ or $10\mu l$ of PWM/ml as determined by RIA.
†Numbers in brackets represent the number of different samples examined.

TABLE 2

PRODUCTION OF POLYMERIC AND MONOMERIC IgA BY CULTURED LYMPHOID CELLS*

	−PWM		+PWM	
Source of Cells†	Percent Polymer	Percent Monomer	Percent Polymer	Percent Monomer
Tonsil [3]	49	51	59	41
	(39–60)	(40–61)	(55–65)	(35–45)
Bone marrow [3]	13	87	26	74
	(12–22)	(78–88)	(23–30)	(70–77)
Mediastinal lymph node [3]	42	58	42	58
	(29–58)	(42–71)	(27–67)	(33–73)
Axillary lymph node [3]	38	62	32	68
	(11–54)	(46–89)	(9.4–46)	(54–91)
Gut mucosa [3]	61	39	55	45
	(60–63)	(37–40)	(51–60)	(40–49)
Spleen [3]	14	86	13	87
	(11–17)	(83–89)	(11–15)	(85–89)
Peripheral blood [3]	61	39	79	21
	(60–63)	(27–40)	(78–81)	(19–22)

*Numbers are presented as average (range) percent polymeric and monomeric IgA determined by measuring the area under each phase of the biphasic elution profile of IgA as determined by RIA on fractions of cell-free supernatants chromatographed on Ultrogel AcA22. Cells were cultured for seven days at 1×10^6 cells/ml either without or with $8\mu l$ or $10\mu l$ of PWM.
†Numbers in brackets indicate the number of different tissue samples examined.

or F(ab')$_2$ fragments of anti-IgA and anti-IgM, revealed that these Igs were present in secondary intracytoplasmic granules of numerous macrophages and polymorphonuclear leukocytes. In addition, IgA and IgM were detectable in miscellaneous globules that were probably derived from the cytoplasm of the epithelial cells that transported polymeric IgA into milk.[32] We have previously shown that these globules do not stain for nonspecific esterase or peroxidase that are associated with macrophages and polymorphonuclear leukocytes. Nevertheless they contain SC and are capable of indirect plaque formation.[30,31] We conclude that colostral macrophages and polymorphonuclear leukocytes acquire immunoglobulin after its transport into milk because macrophages appeared to contain polymeric, SC-associated IgA that is typical of secretions.

RELATIONSHIP BETWEEN EXTRACELLULAR SECRETION OF POLYMERIC IGA AND INTRACELLULAR J-CHAIN

Because extracellular polymeric IgA and IgM are associated with J-chain, it has been speculated that J-chain synthesis is indicative of polymer production.[33,34] The presence of J-chain in IgA-producing cells was determined by an immunofluorescence technique using fluorescein isothiocyanate (FITC)-labeled anti-IgA and tetramethylrhodamine isothiocyanate (TRITC)-labeled anti-J-chain as previously described.[26] Interestingly, cells from tissues producing predominantly monomeric IgA contained fewer J-chain-positive cells, and those from tissues that released more polymers, contained higher numbers of J-chain-positive cells.[23] For example, almost 80% of bone marrow IgA cells were negative for J-chain, whereas in gut mucosa, more than 90% of IgA cells displayed intracellular J-chain (TABLE 3). Similarly, the majority of PWM-stimulated PBL that produced IgA stained for J-chain, which was seen either throughout the entire cytoplasm or was restricted to the perinuclear areas, especially during the early days of culture.[23] The absence of J-chain from Ig-containing cells, as determined by immunofluorescence, should be regarded with caution, because more sensitive techniques such as RIA, pulse-labeling with radioactive amino acids, transcription of total messenger RNA from lymphoid cell lines in a wheat-germ system,[35] and immunoelectron microscopy[36] have revealed that J-chain is expressed in small quantities in lymphoid cells from early stages of differentiation along the B-cell axis. Based on these results, it appears that cells characterized by the presence or absence of intracellular μ-chain and L-chains, and by cell-surface markers as pre-B cells, immature and mature B-cells, and null cells, contain small amounts of intracellular J-chain mostly in a free form and characteristically distributed on cell organelles.[36,37] The function of J-chain in these cells remains undetermined.

OCCURRENCE OF POLYMERIC IGA IN HUMAN SERUM AND BILE

Although production of polymeric IgA can be detected in various human lymphoid tissues, the ratio of polymers to monomers in serum appears to be lower than that implied by the biosynthetic data. Because of the possible role of the liver in the selective transfer of polymeric IgA from the circulation into the bile, we have investigated the distribution of various molecular forms of IgA in serum of normal individuals and patients with various liver diseases, and in serum and hepatic bile of patients with T-tube drainage of the common bile duct.[38]

TABLE 3

PERCENT OF CYTOPLASMIC IgA-POSITIVE CELLS CONTAINING J-CHAIN*

Source of Cells	J-chain Staining								
	Fresh Cell Preparations			Seven Day Cultures†					
				− PWM			+ PWM		
	Cytoplasmic	Perinuclear	Negative	Cytoplasmic	Perinuclear	Negative	Cytoplasmic	Perinuclear	Negative
Tonsils	8.7 (0–16)	23 (4.8–46)	68 (38–95)	16 (11–20)	22 (11–33)	62 (47–78)	37 (28–46)	23 (14–32)	41 (22–59)
Bone marrow	5.6 (1.3–8.1)	17 (12–26)	78 (67–86)	12 (11–12)	21 (2–39)	68 (49–87)	13 (12–14)	22 (9–35)	65 (53–77)
Mediastinal lymph node	40 (14–53)	16 (0–20)	44 (35–50)	76 (70–80)	15 (7.1–20)	9.4 (0–14)	58 (44–70)	20 (14–23)	22 (18–33)
Axillary lymph node	27 (17–32)	36 (20–46)	37 (21–63)	7.2 (0–14)	28 (20–36)	65 (50–80)	22 (7.1–38)	12 (11–12)	66 (50–82)
Gut mucosa	89 (81–96)	8.1 (1–15)	2.8 (1.9–3.8)						
Spleen	38 (29–52)	17 (5–34)	46 (33–64)	12	19	69	14	11	75
Peripheral blood	13 (11–16)	64 (61–69)	23 (16–28)	49 (33–73)	27 (13–42)	24 (13–34)	78 (66–91)	11 (10–18)	.10 (2.9–16)

*Results are presented as the mean (range) percent of cells exhibiting cytoplasmic IgA fluorescence and J-chain fluorescence in entire cytoplasm or parinuclear area.

†Cells were cultured for seven days at 1×10^6 cells/ml in the absence or presence of 10 µl/ml of PWM.

Serum samples from normal individuals, and from patients with alcoholic cirrhosis and with high IgA levels, were chromatographed through a standardized column of Ultrogel AcA 22. The concentration of IgA was measured in each fraction by radioimmunoassay. In serum from normal individuals, only small amounts of IgA eluted at the position of IgA polymers (FIGURE 4). This elution contrasted with the properties of IgA in sera of cirrhotics. Two to four times higher levels of total IgA and three to ten times higher levels of polymeric IgA were detected. Levels of IgG were comparable in both groups of individuals, whereas IgM was slightly reduced in some of the cirrhotic patients.[38] The true polymeric nature of the IgA molecules was confirmed by the presence of J-chain. Further

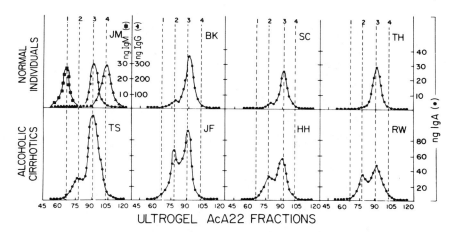

FIGURE 4. Elution profiles of IgA from the sera of four normal individuals and four patients with alcoholic cirrhosis. All sera were diluted 1/100 and fractionated on an Ultrogel AcA 22 column. From each individual fraction, 100 μl was assayed for IgA by radioimmunoassay. Notice that the amounts of polymeric IgA (vertical lines 2) were increased in the sera of patients with alcoholic cirrhosis (bottom) when compared to normal individuals (top row). Small numbers at the top of vertical lines represent ^{125}I-labeled marker proteins used to standardize the Ultrogel AcA 22 column: 1: polymeric IgM; 2: polymeric IgA; 3: monomeric IgA; and 4: IgG. The curves depicted are based on the absolute content of assayed immunoglobulins (in ng/100 μl). For clarity of presentation, only every second point is shown. Symbols: ■ = IgM; ● = IgA; ▲ = IgG. Note that scales of IgA concentration are different for normal individuals and patients.

analyses of this polymeric IgA revealed that approximately 5% of the molecules were associated with SC, which indicates the presence of sIgA in the circulation (6–12 mg%). Although it is possible that patients with liver cirrhosis produce more polymeric IgA than normal individuals, it is also permissible to speculate that the higher levels of polymers in serum may be the result of decreased ability of the cirrhotic liver to transport polymeric forms from serum into the bile.

To examine this possibility we analyzed serum and biliary IgA in patients who had common bile duct obstruction due to cholelithiasis or cholangiocarcinoma. The bile was collected one day to three weeks postoperatively from a T-tube inserted into the common bile duct. Depending on the technique used for IgA

determination (radial immunodiffusion, radioimmunoassay, and fluoroimmu-
nometric assay—FIAX) and the standard used (serum monomeric IgA or sIgA),
we have found[38] that human hepatic bile contains 2.2–17.4 mg% IgA; in one
patient, the level was 77.9 mg% one day after the insertion of the T-tube. Based on
the volume of the hepatic bile secreted, we have estimated that approximately 160
mg of IgA enters the intestinal tract by way of the bile per day. Earlier estimates of
Nagura et al.[39] indicated that the bile may contribute as much as 400 mg of IgA.
These data suggest that approximately 10–40% of intestinal IgA in humans may
be derived from the bile. These values are considerably lower than those
observed in rodents where external bile duct cannulation resulted in a tenfold
reduction in IgA levels of intestinal washings when compared to sham-operated
rats.[40]

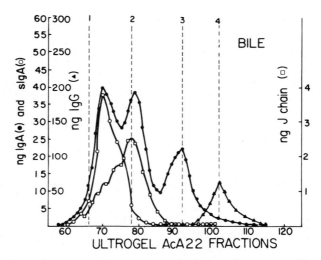

FIGURE 5. Elution profile of an undiluted hepatic bile sample fractionated on an Ultrogel
AcA 22 column. Symbols: ● = IgA; ○ = sIgA: □ = J-chain; and ▲ = IgG. Marker proteins: 1:
polymeric IgM, 2: polymeric IgA; 3: monomeric IgA; 4: IgG. The concentrations of
immunoglobulins and J-chain are expressed in ng per 100 μl sample.

To determine the molecular forms of IgA present, human bile was chromatographed on a standardized Ultrogel AcA 22 column, and the resultant fractions
were analyzed by RIA for IgA, J-chain (after reduction and alkylation), and sIgA
(by precipitation with an anti-SC reagent).[38] Three forms of IgA in various
proportions were detected in all three samples examined (FIGURE 5). Two high
molecular weight fractions eluted in the positions of the dimeric IgA and sIgA
standards; the third form of IgA that occurred in low amounts had an elution
profile like that of monomeric serum IgA. Further analyses of the two high
molecular weight forms revealed that J-chain was present in both fractions,
whereas SC was associated only with the first peak. Monomeric IgA lacked both
J-chain and secretory component. These results indicated that the high molecular
weight IgA that predominates in the bile consists of two forms present in equal
proportions: sIgA containing J-chain and SC, and polymeric IgA with J-chain.

When related to levels of IgG, the concentrations of polymeric IgA in serum and bile indicated active transport of polymers into bile, whereas monomeric IgA could be accounted for by transudation from serum. The origins of the different forms of IgA and the molecular mechanisms involved in their appearance in bile are unclear. Because human hepatocytes seem to lack surface SC, it has been suggested by Nagura *et al.*[39] that either circulating or locally produced IgA may be transported by epithelial cells of the biliary tract using an SC-dependent mechanism. Polymeric IgA lacking SC may be transported by hepatocytes that preferentially bind polymeric IgA through a receptor that is apparently different from secretory component.[41]

It remains to be examined directly whether the human liver participates in the transport of IgA-IC. An increased level of polymeric IgA, and the appearance of IgA-IC and their deposition in the kidneys, and possibly skin, of individuals with diseases that affect the hepatobiliary system suggest the existence of such a pathway.[42-44]

REFERENCES

1. LOBB, C. J. & L. W. CLEM. 1981. Phylogeny of immunoglobulin structure and function XII. Secretory immunoglobulins in the bile of the marine teleost Archosargus probatocephalus. Mol. Immunol **18:** 615–619.
2. PORTIS, J. L. & J. E. COE. 1975. IgM the secretory immunoglobulin of reptiles and amphibians. Nature (London) **258:** 547–548.
3. HEREMANS, J. F. 1974. Immunoglobulin A. *In:* The Antigens, Vol. 2. M. Sela, Ed. p. 365–522. Academic Press. New York.
4. BRANDTZAEG, P. 1981. Transport models for secretory IgA and secretory IgM. Clin. Exp. Immunol. **44:** 221–232.
5. CRAGO, S. S., R. KULHAVY, S. J. PRINCE & J. MESTECKY. 1978. Secretory component on epithelial cells is a surface receptor for polymeric immunoglobulins. J. Exp. Med. **147:** 1832–1837.
6. NAGURA, H., P. K. NAKANE & W. R. BROWN. 1979. Translocation of dimeric IgA through neoplastic colon cells *in vitro.* J. Immunol. **123:** 2359–2368.
7. ORLANS, E., J. PEPPARD, J. REYNOLDS, & J. HALL. 1978. Rapid active transport of immunoglobulin A from blood to bile. J. Exp. Med. **147:** 588–592.
8. LEMAITRE-COELHO, I., G. D. F. JACKSON & J.-P. VAERMAN. 1978. High levels of secretory IgA and free secretory component in the serum of rats with bile duct obstruction. J. Exp. Med. **147:** 934–939.
9. FISHER, M. M., B. NAGY, H. BAZIN & B. J. UNDERDOWN. 1979. Biliary transport of IgA: Role of secretory component. Proc. Natl. Acad. Sci. USA **76:** 2008–2012.
10. SOCKEN, D. J., K. N. JEEJEEBHOY, H. BAZIN & B. J. UNDERDOWN. 1979. Identification of secretory component as an IgA receptor on rat hepatocytes. J. Exp. Med. **150:** 1538–1548.
11. ORLANS, E., J. PEPPARD, J. F. FRY, R. H. HINTON & B. M. MULLOCK. 1979. Secretory component as the receptor for polymeric IgA on rat hepatocytes. J. Exp. Med. **150:** 1577–1581.
12. RUSSELL, M. W., T. A. BROWN & J. MESTECKY. 1981. Role of serum IgA: Hepatobiliary transport of circulating antigen. J. Exp. Med. **153:** 968–976.
13. SOCKEN, D. J., E. S. SIMMS, B. NAGY, M. M. FISHER & B. J. UNDERDOWN. 1981. Transport of IgA antibody-antigen complexes by the rat liver. Mol. Immunol. **18:** 345–348.
14. PEPPARD, J., E. ORLANS, A. W. R. PAYNE & E. ANDREW. 1981. The elimination of circulating complexes containing polymeric IgA by excretion into the bile. Immunology **42:** 83–89.
15. PHILLIPS, J. O., M. W. RUSSELL, T. A. BROWN & J. MESTECKY. 1983. Selective hepatobiliary transport of monoclonal IgG but not IgM anti-idiotypic antibodies by IgA. Ann. N.Y. Acad. Sci. This volume.

16. SOCKEN, D. J., E. S. SIMMS, B. NAGY, M. M. FISHER & B. J. UNDERDOWN. 1981. Secretory component-dependent hepatic transport of IgA antibody-antigen complexes. J. Immunol. **127:** 316-319.
17. RUSSELL, M. W., T. A. BROWN, R. KULHAVY & J. MESTECKY. 1983. IgA-mediated hepatobiliary clearance of bacterial antigens. Ann. N.Y. Acad. Sci. This volume.
18. BROWN, T. A., M. W. RUSSELL & J. MESTECKY. 1982. Hepatobiliary transport of IgA immune complexes: Molecular and cellular aspects. J. Immunol. **128:** 2183-2186.
19. RUSSELL, M. W., T. A. BROWN & J. MESTECKY. 1982. Preferential transport of IgA and IgA-immune complexes to bile compared with other external secretions. Mol. Immunol. **19:** 677-682.
20. BRANDTZAEG, P. 1973. Two types of IgA immunocytes in man. Nature (London) New Biol. **243:** 142-143.
21. RADL, J., H. R. E. SCHUIT, J. MESTECKY & W. HIJMANS. 1974. The origin of monomeric and polymeric forms of IgA in man. Adv. Exp. Med. Biol. **45:** 57-65.
22. CRAGO, S. S. & J. MESTECKY. 1979. Secretory component: Interaction with intracellular and surface immunoglobulins of human lymphoid cells. J. Immunol. **122:** 906-911.
23. KUTTEH, W. H., S. J. PRINCE & J. MESTECKY. 1982. The tissue origins of human polymeric and monomeric IgA. J. Immunol. **128:** 990-995.
24. KAJI, H. & R. M. E. PARKHOUSE. 1974. Intracellular J chain in mouse plasmacytomas secreting IgA, IgM and IgG. Nature (London) **249:** 45-47.
25. BRANDTZAEG, P. 1974. Presence of J chain in human immunocytes containing various immunoglobulin classes. Nature (London) **252:** 418-420.
26. MESTECKY, J., R. J. WINCHESTER, T. HOFFMAN & H. G. KUNKEL. 1977. Parallel synthesis of immunoglobulins and J chain in pokeweed mitogen-stimulated normal cells and in lymphoblastoid cell lines. J. Exp. Med. **145:**760-765.
27. KUTTEH, W. H., W. J. KOOPMAN, M. E. CONLEY, M. L. EGAN & J. MESTECKY. 1980. Production of predominantly polymeric IgA by human peripheral blood lymphocytes stimulated *in vitro* with mitogens. J. Exp. Med. **152:** 1424-1429.
28. GOLDBLUM, R. M., S. AHLSTEDT, B. CARLSSON, L. A. HANSON, U. JODAL, G. LIDIN-JANSON & A. SOHL-AKERLUND. 1975. Antibody-forming cells in human colostrum after oral immunisation. Nature (London) **257:** 797-798.
29. AHLSTEDT, S., B. CARLSSON, L. A. HANSON & R. M. GOLDBLUM. 1975. Antibody production by human colostral cells. Scand. J. Immunol. **4:** 535-539.
30. LAVEN, G. T., S. S. CRAGO, W. H. KUTTEH & J. MESTECKY. 1981. Hemolytic plaque formation by cellular and noncellular elements of human colostrum. J. Immunol. **127:** 1967-1972.
31. CRAGO, S. S., S. J. PRINCE, T. G. PRETLOW, J. R. MCGHEE & J. MESTECKY. 1979. Human colostral cells I. Separation and characterization. Clin. Exp. Immunol. **38:** 585-597.
32. MORO, I., S. S. CRAGO & J. MESTECKY. 1982. Localization of IgA in human colostral elements using immunoelectron microscopy. Fed. Proc. Fed. Am. Soc. Exp. Biol. **41:** 843 (Abstr. #3350).
33. INMAN, F. P. & J. MESTECKY. 1974. The J chain of polymeric immunoglobulins. Contemp. Top. Mol. Immunol. **3:** 111-141.
34. KOSHLAND, M. E. 1975. Structure and function of the J chain. Adv. Immunol. **20:** 41-69.
35. MCCUNE, J. M., S. M. FU & H. G. KUNKEL. 1981. J chain biosynthesis in pre-B cells and other possible precursor B cells. J. Exp. Med. **154:** 138-145.
36. HAJDU, I., J. LEHMEYER, Z. MOLDOVEANU, J. MESTECKY & M. D. COOPER. 1982. Ultrastructural studies of μ- and J chain expression as a function of B cell differentiation. Fed. Proc. Fed. Am. Soc. Exp. Biol. **41:** 305 (Abstr. #217).
37. KUTTEH, W. H., F. ALONSO, Z. MOLDOVEANU & J. MESTECKY. 1982. Synthesis of J chain by human lymphoid cells. Fed. Proc. Fed. Am. Soc. Exp. Biol. **41:** 833 (Abstr. #3293).
38. KUTTEH, W. H., S. J. PRINCE, J. O. PHILLIPS, J. G. SPENNEY & J. MESTECKY. 1982. Properties of immunoglobulin A in serum of individuals with liver diseases and in hepatic bile. Gastroenterology **82:** 184-193.
39. NAGURA, H., P. D. SMITH, P. K. NAKANE & W. R. BROWN. 1981. IgA in human bile and liver. J. Immunol. **126:** 587-595.

40. LEMAITRE-COELHO, I., G. D. F. JACKSON & J.-P. VAERMAN. 1978. Relevance of biliary IgA antibodies in rat intestinal immunity. Scand. J. Immunol. **8:** 459–463.

41. HOPF, U., P. BRANDTZAEG, T. H. HUTTEROTH & K. H. MEYER ZUM BUSCHENFELDE. 1978. *In vivo* and *in vitro* binding of IgA to the plasma membrane of hepatocytes. Scand. J. Immunol. **8:** 543–549.

42. BERGER, J., H. YANEVA & B. NABARRA. 1978. Glomerular changes in patients with cirrhosis of the liver. Adv. Nephrol. Necker Hosp. **7:** 3.

43. EGIDO, J., J. SANCHO, F. MAMPASO, M. LOPEZ-TRASCASA, M. SANCHEZ-CRESPO, R. BLASCO & L. HERNANDO. 1980. A possible common pathogenesis ofthe mesangial IgA glomerulonephritis in patients with Berger's disease and Schönlein-Henoch Syndrome. Proc. Eur. Dial. Transplant Assoc. **17:** 660.

44. SANCHO, J., J. EGIDO, M. SANCHEZ-CRESPO & R. BLASCO. 1982. Detection of monomeric and polymeric IgA-containing immune complexes in serum and kidney from patients with alcoholic liver disease. Clin. Exp. Immunol. **47:** 327–335.

DISCUSSION

R. M. E. PARKHOUSE (*National Institute for Medical Research, London, England*): We showed some time ago, and I know that the Birmingham group has made similar observations, that J-chain is also expressed in plasma cells that do not only produce polymeric immunoglobulins. This production includes cells making IgG, as well as cells that produce only light chains. Today we have heard that J-chain is made in pre-B-cells. Does the presence of J-chain in plasma cells not making polymeric immunoglobulins reflect the fact that J-chain, which is made early on in the B-cell lineage, is never turned off? Alternatively, is J-chain serving another function?

J. MESTECKY (*University of Alabama in Birmingham*): We do not know the function(s) of J-chain. There is a possibility that J-chain may be mediating the disulfide bond-exchange reactions that occur during assembly of intracellular immunoglobulins, whether they are polymeric or monomeric. Polymeric immunoglobulin formation would involve one more step. We found with Dr. Preud'homme, IgA$_1$ myeloma protein that dissociated in the presence of urea and guanidine into H- and L-chains. We could not detect any intracellular J-chain.

There is another possibility that J-chain is a proteolytic enzyme that may process chains during their synthesis. As you know, L- and H-chains are produced as pro-L and pro-H-chains, and it is possible that J-chains may cleave N-terminal sequences of these chains before they are secreted.

T. B. TOMASI (*University of New Mexico, Albuquerque, N. Mex.*): Some time ago, we reported that in alcoholic cirrhosis, there were elevated levels of IgA and an increased percentage of dimers. When we looked at that IgA, it was complexed with albumin. It was a dimer, but we also had albumin in a complex with it.

A similar phenomenon occurs in the bile, and, there seem to be two types of complexes. In one type, the albumin is disulfide-bonded to the IgA; in the other it appears that there is an antibody-like activity, that is an IgA antibody directed against the patient's albumin. Have you done any studies along these lines?

MESTECKY: Several controls were performed to classify the immunoglobulin to establish that it was a polymer. We looked for the presence of J-chain and dissociation in acid buffer. We did not look for albumin specifically; however, an immune complex would dissociate under conditions as you and others have described. We next performed sulfitolysis or reduction and alkylation. These procedures resulted in a decrease in the molecular weight.

E. ORLANS (Chester Beatty Research Center, Surrey, England): When you did your DNP-HSA IgA-mediated transport in mice, did you try labeling the mouse myeloma protein to determine what proportion of the MOPC 315 dimer without antigen was present in the bile?

MESTECKY: There was transport of ^{125}I-labeled IgA. Interestingly, there is some discrepancy with the results of others. We do not see much transport of the circulating polymeric IgA labeled with ^{125}I into other secretions. Bile appears to be unique in this regard.

ORLANS: We have transferred the MOPC 315 into the rat and found that it is not efficiently transported.

R. A. GOOD (Oklahoma Medical Research Foundation, Oklahoma City): I was particularly concerned about the cirrhotic patients, where you observed a decrease in what might be thought of as a clearance mechanism for IgA. One wonders whether or not these patients will have IgA in the dimeric form deposited in other sites, or whether other pathways of clearance are used? We heard at this conference about the stimulation of gastrointesintal production of IgA, the IgA complexes, and their capacity to damage the mesangium. Do the cirrhotic patients have deposits of the dimeric IgA in the mesangium? If you interfere with the liver clearance mechanism, do you get any pathology in the kidneys as a consequence?

MESTECKY: There are some published papers dealing with this topic. Patients with liver cirrhosis may have IgA deposited in their kidneys. There is now a very nice characterization as to the form and subclass of IgA in individuals with alcoholic liver cirrhosis. With regard to liver and blockage of IgA transport, these experiments have been done in animals. If you introduce carbon tetrachloride into rats, they will have selective IgA nephropathy, with selective deposits of IgA in the kidneys.

J. J. CEBRA (University of Pennsylvania, Philadelphia): In supporting your notion that peripheral blood cells stimulated with pokeweed mitogen are more differentiated and possibly on their way to the lamina propria, Dr. Fuhrmann finds that there are clones that come from cells that generate daughters and only make dimeric IgA. Furthermore, the IgA from switching clones, where you have mixed isotypes, that is, IgM and IgG coexpressed, have a high proportion of monomeric IgA. So it may be the increase of synthesis of J-chain that could be related to the state of IgA differentiation.

Are these globules that are in the milk membrane bonded?

MESTECKY: Yes.

ANALYSIS OF THE EFFECTOR FUNCTIONS OF DIFFERENT POPULATIONS OF MUCOSAL LYMPHOCYTES*

D. M. V. Parrott, C. Tait, S. MacKenzie, A. McI. Mowat, M. D. J. Davies, and H. S. Micklem†

Department of Bacteriology and Immunology
Western Infirmary
University of Glasgow
Glasgow, Scotland
†Department of Zoology
University of Edinburgh
Edinburgh, Scotland

INTRODUCTION

The small intestine continually receives a large and varied antigenic load, and one would anticipate that there would be large numbers of very diverse cell-mediated effector cells as well as regulatory mechanisms present, especially among those cells closest to the gut lumen, namely intraepithelial lymphocytes (IEL).

Following the development of methods for the separation of lymphocytes from the lamina propria (LPL) and from the epithelial layer, IEL, and for the subsequent purification of those lymphocytes from contaminating epithelial cells,[1] it became practicable to study mucosal cell-mediated effector cells in small laboratory animals. It was deduced from earlier studies[2-4] that the majority of IEL were T-derived cells, the numbers of which were considerably influenced by the contents of the gut lumen. A distinguishing feature of IEL is that a considerable proportion contains granules that stain with Giemsa or Astra blue. The granules were first observed by Collan in 1972[5] and have given rise to the theory that IEL may be related to mast cells,[6,7] and most recently to the suggestion that they are rich in natural killer (NK) cells.[8] Circumstantial evidence, therefore, led us to anticipate that it should be possible to demonstrate both cytotoxic T and natural killer activity in IEL from the gut mucosa. In this paper we summarize our progress so far. For purposes of comparison, data on lamina propria and lung lymphocytes are also included.

MATERIALS AND METHODS

Animals

C57BL/10ScSn, DBA/A, CBA/Ca, BALB/c, and C57BL/6 bg^j bg^j mice from 6–12 weeks of age were supplied from departmental stocks. A breeding nucleus of C57BL/6 bg^j bg^j was a gift from Dr. H. S. Micklem, Department of Zoology, University of Edinburgh. CBA/nunu and CBA/nu mice were obtained from Olac

*This work was supported by a grant from M.R.C. (U.K.) Grant No. G8011059.

0077-8923/83/0409-307 $1.75/0 © 1983, NYAS

Ltd., Bicester, England. Age and sex-matched mice were used in all experiments.

Cell Preparations

Spleen, lymph node, Peyer's patch, and thymus cell-suspensions were prepared by standard techniques. Lamina propria lymphocytes and IEL were prepared and purified on a two-step discontinuous Percoll (Pharmacia) gradient of densities 1.055 and 1.085g.[1,9]

Care was taken during the preparation of LPL for NK assay in selecting the preparation of collagenase. Previous experience had shown that Worthington preparation CLSPA[1] (Millipore (U.K.) Ltd., Harrow, Middlesex, England) was suitable for most purposes, including the extraction of cytotoxic T-cells, but when this preparation was tested on spleen cells that were then assayed for NK activity, about 40% of NK activity was lost. C2139 (Sigma Chemical Co. Ltd., Poole, Dorset, England) did not reduce spleen NK activity and was used to extract LPL that were to be assayed for NK activity.

Staining Methods for Cytocentrifuge Preparations

Giemsa slides were fixed in methanol and stained overnight in 1:20 dilution of stock Giemsa in pH 6.5 Sörensen's phosphate buffer. Slides were differentiated in 0.25% colophonium resin in methylated spirit and then mounted as usual.

Astra Blue Staining

Slides were fixed in Carnoy's fluid, dried and rehydrated, then stained for 30 minutes in 0.1% Astra blue in 0.7N hydrochloric acid pH 0.3. After washing in 0.7N HCl, slides were lightly counterstained in safranin, dehydrated, and mounted.

Immunofluorescent Staining

Cell-surface antigens were identified by methods detailed elsewhere.[10] Rat monoclonals were used to identify T-cell antigens, and these included Thy-1.2 (Clone No. 30-H12), Lyt-1 (Clone No. 53-7.2), Lyt-2 (Clone No. 53-6.7), and Lyt-3 (Clone No. 53-5.8). A fluoresceinated affinity-purified rabbit anti-rat immunoglobulin (Ig) serum absorbed in solid phase with mouse Ig was used as the second-step reagent for indirect staining. Cell surface Ig was detected with fluoresceinated affinity-purified rabbit anti-mouse serum.

Tumor Cells

P-815 (H-2^d), EL-4 (H-2^b), and YAC-1 (H-2^a) tumor cells were grown in vitro in RPMI-1640 + 10% fetal calf serum (FCS). Cells were always subcultured 24 hours before use. For use in the cytotoxicity assay, tumor cells were labeled at 5×10^6 cells/50 μ Ci ^{51}Chromate/ml of medium for 60 minutes at 37° C. The cells were then washed five times and resuspended at 2×10^5 cells/ml for use in the assay.

Tumor Inoculation

C57BL mice were injected intraperitoneally or subcutaneously with 3×10^7 P-815 or EL-4 cells in 0.5 ml buffered saline. Control animals received buffered saline only.

Cytotoxic Assays

The specific T-cell cytotoxicity assay against P-815 or EL-4 is as described previously.[11]

The NK cytotoxic assay was set up in V-bottomed microtiter plates as previously described[11] for cytotoxic T-cell assays except that the incubation time was 4 hours or 18 hours at 37° C. Effector to target-cell ratios of 25:1, 50:1, and 100:1 were used. For assessing the spontaneous release of ^{51}Chromate, tumour cells were incubated with thymus cells, which have no NK activity, at the appropriate cell densities. When cell mixtures were used, the effector to target ratio expressed was always the spleen to target ratio, and the contribution of the second cell type in the mixture was 1:1 with spleen cells.

Calculation of Results

The percentage specific cytotoxicity induced by each cell type was calculated, using the following formula:

$$\text{Percent specific cytotoxicity} = \frac{\text{Release in presence of effector cells} - \text{spontaneous release}}{\text{Maximum release} - \text{spontaneous release}} \%$$

Maximum release of ^{51}Chromium was assessed by treating labeled cells with 5% Triton X-100. In each experiment, the results were expressed as the mean of quadruplicate cultures of cells derived from a pool of two to four mice. The results shown in the tables are expressed as the median and range of a number of separate experiments.

RESULTS

Histochemistry of Mucosal Lymphocytes

Up to 60% of IEL, depending upon the strain, contain distinct cytoplasmic granules that stain with Giemsa or Astra blue, (those in Beige mice being especially prominent) but there are few, if any, granule-containing cells among lamina propria lymphocytes.[9] In the present experiments, we found that CBA/nunu mice had slightly fewer granule-bearing IEL than heterozygote mice, and the granules were smaller in nunu than in nu$^+$ mice. Treatment with anti-Thy-1.2 and complement reduced the number of granule-staining cells in both C57BL and

TABLE 1

NUMBERS OF GRANULAR IEL AND NK CYTOTOXICITY*

| | Numbers Granular IEL | | NK Cytotoxicity* | |
| | Mean | | Mean | |
Strain	(Range)	[Numbers Estimations]	(Range)	[Numbers Estimations]
C57BL/10ScSn	37 (31–52)	[5]	1.6 (0–4)	[7]
C57BL α Thy-1.2 treated IEL	32 (10–37)	[4]	2, 1	
NIH	52 (52–59)	[4]	4, 4	
CBA/nu⁺	42 (35–50)	[5]	4, 9, 1	
CBA/nunu	27 (18–39)	[6]	4, 11, 10	
C57BL6/bgⁱbgⁱ	52 (49–55)	[4]	<1	
C57BL6/bgⁱbgⁱ α Thy-1.2 treated IEL	19, 17		<1	

*Effector to Target ratio 50:1; 4 hour assay with Yac-1

Beige mice (TABLE 1), and those Thy-1.2 resistant cells had somewhat smaller granules. We have the impression that the numbers of granule-containing IEL fluctuate, and although granules were present in the cytoplasm of medium as well as large IEL, they were more easily seen in large cells. Granule-containing IEL can also be seen in sections of intestine; the proportion appears to be the same as in cell preparations of IEL. We have no reason to suspect that the separation of IEL from the epithelial layer alters the number of granule-containing cells in any way.

The Surface Phenotype of Mucosal Lymphocytes

Previous experience using anti-Thy-1.2 and complement cytotoxicity indicated that 60–65% of IEL and 75–80% of LPL carry T-cell surface markers.[1] More

TABLE 2

SURFACE ANTIGENS ON IEL AND LPL FROM CBA/nu⁺ AND CBA/nunu MICE*

	Thy-1	Lyt-1	Lyt-2	Lyt-3	sIg
IEL					
nu⁺	14, 22	13, 18	62, 57	11, 8	9, 4
nunu	3, 2	3, 0	46, 48	1, 0	6, 4
LPL					
nu⁺	22, 26	15, 14	13, 11	11, 5	40, 36
nunu	7, 5	3, 1	5, 2	7, 5	47, 35
LN					
nu⁺	64, 66	59, 57	22, 18	20, 21	28, 17
nunu	5, 1	4, 0	2, 0	2, 0	92, 87

*Pooled cells from two to three ♀ mice: two pools analyzed

recently, we have analyzed the surface phenotype IEL and LPL, by fluorescence microscopy (TABLE 2, FIGURE 1) and in the fluorescence-activated cell-sorter.[10]

In lymph nodes (TABLE 2, FIGURE 1) and Peyer's patch tissue,[10] virtually all the T-cells stained for both Thy-1 and Lyt-1, whereas a minority of cells stained for Lyt-2 and Lyt-3 in addition to Thy-1 and Lyt-1. Lymph nodes from nude mice contained minimal numbers of cells with any T-cell markers. The distribution of staining among IEL was very different from lymph nodes. The numbers of IEL that stained for Thy-1 and Lyt-1 showed variation between batches of mice of the same strain, although, unlike lymph nodes and Peyer's patches, there were Thy-1$^+$ stained cells that did not stain for Lyt-1 (FIGURE 1). The most consistent and unusual finding was, however, that a majority of cells carried Lyt-2, and

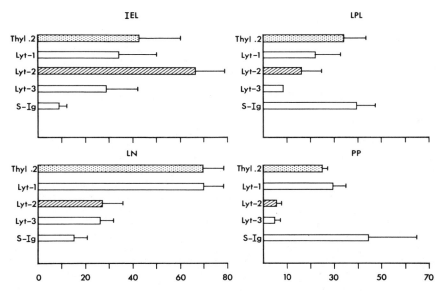

FIGURE 1. The frequency (percent) of cells carrying various membrane antigens, determined by immunofluorescent staining with monoclonal antibodies in CBA/Ca mice. Observations were made on pooled cells from two to three donors. The results are mean ± S.D. from between 5–12 separate pools. Attention is drawn to the results of Thy-1.2 (stippled) and Lyt-2 (crosshatched).

furthermore, that a substantial, but variable proportion of cells carried Lyt-2 antigen, but lacked Lyt-3, Thy-1, or Lyt-1. The Thy 1$^-$, Lyt 1$^-$2$^+$3$^-$ cells were especially obvious among IEL from nude mice (TABLE 2) because very low numbers of cells carried any other T-cell marker. Staining of lamina propria T-cells (FIGURE 1, TABLE 2) showed some variation, and most demonstrated the conventional pattern of a dominance of Thy-1$^+$ and Lyt-1$^+$ stained cells with a minority staining for Lyt-2 and Lyt-3 as well. Nevertheless, there were cells that stained for Thy-1.2, but not for Lyt-1, and a few cells that stained for Lyt-2, but not for Lyt-3. The striking predominance of Lyt-2 staining of IEL from nude mice was not seen among lamina propria lymphocytes. Lamina propria lymphocytes, as expected, contained many more cells that stained for cell surface Ig than for intraepithelial lymphocytes.

TABLE 3

THE EFFECT OF INCREASING ASSAY TIMES ON NK CYTOTOXICITY OF
IEL AND SPLEEN CELLS

| | | Percent Specific Cytotoxicity Against Yac-1 | | | |
| | | 4 hour | | 18 hour* | |
Strain	E:T	IEL	Spleen	IEL	Spleen
C3H/He	50:1	5	27	27	43
	25:1	4	18	9	32
C57BL6/bg^{j}bg^j	50:1	<1	<1	40	5
	25:1	<1	<1	31	3
CBA/nu$^+$	50:1	9	18	68	22
	25:1	<1	14	25	18
CBA/nunu	50:1	11	43	69	55
	25:1	<1	40	20	48

*Cells plus ^{51}Cr-labeled targets cultured overnight. No cytotoxicity was observed when cells were cultured alone overnight and targets added for a 4 hour assay period.

Natural Killer Cytotoxicity in Intraepithelial Lymphocytes

Using the standard four-hour assay against the Yac-1 tumour cell line, we detected only a small level of cytotoxicity in IEL from six different strains of mice as compared with spleen cells (TABLE 1 and 3) and no cytotoxicity at all in Beige mice. CBA/nunu mice (TABLES 1 and 3) also had comparatively modest amounts of NK activity in IEL, and although we, like others,[12,13] found substantially more NK activity in spleen cells from CBA/nunu than in CBA/nu mice, the cytotoxicity of IEL from CBA/nunu mice was not significantly greater than other strains. These low levels of NK cytotoxicity were surprising in view of the findings, by several groups of workers, that NK cytotoxicity was reflected by the numbers of large granular lymphocytes.[8,14-16] This generalization in our experience does not extend to IEL (TABLE 1). Increasing the time of assay to 18 hours did, however, increase the NK activity of IEL very substantially (TABLE 3), and to a much greater extent than in spleen or lymph nodes in all the six strains examined (C57BL, BALB/c, and NIH as well as those detailed in TABLE 3). The observations on Beige mice were interesting because some NK cytotoxicity against Yac-1 appeared after 18 hours incubation, when little activity could be detected elsewhere. Furthermore, although we found significantly more activity in CBA/nunu spleens and lymph nodes than in CBA/nu mice, the NK cytotoxicity was equally high in IEL from CBA/nu and CBA/nunu at 18 hours. Overnight incubation of IEL before

TABLE 4

INCREASE OF NK CYTOTOXICITY IN ALLOGENEIC
TUMOR*—INJECTED C57BL MICE

| | E:T Ratio | Percent Cytotoxicity at Four Hours | | |
		IEL	Spleen	MLN
Four days after	50:1	<1	10	1
P-815 injection	25:1	<1	4	<1
11 days after	50:1	24	56	29
P-815 injection	25:1	22	41	17

*3×10^7 P-815 (H-2^d) injected into C57BL/10ScSn (H-2^b)

subsequent exposure of target cells for four hours did not enhance cytotoxicity. Prior treatment of IEL with anti-Thy-1.2 plus complement did not significantly reduce the 18 hour NK activity of IEL or spleen cells.[17]

Enhancement of Four-Hour NK Cytotoxicity (TABLE 4)

We attempted to boost NK cytotoxicity by injecting mice with syngeneic or allogeneic tumors. The effects upon IEL were trivial in mice injected with syngeneic tumors and early after allogeneic tumors. At 11 days after the injection of an allogeneic tumor (P-815), however, there was considerable enhancement of NK cytotoxicity in C57BL mice, in both IEL and spleen cells; this effect was demonstrable in a four-hour assay.

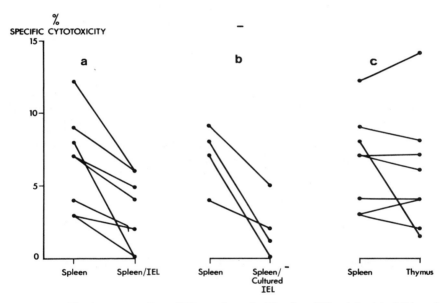

FIGURE 2. The suppressor effect of IEL on 4 hour C57BL spleen NK activity: (a) addition of fresh IEL; (b) addition of IEL cultured for 18 hours; (c) addition of thymus cells. Assayed at 25:1 spleen to target ratio.

Suppression of Spleen Natural Killer Activity by Intraepithelial Lymphocytes

The possibility of suppressor activity in IEL was investigated by coculturing different dilutions of IEL, thymus, or mesenteric lymph node cells with C57BL spleen cells and assaying the cell-mixtures against Yac-1 cells for four hours. Mesenteric lymph node cells had little effect upon spleen NK activity. Addition of thymus cells had variable effects; occasionally, suppression was observed (FIGURE 2c), but usually there was only a little effect. By contrast, IEL consistently inhibited spleen NK activity especially at high-effector to target ratios (FIGURE 2a). Even at 25:1 ratio, there was a mean suppression of 55% in eight experiments (FIGURE 2a). Preculture of IEL for 18 hours before mixing with spleen cells did not reduce the suppressive activity (mean 80%) [FIGURE 2b]. Spleen/IEL mixtures also showed some inhibition in an 18 hour assay, although, at this assay time, the IEL themselves also exhibited NK activity.

The Effect of Removing Macrophages and Anti-Thy-1.2 Treatment of Intraepithelial Lymphocytes on NK Activity and on Suppressor Activity

There are few, if any, macrophages normally present among intraepithelial lymphocytes. Nevertheless, IEL were exposed to two different procedures for removing macrophages, namely, carbonyl iron and G10 Sephadex. Neither of these procedures[17] elevated the four-hour assay NK activity of IEL or decreased the suppressor effect of IEL on spleen NK activity.

In a separate series of experiments, IEL were treated with α Thy-1.2 and complement before testing in coculture assays, but there was no reduction in suppressor effect.

Natural Killer Cytotoxicity and Suppression in Lamina Propria Lymphocytes

In preliminary series of experiments that were directly comparable to those carried out with IEL, we tested the ability of LPL to mediate NK cytotoxicity against Yac targets, and for the ability of LPL to exert suppression on spleen NK activity. Because preparation of LPL requires the use of collagenase for separation of cells, care was taken (see METHODS) to use only that preparation of collagenase that does not contain trypsin and which prior testing on spleen cells had shown did not affect NK activity. Lamina propria lymphocytes had little or no NK activity in either 4 hour assay (data not shown) or 18 hour assay, and there was only slight suppressor effect on spleen cells (TABLE 5).

The Generation of Cytotoxic T-Cells in the Intestinal Mucosa After the Intraperitoneal Injection of P-815 Mastocytoma Cells

C57BL mice, injected with 3×10^7 P-815 tumour cells, were killed at selected time intervals. The LPL and IEL were assayed for the proportion of cytotoxic

TABLE 5

NK CYTOTOXICITY AND SUPPRESSION IN LPL* FROM C57BL/10ScSn MICE

	Percent Specific Cytotoxicity at 18 Hours		
E:T		50:1	25:1
LPL		2	$\leqslant 1$
Spl‡		18	11
MLN†		7	$\leqslant 1$
Spl/LPL		12	6
Spl/Thy		14	7
Spl/MLN		15	12

*Separated by the method of Davies and Parrott,[1] using C-2139 collagenase.
†MLN = mesenteric lymph nodes.
‡Spl = spleen.

TABLE 6

CYTOTOXIC T-CELL ACTIVITY* IN MUCOSAL SITES AFTER INTRAPERITONEAL
OR SUBCUTANEOUS INJECTION OF P-815 CELLS INTO C57BL/10ScSn MICE

Day	Route	Percent Cytotoxicity				
		IEL	LPL	Lungs	MLN†	Spleen
6	ip	16.8 ± 0.6	51.0 ± 8.4	38.7 ± 8.9	19.7 ± 4.7	10.2 ± 5.6
	sc	<1	5.3 ± 3.4	13.4 ± 2.5	3.9 ± 0.7	6.6 ± 2.6
11	ip	50.8 ± 11.1	76.1 ± 2.3	68.9 ± 5.4	39.5 ± 10.9	40.2 ± 3.3
	sc	<1	4.1 ± 1.2	8.1 ± 2.3	<1	2.5 ± 1.4

*Effector: Target ratio 50:1
†MLN - ˉnesenteric lymph nodes.

T-cells, and for the purposes of comparison, spleen and mesenteric lymph node
were also assayed. In some experiments, Peyer's patches and lung were also
assayed. In our first experiments, which did not include IEL, we were surprised to
find that as early as five days after the intraperitoneal injection of tumour cells,
there was a high level of cytotoxicity in lamina propria lymphocytes. The peak
was higher than other tissues sampled and persisted beyond the time (40 days)
when cytotoxicity levels were falling in the spleen and mesenteric lymph node.[11]
Subsequently,[9] comparable levels of cytotoxicity were also found in the lungs and
in IEL (TABLE 6). Cytotoxicity in IEL increased more slowly than in the lungs or
LPL (TABLE 6) and did not attain such high levels, but nevertheless contained as
much cytotoxic activity as the mesenteric lymph node or spleen. There was no
spontaneous cytotoxicity against P-815 cells in IEL, LPL, or lungs from unimmunized control mice. Subcutaneous injection of P-815 cells elicited much lower
levels of cytotoxic activity, and though some activity was detectable among LPL
and lungs (TABLE 6), none could be detected in IEL preparations. Directly
comparable results (data not shown) were obtained when EL-4 tumor cells were
injected in BALB/c mice. We were confident that the cytotoxicity that we were
measuring was specific T-cell cytotoxicity because C57BL mice injected with
P-815 (H-2^d) tumor did not show any activity against EL-4 (H-2^b) or TLX-5 (H-2^k);
mice injected with EL-4 did not show cytotoxicity against P-815 (unpublished),
and specific cytotoxicity was eliminated by prior *in vitro* treatment of effector
cell-populations with α Thy-1.2 antiserum.[11]

DISCUSSION

Intraepithelial lymphocytes are a distinct population of cells adjoining the gut
lumen, whose siting and unusual morphology has aroused interest and speculation as to their function.[4,6,7,9,18] Like others,[5-7] we found that a considerable
proportion of IEL contain Giemsa staining granules, a characteristic shared by the
subset of human lymphocyte T[19] and also by NK cells.[15,16] Unpublished results
show that up to 70% of IEL also stain with ANAE, sharing the distinctive pattern
characteristic of mouse T-lymphocytes. Most previous researchers have agreed
that many, if not all, IEL have some of the characteristics of T-lymphocytes,[2-4,20]
although they are different from small recirculating T-lymphocytes,[20] and recent
work, including that presented here, is beginning to clarify the situation. Selby
and his coworkers[21] have reported that 70% of human IEL are of the suppressor

cytotoxic (OKT8[+]) phenotype. The results of Micklem et al.[10] and those presented here, show that a mean of 66% IEL from CBA mice, carry the Lyt-2 antigen, which is a suppressor cytotoxic marker in mice. Other recent data suggest that a comparable cell population, staining with MRC OX-8, a suppressor cytotoxic marker in rats, is present among IEL from rats.[22] We have shown that more than half of the Lyt-2[+] cells lacked detectable Lyt-3, and a variable percentage (20–30%) lacked detectable Lyt-1 and/or Thy-1. Thy 1[-], Lyt 1[-]2[+]3[-] cells were particularly obvious in IEL from nude mice, and we have speculated that this novel cell type has not been previously described in the literature.[10]

By contrast with IEL, LPL do not have granules that stain with Giemsa or Astra blue. Only a minority (mean 16%) of mouse LPL stain with Lyt-2, whereas a mean of 39% of human LPL were OKT8[+].[21]

It has been suggested that all granular IEL belong to a bone marrow derived population, whereas nongranular IEL are thymus derived.[23] We do not find such a clear separation, because IEL from nude mice often have fewer granular IEL than heterozygote mice, and treatment of IEL from C57BL and Beige mice with anti-Thy-1[+] and complement reduces the number of granule-staining intraepithelial lymphocytes.

In our experience there are, therefore, Thy-1[+] granular IEL and Thy-1[-] granular IEL. Furthermore, although half of Lyt-2 bearing cells are granular, there are nevertheless Lyt-2 bearing cells that do not appear to have granules.[10]

Our findings on the morphology and phenotype of IEL are very relevant to recent observations on the similarities between suppressor-cytotoxic subsets of T-lymphocytes and NK cells in both man and rat. These functionally different categories of lymphocytes both contain a preponderance of cells that are larger than normal and have granular cytoplasm. Many large granular lymphocytes in man react with OKT8[15], and many of these same cells in rats react with OX-8.[16] Large granular lymphocytes are a minority population (up to 6%) in the blood and tissues of man[15] and rat,[16] but a large minority or a majority population among IEL that would, therefore, be expected to have a high level of cytotoxicity, both spontaneous NK and specific T-cell and presumably also suppressor activity.

We tested IEL for NK activity against Yac-1 tumor line, but little or no spontaneous cytotoxicity against Yac-1 was found, using conventional short assay times. This finding was somewhat unexpected because others[18,8] have reported high NK activity among intraepithelial lymphocytes. When, however, the assay period was prolonged to 18 hours, high levels of NK cytotoxicity against Yac-1 was found. It is significant that both Arnaud-Battandier[18] and Tagliabue et al.[8] used prolonged assay times (18–20 hours) to detect NK activity, although they did not comment on this factor. The NK activities of spleen and IEL did not parallel one another in any of the strains of mice that we tested, including nude and Beige, and it is possible that spontaneous cytotoxicity in IEL is mediated by a different type of cell from that in the spleen. In agreement with Arnaud-Battandier et al.,[18] we did not find any NK activity among LPL, even after prolonged assay times.

It is possible that prolonged assay times are required for the demonstration of IEL-NK activity, because the NK cells were damaged during extraction and required time for reconstitution to occur. This situation is unlikely, however, as no enzymes were used to extract IEL, and spleen cells subjected to the same procedure[17] did not lose their NK activity. We have attempted to activate NK activity by prior injection of syngeneic or allogeneic tumors. Activation did occur, and four-hour NK activity appeared in IEL, but only some days after stimulation with an allogeneic tumor. It is possible, however, that this activity could have been mediated by activated T-cells because cytotoxicity against Yac-1 coincided with a peak of specific cytotoxicity against P-815. It has been shown that clones of cytotoxic T-cells and cultured T-cells can kill Yac targets.[24]

Campbell Tait, a student working in my laboratory, obtained evidence for an NK suppressor among intraepithelial lymphocytes. This evidence has been confirmed and expanded.[17] The NK activity of spleen cells was significantly suppressed during coculture experiments, and the suppression was evident during both 4 hour and 18 hour assays. This suppressor effect[17] does not appear to be mediated by macrophages or by T-cells because removal of macrophages or with Sephadex and by carbonyl iron treatment with anti-Thy-1.2 and complement, did not reduce suppression, and IEL from nude mice were able to exert suppression. The suppression is not H-2 restricted,[17] and it is not due to cold target competition or simple crowding. The effect does not appear to be exerted by contaminating epithelial cells, but we are investigating the effects of suppressor substances such as prostaglandin[25] or histamine.[26] Addition of indomethacin to assay cultures did not alleviate suppression, but further work is necessary before we can exonerate prostaglandin.

Histamine is another known inhibitor of cellular immune functions,[26] and there are many mast cells capable of releasing histamine present in the lamina propria. Culturing in the presence of cimetidine, a histamine inhibitor, did not reduce suppression.[17] So far, however, the mode of action of the IEL suppressor effect on spleen NK cells remains unclear.

In a separate series of experiments, we have been studying the arrival, in mucosal surfaces, of specific cytotoxic T-cells against P-815 and El-4 in mice immunized by prior injection of the appropriate allogeneic tumor. There were clear differences in the levels of cytotoxicity detected among IEL compared with adjoining LPL, and a separate mucosal site, that is, the lungs: this difference was dependent on the time after tumor injection and the route of injection. The level of cytotoxicity was substantially lower than in LPL or lung lymphocytes, especially at early times after tumor injection; there was little or no cytotoxicity in either IEL or LPL after subcutaneous injection, although some cytotoxicity was present in lung lymphocytes.[9] These experiments demonstrate clearly, however, that not only are cytotoxic effector T-cells delivered to mucosal sites after systemic priming, but the level of cytotoxicity is higher in the mucosal tissues than in Peyer's patches, mesenteric lymph nodes, or spleen.[11,9] It is known that activated T-lymphoblasts have a very strong propensity to leave the recirculating pool of lymphocytes and to migrate into various tissues, including mucosal surfaces.[27] A particularly relevant example of the migratory behavior of alloactivated T-lymphoblasts is the experiments of Sprent and Miller[28,29] who injected BALB/c lymphocytes into (CBA × BALB/c) F_1 irradiated mice, and found that the resulting anti-H-2^d lymphoblasts had very high cytotoxicity against P-815 tumor cells. Sprent and Miller tested thoracic duct lymphoblasts and not mucosal cells, but it is very likely that the thoracic duct cells tested will have come directly from the intestinal mucosa. Our system and that of Sprent and Miller is, of course, artificial, but the results do acquire sense, if the systems are viewed as models for studying the *in vivo* distribution and migratory pattern of alloreactive cytotoxic T-cells, especially if one regards the ability to generate cytotoxic T-cells as an adaptation designed to eliminate virus-infected cells, rather than allografts of normal or tumor tissue.[30] A separate, but equally important adaptation, would be one that ensured that cytotoxic T-cells, primed against virus-infected cells, should migrate into, and preferentially accumulate in, especially vulnerable tissue, such as the mucosal surfaces. H-2-restricted cytotoxic T-cells do appear in the lungs after intranasal infection with live influenza virus[31] and in the spleen after subcutaneous injection of live virus.[32] On the basis of our experiments, we would predict that some cytotoxic T-cells against influenza virus-infected cells should also appear among intraepithelial lymphocytes and lymphocytes from the lamina propria.

In this paper we have described various morphological and functional characteristics of IEL that differentiate them clearly from lamina propria lymphocytes. Therefore, although IEL must traffic through lamina propria[27,20] in order to reach their epithelial position, they are not casual émigrés who have strayed inadvertently across the basal layer. Some process of selection must take place. As yet we cannot, with complete confidence, ascribe any of the three functions of IEL described, whether NK, NK suppression, or cytotoxic T-cell, to either granular, non-granular, or Lyt-2$^+$ cells, without further experimentation. It is clear, however, that the intestinal mucosa contains populations of immune effector cells that are heterogeneous in nature and function. Analysis of these populations should throw considerable light on the cell-mediated defense mechanisms at mucosal surfaces.

SUMMARY

Lymphocytes separated from the epithelial layer of mouse small intestine, IEL, were tested for their NK cytotoxicity against Yac-1 targets. There was little NK activity in a 4 hour assay, but high activity in an 18 hour assay, and the NK activity of IEL did not parallel that in the spleen in any of the mouse strains tested. Furthermore, IEL exerted a suppressor activity on mouse spleen NK activity. Specific T-cell cytotoxicity appeared in IEL in mice immunized with an intraperitoneal injection of P-815 tumor cells.

By contrast with IEL, LPL had little NK or NK suppressor activity, but higher levels of specific T-cell cytotoxicity in tumor-immunized mice than intraepithelial lymphocytes.

A high proportion of IEL had granules that stained with Giemsa and Astra blue. Furthermore many IEL carried Lyt-2$^+$ phenotype and no other T-cell surface antigen. Intraepithelial lymphocytes appeared, therefore, to have staining and phenotype characteristics of both granular NK cells and suppressor cells. It was clear that the intestinal mucosa contained populations of immune effector cells that were heterogeneous in nature and function.

REFERENCES

1. DAVIES, M. D. J. & D. M. V. PARROTT. 1981. Gut **22**: 481–488.
2. FERGUSON, A. & D. M. V. PARROTT. 1972. Clin. Exp. Immunol. **12**: 477–488.
3. GUY-GRAND, D., C. GRISCELLI & P. VASSALLI. 1974. Eur. J. Immunol. **4**: 435–443.
4. FERGUSON, A. 1977. Gut **18**: 921–937.
5. COLLAN, Y. 1972. Scand. J. Gastroenterol. **7** (Suppl. 18): 1–93.
6. RUDZIK, O., & J. BIENENSTOCK. 1974. Lab. Invest. **30**: 260–266.
7. GUY-GRAND, D., C. GRISCELLI & P. VASSALLI. 1978. J. Exp. Med. **148**: 1661–1677.
8. TAGLIABUE, A., W. LUINI, D. SOLDATESCHI & D. BORASCHI. 1981. Eur. J. Immunol. **11**: 919–922.
9. DAVIES, M. D. J. & D. M. V. PARROTT. 1981. Immunology **44**: 367–371.
10. MICKLEM, H. S., J. M. URE, M. D. J. DAVIES & D. M. V. PARROTT. 1982. Submitted
11. DAVIES, M. D. J. & D. M. V. PARROTT. 1980. Clin. Exp. Immunol. **42**: 273–279.
12. HERBERMAN, R. B., M. E. NUNN, D. H. LAURIN. 1975. Int. J. Cancer **16**: 216–229.

13. KIESSLING, R., E. KLEIN, & H. WIGZELL. 1975. Eur. J. Immunol. **5:** 112–117.
14. LUINI, W., D. BORASCHI, S. ALBERTI, A. ALEOTTI & A. TAGLIABUE. 1981. Immunology **43:** 663–667.
15. TIMONEN, T., J. R. ORTALDO & R. B. HERBERMAN. 1981. J. Exp. Med. **153:** 569–582.
16. REYNOLDS, C. W., T. TIMONEN & R. B. HERBERMAN. 1981 J. Immunol. **127:** 282–287.
17. MOWAT, A. McI., C. TAIT, S. MACKENZIE, M. D. J. DAVIES & D. M. V. PARROTT. 1982. Clin. Exp. Immunol. In press.
18. ARNAUD-BATTANDIER, F., B. M. BUNDY, M. O'NEILL, J. BIENENSTOCK & D. L. NELSON. 1978. J. Immunol. **121:** 1059–1065.
19. GROSSI, C. E., S. R. WEBB, A. ZICCA, P. M. LYDYARD, L. MORETTA, C. MINGARI & M. D. COOPER. 1978. J. Exp. Med. **147:** 1405–1417.
20. PARROTT, D. M. V. 1976. Clinics in Gastroenterol. **5:** 211–228.
21. SELBY, W. S., G. JANOSSY & D. P. JEWELL. 1981. Gut **22:** 169–176.
22. LYSCOM, N. & M. J. BRUETON. 1982. Immunology **45:** 775–783.
23. MAYRHOFER, G. 1980. Blood **55:** 632–635.
24. NABEL, G., L. R. BUCALO, J. ALLARD, H. WIGZELL & H. CANTOR. 1981. J. Exp. Med. **153:** 1582–1603.
25. DROLLER, M. J., M. V. SCHNEIDER & P. PERLMANN. 1978. Cell. Immunol. **39:** 165–177.
26. ROCKLIN, R. E., J. BREARD, S. GUPTA, R. A. GOOD & K. L. MELMON. 1980. Cell. Immunol. **51:** 226–237.
27. PARROTT, D. M. V. & P. C. WILKINSON. 1981. Prog. Allergy **28:** 193–284.
28. SPRENT, J. & J. F. A. P. MILLER. 1976. Cell. Immunol. **21:** 303–313.
29. SPRENT, J. 1976. Cell. Immunol. **21:** 278–302.
30. ZINKERNAGEL, R. M. & P. C. DOHERTY. 1979. Adv. Immunol. **27:** 52–177.
31. ENNIS, F. A., M. A. WELLS, G. M. BUTCHKO & P. ALBRECHT. 1978. J. Exp. Med. **148:** 1241–1250.
32. LEUNG, K. N. & G. L. ADA. 1980. Scand. J. Immunol. **12:** 481–487.

DISCUSSION OF THE PAPER

J. R. McGHEE (*University of Alabama in Birmingham*): The finding of Lyt-2 cells in the IEL population that has lost Lyt-3 and are Thy-1 negative is very interesting. What do you think this discovery means?

D. M. V. PARROTT (*University of Glasgow, Glasgow, Scotland*): I think that these cells are differentiating and possibly losing surface antigens. They may start off with the regular phenotype and may lose other than what they need.

M. D. COOPER (*University of Alabama in Birmingham*): Have you looked at those Lyt-2 IEL to see if they are granular lymphocytes? One reason for asking this is that human natural killer cells identified by a monoclonal antibody often express T-cell antigens, the panspecific T-cell antigen, and the OKT8, the suppressor phenotype.

Would you also comment on the granules you saw in those IEL in the Beige mouse. Did you choose them because they had a single, very large granule that was more easily demonstrable than the multiple granules you usually see in other strains of mice? Humans with the *Chediak-Higashi* syndrome have normal numbers of NK-1 cells. They do not function well, and they are morphologically distinguished by this large single granule that you see in the cytoplasm, as you also see in polymorphonuclear leukocytes and in pigment cells that reflect the problem they suffer.

PARROTT: Yes, I chose to show a picture of the Beige mouse cell because of the single large granule; it's much easier to see in sections. I also intended to mention your work on human T-gamma cells that stain in a similar fashion to that seen in the Beige mouse.

You also asked whether the Lyt-2 cells are the granule cells? One can get, using a cocktail of appropriate antisera, up to 60% of granule cells with an Lyt-2 antigen.

M. R. SZEWCZUK (Queen's University, Kingston, Ontario, Canada): In your studies with the NK, you used the Yac-1 cell line. Did you also use a panel of other tumor cells, and did you perform a marker study of these NK cells?

PARROTT: The answer to both of your questions is no. I hope that you can provide me with your antisera for these studies.

K. E. JENSEN (Pfizer Central Research, Groton, Conn.): I wonder if your IEL cells might be producing prostaglandin (PG) E2. There are a number of reports suggesting that NK cells in peripheral blood or spleen are quite sensitive to prostaglandin E2.

PARROTT: Yes, they might. We have tried to increase suppression by adding exogenous PG E2; this attempt did not succeed. We also tried to offset suppression by treatment with indomethacin and this also did not work. These are, however, preliminary experiments and your point is well-taken. These experiments should be repeated, and we should do more work in this area.

R. A. GOOD (Oklahoma Medical Research Foundation, Oklahoma City): Have you tried interferon as a means of enhancing that rather delayed function of the intraepithelial natural killer activity?

PARROTT: No. We plan, however, to use interferon as well as IL-2.

M. F. KAGNOFF (University of California at San Diego, La Jolla): A few years ago, we showed that when you feed mice cells that bear major and minor histocompatibility differences, you induce cytotoxic T-cells or precursors of the cells in Peyer's patches. Have you had an opportunity to look at where the cytotoxic T-cells arise? Do you think they are arising in those local sites, or is it possible that they are induced in Peyer's patches?

PARROTT: I really do not know the origin of these cells. I do not think that they are induced in the Peyer's patches, although this idea would be a logical conclusion. Anatomically, however, that would be difficult for me to envisage. We have tried to feed tumor cells; however, the results are not clear.

B. H. WAKSMAN (National Multiple Sclerosis Society, New York, N.Y.): You have shown us several very exciting new things, and I hate to add a criticism at the end of a very beautiful study. The criticism concerns the question of numbers and the suggestion that one is seeing a real suppressor effect. Your conclusion about suppressor cells is based essentially on two points. The first, delay in the apparent natural killer effect, and the second, the result of a series of experiments with mixtures of two types of cells. In every instance, however, the amount of killing that you saw with the mixture fell between the values for what one observed with the two cell types used alone. There is a great problem with drawing any inferences from the use of that kind of mixture? Supposing, at a ratio of 50 to 1, you have among the 50 only 3 or 4 cells that had natural killer action. You begin to have rather difficult stochastic effects coming in as to whether killing is going to take place. If you dilute a slightly more active population with a slightly less active population, I think you would get the kinds of numbers that you observe, just on stochastic grounds alone. So, I am not sure you have an adequate numerical basis for saying there is any suppressor effect at all.

PARROTT: That is a valid point and I realize much more work must be performed. Nevertheless, I wanted to present our most recent studies at this meeting.

THE ROLE OF IgE IN PATHOGENESIS OF MUCOSAL VIRAL INFECTIONS*

Robert C. Welliver† and Pearay L. Ogra

*Department of Pediatrics and Microbiology,
State University of New York at Buffalo,
and
Division of Infectious Diseases
Children's Hospital
Buffalo, New York 14222*

INTRODUCTION

Immunoglobulin E antibody against a variety of inanimate substances plays an important role in mediating atopic disease, but the function of IgE antibodies to infectious agents in immunity to or pathogenesis of illnesses has not been studied extensively. Several studies suggest that IgE assists macrophages,[1,2] lymphocytes,[3] and eosinophils[2,4] in clearing intestinal parasites, and pseudomonas-specific IgE antibodies have been demonstrated in patients with cystic fibrosis, although their significance is uncertain.[5] Respiratory viral infections are common causes of episodes of wheezing in infants and young children, particularly in families with histories of atopic disease.[7] Respiratory syncytial virus (RSV) is the most important cause of severe respiratory illness in infancy.[8] We attempted to determine the potential role of RSV-specific IgE antibody in the pathogenesis of wheezing-associated respiratory illness due to respiratory syncytial virus.

MATERIALS AND METHODS

Study Population

The study population consisted of infants enrolled in an ongoing study of respiratory illness in childhood. These children were recruited either at birth or in the first few months of life at the time of hospitalization with respiratory illness due to infection with respiratory syncytial virus. Study objectives were explained to the parents, and signed statements of informed consent were obtained. After being recruited into the study, these infants were seen at the time of each episode of respiratory illness.

Collection of Samples

At the time of each illness, samples of nasopharyngeal secretions (NPS) were obtained by aspiration into plastic catheters as previously described.[9] Samples of

*The original studies were supported in part by grants from the National Heart, Lung, and Blood Institute (HL-21829) and the National Institute of Allergy and Infectious Diseases (AI-15939).

†Address for correspondence: Dr. Robert Welliver, Children's Hospital of Buffalo, 219 Bryant Street, Buffalo, New York 14222.

0077–8923/83/0409–0321 $1.75/0 © 1983, NYAS

NPS were centrifuged to sediment exfoliated airway epithelial cells. Supernatants were decanted.

Detection of Cell-Bound IgE

Using immunofluorescence microscopy, sedimented cells were studied simultaneously for the presence of RSV antigen and cell-bound IgE, as previously described.[8] In brief, RSV-infected cells were identified by staining with rabbit anti-RSV antibody (Wellcome, Beckenham, England) and rhodamine-conjugated goat anti-rabbit globulin (Cappel Laboratories, Cochranville, Pa.). The same cells were then studied for the presence of cell-bound IgE by staining with fluorescein-conjugated goat anti-human IgE (Meloy, Springfield, Va.). Slides were then examined by fluorescence microscopy using separate filter systems to reveal positive staining for rhodamine and fluorescein. Controls consisted of uninfected human epithelial tissue culture cells and samples of cells obtained from patients with infection due to other viruses. Control cells, examined in a blind fashion by the microscopist, revealed neither positive staining for RSV nor for IgE. Preincubation of anti-RSV serum with purified RSV and preincubation of anti-IgE conjugates with purified human IgE (Kallestad, Chaska, Minn.) before testing resulted in blocking of fluorescence.

Detection of Virus-Specific IgE in Secretions

Quantities of RSV-specific IgE in secretions were determined by enzyme-linked immunosorbent assays (ELISA) as previously described.[9] Supernatants of centrifuged NPS specimens were decanted and held at $-70°C$ before testing. In brief, the assay was performed after adhering sucrose gradient-purified RSV to the bottom of microELISA wells. Serial two-fold dilutions of NPS in buffer were incubated with the virus antigen, and were overlayed with horseradish peroxidase-conjuated goat anti-human IgE (Miles Laboratories, Elkhardt, Ind.). Next, 5-aminosalicylic acid (Sigma, St. Louis, Mo.) was added with hydrogen peroxidase, and the optical density of the mixture was read after 30 minutes at 488 nanometers. Protein concentrations of NPS samples were determined by standard methods,[9] and measured titers of RSV-IgE were corrected to a protein content of 10 mg per milliliter.

Control for the specificity of the assay included concurrent study of test wells of virus-coated wells incubated with secretions and substrate without conjugate, of virus-coated wells incubated with phosphate-buffered saline (instead of secretions) with conjugate and substrate, and of the uninfected-cell controls mentioned above. All control wells remained colorless for several hours after plates were read, indicating that neither the conjugate nor the RSV-IgE was adhering nonspecifically to any substance in the wells. The substrate itself eventually developed a brown color on prolonged exposure to light.

Additional controls consisted of blocking experiments designed to ensure the specificity of the assay for IgE isotype and the specificity for IgE for respiratory syncytial virus. Aliquots of the conjugate were incubated with an equal volume of phosphate-buffered saline or of purified human IgE (Kallestad Laboratories, Chaska, Minn.). This purified IgE is normally used for competitive binding in radioimmunoassays for detection of human IgE levels. After preincubation of conjugates with human IgE, reactions between the conjugate and secretions known to be positive were completely blocked, indicating that the conjugate was in fact measuring IgE in secretions. The purified human IgE was not capable of blocking the reaction of horseradish peroxidase-conjugated goat anti-human IgA or anti-human IgG, indicating that the human IgE compound was not contaminated with other immunoglobulins. Also, the conjugated anti-human IgE developed no precipitin lines when tested by immunoelectrophoresis against human light chains or normal human serum. By contrast, a single precipitin line formed when the anti-human IgE was run against purified human IgE. Finally, aliquots of the secretions were preincubated overnight with either RSV-infected or uninfected tissue-culture cells. Incuation of known positive secretions with RSV-infected cells, followed by centrifugation and testing of the supernatant fluid in the ELISA assay, resulted in detection of titers below 4, whereas similar exposure of positive secretions to uninfected cells did not result in blocking, demonstrating that the IgE was virus-specific.

Secretions were also available from eight patients with influenza or parainfluenza virus infections but without documented previous RSV infection. Testing of these secretions for RSV-IgE indicated titers below four in all eight patients, even though three of them had wheezing at the time of influenza or parainfluenza virus infection.

Histamine Content of Secretions

Specimens of nasopharyngeal secretions for detection of histamine were obtained from 49 unselected study patients within 20 days (usually within seven days) of the onset of illness, by aspiration into mucus traps as described above, except that catheters were rinsed throughout with 2.5 ml of phosphate-buffered saline. Cells were separated by centrifugation; the supernatant fluids were decanted, acidified by adding two drops of 1 N hydrochloric acid, and frozen at $-20°C$ before testing. Histamine content was determined with minor modifications of automated fluorometric methods previously described.[9] Histamine concentrations below 1 ng per ml (before standardization) were considered negative for the presence of histamine. Reassurance that the fluorometric material was indeed histamine was obtained by demonstrating that the quantity of histamine measured could be reduced by exposure to diamine oxidase, an enzyme that degrades histamine. The nondegradable fraction of histamine probably represents 1-methylhistamine (the major metabolite of histamine), which is not oxidized by diamine oxidase. Final histamine concentrations were standardized to a protein content in the mixtures containing secretions and phosphate-buffered saline (1 mg per milliliter).

Arterial Blood Gas Determinations

Arterial blood gases, with the patient breathing room air, are routinely obtained by house officers on at least one occasion before administering oxygen as part of the routine care of patients with respiratory illness at our institution. The lowest arterial partial pressure of oxygen (pO_2) with the patient breathing room air was used as an indicator of severity of illness.

Statistical Analysis

Differences in titers of RSV-IgE or of histamine content in nasopharyngeal secretions among patients in the four illness groups were calculated by Student's *t*-test. Chi-square analysis was used to compare the rates of detection of RSV-IgE and histamine among illness groups. Regression lines demonstrating the correlation of degree of hypoxia with either IgE titer or histamine concentration were calculated with the least-squares method, and correlation coefficients (r-values) were calculated according to standard methods.

RESULTS

Appearance of Cell-Bound IgE

The results of immunofluorescence testing for the presence of RSV antigen and IgE are shown in FIGURE 1. Viral antigen could be detected in samples of nasopharyngeal epithelial cells (NPEC) in all patients tested up to 10 days after the onset of illness. Viral antigen could be detected in approximately 40 to 50% of samples taken from patients 21 to 55 days after the onset of illness, but the antigen was not detectable more than 8 weeks after infection. The persistence of viral antigen in NPEC was not related to the form of illness present. Cell-bound IgE was demonstrated in NPEC from 50 to 70% of patients in the first 10 days of illness, in 30 to 35% of patients from 21 to 55 days after the onset of illness, and in 3 patients (23%) 8 weeks or more after the illness. In these patients, over one half of the RSV-infected cells showed cell-bound IgE early in the illness. This proportion decreased over the course of the illness. In most patients, the period after infection when virus antigen could be detected was longer than the period of detection of IgE. In three patients, however, IgE, which was previously found only on RSV-infected cells, was still detectable 56 days or more after infection, when viral antigen was no longer detectable.

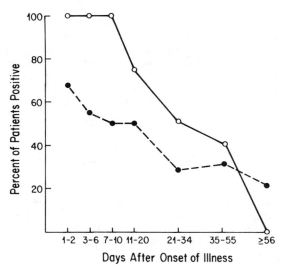

FIGURE 1. Detection of RSV antigen (open circles) and cell-bound IgE (solid circles) on exfoliated nasopharyngeal epithelial cells at various intervals after the onset of illness due to respiratory syncytial virus. (R.C. Welliver, T.N. Kaul, & P.L. Ogra.[9] With permission from the *New England Journal of Medicine*).

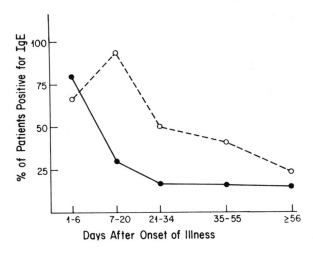

FIGURE 2. Relation of form of illness to persistence of cell-bound IgE in the respiratory tract after respiratory syncytial virus infection. The solid line indicates results in patients with upper-respiratory tract illness or pneumonia; the broken line indicates results in patients with bronchiolitis or asthma (R.C. Welliver, *et al.*[9] With permission from the *New England Journal of Medicine*).

The relation of the form of clinical illness experienced to the presence and persistence of cell-bound IgE is shown in FIGURE 2. Between 70 and 80% of patients had demonstrable cell-bound IgE in the first 6 days of illness, regardless of the form of clinical illness present. When we studied samples, however, taken 7 to 20 days after the onset of illness, we found that all patients with bronchiolitis or asthma and 33% of patients with upper-respiratory tract illness or pneumonia had evidence of cell-bound IgE. In samples taken 21 to 34 days after the onset of illness, 50% of patients with bronchiolitis or asthma and 17% of patients with upper-respiratory tract illness or pneumonia had cell-bound IgE present. When we pooled the results from samples taken 7 to 34 days after the onset of illness, cell-bound IgE was found in 16 of 22 patients with bronchiolitis or asthma (73%), but in only 4 of 15 patients with upper-respiratory-tract illness or pneumonia (27%)—a difference that was statistically significant (chi-square with Yates' correction = 4.18; $p < 0.05$). When we studied samples taken 35 to 55 days after the onset of illness, we found cell-bound IgE present in 45% of 22 subjects with bronchiolitis or asthma and in 20% of 10 patients with upper-respiratory tract illness or pneumonia. This difference however, was not statistically significant.

Kinetics of the RSV-IgE Response Free in Secretions

The development of RSV-IgE in the respiratory tracts of all patients at various times after the onset of illness is shown in FIGURE 3. Each point represents the RSV-IgE titer in one patient. Samples were taken on no more than three occasions per patient. RSV-IgE could be detected in secretions as early as one to three days after the onset of illness. The mean titer for the entire group increased over the study period, and RSV-IgE persisted in many patients throughout the first 5 to 13 weeks of the follow-up period.

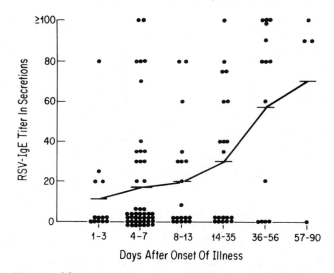

FIGURE 3. Kinetics of the RSV-IgE secretory antibody response. Each point represents the RSV-IgE titer determined in secretions from a single patient at various times after the onset of illness; no patient is represented by more than three determinations. The solid line connects the arithmetic mean at each time point. The observed titers are standardized to a protein concentration in fluid of 10 mg per milliliter. (Reprinted, by permission of the *New England Journal of Medicine*. 1981. **305**: 843).

RSV-IgE Response According to Illness Group

In this phase of the study, patients were classified as having upper-respiratory illness alone (Group I, 9 patients), pneumonia without wheezing (Group II, 9 patients), pneumonia with wheezing (Group III, 10 patients) and bronchiolitis without pneumonia (Group IV, 43 patients) according to criteria previously described.[9]

RSV-IgE responses in the four illness groups are shown in FIGURE 4. Antibody titers in secretions obtained 1 to 7 days and 14 to 90 days after the onset of illness were pooled to represent the acute and convalescent phases. Results are represented no more than once per patient, in the one-to-seven-day period, and no more than twice per patient in the 14-to-90 day period. Over 80% of patients had only one convalescent-phase sample taken, regardless of illness group. In the acute phase, RSV-IgE antibody could not be detected in any patient in Group I or II; but the antibody was detected in 3 of 10 patients in Group III (the mean titer was 22) and in 21 of 43 patients (49%) in Group IV (mean titer, 19.8). Statistically significant differences were observed when comparing the mean RSV-IgE titer in patients in Group IV with that in patients in either Group I or Group II (in either compaison, $t > 3.80$, $p < 0.005$), and the mean RSV-IgE titer in patients in Group III and IV combined (wheezing) with that in Groups I and II combined (no wheezing) ($t = 2.48$, $p < 0.05$). Furthermore, the incidence of RSV-IgE among patients in Group III or IV combined was significantly increased, as compared with that among patients in Groups I and II combined (chi-square = 6.82, $p < 0.01$).

In the convalescent phase, RSV-IgE was undetectable in Group I and was present in only 14% of the patients in Group II (mean titer, 8). By contrast, RSV-IgE was detectable in 60% of the patients in Group III (mean titer, 44.6) and in 68% of those in Group IV (mean titer, 60.1). Statistically significant differences were observed when comparing the mean RSV-IgE titer in Group IV with that in Groups I and II combined (t = 2.27, p < 0.05), the mean RSV-IgE titer in Group IV with that in Group I and II combined (t = 3.98, p < 0.01), the mean RSV-IgE titer in Groups III and IV combined (wheezing) with that of Groups I and II combined (no wheezing) (t = 3.28, p < 0.01), and the incidence of RSV-IgE in Groups III and IV combined with that in Groups I and II combined (chi-square = 4.03, p < 0.05).

Relation of Peak RSV-IgE Response to Degree of Hypoxia

The relation between the peak RSV-IgE response and the lowest arterial partial pressure of oxygen is shown in FIGURE 5, as determined in each patient studied. Only data from patients in whom samples were taken for RSV-IgE determination at least 14 days after the onset of illness (to allow detection of peak responses) are included in the figure. Patients, however, with all forms of illness are included. A high significant correlation between peak RSV-IgE response and severity of illness, as determined by the degree of hypoxia, was observed (r= −0.47, p < 0.01).

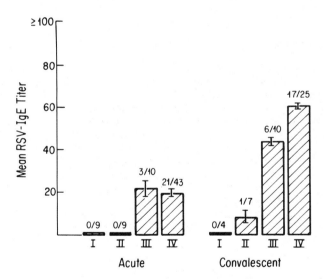

FIGURE 4. The RSV-IgE response analyzed according to illness group. The fractions represent the number of patients positive for RSV-IgE per number tested. Bars represent arithmetic mean for the RSV-IgE titer (±1 S.E.). Group I had upper-respiratory tract disease only; group II—pneumonia without wheezing; group III—pneumonia with wheezing; and group IV—bronchiolitis without pneumonia. The acute phase represents the first seven days after the onset of illness, and the convalescent phase the 14th through the 90th day after the onset of illness. (Reprinted, by permission of the *New England Journal of Medicine* 1981. **305:** 843).

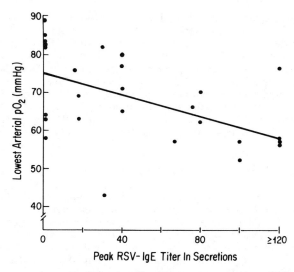

FIGURE 5. Relation of peak RSV-IgE titer to degree of hypoxia. The solid line was calculated by the method of least squares. Coefficient of correlation, $r = -0.47$; $p < 0.01$; pO_2 denotes partial pressure of oxygen. (Reprinted, by permission of the *New England Journal of Medicine* 1981. **305**: 844).

Analysis of Histamine Content According to Illness Group

Samples of nasopharyngeal secretions were obtained for analysis of histamine content at various times for up to 20 days after the onset of illness. In patients from whom sequential samples were obtained, the concentration of histamine measured did not vary over this period. Mean peak concentrations of histamine in the four illness groups are shown in TABLE 1. Histamine levels above one ng per milliliter of secretion-buffer mixture were present in all illness groups. Statistically significant differences in the mean concentrations of histamine were observed when either Group III or Group IV was compared with Groups I and II

TABLE 1

HISTAMINE CONTENT IN NASOPHARYNGEAL SECRETIONS

Illness Group*	No. Patients Positive/No. Tested	Histamine Content ng/ml of mixture† (mean ± S.E.)
I	1/2	1.1 ± 1.0
II	2/10	0.6 ± 0.02
III	7/8	2.7 ± 0.3
IV	20/29	2.8 ± 0.2

*When Groups III and IV (wheezing) were compared with Groups I and II (no wheezing), there were statistically significant differences in the incidence of detectable histamine and mean histamine concentrations.

†Mixture of nasopharyngeal secretions and phosphate-buffered saline.

combined (in either comparison, t ≥ 2.1, p < 0.05). Statistically significant differences were also observed when the incidence of detectable histamine in Groups III and IV combined was compared with this incidence in Groups I and II combined (chi-square = 6.88, p < 0.001).

Relationship of Histamine Concentration to Degree of Hypoxia

A statistically significant correlation (r = − 0.34, p = 0.05) between peak histamine concentration and degree of hypoxia was observed (data not shown).

DISCUSSION

The present study demonstrates the appearance of IgE immunoglobulin both on the surface of exfoliated airway epithelial cells, and free in NPS following infection with RSV in infancy. We believe that the cell-bound IgE is specific for RSV in that it was found almost exclusively on those cells that simultaneously could be shown to be expressing RSV antigen. In the three instances in which cells were positive for IgE and negative for RSV, samples were obtained eight weeks after the onset of illness, at which time the amount of antigen expressed on the cell surface may have been so small that it could not have been detected by immunofluorescence. Another possibility is that the IgE was bound nonspecifically to an RSV-induced receptor for IgE. Attempts, however, to induce such a receptor through infection of human epithelial cells *in vitro* were unsuccessful. That the IgE antibody free in secretions was indeed specific for RSV was confirmed by the blocking experiments described above.

Cell-bound IgE was observed in samples obtained from patients with all forms of clinical illness due to respiratory syncytial virus. Because assays for RSV-IgE free in secretions were uniformly negative in patients with upper-respiratory infection alone, this finding suggests that the amount of RSV-IgE produced in these patients was comparatively small. The overall kinetics of the appearance of cell-bound and cell-free IgE (FIGURES 2 and 3) would also suggest that small amounts of IgE initially produced are bound to cell surfaces, presumably to viral antigen, whereas RSV-IgE appears free in secretions only after all such binding sites have been saturated.

It is unclear whether the lesser amount of IgE found in patients without wheezing plays a role in eradication of RSV from the respiratory tract, or alternatively, is present in such small amounts so as not to result in clinically evident airway obstruction. The presence of small amounts of histamine in secretions of patients with upper-respiratory infection alone or pneumonia without wheezing suggests that minor quantities of IgE produced in these patients may have resulted in the release of modest quantities of histamine. Also, it has been observed[10] that patients with RSV pneumonia often have radiographic evidence of hyperinflation of the chest in the absence of audible wheezing. It seems possible that this minor degree of airway obstruction may result from production of low titers of IgE and release of small quantities of histamine. The appearance of larger quantities of RSV-IgE and of histamine seems to play a major role in lower respiratory illness due to RSV infection, in that both compounds were present more frequently and in greater quantities in patients with RSV-induced wheezing than in infected patients without wheezing. Peak levels of RSV-IgE and histamine were also correlated with the degree of arterial hypoxemia. In subsequent studies from our laboratory (data not shown) it has been observed that RSV-IgE persists in NPS in detectable quantities for two to three months after the onset of illness, and that measurable amounts of histamine are present for roughly the same period. It is currently unclear what role the persistence of histamine in NPS plays in predisposing the development of subsequent episodes of wheezing after RSV infection. The results of our studies to date identify a mechanism by which viral infections may result in wheezing, and may explain the recognized association of a family history of atopy with the development of recurrent episodes of wheezing after RSV infection in infancy.[11]

REFERENCES

1. CAPRON, A., A. J. DESSEIN, M. CAPRON, H. BAZIN. 1975. Specific IgE antibodies in immune adherence of normal macrophages to S. mansoni echistosomulas. Nature (London) **253**: 474.
2. HAQUE, A., A. OUAISSI, M. JOSEPH, M. CAPRON & A. CAPRON. 1981. IgE antibody in eosinophil-and macrophage-mediated in vitro killing of dipetalonema viteae microfilariae. J. Immunol. **127**: 716–725.
3. RUITENBERG, J., P. A. STEERENBERG. 1974. Intestingal phase of Trichinella spiralis in congenitally athymic mice. J. Parasit. **60**: 1056.
4. DESSEIN, A. J., W. L. PARKER, S. L. JAMES, J. R. DAVID. 1981. IgE antibody and resistance to infection. I. Selective suppression of the IgE response in rats diminishes the resistance and the eosinophil response to T. spiralis infection. J. Exp. Med. **193**:423–436.
5. SHEN, J., P. BRACKETT, T. FISCHER, A. HOLDER, F. KELLOGG & J. G. MICHAEL 1981. Specific Pseudomonas immunoglobulin E antibodies in sera of patients with cystic fibrosis. Infect. Immunity **32**: 967–968.
6. HENDERSON, F. W., W. A. CLYDE Jr., A. M. COLLIER, F. W. DENNY. 1979. The etiologic and epidemiologic spectrum of bronchiolitis in pediatric practice. J. Pediatr. **95**: 183–190.
7. SIMS, D. G., 1979. Infections in the wheezy child. J.R. Soc. Med. **72**: 54–56.
8. KIM, H. W., J. O. ARROBIO, C. D. BRANDT et al. 1973. Epidemiology of respiratory syncytial virus infection in Washington, D.C. I. Importance of the virus in different respiratory tract disease syndromes and temporal distribution of infection. Am. J. Epidemiol. **98**: 216–225.
9. WELLIVER, R. C., T. N. KAUL & P. L. OGRA. 1980. The appearance of cell-bound IgE in respiratory-tract epithelium after respiratory-syncytial-virus infection. N. Engl. J. Med. **303**: 1198–1202.
10. RICE, R. P., & F. LODA. 1966. A roentgenographic analysis of respiratory syncytial virus pneumonia in infants. Radiology **87**: 1021–1027.
11. ROONEY, J. C., & H. E. WILLIAMS. 1971. The relationship between proved viral bronchiolitis and subsequent wheezing. J. Pediatr. **79**: 744–747.

DISCUSSION OF THE PAPER

B. H. WAKSMAN (National Multiple Sclerosis Society, New York, N.Y.): I have two questions and a comment. You have emphasized what you might call the immunopathological effector arm of the response and have not stressed at all the question of whether this is a mucosal immune system. When you performed blood gas analyses, did you also measure blood antibody (IgE) levels. This information would give us an opportunity to know if some of these patients had a purely mucosal response.

The second question has to do with the effector role of IgE in immunity. Was there any evidence to show correlation between the development of a local IgE antibody response and some diminution in the amount of virus that was present at particular times in these patients?

The third point is simply a comment. You showed a slide that left an impression that is perhaps slightly misleading. It was the slide in which you showed the time course of IgE-antibody formation. There were many points along the bottom line at zero, and then there was a scattering of points above zero. You drew a line that averaged all these things and conveyed the impression that this response is a slow and late one. Nevertheless, what the slide really showed was that in those patients who do respond, the response begins by three days. You might wish a comment on this point.

R. C. WELLIVER (*State University of New York at Buffalo*): Subsequent to this study we have looked at virus specific IgE in serum. It does occur there, but it appears to occur at least a week later than we can detect RSV IgE in secretions. Based upon this information and data of others, where IgE-forming cells appear to be localized primarily at mucosal surfaces, we would suggest that this response is a mucosal one, and that IgE appears in the serum only after a large volume of IgE has been produced at the mucosal surface. With regard to the second question, we found no differences in the patients' responses. In fact, these patients continued to show virus long after secretory antibodies were present in good titers. IgE really did not play much role in reduction of shedding of the virus.

G. H. LOWELL (*Walter Reed Army Institute of Research, Washington, D.C.*): Your ELISA system offers you a nice method to measure IgE, as well as IgA and IgG antibody titers in the same secretion. Have you looked at the ratio of IgE to IgG or IgA, and can this be correlated with the clinical course of the disease? Certainly, the increase in IgE in convalescent secretions would suggest that IgE might be playing a good role for the host.

WELLIVER: Yes, we have done this correlation. The overall kinetics of appearance of IgA, IgG, IgM, and IgE in secretions is about the same, and the ratio of IgA to IgE remains the same throughout the course of the illness. They both peak at roughly the same time and disappear at approximately the same time. Both can be present at the same time that cultivable virus is present in secretions. So, if IgE is particularly good for you, you can not prove it on the basis of that data.

D. E. BOCKMAN (*Medical College of Georgia, Augusta, Ga.*): You indicated that you were looking at surface IgE, yet you use fixed cells in these studies. Did you actually perform studies to determine whether the IgE was on the surface or intracellular? This is important because the functional implications would be different.

WELLIVER: That is a good point, and because the cells in my studies were acetone-fixed, I cannot differentiate surface from intracytoplasmic IgE.

R. M. GOLDBLUM (*University of Texas, Galveston, Tex.*): How do you perceive the relationship between the virus, the epithelial cell, and the IgE antibody? I know of no information that would say that epithelial cells have a specific receptor for the Fc portion of IgE. Are these really epithelial cells, or could they be basophils that have been infected with viruses and thus cause the release of mediators that then lead to clinical problems? Once the basophils have released their granules, it might be much more difficult to distinguish them from epithelial cells.

WELLIVER: These cells have the size and morphology of epithelial cells and when one examines recovered cells, no basophils are present. One primarily sees an epithelial cell. Regarding the Fc receptor, we have infected epithelial tissue culture cells with RSV and incubated them with human IgE, and there is no adherence by ways of the Fc receptor.

GOLDBLUM: Are you suggesting that binding is occurring by way of, for example, specific Fab binding to RSV?

WELLIVER: Yes.

P. BRANDTZAEG (National Hospital, Oslo, Norway): I am not sure we should agree that IgE is a mucosal antibody in terms of it being a secretory antibody such as IgA and IgM. There is no evidence for a specific secretion of IgE through glandular structures. I also do not think there are any studies showing a particular prominence of IgE responses at mucous membranes. On the other hand, we have looked at tissues from patients with atopic rhinitis and milk allergies, and we do not find any accumulation of IgE-producing cells. I think Maeyerhofer showed several years ago with his model of Nippostrongylus infection that the IgE response was located in the mesenteric lymph nodes and not in the mucosa. Nevertheless, we find numerous mast cells appearing in mucous membranes that may contain IgE. But, IgE does not seem to be synthesized in the mucous membrane.

WELLIVER: Although there may be some species differences, the studies that I am aware of have looked for IgE-producing B-cells and have found them at mucosal surfaces but not in peripheral lymph nodes, or in mesenteric lymph nodes. From that data, you would presume that we are dealing with mucosal process.

BRANDTZAEG: These are B-cells with membrane IgE; however, I was referring to cytoplasmic production of IgE.

WAKSMAN: These are, of course, very important issues that Dr. Brandtzaeg raises and I would like to add two more words on this subject. First of all, in the Tada-Ishizaka paper, which first described localization of IgE cells in mucosae, those were plasma cells, not B-cells. This point was again demonstrated in later studies. I did not imply that IgE is secretory, but instead, that it is a mucosal response, that is, the antibody is synthesized at mucosal sites.

BRANDTZAEG: Of course, I do not refute that IgE responses may take place in the mucous membranes, like IgG, IgM, and IgD responses may take place in mucous membranes. I do not agree with this concept, however, that IgE follows IgA responses in particular, as in the paper you mentioned on tonsils. This data cannot be reproduced using specific antisera. We have looked at this problem many times, and we do not find IgE-producing cells in tonsils. I think the balance of evidence on mucous membranes and IgE-producing cells would favor that there is no particular tendency for an IgE response in mucous membranes.

AGING AND THE MUCOSAL-ASSOCIATED LYMPHOID SYSTEM*

Myron R. Szewczuk† and Andrew W. Wade

Department of Microbiology and Immunology
Queen's University
Kingston, Ontario, Canada K7L 3N6

INTRODUCTION

It is becoming increasingly accepted that immune function declines with age in man and experimental animals. This decline in the immune system during aging has been related to changes that involve the cells themselves, the properties of such cells, and the environmental influences in which these cells must function.[1] We understand little of the mechanisms underlying this decline. Efforts have been concentrated on the rate and the degree of decline of the major components of the systemic immune system.[2] Moreover, there is no information on the effect of aging on the immune function at different local sites of the immune system, for an example, the mucosal lymphoid apparatus.

It is well known that the ability to produce a humoral immune response is dependent on the interaction or collaboration of T-lymphocytes (both T-helper cells and T-suppressor cells), macrophages, and B-cells. The decline in antibody-forming capacity seen with aging could be attributed to an alteration in the number or function of any or all of these three cell types. Such an alteration might consist of an absolute decrease in cell number, for example, cell death, a relative decrease in cell number, for example, increase in suppressor-cell activity, and/or a decrease in the functional efficiency of any or all of the above individual cells. Interplay of cellular components is essential for efficient immune function, and any disturbance of this cell-cell communication might arise as a result of several factors. The decrease in immune function of the aged may be expressed quite differently from one individual to another, and this expression may account for the great variability seen in the immunological studies on aging.

AGING AND THE IMMUNE SYSTEM

There is considerable evidence to suggest a relationship between aging and a decline in B-cell function. For example, thymic (T)-dependent splenic B-cell responses are most affected by age, as manifested by a depressed splenic response to T-dependent antigens.[3-7] In addition, splenic B-cell responses to T-cell-independent antigens have been shown to decrease with age.[8,9] Studies by Singhal and coworkers[10] showed that the intrinsic proliferative capacity of bone marrow B-cells from old mice to B-cell mitogens is normal and have suggested that the decline in antibody production in old animals may be due in part to a decline in proliferative potential of the antibody-forming cell precursors. By

*This work was supported in part by the Medical Research Council of Canada, Grant No. MA-7347, the Muscular Dystrophy Association of Canada, and the Gerontology Research Council of Ontario.

†Gerontology Research Council of Ontario Scholar.

333

contrast to that found with bone marrow B-cells, Callard[11] found that spleen cells from old mice responded less well to mitogens than those from young mice.

On the other hand, others have found that the number of B-cells in lymph nodes and spleen do not change appreciably with age[12] but that there is an increase in the number of plasma cells, especially in mice of certain autoimmune-prone strains.[13] Studies on the total number of stem cells from mouse bone marrow have shown that they remain quite constant with age[14] and appear not to lose their lymphohematopoietic activity.[15] The rate of B-cell formation appeared to decline with age.[16] More recently, Woda and Feldman[17] have found that there is a loss with age of splenic cells with a high density of surface Ig. It is still unclear whether this age-associated decline in B-cell immunocompetence includes a relative decrease in cellular activity or a loss of functional efficiency.

To explain these observations of B-cell functions that accompany aging, it has been suggested[18] that the environment in which the cells find themselves might induce changes in these cells that in turn affect their responsiveness essential to their differentiation. Other explanations may lie in the intrinsic nature of the cells or their properties.

Results of studies on macrophages have shown that their handling of antigens is not affected with age, both during the induction of immune responses and by ingestion of antigenic aggregates.[11,19,20]

The decline in immune function that accompanies aging has also been shown to be due to changes in T-cell functions. Some functional studies include several topics: age-related decline in delayed hypersensitivity in man[21] and in mice,[22] which has been attributed to T-suppressor cells; decreased ability to mount a vigorous graft-versus-host reaction;[23] a decline in proliferative capacity of human T-cells[24,25] and rodent splenic T-cells in response to mitogens;[26] a decline in generation of cytotoxic cells against tumors;[23] a decrease in T-helper cell functions as is revealed by in vivo and in vitro assays;[3-8] and a decline in suppressor cell activity on T-cell functions[27] or an increase in suppressor-cell activity that influences antibody production.[8,28] It is still not clear, however, whether a defect in T-lymphocyte function in aging animals represents a reduction in T-helper cell activity or an increase in T-suppressor cell activity.

MUCOSAL-ASSOCIATED LYMPHOID SYSTEM

Other than the observations of Singhal and coworkers,[10] that bone marrow B-cells of old mice have a normal proliferative response to B-cell mitogens in vitro as compared with young mice, relatively little is known of the effects of aging on the immune function at various lymphatic sites, for example, the peripheral lymph nodes and the mucosal lymphoid apparatus. It has been suggested that the mucosal lymphoid apparatus differs from the systemic lymphoid system.[29,30] For example, Peyer's patch cells have IgA surface receptors but little intracellular IgA, that is, they are not at the stage of secreting IgA, although they can do so if cultured in vitro.[31] In addition, it has been shown that Peyer's patch cells do not respond to antigen applied intraluminally,[32] but respond minimally to antigen given directly.[33] Cells of the mesenteric lymph node and thoracic duct have large numbers of cells already secreting IgA.[29] The primary interaction of antigen with lymphocytes may take place in the Peyer's patches; the primed cells start differentiating, then may migrate by way of efferent lymphatics to the mesenteric lymph nodes. Efferent lymphatics from the mesenteric nodes empty into the thoracic duct and the contents of the duct are emptied into the general circulation at the subclavian vein.[29]

Cebra et al.[34,35] looked at the antigen sensitivity of Peyer's patch cells and compared these with cells from peripheral lymph nodes and spleen from young animals. They found that the frequency of clonal precursor cells in Peyer's patches reactive with phosphorylcholine was no different than that found for B-cells from peripheral lymph nodes, spleen, and mesenteric lymph nodes. The proportion of precursors, however, that gave rise to clones expressing anti-phosphorylcholine was much lower in Peyer's patches and mesenteric lymph nodes (39–48%) than in peripheral lymph nodes and spleen (70–74%). In addition, the clonal precursor population derived from Peyer's patches is also strikingly different from that derived from spleen, because Peyer's patch B-cells make more IgA antibody than splenic-derived clones (84 as compared to 50%, respectively), and the frequency of clones making only IgA antibody is much higher in Peyer's patches (42%) than in spleen (4%).

No correlation was observed between clone size (total antibody produced) and the isotypes of Ig expressed. These findings were interpreted as indicating that Peyer's patch cells are under different stimulation from their microenvironment than are cells found in peripheral lymph nodes or spleen. There may be other alternatives to explain these differences, for example, initial localization of specialized cells in those sites.

SITE PREFERENCE FOR A DECLINE IN IMMUNE COMPETENCE WITH AGING

We have looked at the effect of aging on immune reactivity to trinitrophen-ylated bovine gamma globulin (TNP-BGG) immunization in C57BL/6J male mice. The magnitude of the immune response in old and young mice was measured in various lymphatic sites using the plaque-forming cell (PFC) assay as a probe for changes in humoral immune reactivity at a cellular level. Age kinetic studies[36] revealed that the number of IgM, IgG, and IgA anti-TNP PFC in the spleen reached a peak response at four months of age. After four months, there was a significant decline in the number of PFC as compared with the peak response of mice at four months of age (FIGURE 1). We have also shown[36] that old mice given antigen in the footpads and the base of the tail produced a reduced number of IgM, IgG, and IgA PFC responses in the draining peripheral lymph nodes (FIGURE 1). These results strongly support the view that the systemic lymphoid system declines in immune function with increasing age of the animal.

By contrast, no significant decline in the number of IgM, IgG, and IgA anti-TNP PFC in the mesenteric and mediastinal (or bronchial) lymph nodes[36] of mice over four months of age was observed (FIGURE 1). When TNP-BGG in complete Freund's adjuvant (CFA) was given by way of gastric intubation,[36] the anti-TNP PFC responses in the draining mesenteric lymph node as well as in the spleen from old mice were significantly enhanced as compared with the responses of the young control group (FIGURE 2). It is interesting that splenic PFC responses of old mice to TNP-BGG immunized by way of gastric intubation were in contrast to the findings of antigen presented intraperitoneally. The exact nature of these differences due to route of immunization remains unclear.

The findings in these studies suggest a lack of age-associated immune dysfunction in the mucosal-associated lymph nodes. Explanations may be a result of the following: (a) Shifts in subpopulations of T-helper and suppressor lympho-cytes may occur between mucosal and systemic tissues with age. Evidence for support of this view comes from studies by Mattingly and Waksman,[37] who have shown that young adult rats given sheep red blood cells (SRBC) orally had specific suppressor cells to the antigen in their Peyer's patches and mesenteric lymph

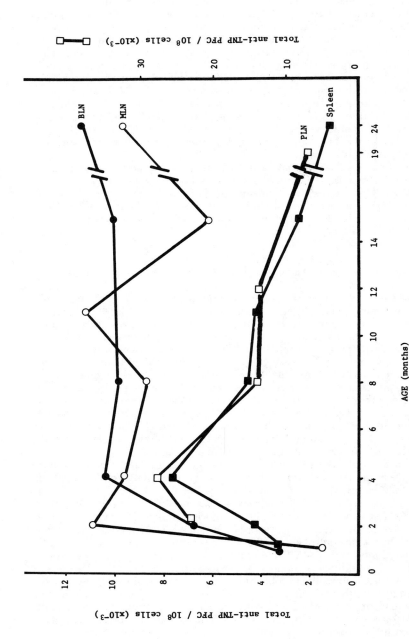

FIGURE 1. Effect of age on the total number of anti-TNP PFC responses of C57BL/6J mice. Male mice received 500 µg TNP-BGG in CFA intraperitoneally. Splenic (■), mediastinal (or bronchial) lymph node (BLN, ●), and mesenteric lymph node (MLN O) anti-TNP PFC per 10^8 nucleated cells were assayed two weeks after immunization. For peripheral lymph node (PLN, □) responses, mice received TNP-BGG in CFA distributed in the four footpads and the base of the tail. PLN including axillary, brachial, popliteal, sciatic, inguinal, caudal, and lumbar were pooled from individual mice. The total number of PFC as a function of age are the sum total of the number of IgM, IgG, and IgA anti-TNP PFC. [M.R. Szewczuk, R.J. Campbell & L.K. Jung.[36] With permission from the *Journal of Immunology*].

nodes after two days of feeding. After four days of feeding, similar suppressor cells were found in the thymus and spleen, but were missing in Peyer's patches or mesenteric lymph nodes. Similar findings were obtained using soluble ovalbumin given by gastric intubation.[38] Kagnoff[39] and Kiyono et al.,[40] on the other hand, have shown that feeding mice with SRBC primes Peyer's patch lymphocytes for T-helper cell activity. (b) Memory cells may reside in mucosal areas as a result of gut antigen priming and thus give secondary-type responses. In support of this view, Gearhart and Cebra[41] found that animals immunized with phosphorylcholine and inulin, which are found on intestinal bacteria, produced secondary-type

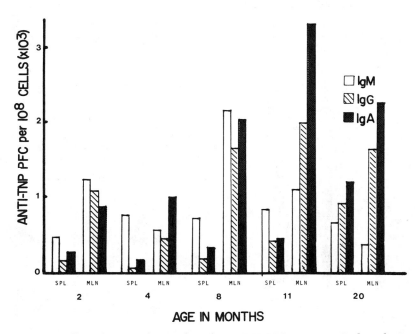

FIGURE 2. Effect of age on the number of anti-TNP PFC responses in the spleen and mesenteric lymph nodes by way of gastric intubation immunization. Male mice received 500 μg TNP-BGG in CFA by gastric intubation. Splenic (SPL) and mesenteric lymph node (MLN) anti-TNP PFC per 10^8 nucleated cells were assayed two weeks after immunization.

responses. It is unclear, however, what the "primary" antigens are in the mucosal areas of old animals that give rise to an elevated PFC response to TNP-BGG.

This differential effect of aging on immune responses *in vivo* of mucosal and systemic lymphoid tissues suggests a site preference for an age-related decline in immune function.

HETEROGENEITY OF AFFINITY OF THE PRIMARY PLAQUE-FORMING CELL
RESPONSE IN MUCOSAL LYMPH NODES OF MICE OF DIFFERENT AGES

Male C57BL/6J mice of different ages were immunized i.p. with TNP-BGG in complete Freund's adjuvant. The number of IgM, IgG, and IgA anti-TNP PFC

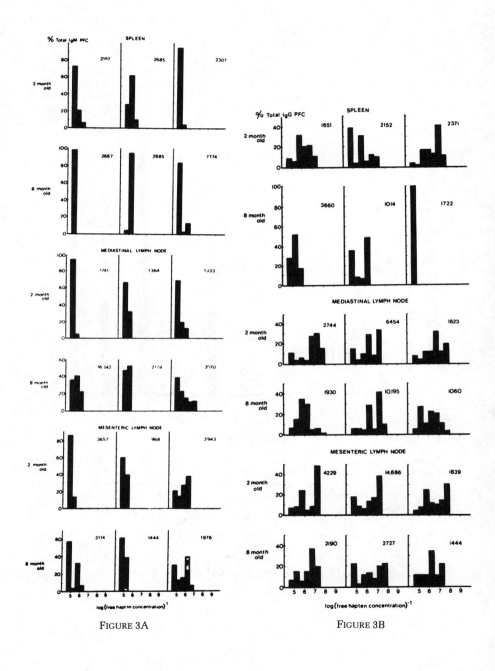

FIGURE 3A

FIGURE 3B

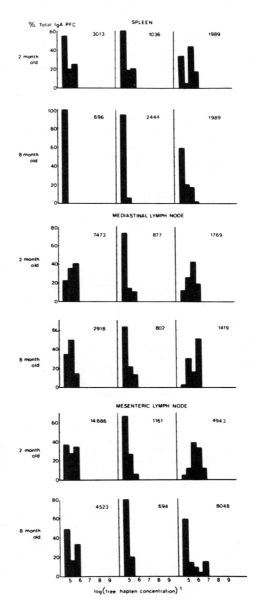

FIGURE 3. Affinity distributions of the primary IgM (left), IgG (center), and IgA (right) PFC responses in the spleen, mediastinal, and mesenteric lymph nodes of C57BL/6J male mice of different ages. Each histogram illustrates the distribution of anti-TNP PFC with respect to affinity in pooled tissues from mice 14 days after immunization with 500 μg TNP-BGG in CFA i.p. In the first (upper) and second rows are data on the splenic PFC responses. In the third and fourth rows are the data on the mediastinal lymph node PFC responses. In the fifth and sixth rows are data on the mesenteric lymph node PFC responses. The abscissa represents the log of the inverse of the free hapten concentration used in the plaque inhibition assay. The ordinate represents the percentage of the total population of PFC present in each subpopulation. Affinity increases to the right. The number of PFC per 10^8 nucleated cells is indicated to the right upper corner of each histogram. (M.R. Szewczuk & R.J. Campbell.[43] With permission from the *Journal of Immunology*).

FIGURE 3C

and the distribution of the PFC with regard to avidity in the spleen, mesenteric, and mediastinal lymph nodes, were determined two weeks after immunization. The distribution of IgM, IgG, and IgA PFC with regard to avidity was determined by hapten inhibition of plaque formation. The distribution of affinity may be quantitated using the Shannon heterogeneity index,[42] thereby permitting a simple statistical evaluation of the data. This index is expressed as a $\log_2$ term and multiplies with increasing heterogeneity of the PFC distribution. The results are presented in FIGURE 3 and TABLE 1. Plaque-forming cells from all lymphoid tissues of two-month-old mice were highly heterogeneous and were of high average avidity. With aging, the primary splenic PFC response was found to be markedly restricted in heterogeneity, with a preferential loss of IgM, IgG, and IgA high avidity plaque-forming cells.[43] The draining peripheral lymph node IgG PFC response of old mice exhibited similar restriction in heterogeneity, with a preferential loss of high avidity plaque-forming cells.[43] By contrast, mesenteric

TABLE 1

EFFECT OF AGE ON THE HETEROGENEITY OF AFFINITY OF ANTI-TNP PFC RESPONSES IN DIFFERENT LYMPHATIC SITES OF $C_{57}BL/6J$ MICE[43]

Age	Tissues*	Affinity Index for		
		IgG PFC	IgM PFC	IgA PFC
2 months	SPL	2.27 ± 0.13	0.88 ± 0.52	1.50 ± 0.18
	PLN	2.00 ± 0.16	N.D.	N.D.
	BLN	2.43 ± 0.21	0.80 ± 0.46	1.49 ± 0.39
	MLN	2.31 ± 0.25	1.15 ± 0.68	1.57 ± 0.43
4 months	SPL	2.04 ± 0.27 $p < 0.02$	1.64 ± 0.49	2.12 ± 0.20
	PLN	2.12 ± 0.17	N.D.	N.D.
	BLN	2.62 ± 0.01	0.92 ± 0.66	1.71 ± 0.03
	MLN	2.53 ± 0.52	0.75 ± 1.05	1.77 ± 0.47
8 months	SPL	1.22 ± 0.83 $p < 0.001$	0.37 ± 0.34	0.52 ± 0.27 $p < 0.001$
	PLN	1.53 ± 0.41 $p < 0.05$	N.D.	N.D.
	BLN	2.53 ± 0.18	1.57 ± 0.58	1.44 ± 0.15
	MLN	2.45 ± 0.15	1.49 ± 0.55	1.30 ± 0.52
15–19 months	SPL	1.15 ± 0.91 $p < 0.02$	0.33	0.37
	PLN	1.28 ± 0.21 $p < 0.001$	N.D.	N.D.
	BLN	2.26 ± 0.36	1.46 ± 0.05	2.04 ± 0.19
	MLN	2.03 ± 0.42	1.86 ± 0.47	1.50 ± 0.08

*SPL = spleen; PLN = draining peripheral lymph nodes; BLN = mediastinal (or bronchial) lymph nodes; MLN = mesenteric lymph nodes. N.D. = not determined.

and mediastinal lymph node PFC response of old mice remained highly heterogeneous with respect to antibody affinity in the three isotypes studied.[43] The results of these studies imply that T-helper cell activity is unimpaired in the mucosal-associated lymphoid system of old animals, because it has been suggested[49] that impaired T-helper cell activity may contribute to the preferential loss of high affinity plaque-forming cells. The findings provide further support for the notion that the mucosal-associated lymphoid system differs from the systemic system with regard to its immune competence with age.

DIVISION OF THE IMMUNE SYSTEM INTO REGULATORY COMPARTMENTS

Autoanti-idiotypic (Id) antibodies have been shown to be responsible for a decline in the number of PFC, a reduction in the heterogeneity of avidity of PFC, and the occurrence of anti-Id-blocked, hapten-augmentable plaque-forming cells.[44] This autoanti-Id antibody, produced during the course of the immune response was explained, perhaps, by combining with B-cell surface antigen receptors and thus inhibiting antibody secretion. In a recent report, we have demonstrated that the decline in the number of PFC, loss of high-affinity PFC and occurrence of hapten-augmentable PFC with age in the splenic B-cell population was due to autoanti-Id antibody regulation.[45] This finding was subsequently confirmed by Goidl *et al.*[46]

Therefore, we have examined the hypothesis that the lack of age-associated immune dysfunction in the mucosal-associated lymph nodes may be due to a lack of this type of immunoregulation as seen in the spleen. We investigated the appearance of anti-Id-blocked, hapten-augmentable, anti-TNP PFC during the normal immune response to TNP-BGG in C57BL/6J male mice at different ages. It was found[47] that the mesenteric and mediastinal lymph node PFC responses of old mice exhibited no appreciable appearance of anti-Id-blocked, hapten-augmentable anti-TNP PFC (see FIGURE 4). By contrast, eight months or older mice produced a significantly high percentage of hapten-augmentable IgM, IgG, and IgA PFC in the spleen.[45] Furthermore, mice receiving antigen in the footpads and base of the tail also produced a significantly high percentage of hapten-augmentable PFC in the draining peripheral lymph nodes.[47] To verify the specificity of the anti-Id-blocked, hapten-augmentable PFC, TNP-ϵ-amino-n-caproic acid as hapten was found to specifically augment anti-TNP plaque-forming cells.[47] These results are consistent with the hypothesis that a lack of age-associated autoanti-Id antibody regulation occurs in the mucosal-associated lymph nodes from C57BL/6J male mice. On the other hand, regulation of autoanti-Id antibodies was prevalent in the spleen and draining peripheral lymph nodes of the same old animals. These findings introduce an important issue, namely a division of the immune system into regulatory compartments.

SUMMARY AND CONCLUSIONS

Several lines of evidence support the notion that the mucosal-associated lymphoid system differs from the systemic. It is possible that the mucosal lymphoid system may also differ from the systemic system with regard to immune competence with age.

Our findings in these studies indicate a lack of age-associated immune dysfunction in the mucosal-associated lymph nodes: that is, mesenteric and mediastinal lymph node PFC responses of old mice that revealed no decline in magnitude were found to be highly heterogeneous with regard to antibody affinity and revealed no appreciable anti-idiotype-blocked, hapten-augmentable plaque-forming cells. By contrast, the number of splenic and, as well, draining peripheral lymph node IgM, IgG, and IgA anti-TNP PFC responses to TNP-BGG was found to decrease with age with a preferential loss of high affinity plaque-forming cells. This decline in immune activity in the systemic tissues coincided with the increased appearance of anti-idiotype-blocked, hapten-augmentable plaque-forming cells. This differential effect of aging on immune responses *in vivo* of mucosal and systemic lymphoid tissues imply a site preference for an age-related decline in immune function,[36] and a division of the immune system into regulatory compartments during the normal immune response to antigen in old mice.[47]

The present demonstration of a differential effect of aging on immune function *in vivo* raises an important issue with regard to age-related host defense

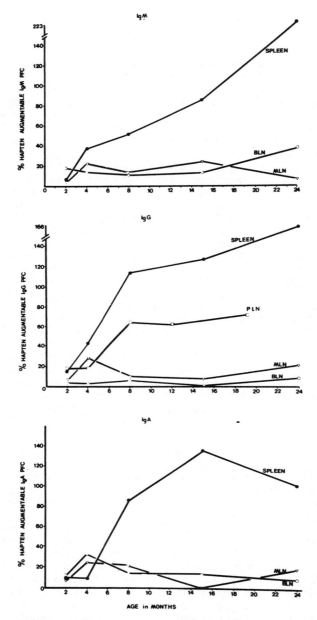

FIGURE 4. Effect of age on the appearance of anti-idiotype-blocked, hapten-augmentable IgM, IgG, and IgA anti-TNP PFC during the normal immune response to TNP-BGG in C57BL/6J mice. Male mice received 500 μg TNP-BGG in CFA i.p. Splenic (●), mediastinal (BLN, ○), and mesenteric (MLN, ▽) lymph node anti-TNP PFC per 10^8 nucleated cells were assayed two weeks after immunization. For peripheral lymph node (PLN, □) responses, mice were immunized with the same antigen, equally distributed in the four footpads and the base of the tail. PLN anti-TNP PFC were assayed 14 days after immunization. Percentage augmentation of PFC by optimal hapten concentration (1×10^{-9} to 1×10^{-7} M TNP-EACA) is calculated as: $100 \times$ (PFC in the presence of hapten − PFC in the absence of hapten)/PFC in the absence of hapten. (M.R. Szewczuk & R.J. Campbell.[45,47] With permission from *Nature* and the *European Journal of Immunology*).

mechanisms. For example, it would seem reasonable to predict that if immune function totally wanes with age, old individuals would be greatly susceptible to disease and infection. On the contrary, host defense mechanisms relevant to infection show minimal alterations in healthy aged individuals.[48] Thus, we believe that mucosal immunity may play a very important role in host defenses in elderly individuals.

REFERENCES

1. YUNIS, E. J., G. FERNANDES & R. A. GOOD. 1978. Aging and involution of the immunological apparatus. *In* The Immunopathology of Lymphoreticular Neoplasms. J. J. Twomey & R. A. Good, Eds.: p. 53. Plenum Publishing Corp. New York.
2. MAKINODAN, T., R. A. GOOD & M. M. B. KAY. 1977. Cellular basis of immunosenescence. *In* Immunology and Aging. T. Makinodan & E. Yunis, Eds.: p. 9. Plenum Publishing Corp. New York.
3. GOIDL, E. A., J. B. INNES & M. E. WEKSLER. 1976. J. Exp. Med. **144:** 1037.
4. KROGSRUD, R. L. & E. H. PERKINS. 1977. J. Immunol. **118:** 1607.
5. WEKSLER, M. E., J. B. INNES & G. GOLDSTEIN. 1978. J. Exp. Med. **148:** 996.
6. CALLARD, R. D. & A. BASTEN. 1978. Eur. J. Immunol. **8:** 552.
7. MAKINODAN, T. & W. J. PETERSON. 1962. Proc. Natl. Acad. Sci. U.S.A. **48:** 234.
8. PRICE, G. B. & T. MAKINODAN. 1972. J. Immunol. **108:** 403.
9. CALLARD, R. E., A. BASTEN & L. K. WATERS. 1977. Cell Immunol. **31:** 26.
10. DUWE, A. K., J. C. RODER & S. K. SINGHAL. 1979. Immunology **37:** 293.
11. CALLARD, R. E. 1978. Eur. J. Immunol. **8:** 697.
12. MAKINODAN, T. & W. H. ADLER. 1975. Fed. Proc. Fed. Am. Soc. Exp. Biol. **34:** 153.
13. GOOD, R. A. & E. J. YUNIS. 1974. Fed. Proc. Fed. Am. Soc. Exp. Biol. **33:** 2040.
14. CHEN, M. G. 1971. J. Cell. Physiol. **78:** 228.
15. HARRISON, D. E. & J. W. DOUBLEDAY. 1975. J. Immunol. **114:** 1314.
16. FARRAR, J. J., B. E. LOUGHMAN & A. A. NORDIN. 1974. J. Immunol. **112:** 1244.
17. WODA, B. A. & J. D. FELDMAN. 1979. J. Exp. Med. **149:** 416.
18. MAKINODAN, T., J. W. ALBRIGHT, P. I. GOOD, C. P. PETER & M. L. HEIDRICK. 1976. Immunology **31:** 903.
19. PERKINS, E. H. & T. MAKINODAN. 1971. Nature of humoral immunologic deficiencies of the aged. *In* Proceedings of Rocky Mountain Symposium on Aging. p. 80. Colorado State University. Fort Collins, Colorado.
20. HEIDRICK, M. L. 1972. Gerontologist **12:** 28.
21. MACKAY, I. R. 1972. Gerontologia **18:** 285.
22. MITSUOKA, A., S. MORIKAWA, M. BABA & T. HARADA. 1979. J. Exp. Med. **149:** 1018.
23. GOODMAN, S. A. & T. MAKINODAN. 1975. Clin. Exp. Immunol. **19:** 533.
24. TICE, R. R., E. I. SCHNEIDER, D. KROM & P. THORNE. 1979. J. Exp. Med. **149:** 1029.
25. WEKSLER, M. E. & H. HUTTEROTH. 1974. J. Clin. Invest. **53:** 99.
26. MATHIES, M., L. LIPPS, G. S. SMITH & R. L. WALFORD. 1973. J. Gerontol. **28:** 425.
27. HALLGREN, H. M. & E. YUNIS. 1977. J. Immunol. **118:** 204.
28. FERNANDES, G., P. FRIEND & E. J. YUNIS. 1977. Fed. Proc. Fed. Am. Soc. Exp. Biol. **36:** 1313a.
29. PARROTT, D. M. V. 1976. Clinics in Gastroenterol. **5:** 211.
30. BEFUS, A. & J. BIENENSTOCK. 1981. The mucosa-associated immune system of the rabbit. *In* Animal Models of Immunological Processes. J. Hay, Ed.: 167. Academic Press. New York.
31. CEBRA, J. J., S. W. CRAIG & P. P. JONES. 1974. Cell types contributing to the biosynthesis of IgA. *In* The Immunoglobulin A System. J. Mestecky & A. R. Lawton, Eds.: 23. Plenum Press. New York.
32. BIENENSTOCK, J. & J. DOLEZEL. 1971. J. Immunol. **106:** 938.
33. VELDKAMP, J., K. VANDER GORAG & J. M. N. WILLERS. 1973. Immunology **25:** 761.
34. CEBRA, J. J., P. J. GEARHART, R. KAMAT, S. M. ROBERTSON & J. TSENG. 1977. Biochem. Soc. Trans. **5:** 1076.

35. CEBRA, J. J., P. J. GEARHART, R. KAMAT, S. M. ROBERTSON & J. TSENG. 1977. Cold Spring Harbor Symp. Quant. Biol. **41:** 201.
36. SZEWCZUK, M. R., R. J. CAMPBELL & L. K. JUNG. 1981. J. Immunol. **126:** 2200.
37. MATTINGLY, J. A. & B. H. WAKSMAN. 1978. J. Immunol. **121:** 1878.
38. RICHMAN, L. K., J. M. CHILLER, W. R. BROWN, D. G. HANSON & N. M. VAZ. 1978. J. Immunol. **121:** 2429.
39. M. F. KAGNOFF. 1975. J. Exp. Med. **142:** 1425.
40. KIYONO, H., J. L. BABB, S. M. MICHALEK & J. R. MCGHEE. 1980. J. Immunol. **125:** 732.
41. GEARHART, P. J. & J. J. CEBRA. 1979. J. Exp. Med. **149:** 216.
42. BRILLOUIN, L. 1956. Science and Information Theory. Academic Press. New York.
43. SZEWCZUK, M. R. & R. J. CAMPBELL. 1981. J. Immunol. **126:** 472.
44. SCHRATER, A. F., E. A. GOIDL, G. J. THORBECKE & G. W. SISKIND. 1979. J. Exp. Med. **150:** 138.
45. SZEWCZUK, M. R. & R. J. CAMPBELL. 1980. Nature (London) **286:** 164.
46. GOIDL, E. A., G. J. THORBECKE, M. E. WEKSLER & G. W. SISKIND. 1980. Proc. Natl. Acad. Sci. USA **77:** 6788.
47. SZEWCZUK, M. R. & R. J. CAMPBELL. 1981. Eur. J. Immunol. **11:** 650.
48. PHAIR, J. P. 1979. J. Chronic Dis. **32:** 535.

DISCUSSION OF THE PAPER

N. F. PIERCE (*Johns Hopkins University, School of Medicine, Baltimore, Md.*): Have you considered the possibility that these mice have naturally acquired, during the aging process, sensitization at the mucosal surface to the antigens you have employed and thereby have been primed for a mucosal IgA response. This naturally acquired antigen could also lead to a concurrent suppression or tolerance to your parenterally administered antigen.

M. R. SZEWCZUK (*Queen's University, Kingston, Ontario, Canada*): The reasons for the difference between mucosal associated lymph nodes and the spleen responses could be due to a number of factors. One is probably gut antigen priming, so what we see in the mucosal-associated lymph nodes would be a secondary immune response. It could also be due to a shift in subpopulations of T-cells or to other causes. There are numerous explanations and we are looking at this aspect.

J. A. MATTINGLY (*Ohio State University, Columbus, Ohio*): Have you looked for T-suppressor cells?

SZEWCZUK: Others have looked at suppressor cells in the spleen and have actually found that suppressor cells increase with age in the spleen.

MATTINGLY: Your results could be explained by an increasing amount of nonspecific suppressor cells with age.

SZEWCZUK: Yes, and another possibility could be due to these autoantiidiotypic antibodies.

J. A. BASH (*Georgetown University, Washington, D.C.*): In keeping with this autoanti-idiotypic mechanism, have you looked to see if the mesenteric lymph node plaques are inhibitable with anti-idiotypic antibody?

SZEWCZUK: Although that experiment is planned, we have not yet performed it.

M. W. RUSSELL (*University of Alabama in Birmingham*): Why do you suggest that the auto-idiotypic antibody only acts in the spleen and not in the peripheral lymph nodes? It would seem that anti-idiotypic antibodies should be in all sites.

SZEWCZUK: I can not answer that question at the present time.

MUCOSAL IMMUNE RESPONSES IN MALNUTRITION

R. K. Chandra

Department of Pediatrics
Memorial University of Newfoundland
St. John's, Newfoundland, Canada

Diet and health are intimately linked with each other. Epidemiologic, clinical, and autopsy data have confirmed the mutually aggravating interaction between malnutrition and infection. The Pan American Health Organization study of mortality patterns revealed that 57% of the children who died before they were five years of age showed evidence of nutritional deficiencies as either the underlying or an associated cause of death.[1] Complications and mortality associated with common infectious diseases and diarrhea are increased several-fold in malnourished populations. These data have led to the investigation of immunocompetence of undernourished children and adults.[2-5]

CELL-MEDIATED IMMUNITY

The rapid involution of the thymus in malnutrition has been recognized for more than a century. Protein-energy malnutrition results in marked histomorphological derangements in the thymus, including reduction in its size and weight, depletion of lymphocytes, loss of corticomedullary differentiation, and swelling and degeneration of Hassall's corpuscles. Paracortical regions of the lymph node and periarteriolar tissue in the spleen exhibit similar changes. The tissue changes may be the result of one or both of the following: impaired cellular proliferation and elevated free cortisol concentrations. Concomitant infection, such as measles, produces additional lymphoid atrophy. Nutritional recovery is associated with gradual return of the thymus histology to normal in deprived experimental animals.

Lymphoid atrophy and impaired maturation result in a decreased number of rosetting T-lymphocytes in the peripheral blood in malnutrition. About 15% of children with moderate-severe protein-energy malnutrition show lymphopenia. In malnutrition, the number of precursor cells may be reduced, but more likely, there is impaired differentiation as a result of decreased thymic hormone activity. Thymus extracts mixed with peripheral blood mononuclear cells of malnourished children increases the number of rosetting cells *in vitro*. There is an increase in the number of "null" cells that bear neither B- nor T-lymphocyte markers. Many of these "null" cells are immature T-lymphocytes containing large amounts of terminal deoxynucleotidyl transferase.

Delayed cutaneous hypersensitivity reactions, following primary immunization or recall challenge with antigens to which individuals are often sensitized by prior exposure, are decreased in protein-energy malnutrition and improve after appropriate feeding. The mechanisms underlying the deficit in delayed cutaneous hypersensitivity in malnutrition are not clear. Defects in the afferent limb of antigen recognition and processing, in the number and function of the subpopulation of T-lymphocytes responsible for delayed hypersensitivity, in lymphokines and other chemotactic mediators, and in mobilization of polymor-

0077-8923/83/0409-0345 $1.75/0 © 1983, NYAS

phonuclear leukocytes and macrophages may be present singly or in combination.

T-cell-mediated immune responses in malnutrition are rapidly corrected on nutritional recovery, unless the nutritional deficiency occurred in the prenatal or early postnatal life, in which case the deficit may be prolonged or even permanent. Deficiency of single nutrients, such as zinc, iron, pyridoxine, and vitamin A cause profound alterations in cell-mediated immunity and probably contribute to the immunoincompetence of children with marasmus and kwashiorkor.

OTHER IMMUNE RESPONSES

Serum immunoglobulins are normal or increased, the result of concurrent infection or decreased T-suppressor cell activity. IgG turnover is usually increased. IgE levels are elevated, especially in those with parasite disease. Antibody response is generally normal, provided adequate amounts of antigen are used, sometime in adjuvant. The exception is the response to those antigens that require the cooperation of T-helper lymphocytes.

The total number of leukocytes and neutrophils is generally normal, but there are changes in phagocyte function in malnutrition. Chemotactic migration is normal or slightly delayed, unless nutritional deficiency is complicated by infection when the mobilization is markedly reduced. Ingestion is normal but the intracellular killing of bacteria and fungi is reduced. The resting activity of the hexose monophosphate shunt is increased, but it fails to rise significantly following phagocytosis. Iodination is decreased. Intracellular killing is also reduced in iron deficiency with or without anemia. These abnormalities are reversed within a few weeks of appropriate nutritional supplements.

Several studies have demonstrated consistent changes in the complement system in malnutrition. Many of the complement components are produced in the liver, which is often affected in protein deficiency. Undernourished children show reduced levels of C3, C1, C2, and C5, and occasionally of other complement components. In one study, split products of C3 were demonstrated by immunoelectrophoresis, particularly in patients with infection. There are limited data on the alternative pathway of complement. Factor-B concentration may also be decreased in moderate protein-energy malnutrition.

There are significant changes in several nonspecific host defenses in nutritional deficiency. The production of lysozyme is decreased resulting in lower levels in the plasma, tears, saliva, and other secretions. Tissue changes, alterations in the complicated process of mucus trapping and ciliay movement, and metaplasia of mucosal epithelia observed in malnutrition probably influence susceptibility to infection. Many acute-phase reactants, such as C-reactive protein, inhibit cellular immunity and are often elevated in malnourished infected individuals. Interferon production is decreased in malnutrition. These aspects of nutrition-immunity interactions have been reviewed.[2-5]

MUCOSAL IMMUNE RESPONSES

Dietary factors play a critical role in gastrointestinal structure and function.[6] Tonsils are small in size. Atrophy of gut-associated lymphoid aggregates is a

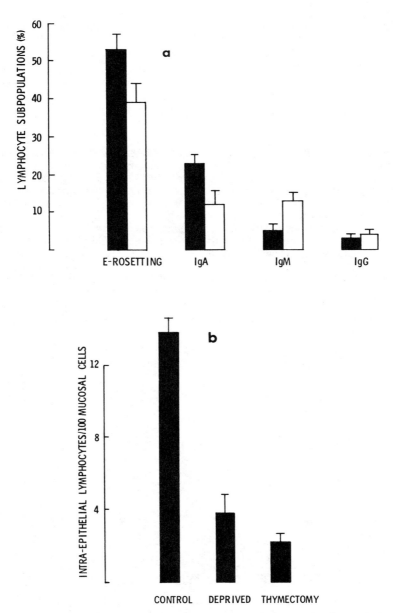

FIGURE 1a and b. Proportion of lymphocytes in intestinal mucosa of malnourished (open columns) and undernourished (closed columns) children, (Fig. 1a), and effects of protein-calorie deprivation and neonatal thymectomy on intraepithelial lymphocytes in rats (Fig. 1b).

TABLE 1

IMMUNOGLOBULIN-A CONCENTRATION IN NASOPHARYNGEAL SECRETIONS*

Group	Total Protein (mg/dl)	IgA (mg/dl)
Well nourished	180 ± 37	35 ± 7†
Malnourished	162 ± 29	11 ± 5†

*Data are shown as mean ± S.D.
†Significantly different, p < 0.01

prominent finding in autopsy studies of children dying of severe protein-energy malnutrition. There is a decrease in the number of rosette-forming T-lymphocytes, including intraepithelial cells,[7] and a selective reduction in sIgA-bearing B-cells (FIGURE 1). IgM-bearing B-cells are increased, as also seen in congenital selective IgA deficiency. There are similar changes in plasma cells producing the two immunoglobulin isotypes.

Secretory IgA concentration is reduced in mucosal secretions in malnutrition[8,9] (TABLE 1), and the specific antibody response is blunted[8] (FIGURE 2). There are limited data on the functional attributes of intestinal lymphocytes in malnutrition. We have found moderate reduction in *in vitro* responses to phytohemagglutinin and concanavalin A as compared with peripheral blood lymphocytes (FIGURE 3) and an increase in spontaneous cytotoxicity (FIGURE 4). Antibody-dependent cell-mediated cytotoxicity was unchanged (FIGURE 5). In vitamin A deficiency, the homing of lymphocytes to mucosal sites is altered dramatically (R. K. Chandra, unpublished data).

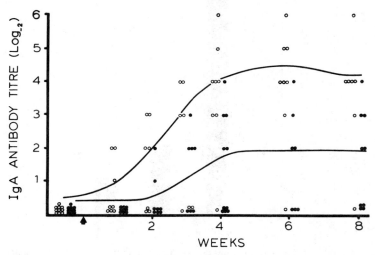

FIGURE 2. Secretory IgA antibody in nasopharyngeal secretions in malnourished (●) and healthy (O) children, given one dose of line-attenuated measles vaccine (arrow).

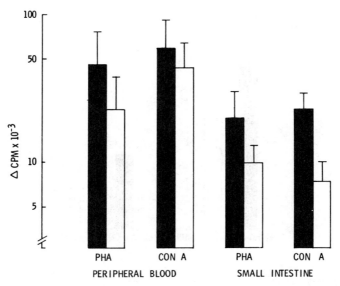

FIGURE 3. *In vitro* intestinal lymphocyte response to phytohemagglutinin (PHA) and concanavalin A (Con A), in malnourished (open columns) and well nourished (closed columns) subjects.

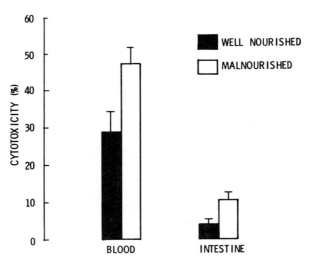

FIGURE 4. Spontaneous cell-mediated cytotoxicity of gut lymphocytes using Chang tissue culture liver cells as targets in undernourished children.

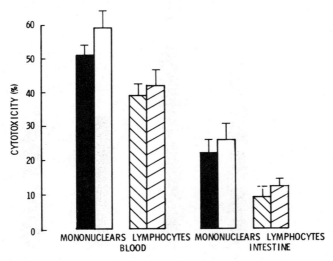

FIGURE 5. Antibody-dependent cell-mediated cytotoxicity using chicken red blood cells as targets. There were no differences between responses of intestinal lymphocytes obtained from well-nourished and malnourished children.

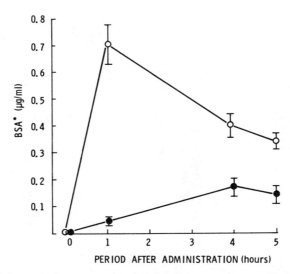

FIGURE 6. Enhanced absorption of radiolabeled bovine serum albumin (BSA) after intragastric gavage in protein-deprived rats (O) compared with controls (●).

IMPLICATIONS

The practical significance of impaired mucosal immunity in the gastrointestinal tract and other mucosal surfaces is not clear. There is increased colonization and enhanced susceptibility to enteral infections, which are often more frequent and severe in protein-calorie malnutrition. Mucosal binding of enterotoxin is reduced, thereby allowing metabolic and secretory changes preceding diarrhea. The inefficient barrier permits septicemic spread of enteric microorganisms. Macromolecular absorption is increased (FIGURE 6). In children, the enhanced uptake of food antigens did not appear to be of harmful consequence.[10] It is not known if other immunopathologic disorders known to be associated with defective mucosal immunity, for example, autoimmunity, are increased in undernourished subjects.

There is little doubt that protein-energy malnutrition and deficiencies of several individual nutrients produce significant effects on mucosal immune responses, cell-mediated immunity, and nonspecific protective factors. The mechanisms involved, however, and the practical significance of these findings are not completely understood.

REFERENCES

1. PUFFER, R. R. & C. V. SERRANO. 1973. Patterns of mortality in childhood. Pan Am. Health Organ. Washington, D.C.
2. SCRIMSHAW, N. S., C. E. TAYLOR & J. E. GORDON. 1968. Interactions of Nutrition and Infection. WHO Monogr. Ser. 57.
3. CHANDRA, R. K. & P. M. NEWBERNE. 1977. Nutrition, Immunity and Infection. Mechanisms of Interactions. Plenum Press. New York.
4. SUSKIND, R. M. (Ed.) 1977. Malnutrition and the Immune Response. Raven Press. New York.
5. CHANDRA, R. K. 1980. Immunology of Nutritional Disorders. Edward Arnold Publishers. London.
6. CHANDRA, R. K. 1979. Nutrition and the Gastrointestinal Tract. In Practice of Pediatrics. V. C. Kelly, Ed. Harper & Row. New York.
7. CHANDRA, R. K. 1981. Mucosal immunity in nutritional deficiency. In The Mucosal Immune System in Health and Disease. P. L. Ogra & J. Bienenstock, Eds. 81st Ross Conference on Pediatric Research. Columbus, Ohio.
8. CHANDRA, R. K. 1975. Reduced secretory antibody response to live attenuated measles and poliovirus vaccines in malnourished children. Brit. Med. J. 2: 583-585.
9. SIRISINHA, S., R. M. SUSKIND & R. EDELMAN. 1975. Secretory and serum IgA in children with protein-calorie malnutrition. Pediatrics 55: 166-170.
10. CHANDRA, R. K. 1975. Food antibodies in malnutrition. Arch. Dis. Child. 50: 225-228.

DISCUSSION OF THE PAPER

R. A. GOOD (*Oklahoma Medical Research Foundation, Oklahoma City*): These studies are very interesting. The only question that I have relates to what was mentioned concerning zinc metabolism. It is not possible to get protein-calorie malnutrition without getting profound zinc deficiency at the same time. With respect to cell-mediated immunity, it has been shown that one can correct the cell-mediated immunological deficits of protein-calorie malnutrition by giving zinc alone and without the restoration of the protein-calorie deficits. The question I have is, Can these abnormalities of intestinal or mucosal immunity function be corrected simply with zinc?

R. K. CHANDRA (*Memorial University of Newfoundland, St. John's, Newfoundland, Canada*): Other groups have not been able to confirm Golden's observation that giving zinc to children with protein-calorie malnutrition would completely correct the cell-mediated immune function. Certainly, in about 30–40% of children that is true, but not in the majority. Second, we have looked at the correction of the secretory immune system by giving just zinc, and this procedure has had very minimal effect on this aspect of immunity, as opposed to the more dramatic effects on cell-mediated immunity.

THE SECRETORY IMMUNE SYSTEM OF LACTATING HUMAN MAMMARY GLANDS COMPARED WITH OTHER EXOCRINE ORGANS*

Per Brandtzaeg

Histochemical Laboratory
Institute of Pathology
The National Hospital
Oslo, Norway

It is well known that human colostrum and milk are much richer in IgA than other exocrine secretions. Thus, colostrum contains about 300 times more IgA than stimulated parotid secretion and about 60 times more than normal unstimulated whole saliva.[1] The idea has therefore emerged that lactating mammary glands either harbor a remarkably active secretory immune system or, alternatively, by some unknown mechanism, drain selectively dimeric IgA from serum.[2] The former possibility appears paradoxical because the mammary glands, like the major salivary glands, are sheltered from a continuous exposure to antigens and mitogens, in contrast to the secretory immune systems of respiratory and gastrointestinal mucosae. Elucidation of the mentioned possibilities, however, has not been feasible because no previous study has characterized quantitatively the secretory immune system of lactating mammary glands with reference to data available for other secretory tissues. This lack of basic information concerns all mammalian species; although some immunohistochemical investigations have been carried out on lactating mammary glands from sheep,[3] pig,[4] rabbits,[5,6] mice,[7] rats,[8] and cows,[9] the results have not been compared on a quantitative basis with the situation in other exocrine glands. The only immunohistochemical study of human lactating glands that I am aware of, likewise provided no quantitative information.[10]

The purpose of the present investigation was twofold. First, I wanted to characterize in situ the cellular aspects of the secretory immune system of human lactating mammary glands and to relate the findings to information about other glandular tissues subjected to comparable studies in our laboratory. The number of lactating glands available for investigation was unfortunately small, because of the difficulties involved in obtaining such fresh material; but the studied specimens are collectively thought to afford a representative map of the activated mammary gland immune system. Second, by applying available information about the secretion of IgA by parotid and lactating mammary glands, I wanted to compare the secretory capacity of these organs in relation to tissue wet weight and complements of immunoglobulin (Ig)-producing cells.

*This work was supported by the Norwegian Research Council for Science and the Humanities, the Norwegian Cancer Society, and Anders Jahre's Fund.

0077-8923/83/0409-353 $01.75/0 © 1983, NYAS

Mammary Specimens

From each of two breasts, 16 specimens (about 2 × 3 × 5 mm) were excised during mammary surgery. The first series of samples (coded M_1) was obtained from a 26-year-old woman who had been breast-feeding regularly for eight months. She was admitted to the hospital because of a localized tumor; it was excised from her right breast and diagnosed as benign. The second series (coded M_2) was obtained from a 31-year-old woman, who early in her eighth month of pregnancy was subjected to total mastectomy because of a carcinoma in her right breast. All samples were taken well away from the tumors and could histologically be characterized as normal lactating mammary gland tissue containing greatly expanded lobules packed with secretory alveoli. Conspicuous alveolar and ductal accumulations of secretion were noted in M_2 in contrast to M_1. The latter breast had been emptied by natural suction about one hour before surgery.

Control specimens of nonlactating mammary tissue were obtained from women with carcinoma (44 and 52 years old) or fibroadenoma (31 years old) of the breast, and from a man with gynecomastia (46 years old).

Reference Material of Exocrine Tissues

Histologically normal specimens were obtained from human parotid ($n = 10$), submandibular ($n = 7$), and lacrimal glands ($n = 13$), and from colonic mucosa ($n = 19$). A more detailed description of this material can be found in previous publications from our laboratory.[11-13]

Reference Substrate for Extracellular Dimeric IgA

A dermal biopsy specimen from a patient with excessive intestinal production of IgA was used as a substrate for extracellularly distributed dimeric IgA. The serum of this patient contained about 50 g/l of polyclonal polymeric (about 80% dimeric) IgA as reported in detail previously.[14]

Tissue Preparation Methods

The tissue specimens were placed directly in ice-chilled phosphate-buffered saline (PBS), pH 7.5 and brought to the laboratory within one hour. Half of each series of mammary samples was immediately transferred to cold 96% ethanol for fixation and further processing, including paraffin embedding as described previously.[15] Before ethanol fixation the remaining samples were washed for 48 hours in PBS at 4° C to remove diffusible immunoglobulins from the tissues.[15]

Histochemical Procedures

From every paraffin block, serial tissue sections were cut at 6 μm on a Jung Rotary Microtome 1130. One section from each series was stained with hematoxylin and eosin for morphological evaluation. Another section was stained for nonspecific esterase employing α-naphthyl butyrate, which is considered to be the most selective substrate for the demonstration of cells belonging to the monocyte series.[16] This substrate (Sigma) was used at a final concentration of one g/l and the incubation time was one hour at 37° C.

The remaining sections were subjected to paired immunofluorescence staining by incubation with mixtures of rabbit IgG-fluorochrome conjugates prepared in our laboratory.[17,18] The specificities included the different human Ig-isotypes (γ, α, μ, δ, and ε heavy chains), secretory component (SC), and J-chain. The same fluorescein isothiocyanate (FITC) and tetramethylrhodamine isothiocyanate (TRITC) conjugates were used for all tissue categories; their characteristics have been reported elsewhere.[15,19,20] In addition, a TRITC conjugate specific for a leukocyte antigen was used for tracing of macrophages.†

For the demonstration of cytoplasmic J-chain, dewaxed sections were alternatively incubated with the conjugates, both directly and after pretreatment in 6M urea, pH 3.2, for one hour at 4° C, to expose hidden antigenic determinants.[19]

For the demonstration of cytoplasmic SC-binding activity, the sections were first incubated with free SC at 15 μg/ml (dissolved in a solution of normal rabbit IgG, 10 g/l in PBS) for one hour at 22° C, and next with a mixture of FITC-labeled isotype-specific conjugate and TRITC-labeled anti-SC conjugate.[21,22] Control sections were incubated with the rabbit IgG alone for one hour before the application of conjugates.

Fluorescence Microscopy and Cell Enumeration

Fluorescence features were evaluated in a Leitz Orthoplan microscope equipped with an Osram HBO 200W lamp for TRITC excitation, an XBO 150W lamp for FITC, Leitz 10X, 25X, 40X, and 54X immersion objectives, and an X10 ocular. A Ploem-type vertical illuminator with interference filters was used for selective evaluation of green and red fluorescence. Both selective and double-exposed color slides (Ektachrome ASA 400 daylight film) were used for evaluation of paired staining results.

Fluorescing cells were examined in sections of washed tissues. Counting was done with the X25 objective in "tissue units" as defined by the outer frame of an ocular grid (Leitz code No. 519902), representing a section area of 0.08 mm². Such recording was carried out in a systematic manner throughout each section of glandular tissue, omitting compact fat and large peripheral bands of dense connective tissue devoid of epithelial elements. At least 30 tissue units were included for every section to obtain representative counts.[11] Alternatively, for the intestinal mucosa, cell counts were based on double-exposed color slides as described previously.[13]

For enumeration of immunocytes according to isotype, all cells with a discernible nucleus, and cell-like bodies (diameter 8–12 μm) with a pure green or red cytoplasmic color, were included. For evaluation of cytoplasmic J-chain expression or SC-binding, the immunocyte was labeled with respect to isotype by green fluorescence, and the studied function was identified by red fluorescence. The intensity of the latter was subjectively graded from negative through

---

†This leukocyte antigen (L₁) is present in the granulocyte and monocyte series of cells including tissue macrophages but disappears in epithelioid cells forming granulomas. In addition, it is present in certain epithelia, mainly of the squamous type (P. Brandtzaeg & I. Dale, unpublished observations).

moderate (+) to strong (+ +), taking as a reference the overall impression of the positive cells in the actual tissue section.

Evaluation of the extracellular and epithelial distribution of immunoglobulin components was performed in sections of directly ethanol-fixed material. Comparisons of results of J-chain staining in urea-treated and untreated tissue sections were carried out to obtain information about the distribution of dimeric IgA.

TABLE 1

IMMUNOGLOBULIN CONCENTRATIONS IN LACTEAL SECRETIONS MATCHING
THE TWO STUDIED MAMMARY GLANDS (M_1 AND M_2) COMPARED
WITH SERUM DATA AND REFERENCE VALUES

Sample Category	IgG (g/l)	IgA (g/l)	IgM (g/l)	Concentration Ratios	
				IgG/IgA	IgG/IgM
Serum M_1	10.6	2.34	2.46	4.5	4.3
Serum M_2	9.0	0.92	1.96	9.8	4.6
Reference values for normal serum (mean ± S.D.)*	13.0 ± 3.4	2.96 ± 1.36	1.26 ± 0.55	4.4	10.3
Milk M_1	0.11	3.73	0.10	0.029	1.14
Colostrum M_2	1.22	85.87	3.52	0.014	0.35
Reference values for pooled colostrum (mean ± S.D.)*	0.11 ± 0.05	11.40 ± 5.52	0.58 ± 0.25	0.010	0.20
Reference values for stimulated parotid secretions (mean ± S.D.)*	0.0004 ± 0.0003	0.0395 ± 0.0137	0.0004 ± 0.0004	0.009	0.84

*Reference values were based on 21 adult serum samples, 4 pools of defatted colostrum (each comprising 3–7 individual samples), and 9 stimulated parotid fluids.[1]

Quantitation of Immunoglobulins in Serum and Exocrine Secretions

The blood samples were allowed to clot at room temperature, and the separated serum was stored at −60° C. IgG, IgA, and IgM were quantified by single radial immunodiffusion (SRID) with reference to defined standard proteins.[1]

Just before surgery, small samples of lacteal secretions were obtained by manual expression from the breasts, collateral to the two studied by immunohistochemistry. Pooled colostrum was collected by a standard breast pump from several women on the first and second postpartum day. All samples were defatted by centrifugation of 27,000 g for one hour at 4° C and further stored at −60° C until quantitation of immunoglobulins. This procedure was done by SRID—the results for IgA being converted from percentage of serum standard values to secretory IgA by the factor 6.8 as determined previously.[1]

Parotid secretions were collected from nine healthy adults by placing a Curby cap over one of the Stensen's ducts. The fluid was collected into ice-cooled, graduated cylinders and the volume measured to the nearest 10 μl. The average flow rate could thus be calculated for each sample. The samples were immediately stored at −20° C, which was shown not to affect the content of IgA in stimulated secretions.[23] The IgA concentration was quantified by SRID with reference to a purified parotid IgA standard.[1] On the basis of individual samples collected over two 30-minute periods from 7 of the subjects (10th–40th minute and 45th–75th minute of stimulation), duplicate figures were determined for the maximum physiological IgA-secretion rate (μg/min/gland).[1,23] For four of the individuals, parotid sampling was prolonged for three hours with continuous gustatory stimulation.

Data Analyses

The results are given as means ± standard deviation (S.D.), both for cell counts and for Ig measurements. The reproducibility of the methods has been reported before.[1,11] The densities of Ig-producing cells are expressed as numbers/mm² of sections cut at 6 μm. The percentage isotype distribution of the cells was calculated for each specimen to obtain equal statistical weight in the mean figure. Because IgE immunocytes were extremely rare, these were not included in the calculations. Statistical comparisons were based on the Student's *t*-test (two-tailed two sample test).

RESULTS

Exocrine Secretions

The concentrations of IgG, IgA, and IgM in the serum samples obtained from the two donors of breast tissue fell well within the ranges of normal reference values (TABLE 1). The milk sample contained more IgA than the corresponding serum sample, and the concentration was in the upper range reported for Norwegian mother's milk collected eight months after parturition.[24] The levels of IgG and IgM were in good agreement with those reported previously for milk collected after five months of lactation.[24] The prepartum sample of colostrum contained almost five times more IgA than the richest of the four postpartum pools (TABLE 1), and the concentration fell in the upper range reported for Norwegian colostrum collected three to four days after delivery.[24] Also the levels of IgG and IgM in the prepartum sample were relatively high (TABLE 1). Ultracentrifugation showed normal sedimentation properties of secretory IgA in this sample, although free SC was mostly degraded to different fragments.[25]

Pooled colostrum contained on an average almost 300 times more IgA than stimulated parotid secretion (TABLE 1). Despite this striking difference, the ratio between the IgG and IgA levels was remarkably similar in the two fluids and more than 400 times reduced, compared with the same ratio in serum (TABLE 1). The prepartum sample of colostrum showed an IgG:IgA ratio similar to that of pooled colostrum and it was 700 times reduced, compared with the same ratio in the corresponding serum sample (TABLE 1).

The pre- and postpartum colostral IgG:IgM ratios were similar and corresponded to figures previously reported for the first week after delivery.[24] Haneberg noted an increase in this ratio to 1.7 after five months of lactation. The milk sample included in the present study likewise showed a higher IgG:IgM ratio than colostrum (TABLE 1), but it was 3.8 times lower than the same ratio in the corresponding serum sample. The IgG:IgM ratio in parotid secretion fell between those in colostrum and milk (TABLE 1).

Estimation of Maximum Glandular IgA Output

Based on determination of the IgA secretion rate (μg/minute/gland) in seven subjects, it could be calculated that the maximum daily output of IgA from a normal parotid gland amounts to about 0.04 grams. This extrapolation seemed justified because the result was similar, whether the estimation was based on

TABLE 2

ESTIMATED MAXIMUM OUTPUT OF IgA FROM ADULT HUMAN PAROTID AND LACTATING MAMMARY GLANDS IN RELATION TO ORGAN WEIGHT

Type of Gland	IgA Output/24 hours (g/gland)		Organ Weight (g)*
	Mean ± S.D.	Observed range	
Normal parotid (n = 7)†	0.040 ± 0.012	(0.030–0.062)	20–30
Normal parotid (n = 7)‡	0.038 ± 0.013	(0.026–0.062)	
Lactating mammary (n = 18)§	0.727 ± 0.582	(0.14–2.49)	560–1800¶

*Data from Report of the Task Group on Reference Man.[26]
†Data based on samples of parotid fluid obtained from healthy individuals between the 10th and 40th minute of gustatory stimulation (see text).[23]
‡Data based on samples obtained from the same individuals between the 45th and 75th minute of gustatory stimulation (see text).[23]
§Data based on milk samples collected between one week and six months postpartum.[24]
¶Contains about 12% wet weight of fat.[26]

secretions collected between the 10th and 40th minute or between the 45th and 75th minute of persistent gustatory stimulation (TABLE 2). Moreover, there was no indication of a lowering of the parotid IgA level when the secretion was continuously stimulated for three hours in four of the subjects.

Figures for total daily amounts of IgA secreted per mammary gland were obtained from a study of Haneberg based on lacteal samples from Norwegian women.[24] The quantitations of IgA were performed by a method similar to that used in our laboratory. He found no consistent differences in total IgA output between one week and six months after parturition—the mean value being 18.6 times higher than the theoretical maximum parotid IgA output (TABLE 2).

When the figures thus obtained for IgA output are related to reference data for organ weight (TABLE 2), it is apparent that despite large individual variations, parotid and lactating mammary glands show a remarkably similar daily secretion of IgA per kilogram wet weight of tissue (parotid, 1.3–2.0 g and mammary gland

TABLE 3

Densities and Percentages of Immunoglobulin-Producing Cells in the Two Mammary Glands Studied Compared with Reference Material from Salivary and Lacrimal Glands and Colonic Mucosa

Tissue Category	Number of cells/mm² (mean + S.D.)				Isotype percentages			
	IgG	IgA	IgM	IgD	IgG	IgA	IgM	IgD
Mammary glands:								
M_1	2.8 ± 1.3	65.9 ± 11.7	7.5 ± 1.1	0.5 ± 0.4	3.7	85.9	9.9	0.7
M_2	14.9 ± 4.5	70.3 ± 18.7	10.4 ± 2.4	1.9 ± 0.8	15.5	71.5	11.1	2.1
Parotid glands*	2.9 ± 1.8	58.4 ± 26.1	4.1 ± 4.1	2.9 ± 4.1	4.5	86.5	5.9	3.1
Submandibular glands*	5.8 ± 4.9	122.9 ± 54.7	10.0 ± 4.4	2.2 ± 2.2	3.7	86.9	7.9	1.6
Lacrimal glands†	33 ± 21	457 ± 121	49 ± 31	57 ± 35	5.5	77.4	7.4	9.7
Colonic mucosa‡	24 ± 12	516 ± 208	32 ± 28	<1	4	90	6	<1

*Based on cell counts in normal specimens from 10 parotid and 7 submandibular glands.[11]
†Based on cell counts in specimens from 13 normal lacrimal glands.[12]
‡Based on cell counts in 19 normal colonic mucosal specimens.[13]

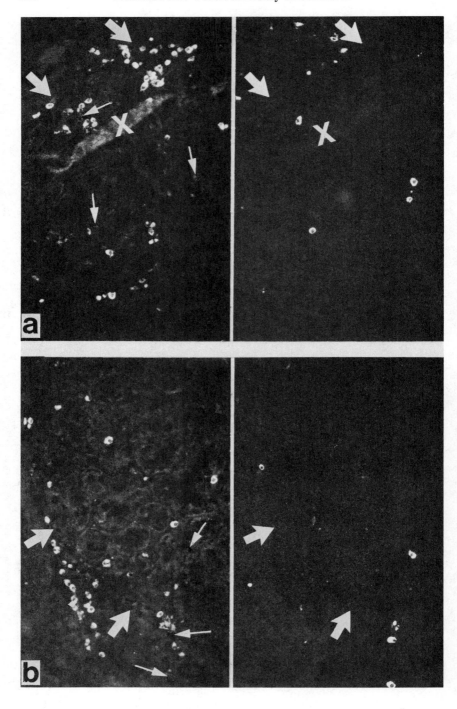

when fat subtracted, 0.5–1.5 g). Applying medians instead of means in these calculations give comparable results (parotid, 1.1–1.7 g and mammary, 0.3–1.1 g).

Immunocyte Densities in Breast Tissue and Reference Material

Ig-producing cells were enumerated in two histologically representative washed specimens from each lactating mammary gland. From every tissue block, two sections were examined for the IgA isotype, three for IgG and IgM, and five for IgD. In the postpartum breast (M_1), the variation between different sections from the same block was as large as between the two specimens, whereas in the prepartum breast (M_2), the density of IgA immunocytes was much higher in one of the samples (86 compared to 54 cells/mm²). The mean figure, however, was similar for the two glands with regard to IgA-positive cells, whereas M_2 contained significantly more IgG ($p < 0.001$), IgM ($p < 0.05$), and IgD ($p < 0.001$) cells than M_1. Thus, the representation expressed as percentage was considerably higher for the IgG and IgD isotypes in M_2 than in M_1 (TABLE 3).

In M_2, the Ig-producing cells were distributed singly or in small clusters, both throughout the lobules and in the interlobular septa particularly adjacent to ducts. In M_1 most immunocytes occurred at the periphery of the lobules (FIGURE 1). The IgG-, IgM-, and IgD-positive cells seemed to be located randomly among the IgA immunocytes (FIGURE 1). Altogether, only three IgE-producing cells were seen in a section from one of the two M_2 specimens; both M_1 specimens were apparently devoid of cells belonging to this isotype.

Lobules containing SC-positive alveolar epithelium were found in one specimen from one of the breasts with carcinoma and in several from the one with fibroadenoma. The density of IgA-producing cells within the lobules varied from 46–284/mm² (mean, 165/mm²), and that of IgM cells from 2–20/mm² (mean, 12/mm²). The intralobular density of IgG cells was, on an average, 9/mm² in the breast with fibroadenoma, but 195/mm² in that with carcinoma; a marked preponderance of IgG immunocytes was seen adjacent to SC-negative clearly malignant epithelial elements. Nevertheless, the other carcinoma, that also was SC-negative, contained in areas with neoplastic epithelium 120 IgA-cells, 16 IgG-cells, and 9 IgM-cells/mm². Despite faint apical SC-positivity in the hyperplastic duct elements, no Ig-producing cells were found in the breast with gynecomastia.

The mean density of IgA immunocytes only tended to be lower in the parotid than in the lactating mammary glands. The density of IgG cells, moreover, was similar in the parotid and in M_1 (TABLE 3). IgM immunocytes, on the other hand, were significantly more frequent in the two mammary glands considered together

---

FIGURE 1. Paired immunohistochemical staining for IgA/IgM and IgA/IgG in two sections of washed tissue from the postpartum lactating mammary gland (left panel: green fluorescence for IgA; right panel: red fluorescence for IgM or IgG). Large arrows indicate border between lobulus and extralobular connective tissue. Magnification: ×155.

a: A lobule where most IgA-producing cells are present between the peripheral alveoli. A few IgM-producing cells in the same field (some of their positions indicated by small arrows) are scattered among the IgA immunocytes. X = a fold in the section crossing the lobule.

b: A cluster of IgA immunocytes at the periphery of a lobule. Three of the four IgG-producing cells in the same field (their positions indicated by small arrows) are located between the alveoli.

than in the parotid (p < 0.005), whereas the reverse trend was noted for IgD cells (0.05 < p < 0.10).The submandibular glands contained significantly more IgA immunocytes than the lactating mammary glands (p < 0.02), whereas there were no significant differences with regard to the frequencies of IgG-, IgM-, and IgD-cells (TABLE 3).

All isotypes were strikingly more frequent in lacrimal glands than in both salivary and lactating mammary glands (TABLE 3). The factors of density increase were 3.8–11.5 for IgG-cells (depending on the category of gland), 3.7–7.8 for IgA-cells, 4.9–12.0 for IgM-cells, and as high as 20–48 for IgD-cells. This increase resulted in a significantly raised percentage of the IgD-isotype in lacrimal compared with both mammary and salivary glands (p < 0.005). The densities of IgG, IgA, and IgM immunocytes were comparable in lacrimal glands and colonic mucosa, but only a negligible number of the IgD isotype could be found in the latter type of exocrine tissue (TABLE 3).

Characterization of Glandular Immunocytes with Regard to J-Chain Expression and Nature of Cytoplasmic Immunoglobulin

The expression of cytoplasmic J-chain by the different isotypes of Ig-producing cells was similar in the two mammary glands (TABLE 4). In tissue sections treated with acid urea, 90–100% of the IgA immunocytes were positive. This positivity was significantly higher (p < 0.01) than without such pretreatment (64–78%). Also, there was a significant shift from moderate to strong J-chain staining of IgA cells (p < 0.001)—the respective figures being 59% and 15% without, compared to 31% and 62% with urea pretreatment (FIGURE 2a). The staining intensity of IgM immunocytes was likewise significantly enhanced by acid urea (p < 0.02), although these cells were 100% J-chain positive also in undenatured sections.

The J-chain staining of IgG and IgD cells was apparently unaffected by pretreatment with acid urea (FIGURE 2b). These results agreed with those obtained in sections of salivary glands and intestinal mucosa (TABLE 4). The large interspecimen variability in the results for IgG and IgD cells was not unexpected because relatively few such immunocytes were available for evaluation in the sections. Nevertheless, for all glandular tissues studied, the average percentage of J-chain positivity fell within 37–68% for IgG cells, but was 84–100% for the IgD cells, which represents a highly significant difference. Moreover, the proportion of J-chain positive cells with strong staining was always much larger for the IgD than for the IgG isotype.

Results of SC-binding tests on tissue sections confirmed that most IgA immunocytes in the mammary glands produced dimers or larger polymers with affinity for SC (FIGURE 3). In M_1, 74–75% of the IgA cells were positive (TABLE 5); this result corresponded to the figure obtained for IgA cells expressing sufficient J-chain to be revealed without pretreatment in acid urea (TABLE 4). The SC-binding test is apparently not sufficiently sensitive to detect small amounts of intracellular dimers, and it is probably vulnerable to variations in tissue processing or adversely affected by epithelial elements rich in SC, which may compete for the fluorescent antibody. Thus, despite conformity in the staining for J-chain, M_2 (in which SC-positive epithelium abounded; see below) showed lower binding activity and less bright staining of the positive cells than M_1 (TABLE 5). A large proportion of the IgM immunocytes in M_1 likewise bound SC (56–74%).

TABLE 4

PERCENTAGE J-CHAIN POSITIVITY OF MAMMARY GLAND IMMUNOCYTES OF DIFFERENT ISOTYPES
COMPARED WITH REFERENCE VALUES

Tissue Category	Tissue Sections Treated with Acid Urea				Untreated Tissue Sections			
	IgG	IgA	IgM	IgD	IgG	IgA	IgM	IgD
Mammary gland specimens (n = 4)	57% ± 17% (89)*	93% ± 5% (1301)	100% (159)	100% (11)	51% ± 16% (128)	74% ± 7% (1042)	100% (143)	96% ± 7% (14)
Parotid glands†	35% (17)	93% (375)	100% (26)	92% (13)	39% (31)	54% (353)	80% (39)	95% (19)
Submandibular glands†	47% (114)	80% (507)	99% (92)	81% (21)	32% (108)	52% (403)	93% (101)	86% (22)
Intestinal mucosa‡	67% (49)	97% (244)	100% (46)	N.D.§	69% (42)	67% (304)	100% (48%)	N.D.

*Figures in parentheses show total number of cells evaluated by paired immunofluorescence staining for isotype and J-chain.
†Based on cell counts in sections from normal specimens of three parotid and three submandibular glands.[11]
‡Based on cell counts in sections from jejunal mucosa of a patient with an intensified intestinal production of IgA.[14]
§Not determined because of insufficient number of cells.

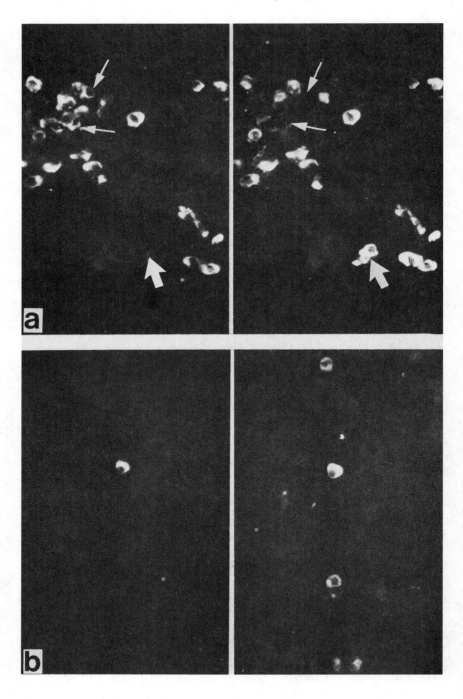

Biological Characteristics of Mammary Gland Epithelium

The postpartum (M_1) and prepartum (M_2) mammary gland specimens were strikingly different with regard to the epithelial distribution of immunoglobulins and secretory component. In M_1, the alveolar cells showed very faint staining for SC with some accentuation close to the nucleus and along the lateral borders, where also traces of IgA were detected (FIGURE 4a, b). Apical granular staining for SC and IgA were occasionally seen in addition. The collecting ductules usually showed brighter cytoplasmic staining than the alveoli (FIGURE 4c), and luminal accumulations of SC- and IgA-positive material were often seen in the larger ducts.

In M_2, accumulations that stained brightly for SC and IgA, and faintly for IgM, were commonly present in alveoli and ducts (FIGURE 5). This content usually had a globular appearance (FIGURES 6b and 7b), and fluorescent cells could sometimes clearly be identified in the lumen (FIGURE 6a). The intracellular alveolar staining showed remarkable differences in intensity, both between and within lobules. Even within the same alveolus both intense and faint epithelial cells were found (FIGURE 5). Positivity for IgA and SC was not completely congruent because selective staining for SC usually occurred adjacent to the nucleus (FIGURE 6). Staining for both components often had a granular or vesicular appearance, especially apically in the cells where the fluorescence sometimes merged with the double-stained globular accumulations in the lumen (FIGURE 6). The duct epithelium usually showed a distinct apical positivity both for SC and IgA (FIGURE 7b). The epithelium of some of the large ducts, however, appeared completely negative, although apical fluorescence was difficult to exclude because positive luminal content adhered to the cells (FIGURE 7b).

In M_1, staining for nonspecific esterase of varying strength was seen in the ductal epithelium, whereas the alveoli were mostly negative. Conversely, in some lobules from M_2, the alveolar epithelium was positive for nonspecific esterase. The globular accumulations in the lumina were particularly intense, but only occasional positive intraluminal cells with the morphology of macrophages were seen. Cells positive for nonspecific esterase were virtually absent from the glandular stroma, and immunofluorescence marker studies revealed only a few scattered macrophages in stroma and alveoli except for occasional interlobular accumulations in M_2. Ducts adjacent to these collections contained some intraepithelial and intraluminal IgA-positive macrophages.

Extracellular Distribution of Immunoglobulins in Mammary Glands

In both mammary glands, diffuse intense staining in directly ethanol-fixed specimens demonstrated an abundance of both IgG and IgA in the intra- and

---

FIGURE 2. Paired immunohistochemical staining for IgA/J-chain and IgD/J-chain in two sections of washed tissue from the postpartum mammary gland (left panel: green fluorescence for IgA or IgD; right panel: red fluorescence for J-chain). Magnification ×400.

a: A cluster of intralobular IgA immunocytes is shown in this section that was pretreated in acid urea; most of them are J-chain positive. Two negative cells are indicated by small arrows, whereas two J-chain positive cells of another isotype are indicated by a large arrow.

b: An intralobular IgD-producing cell, strongly positive for J-chain, is found among other immunocytes (probably of the IgA-isotype), which are faintly stained in this section that had not been pretreated in acid urea.

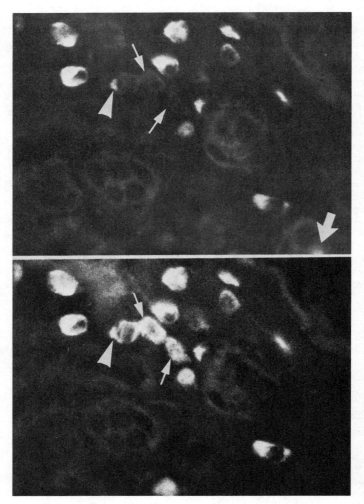

FIGURE 3. Immunohistochemical demonstration of *in vitro* binding of SC to the cytoplasm of IgA immunocytes in a section of washed tissue from the postpartum mammary gland (left: green fluorescence for IgA; right: red fluorescence for SC). Magnification: ×620. The section was incubated with free SC prior to the paired staining for SC and IgA. IgA immunocytes in intralobular stroma show variable cytoplasmic binding of SC; two cells (small arrows) are completely negative. In one cell, SC has become bound to a restricted area adjacent to the nucleus, probably representing the Golgi zone (arrowhead). The alveolar epithelium shows little or no staining for innate SC in this case, but one alveolus contains some SC-positive material (large arrow).

interlobular connective tissue (FIGURE 7). The staining was accentuated in vascular and epithelial basement membrane zones, but the epithelial cells and the luminal accumulations were completely negative for IgG (FIGURE 7). IgM was found in an extracellular distribution similar to that of IgG and IgA, but the staining intensity was considerably lower (FIGURE 8c).

In an attempt to determine if the extravascular IgA was mainly dimeric, staining for J-chain was compared in adjacent sections with and without pretreatment in acid urea. In the undenatured sections, faint J-chain staining was restricted to immunocytes and luminal accumulations of IgA (FIGURE 8a). After urea treatment, the staining was strikingly intensified both in epithelium and immunocytes, and there was also diffuse J-chain positivity of varying intensity in the connective tissue (FIGURE 8b). The distribution of extracellular J-chain, however, corresponded to that of IgM (FIGURE 8c). By contrast, in dermal control sections rich in extravascular dimeric IgA, bright J-chain staining was produced in the connective tissue without denaturation in acid urea (FIGURE 9a) and despite virtual absence of IgM (FIGURE 9b).

TABLE 5

PERCENTAGE OF MAMMARY GLAND IgA IMMUNOCYTES EXPRESSING SC AFFINITY

Specimen*	Total Number†	Positive	(++)	(+)
M_1	324	74%	(42%)	(32%)
M_1	345	75%	(34%)	(41%)
M_2	190	69%	(18%)	(51%)
M_2	91	53%	(12%)	(41%)

*Two sections from each of the two mammary glands (M_1 and M_2) were subjected to SC-binding test.

†Total number of cells evaluated by paired immunofluorescence for SC bound in vitro. The staining intensity of positive cells was graded subjectively as strong (++) or moderate (+).

DISCUSSION

The data presented show that there is a remarkable similarity between human salivary and lactating mammary glands; this holds true for the estimated daily output of IgA per kilogram wet weight, the density of Ig-producing immunocytes, and the isotype distribution of these cells.

As pointed out in the introduction, no previous quantitative information on the presence of Ig-producing cells in mammary glands is available for comparison with other exocrine tissues. The consensus, based on animal studies, seems to be that the lactating mammary glands contain few immunocytes. Nevertheless, a recent comparative histological investigation indicated large interspecies variations with regard to the occurrence of plasma cells in mammary glands, and the human lactating tissue was reported to be relatively rich in such cells.[27] Findings for other exocrine sites of animals should likewise not be extrapolated to the human situation. Thus, lacrimal glands of sheep have been claimed by Hall et al.[28] to contain few plasma cells; this statement has subsequently been cited without reference to species.[2] By contrast, as reported above, the density of Ig-producing cells in human lacrimal glands is almost the same as in the colonic mucosa, that is,

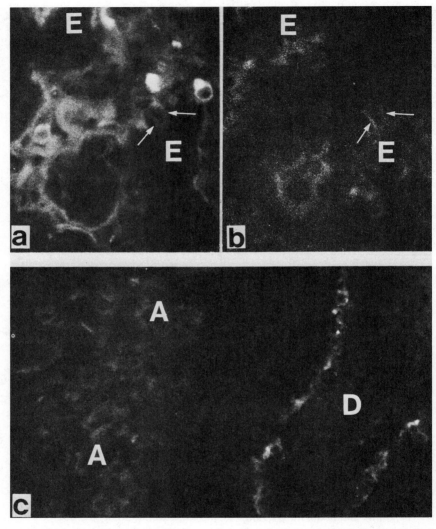

FIGURE 4. Immunohistochemical staining for IgA and SC in sections of directly ethanol-fixed tissue from the postpartum mammary gland.

a: Green fluorescence demonstrates extracellular IgA in the intralobular stroma and a few IgA-producing cells. Only traces of IgA can be detected in the alveolar epithelium (E), mainly along the lateral cell borders (arrows). Magnification: ×390.

b: In the same field, the alveolar epithelium likewise contains very little SC, as shown by faint red fluorescence, mainly adjacent to the nuclei and along the lateral cell borders (arrows). Magnification: ×390.

c: Faint staining for SC is seen in the alveolar epithelium (A), whereas the epithelium of an interlobular collecting duct (D) contains more SC in some of its cells. Magnification: ×150.

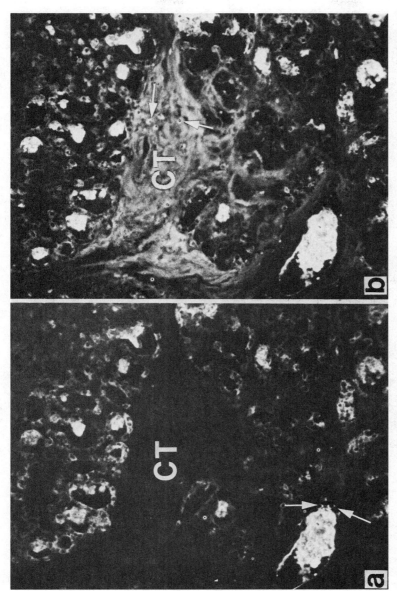

FIGURE 5. Paired immunohistochemical staining for SC (a: red fluorescence) and IgA (b: green fluorescence) in a section of directly ethanol-fixed tissue from the prepartum mammary gland. Magnification: ×155.

a: Ducts and distended alveoli contain SC-positive accumulations, and the epithelium shows varying degrees of positivity. Note that there is often variability from cell to cell within a single alveolus. The epithelium of a large collecting duct (to the lower left) is negative except for a few cells (arrows), but the luminal content adheres to the apical face of the cells. b: The alveolar and ductal distribution of IgA is similar to that of SC, but IgA is, in addition, present in the connective tissue (CT) and in some immunocytes (arrows).

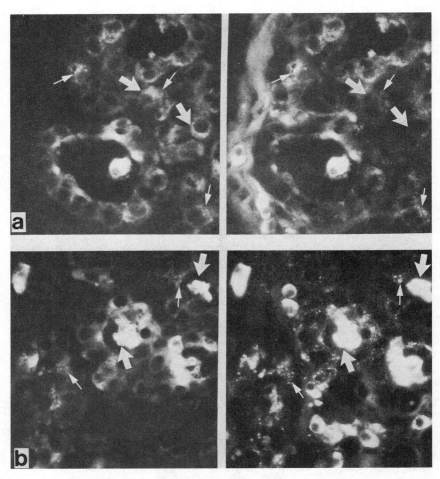

FIGURE 6. Paired immunohistochemical staining for SC and IgA in two sections of directly ethanol-fixed tissue from the prepartum mammary gland (left panel, red fluorescence for SC; right panel, green fluorescence for IgA). Magnification: ×480.

a: SC and IgA are distributed similarly throughout the cytoplasm of the alveolar cells, the staining often giving a granular or vesicular appearance (small arrows). This feature is more distinct for IgA because some cells contain additional cytoplasmic SC, especially adjacent to the nucleus (large arrows). A double-stained cell is present in the lumen of a distended alveolus. IgA is, in addition, present in the intralobular connective tissue and in three immunocytes to the far left.

b: In this field the vesicular appearance of the epithelial staining is particularly prominent (small arrows), and is also shown by the luminal accumulations (large arrow). Preferential diffuse epithelial staining for SC is seen close to the nuclei. Several IgA-producing immunocytes are present in the intralobular connective tissue.

FIGURE 7. Paired immunohistochemical staining for IgA and IgG in two sections of directly ethanol-fixed tissue from the prepartum mammary gland (left panel, green fluorescence for IgA; right panel, red fluorescence for IgG). Magnification: ×110.

a: The intralobular connective tissue contains extracellular IgA and IgG in an identical distribution, the staining being particularly intense in vascular and epithelial basement membrane zones. Intraluminal and epithelial staining in alveoli and ducts is selective for IgA.

b: The interlobular connective tissue is also positive for both IgA and IgG, whereas IgG is absent from epithelium and lumina. The small interlobular collecting duct (at the top) shows apical epithelial staining for IgA. The large duct (to the right) contains globular accumulations of IgA, which in some places adhere to the apical face of the epithelium; in other places the epithelium is clearly unstained (arrows).

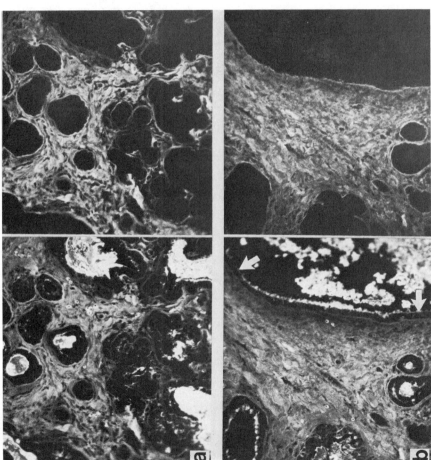

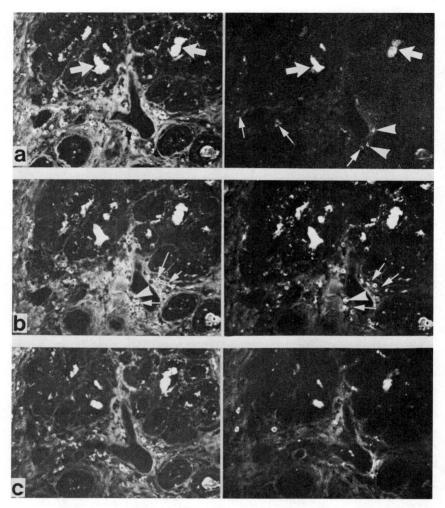

FIGURE 8. Paired immunohistochemical staining for IgA/J-chain or IgA/IgM in comparable fields showing the same lobule in three serial sections from directly ethanol-fixed tissue
from the prepartum mammary gland (left panel, green fluorescence for IgA; right panel, red
fluorescence for J-chain or IgM). Magnification: ×120.

a: Despite large concentrations of extracellular IgA in the connective tissue, faint staining
for J-chain in this undenatured section is restricted to IgA-producing cells (small arrows) or
occasional immunocytes of another isotype (arrowheads), and to the most prominent
luminal accumulations of secretory IgA (large arrows).

b: This section had been treated in acid urea, and with few exceptions (small arrows),
there is intensified J-chain staining of IgA-producing cells, rare immunocytes of another
isotype (arrowheads), and intraepithelial and intraluminal secretory IgA. There is also faint
staining for extracellular J-chain in the connective tissue.

c: Paired staining for IgA and IgM shows that less IgM is present in the epithelium and
luminal accumulations, and there are only a few IgM immunocytes in the stroma. The
extracellular staining for IgM in the connective tissue is similar to that shown for J-chain in
b. The exposure times were identical within each panel to render comparisons valid.

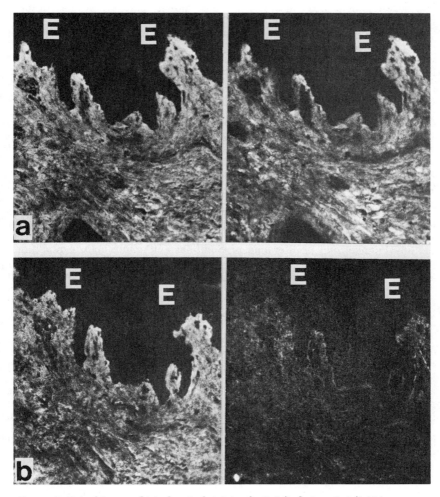

FIGURE 9. Paired immunohistochemical staining for IgA/J-chain or IgA/IgM in comparable fields in two serial sections of a directly ethanol-fixed skin specimen from a patient who had about 60 g/l of dimeric IgA in his serum (left panel, green fluorescence for IgA; right panel, red fluorescence for J-chain or IgM). Magnification: ×150.

a: Extravascular dimeric IgA in the dermis contains sufficient J-chain to be demonstrated without pretreating the section in acid urea.

b: Paired staining for IgA and IgM shows that IgM is virtually absent from the dermis. The epidermis (E) at the top is negative for both immunoglobulins. The exposure times were identical to those in FIGURE 8.

four to nine times higher than in salivary and lactating mammary glands. This finding agrees with the fact that the concentrations reported for IgA (converted to secretory IgA by a factor of 3) in stimulated human tears, are at least 15 times higher than in stimulated parotid secretions.[29,30]

Hochwald et al.[31] reported almost 20 years ago that specimens of human mammary glands kept in culture seemed to synthesize IgA selectively, compared with IgG and IgM. This observation was confirmed 12 years later by Drife et al.;[32] they detected preferential IgA synthesis in 81% of "resting" breasts from both parous and nulliparous women. Immunohistochemistry showed intralobular IgA-producing cells, and luminal deposits of IgA. The secretory immune system of the mammary glands, therefore, does not depend on pregnancy to come into function. This observation was confirmed in the present study because lobules with alveolar elements occurring in breasts of nonpregnant women with fibroadenoma or carcinoma, were shown to contain a density of IgA-producing cells that on an average was twice the overall density in lactating mammary glands. Moreover, the percentage representation of IgM immunocytes was similar. Conversely, the IgG-cell percentage was strikingly increased in the presence of carcinoma.

In many species, including the human, the overall number of plasma cells has been found to be much higher in the lactating than in the resting breast.[27] After pregnancy, the increment of local IgA-producing cells has been found to parallel the development and proliferation of glandular epithelium both in rabbit and mouse mammary glands.[5-7] A similar hormonal expansion of the secretory immune system has been indicated in the human counterpart.[10] Experiments in mice have demonstrated a hormonal influence on the migration of immunological precursor cells into the glandular tissue,[33] but this effect is probably mediated through the development of nonlymphoid (vascular or epithelial) elements of the mammary gland.

It has been directly shown in mice that precursors for the IgA-producing cells appearing in mammary and salivary glands are derived, at least in part, from gut-associated lymphoid tissue (GALT).[33-36] Conversely, Hall et al.[28] found no homing of precursors from GALT to the lacrimal glands in sheep, although there is indirect evidence that such homing may take place in man.[37] Different results may reflect the fact that GALT is probably not the only mucosa-associated lymphoid tissue from which distribution of stimulated B-cells takes place. Thus, precursor cells are able to migrate from bronchial-associated lymphoid tissue (BALT) to the intestinal mucosa, although a certain tendency for regional localization according to origin has been reported.[38]

It has been claimed that the hormone-dependent migration of precursors from GALT into mammary glands is specific for IgA-producing immunocytes.[7,33] This claim can not be true in the human species, because about 20% of the Ig-producing cells in the lactating mammary glands were found to contain other isotypes. Like the IgA immunocytes, most of the local IgM- and IgD-producing cells were also J-chain positive, and the same held normally true for about 50% of the IgG-producing cells. We have previously proposed that circulating J-chain expressing B-cell blasts, regardless of isotype, continuously contribute to the gland-associated immunocyte populations throughout the body.[39] Expression of J-chain is apparently a sign of clonal immaturity,[40] which also according to other lines of evidence seems to be a feature of B-cells accumulating in glandular sites.[41] Moreover, GALT has been shown to be a major source of IgG- and IgM-producing cells normally appearing in the intestinal mucosa of mice.[38]

Altogether, the attraction of B-cell blasts to glandular sites is clearly independent of a precommitment to IgA expression. Thus, glandular complements of IgM-, IgG-, and IgD-producing cells developing in selective IgA deficiency add up to a size comparable to that of the normal IgA-predominant immunocyte population.[12] A striking observation, probably reflecting a dichotomy in the homing of precursors, is that the lack of IgA immunocytes in such patients is replaced with IgM- and IgG-producing cells in the gastrointestinal mucosa, but mainly with IgD-producing cells in lacrimal, nasal, and parotid glands.[12] This finding accentuates the relatively high proportion of IgD immunocytes that

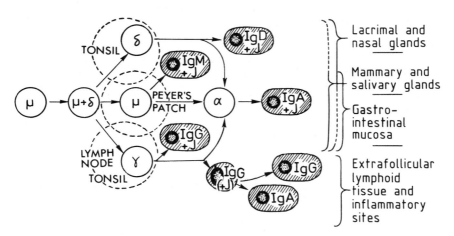

FIGURE 10. Schematic illustration of maturational pathways proposed for B-cells originating in tonsils, Peyer's patches, or lymph nodes, and the partially selective retention of these cells in various tissue sites. The hatched cells represent locally retained immunocytes with cytoplasmic IgM, IgG, IgD, or IgA, which in the exocrine tissues are expressed along with J-chain as a sign of clonal immaturity (cells labeled +J). Parenthesized +J symbolizes repression of J-chain synthesis, perhaps due to accumulation of J-chain in IgG-producing cells during clonal maturation. The solid and broken clasps to the right indicate that differentiation through IgD expression is a sign of tonsillar derivation and that such cells migrate mainly to lacrimal and nasal glands but also to salivary and mammary glands. Differentiation through IgM expression is particularly a sign of derivation from Peyer's patches; such cells migrate to all exocrine tissues, but less to lacrimal and nasal glands than to the others. Differentiation through IgG expression may take place to some extent for cells normally retained in all exocrine tissues. Extrafollicular lymphoid tissue and inflammatory sites retain mainly mature clones with at least partially repressed J-chain synthesis. Findings supporting the proposed scheme are discussed in the text (modified from reference 12).

normally prevails in the latter sites—amounting to more than 9% in both lacrimal (TABLE 3) and nasal glands.[12]

Because tonsillar cells, at least in situ, show a greater tendency to IgD-expression than that shown by B-cells during differentiation in other lymphoid tissues,[42,43] various maturational pathways leading to the development of glandular-associated immunocyte populations may be visualized (FIGURE 10). The intermediate representation of IgD cells in both salivary and mammary glands (TABLE 3) may, accordingly, suggest that these sites receive precursor cells both from the Peyer's patches and from the tonsils. This view is supported by the fact that human colostrum contains antibodies not only to enteric antigens, but also to respiratory syncytial virus.[44]

Although many uncertainties are involved in estimating the daily glandular output of IgA, the results (TABLE 2) indicate, in view of the immunocyte density figures (TABLE 3), that salivary and lactating mammary glands function similarly with regard to the external translocation of locally synthesized IgA and the additional putative transfer of dimeric IgA from serum. The quantitative relationship between these two possibilities for the origin of lacteal and salivary IgA is unknown. That an SC-mediated transfer of polymeric IgA and IgM from serum can take place through the salivary glands has been shown in patients with myelomatosis or Waldenström's macroglobulinemia.[45,46] There is reason to believe that such transfer may similarly take place through the mammary glands, as previously documented experimentally in mice.[2,47] Compared with the situation, however, in several other mammalian species, including the murine, human blood normally receives relatively little polymeric IgA from lymph.[48] The secretory immune system of human mammary glands is therefore, in teleological terms, dependent on a relatively rich complement of local immunocytes. Nevertheless, in the rat, where only few plasma cells are found in lactating mammary glands,[27] a transfer of dimeric IgA from serum to milk has not been revealed.[49] In this context it may be relevant that the hepatic transport of polymeric IgA from blood to bile apparently is much more efficient in the rat than in most other species.[50]

Immunofluorescence studies of the connective tissue stroma of human mammary glands showed an abundance of extracellular IgG and IgA and smaller amounts of IgM. Nevertheless, the IgA seemed to be mainly monomeric, even in the prepartum state. Thus, there is no evidence that the glandular stroma may act as a selective depot for polymeric IgA. It remains to be clarified how the locally produced IgA is passed from the immunocytes to the epithelium without being lost to the lymph. As discussed elsewhere,[50,51] one has to consider that there is a directional diffusion—perhaps through small rivulets, which have been described in the connective tissue ground substance.[52]

As in other exocrine tissues,[11,14] the IgA immunocytes of lactating mammary glands were heterogenous with regard to cytoplasmic J-chain expression. This heterogeneity probably indicates that they produce varying proportions of monomeric and polymeric IgA. The fact that denaturation of the tissue sections significantly enhanced J-chain positivity (from 74% to 93%) and cytoplasmic staining intensity, documents that polymerization of IgA takes place in the endoplasmic reticulum of the glandular immunocytes as discussed previously.[53] This possibility was further attested to by the cytoplasmic SC affinity shown by about 75% of the cells in the postpartum specimen. Most of the locally produced IgA can therefore be subjected to external translocation by an SC-mediated mechanism, as proposed for other exocrine tissues.[50,51] There was evidence in the mammary glands that such selective transport, including only J-chain-containing IgA (and some IgM), takes place both through alveolar and ductal epithelium, with the exception of the larger collecting ducts.

Secretory component-bound IgA and IgM are most likely carried through the mammary gland epithelium in the secretory vesicles that have been shown to contain caseins and major milk whey proteins.[54] The presence of osmotically active compounds such as lactose in the same vesicles, causes water to be drawn into them and explains their swollen and distended appearance.[54] Large SC- and IgA-positive vesicular bodies were localized apically in the alveolar epithelium of many lobules in the prepartum specimen. A considerable capacity for intraepithelial storage of secretory IgA was thus indicated, but there was marked functional heterogenity from lobule to lobule, and even from cell to cell within the same alveolus. Much less secretory IgA was present in the epithelium of the postpartum specimen–perhaps reflecting a faster external transport during milk production. In the bovine mammary gland, a similar distinction has been observed between pre- and postpartum specimens with regard to epithelial staining for IgG_1, that is selectively transferred into lacteal secretions in that species.[55]

There was no evidence for a significant role of macrophages in the translocation of IgA into colostrum. Such a function has recently been proposed for these cells.[56] As a matter of fact, relatively few stromal and intraepithelial macrophages were identified, after the use of an antigenic marker and staining for nonspecific esterase. The latter approach has been applied for identification of colostral macrophages in several previous studies.[56-59] Nevertheless, the presence of these esterases in both alveolar and ductal epithelium of lactating mammary glands, as shown here and elsewhere,[58] renders identification of macrophages in colostrum by this criterion unreliable. The natural shedding from alveoli and ducts will obviously bring numerous IgA- and esterase-containing epithelial cells into the secretions. It is likewise possible that such shed epithelial elements are responsible for the reported production of IgA and antibodies by colostral cells.[60,61]

CONCLUSIONS

1. The density of IgA-producing cells is similar in human salivary and lactating mammary glands, but six to seven times less than in lacrimal glands and colonic mucosa.

2. The daily output of IgA/kilogram of wet weight is similar for salivary and lactating mammary glands.

3. The transport of IgA (and IgM) into colostrum and milk apparently takes place mainly by exocytosis of SC-containing vesicles, although additional holocrine and apocrine secretion may take place. Few true macrophages were identified, and these cells do not seem to play a significant role in the external translocation of IgA.

4. Large capacity for storage of IgA in the mammary gland epithelium and duct system apparently explains the striking output of IgA during feeding; there is no evidence for a selective extracellular accumulation of dimeric IgA in the glandular stroma.

5. Precursor cells for the secretory immune system of mammary and salivary glands are most likely derived both from tonsils and Peyer's patches; dual derivation was indicated by the intermediate representation of IgD immunocytes in these glands as compared with lacrimal and nasal mucosal glands on the one hand, and the gastrointestinal mucosa on the other.

ACKNOWLEDGMENTS

I would like to thank Dr. F.R. Korsrud, Dr. S.T. Gjeruldsen, and Dr. K. Baklien for collaboration in the establishment of reference data for Ig-producing cells, and the technicians of our laboratory for careful work. I am also grateful to Dr. B. Haneberg for allowing me to use his data on the daily secretion of lacteal IgA. The surgical staff of the Norwegian Radium Hospital, and particularly Dr. A. Engeset, are acknowledged for cooperation in obtaining lactating mammary gland specimens. The secretarial staff and the Phototechnical Department gave invaluable assistance in the preparation of the manuscript.

REFERENCES

1. BRANDTZAEG, P., I. FJELLANGER & S. T. GJERULDSEN. 1970. Human secretory immunoglobulins. I. Salivary secretions from individuals with normal or low levels of serum immunoglobulins. Scand. J. Haematol. Suppl. No. **12:** 1-83.
2. HALSEY, J. H., B. H. JOHNSON & J. J. CEBRA. 1980. Transport of immunoglobulins from serum to colostrum. J. Exp. Med. **151:** 767-772.
3. LEE, C. S. & A. K. LASCELLES. 1970. Antibody-producing cells in antigenically stimulated mammary glands and in the gastro-intestinal tract of sheep. Aust. J. Exp. Biol. Med. Sci. **48:** 525-535.
4. PORTER, P., D. E. NOKAES & W. D. ALLEN. 1970. Secretory IgA and antibodies to *Escherichia coli* in porcine colostrum and milk and their significance in the alimentary tract of the young pig. Immunology **18:** 245-257.
5. LEE, H., W. C. HANLEY & K. L. KNIGHT. 1977. Kinetics of the appearance of IgA containing cells in mammary glands of pregnant rabbits. Fed. Proc. Fed. Am. Soc. Exp. Biol. **36:** 1310 (abstr.).
6. LEE, H. & W. C. HANLEY. 1978. Relationship of glandular development to development of Ig cell systems in rabbit mammary tissue. Fed. Proc. Fed. Am. Soc. Exp. Biol. **37:** 1744 (Abstr.).
7. WEISZ-CARRINGTON, P., M. E. ROUX & M. E. LAMM. 1977. Plasma cells and epithelial immunoglobulins in the mouse mammary epithelium during pregnancy and lactation. J. Immunol. **119:** 1306-1309.
8. LEE, C. G., P. W. LADDS, D. L. WATSON & M. E. GODDARD. 1979. Immunofluorescence studies of the local immune response in the mammary glands of rats. Infect. Immun. **23:** 453-459.
9. BUTLER, J. E. 1981. A concept of humoral immunity among ruminants and an approach to its investigation. *In* Advances in Experimental Medicine and Biology. The Ruminant Immune System. J. E. Butler, Ed.: **137:** 3-55. Plenum Press. New York.
10. FUJIMURA, M., S.-T. CHEN, T. SUDO, T. KUYAMA & T. SAITO. 1981. Cellular aspects of immunoglobulins. VII. Localization of immunoglobulins in female mammary gland. Acta Histochem. Cytochem. **14:** 163-167.
11. KORSRUD, F. R. & P. BRANDTZAEG. 1980. Quantitative immunohistochemistry of immunoglobulin- and J-chain-producing cells in human parotid and submandibular salivary glands. Immunology **39:** 129-140.
12. BRANDTZAEG, P., S. T. GJERULDSEN, F. KORSRUD, K. BAKLIEN, P. BERDAL & J. EK. 1979. The human secretory immune system shows striking heterogeneity with regard to involvement of J chain-positive IgD immunocytes. J. Immunol. **122:** 503-510.
13. BAKLIEN, K. & P. BRANDTZAEG. 1975. Comparative mapping of the local distribution immunoglobulin-containing cells in ulcerative colitis and Chrohn's disease of the colon. Clin. Exp. Immunol. **22:** 197-209.
14. BRANDTZAEG, P. & K. BAKLIEN. 1977. Characterization of the IgA immunocyte population and its product in a patient with excessive intestinal formation of IgA. Clin. Exp. Immunol. **30:** 77-88.
15. BRANDTZAEG, P. 1974. Mucosal and glandular distribution of immunoglobulin components. Immunohistochemistry with a cold ethanol-fixation technique. Immunology **26:** 1101-1114.
16. LI, C. Y., K. W. LAM & L. T. YAM. 1973. Esterases in human leukocytes. J. Histochem. Cytochem. **21:** 1-12.
17. BRANDTZAEG, P. 1973. Conjugates of immunoglobulin G with different fluorochromes.

I. Characterization by anionic-exchange chromatography. Scand. J. Immunol. **2:** 273–290.

18. BRANDTZAEG, P. 1973. Conjugates of immunoglobulin G with different fluorochromes. II. Specific and non-specific binding properties. Scand. J. Immunol. **2:** 333–348.
19. BRANDTZAEG, P. 1976. Studies of J chain and binding site for secretory component in circulating human B cells. I. The surface membrane. Clin. Exp. Immunol. **25:** 50–58.
20. BRANDTZAEG, P. 1981. Prolonged incubation time in immunohistochemistry: Effects on fluorescence staining of immunoglobulins and epithelial components in ethanol- and formaldehyde-fixed paraffin-embedded tissues. J. Histochem. Cytochem. **29:** 1302–1315.
21. BRANDTZAEG, P. 1973. Two types of IgA immunocytes in man. Nature (London) New Biol. **243:** 142–143.
22. BRANDTZAEG, P. 1974. Characteristics of SC-Ig complexes formed in vitro. In Advances in Experimental Medicine and Biology. The Immunoglobulin A System. J. Mestecky & A. R. Lawton, Eds.: **45:** 87–97. Plenum Press. New York.
23. BRANDTZAEG, P. 1971. Human secretory immunoglobulins. VII. Concentrations of parotid IgA and other secretory proteins in relation to the rate of flow and duration of secretory stimulus. Arch. Oral Biol. **16:** 1295–1310.
24. HANEBERG, B. 1974. Human milk immunoglobulins and agglutinins to rabbit erythrocytes. Int. Arch. Allergy Appl. Immunol. **47:** 716–729.
25. BRANDTZAEG, P. 1975. Human secretory component. IV. Aggregation and fragmentation of free secretory component. Immunochemistry **12:** 877–881.
26. SNYDER, W. S., M. J. COOK, E. S. NASSET, L. R. KARHAUCEN, G. P. HOWELLS & I. H. TIPTON. 1975. Report of the Task Group on Reference Man. The International Commission on Radiological Protection. **23:** 124, 195. Pergamon Press. Oxford.
27. PUMPHREY, R. J. H. 1977. A comparative study of plasma cells in the mammary gland in pregnancy and lactation. Symp. Zool. Soc. London **41:** 261–276.
28. HALL, J. G., J. HOPKINS & E. ORLEANS. 1977. Studies on the lymphocytes of sheep. III. Destination of lymph-borne immunoblasts in relation to their tissue of origin. Eur. J. Immunol. **7:** 30–37.
29. LITTLE, J. M., Y. M. CENTIFANTO & H. E. KAUFMAN. 1969. Immunoglobulins in human tears. Am. J. Ophthalmol. **68:** 898–905.
30. KÜHL, W. 1971. Der Immunoglobulingehalt der menschlichen Tränflüssigkeit. Albrecht von Graefes Arch. Klin. Exp. Ophthalmol. **182:** 76–81.
31, HOCHWALD, G. M., E. B. JACOBSON & G. J. THORBECKE. 1964. C^{14}-amino acid incorporation into transferrin and β_{2A}-globulin by ectodermal glands. Fed. Proc. Fed. Am. Soc. Exp. Biol. **23:** 557 (abstr.).
32. DRIFE, J. O., D. B. L. McCLELLAND, A. PRYDE, M. M. ROBERTS & I. I. SMITH. 1976. Immunoglobulin synthesis in the "resting" breast. Brit. Med. J. **2:** 503–506.
33. WEISZ-CARRINGTON, P., M. E. ROUX, M. McWILLIAMS, J. M. PHILLIPS-QUAGLIATA & M. E. LAMM. 1978. Hormonal induction of the secretory immune system in the mammary gland. Proc. Natl. Acad. Sci. USA **75:** 2928–2932.
34. ROUX, M. E., M. McWILLIAMS, J. M. PHILLIPS-QUAGLIATA, P. WEISZ-CARRINGTON & M. E. LAMM. 1977. Origin of IgA-secreting plasma cells in the mammary gland. J. Exp. Med. **146:** 1311–1322.
35. ROSE, M. L., D. M. V. PARROTT & R. G. BRUCE. 1978. The accumulation of immunoblasts in extravascular tissues including mammary gland, peritoneal cavity, gut and skin. Immunology **34:** 415–423.
36. JACKSON, D. E., E. T. LALLY, M. C. NAKAMURA & P. C. MONTGOMERY. 1981. Migration of IgA-bearing lymphocytes into salivary glands. Cell. Immunol. **63:** 203–209.
37. MESTECKY, J., J. R. McGHEE, R. KULHAVY, S. MICHALEK, S. CRAGO & R. R. ARNOLD. 1978. Synthesis of IgA and the induction of local immunity. Protides Biol. Fluids Proc. Colloq. **25:** 811–818.
38. McDERMOTT, M. R. & J. BIENENSTOCK. 1979. Evidence for a common mucosal immunologic system. I. Migration of B immunoblasts into intestinal, respiratory, and genital tissues. J. Immunol. **122:** 1892–1898.
39. BRANDTZAEG, P. 1981. The humoral immune systems of the human gastrointestinal tract. Monogr. Allergy **17:** 195–221.

40. KORSRUD, F. R. & P. BRANDTZAEG. 1981. Immunohistochemical evaluation of J-chain expression by intra- and extra-follicular immunoglobulin-producing human tonsillar cells. Scand. J. Immunol. **13:** 271–280.
41. CEBRA, J. J., G. J. GEARHART, J. F. HALSEY, J. L. HURWITZ & R. D. SHAHIN. 1980. Role of environmental antigens in the ontogeny of the secretory immune response. J. Reticuloendothelial Soc. **28:** 61s–71s.
42. BRANDTZAEG, P., L. SURJAN & P. BERDAL. 1978. Immunoglobulin systems of human tonsils. I. Control subjects of various ages. Quantification of Ig-producing cells, tonsillar morphometry, and serum immunoglobulin levels. Clin. Exp. Immunol. **31:** 367–381.
43. KORSRUD, F. R. & P. BRANDTZAEG. 1980. Immune systems of human nasopharyngeal and palatine tonsils: histomorphometry of lymphoid components and quantification of immunoglobulin-producing cells in health and disease. Clin. Exp. Immunol. **39:** 361–370.
44. DOWNHAM, M. A. P. S., R. SCOTT, D. G. SIMS, J. K. G. WEBB & P. S. GARDNER. 1976. Breast-feeding protects against respiratory syncytial virus infections. Brit. Med. J. **2:** 274–276.
45. VIRELLA, G., P. C. MONTGOMERY & I. M. LEMAITRE-COELHO. 1978. Transport of oligomeric IgA of systemic origin into external secretions. In Advances in Experimental Medicine and Biology. Secretory Immunity and Infection. J. R. McGEE, J. MESTECKY and J. L. BABB, Eds.: **107:** 241–251. Plenum Press. New York.
46. BRANDTZAEG, P. 1971. Human secretory immunoglobulins. II. Salivary secretions from individuals with selectively excessive or defective synthesis of immunoglobulins. Clin. Exp. Immunol. **8:** 69–85.
47. JACKSON, G. D. F., I. LEMAITRE-COELHO, & J. P. VAERMAN. 1978. Transfer of MOPC-315 IgA to secretions in MOPC-315 tumour-bearing and normal BALB/c mice. Protids Biol. Fluids Proc. Colloq. **25:** 919–922.
48. KAARTINEN, M., T. IMIR, M. KLOCKARS, M. SANDHOLM & O. MÄKELÄ. 1978. IgA in blood and thoracic duct lymph: concentration and degree of polymerization. Scand. J. Immunol. **7:** 229–232.
49. DAHLGREN, U., S. AHLSTEDT, L. HEDMAN, C. WADSWORTH & L. Å. HANSON. 1981. Dimeric IgA in the rat is transferred from serum into bile but not into milk. Scand. J. Immunol. **14:** 95–98.
50. BRANDTZAEG, P. 1982. Review and discussion of IgA transport to mucosal surfaces. In Recent Advances in Mucosal Immunity. W. STROBER, L. Å. HANSON, K. W. SELL, Eds.: 267–285. Raven Press. New York.
51. BRANDTZAEG, P. 1981. Transport models for secretory IgA and secretory IgM. Clin. Exp. Immunol. **44:** 221–232.
52. GUYTON, A. C. 1975. Interstitial fluid pressure and dynamics of lymph formation. Fed. Proc. Fed. Am. Soc. Exp. Biol. **35:** 1861–1862.
53. BRANDTZAEG, P. 1976. Structural, functional and cellular studies of human J chain. Ric. Clin. Lab. **6.** Suppl. No. 3: 15–38.
54. SASAKI, M., W. N. EIGEL & T. W. KEENAN. 1978. Lactose and major milk proteins are present in secretory vesicle-rich fractions from lactating mammary gland. Proc. Natl. Acad. Sci. USA **75:** 5020–5024.
55. LEARY, H. L. & B. L. LARSON. 1981. Immunoglobulin G transport by the bovine mammary gland—an immunocytochemical approach. In Advances in Experimental Medicine and Biology. The Ruminant Immune System. J. E. Butler, Ed.: **137:** 802 (Abstract). Plenum Press. New York.
56. PITTARD, W. B., S. H. POLMAR & A. A. FANAROFF. 1977. The breast milk macrophages: a potential vehicle for immunoglobulin transport. J. Reticuloendothelial Soc. **22:** 597–603.
57. CRAGO, S. S., S. J. PRINCE, T. G. PRETLOW, J. R. McGHEE & J. MESTECKY. 1979. Human colostral cells. I. Separation and characterization. Clin. Exp. Immunol. **38:** 585–597.
58. HO, C. S., L. C. WONG & J. W. M. LAWTON. 1979. Human colostral and breast milk cells. A light and electron microscopic study. Acta Paediatr. Scand. **68:** 389–396.
59. WEAVER, E. A., R. M. GOLDBLUM, C. P. DAVIS & A. S. GOLDMAN. 1981. Enhanced

immunoglobulin A release from human colostral cells during phagocytosis. Infect. Immun. **34**: 498–502.

60. MURILLO, G. J. & A. S. GOLDBLUM. 1970. The cells of human colostrum. II. Synthesis of IgA and β_{1c}. Pediatr. Res. **4**: 71–75.

61. AHLSTEDT, S., B. CARLSSON, L. Å. HANSON & R. M. GOLDBLUM. 1975. Antibody production by human colostral cells. I. Immunoglobulin class, specificity, and quantity. Scand. J. Immunol. **4**: 535–539.

DISCUSSION OF THE PAPER

J. MESTECKY (*University of Alabama in Birmingham*): I was surprised by the number of IgD cells in the mammary gland, and I would like Dr. Leslie to comment on his findings of IgD in milk.

G. LESLIE (*University of Oregon, Portland, Oreg.*): Dr. Olsen, who works in my laboratory has shown that in rat and in human milk, there are high concentrations of IgD. Preliminary studies suggest that it is of high molecular weight. In rats, the levels of IgD are up to 200 times higher than in serum. In view of your studies of localization of IgD-plasma cells, we might think about IgD as being one of the secretory immunoglobulins. Do you have any comments that concern the distribution and origin of IgD in milk? Is IgD transported from serum or derived from plasma cells found in the mammary gland?

P. BRANDTZAEG (*The National Hospital, Olso, Norway*): We have no evidence indicating that IgD is transported through the epithelium along with IgA and IgM. According to the immunoflurescent pictures, it leaks out between epithelial cells along with IgG.

In the case of IgA deficiency, IgA cells are replaced with more than 60% IgD-plasma cells in lacrimal and nasal glands. This phenomenon contrasts with the gastrointestinal tract, where there is no IgD replacement when IgA is lacking.

LESLIE: Both in the human and the rat, milk and colostrum IgD appear to be of high molecular weight. We have not done the characterization of IgD as to the presence of J-chain or secretory component.

R. GOLDBLUM (*University of Texas, Galveston, Tex.*): I would like to comment about the cells that are in colostrum. There is evidence, in addition to the presence of the nonspecific esterase, to indicate that these cells are probably macrophages. They will take up particles. Monoclonal antibodies to the fat globule membranes do not react with milk cells that we consider to be macrophages.

Another point concerns the milk cells as carriers of IgA. Dr. Weaver in our laboratory has been studying the compartmentalization of IgA in the particulate fraction of milk, and she has shown that IgA is inside of milk cells. The majority of these cells are macrophages and neutrophils. Opsonized particles are taken up, and there is a correlation between uptake of particles, as demonstrated by microscopy, and release of IgA; 75% of IgA is secretory IgA. Therefore, the cells that are phagocytic, seem also to be carrying IgA, and that IgA can be specifically released from the cells upon phagocytosis.

BRANDTZAEG: My point was that you cannot trust nonspecific esterase alone as a marker for macrophages in milk and colostrum. We also used immunofluorescence marker antigens. In prepartum samples, and postpartum samples, we find few true macrophages. Most of them are located in the interlobular connective tissue, and few migrate into the epithelium. I think a better identification of macrophages should be performed because nonspecific esterase is not of the best criterion for characterization of cells as macrophages.

FUNCTION OF THE HUMAN LIVER IN IgA
HOMEOSTASIS IN PLASMA*

D. L. Delacroix and J. P. Vaerman†

Gastroenterology Laboratory
University Clinic of St. Luke
International Institute of Cellular and Molecular Pathology
Experimental Medicine Unit
Catholic University of Louvain
Brussels, Belgium

INTRODUCTION

Polymeric IgA (pIgA) is the predominant immunoglobulin in most mammalian secretions, where it occurs bound to secretory component (SC) to form secretory IgA (sIgA), whose protective function through "immune exclusion" is largely admitted.[1-4] The role of epithelial-cell membranous SC in the vesicular transcellular transport of pIgA (and IgM) into secretions is now well documented.[5-13] Local mucosal synthesis of IgA, rather than its transfer from plasma, was long regarded[14,15] as the major source of sIgA in all exocrine secretions. Recently, however, the murine liver was shown to actively transport large amounts of pIgA from plasma into bile, pointing to a crucial link between plasma IgA, and IgA in bile and intestinal secretions, hence, to a unique role of the murine liver in the gut secretory immune system.[16-18] Such a SC-dependent plasma-to-bile transfer of pIgA, first suggested by our research with mice intravenously (i.v.) injected with MOPC-315 IgA,[19] was later clearly demonstrated in rats on the following grounds. Rat bile contains much free SC, and much higher levels of IgA than rat serum.[20,21] Intravenously injected pIgA, but not monomeric IgA (mIgA), is rapidly removed from the circulation and transported in bile where it appears bound to secretory component.[22-28] Bile-duct ligation results in a rapid and selective increase of both pIgA and SC in serum.[29] Rat hepatocytes synthetize[30-32] and express SC on their membrane.[30,32-35] Binding of pIgA, or of anti-SC antibodies[24,28,36] with this SC results in their vesicular uptake and transport across the hepatocyte.[37-43] More recently, several groups also showed that i.v. injected antigens complexed with pIgA antibodies were actively transported from plasma to bile.[44-49] Active plasma-to-bile transfer of pIgA also occurs in rabbits[40,50,51] and in fowl,[52] but cannot be generalized to all animal species.[40,50,53]

In humans, pIgA is present in serum[54,55] at roughly similar concentrations as in other mammals.[3,56] Large additional amounts of mIgA in human serum, however, render the separate consideration of mIgA and pIgA mandatory when studying the role and fate of serum IgA. Because of serious problems of standardization of the assays, separate changes in levels of mIgA and pIgA were rarely reported. Although increased total serum IgA levels, with a preferential contribution of

*This study was supported by grants No. 4.4504.70 and No. 220992 from the Medical Science Research Foundation, Brussels. D. L. Delacroix is Senior Research Assistant at the National Scientific Research Foundation, Brussels. Financial support was also given by the Medical Science Liaison, Puurs, Belgium.

†Correspondence to: J. P. Vaerman, UCL—ICP—MEXP, 75, avenue Hippocrate, B—1200 Brussels, Belgium.

0077-8923/83/0409-0383 $1.75/0 © 1983, NYAS

pIgA[2,57,58] were reported in cirrhosis, such data do not exist for biliary obstruction (BO), and nothing suggests a relationship between the high serum levels of pIgA in cirrhosis and an impaired plasma-to-bile transfer by the diseased liver. High levels of serum SC, putatively bound only to pIgA,[59] have also been found in liver diseases (LD),[60-63] but the specificity and the explanation of this phenomenon remain unclear. Immunohistochemical detection of SC in human liver is discordant: some[64,65] only detected SC in or on bile-duct cells, whereas others found intense SC-staining in hepatocytes,[66] even more than in bile-duct cells as in rats.[41,67] The presence in human hepatic bile of substantial amounts of sIgA was shown by Dive & Heremans[68] who suggested a local production of IgA in addition to a passive transudation from plasma. Recently, Kutteh et al.,[58] while examining three hepatic biles, found the bile-to-serum pIgA concentration ratio 1.7–11.0 times higher than the corresponding ratio for IgG. They did not, however, determine the origin of this IgA in relative excess.[58]

In our attempts to examine the role of the human liver in plasma IgA homeostasis, we first scrutinized the influence of the size of IgA in various immunoassays[69-71] in order to quantitate separately mIgA, pIgA, and sIgA in various fluids at a high level of sensitivity and with a minimum of methodological error. Different clinical and technical approaches were used to assess the relationships between human serum, liver, and bile with respect to mIgA, pIgA, and SC. These studies are reviewed here.

MATERIALS, METHODS, AND RESULTS

High Concentrations of SC in Serum During Liver Disease

A competition radioimmunoassay (RIA) using [^{125}I]sIgA and insolubilized goat anti-SC IgG was used to measure total SC in sera; results were expressed in μg/ml of equivalent of 11S sIgA.[72]

Specificity of High Serum SC Levels in Liver Disease[73]

In 120 healthy controls, SC levels ranged between 3 and 28 μg/ml. No significant increases were found in 46 patients with combined high total serum IgA, inflammatory syndrome, and normal liver function tests (not shown). Mean levels in patients with epithelial cancers (11.4 μg/ml), IgA myeloma (10.7 μg/ml), Crohn's disease (16.1 μg/ml), or rheumatoid arthritis (12.7 μg/ml) were only slightly elevated, in contrast with patients with cirrhosis (52 μg/ml), or epithelial cancer with liver metastasis, who showed marked elevations of serum SC, higher than those in lactating women (19.4 μg/ml) (FIGURE 1).

Clinical and Biochemical Relationships between High Serum SC and Cholestasis or Regeneration of the Liver[74]

Among 147 patients with well classified LD, the highest mean levels of serum SC were found in primary biliary cirrhosis (PBC) (112 μg/ml), BO (101 μg/ml), and acute hepatitis (AH) (99 μg/ml), higher (p < 0.001) than those in other forms of parenchymal LD (FIGURE 2). The particular influence of cholestasis on high serum

SC levels, suggested by results in BO and PBC as previously reported,[60,62] was confirmed in other forms of chronic parenchymal LD, where serum SC levels strongly correlated with serum concentrations of alkaline phosphatase and leucine aminopeptidase (FIGURE 3), but not with parameters of the functional parenchymal mass, such as prothrombin time and aminopyrine breath test, or with the presence of a portacaval shunt (FIGURE 2). No correlation was found between serum levels of SC and of total IgA. In seven cases of fulminant massive

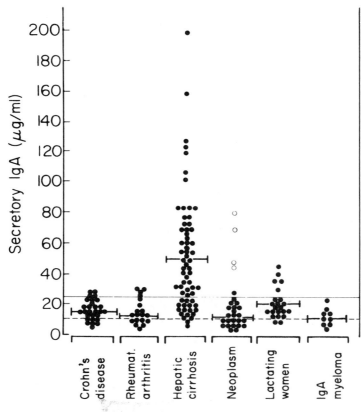

FIGURE 1. Serum SC levels, expressed as 11S sIgA equivalents, in various groups of subjects. Means are indicated by ⊢. Open circles: neoplasms with liver metastases. Horizontal line and dashed line represent the upper 97th percentile and mean level of 120 normal controls, respectively. (D. L. Delacroix & J. P. Vaerman.[73] With permission from *Clinical and Experimental Immunology*).

necrosis of the liver, when coma (stage four) and a fall of the prothrombin time occurred, high SC levels could not be maintained and dropped to the upper limit of the normal range (FIGURE 4, left). In three cases, SC levels rose again when clinical and biochemical evidence of liver regeneration, that is disappearance of

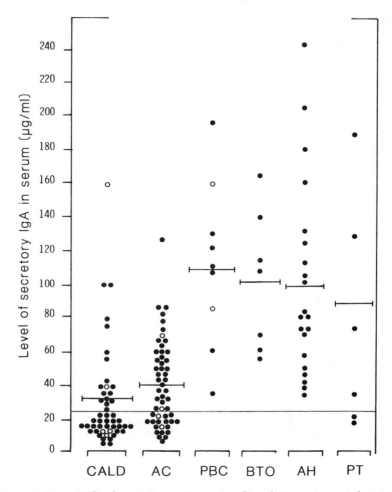

FIGURE 2. Serum SC levels, as in FIGURE 1, in various liver diseases. Open circles: patients with surgical portacaval shunt. CALD: chronic active liver disease; AC: alcoholic cirrhosis; PBC: primary biliary cirrhosis; BTO: biliary tract obstruction; AH: acute hepatitis; PT: primary liver tumor. (D. L. Delacroix, M. Reynaert, S. Pauwels, A. P. Geubel & J. P. Vaerman.[74] With permission from *Digestive Diseases and Sciences*).

the encephalopathy and correction of the prothrombin time, occurred (FIGURE 4, right). A decreased liver catabolism of circulating sIgA, as previously suggested by others,[59,60] is thus unlikely to explain the high serum SC in liver disease. A direct release of free SC from undefined regenerating liver cells into the circulation is likely to occur in acute hepatitis. In this hypothesis, and according to the high affinity of human free SC for human IgM,[75,76] IgM-bound SC should also be found in AH serum.

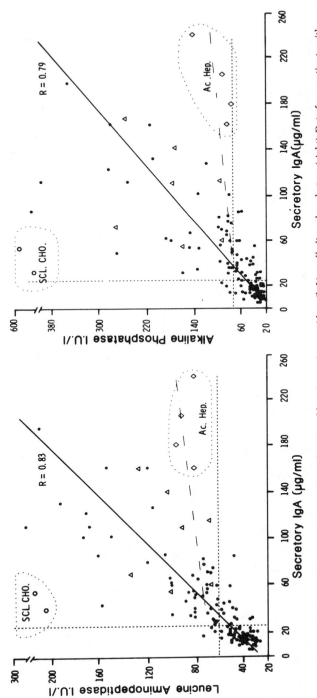

FIGURE 3. Correlations between serum values of sIgA and leucine aminopeptidase (left) or alkaline phosphatase (right). Data from patients with sclerosing cholangitis (O), acute hepatitis (◊) and biliary obstruction (△) are not involved in the calculations of the correlation coefficients (R). Dotted lines represent the upper limits of control ranges. The dashed lines represent the linear regression in the whole group of acute hepatitis from which only the four patients with the highest SC values are represented. (D. L. Delacroix, M. Reynaert, S. Pauwels, A. P. Geubel & J. P. Vaerman.[74] With permission from *Digestive Diseases and Sciences*).

Molecular State of Serum SC in Liver Disease

A more sensitive RIA for SC was set up with a sensitivity at 2 μg/ml.[77] Sera with high SC levels were fractionated by sucrose density gradient ultracentrifugation (SDGU) for 16 hours at 34,000 rpm at 20° C in a Beckman SW-41 Ti rotor; SC, IgM, and IgA were quantitated in the 31 gradient fractions. IgM-bound SC (sIgM) was found in all sera; it constituted less than 15% of the total SC in sera of BO and postnecrotic or alcoholic cirrhosis. By contrast, high proportions of sIgM (up to 91%), were found in AH (FIGURE 5) and PBC sera, and correlated significantly with serum IgM/pIgA molar ratios.[77,78]

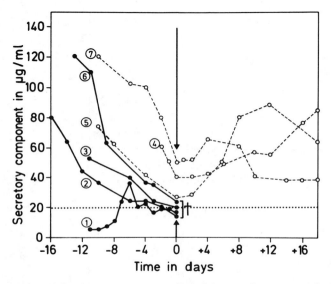

FIGURE 4. Serum SC levels in seven patients with fulminant hepatitis. At the left of the arrows, all patients were in coma stage four for at least a few days. At day 0, patients one, two, three, and six died, whereas patients four, five, and seven started to recover from coma with progressive correction of their prothrombin time.

Plasma-To-Bile Transport of IgA

Molecular State of Human IgA and SC in Bile Compared to Other Secretions

The sedimentation profiles of IgA and SC were studied in six different secretions, using specific immunoradiometric assays (IRMA)[70] for IgA and for SC, after SDGU of a pool (n ≥ 6) of each secretion. Results are shown in FIGURE 6. Substantial amounts (>5% of total IgA) of mIgA were found only in bronchial secretions (18%) and hepatic bile (35%), the latter displaying a unique peak of dimeric IgA devoid of SC in addition to 11S sIgA. Free SC occurred in bile as in other secretions (FIGURE 6); it was also present in a bile sample from an IgA-deficient patient (not shown).[78]

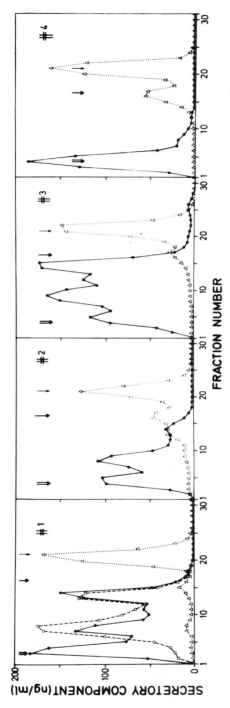

FIGURE 5. Sucrose density gradient ultracentrifugation profiles of IgA ($\triangle \cdots \triangle$), total SC ($\bullet\!\!-\!\!\bullet$), and IgA-bound SC ($\bigcirc\!\!-\!\!-\bigcirc$), all measured by immunoradiometric assays, in serum of four patients with acute hepatitis and high serum SC levels. Sedimentation from right to left. Double arrow: position of IgM measured by IRMA; thick arrow: position of marker ^{125}I-labeled dimeric IgA; thin arrow: position of IgG measured by optical density. Patients one and four had high serum IgM levels.

Selectivity of the Excretion of pIgA in Bile Compared to Other Human Secretions

Using the same secretion pools and their corresponding serum pools, the secretion-to-serum concentration ratios (S/S-CR) for mIgA, pIgA, IgG, and IgM were measured using specific IRMA[79] and SDGU. The S/S-CR for mIgA, pIgA,

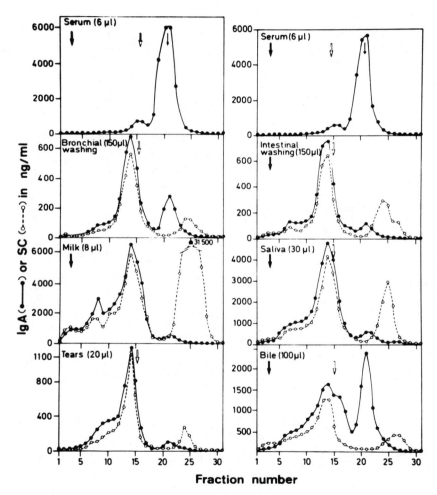

FIGURE 6. Sucrose density gradient ultracentrifugation profiles of IgA (●—●) and SC (O---O) in two normal sera and in six different pools of exocrine secretions. Volume of each fluid applied on the gradient is indicated between parentheses. Sedimentation from right to left. Thick arrow: position of IgM measured by IRMA; open arrow: position of marker [125I]dimeric IgA; thin arrow: position of IgG by optical density. Free SC is seen in all secretions around fraction number 25. Note significant amounts of mIgA in bronchial washing and bile, and dimeric IgA devoid of SC in bile.

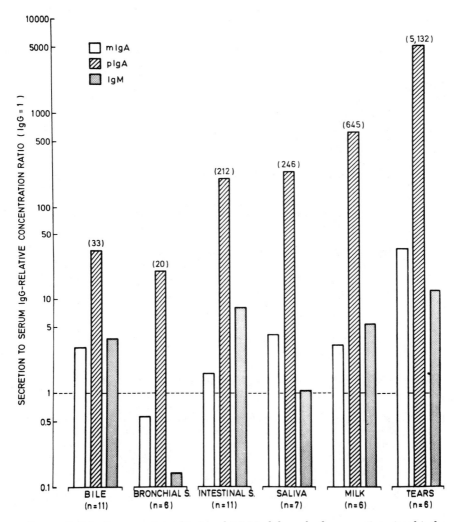

FIGURE 7. Selective excretion of IgA and IgM in bile and other secretions (pools): the columns are secretion-to-serum concentration ratios relative to those for IgG taken as reference (dashed line-1): IgA and IgM were measured by IRMA, and mIgA and pIgA were separated by density gradient centrifugation. n = number of individual secretions, or sera, used for making pools. Note log scale.

and IgM were expressed relatively to those for IgG taken as reference. These IgG-relative S/S-CR (FIGURE 7) indicate a selective excretion of pIgA in all secretions, smaller in bile and bronchial secretions and highest in milk and tears (FIGURE 7). Except in bronchial secretions, IgM was also more selectively excreted than IgG, even in saliva, if one considers its high molecular weight. In all secretions, mIgA was excreted at least tenfold less selectively than pIgA, but was still in excess when compared to IgG. A passive transport of locally produced mIgA could explain this excess.

Selective Secretion of pIgA in Human Hepatic Bile Compared to Rat and Rabbit Bile

The selective excretions of pIgA, IgG, and IgM in 17 individual samples of human hepatic bile (T-tube or retrograde cholangiography) were compared to those in 8 individual rabbit hepatic biles[51] or in 9 rat biles. The bile-to-serum concentration ratios (B/S) were, this time, expressed relatively to the corresponding B/S for albumin taken as reference. For rabbits[51] and rats (unpublished data kindly provided by Dr. I. Lemaître-Coelho), the protein levels were measured by radial immunodiffusion, the amount of mIgA being considered unsignificant, or by IRMA for IgM. In human hepatic bile, the levels of total IgA ranged from 37 to 159 μg/ml($\bar{x}$ = 77 μg/ml), close to the IgG levels ($\bar{x}$ = 89 μg/ml), and much lower than IgA levels reported by others[64] who did not find detectable IgG and IgM. Polymeric IgA comprised 43 to 89% of total IgA ($\bar{x}$ = 70%). Concentrations of pIgA in human bile were always lower than in serum ($\bar{x}$ = 25% of serum value), whereas IgA levels in rat and rabbit biles always largely exceeded those in corresponding sera (up to 37-fold). The mean albumin-relative B/S indicated a 14-fold and 50-fold less important selective excretion of pIgA in human bile than in rabbit or rat bile, respectively (FIGURE 8). In contrast, the slight selective excretion of IgM was roughly similar in the three species (FIGURE 8).

Plasma Versus Local Contribution to IgA in Human Bile

In 5 of the 17 patients studied for B/S ratios, 2-10 μCi of [^{125}I]pIgA and (or in one case) of [^{131}I]mIgA of polyclonal origin[69] were i.v. injected. Simultaneous measurements of the specific activities of mIgA and pIgA were made in serum, bile (T-tube drainage or transhepatic catheter in one case), and whole mixed saliva, using the anti-α-precipitable radioactivities as described.[79] Comparisons of specific activities indicated that 37-69% of pIgA in bile derived from plasma, compared to 0.6-3.7% in saliva. Most of bile mIgA (73-100%) derived from plasma, compared to less than 77% in saliva. Mean albumin-relative S/S-CR for mIgA and pIgA in the five patients studied are shown in FIGURE 9, with the shaded columns representing the ratios obtained when considering only bile IgA of plasma origin. Although about half of pIgA in bile derived from plasma, the selectivity of this transport from plasma was not much different in bile and saliva when expressed relatively to albumin (FIGURE 9). Most of the difference between the selective enrichment in pIgA in these two secretions was related to a major contribution of locally produced pIgA in the salivary glands, but not in the liver. In terms of absolute amounts, and according to mean 50% or 2% of pIgA of plasma origin in bile or saliva respectively, about 27 mg of pIgA were transported daily from plasma to bile in our 17 patients for a bile output of about one liter. For a similar output of saliva, only three mg of pIgA would originate from plasma. This low value for human bile agrees with the very small recoveries ($\pm$2%) of i.v. injected [^{125}I]pIgA in a 24-hour bile collection in our patients,[79] and contrasts with the large recoveries in hepatic bile of rats and rabbits (30-70% in three hours) injected with the same labeled pIgA.

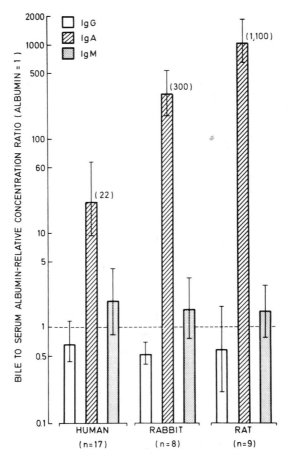

FIGURE 8. Comparative selective excretion of pIgA, IgG, and IgM in human, rabbit, and rat hepatic biles. Columns give means ± SD of bile-to-serum concentration ratios relative to those of albumin taken as reference (dashed line-1). All proteins were measured by IRMA except IgA and IgG in rats and rabbits (radial immunodiffusion). n = number of individual pairs of bile and serum analyzed.

Immunohistochemical Detection of SC in Human Liver

A rabbit anti-SC antiserum and the peroxidase-anti-peroxidase complex technique were used to detect SC in human liver sections (surgical biopsies). Ileal mucosa was used as positive control, and the inhibition of staining by SC, but not by IgA, was demonstrated. By optical microscopy, SC was clearly detected in liver only in and on bile duct cells; in gut also, only nonmucinous epithelial cells were stained. No SC-staining was found in or on hepatocytes (FIGURE 10), as others have found.[64,65]

Lack of Selective Increase of Serum pIgA During Biliary Obstruction

Serum levels of mIgA, pIgA, and SC were measured by SDGU and RIA in 34 clinically healthy adults, in 14 patients with complete tumorous extrahepatic BO, and in 35 patients with alcoholic cirrhosis.[80] Means (±SD) of results are shown in FIGURE 11. No significant increases in serum pIgA were found in BO (248 ± 126 μg/ml), compared to (224 ± 93 μg/ml) controls; there was also no change in its contribution to total IgA ($\bar{x}$ = 12%, range 4–21% compared to $\bar{x}$ = 13%, range

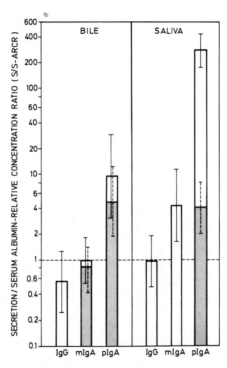

FIGURE 9. Secretion-to-serum albumin-relative concentration ratios (S/S-ARCR) (means ± SD) of IgG, mIgA, and pIgA for bile and saliva of five patients i.v. injected with [^{125}I]pIgA and [^{131}I]mIgA. Shaded columns represent the S/S-ARCR calculated only from their serum-derived fractions. The horizontal dashed line represents the S/S-ARCR of albumin taken as unit. Note log scale. (D. L. Delacroix, H. F. Hodgson, A. McPherson, C. Dive.[79] & J. P. Vaerman. With permission from *The Journal of Clinical Investigation*).

5–22% in controls). This situation contrasted with the marked and preferential increase (p < 0.001) of pIgA in cirrhosis (985 ± 696 μg/ml), with also the proportion of pIgA significantly increased ($\bar{x}$ = 21%, range 9–40%). Larger increases of SC were found in sera of BO than of cirrhosis (p < 0.001), without correlation to changes in pIgA levels, in discordance with a previous suggestion.[58] Again, these data contrast with the rapid and selective increases of both pIgA and SC in sera of rats[29] and rabbits[51] after bile duct ligation.

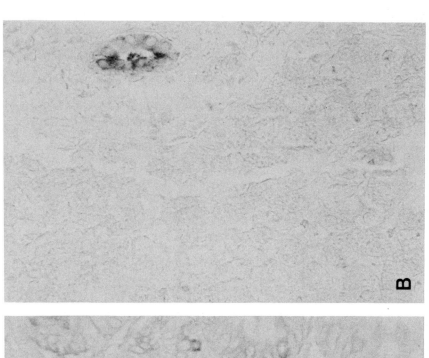

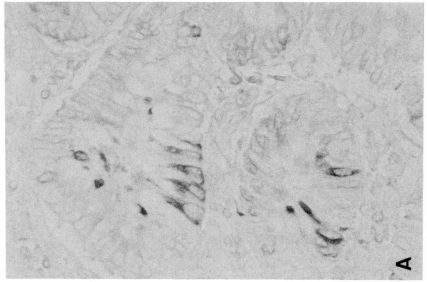

FIGURE 10. Immunohistochemical localization of SC in human liver (B) and ileal mucosa (A). Kindly performed by Dr. J. Rahier, University of Louvain, Brussels.

*Indirect Evidence for an SC-Independent Mechanism of Selective Removal of
Circulating pIgA by the Human Liver*

Recently, we compared the plasma survivals of i.v. injected [^{131}I]mIgA and
[^{125}I]pIgA in healthy subjects and in cirrhotics.[80] As reported in controls,[79] the
fractional catabolic rate (FCR) of pIgA was 1.8 times larger than that of mIgA
(FIGURE 12). Preliminary results in cirrhotics indicated a significant reduction of
the FCR of pIgA but not of mIgA, whereas such a reduction was not found in a
case of complete biliary obstruction. In cirrhotics, a significant correlation was
found between the increase of the i.v. pool of pIgA and the reduction of the pIgA
fractional catabolic rate. This correlation suggests a direct linkage between the
preferential elevation of serum pIgA and a reduction of its catabolism during
cirrhosis, whereas such changes would not occur, or at a much lesser degree,
during biliary obstruction. A selective removal of circulating pIgA by some liver
cells could thus occur in humans, but it would be quite different from the
SC-dependent plasma-to-bile transport of pIgA by rat and rabbit hepatocytes.
The occurrence of such a mechanism seems supported by the reported affinity of
human hepatocytes for pIgA, but not for mIgA, independently from the presence
of secretory component.[65]

CONCLUSIONS

In humans, a particular relationship between serum, liver, and bile was
demonstrated with respect to pIgA and secretory component. 1) High serum
concentrations of SC occur during liver disease and correlate with cholestasis and
liver regeneration. The evolution of serum SC levels in AH and the occurrence of
substantial amounts of IgM-bound SC in these cases support a direct release of
free SC by the liver in the circulation. 2) Polymeric IgA is transported from plasma
to bile 7 or 10 times more selectively than mIgA or IgG, and is found at least partly

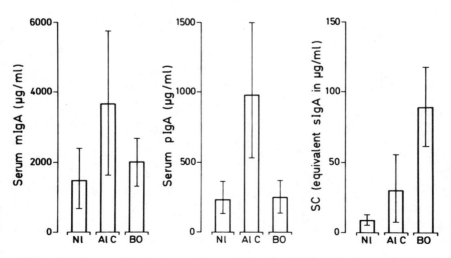

FIGURE 11. Comparative mean serum concentrations ± SD of mIgA, pIgA, and SC in 34
normal controls (NI), 35 patients with alcoholic cirrhosis (AlC), and 14 patients with biliary
obstruction (BO).

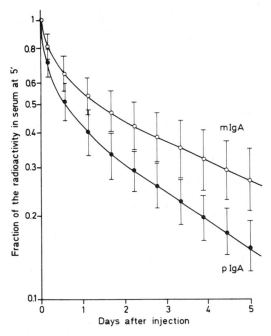

FIGURE 12. Survival in plasma of i.v. injected I-labeled mIgA and pIgA; note faster catabolism of pIgA. Radioactivities in serum are means ± SD in nine healthy volunteers.

associated with SC in bile. 3) Secretory component in liver is found selectively in or on bile-duct cells, suggesting its synthesis by these cells and their predominant role in this selective pIgA transport.

The role of this transport mechanism in the homeostasis of pIgA in plasma is, however, much less important in humans than in rats and rabbits. 1) Compared to these mammals, the selectivity of the excretion of pIgA in bile (relative to albumin) is 50 and 14 times smaller in humans, and seems similar to that in saliva. 2) Only about 2% of the injected pIgA is recovered in bile over 24 hours in humans. 3) The lack of detectable SC in or on human hepatocytes is likely to explain the smaller plasma-to-bile transport of pIgA in humans. 4) Biliary obstruction in humans does not result in a significant increase of circulating pIgA, as is found in rats and rabbits.

Human liver could play a significant role, however, in the selective removal of pIgA from plasma by another SC-independent mechanism, because unlike in BO, preferential increases of serum pIgA and a selective reduction of the FCR of pIgA occur during parenchymal liver disease.

ACKNOWLEDGMENTS

We thank Drs. P. J. Kestens, J. B. Otte, A. P. Geubel, M. Reynaert, and C. Dive from the University Clinic of St. Luke, Brussels, and H. J. F. Hodgson, from the

Royal Postgraduate Medical School, London, for having allowed us to study their patients. The excellent technical assistance of J. P. Dehennin, R. Meykens, and J. Naze-De Mets is gratefully acknowledged.

REFERENCES

1. TOMASI, T. B. & J. BIENENSTOCK. 1968. Adv. Immunol. **9:** 1–96.
2. TOMASI, T. B. & H. M. GREY. 1972. Prog. Allergy **16:** 81–213.
3. HEREMANS, J. F. 1974. *In* The Antigens. M. Sela, Ed.: Vol. 2: 365–522. Academic Press. New York.
4. HANSON, L. Å. & P. BRANDTZAEG. 1980. *In* Immunological Disorders in Infants and Children. R. E. Stiehm and V. A. Fulginiti, Eds.: 2nd edit.: 137–164. W. B. Saunders Co. London.
5. BRANDTZAEG, P. 1974. J. Immunol. **112:** 1553–1559.
6. POGER, M. E. & M. E. LAMM. 1974. J. Exp. Med. **139:** 629–642.
7. BRANDTZAEG, P. 1978. Scand. J. Immunol. **8:** 39–52.
8. CRAGO, S. S., R. KULHAVY, S. J. PRINCE & J. MESTECKY. 1978. J. Exp. Med. **147:** 1832–1837.
9. BROWN, W. R., K. ISOBE, P. K. NAKANE & B. PACINI. 1977. Gastroenterology **73:** 1333–1339.
10. NAGURA, H., P. K. NAKANE & W. R. BROWN. 1979. J. Immunol. **123:** 2359–2368.
11. KÜHN, L. C. & J. P. KRAEHENBUHL. 1979. J. Biol. Chem. **254:** 11072–11081.
12. KÜHN, L. C. & J. P. KRAEHENBUHL. 1981. J. Biol. Chem. **256:** 12490–12495.
13. BRANDTZAEG, P. 1981. Clin. Exp. Immunol. **44:** 221–232.
14. BUTLER, W. T., R. D. ROSSEN & T. A. WALDMANN. 1967. J. Clin. Invest. **46:** 1883–1893.
15. STROBER, W., R. M. BLAESE & T. A. WALDMANN. 1970. J. Lab. Clin. Med. **75:** 856–862.
16. VAERMAN, J. P., I. LEMAÎTRE-COELHO & G. D. F. JACKSON. 1978. *In* Secretory Immunity and Infection. J. R. McGhee, J. Mestecky and J. L. Babb, Eds.: Adv. Exp. Med. Biol. **107:** 233–240. Plenum Press. New York.
17. LEMAÎTRE-COELHO, I., G. D. F. JACKSON & J. P. VAERMAN. 1978. Scand. J. Immunol. **8:** 21–28.
18. HALL, J. G. & E. ANDREW. 1980. Immunology Today **1:** 100–104.
19. JACKSON, G. D. F., I. LEMAÎTRE-COELHO & J. P. VAERMAN. 1977. Protides Biol. Fluids Proc. Colloq. **25:** 912–922.
20. LEMAÎTRE-COELHO, I., G. D. F. JACKSON & J. P. VAERMAN. 1977. Eur. J. Immunol. **7:** 588–590.
21. MULLOCK, B. M., M. DOBROTA & R. H. HINTON. 1978. Biochim. Biophys. Acta **543:** 497–507.
22. JACKSON, G. D. F., I. LEMAÎTRE-COELHO, J. P. VAERMAN, H. BAZIN & A. BECKERS. 1978. Eur. J. Immunol. **8:** 123–126.
23. ORLANS, E., J. PEPPARD, J. REYNOLDS & J. HALL. 1978. J. Exp. Med. **147:** 588–592.
24. FISHER, M. M., B. NAGY, H. BAZIN & B. J. UNDERDOWN. 1979. Proc. Natl. Acad. Sci. USA **76:** 2008–2012.
25. VAERMAN, J. P. & I. LEMAÎTRE-COELHO. 1979. *In* Transmission of Proteins through Living Membranes. W. A. Hemmings, Ed.: 383–398. Elsevier/North Holland Biomedical Press. Amsterdam.
26. REYNOLDS, J., L. GYURE, E. ANDREW & J. G. HALL. 1980. Immunology **39:** 463–467.
27. DAHLGREN, U., S. AHLSTEDT, L. HEDMAN, C. WADSWORTH & L. Å HANSON. 1981. Scand. J. Immunol. **14:** 95–98.
28. LEMAÎTRE-COELHO, I., G. ACOSTA-ALTAMIRANO, C. BARRANCO-ACOSTA, R. MEYKENS & J. P. VAERMAN. 1981. Immunology **43:** 261–270.
29. LEMAÎTRE-COELHO, I., G. D. F. JACKSON & J. P. VAERMAN. 1978. J. Exp. Med. **147:** 934–939.
30. SOCKEN, D. J., K. N. JEEJEEBHOY, H. BAZIN & B. J. UNDERDOWN. 1979. J. Exp. Med. **150:** 1538–1548.

31. ZEVENBERGEN, J., C. MAY, J. C. WANSON & J. P. VAERMAN. 1980. Scand. J. Immunol. **11:** 93-97.
32. LIMET, J. N., Y.-J. SCHNEIDER, J. P. VAERMAN & A. TROUET. 1980. Toxicology **18:** 187-194.
33. ORLANS, E., J. PEPPARD, J. F. FRY, R. H. HINTON & B. M. MULLOCK. 1979. J. Exp. Med. **150:** 1577-1581.
34. LIMET, J. N., Y.-J. SCHNEIDER, A. TROUET & J. P. VAERMAN. 1981. In The Mucosal Immune System. F. J. Bourne, Ed.: Curr. Top. Veterin. Med. & Anim. Sci. **12:** 49-68. Martinus Nijhoff, London & Den Haag.
35. LIMET, J. N., Y.-J. SCHNEIDER, A. TROUET & J. P. VAERMAN. 1981. Protides Biol. Fluids Proc. Colloq. **29:** 423-426.
36. LEMAÎTRE-COELHO, I., R. MEYKENS & J. P. VAERMAN. 1981. Protides Biol. Fluids Proc. Colloq. **29:** 419-422.
37. BIRBECK, M. S. C., P. CARTWRIGHT, J. G. HALL, E. ORLANS & J. PEPPARD. 1979. Immunology **37:** 477-484.
38. MULLOCK, B. M., R. H. HINTON, M. DOBROTA, J. PEPPARD & E. ORLANS. 1979. Biochim. Biophys. Acta **587:** 381-391.
39. RENSTON, R. H., A. L. JONES, W. D. CHRISTIANSEN, G. T. HRADEK & B. J. UNDERDOWN. 1980. Science **208:** 1276-1278.
40. VAERMAN, J. P., I. M. LEMAÎTRE-COELHO, J. N. LIMET & D. L. DELACROIX. 1982. In Recent Advances in Mucosal Immunity. W. Strober, L. Hanson, and K. Sell, Eds.: 233-250. Raven Press. New York.
41. TAKAHASHI, I., P. K. NAKANE & W. R. BROWN. 1982. J. Immunol. **128:** 1181-1187.
42. LIMET, J. N., Y. J. SCHNEIDER, A. TROUET & J. P. VAERMAN. 1982. Eur. J. Biochem. **125:** 437-443.
43. COURTOY, P. J., J. N. LIMET, P. BAUDHUIN, J. QUINTART, Y.-J. SCHNEIDER & J. P. VAERMAN. 1983. Ann. N.Y. Acad. Sci. This volume.
44. PEPPARD, J. V., E. ORLANS, A. W. R. PAYNE & E. ANDREW. 1981. Immunology **42:** 83-89.
45. SOCKEN, D. J., E. S. SIMMS, B. NAGY, M. M. FISHER & B. J. UNDERDOWN. 1981. Mol. Immunol. **18:** 345-348.
46. RUSSEL, M. W., T. A. BROWN & J. MESTECKY. 1981. J. Exp. Med. **153:** 968-976.
47. SOCKEN, D. J., E. S. SIMMS, B. NAGY, M. M. FISHER & B. J. UNDERDOWN. 1981. J. Immunol. **127:** 316-319.
48. PEPPARD, J. V., E. ORLANS, E. ANDREW & A. W. R. PAYNE. 1982. Immunology **45:** 467-472.
49. RUSSEL, M. W., T. A. BROWN & J. MESTECKY. 1982. Mol. Immunol. **19:** 677-682.
50. HALL, J. G., L. A. GYURE & A. W. R. PAYNE. 1980. Immunology **41:** 899-902.
51. DELACROIX, D. L., A. M. DENEF, G. A. ACOSTA, P. C. MONTGOMERY & J. P. VAERMAN. 1982. Scand. J. Immunol. **16:** 343-350.
52. ROSE, M. E., E. ORLANS, A. W. R. PAYNE & P. HESKETH. 1981. Eur. J. Immunol. **11:** 561-564.
53. DIVE, C., R. A. NADALINI, J. P. VAERMAN & J. F. HEREMANS. 1974. Eur. J. Clin. Invest. **4:** 241-246.
54. HEREMANS, J. F., M. T. HEREMANS & H. E. SCHULTZE. 1959. Clin. Chim. Acta **4:** 96-102.
55. CUADRADO, E. & J. P. VAERMAN. 1977. Protides Biol. Fluids Proc. Colloq. **25:** 915-918.
56. VAERMAN, J. P. 1973. In Research in Immunochemistry and Immunobiology. J. B. G. Kwapinski, Ed.: Vol. 3: 91-183. University Park Press. London.
57. ANDRÉ, F. & C. ANDRÉ. 1976. Biol. Gastroentérologie (Paris) **9:** 147-150.
58. KUTTEH, W. H., S. J. PRINCE, J. O. PHILLIPS, J. G. SPENNEY & J. MESTECKY. 1982. Gastroenterology **82:** 184-193.
59. ISCAKI, S., C. GENESTE & J. PILLOT. 1980. Immunology Letters **1:** 217-221.
60. THOMPSON, R. A., R. CARTER, R. P. STOKES, A. M. GEDDES & J. A. D. GOODALL. 1973. Clin. Exp. Immunol. **14:** 335-346.
61. THIERRY, R. C., S. ISCAKI & J. PILLOT. 1979. Pathol. Biol. **27:** 483-486.
62. GOLDBLUM, R. M., G. K. POWELL & G. VAN SICKLE. 1980. J. Pediatr. **97:** 33-36.
63. ISCAKI, S., C. BUFFET, M. J. BRIANTAIS, C. GENESTE, J. P. ETIENNE & J. PILLOT. 1981. Gastroentérologie Clin. Biol. **5:** 305-313.

64. NAGURA, H., P. D. SMITH, P. K. NAKANE & W. R. BROWN. 1981. J. Immunol. **126:** 587–595.
65. HOPF, U., P. BRANDTZAEG, T. H. HÜTTEROTH & K. H. MEYER ZUM BÜSCHENFELDE. 1978. Scand. J. Immunol. **8:** 543–549.
66. HSU, S. M. & P. L. HSU. 1980. Gut **21:** 985–989.
67. WILSON, I. D., M. WONG & S. L. ERLANDSEN. 1980. Gastroenterology **29:** 924–930.
68. DIVE, C. & J. F. HEREMANS. 1974. Eur. J. Clin. Invest. **4:** 235–239.
69. DELACROIX, D. L., R. MEYKENS & J. P. VAERMAN. 1982. Mol. Immunol. **19:** 297–305.
70. DELACROIX, D. L., J. P. DEHENNIN & J. P. VAERMAN. 1982. J. Immunol. Meth. **48:** 327–337.
71. DELACROIX, D. L. & J. P. VAERMAN. 1982. J. Immunol. Methods **51:** 49–55.
72. DELACROIX, D. L. & J. P. VAERMAN. 1981. J. Immunol. Methods **40:** 345–358.
73. DELACROIX, D. L. & J. P. VAERMAN. 1981. Clin. Exp. Immunol. **43:**633–640.
74. DELACROIX, D. L., M. REYNAERT, S. PAUWELS, A. P. GEUBEL & J. P. VAERMAN. 1982. Digest. Dis. Sci. **27:** 333–340.
75. BRANDTZAEG, P. 1977. Immunochemistry **14:** 179–188.
76. SOCKEN, D. J. & B. J. UNDERDOWN. 1978. Immunochemistry **15:** 499–506.
77. DELACROIX, D. L. & J. P. VAERMAN. 1982. Clin. Exp. Immunol. **49:** 717–724.
78. DELACROIX, D. L., P. JONARD, C. DIVE & J. P. VAERMAN. 1982. J. Immunol. **129:** 133–138.
79. DELACROIX, D. L., H. F. HODGSON, A. McPHERSON, C. DIVE & J. P. VAERMAN. 1982. J. Clin. Invest. **70:** 230–241.
80. DELACROIX, D. L., K. B. ELKON, A. P. GEUBEL, H. J. F. HODGSON & J. P. VAERMAN. 1983. J. Clin. Invest. In press.

DISCUSSION OF THE PAPER

R.M.E. PARKHOUSE (*National Institute for Medical Research, London, England*): I would like to ask you two questions about the association between secretory component and IgM. First, are they covalently linked? Second, is the complex between 19S IgM pentamer and one secretory component, or do you have two 19S pentamers and one secretory component?

J. P. VAERMAN (*Catholic University of Louvain, Brussels, Belgium*): Because we have no standard for secretory IgM, we can not quantitate it. There was binding, by the radiometric assay, of the labeled anti-μ reagent but we have not purified sIgM. I doubt that there is a covalent binding between SC and IgM. Because of the presence of bile salts, we frequently found that IgM in bile lacks SC. We have, however, only indirect evidence and no more data on this point.

M. W. RUSSELL (*University of Alabama in Birmingham*): In one of your earlier slides you indicated that levels of secretory component were increasing in cirrhotic patients who were recovering.

VAERMAN: These were not cirrhotics. These were patients with fulminating massive liver necrosis.

RUSSELL: Have you had the opportunity to examine samples from very young children, fetuses, or abortuses for the presence of secretory component in serum?

D. L. DELACROIX (*Catholic University of Louvain, Brussels, Belgium*): We suspect that some of the secretory component we find in serum of several patients with fulminating hepatitis is coming from regenerative cells in the liver. By immunochemical procedures, we examined the liver of a six-month-old fetus, and we did not find secretory component in hepatocytes. We are currently studying, by histochemistry, the precise nature of the cells that produce the secretory component in the liver during regeneration.

P. BRANDTZAEG (*The National Hospital, Oslo, Norway*): I would like to comment on the binding between SC and IgM. We cannot find more than one binding site for SC on 19S IgM. I am glad that you have raised the question of an additional binding site for IgA on human hepatocytes. This possibility was suggested on the basis of experiments performed in cooperation with Dr. Hopf from Berlin. We have also found that there is, in addition to secretory component, another binding site for IgA on rat hepatocytes.

VAERMAN: You also reported the binding of monomeric IgA.

BRANDTZAEG: Yes, but not to the same extent as polymeric IgA. Could you make the assertion that there is a less efficient transport of IgA by human liver because of a lack of SC-dependent transport?

VAERMAN: Secretory component and IgA can be found in bile duct cells. Although we would have liked to find SC on human hepatocytes, the immunohistochemical staining in our hands was negative. Nevertheless, there are reports indicating that SC is present in human hepatocytes. We believe that perhaps the staining intensity limits the detection. If one considers the number of hepatocytes compared to the number of bile-duct cells, one can explain the relatively low transfer of polymeric IgA that we find in humans.

DIFFERENCES IN PROCESSING OF POLYMERIC IgA AND ASIALOGLYCOPROTEINS BY THE RAT LIVER*

Brian J. Underdown, J. Michael Schiff, Barbara Nagy, and
Murray M. Fisher

Institute of Immunology
Department of Medicine and Medical Genetics
University of Toronto
Toronto, Ontario, M5S 1A8
Canada

The original observations of Vaerman and colleagues that polymeric IgA traverses the liver from blood to bile,[1,2] led our group, as well as others, to study the mechanism of transport.[3,4] In the rat, polymeric IgA is taken up specifically by a receptor that has been identified as membrane-bound secretory component.[5-8] Uptake and transport is controlled by receptor-ligand binding and is not dependent on other properties of polymeric IgA, because IgG antibodies to secretory component (SC) or their Fab fragments are also taken up and delivered to bile.[4,9] There is general agreement that in the rat, the hepatocyte is responsible for the transport of pIgA, and electron microscopic and subcellular fractionation studies indicate that transport proceeds by way of endocytic vesicles.[10-12]

The liver also takes up a large number of different proteins from blood, but by contrast to the processing of pIgA, most proteins taken up by the hepatocyte are degraded in lysosomes.[13]

The mechanisms by which the hepatocytes can sort proteins into the transport pathway, in the case of pIgA, or the degradative pathway, in the case of asialoglycoproteins, are not known. The experiments described in this paper are part of an approach to elucidate the factors controlling the processing of proteins by the rat liver.

A diagram illustrating some of the elements of the degradative and transport pathways is presented in FIGURE 1. The hepatocyte must at some stage be capable of sorting proteins destined for degradation in lysosomes from those such as pIgA destined for transport to bile. In our studies we have compared the processing of human asialo orosomucoid (ASOr) to rat pIgA. Both ligands are thought to be taken up by receptor-mediated endocytosis.[10-12,14] Clearly, the asialoglycoproteins and pIgA could be taken up in the same endocytic vesicles around coated pits[14] or the proteins could be independently sorted into different endocytic vesicles through the differential localization of their respective receptors at the sinusoidal membrane. Differential sorting at the surface of the hepatocyte would allow entry of each ligand onto separate endocytic pits. The different endocytic vesicles would then require different intracellular controlling elements, one set shuttling asialoglycoprotein-containing vesicles to the lysosomes, the other set shuttling pIgA-containing vesicles to the bile canaliculus. If on the other hand, asialoglycoproteins and pIgA are taken into the same endocytic vesicles, then a mechanism for intracellular sorting would be required to direct pIgA away from the lysosomes and toward the bile canaliculus.

The available electron microscopic evidence has provided limited data to answer the questions posed above. Data indicate that asialoglycoproteins are

*This work was supported by grants from the Medical Research Council of Canada.

0077–8923/83/0409–0402 $1.75/0 © 1983, NYAS

taken up around coated pits into 100nm endocytic vesicles.[14] The endocytosed asialoglycoproteins may be transferred to somewhat larger vesicles similar to those described by Pasten and colleagues as receptosomes.[15] Asialoglycoproteins are then found within lysosomes where they are degraded.[16,17] Polymeric IgA is also taken up in 100nm endocytic vesicles. Data presented in this volume (Courtoy *et al.*) indicate that pIgA is observed in coated vesicles as well as in larger receptosome-like vesicles. Unfortunately, double-labeling electron microscopic data is not available to indicate whether asialoglycoproteins and pIgA share a common pathway at any stage during their processing by the liver.

To approach this problem, we have carried out a series of experiments with

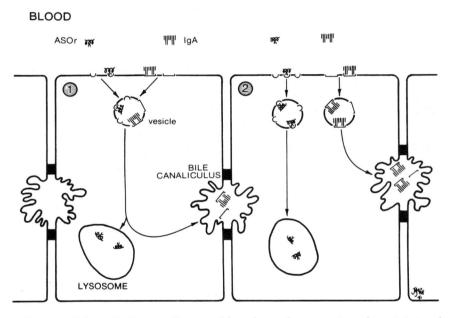

FIGURE 1. Schematic diagram of two possible pathways for processing polymeric IgA and asialoglycoproteins. The hepatocyte on the left side is depicted endocytosing both ASOr and pIgA into a common vesicle. In this model the two ligands would be sorted intracellularly. The hepatocyte on the right side is depicted endocytosing ASOr and pIgA into two separate vesicles followed by independent handling of the two ligands within the cell.

various compounds that are thought to affect different stages of hepatic processing, in an attempt to gain evidence for differences in the processing of asialoglycoproteins and pIgA by the rat liver.

INTERFERENCE WITH LYSOSOMES DOES NOT AFFECT TRANSPORT OF pIgA

Chloroquine is a lysosomotropic agent that is thought to inhibit lysosomal degradation by raising pH.[18] More recent data indicate that chloroquine also prevents the delivery of protein ligands from intermediate Golgi-associated vesicles to lysosomes. Accordingly, we examined the ability of the isolated perfused liver to take up and process [125I]pIgA and [131I]asialo orosomucoid in the absence or presence of chloroquine. Isolated livers were perfused as previously described.[4,20] Control perfusions were carried out in which [125I]pIgA and [131I]ASOr were simultaneously added to the perfusate following a two-hour stabilization period. In experiments with chloroquine, 25 μmoles of the drug were added 0.5 and 0.25 hour prior to addition of [125I]pIgA and [131I]ASOr. The results of a representative experiment are presented in FIGURE 2. Chloroquine markedly affected the uptake and processing of [131I]ASOr, whereas chloroquine had no effect on the uptake or appearance of [125I]pIgA. Following uptake of [131I]ASOr, the isolated liver normally degrades the ASOr, and free iodide is returned to the blood perfusate[6] (FIGURE 2, ▲——▲). The effect of chloroquine on lysosomal processing in these experiments may be inferred by the delayed return of free iodide to blood (FIGURE 2, △——△) and the marked accumulation of [131I] in the liver. (In the absence of chloroquine, 3.0% was retained by the liver; in the presence of chloroquine 103% was retained by the liver.) By contrast, the clearance of [125I]pIgA from blood was not affected by chloroquine (FIGURE 2), nor was its transport to bile. Additional experiments indicated that the effect of chloroquine was reproducible and dose dependent. The above experiments are consistent with the hypothesis that processing of pIgA by the isolated rat liver does not involve lysosomes. It should also be noted that chloroquine has been found to affect a set of vesicles associated with the Golgi region that have been implicated in the processing of asialoglycoproteins prior to their entry into lysosomes.[19] The lack of effect of chloroquine on the transport of pIgA is

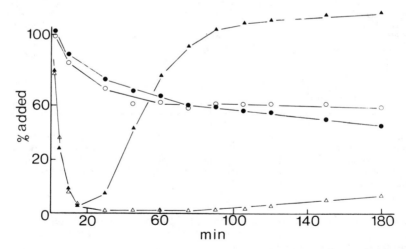

FIGURE 2. Effect of chloroquine on the processing of [125I]pIgA and [131I]ASOr. Approximately 2×10^5 cpm of each protein was added to the perfusate at t = 0 minutes which was two hours after an initial equilibration period. Blood samples were taken and counted at the time shown and plotted as percent remaining of total added. The solid symbols represent the radioactivity observed in a control experiment in which no chloroquine was added: ●——● = [125I]pIgA; ▲——▲ = [131I]ASOr. The open symbols represent an experiment in which 25 μmoles of chloroquine were added to the perfusate 0.5 and 0.25 hour before addition of radiolabeled proteins: ○——○ = [125I]pIgA; △——△ = [131I]ASOr.

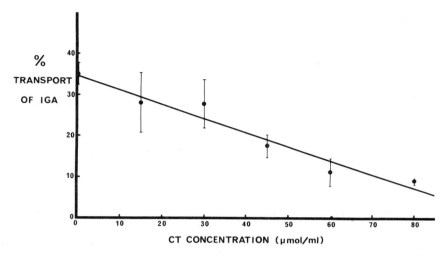

FIGURE 3. Dose-dependent inhibition of [^{125}I]pIgA transport by taurocholic acid. The mean transport was 35 ± 2.6 (S.E.M.) percent in 15 control experiments. Each of the other data points represents a minimum of three experiments. Taurocholic acid (CT) was added simultaneously with [^{125}I]pIgA.

consistent with a hypothesis that places sorting before the delivery of ASOr to such vesicles.

CONJUGATED BILE ACIDS AFFECT pIgA TRANSPORT
WITHOUT AFFECTING PROCESSING OF ASIALO OROSOMUCOID

We turned our attention to the effect of bile acids on the processing of ASOr and pIgA, because bile acids influence bile flow. In the isolated perfused liver, both cholic acid and taurocholic acid increase bile flow during the first 30 minutes following addition of either bile acid. Whereas cholic acid had no effect on the processing of pIgA, taurocholate had a marked inhibiting effect on the uptake of pIgA. The effect of taurocholate was specific, because transport of pIgA was affected without any effect on the processing of ASOr (FIGURE 3). As can be seen from FIGURE 3, the clearance time of pIgA from the blood perfusate in the presence of taurocholate was markedly reduced, and the transport to bile was reduced accordingly. The inhibition of pIgA was found to be dose dependent (FIGURE 4) and was greater when given one hour prior to addition of pIgA compared to simultaneous addition of pIgA and taurocholate. Inhibition was specific, because uptake and processing of asialoglycoprotein was not affected. In a series of additional experiments, we obtained evidence indicating that tauro-cholate was not altering the structure of the [^{125}I]pIgA, at least in its ability to bind SC *in vitro*, or to be transported by the liver.

The above experiments suggested to us that taurocholate might be interfering with secretory component (SC) turnover in the isolated perfused liver while having little effect on the receptor for asialo orosomucoid. Accordingly, free SC and secretory IgA were measured in the bile produced by livers perfused in the

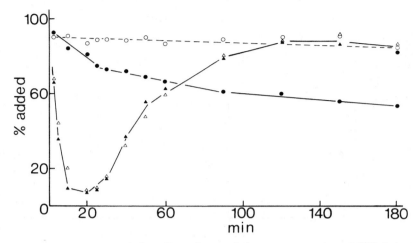

FIGURE 4. Comparison of the effect of taurocholate on processing of [¹²⁵I]pIgA and [¹³¹I]ASOr. Taurocholic acid (70 μmoles) was added to the perfusate at t = 0 minutes along with [¹²⁵I]pIgA and [¹³¹I]ASOr. The control perfusion (no taurocholate added) is represented by the closed symbols: ●——● = [¹²⁵I]pIgA; ▲——▲ = [¹³¹I]ASOr. The perfusion with taurocholate is represented by the open symbols: ○——○ = [¹²⁵I]pIgA; △——△ = [¹³¹I]ASOr. The data represent percent remaining in blood perfusate at the times shown.

presence of a bolus of 0.45 μmoles taurocholate and compared to bile from control perfusions. The results obtained from four perfusions are shown in TABLE 1. In control experiments, the quantity of secretory IgA produced in bile decreased with time as the liver removed pIgA from blood to bile. The quantity of free SC increased as IgA available for transport decreased and the system shifted to receptor excess. In perfusions where a bolus of taurocholate was added at two hours, the quantity of secretory IgA in bile relative to control experiments decreased as previously observed with the radiolabeled tracer studies. Of interest

TABLE 1

EFFECT OF TAUROCHOLATE ON BILIARY IgA AND SC*

	Free SC		Biliary IgA		Total SC	
	Hours		Hours		Hours	
	0–2	3–5	0–2	3–5	0–2	3–5
Control	0.09	0.28	0.60	0.25	0.21	0.33
Taurocholate	0.06	0.15	0.64	0.10	0.18	0.17
(0.45 mM)						
Percent Difference†		−18%		−62%		−40%
(T.C. vs. Control)						

*Each number represents the mean of two experiments expressed as mg produced in the time period indicated. Taurocholate (T.C.) added (45 μmoles/100 ml perfusion fluid) at two hours.

†Percent difference calculated after normalization to zero to two hours and calculated as the difference in normalized values of protein produced between three and five hours.

was the finding that the quantity of free SC produced in the presence of taurocholate was also reduced. The total quantity of SC produced in bile was calculated from the quantity of biliary IgA assuming a molecular weight of 380,000 and molar content of bound SC to be one (molecular weight = 70,000) per mole of biliary IgA. The total SC was calculated by addition of free SC and bound SC. The results indicate that in the presence of taurocholate, the secretion of SC (bound and free) into bile was reduced. These results indicate, therefore, that taurocholate interferes with the secretion of SC into bile and suggested to us that the decreased transport of polymeric IgA in the presence of taurocholate may be due to an altered expression of SC at the sinusoidal surface of the hepatocyte,

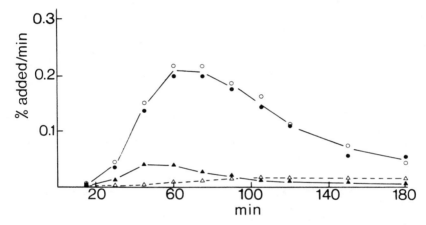

FIGURE 5. Comparison of the effect of dansyl cadaverine on processing [^{125}I]pIgA and [^{131}I]ASOr: comparison of radioactivity appearing in bile. The small quantity of ^{131}I counts appearing in bile (▲ and △) consisted of approximately 50% intact [^{131}I]ASOr and 50% low molecular weight counts (see text). The control experiment is represented by closed symbols; the open symbols represent an experiment in which 25 μmoles of dansyl cadaverine was added at 1, 0.5 and 0 hour prior to addition of radiolabeled proteins. A single line joins the points for [^{125}I]pIgA perfused in the absence (●——●) or presence (○——○) of dansyl cadaverine indicating no difference in the data points. By contrast, dansyl cadaverine delayed the appearance of ^{131}I counts. The gel filtration analysis (not shown) combined with the kinetic profile implies that dansyl cadaverine delayed the appearance of both intact [^{131}I]ASOr and the low molecular weight degradation products.

either resulting from altered turnover or synthesis of secretory component. The results obtained with chloroquine and taurocholate illustrate the differences in the processing of ASOr and pIgA.

DANSYL CADAVERINE INHIBITS PROCESSING OF ASOr BUT NOT pIgA

To investigate whether early endocytic events may be common to both pathways, we used dansyl cadaverine as a probe, because this compound has been reported to inhibit the endocytosis of ligands by fibroblasts, possibly through its action in inhibiting transglutaminase.[21] We postulated that transglutaminase was associated in receptor aggregation during collection of ligand-receptor complexes over coated pits.

Twenty-five μmoles of dansyl cadaverine were added to the perfusate one hour and 0.5 hour prior to addition of radiolabeled proteins as well as simultaneously with the radiolabeled proteins. The results of a representative experiment are shown in FIGURE 5. Dansyl cadaverine had no effect on the transport of [^{125}I]pIgA to bile. By contrast, dansyl cadaverine markedly delayed the processing of ASOr that was observed by a slower return of free iodide to blood (not shown) and a delayed appearance of [^{131}I]ASOr in bile (shown in FIGURE 5 for comparison to [^{125}I]pIgA).

These results indicate that similar to its effect on uptake and degradation of various protein ligands by macrophage and fibroblasts, dansyl cadaverine also delays the processing of asialoglycoprotein for degradation in hepatocytes as well as the small quantity of ASOr that appears in bile. By contrast, no effect was observed on the transport of [^{125}I]pIgA to bile, perhaps because receptor cross-linking is not a requirement for IgA uptake. Because dansyl cadaverine is thought to affect receptor-mediated endocytosis at the cell surface, we believe this experiment demonstrates that the ASOr and IgA pathways are independent, even at the point of initial uptake.

The differential effect of all three drugs described in this paper illustrates that the lysosomal degradation of ASOr and biliary transport of IgA are subject to different controlling mechanisms throughout the respective pathways, which may in fact share no metabolic step. Whether the IgA pathway shares any common step with the biliary transport of the small amount of intact ASOr after endocytosis is less clear.

Specific transport or degradation of different ligands subsequent to endocytosis undoubtedly takes place in other cell types. Transport of undegraded immunoglobulin G takes place across the placenta or the intestine of the suckling infant as well as the mammary epithelium of ruminants. A small fraction of dietary antigens reach the circulation intact, and it is possible that such antigens follow a route analogous to that taken by pIgA in the rat liver or across intestinal epithelial cells. The ability of cells to sort ligands into the degradative or transport pathways is a fundamental process deserving further study.

REFERENCES

1. LEMAITRE-COELHO, I., G. D. F. JACKSON & J. P. VAERMAN. 1977. Rat bile as a convenient source of secretory IgA and free secretory component. Eur. J. Immunol. 7: 588–590.
2. JACKSON, G. D. F., I. LEMAITRE-COELHO, J. P. VAERMAN, H. BAZIN & A. BECKERS. 1978. Rapid disappearance from serum of intravenously injected rat myeloma IgA and its secretion into bile. Eur. J. Immunol. 8: 123–126.
3. ORLANS, E., J. PEPPARD, J. REYNOLDS & J. HALL. 1978. Rapid active transport of immunoglobulin A from blood to bile. J. Exp. Med. 147: 588–592.
4. FISHER, M. M., B. NAGY, H. BAZIN & B. J. UNDERDOWN. 1979. Biliary transport of IgA: role of secretory component. Proc. Natl. Acad. Sci. USA 76: 2008–2012.
5. SOCKEN, D. J., K. N. JEEJEEBHOY, H. BAZIN & B. J. UNDERDOWN. 1979. Identification of secretory component as an IgA receptor on rat hepatocytes. J. Exp. Med. 150: 1538–1548.
6. ORLANS, E., J. PEPPARD, J. F. FRY, R. H. HINTON & B. M. MULLOCK. 1979. Secretory component as the receptor for polymeric IgA on rat hepatocytes. J. Exp. Med. 150: 1577–1581.
7. MOSTOV, K. E., J. P. KRAHENBUHL & G. BLOBEL. 1980. Receptor-mediated transcellular

transport of immunoglobulin: synthesis of secretory component as multiple and larger transmembrane forms. Proc. Natl. Acad. Sci. USA **77**: 7257–7261.

8. KUHN, L. C. & J. P. KRAEHENBUHL. 1981. The membrane receptor for polymeric immunoglobulin is structurally related to secretory component. Isolation and characterization of membrane secretory component from rabbit liver and mammary gland. J. Biol. Chem. **256**: 12490–12495.

9. LEMAITRE-COELHO, I., G. A. ALTAMIRANO, C. BARRANCO-ACOSTA, R. MEYKENS & J. P. VAERMAN. 1981. *In vivo* experiments involving secretory component in the rat hepatic transfer of polymeric IgA from blood into bile. Immunology **43**: 261–270.

10. BIRBECK, M. S. C., P. CARTWRIGHT, J. G. HALL, E. URLANS & J. PEPPARD. 1979. The transport by hepatocytes of immunoglobulin A from blood to bile visualized by autoradiography and electron microscopy. Immunology **37**: 477–484.

11. RENSTON, R. H., A. L. JONES, W. D. CHRISTIANSON, G. T. HRADEK & B. J. UNDERDOWN. 1980. Evidence for a vesicular transport mechanism in hepatocytes for biliary secretion of immunoglobulin A. Science **208**: 1276–1278.

12. TAKAHASHI, I., P. K. NAKANE & W. R. BROWN. 1982. Ultrastructural events in the translocation of polymeric IgA by rat hepatocytes. J. Immunol. **128**: 1181–1187.

13. EVANS, W. H. 1981. Membrane traffic at the hepatocyte's sinusoidal and canalicular surface domains. Hepatology **1**: 452–457.

14. WALL, D. A., G. WILSON & A. L. HUBBARD. 1980. The galactose-specific recognition system of mammalian liver: the route of ligand internalization in rat hepatocytes. Cell **21**: 79–93.

15. WILLINGHAM, M. C. & I. PASTAN. 1980. The receptosome: an intermediate organelle of receptor-mediated endocytosis in cultured fibroblasts. Cell **21**: 67–77.

16. LABADIE, J. H., K. PETERSON CHAPMAN & N. N. ARONSON JR. 1975. Glycoprotein catabolism in rat liver. Lysosomal digestion of iodinated asialo-fetuin. Biochem. J. **152**: 271–279.

17. DUNN, W. A., J. H. LABADIE & N. N. ARONSON, JR. 1979. Inhibition of ^{125}I-asialofetuin catabolism by leupeptin in the perfused rat liver and *in vivo*. J. Biol. Chem. **254**: 4191–4196.

18. LIE, S. O. & B. SCHOFIELD. 1973. Inactivation of lysosomal function in normal cultured human fibroblasts by chloroquine. Biochem. Pharmacol. **22**: 3109–3114.

19. POSNER, B. I., B. A. PATEL, M. N. KHAN & J. M. BERGERON. 1982. Effect of chloroquine on the internalization of ^{125}I-Insulin into subcellular fractions of rat liver. J. Biol. Chem. **257**: 5789–5799.

20. FISHER, M. M., R. MAGNUSSON & K. MIYAI. 1971. Bile acid metabolism in mammals. I. Bile acid-induced intrahepatic cholestasis. Lab. Invest. **25**: 88–91.

21. DAVIES, P. J. A., D. R. DAVIES, A. LEVITZKI, F. R. MAXFIELD, P. MILHAUD, M. C. WILLINGHAM & I. H. PASTAN. 1980. Transglutaminase is essential in receptor-mediated endocytosis of α_2-macroglobulin and polypeptide hormones. Nature (London) **283**: 162–167.

22. THOMAS, P. & J. W. SUMMERS. 1978. The biliary excretion of circulating asialoglycoproteins in the rat. Biochem. Biophys. Res. Commun. **80**: 335–339.

DISCUSSION OF THE PAPER

J. MESTECKY (*University of Alabama in Birmingham*): If you remove sialic acid from IgA, through which pathway would IgA be processed?

B. J. UNDERDOWN (*University of Toronto, Toronto, Ontario, Canada*): The approach we were going to pursue, was to add galactose to IgA, in an attempt to see how the cells would be able to handle this situation. We have not done the experiment with the removal of sialic acid.

J. P. VAERMAN (*Catholic University of Louvain, Brussels, Belgium*): In a limited number of experiments, we examined the transport of human polymeric IgA treated with sialidase. The transfer was reduced, but not in a significant way; it was reduced from 50% to 40 percent. Because large variations were seen, we felt that the reduction was not significant.

UNIDENTIFIED SPEAKER: Leupeptin is quite specific for cystine or thialoproteases. Did you observe the same effect when you used serine protease inhibitors?

UNDERDOWN: We have not used serine protease inhibitors and there are several other probes that we would like to use.

D. E. BOCKMAN (*Medical College of Georgia, Augusta, Ga.*): When you look at the region where the difference between high and low molecular weight material is evident, you will be forced to look at the cell membrane, perhaps with its associated glycocalyx. In that region, the endothelial cells have fenestrae large enough so that none of the molecules in question would be retarded. The basal lamina does not exist in that area, and the selectivity of transport would not exist.

UNDERDOWN: In advancing the hypothesis for molecular weight sieving, I am unable to identify where the sieve exists. Yet, the data from several laboratories, including ours are clear. I think Dr. Rifai also examined the clearance of asialoglycoproteins and showed an effect of molecular weight of transported substances. Dr. Mestecky and his colleagues have shown the same.

M. BLAKE (*Rockefeller University, New York, N.Y.*): Does anyone know the initial triggering event of that endocytosis?

UNDERDOWN: Mullock has shown in the IgA system and Hubbard in the asialoglycoprotein system that the process is constitutive. The vesicles are formed and the process proceeds whether the ligand is there or not. This may explain the occurrence of free SC in bile in the absence of any IgA.

COMPARATIVE ASPECTS OF THE HEPATOBILIARY TRANSPORT OF IgA*

E. Orlans,† J. V. Peppard,† A. W. R. Payne,† B. M. Fitzharris,†
B. M. Mullock,‡ R. H. Hinton,‡ and J. G. Hall†

†Department of Tumour Immunology
Institute of Cancer Research
Belmont, Sutton, Surrey, England
‡Robens Institute of Industrial
and Environmental Health and Safety
University of Surrey, Guildford, England

Clear demonstration that macromolecules can move across cells is relatively recent. In 1972, proteins were first shown to cross capillary endothelia in vesicles,[1] and vesicle-mediated transfer of IgA across the enterocytes of the intestine was first described[2] and has been the subject of much further work.[3] Ultrastructural methods, however, were the only ones used, so that it was impossible to be completely certain that the material was within the cell. Moreover, even if the material was conceded to be within a vesicle in the cell, in both capillary endothelium and enterocytes, the geometry of the cells is such that endocytic vesicles carrying the protein are unlikely to be in the vicinity of lysosomes and might simply be nonspecific endocytic vesicles rather than specialized and protected transport vesicles.

This situation changed when studies in laboratories, including ours, showed that IgA is transported across rat hepatocytes from serum into bile[4,5] by a mechanism that involves receptor-mediated endocytosis at the sinusoidal face of the hepatocyte,[6-8] transfer across the cells in specialized "shuttle" vesicles that do not fuse with lysosomes,[9,10] and discharge at the bile canalicular face of the cell.[11] The geometry of the hepatocyte ensures that vesicles carrying material to bile must pass through the lysosomes clustered around the bile canalicular face of the cell. Comparison of protein concentrations in rat blood and bile showed that the biliary IgA concentration was too high relative to blood to be accounted for by filtration through the tight junctions between hepatocytes, whereas cell fractionation experiments revealed that endogenous IgA was tightly bound to the membrane of small vesicles that differed from lysosomes or plasma membrane vesicles. Hence, in the rat liver system, transport of IgA through hepatocytes in specialized endocytic vesicles is clearly established. Haptoglobin-hemoglobin complexes are similarly transferred[12] and polypeptide hormones have been demonstrated in distinctive vesicles from hepatocytes;[13] it would, therefore, appear that vesicle-mediated transport is not confined to IgA. Furthermore, because vesicle-mediated transfer certainly occurs in liver, it seems very likely that the vesicles observed in gut enterocytes[3] are indeed also specifically transferring IgA and that similar vesicles are involved in the transfer of IgG across the placenta from mother to young[14] and across the gut lining in very young rats.[15]

Transfer of IgA across liver from blood to bile is therefore a convenient model

*Financial support was provided by the Medical Research Council and the Cancer Research Campaign.

411

of a transit system that occurs in many tissues of higher organisms. Moreover, in the rat liver IgA transport system, unlike the IgG system, the receptor has been identified as secretory component,[6,7] which hepatocytes, like most other epithelial cells, synthesize. By following the movements of a fucose label, it was shown that newly synthesized secretory component was glycosylated in the Golgi apparatus and from there passed to the sinusoidal plasma membrane,[8] where it was displayed on the surface of the cell and could bind polymeric IgA from the blood. Endocytic vesicles formed from the sinusoidal plasma membrane, then transferred secretory component to the biliary face of the cell. IgA that had bound was also transferred to the biliary face, but the process did not depend on IgA binding, because in vitro perfusion experiments showed that secretory component was transported efficiently in the absence of IgA.[16]

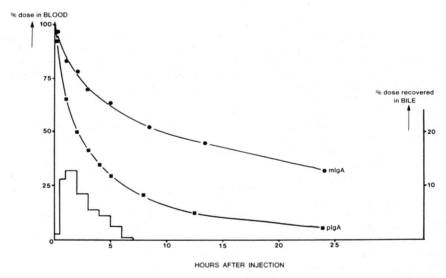

FIGURE 1. Radioactivity in blood and bile of rats after the i.v. injection of ^{125}I-labeled human IgA. Monomeric (mIgA) and polymeric (pIgA) IgA purified from the same myeloma serum were used. The histogram shows the appearance of intact polymeric IgA in the bile.

Thus the transfer of polymeric IgA from blood to bile in rats has provided a relatively simple experimental system for showing that large, intact protein molecules cross cells. Rats with cannulae inserted into the common bile duct can be given radiolabeled polymeric IgA i.v., and the bile can be collected quantitatively. Blood samples may be taken from the tail at appropriate intervals. The procedure can be done on anaesthetized animals, on conscious rats in restraining cages, or by in vitro perfusion methods.[17]

The kind of result obtained from such experiments is shown in FIGURE 1 where monomeric and dimeric IgA, isolated from the same human[18] paraprotein were used, and in TABLE 1 where rat IgA was injected.[4] This type of result provides four criteria for judging whether or not active transfer is occurring: 1. the relative rates at which the monomeric and polymeric IgA disappear from the blood; 2. the total recovery of protein-bound radioactivity, usually expressed as the percentage of

TABLE 1

RADIOACTIVITY IN SERUM AND BILE AFTER I.V. INJECTION OF [^{125}I]IgA*

Time After Injection	Blood Serum	Bile	Bile
Hour	cpm/ml	cpm/ml	cpm/sample
0.25	8.2×10^5		
		4.2×10^6	1.5×10^6
1	4.5×10^5		
		5.4×10^6	2.9×10^6
2	3.3×10^6		
		1.6×10^6	1.0×10^6
3	2.8×10^5		
		0.4×10^6	0.4×10^6
5	2.2×10^5		
Total			5.8×10^6

*Measurements made during the five hours after i.v. injection of 2×10^7 cpm of [^{125}I]IgA. The values for serum are from samples taken at the beginning and end of each period of bile collection, and are means from assays on seven rats, three of which had been cannulated.[4]

the injected dose; 3. a comparison of the radioactivity per gram (specific activities) of blood and bile (especially important when the total recovery is low, or in work with, for example, mice where bile duct cannulation or repeated blood sampling are extremely difficult); and 4. the time course of these events—the time after i.v. injection at which biliary excretion of specifically transported proteins is at a peak is highly characteristic, namely 30–120 minutes later. (Any proteins damaged during preparation and labeling will be taken up into liver lysosomes and

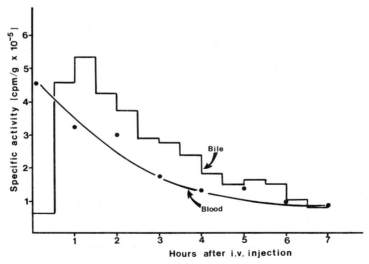

FIGURE 2. The mean protein-bound radioactivity in the blood and bile of five rabbits after i.v. injection of ^{125}I-labeled polymeric rat IgA. About 35% of the injected dose appeared in the bile within seven hours. Very similar results were obtained after the injection of ^{125}I-labeled human polymeric IgA.

degraded. In our experience, bile collected more than three hours after injection tends to have increasing amounts of radioactivity that is not protein-bound and in any case contributes little to the total recovery value.)

Another general feature of the rat system is that the incubation with secretory component of polyclonal as well as monoclonal polymeric IgA inhibits its transport[19] into bile and that isolated biliary IgA does not obey the criteria outlined above.

ANIMAL SPECIES OTHER THAN RAT

Rabbits injected with rat or human polymeric IgA transported both (FIGURE 2), whereas guinea pigs transported neither, with the radiolabeled antigen remaining

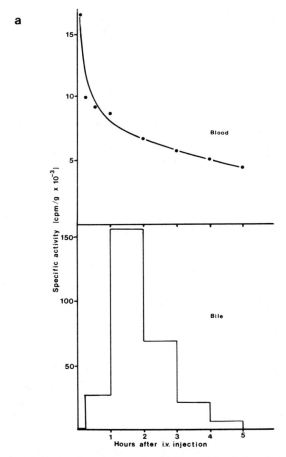

FIGURE 3. Protein-bound radioactivity in the blood and bile of sheep (a) and rats (b) after i.v. injection of ^{125}I-labeled polymeric sheep IgA prepared from lymph. The percent of the injected dose recovered in bile 5 hours after injection was 5% in sheep and 20% in rats.

TABLE 2

IgG, IgA, AND ALBUMIN IN SHEEP BILE

| Sheep No. | Relative Amounts in Bile (Bile/Serum Ratios × 100) OF | | |
	Albumin	IgG	IgA
637	4	4	1619
300	1.5	1	1541
101	5	6	1200
808	2	2	600
161	8	1	305
350	2	0.3	167
164	2	2	82
815	4	0.4	55
Mean values:	3.6	2.1	696

in the circulation.[20] Bile flow in guinea pigs was about 20 times greater than that in rats, and the bile was also consequently dilute.

In sheep given either rat or human polymeric IgA, the radioactivity remained in the blood with less than 1% appearing in bile. Because of our group's special interest in the lymphatic physiology of sheep, IgA, both from colostrum and intestinal lymph, and antiserum specific for sheep α-chains, were prepared. Estimations of IgG, serum albumin, and IgA in paired samples of blood and bile

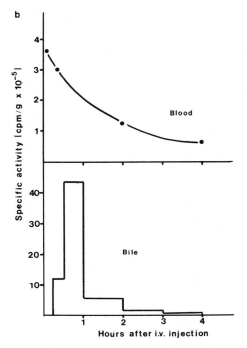

FIGURE 3. Continued

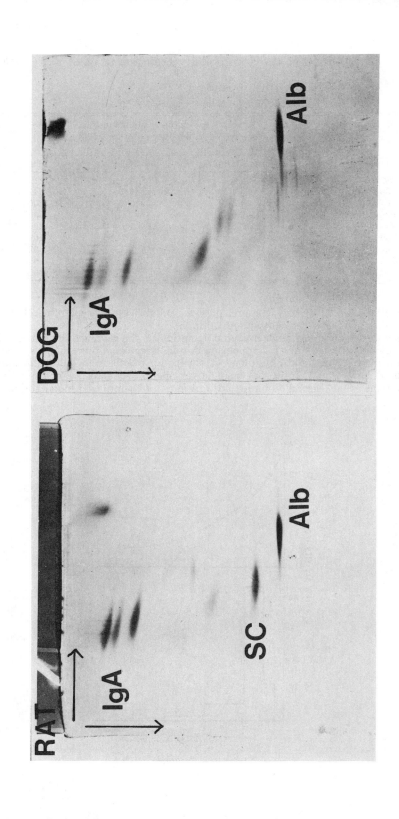

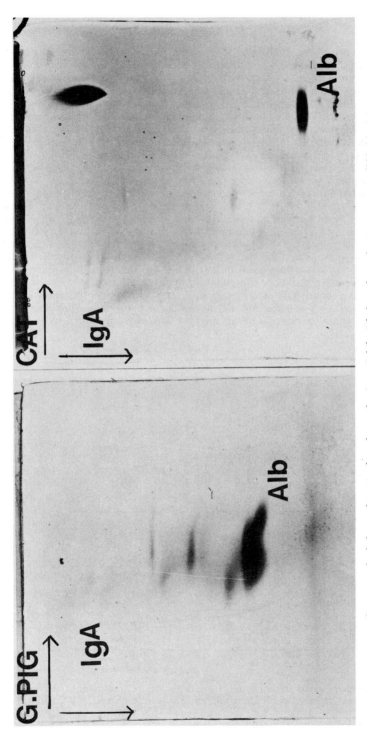

FIGURE 4. Two-dimensional gel electrophoresis of rat, dog, and guinea pig bile. Bile from dog and guinea pig was gall bladder bile, and that from guinea pig had been concentrated 12-fold. The first dimension (horizontal arrow) was run in agarose gel (origin to the left) and the second (vertical arrow) in a gradient (2.5 to 27%) polyacrylamide gel (Gradipore Gel, Universal Scientific Ltd.). The positions of IgA, albumin (Alb) and, where known, secretory component (SC) are marked.

from eight sheep (TABLE 2) showed that despite large variations in the protein composition of sheep bile, IgG and serum albumin were on average no more than 4% of the serum values, whereas the corresponding value for IgA was 700% — unequivocal evidence for selective transfer into bile.

The injection of radiolabeled sheep IgA from lymph into a sheep showed that it was transported into bile, and although recovery of the injected dose was only 5%, the other criteria for active transport were fulfilled (FIGURE 3a). With the same preparation of sheep IgA injected into rats (FIGURE 3b), the recovery was 20%, showing that the sheep IgA had not been damaged by the isolation procedures. Thus sheep provide an example of a species that transports homologous, but not human or rat IgA.

Radiolabeled human IgA injected i.v. into one cat, one dog, and one piglet was not transported into bile. Results from these single experiments, however, should be interpreted with caution in species where normal rate of bile flow is not known. In some experiments with cannulated rats in which bile was flowing irregularly or scantily, IgA transport was grossly inhibited, that is, to a much greater degree than could be accounted for by the smaller volume of bile collected. The inhibition may well be attributed to trauma of the biliary tract, resulting in release of secretory component into the circulation.

To have to prepare polyclonal polymeric IgA, and a specific anti-α-chain antiserum, from every species that did not transport heterologous myeloma IgA would be extremely tedious. Another method, however, involving two-dimen-

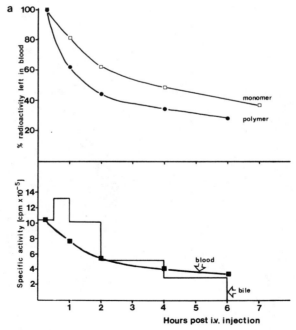

FIGURE 5. Protein-bound radioactivity in blood and bile of rats after injection i.v. of ^{125}I-labeled mouse IgA from two different myelomas. Monomeric MOPC 315 did not appear in bile. The recoveries in bile of both TEPC 15 (b) and MOPC 315 polymeric IgA (a) were similar at about 15% of the injected dose.

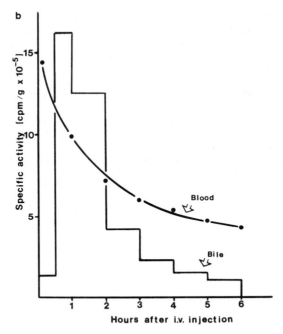

FIGURE 5. Continued

sional electrophoresis, makes it possible to identify IgA in bile, but only when it is relatively abundant (approx. 250–300 μg/ml).[21] Polymeric IgA can be identified in rat bile as a group of three bands lying close to the origin. In rats, dogs, cats (FIGURE 4), and chickens it is clear that polymeric IgA is one of the major proteins of bile. Polymeric IgA could be identified in some guinea pig biles (FIGURE 4) and human biles, but the amounts were small compared with other proteins. No bands corresponding to IgA were seen in pig or sheep bile.

From the limiting existing information on α-chain homologies in different species as detected by cross reactions (for example 22), on the relative *in vitro* binding affinities of the free secretory component and polymeric IgA preparations from different species (for example 23), there appears to be no correlation between either of these factors and transport of heterologous IgA. To illustrate this point the transport of two different mouse IgA myeloma proteins in the rat system is shown in FIGURE 5a and b: the mouse proteins are transported by rats, but mouse proteins are not transported as efficiently as human or rat IgA. By contrast, the most spectacular instance of blood to bile transport was that of human IgA by chickens[24] (FIGURE 6), where recovery of the injected dose was never less than 40 percent. Recoveries of injected heterologous IgA are summarized in FIGURE 7.

MAN

IgA physiology in man has received more attention and generated more controversy than that in other species, both because of possible clinical implications and much greater technical problems. The latter include the fact that one cannot inject radiolabeled myeloma proteins into healthy individuals, the huge variations in the protein composition of the bile, and the uniquely high levels of total, and particularly, monomeric IgA in the blood. There are at least three separate questions to be answered in connection with the human IgA problem: (1) Is the polymeric form synthesized in large amounts? (2) Is the polymer removed from the blood into the bile, thus leaving primarily monomer in the blood? (3) If so, is the transport mechanism the same as in rats?

There is general agreement among all who have studied the IgA formed by submucosal plasma cells that it is polymeric, but its contribution to the serum pool is not known. In man, the incidence of myeloma proteins of a given heavy or light chain type is accepted as being representative of the normal pool.[25] We have examined all the sera received in our laboratory from patients with IgA myeloma in gradient gel electrophoresis; in some cases, samples taken at long intervals from the same patient were available.

The examples shown in FIGURE 8a and b, and a summary of results in TABLE 3,

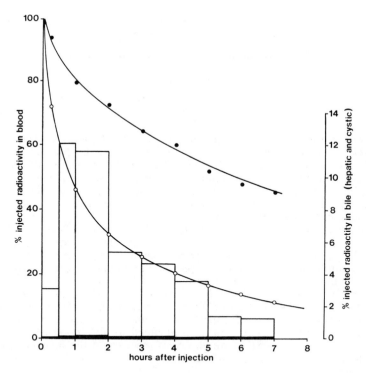

FIGURE 6. The decline in radioactivity with time in the blood of chickens after i.v. injection of either dimeric (O——O) or monomeric (●——●) human [^{125}I]IgA; the protein-bound radioactivity recovered in bile (hepatic + cystic) at the intervals marked on the abscissa is shown by the open and solid bars for birds given dimer and monomer, respectively. The 100% value for radioactivity in the blood was taken as the injected dose (4.9 × 10^7 cpm) divided by the volume of blood. (With permission from the *European Journal of Immunology*.)[24]

IgA obtained from	IgA injected into →	RAT	SHEEP	GUINEA PIG	RABBIT	CHICKEN
RAT		30%	<1%	<1%	35%	ND
HUMAN		40%	<1%	<1%	35%	40%
* MOUSE		15%	ND	ND	ND	ND
SHEEP		20%	5%	ND	ND	ND

*MOPC 315 or TEPC 15 myeloma.

FIGURE 7. Recoveries (percent of dose injected i.v.) of polymeric IgA in bile.

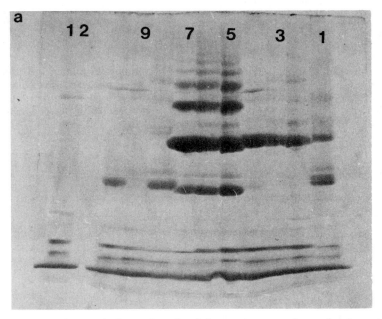

FIGURE 8a. Gradient gel electrophoresis of three serum samples each taken at long intervals from three patients with IgA myeloma, together with serum Lev (track 1) and pooled normal human serum (track 12). Dates of serial samples; tracks 2–4 April 1977–February 1980; tracks 5–7 May 1978–August 1979; tracks 8–10 September 1976–November 1979.

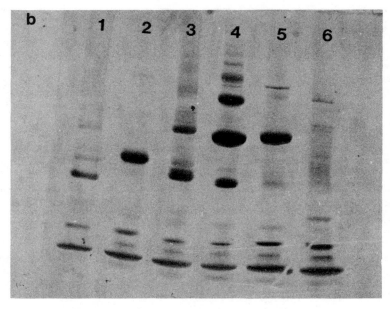

FIGURE 8b. Gradient gel electrophoresis of five IgA myeloma sera: Hal (1), Sau (2), Lev (3), Fry (4), and Des (5). Track 6 is normal human serum. The two main Lev paraproteins were purified and their size was determined by ultracentrifugation as 354,000 ± 1,000 and 162,000 ± 600.

demonstrate that size heterogeneity is a common feature of human IgA proteins, that the heterogeneity is not due to polymerization or disaggregation on storage, and in particular that most of the myeloma sera contain a much higher proportion of oligomeric IgA than the 10% generally quoted as being the proportion in normal serum.

TABLE 3

SIZE DISTRIBUTION OF THE MONOCLONAL IgA IN 10 RANDOMLY CHOSEN HUMAN MYELOMA SERA*

IgA Myeloma	Monomer	Dimer	>Dimer
Des	(+)	+++	?+
Edw	++	+	+/−
Fry	++	++++	+++
Hal	++	(+)	?+
Lev	++	++	?+
Sau	++		
Smi	+	+	+/−
Ric	+	−	−
Win	?+	+	+/−
Woo	++	+++	(+)

*The sera were examined in gradient gel electrophoresis, showing that 8/10 human IgA myeloma sera contain some oligomeric paraproteins. Protein Sau was of a mobility intermediate between those normally observed for monomer and dimer.

TABLE 4

ORIGINS OF THE BILE SAMPLES ANALYZED

Sample Nos.	Method of Collection	Clinical Source
1–9	Endoscopic retrograde choledo-chopancreatography	Patients after cholecystectomy
10–15	T-tube drainage	Patients after cholecystectomy
16–27	Needle aspiration from biliary tract at laparotomy	Patients with no known hepato-biliary disease
28–29	Aspiration from duodenum	Patients with no known hepato-biliary disease
30	Aspiration from duodenum	Pool from twelve normal volunteers

In an attempt to answer question 2, the concentrations of IgG, serum albumin, and sIgA were measured in 30 samples of bile whose origins are listed in TABLE 4. The reason for measuring sIgA rather than total IgA is its lesser degree of heterogeneity and the virtual certainty that having acquired secretory component, it must have passed through the liver. Human bile contains large amounts of IgA, both polymeric and monomeric, devoid of secretory component,[26] some of which will be present due to transudation. Free secretory component, which would cause errors in the sIgA estimations, measured by split-gel rocket electrophoresis, was detected in only a minority of the 30 bile samples and never amounted to more than 15% of the material reacting with the anti-secretory component serum. The concentrations of IgG and serum albumin plotted in FIGURE 9 exhibit large

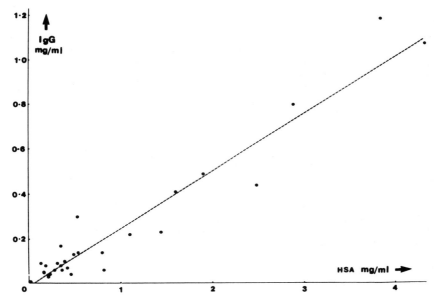

FIGURE 9. Graph showing a positive correlation between concentration of IgG and albumin in 30 samples of human bile.

variations and both are obviously a function of total protein concentration. A similar pattern is observed when the concentrations of other major serum proteins such as hemopexin and transferrin are plotted against the concentration of albumin, but there is little if any correlation between the concentration of sIgA and other proteins in bile. With the exception of samples 28–30, (TABLE 4) obtained from normal subjects by duodenal aspiration and which contained large amounts of sIgA and barely detectable amounts of the other proteins, there was no correlation between the origin of the bile samples and their protein composition. The results in TABLE 5 clearly show that in man as well, there is selective concentration of sIgA in the bile.

The third question is currently the most difficult to answer, because there is disagreement as to whether secretory component is detectable on human hepatocytes. Experiments using hepatocytes in short-term culture that demonstrated the presence of secretory component on rat hepatocytes have not yet been reported for human material. In view of the variation observed in other species and the ability to transport human IgA exhibited by other animals, however, we think it probable that the transport mechanism in man and rat is similar.

TABLE 5

MEDIAN CONCENTRATIONS OF IgG, sIgA, AND ALBUMIN IN 30 SAMPLES OF HUMAN BILE

	Protein in μg/ml			$\dfrac{sIgA}{Albumin} \times 10^3$
	IgG	Albumin	sIgA	
Serum	12,000	40,000	18	0.45
Bile	90	405	72	160
(Ranges)	(10–1,190)	(10–4,320)	(9–556)	(23–30,000)

GENERAL CONCLUSIONS

All the species that we have examined, with the possible exception of the pig, do transfer at least homologous IgA from blood to bile. There are marked differences in the amounts of IgA relative to other plasma proteins in bile, both within and between species. In rats, mice, rabbits, cats, dogs, and chickens, IgA is one of the major bile proteins, whereas in guinea pigs and sheep, IgA is a minor constituent of the bile. We have shown that active transport of IgA from blood to bile does occur in the sheep and have provided some evidence that it also takes place in humans.

It seems likely, therefore, that the transfer of homologous IgA from blood to bile is a common phenomenon among higher vertebrates. The results of cross-species comparisons of IgA transfer are confusing and show no obvious phylogenetic relationship: one rodent (guinea pig) fails to transport the IgA of another rodent, whereas chickens transport human IgA. Moreover, the results can be viewed another way: "vigorous" transporters, such as the rat, do transfer heterologous IgA, whereas "poor" transporters, like sheep, do not. The explanation for this is unknown, but is possibly related to the density of secretory component molecules on the cell surface. The presence of substantial amounts of free secretory component in the bile of rats suggests that in such animals there is a considerable excess of these receptor molecules over the amount of polymeric IgA present in the blood. In poor transporters, there may be smaller numbers of secretory component molecules at the sinusoidal surface of the hepatocyte, so that these become saturated with IgA before formation of the endocytic vesicles.

Hence, in poor transporters, the heterologous IgA must compete with the animal's own IgA for binding sites, whereas this competition does not occur in vigorous transporters where there is an excess of receptor sites. Until the amounts of free secretory component in the bile of other species have been measured, however, this explanation can only be tentative.

Finally, there remains the question of the physiological importance of IgA transfer into bile. Cross-species comparisons have frequently shed light on similar problems. Two roles have been suggested.[27,28] First, the presence of IgA in bile will help prevent adhesion to the bile duct and the upper part of the intestine of any pathogens that escape being killed by the stomach acid. Second, potentially harmful IgA antibody antigen complexes are transferred from blood to bile so that this transfer system provides a means for removing antigens from the circulation without allergic consequences.

The relative importance of these two functions is impossible to evaluate and may vary according to the nature of the animal's diet and its contamination with microbial pathogens.

ACKNOWLEDGMENTS

We would like to thank Miss L. Shaw for her excellent technical assistance, Dr. R. Binns, Mr. R. White, and Dr. D. Denham for carrying out the pig, dog, and cat surgery, and Dr. Claudia Berek for providing the specifically purified TEPC 15 mouse IgA myeloma. The determinations of sheep bile proteins were carried out by Mrs. Christine Winstanley and the ultracentrifugation of purified Lev IgA proteins by Dr. Ken Shooter. Bile samples were kindly provided by Dr. Mary Hinton, Dr. Parveen Kumar, Dr. Tim Cooke, Dr. John Thornton, and Dr. Mary Calladine. IgA myeloma sera were provided by Drs. Ray Powles, Hugh Clink, and George Stevenson.

REFERENCES

1. SIMIONESCUE, N., M. SIMIONESCUE & G. E. PALADE. 1972. Permeability of intestinal capillaries—pathway followed by dextrans and glycogens. J. Cell. Biol. **53:** 365–392.
2. PORTER, P., D. E. NOAKES & W. D. ALLEN. 1972. Intestinal secretion of immunoglobulins in the pre-ruminant calf. Immunology **23:** 299–312.
3. BROWN, W. R. 1978. Relationships between immunoglobulins and the intestinal epithelium. Gastroenterology **75:** 129–138.
4. ORLANS, E., J. PEPPARD, J. REYNOLDS & J. HALL. 1978. Rapid active transport of immunoglobulin A from blood to bile. J. Exp. Med. **147:** 588–592.
5. JACKSON, G. D. F., I. LEMAÎTRE-COELHO, J. P. VAERMAN, H. BAZIN & A. BECKER. 1978. Rapid disappearance from serum of intravenously injected rat myeloma IgA and its secretion into bile. Eur. J. Immunol. **8:** 123–126.
6. ORLANS, E., J. PEPPARD, J. F. FRY, R. H. HINTON & B. M. MULLOCK. 1979. Secretory component as the receptor for polymeric IgA on rat hepatocytes. J. Exp. Med. **150:** 1577–1581.
7. SOCKEN, D. J., K. N. JEEJEEBHOY, H. BAZIN & B. J. UNDERDOWN. 1979. Identification of secretory component as an IgA receptor on rat hepatocytes. J. Exp. Med. **150:** 1538–1548.
8. MULLOCK, B. M., R. H. HINTON, M. DOBROTA, J. PEPPARD & E. ORLANS. 1980. Distribution of secretory component in hepatocytes and its mode of transfer into bile. Biochem. J. **190:** 819–826.
9. MULLOCK, B. M., R. H. HINTON, M. DOBROTA, J. PEPPARD & E. ORLANS. 1979. Endocytic vesicles in liver carry polymeric IgA from serum to bile. Biochim. Biophys. Acta **587:** 381–391.

10. TAKAHASHI, I., P. K. NAKANE & W. R. BROWN. 1982. Ultrastructural events in the translocation of polymeric IgA by rat hepatocytes. J. Immunol. **128:** 1181–1187.
11. MULLOCK, B. M., R. S. JONES, J. PEPPARD & R. H. HINTON. 1980. Effect of colchicine on the transfer of IgA across hepatocytes into bile in isolated perfused liver. FEBS Lett. **120:** 278–282.
12. HINTON, R. H., M. DOBROTA & B. M. MULLOCK. 1980. Haptoglobin-mediated transfer of haemoglobin from serum into bile. FEBS Lett. **112:** 247–250.
13. SMITH, G. D., W. H. EVANS & T. J. PETERS. 1980. Ligand-induced changes at the hepatocyte sinusoidal plasma membrane. FEBS Lett. **112:** 104–106.
14. PEARSE, B. M. F. 1982. Coated vesicles from human placenta carry ferritin, transferrin and immunoglobulin G. Proc. Nat. Acad. Sci. USA **79:** 456–460.
15. RODEWALD, R. 1980. Distribution of Immunoglobulin G receptors in the small intestine of the young rat. J. Cell Biol. **85:** 18–32.
16. MULLOCK, B. M., R. S. JONES & R. H. HINTON. 1980. Movement of endocytic shuttle vesicles from the sinusoidal to the bile canalicular face of hepatocytes does not depend on occupation of receptor sites. FEBS Lett. **113:** 201–205.
17. FISHER, M. M., B. NAGY, H. BAZIN & B. J. UNDERDOWN. 1979. Biliary transport of IgA: Role of secretory component. Proc. Natl. Acad. Sci. USA **76**(4): 2008–2012.
18. PEPPARD, J., E. ORLANS, A. W. R. PAYNE & E. ANDREW. 1981. The elimination of circulating complexes containing polymeric IgA by excretion in the bile. Immunology **42:** 83–89.
19. REYNOLDS, J., L. GYURE, E. ANDREW & J. G. HALL. 1980. Studies of the transport of polyclonal IgA antibody from blood to bile in rats. Immunology. **39:** 463–467.
20. HALL, J. G. H., L. A. GYURE, A. W. R. PAYNE & E. ANDREW. 1981. Comparative aspects of secretory immunity: the transport of heterologous IgA from blood to bile in experimental animals. *In* The Mucosal Immune System. F. J. Bourne, Ed.: 31–44. Martinus Nijnoff Publishers. The Hague.
21. MULLOCK, B. M., M. DOBROTA & R. H. HINTON. 1978. Sources of the proteins of rat bile. Biochim. Biophys. Acta. **543:** 497–507.
22. ORLANS, E. & A. FEINSTEIN. 1971. Detection of alpha, kappa and lambda chains in mammalian immunoglobulins using fowl antisera to human IgA. Nature (London) New Biology. **233**(36): 45–47.
23. UNDERDOWN, B. J. & D. J. SOCKEN. 1978. A comparison of secretory component—immunoglobulin interactions amongst different species. *In* Secretory Immunity and Infection. J. R. McGhee, J. Mestecky and J. L. Babb, Eds.: 503–511. Plenum Press. New York.
24. ROSE, M. E., E. ORLANS, A. W. R. PAYNE & P. HESKETH. 1981. The origin of IgA in chicken bile: its rapid active transport from blood. Eur. J. Immunol. **11:** 561–564.
25. MILSTEIN, C. & J. A. L. PINK. 1970. Structure and evolution of immunoglobulins. *In* Progress in Biophysics and Molecular Biology. J. A. V. Butler and D. Noble, Eds.: Vol. 21: 209–263. Pergamon Press. New York.
26. KUTTEH, W. H., S. J. PRINCE, J. O. PHILLIPS, J. G. SPENNEY & J. MESTECKY. 1982. Properties of immunoglobulin A in serum of individuals with liver diseases and in hepatic bile. Gastroenterology. **85:** 184–193.
27. PEPPARD, J. V., E. ORLANS, E. ANDREW & A. W. R. PAYNE. 1982. Elimination into bile of circulating antigen by endogenous IgA antibody in rats. Immunology **45:** 467–472.
28. MULLOCK, B. M. & R. H. HINTON. 1981. Transport of proteins from blood to bile. Trends. Biochem. Sci. **6:** 188–190.

DISCUSSION OF THE PAPER

J. MESTECKY (*University of Alabama in Birmingham*): You raised an interesting point that concerns the incidence of IgA polymers and monomers in normal versus myeloma serum. I do not think that there is much correlation. Most of the

IgA myeloma proteins are polymeric, but there is always an admixture of a monomer. IgA in serum of myeloma patients contains a whole spectrum of polymers that does not correspond to the distribution of molecular forms of IgA in normal human serum.

A. J. HUSBAND (*The University of Newcastle, Newcastle, Australia*): I am not sure where you leave the status of the sheep with respect to IgA-bile transport. You mentioned that IgA levels in bile are 700% higher than in serum. This high percentage could be due to local production, because there are IgA-plasma cells in the biliary tree. When you injected the radiolabeled IgA intravenously, you only collected about 5% in bile. Could you clarify the position as to whether bile transport of IgA in sheep is analogous to the rodent species?

E. ORLANS (*Institute of Cancer Research, Belmont, Sutton, Surrey, England*): I do not think that anyone has seen plasma cells in normal sheep liver.

HUSBAND: We have seen IgA-plasma cells in the mucosa of the bile duct and in other components of the biliary tree.

D. L. DELACROIX (*Catholic University of Louvain, Brussels, Belgium*): You find more secretory IgA in human bile ducts than in human serum. Is that correct?

ORLANS: Yes.

DELACROIX: This finding does not mean that the total polymeric IgA in bile is higher than the total polymeric IgA in serum, because secretory IgA in serum is a very small part of total polymeric IgA and probably does not involve transport by a secretory component dependent system, because it is already bound to secretory component.

ORLANS: We know the values for IgA in human serum. I think that secretory IgA is rather less heterogeneous. There is general disagreement as to the percentage of secretory IgA in the bile. Mestecky's group reported that about 50% of the total IgA was bound to secretory component, and Brown and his colleagues reported that there was 70 to 90 percent.

MESTECKY: I think there is no disagreement. Dr. Vaerman and his associates detect secretory IgA roughly in the same amount and the same proportion as we do.

ORLANS: I believe that the reason that we do not see much polymeric IgA in human serum is because it is transported into bile and acquires secretory component in transit.

J. E. BUTLER (*University of Iowa, Iowa City, Iowa*): I was happy to see that you were able to demonstrate biliary transport in the sheep, because several years ago we did some preliminary studies that showed that when we use labeled IgA, IgM, IgG_1 or IgG_2 and studied their transporting in cattle, there was, indeed, a selective appearance of the IgA and IgG_1 in bile. IgG_1 was present, however, only in fragments. There was no transport of these immunoglobulins into saliva. The most curious aspect of this study was that secretory IgA, which by several immunochemical criteria contains greater than 95% secretory component, selectively appeared in bile. We were happy to hear the work of Vaerman that suggests that there may be a secretory component independent mechanism for transport of IgA.

MESTECKY: Dr. Phillips from our laboratory studied the transport of human secretory IgA through the mouse liver, and some secretory IgA was also transported into the bile apparently by a secretory component-independent mechanism.

INDUCTION AND EXPRESSION OF ANTIBODIES IN SECRETIONS: THE OCULAR IMMUNE SYSTEM*

Paul C. Montgomery†, Ahmet Ayyildiz,†
Isabel M. Lemaitre-Coelho,§ Jean-Pierre Vaerman,§
and John H. Rockey‡

†Department of Microbiology
Center for Oral Health Research
School of Dental Medicine
‡Scheie Eye Institute
Department of Ophthalmology
School of Medicine
University of Pennsylvania
Philadelphia, Pennsylvania 19104
§Experimental Medicine Unit
International Institute of Cellular and Molecular Pathology
Faculty of Medicine
Catholic University of Louvain
Brussels, Belgium

INTRODUCTION

The concept of a common mucosal immune system linked by emigrating populations of IgA-precursor cells has been supported by two major types of investigations: antibody induction studies and cell migration experiments. Antibody induction studies have not only shown the effectiveness of local antigen stimulation[1-7] as one means of triggering secretory antibody responses, but also have documented antigen ingestion as an effective alternative approach to elicit antibody (in particular, IgA) responses in secretions[8-11] (including milk, saliva, bronchial, and intestinal fluid). In many cases the induction of IgA antibodies in secretions occurred in the absence of measurable serum antibody responses.

Early cellular analysis showed that Peyer's patches were enriched sources of IgA-precursor cells[12] that migrated to the mesenteric lymph nodes (MLN) and eventually seeded the lamina propria of the small intestine and bronchial areas.[13] Subsequent studies documented that MLN blasts also homed to gestational mammary glands[14] and genital areas[15] giving rise to cells expressing the IgA isotype. Recently, these investigations have been extended to include the salivary glands.[16] In addition, antibody-producing cells have been found in the milk of humans following oral immunization[17] and specific IgA antibody-producing cells have been documented in lactating mammary glands and other secretory sites following transfer of MLN cells from orally immunized animals.[18]

Initial evidence from the ocular system suggests that certain compartments of the eye may be linked to the secretory immune system. Although IgA-containing plasma cells have been shown to predominate in rabbit conjunctiva,[19] it is not clear if secretory component is produced by conjunctival epithelium.[20] Secretory component is present, and IgA predominates in tears, with a corresponding

*This work was supported by United States Public Health Service Grant EY-03894 and DE-02623.

0077-8923/83/0409-0428 $1.75/0 © 1983, NYAS

predominance of IgA-plasma cells in both human[21] and rabbit[22] lacrimal glands. Furthermore, secretory component producing epithelial cells appear in acini, ducts, and tubules of the lacrimal gland.[21] These data taken together with evidence on the appearance of IgA antibodies in tears following oral immunization in humans[23] have argued in favor of extending the concept of the common mucosal immune system to one compartment of the ocular area. In an attempt to further test this hypothesis, the present investigation has studied methods of inducing IgA-antibody responses in tears, compared IgA-antibody expression in tears with other secretions, and assessed the capacity of IgA-bearing gut-derived cells to home in lacrimal glands.

MATERIALS AND METHODS

Antigen Preparation and Immunization

The preparation of dinitrophenylated type III-pneumococcal (DNP-Pn) vaccine has been detailed elsewhere.[24] The protein content of the preparations was determined by either micro-Kjeldahl or Nessler analysis; 1 mg of DNP-Pn vaccine represents approximately 3.2×10^8 organisms. Female Fischer 344 CDF/CrlBR rats (150 g, Charles River Breeding Laboratories, Wilmington, Mass.) were immunized with DNP-Pn by one of four protocols: intravenous injection, subcutaneous injection, gastric intubation, or topical application to the eye (ocular/topical). Immunization was carried out at biweekly (14 day) intervals over a period of 12 weeks. Each animal received 2000 μg of DNP-Pn vaccine diluted in sterile saline. Subcutaneous injections were administered at four ventral sites. For topical application to the ocular area, the antigen was suspended in 20 μl and the dosage divided equally between each eye. Care was taken to insure that the antigen was applied to and contained within the conjunctival sac. In all cases animals were lightly anesthetized with anesthesia grade ether.

Sample Collection

Blood, tears, and saliva were collected prior to immunization and seven days after the sixth injection. For these procedures animals were anesthetized by intraperitoneal injection of Myothesia (Beecham Laboratories, Bristol, Tenn., 0.15 ml of a 1:1 stock dilution). Following anesthesia, an intraperitoneal injection of pilocarpine hydrochloride (4% isoptocarpine, Cooper Laboratories, San German, P.R., 0.07 ml of a 1:1 stock dilution) was administered. Saliva was allowed to flow into a collection tube, and tears were sampled using precalibrated (50 or 100 μl) paper wicks (Whatman No. 3 filter paper) with care taken to avoid cross contamination of tear and saliva samples. Subsequently, animals were sacrificed by an anesthesia overdose with bronchial and intestinal lavage carried out using phosphate buffered saline (2 and 10 ml, respectively). Intestinal washings were immediately subjected to centrifugation at 5,000 g to remove particulate matter, and with saliva and bronchial washings, frozen, thawed, and subjected to centrifugation at 12,000 g to remove mucins. Tear collection strips were soaked overnight in 0.15 M NaCl (0.75 ml for 50 μl, or 1.00 ml for 100 μl wicks) at 4° C. Tear eluates were subjected to centrifugation and stored frozen with the other samples. Serum, tears, saliva, and bronchial and intestinal washings were collected from unimmunized rats in an identical manner.

Radioimmunoassays

Solid-phase radioimmunoassay procedures were used to quantitate IgA, IgG, and IgM anti-DNP antibodies in serum, tears, saliva, and bronchial and intestinal fluids. These procedures as well as the calibration assay have been detailed elsewhere.[25,26] The sensitivity limit for IgA, IgG, and IgM anti-DNP antibodies was 0.5, 1.0, and 0.8 ng, respectively. In addition, the radioimmunoassay procedure was used to assess the distribution of IgA anti-DNP antibodies in fractions obtained in the isoelectric focusing system.

Isoelectric Focusing

The microscale isoelectric focusing method has been described previously.[25] The concentrations of the sucrose solutions used to form the discontinuous support gradient were modified (0.2 ml 50%; 0.2 ml 40%; 0.1 ml 30%; 0.3 ml 25%, containing a 1:1 mix of sample; 0.2 ml 10%) to achieve a larger sample load. The radioimmunoassay was employed to assess the distribution of IgA anti-DNP antibodies in fractions obtained after focusing was completed. The binding data were corrected for machine background and the cpm/50 μl of test fraction was plotted against the individual pH values. All samples were focused a minimum of three to four times to ensure spectrotype reproducibility. Fractions obtained from normal tears, bronchial fluid, or saliva were assayed, and these data are expressed as a horizontal bar representing the calculated average background binding over the relevant pH range.

Adoptive Transfer System

C57BL/6J mice were obtained from the Jackson Laboratory (Bar Harbor, Maine) at six to eight weeks of age. Suspensions of cells from MLN or peripheral lymph nodes (PLN; surface and deep cervical, axillary, brachial, inguinal) were prepared in ice cold RPMI-1640 medium (pH 7.2) with 20 mM N-2-hydroxyethyl piperazine-N'-2-ethane sulfonic acid (HEPES) buffer and 10% newborn calf serum (Microbiological Associates Bioproducts, Walkersville, Md.) as detailed elsewhere.[16] Cells were incubated for 90 minutes at 37° C at 5 × 10^7/ml in medium containing 4 μCi/ml of [^{125}I]iododeoxyuridine (^{125}IUDR, Amersham/ Searle Corp., Arlington Heights, Il.) to label those cells synthesizing DNA. The cells were washed three times in cold medium and filtered rapidly through nylon wool to yield suspensions of individual, viable cells, free of unbound radiolabel. Between 2 × 10^7 and 5 × 10^7 viable cells were transferred intravenously. In some experiments, selectively depleted populations of MLN were prepared following procedures detailed elsewhere.[16] Radiolabeled MLN cells were incubated with rabbit antisera specific for mouse IgG$_{1,2}$ (anti-γ) and IgM (anti-μ, Litton Bionetics, Kensington, Md.) or with goat antiserum to mouse IgA (anti-α, Meloy Laboratories, Inc., Springfield, Va.) plus guinea pig complement (BBL, Cockeysville, Md.) at 37° C for 45 minutes. Cells to be transferred were washed in RPMI and filtered as above. The details of the antisera absorption protocols, specificity, and cytotoxicity have been reported earlier.[16]

Eighteen to twenty-four hours after cell transfer, PLN, MLN, small intestine, and salivary and lacrimal glands were removed from recipients and weighed. Radioactivity was measured in an Intertechnique gamma counter (70% efficiency for ^{125}I). Recovered radioactivity was expressed as a percentage of that injected per gram of recipient tissue ± standard deviation. Following calculation of means and standard deviations, P values were determined by the unpaired, two-tailed Student's t-test.

RESULTS

IgA Anti-DNP Antibody Responses in Animal Groups
following Various Immunization Routes

The IgA anti-DNP antibody responses of rats receiving six biweekly dosages of DNP-Pn by the intravenous, subcutaneous, gastric, or ocular/topical (application to the eye) routes were assessed by solid phase radioimmunoassay. The response frequencies and IgA antibody levels in serum, intestinal fluid, bronchial fluid, saliva, and tears are shown in TABLE 1. None of the immunization routes elicit serum IgA responses. The response frequencies and antibody titers of intestinal fluid samples are comparable in all animal groups. With the exception

TABLE 1

IgA Anti-DNP Antibody Responses Following Various Immunization Routes

Route	Serum		Intestinal Fluid	Bronchial Fluid	Saliva	Tears
Intravenous	0* (0/5)†	0‡	100 (5/5) 3058	40 (2/5) 418	80 (4/5) 159	20 (1/5) 52§
Sub-cutaneous	0 (0/6)	0	100 (6/6) 2819	100 (6/6) 106	50 (3/6) 157	50 (3/6) 167
Gastric	0 (0/16)	0	100 (16/16) 2766	75 (12/16) 580	71 (12/17) 252	71 (12/17) 196
Ocular/Topical	0 (0/9)	0	100 (9/9) 3170	78 (7/9) 196	89 (8/9) 338	22 (2/9) 108

*Percentage of animals displaying IgA anti-DNP anbibody responses.
†Responding animals/total animals immunized.
‡Nanograms IgA anti-DNP antibodies/ml of fluid; average IgA values calculated for all responding rats using solid phase radioimmunoassay data.
§Nanograms IgA anti-DNP antibodies/ml of eluate obtained from a precalibrated filter paper strip saturated with 100 μl of tears.

of the response frequency in the subcutaneous and intravenous groups, the percentage of bronchial and saliva samples displaying IgA responses is greater in gastric and ocular/topical groups. The highest antibody levels for bronchial fluid and saliva appear in gastric and ocular/topical animals, respectively. Gastric immunization gives both higher response frequencies and IgA-antibody levels in tears. It is interesting to note that the response frequencies match, and antibody levels are comparable for saliva and tears of the subcutaneous and gastric groups, whereas for the intravenous and ocular/topical groups, both the response frequencies and antibody levels in tears are markedly lower than saliva.

IgA, IgG, and IgM Anti-DNP Antibody Responses in Individual Rats

Individual animals from the subcutaneous, gastric, and ocular/topical group were selected for more detailed analysis. The IgA, IgG, and IgM anti-DNP antibody responses in the serum, intestinal fluid, bronchial fluid, saliva, and tears of these rats are presented in TABLE 2. It is readily apparent that the presence, absence, or level of IgA antibodies in tears, as in secretions and serum, is independent of the occurrence of antibody responses in the other isotypes. Under the conditions of our study, these data indicate that the gastric route is not as effective as the subcutaneous, intravenous (data not shown), or ocular/topical route at triggering IgG or IgM responses in serum, tears, and other secretions. It is particularly interesting to note the appearance of IgG antibodies in serum and secretions of animals receiving antigen by the ocular/topical route.

IgA Anti-DNP Antibody Spectrotypes in Tears and Secretions
of Individual Rats

The expression of IgA anti-DNP antibodies in tears, saliva, and bronchial fluid of individual rats was assessed using isoelectric focusing. FIGURE 1 shows the

TABLE 2

IGA, IGG, AND IGM ANTI-DNP ANTIBODY RESPONSES OF INDIVIDUAL RATS FOLLOWING VARIOUS IMMUNIZATION ROUTES

Route/Animal		Serum	Intestinal Fluid	Bronchial Fluid	Saliva	Tears
Subcutaneous						
I SC-6	IgA	0*	3292	46	142	264
	IgG	16951	33	1049	4	54
	IgM	0	0	0	37	28
Gastric						
I GI-4	IgA	0	1037	570	388	263
	IgG	0	0	0	0	0
	IgM	0	0	0	0	0
II GI-3	IgA	0	2683	244	55	202
	IgG	0	0	141	0	0
	IgM	0	0	0	0	0
Ocular/Topical						
II OT-2	IgA	0	848	212	0	102
	IgG	17931	0	907	238	0
	IgM	0	0	0	46	0

*Anti-DNP antibodies, ng/ml fluid or eluate from a precalibrated filter paper strip saturated with 100 μl of tears, using the solid phase radioimmunoassay (anti-isotype specific reagents).

antibody spectrotypes of rat I SC-6, receiving subcutaneous immunization. The overall complexity of the tear (T), saliva (S), and bronchial (B) spectrotypes vary, showing components with different pI's ($\downarrow$). The tear spectrotype displays six major components (pI 4.18, 4.55, 5.05, 5.23, 5.50, and 5.75), the saliva spectrotype five major components (pI 4.30, 4.61, 4.95, 5.12, and 5.33), the bronchial spectrotype three major components (pI 5.17, 5.30, and 5.57).

FIGURES 2 and 3 show the IgA-antibody spectrotypes of rats I GI-4 and II GI-3 that received antigen by the gastric route. The spectrotypes for both animals are complex with I GI-4 displaying seven major components (pI 4.08, 4.53, 4.90, 5.21,

FIGURE 1. IgA anti-DNP antibody spectrotypes in tears (T), saliva (S), and bronchial fluid (B) of rat I SC-6 immunized by subcutaneous injection. For this and subsequent figures the pH range was obtained by mixing 0.25 ml pH 3–6, 1.0 ml pH 4–6, and 1.25 ml pH 5–8 Ampholines. IgA-antibody content of individual fractions was assessed by solid phase radioimmunoassay (^{125}I-labeled anti-α chain reagent). The arrows indicate spectral components with different pI's; the horizontal bar represents the calculated average background binding when the appropriate normal fluid was focused in an identical manner.

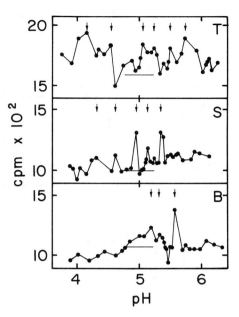

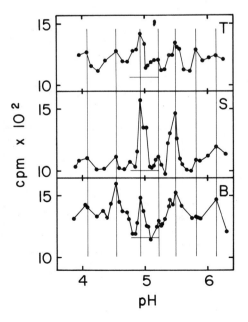

FIGURE 2. IgA anti-DNP antibody spectrotypes in tears (T), saliva (S), and bronchial fluid (B) of rat I GI-4 immunized by gastric intubation. The vertical bars represent spectral components with identical pI's.

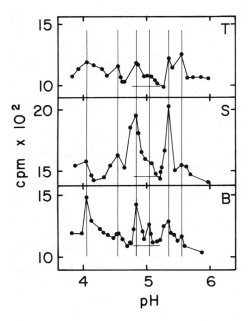

FIGURE 3. IgA anti-DNP antibody spectrotypes in tears (T), saliva (S), and bronchial fluid (B) of rat II GI-3 immunized by gastric intubation. The vertical bars represent spectral components with identical pI's.

FIGURE 4. IgA anti-DNP antibody spectrotypes in tears (T) and bronchial fluid (B) of rat II OT-2 immunized by topical application to the eye. The vertical bars represent spectral components with identical pI's, the arrows spectral components with different pI's.

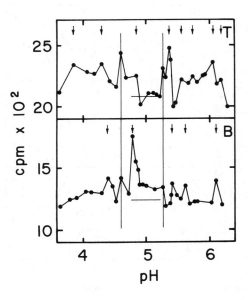

5.48, 5.80, and 6.12) and II GI-3 displaying six major components (pI 4.05, 4.55, 4.84, 5.04, 5.36, and 5.57). Whereas spectral components of the individual rats do not match, the pI's of the tears (T), saliva (S), and bronchial fluid (B) for each individual rat are identical (indicated by the vertical bars).

The IgA-antibody spectrotype of rat II OT-2, immunized by the ocular/topical route, is shown in FIGURE 4. As in the case of the subcutaneous route animal (FIGURE 1), the overall complexity of the tear and bronchial spectrotypes differ, with the bronchial being somewhat less complex. The tear (T) spectrotype displays 10 major components (pI 3.84, 4.30, 4.60, 4.84, 5.28, 5.37, 5.56, 5.72, 6.04, and 6.18), and the bronchial spectrotype seven major components (pI 4.39, 4.60, 4.78, 5.28, 5.41, 5.61, and 6.11). It is interesting to note that whereas the majority of the spectral components possess different pI's ($\downarrow$), two components with identical pI's (vertical bars) appear in each spectrotype.

TABLE 3

PERCENTAGE OF INJECTED LABEL RECOVERED FROM RECIPIENT ORGANS FOLLOWING
TRANSFER OF ^{125}IUDR-LABELED MLN AND PLN CELLS

Recipient Organs	Donor Cells	Number of Recipients	Label Recovered*	Preference Index†	p‡
PLN	MLN	9	5.25 ± 2.08		
	PLN	6	5.07 ± 0.72	1.03	>.9 (N.S.)§
MLN	MLN	9	4.26 ± 0.75		
	PLN	6	2.30 ± 0.45	1.85	0.005 < P < 0.01
Small Intestine	MLN	9	4.22 ± 1.52		
	PLN	6	1.46 ± 0.46	2.89	0.025 < P < 0.05
Salivary Glands	MLN	9	1.60 ± 0.52		
	PLN	6	0.70 ± 0.29	2.29	0.025 < P < 0.05
Lacrimal Glands	MLN	9	0.42 ± 0.19		
	PLN	6	0.15 ± 0.05	2.80	0.05 < P < 0.10

*Recovery expressed as mean percent injected cpm/g tissue ± SD.
†Preference index = percent injected cpm/g in MLN recipients ÷ percent injected cpm/g in PLN recipients.
‡Two-tailed Student's t-test.
§Not significant.

Relative Migratory Properties of MLN and PLN Cell Populations

In order to directly establish the linkage of tissue in the ocular area to other components of the common mucosal immune system, the relative migratory properties of MLN and PLN cells into lacrimal glands were studied using the murine adoptive transfer model. The percentages of ^{125}IUDR-labeled MLN and PLN cells are shown in TABLE 3. As documented by the preference indices[14,16] (values above one, calculated from statistically significant label recovery data, indicate a greater tendency of MLN cells to migrate to the recipient organ when compared to PLN cells), MLN cells have a greater propensity to selectively localize in MLN, small intestine, salivary (submandibular and sublingual), and lacrimal glands, but not in peripheral lymph nodes.

Effect of Antisera Pretreatment on the Migratory Patterns of MLN Cells

In order to determine if the preferential homing of MLN cells was due to an IgA-bearing population, we studied the migratory properties of MLN cells to recipient organs following selective depletion with isotype specific antisera. Cytolysis was carried out using anti-α or anti-γ, and anti-μ plus complement. The results of these experiments are summarized in TABLE 4. These data show that the migration of MLN cells to MLN, small intestine, and salivary and lacrimal glands is reduced by a significant percentage by pretreatment with anti-α and complement. It is important to note that previous control studies comparing the effect of pretreatment with this anti-γ and anti-μ antiserum with the appropriate normal serum showed no differences in homing.[16] Furthermore, absorption of the anti-α antisera used in these studies with an IgA immunoabsorbent prior to pretreatment documented that the abrogation of the MLN cell migration was due to the specificity of the serum for IgA.[16] Interpreting these data in the context of previous

TABLE 4

EFFECT OF ANTISERA PLUS COMPLEMENT ON HOMING OF [125]IUDR-LABELED MLN CELLS
TO RECIPIENT ORGANS

Recipient Organs	Treatment of MLN Cells	Number of Recipients	Label Recovered	Percentage Reduction In Recovery	p^*
MLN	Anti-μ + Anti-γ	4	5.44 ± 0.57		
	Anti-α	4	4.05 ± 0.99	25.6	$0.05 < P < 0.10$
Small Intestine	Anti-μ + Anti-γ	4	5.47 ± 1.17		
	Anti-α	4	3.39 ± 0.74	38.0	$0.05 < P < 0.10$
Salivary Glands	Anti-μ + Anti-γ	4	1.79 ± 0.47		
	Anti-α	4	0.82 ± 0.15	54.2	$0.005 < P < 0.01$
Lacrimal Glands	Anti-μ + Anti-γ	4	0.80 ± 0.12		
	Anti-α	4	0.33 ± 0.15	58.7	$0.005 < P < 0.01$

*Two-tailed Student's t-test.

control studies indicates that the selective localization displayed by the MLN cells is due to an IgA-bearing population.

DISCUSSION

Previous investigations using the DNP-Pn antigen have indicated that the gastric (gastrointestinal) route is an effective means of eliciting IgA antibodies in secretions, generally in the absence of serum IgA and IgG responses.[11,27] The current data show that the gastrointestinal route also is an effective method of inducing IgA antibodies in tears. Despite differences in the antigenic stimulus and frequency of gastrointestinal stimulation, our findings agree with earlier observations, showing the simultaneous occurrence of IgA antibodies in tears and saliva of humans.[23] The relative ineffectiveness of the ocular/topical route (percentage of responders) in eliciting tear IgA-responses is interesting in view of the high response frequencies and levels of IgA-antibodies in saliva. The variability and patterns of appearance of IgA-, IgG-, and IgM-antibody responses in serum and secretions of animals immunized by the subcutaneous (as well as intravenous route, unpublished observations) and ocular/topical routes suggest that antigen dissemination may be occurring in these animals. The antibody response patterns of DNP-Pn introduced topically in the eye differ from those obtained with another particulate antigen, DNP-*Streptococcus mutans*, which does not evoke salivary IgA-antibody responses when injected in the mammary gland area.[28] Although it is not clear if these differences reflect a differential capacity of these tissues to deal with antigenic stimuli, our data, taken together with studies showing antibody induction following ocular/topical immunization,[29] support the hypothesis that conjunctival-associated lymphoid tissue may function in an antigen sampling, processing,[30] and dissemination capacity. By contrast, the lack of IgG and IgM responses and the consistent induction of IgA antibodies in tears and secretions of animals immunized by the gastrointestinal route support the idea that committed IgA-precursor cells migrate to the lacrimal gland.

The spectrotype data show clear differences in the IgA-antibody expression in secretions of animals immunized by different routes. Subcutaneous immunization resulted in spectral components possessing different pI's in tears, saliva, and bronchial fluid. In this case, the lack of homology appears to result from antigen dissemination to the various secretory sites, with the differences reflecting variations in IgA-precursor cells resident in each site. Ocular/topical immunization resulted in spectrotypes displaying components with both different and identical pI's in tears and bronchial fluid. As in the subcutaneous animal, the lack of homology may be due to antigen dissemination and presentation to different IgA-precursor cells resident in the two sites. The expression of two components with identical pI's could reflect either the triggering of identical IgA-precursor-cell populations already present in the lacrimal gland and bronchial tissue or the movement of IgA-precursor cells, triggered in the lacrimal gland to the bronchial tissue. Further experimentation will be required to distinguish between these two possibilities. On the other hand, gastrointestinal stimulation resulted in spectrotypes possessing complete homology in tears, saliva, and bronchial fluid. In this case, assuming that antigen remains confined to the intestinal area, the identity of the spectral components suggest that IgA-precursor cells with identical clonotype potentials seed secretory sites. These data are entirely consistent with our previous observations[27,31] and, in view of the antibody-induction studies, lend support to the migration of committed IgA-precursor cells with identical clonotype potentials to the lacrimal gland as well as other secretory sites.

The selective localization of IgA-bearing MLN cells in lacrimal glands represents an extension of previous studies documenting homing to the lamina propria of the small intestine,[13] bronchus,[13] gestational mammary glands,[14] genital areas,[15] and salivary glands.[16] Although it is known that the homing phenomenon can occur in the absence of antigenic stimulation,[13-16,32] other investigations have documented the homing capacity of IgA-antibody-producing cells to distal mucosal areas following antigen ingestion.[18] Furthermore, intraduodenal immunization generates the dissemination of antigen-specific memory cells to mucosal sites distal from antigen application.[33,34] Thus, in the context of these observations, our cell-homing and antibody-response data indicate that one compartment of the ocular area, the lacrimal gland, is linked to the common mucosal immune system by emigrating, gut-derived IgA-bearing cells.

Conclusions

Gastric (gastrointestinal) immunization has been shown to be an effective method of eliciting IgA antibodies in tears. The spectral identities of IgA antibodies present in tears and other secretions suggest that lacrimal glands and other secretory sites are seeded by identical gut-derived cell populations. Adoptive transfer data indicate that MLN cells bearing the IgA isotype home to lacrimal glands as they do to other secretory sites. These data indicate that the common mucosal immune system extends to one compartment of the ocular area.

Acknowledgment

We thank Mrs. Mary Ann Webster for skillful technical assistance.

References

1. OGRA, P. L., D. T. KARZON, F. RIGHTHAND & M. MACGILLIVRAY. 1968. New Engl. J. Med. **279:** 893–900.
2. HEREMANS, J. F. & H. BAZIN. 1971. Ann. N. Y. Acad. Sci. **190:** 268–274.
3. GENCO, R. J. & M. A. TAUBMAN. 1969. Nature (London) **221:** 679–681.
4. WALDMAN, R. H. & R. GANGULY. 1974. J. Infect. Dis. **130:** 419–440.
5. MONTGOMERY, P. C., J. COHN & E. T. LALLY. 1974. *In* The Immunoglobulin A System. J. Mestecky and A. R. Lawton, Eds.: 453–462. Plenum Press. New York.
6. PIERCE, N. F. & J. L. GOWANS. 1975. J. Exp. Med. **142:** 1550–1563.
7. COX, D. S., M. A. TAUBMAN, J. L. EBERSOLE & D. J. SMITH. 1980. Mol. Immunol. **17:** 1105–1115.
8. ALLARDYCE, R. A., D. J. C. SHEARMAN, B. B. L. MCCLELLAND, K. MARWICK, A. J. SIMPSON & R. B. LAIDEAU. 1974. Brit. Med. J. **3:** 307–309.
9. MICHALEK, S. M., J. R. MCGHEE, J. MESTECKY, R. R. ARNOLD & L. BOZZO. 1976. Science. **192:** 1238–1240.
10. SAIF, L. J. & E. H. BOHL. 1977. Infect. Immun. **16:** 961–966.
11. MONTGOMERY, P. C., K. M. CONNELLY, J. COHN & C. A. SKANDERA. 1978. *In* Secretory Immunity and Infection. J. R. McGhee, J. Mestecky and J. L. Babb, Eds.: 113–122. Plenum Press. New York.
12. CRAIG, S. W. & J. J. CEBRA. 1971. J. Exp. Med. **134:** 188–200.
13. RUDZIK, O., R. J. CLANCY, D. Y. E. PEREY, R. P. DAY & J. BIENENSTOCK. 1975. J. Immunol. **114:** 1599–1604.
14. ROUX, M. E., M. MCWILLIAMS, J. M. PHILLIPS-QUAGLIATA, P. WEISZ-CARRINGTON & M. E. LAMM. 1977. J. Exp. Med. **146:** 1311–1322.
15. MCDERMOTT, M. & J. BIENENSTOCK. 1979. J. Immunol. **122:** 1892–1898.
16. JACKSON, D. E., E. T. LALLY, M. C. NAKAMURA & P. C. MONTGOMERY. 1981. Cell. Immunol. **63:** 203–209.
17. GOLDBLUM, R. M., S. AHLSTEDT, B. CARLSSON, L. HANSON, V. JODAL, G. LINDIN-JANSON & A. SOHL-AKERLUND. 1975. Nature (London) **257:** 797–798.
18. WEISZ-CARRINGTON, P., M. ROUX, M. MCWILLIAMS, J. M. PHILLIPS-QUAGLIATA & M. E. LAMM. 1979. J. Immunol. **123:** 1705–1708.
19. FRANKLIN, R. M., R. A. PRENDERGAST & A. M. SILVERSTEIN. 1973. *In* Immunology and Immunopathology of the Eye. A. M. Silverstein and G. R. O'Connor, Eds.: 302–308. Masson Publishing. New York.
20. COHEN, E. J. & M. R. ALLANSMITH. 1981. Am. J. Ophthalmol. **91:** 789–793.
21. FRANKLIN, R. M., K. R. KENYON & T. B. TOMASI. 1973. J. Immunol. **110:** 894–992.
22. SHIMADA, K. & A. M. SILVERSTEIN. 1975. Invest. Ophthalmol. **14:** 573–583.

23. MESTECKY, J., J. R. McGHEE, R. R. ARNOLD, S. M. MICHALEK, S. J. PRINCE & J. L. BABB. 1978. J. Clin. Invest. **61:** 731–737.
24. MONTGOMERY, P. C. & J. H. PINCUS. 1973. J. Immunol. **111:** 42–51.
25. MONTGOMERY, P. C. & C. A. SKANDERA. 1978. J. Immunol. **121:** 111–114.
26. VAN SNICK, J. L. & P. L. MASSON. 1979. J. Exp. Med. **149:** 1519–1530.
27. MONTGOMERY, P. C., I. M. LEMAITRE-COELHO & J. P. VAERMAN. 1981. Scand. J. Immunol. **13:** 587–595.
28. COX, D. S. & M. A. TAUBMAN. 1982. Mol. Immunol. **19:** 171–178.
29. HALL, J. M. & J. M. PRIBNOW. 1981. Invest. Ophthalmol. **21:** 753–756.
30. CHANDLER, J. W. & A. J. AXELROD. 1980. *In* Immunologic Diseases of the Mucous Membranes. Pathology, Diagnosis and Treatment. G. R. O'Connor, Ed.: 63–70. Masson Publishing. New York.
31. MONTGOMERY, P. C., I. M. LEMAITRE-COELHO & J. P. VAERMAN. 1980. Immunol. Commun. **9(7):** 705–713.
32. HUSBAND, A. J. & J. L. GOWANS. 1978. J. Exp. Med. **148:** 1146–1160.
33. PIERCE, N. F. & W. C. CRAY. 1981. J. Immunol. **127:** 2461–2464.
34. FUHRMAN, J. A. & J. J. CEBRA. 1981. J. Exp. Med. **153:** 534–544.

DISCUSSION OF THE PAPER

J. R. McGHEE (*University of Alabama in Birmingham*): Have you performed your experiment with systemic hyperimmunization followed by gastric intubation and examination of tears for the presence of antibodies.

P. C. MONTGOMERY (*University of Pennsylvania, Philadelphia, Pa.*): No, I have not done that experiment.

McGHEE: Do you know whether there are antibody-producing plasma cells in lacrimal glands?

MONTGOMERY: We have started to set up the double immunofluorescence technique. We observed in the lacrimal gland anti-DNP producing IgA-isotype plasma cells.

S. J. CHALLACOMBE (*Guy's Hospital, London, England*): One of the surprising observations about topical application of antigens in the eye was that it seemed to be more effective.

MONTGOMERY: It is possible that antigen can reach the oral cavity through the naso-lacrimal canal. There are results I did not present. If you examine the immune response induced by topical immunization after three weeks, the ocular responses are comparable to the responses from gastric immunization.

N. F. PIERCE (*The Johns Hopkins University, Baltimore, Md.*): I have a comment with respect to interpretation of your data. While your studies support the idea of tying together the lacrimal gland with the rest of the mucosal immune system, it is important to view this tie as a qualitative, and not necessarily a quantitative, one. Although one can elicit a vigorous response in the gut, this response does not mean that the immune response in the lacrimal gland will be of the same magnitude. In our studies in which we examined, for example, the immune response in the gut and trachea, the response in the trachea was only about 5% of that seen in the gut, which was the primary site of immunization. The other possibility is that after eliciting a vigorous response in the gut, a portion of serum-derived antibodies may find its way into tears.

MONTGOMERY: To address this point we are developing the system to allow us to enumerate antibody-producing cells in the lacrimal glands.

M. D. COOPER (*University of Alabama in Birmingham*): I am really impressed with your demonstration of seeding of cells of the same clone from the gut to the lacrimal and salivary glands. Have you examined to see if the clones that are triggered by the oral route of immunization are similar from animal to animal? How does this repertoire of cells develop in the gut with age and as a function of previous exposure to antigen?

MONTGOMERY: The isoelectric focusing experiments indicate that we are inducing antibodies with identical isoelectric points. This phenomenon is suggestive of cells with identical clonal types. Currently we are examining idiotypes and spectrotypes of antibodies from different animals.

TRANSCELLULAR TRANSPORT OF POLYMERIC IMMUNOGLOBULIN BY SECRETORY COMPONENT: A MODEL SYSTEM FOR STUDYING INTRACELLULAR PROTEIN SORTING

Keith E. Mostov and Günter Blobel

Laboratory of Cell Biology
The Rockefeller University
New York, New York 10021

Nucleated cells have a number of specialized membranes, each containing a particular set of proteins. The location of proteins is not fixed; there is movement between membranes. Such movement may occur by diffusion within the plane of the bilayer or by cytoplasmic vesicles traveling between membranes. Each cell faces two related problems of protein sorting.[1] First, after synthesis, proteins must be directed to their proper location. A given protein may travel through a succession of locations during its lifetime. Second, the differentiation of the various membranes must be maintained even though vesicles are constantly carrying pieces of membrane from one compartment to another.

As a model system for studying sorting, we chose to examine the transepithelial transport of polymeric IgA and IgM (pIg) by secretory component (SC). Certain epithelial cells produce SC, a glycoprotein that is found in association with pIg in many external secretions[5] and is believed to be the receptor mediating the transepithelial transport of pIg into these secretions.[6,7] Two unusual features attracted us to study secretory component.

First, it has a complex intracellular pathway, as revealed by cytochemical and uptake studies:[8-12] Secretory component is made on the rough endoplasmic reticulum and travels through the Golgi apparatus to the basolateral (or in hepatocytes, sinusoidal) surface of the cell. On this surface, pIg, produced by plasma cells, binds to the SC, and the SC-pIg complex is endocytosed. These endocytotic vesicles apparently do not fuse with lysosomes, but instead carry the complex to the apical (or in hepatocytes, bile canalicular) surface where the SC-pIg is released into the glandular secretion by exocytosis. This process may be termed receptor-mediated transcytosis.

The second paradoxical aspect is: How can a soluble secreted protein such as SC function as a membrane receptor,[13-15] when such receptors are usually integral membrane proteins? One possibility is that SC is secreted and then binds to an unidentified integral membrane protein on the basolateral surface.[16] Secretory component would then be a linker between pIg and this unidentified membrane protein.

We found, however, that SC is made as a larger transmembrane precursor, and proposed that this precursor functions as the receptor for pIg.[17] As depicted in FIGURE 1, this transmembrane protein is made on the rough endoplasmic reticulum with a portion, the ectoplasmic domain, translocated into the lumen of the endoplasmic reticulum. After going through the Golgi, SC reaches the basolateral surface, where the ectoplasmic domain is exposed on the outside of the cell. pIg binds to the ectoplasmic domain and the transmembrane protein-pIg complex is endocytosed. This transcytotic vesicle traverses the cell and is

0077-8923/83/0409-0441 $1.75/0 © 1983, NYAS

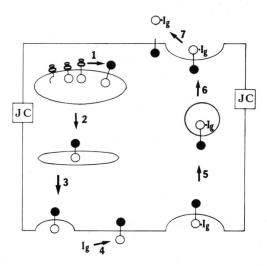

FIGURE 1. Hypothetical model for the intracellular pathway of SC in a glandular cell. The luminal or apical portion of the plasma membrane (upper half) is separated from the basolateral region of the plasma membrane (lower half) by the junctional complex (JC). In parenchymal liver cells, the bile canalicular region of the plasma membrane corresponds to the apical surface, and the sinusoidal region of the plasma membrane is equivalent to the basolateral region. SC is synthesized by membrane-bound polysomes as a transmembrane form(s) and is cotranslationally and asymmetrically integrated into the rough endoplasmic reticulum (step 1) as follows. A distinct ectoplasmic domain (open circle) is translocated into the rough endoplasmic reticulum lumen, another distinct cytoplasmic domain (solid circle) remains untranslocated, and a membrane-spanning segment(s) (bar) links the two domains. After transport to the Golgi complex (step 2), and subsequently to the basolateral region of the plasma membrane (step 3), the ectoplasmic domain of the SC binds to pIg (step 4). The transmembrane SC-pIg complex is then removed from the basolateral region of the plasma membrane through endocytosis (step 5). The endocytotic vesicle traverses the cell and fuses with the apical region of the plasma membrane (step 6). The ectoplasmic domain of transmembrane SC is endoproteolytically cleaved (step 7), most likely either in the endocytotic vesicle or at the apical surface, generating a soluble SC-pIg complex and a membrane bound remainder of transmembrane SC that includes the cytoplasmic domain and transmembrane segment(s). Various different intermediate transmembrane forms of SC resulting from sequential proteolytic or other modifications during its intracellular pathway may exist. Our model is similar to that proposed by Brandtzaeg except that it distinguishes between the larger, intracellular transmembrane form(s) of SC and the smaller, proteolytically generated, secreted form(s) of SC. See K. E. Mostov, et al.[17]

exocytosed at the apical surface. At some unknown point, most likely in the transcytotic vesicle or after exocytosis, the ectoplasmic domain is endoproteolytically cleaved from the transmembrane precursor, so that it can be released with the pIg. Secretory component isolated from secretions is thus a proteolytic fragment that constitutes most, if not all, of the ectoplasmic domain of the transmembrane precursor. The cytoplasmic domain of the transmembrane precursor is probably the effector domain of the receptor, containing information for guiding the SC through its complex intracellular pathway. The cytoplasmic effector domain is thus linked to the ectoplasmic ligand binding domain by a membrane spanning segment(s). The fate of this segment(s) and the cytoplasmic domain after cleavage of the ectoplasmic domain is unknown; probably they are rapidly degraded.

To test this model, we began by investigating the earliest steps in the biosynthesis of rabbit SC, using a cell-free protein synthesis and membrane integration system.[17] Rabbit SC was used because we could obtain ample amounts of SC mRNA from lactating mammary gland and liver. Rabbit SC, however, is heterogeneous, with two or three polypeptides of approximate M_r 70,000 (FIGURE 2, lane 1) and two minor species of approximate M_r 50,000 (not seen in FIGURE 2, lane 1). The exact M_r varies among individuals. When we translated lactating mammary mRNA in the wheat germ cell-free system and immunoprecipitated with goat antiserum to rabbit milk SC (the kind gift of J.-P. Kraehenbuhl), we found two major bands of approximate M_r 90,000 (upper doublet), and two minor bands of approximate M_r 70,000 (lower doublet), as shown in FIGURE 2, lane 2. A slightly different pattern was obtained when we used mammary mRNA from a second rabbit (FIGURE 2, lane 3); the lower band is probably a poorly resolved doublet.

We considered whether all four of the observed bands were primary translation products of SC, or whether they were artifacts of immunoprecipitation or in vitro translation. Because the total translation products of liver differ from that of mammary gland, it is unlikely that the same four bands would be immunoprecipitated from a liver mRNA translation, if any of them were contaminants. Yet we clearly found the same pattern of immunoprecipitated products from translations of liver and mammary mRNAs (FIGURE 3, compare lanes 1 and 2). Furthermore, using a sucrose gradient, we were able to partially separate the mRNAs coding for the upper and lower doublets (FIGURE 4). Hence the lower doublet is not a proteolytic breakdown product of the upper doublet. Additionally, because the mRNAs contain 3' poly (A) tails and intact 5' initiation sites, the lower doublet is not the result of nucleolytic degradation of the mRNAs coding for the upper doublet.

Events that occur cotranslationally at the rough endoplasmic reticulum, such as translocation or integration of proteins across or into the membrane, and core glycosylation of glycoproteins, can be reproduced in vitro by including dog pancreas rough microsomes in the translation reaction.[18] Because SC is a glycoprotein, it was not surprising that when it was translated in the presence of these microsomes, the SC bands shifted up, indicating the cotranslational addition of core sugars (FIGURE 2, lane 5, and FIGURE 3, lane 3). These glycosylated forms are able to bind to concanavalin A-Sepharose.

If SC is a secretory protein, then in vitro we would expect it to be cotranslationally translocated completely into the lumen of the dog pancreas microsomal vesicles, and hence totally protected from digestion by proteases added later. If, however, SC is made as a transmembrane precursor, then a portion would not be translocated into the lumen of the microsomal vesicles and would remain accessible to proteolytic digestion. When the translations performed in the presence of vesicles were subsequently digested with trypsin, all four of the bands were reduced in size by about 15 kilodaltons (FIGURE 2, lane 5, and FIGURE 3, lane 4). This reduction suggests that all four forms are transmembrane proteins with a substantial portion exposed on the cytoplasmic side of the microsomal membrane.

If indeed these larger precursors of SC are the membrane receptors for pIg, they might be able to bind to IgA. We translated SC mRNA in the presence of dog pancreas microsomes, reisolated the membranes, and solubilized them with

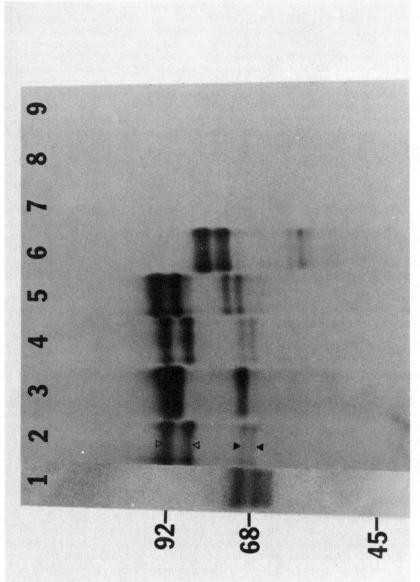

See Legend facing page

Triton X-100. The solubilized mixture was incubated with human IgA coupled to Sepharose, and the bound proteins were examined (FIGURE 5). Although there were some nonspecific contaminants, only the SC bands were bound specifically, because their binding was blocked by either excess cold SC or excess soluble IgA.

We next investigated the biosynthesis of human SC for two reasons. First, unlike the heterogeneity of rabbit SC, human SC consists of only one type of polypeptide. Second, a human colon adenocarcinoma-derived cell line (HT29) was known to make SC[19] and to transport SC and IgA by the normal pathway.[8] We found that the amount of SC produced by these cells was rather small. Fortunately, we were able to isolate a clone of these cells, HT29.E10, that produces significantly larger amounts of secretory component.

In studies to be published elsewhere, we translated mRNA from these cells and found a single primary translation product of SC of M_r 80,000. When translation was performed in the presence of dog pancreas microsomal vesicles, this band shifted up to a M_r of 95,000. Similar to what was observed with rabbit SC, posttranslational trypsinization can remove about 15 kilodaltons of this weight, indicating that human SC is a transmembrane protein.

We also performed pulse and pulse-chase experiments with these cells. With pulses of up to 30 minutes, a single band of M_r 95,000 is seen, which comigrates with the *in vitro* translated and membrane integrated form. Over the next one to two hours, this band shifts up to a form of M_r 100,000, which has complex carbohydrates, as revealed by its resistance to endoglycosidase H degradation. Slowly, this form is proteolytically cleaved to a form of M_r 80,000, and this form is gradually released into the medium.

We know that the pulse-labeled M_r 95,000 form is a transmembrane protein, because when the cells are homogenized and digested with pronase, about 15 kilodaltons are removed. Mature SC is derived from the NH_2-terminal portion of the precursor, because the various precursor forms found in the cells have the

---

FIGURE 2. Cell-free translation and transmembrane integration of rabbit mammary SC. Lane 1: is a Coomassie Blue-stained gel of authentic rabbit milk SC. The remaining lanes are from a fluorograph of cell-free synthesized and immunoprecipitated products. Lane 2: mammary mRNA from rabbit A translated in the wheat germ system; lane 3: as in 2, except the mRNA was from rabbit B; lane 4: as in 2, except that after translation was completed (90 minutes incubation at 25° C), dog pancreas microsomal vesicles were added and the incubation continued for an additional 90 minutes; lane 5: as in 2, except that the microsomal vesicles were present at the start of translation (all four bands are shifted upward, due to cotranslational glycosylation by the membranes); lane 6: as in 5, except that after translation was completed, trypsin was added to the reaction (all four bands are apparently shifted downward by about 15 kilodaltons; each of the two bands of the upper doublet appears to give rise to two closely spaced bands, which could be due to the presence of two nearby tryptic sites of which only one is cleaved in any given molecule—other explanations are possible); lane 7: as in 2, except that immunoprecipitation was carried out in the presence of 1 μg of the SC shown in lane 1 (the added SC completely blocked immunoprecipitation of all four bands); lane 8: as in 4, except that trypsin was added after translation was completed (because membranes were added after translation, the *in vitro* synthesized proteins were not translocated and were digested by trypsin); lane 9: as in 6, except that when trypsin was added, the sample was also adjusted to 1% in Triton X-100 [even though the proteins were translocated, they were degraded when the microsomal vesicles were solubilized by detergent). The positions of the M_r marker proteins are indicated at the left margin, shown as $M_r \times 10^{-3}$ (rabbit muscle phosphorylase B, 92,000; bovine serum albumin, 68,000; hen ovalbumin, 45,000). See K. E. Mostov, *et al.*[17]

same NH$_2$-terminal sequence as colostral secretory component. More importantly, SC is derived from the ectoplasmic, (noncytoplasmic) portion of these
precursors, because the protected fragment generated by pronase digestion of
homogenized cells also has the same NH$_2$-terminal sequence. The proteolytic
cleavage of the transmembrane precursor seems to take place more slowly in cells

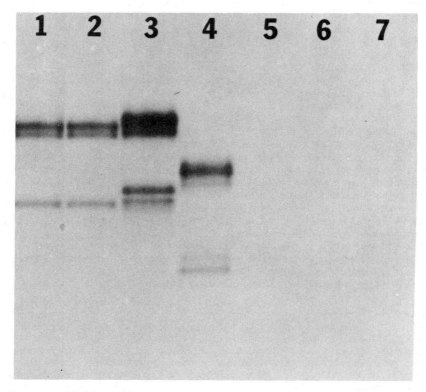

FIGURE 3. Cell-free translation and transmembrane integration of liver SC. Lane 1: as in
lane 3 of FIGURE 2 (to give the positions of the mammary SC bands of rabbit B); lane 2: liver
mRNA from rabbit B translated in the wheat germ system; lane 3: as in 2, except that dog
pancreas microsomal vesicles were present during translation; lane 4: as in 3, except that the
sample was treated with trypsin after translation; lane 5: as in 2, except that immunoprecipitation was performed in the presence of 1 μg of SC; lane 6: as in 2, except that after
translation, microsomal vesicles were added and the incubation was continued for 90
minutes before the sample was treated with trypsin; lane 7: as in 4, except that when trypsin
was added, the sample was also adjusted to 1% in Triton X-100. See K. E. Mostov, et al.[17]

that have been passaged many times in culture. This slowing down may also
occur in animals as they age.
    Taken together, these data provide strong support for our model of how SC
transports pIg through the cell. Viewed from the perspective of this model, one
can see how studies on the intracellular pathway of SC are particularly relevant

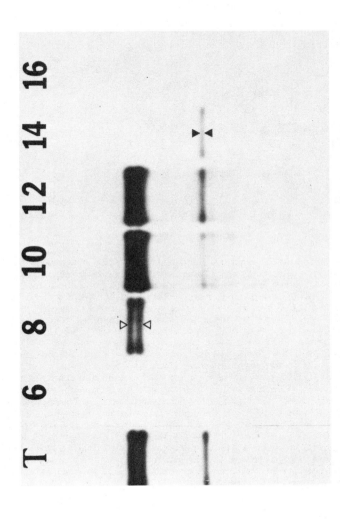

FIGURE 4. Partial purification of mRNAs coding for SC. Poly(A)-containing mRNA from rabbit B was fractionated on a sucrose gradient. Twenty-two fractions were collected and the mRNA from every second fraction was translated. In vitro synthesized products were immunoprecipitated and analyzed. The top of the gradient is toward the right. Only selected fractions are presented. The fraction number from which each lane is derived is indicated at the top of each lane. Lane T is an immunoprecipitate of a translation of total poly(A)-containing mRNA. The upper doublet is indicated by open arrowheads; the lower, unresolved, doublet by closed arrowheads. Note that fraction 8 is enriched for the upper doublet, whereas fraction 14 is enriched for the unresolved lower doublet. The faint band beneath the unresolved lower doublet in fractions 10 and 12 is probably a contaminant. See K. E. Mostov et al.[17]

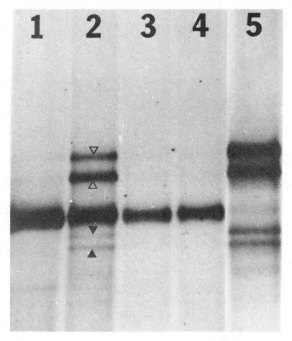

FIGURE 5. *In vitro* translocated SC forms are competent to bind human polymeric IgA. Translations (100 μl) were performed in the presence of microsomal vesicles. After translation was completed, membranes were recovered from the translation mixture by layering it in a Beckman Airfuge tube over a two-step sucrose gradient consisting of 80 μl of 0.5 M sucrose and 25 μl of 2.0 M sucrose. Both sucrose solutions also contained 150 mM NaCl and 20 mM Na phosphate (pH 6.5). After centrifugation for 15 minutes at 160,000 × g, membranes were recovered at the 0.5/2.0 M interface in a volume of 25 μl. They were diluted to 200 μl with 150 mM NaCl/20 mM Na phosphate, pH 6.5, and adjusted to 1% in Triton X-100. A 2 μl aliquot of this mixture was analyzed in lane one. This lane, therefore, represents 1% of the total *in vitro* synthesized products that cosedimented with the membranes. IgA-Sepharose (20 μl) was added to the 198 μl of solubilized membranes and the samples were agitated for 16 hours at 4° C. The beads were then washed five times with 1.2 ml of 1% Triton X-100/150 mM NaCl, and 20 mM Na phosphate, pH 6.5. Bound proteins were eluted by boiling in loading buffer, and the sample was analyzed by electrophoresis and fluorography (lane 2; arrowheads as in FIGURE 2, lane 2). Lane 3: as in 2, except that 10 μg of IgA, not bound to Sepharose, was added at the same time as the IgA-Sepharose; lane 4: as in 2, except that 20 μg of SC was added at the same time as the IgA-Sepharose; lane 5: the material that did not bind to IgA-Sepharose (i.e. the supernatant from the IgA-Sepharose incubation) was adjusted to pH 8.1 and immunoprecipitated without prior denaturation with sodium dodecyl sulfate. See K. E. Mostov, *et al.*[17]

to two general problems of protein sorting, those of receptor-mediated endocytosis and cell polarity.

     Cells constantly internalize polypeptide ligands by receptor mediated endocytosis. Many receptors deliver their ligands (e.g. low density lipoproteins) to lysosomes and then recycle back to the cell surface for reuse.[2] By contrast, some receptors (e.g. for epidermal growth factor) do not recycle after endocytosis, but are probably degraded with their ligands in lysosomes. Still other receptors (e.g. SC and other receptors involved in the transport of immunoglobulins[3]) are believed to avoid the lysosomes, and instead carry their ligands across the cell and release them by exocytosis. It has been suggested that the receptor in the neonatal rat that transports maternal IgG from the intestinal lumen to the blood may recycle.[3] Secretory component, on the other hand, clearly can be used only once, as a large portion is cleaved off and released with the pIg. Although this phenomenon appears to be wasteful, SC may also serve to protect the pIg from degradation. Another possible function for SC may be that it serves to bind pIg to another receptor. Such a receptor might be present on the apical surface of duct rather than acinar cells and thus would function in keeping much of the externally exposed glandular epithelial surfaces "coated" with SC-pIg. In fact, after it has been transported by hepatocytes, pIg seems to remain associated with the biliary epithelium.[22] Furthermore, the binding sites for SC found in rabbit mammary cells[16] may represent binding to tubular cells and not to the membranes of acinar cells.

The transcellular movement of SC is also a useful model system for studying the generation and maintenance of differentiated regions of plasma membrane in polarized cells. Epithelial cells typically have two specialized regions of plasma membrane, the basolateral and apical surface, which are separated by tight junctions. Many proteins are found predominantly or exclusively in one membrane or the other, and certain enveloped viruses bud from only one surface or the other.[4] Secretory component, by contrast, is sent first to the basolateral surface and then to the apical surface.

Several steps may be involved in sorting: first, clustering of proteins to be sorted in the donor membrane and removal by vesicles; second, targeting of vesicles to a specific recipient membrane; third, redistribution of proteins by diffusion in the recipient membrane. In the case of transmembrane proteins, the information for directing the protein may reside in discrete regions (sorting sequences), most likely contained in the cytoplasmic portion of the protein.[1]

Despite the insight into the pathway of SC provided by our data, we still do not understand the mechanisms that guide SC through the cell. Perhaps the key to understanding this mechanism lies in the unusually large cytoplasmic domain of the transmembrane SC precursor.

The one step in protein sorting whose mechanism is fairly well understood is the initial translocation of secretory and membrane proteins across the rough endoplasmic reticulum.[18] The information for sorting in that process is usually contained in a transient NH_2-terminal extension of the protein, called the signal sequence. The signal peptide is recognized by a protein complex, signal recognition protein that causes the ribosome synthesizing the protein to bind to the rough endoplasmic reticulum membrane.[20,21] This binding results in the nascent chain being translocated across the membrane. This "signal hypothesis" led to the general concept that the information for directing a protein resides in a specific sequence or structural feature of the protein that interacts with a specific receptor in the cell.[1]

Where then, does the information for guiding SC reside? The most likely possibility is in the cytoplasmic domain of the transmembrane precursor.[1,17] It is accessible to interact with whatever machinery in the cytoplasm is involved in sorting proteins. Because SC undergoes several sorting steps in its pathway, it is plausible that this cytoplasmic domain contains several discrete sorting signals, each of which specifies a particular step. The existence of several relatively discrete signals may explain why the cytoplasmic tail of the SC precursor is much larger than the cytoplasmic tails of most other integral membrane proteins (other than ion transport proteins) that are found in the plasma membrane. Some of these signals may have homologues in other proteins that undergo sorting steps in common with secretory component. Similarly, the pIg binding domain of SC may be homologous to other receptors for immunoglobulins, especially those receptors involved in transcellular transport.

REFERENCES

1. BLOBEL, G. 1980. Proc. Natl. Acad. Sci. USA **77:** 1496-1500.
2. GOLDSTEIN, J. L., R. G. ANDERSON & M. S. BROWN. 1979. Nature (London) **279:** 679-685.
3. RODEWALD, R. 1979. J. Cell Biol. **85:** 18-32.
4. RODRIGUEZ-BOULAN, E. R. & D. D. SABATINI. 1978. Proc. Natl. Acad. Sci. USA **75:** 5071-5075.
5. TOMASI, T. B., E. M. TAN, A. SOLOMON & R. A. PRENDERGAST. 1965. J. Exp. Med. **121:** 101-124.
6. BRANDTZAEG, P. 1974. J. Immunol. **112:** 1553-1559.
7. BRANDTZAEG, P. & K. BAKLIEN. 1977. In Immunology of the Gut. R. Porter and J. Knight, Eds.: 77-108. Elsevier. Amsterdam.
8. NAGURA, H., P. NAKANE & W. R. BROWN. 1979. J. Immunol. **123:** 2359-2368.
9. RENSTON, R. H., A. L. JONES, W. D. CHRISTIANSEN, G. T. HRADEK & B. J. UNDERDOWN. 1980. Science **208:** 1276-1278.
10. BROWN, W. R., Y. ISOBE & P. NAKANE. 1976. Gastroenterology **71:** 985-995.
11. FISHER, M. M., B. NAGY, H. BAZIN & B. J. UNDERDOWN. 1979. Proc. Natl. Acad. Sci. USA **76:** 2008-2012.
12. MULLOCK, B. M., R. H. HINTON, M. DOBROTA, J. PEPPARD & E. ORLANS. 1980. Biochem. J. **190:** 819-826.
13. ORLANS, E., J. PEPPARD, J. F. FRY, R. H. HINTON & B. M. MULLOCK. 1979. J. Exp. Med. **150:** 1577-1581.
14. SOCKEN, D. J., K. N. JEEJEEBHOY, H. BAZIN & B. J. UNDERDOWN. 1979. J. Exp. Med. **150:** 1538-1548.
15. CRAGO, S. S., R. KULHAVY, S. J. PRINCE & J. MESTECKY. 1978. J. Exp. Med. **147:** 1832-1837.
16. KÜHN, L. C. & J.-P. KRAEHENBUHL. 1979. J. Biol. Chem. **254:** 11072-11081.
17. MOSTOV, K. E., J.-P. KRAEHENBUHL & G. BLOBEL. 1980. Proc. Natl. Acad. Sci. USA **77:** 7257-7261.
18. BLOBEL, G., P. WALTER, C. N. CHANG, B. GOLDMAN, A. ERICKSON & V. R. LINGAPPA. 1979. Symp. Soc. Exp. Biol. **33:** 9-36.
19. HUANG, S. W., J. FOGH & R. HONG. 1976. Scand. J. Immunol. **5:** 263-268.
20. WALTER, P., I. IBRAHIM & G. BLOBEL. 1981. J. Cell. Biol. **91:** 545-550.
21. WALTER, P. & G. BLOBEL. 1981. J. Cell Biol. **91:** 551-556.
22. TAKAHASHI, I., P. K. NAKANE & W. R. BROWN. 1982. J. Immunol **128:** 1181-1187.

DISCUSSION OF THE PAPER

M. LAMM (*Case Western Reserve University, Cleveland, Ohio*): Can you rule out the possibility that you are not detecting a cleavage of the larger forms of SC, but instead are detecting an additional smaller form that is secreted?

K. E. MOSTOV (*The Rockefeller University, New York, N.Y.*): Pulse chase experiments clearly indicate that you do not see a smaller form at early times; our kinetics are completely consistent with the precursor product relationship. If there were two forms of secretory component, one transmembrane and a separate unrelated form, you would expect a separate unrelated smaller form to be detectable at an early time.

L. C. KÜHN (*University of Lausanne, Epalinges, Switzerland*): Mature secretory component appears in approximately six hours on the cell. Do you have any idea whether this appearance is inside the cell or on the surface of the cell? Would the release of free secretory component from cells be enhanced by the presence of IgA?

J. MESTECKY (*University of Alabama in Birmingham*): Where does the SC-cleaving protease come from? Where does it cleave, and at what point of the transport does it cleave?

MOSTOV: I do not know. These are problems that we are currently investigating.

THE ORIGINS OF SECRETORY IgA IN MILK: A SHIFT DURING LACTATION FROM A SERUM ORIGIN TO LOCAL SYNTHESIS IN THE MAMMARY GLAND*

John F. Halsey, Craig S. Mitchell, and Sara J. McKenzie

Department of Biochemistry
University of Kansas
College of Health Sciences
Kansas City, Kansas 66103

INTRODUCTION

Milk and other exocrine secretions such as saliva and intestinal fluid contain immunoglobulins that are believed to provide important protection at the host's mucosal surfaces.[1] In many of these secretions the major immunoglobulin is IgA. During transfer from the interstitial fluid in the lamina propria to a particular secretory fluid the oligomeric forms of IgA acquire an additional polypeptide, called secretory component that is synthesized by local epithelial cells lining the lumen.[2-5] It is generally assumed that the IgA found in a particular exocrine secretion is synthesized locally by plasma cells residing in the glandular submucosa because of the conspicuous presence of IgA-containing cells in glandular interstitia[6,7,8] and the ability of lymphocytes[9,10] and IgA lymphoblasts[11,12] to preferentially migrate to various mucosal tissues. It has also been proposed, however, that the IgA in a particular secretion might in part originate from distant mucosal tissue and be transported by way of the blood to various exocrine secretions.[13-16] The dominant IgA-producing tissue of the body is the gut-associated lymphoreticular tissue where the IgA-cell density is high and the total tissue mass is greatest. A manifestation of this dominance is seen in the specificity of the antibody responses in the various other secretory fluids that usually reflect intestinal antigen exposure.[17,18,19]

Milk contains a variety of proteins, some of which are produced locally by the mammary gland and others that are derived from the serum.[20-22] The predominant immunoglobulin in the milk of most species is IgA and the antibody activity present in this IgA is believed to be part of a response at the gut mucosa. The location of the plasma cells producing the IgA in milk is generally not known.[22] This antibody might be derived from mammary lymphoid cells that have migrated to the gland from the gut or it might be synthesized in distant mucosal tissue. (The mouse mammary gland can efficiently remove dimeric IgA from the serum.)[16,23] In this report, we evaluated the quantitative contribution of these two proposed sites of origin at different times in lactating BALB/c mice. In addition, we compared the ability of several nonreplicating antigens to induce a serum IgA response when administered mucosally or parenterally to mice.

MATERIALS AND METHODS

The BALB/c strain of mice was used for all experiments. In the metabolism studies reported here mice were injected with iodinated protein subcutaneously

*This work was supported in part by National Institutes of Health Grant R01-HD-12416 and a grant from Ross Laboratories, Inc.

in the back. For the period immediately following the injections, they were given drinking water containing 0.01% KI. The TEPC-15 plasmacytoma was grown in pristane (2,6,10,14-tetramethylpentadecane) primed BALB/c mice from cells supplied by Litton Bionetics, Inc., Kensington, Md. (NCI Contract N01-CB-94326).

The TEPC-15 myeloma protein was purified from ascites as previously described.[16,24] The polymeric form of TEPC-15 was isolated by filtration through a calibrated Bio-Gel A-5m (Bio-Rad Laboratories, Richmond, Calif.) column. The purity of the TEPC-15, mouse IgG and mouse albumin was assessed by immunoelectrophoresis, Ouchterlony, and sodium dodecyl sulfate (SDS) polyacrylamide gel electrophoresis analysis. The cholera toxin B subunit (CT-B) and ovalbumin were purchased from Sigma Chemical Co. (St. Louis, Mo.). Both proteins gave one band when examined by SDS-polyacrylamide gel electrophoresis under reducing conditions. Peanut agglutinin was obtained from Bethesda Research Laboratories, Inc. (Bethesda, Md.). Proteins were dinitrophenylated with dinitrobenzene sulfonate according to methods previously described.[25] The proteins were iodinated with carrier-free Na^{125}I (Amersham Corp., Arlington Heights, Ill.) using the iodine monochloride[26] or the chloramine T method.[27] The specific activities of the proteins after exhaustive dialysis were usually in the 0.1 μCi/μg range. The isotopic label was found to be at least 90% precipitable by 8% cold trichloroacetic acid, 20% polyethylene glycol, or the appropriate specific antiserum. In addition, labeled proteins comigrated with native material when examined by SDS-polyacrylamide gel electrophoresis and when filtered through a Sephadex G-100 column.

The serum decay studies were performed by injecting radiolabeled albumin or polymeric IgA into the mother and monitoring protein bound isotope levels in 25 μl samples of blood taken from the tail vein. Serum levels were followed from 2 to 60 hours post injection. To allow time, however, for tissue equilibration following subcutaneous injection, only values after 20 hours were used to calculate half-lives from a plot of log isotope versus time. It should be noted that this method would not be able to detect any very rapid clearance of degraded protein. Radial immunodiffusion was used to determine IgA, albumin, and IgG concentrations in serum and milk samples.[24]

An isotope dilution protocol was used to assess the serum contribution to the proteins found in milk. Lactating mice were injected subcutaneously with 5 μg of iodinated polymeric IgA or other protein. After several hours equilibration, a 25 μl blood sample was taken from the tail vein and a 10–25 μl milk sample was removed from several nipples by manual expression into a precision bore capillary tube. The neonates were allowed to nurse between collection times. The isotope in the samples was counted to obtain the cpm/ml of milk or blood. To estimate the percentage of serum-derived polymeric IgA in milk, the ratio of specific activities in the two fluids was calculated, (dpm = disintegrations per minute):

$$\text{Ratio} = \frac{\dfrac{\text{dpm}}{\text{ml milk}}}{\dfrac{\text{dpm}}{\text{ml blood}}} \times \frac{[\text{IgA}]_{\text{blood}}}{[\text{IgA}]_{\text{milk}}} \times \frac{\%\ \text{polymeric in blood}}{\%\ \text{polymeric in milk}}$$

The proportion of monomeric and polymeric IgA in BALB/c serum and milk was estimated with a Bio-Gel A-1.5 m (47 × .75 cm) chromatography column equilibrated with phosphate buffered saline containing 0.03 M ethylenediamino-tetraacetate (EDTA), 0.1 mg/ml ovalbumin, and 0.05% sodium azide. The column was calibrated with iodinated human IgM, mouse IgG, mouse serum albumin, free iodine, and mouse IgA (monomeric and polymeric). The column chromatography was performed at 4°C with 300 μl samples. Milk samples were clarified with EDTA before applying to the column. Six drop (210 μl) fractions were collected and the IgA concentration determined by radioimmune assay. The elution profiles of milk and serum IgA from the A-1.5 m columns were traced onto transparent paper and the monomer and polymer sections of the profile were cut out and weighed. Fractions from the A-1.5 m column were analyzed in duplicate for IgA content by a competitive binding radioimmune assay as previously described.[24]

Mice to be immunized mucosally were fasted for 12-15 hours. A small laparotomy was used to immunize anesthetized mice intraduodenally. Approximately 100 μl of antigen in buffered saline was injected with a 27 gauge needle into the lumen of the intestine within the first centimeter distal from the pylorus. Oral immunization was performed by gastric intubation of antigen in 0.2 M bicarbonate buffer at pH 8.6.

Antigen-specific antibody was evaluated in sera and other fluids with a solid phase sandwich assay. Small (3⁄16″) polystyrene beads with a specular finish (Precision Plastic Ball, Chicago, Ill.) were washed with water and covered with a solution of 2.5% glutaraldehyde in saline buffered at pH 5.0. After two hours at room temperature this solution was aspirated, and the beads were washed five times with phosphate buffered saline, pH 7.3. A freshly made solution of the desired antigen, 10 μg/ml in 0.1 M NaHCO$_3$, pH 9.5, was added, and this was incubated overnight at 4°C. For control beads, some of the beads were incubated with only the bicarbonate buffer overnight. After the incubation, the beads were washed three times with washing solution (.05% Tween-20, .05 M NaH$_2$PO$_4$, pH 7.3). The beads were stored in a storage buffer (1 mg/ml bovine serum albumin, 0.05 M phosphate, 0.05% sodium azide, pH 7.4) until used.

The experimental serum (diluted in 5 mg/ml bovine serum albumin) was incubated for two hours at 4°C with the antigen-coated beads. Normal serum was used as a control with both the protein-coated and the control plastic beads. After incubation, the beads were washed three times with the washing solution. Iodinated goat anti-mouse immunoglobulin (diluted in 5% normal goat serum), either α-chain or γ-chain specific, was added to each bead and incubated at 4°C overnight. The beads were then washed three times with the washing solution, and each bead was transferred to a clean tube for counting in a gamma counter.

RESULTS

We observed in previous studies that polymeric IgA appeared to be transferred rapidly to the neonate.[16] This observation led us to compare the metabolic turnover of IgA in lactating and nonlactating mice. A tracer amount (5-15 μg) of radiolabeled polymeric IgA was injected into mice and the disappearance of the protein-bound isotope was followed by withdrawing blood samples from the tail vein at various times after injection. From plots of log dpm versus time the serum IgA half-lives in TABLE 1 were obtained. The serum half-life of IgA in normal mice was found to be 35 hours, whereas in lactating mice it was 14-17 hours.

The proportion of IgA present as monomer or polymer in both serum and milk

TABLE 1

IGA IN THE SERUM AND MILK OF BALB/C MICE*

	Serum IgA			Milk IgA	
	Concentration (mg/ml)†	Percent Polymeric	Half-life (hours)	Concentration (mg/ml)†	Percent Polymeric
Normal Female	0.70 ± .03	37 ± 3(4)	35 ± 4(4)	—	—
Four-Day Lactating	0.57 ± .08	50 ± 7(3)	14 ± 1(3)	0.54 ± .06	65 ± 13(4)
Eight-Day Lactating	0.60 ± .07	47 ± 3(3)	17 ± 0(2)	1.10 ± .10	66 ± 11(5)

*All errors shown refer to standard deviations. The numbers in parentheses indicate the number of different samples analyzed.

†Determined in duplicate or triplicate on reduced and alkylated samples by radial immunodiffusion on four to seven different sera or milk samples.

was evaluated by analysis of molecular sieve chromatography profiles. A summary of an analysis of 19 different elution profiles is reported in TABLE 1. The IgA profiles in normal BALB/c serum indicate that about 37% of the IgA is polymeric and the remainder monomeric. These profiles are similar to those observed for CBA mouse serum.[28] The proportion of serum IgA in the polymeric form was found to be somewhat higher in lactating mice (47–50% polymer). The majority of the IgA in milk (65–66%) is polymeric, and this percentage did not change during lactation.

To provide an estimate of the portion of IgA in milk that is serum derived, the ratio of specific activities in milk and serum were determined following the injection of labeled protein. Local synthesis of a protein by cells in the mammary gland will dilute the isotope-labeled protein reaching the mammary duct from the serum.[15,29] Thus the specific activity (μCi/μg of protein) in milk relative to that in the blood serum may be used to assess the origin of a protein. If the ratio of specific activities (milk/serum) is one, then all the protein is considered to be serum-derived, whereas values less than one imply that locally synthesized components contribute to the protein in the secretion. The ratio of specific activities was equal to or greater than 1.0 for albumin and IgG (TABLE 2). This finding indicates that these milk proteins are serum derived. The origin of polymeric milk IgA was evaluated at two different stages of lactation. Based on

TABLE 2

SPECIFIC ACTIVITY RATIOS FOR MOUSE MILK PROTEINS

Protein	Days post partum	Specific Activity Ratio (milk/serum)*
Polymeric IgA	4 days	1.50 ± .11
	8 days	0.23 ± .03
Mouse serum albumin	4 days	1.08 ± .08
	8 days	1.18 ± .45
Mouse IgG	8 days	1.08 ± .04

*The error shown is the standard deviation for milk and serum samples obtained six hours after the injection of labeled protein into three mice.

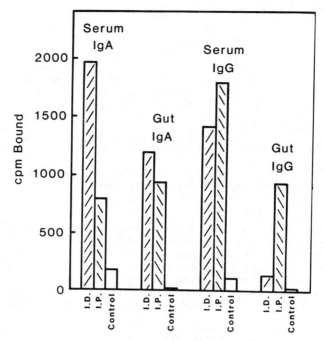

FIGURE 1. Immune response to the B subunit of cholera toxin. Antibody activity in serum or gut washing fluids was assayed with CT-B coated plastic beads and iodinated anti-mouse IgA or IgG. The controls shown represent binding in the presence of normal serum or the gut washing fluid (buffered saline) containing 5 mg/ml bovine serum albumin. The counts bound to the control beads are the same when uncoated beads are used and thus represent nonspecific binding of the labeled anti-immunoglobulin.

this method of analysis, a major portion of the IgA in early milk (day 4) appeared to be serum derived because the specific activity ratio was greater than one. The relative contribution of serum-derived IgA decreased later in lactation (day 8) when local synthesis and direct secretion appeared to become predominant.

Antigenic exposure in the gut may result in secretory IgA in the secretions of remote tissues such as the mammary gland.[17,18,19] If the sIgA in milk is derived from antibody synthesized in the gut-associated lymphoreticular tissues, then the serum IgA should reflect the antigenic exposure of the gastrointestinal tract. To test this hypothesis, mice were immunized intraduodenally at days 0 and 14 with 25 μg of the cholera toxin B subunit. Serum and gut washings were obtained on day 20, and these were assayed for specific antibody of the IgA or IgG class. The results, shown in FIGURE 1, indicate that a mucosal immunization with CT-B gave a significant serum IgA response. This serum IgA response is higher in animals given CT-B mucosally when compared with those immunized parenterally. It was also of interest that mucosal immunization with 25 μg of the CT-B gave a better serum IgA response than either a mucosal or parenteral immunization with 100 μg of ovalbumin or DNP-peanut agglutinin (TABLE 3).

DISCUSSION

The transfer of IgA from serum into mucosal secretions such as milk and saliva has been demonstrated for several species including the sow,[15] cow,[30] dog,[31] and mouse.[16,23] Jackson et al.[23] showed that an IgA-myeloma protein (MOPC-315) was efficiently transferred from serum into the milk and bile of mice. In these studies, the transfer of the injected IgA was quantified with an idiotype-specific immunoassay. Their data suggest that secretion into milk may be a major pathway in the clearance of IgA in lactating mice, particularly if one takes into consideration the larger volume of milk versus bile. Also of interest in this same report was the observation that lactating mice, carrying the MOPC-315 tumor, transfer high titers of this idiotype to their milk. In other studies with a variety of different mouse immunoglobulins, a significant transfer to the milk was observed.[16,24] When tracer amounts of labeled oligomeric IgA were injected subcutaneously, the molecules were transferred with high efficiency ($\geq 30\%$ of injected protein). That this transfer to milk may have a significant effect on IgA metabolism is apparent from the half-lives reported in TABLE 1. Lactating mice turn over their pool of oligomeric IgA twice as fast as normal females. These observations in mice are at variance with what has been reported for rats. Although the experimental approach was quite different, the studies of Dahlgren et al.[32] showed that serum IgA was not transferred into rat milk within the first hour following intravenous injection of antibody-containing lymph. Liver transfer may be much more efficient in rats that, unlike mice, lack a gall bladder.

Previous investigators have shown that milk contains IgA antibodies that are specific for antigens encountered in the gastrointestinal tract.[18,33,34] These observations have led to the concept of a common mucosal immune system, in which antibodies may appear at mucosal sites other than the original point of contact by virtue of the migration of cells or antibody or both. Cholera toxin B subunit, when administered mucosally in the gut, stimulated an IgA response in the serum of mice (FIGURE 1). It is therefore possible that this serum IgA may represent

TABLE 3

SERUM IgA AND IgG RESPONSES TO MUCOSAL AND PARENTERAL IMMUNIZATION

Immunogen	Route of Immunization*		Antibody (CPM Bound)†	
			IgG	IgA
Cholera toxin B Subunit (25 μg)	i.d.	i.d.‡	1306	1767
	i.p.	i.p.	1686	605
DNP-Ovalbumin (100 μg)	i.d.	i.g.	1213	0
	i.d.	i.p.	1527	0
	i.p.	i.p.	1202	0
DNP-Peanut Agglutinin (100 μg)	i.d.	i.g.	2068	145
	i.d.	i.p.	1984	143
	i.p.	i.p.	1842	144

*Groups of three BALB/c mice were immunized by the route indicated on days 0 and 14, and sera were collected on day 20.

†Antibody assayed with antigen-coated plastic beads and iodinated anti-mouse IgA or IgG (heavy chain specific). The specific activities of these two labeled antibodies were similar. The sera were analyzed in duplicate with errors of approximately ±4%.

‡i.d. = intraduodenal; i.p. = intraperitoneal, i.g. = intragastric.

oligomeric IgA in transit to regions of the mucosal immune system distant from the site of antigen contact in the gut.

A number of groups have studied the local and systemic immune response to cholera toxin.[35-39] Svennerholm et al.[36] reported that four oral immunizations with cholera toxin, a protocol that induces IgG and IgA in the intestine and serum, provides for protection from experimental cholera. This group, however, observed that the serum IgG antibody levels were higher than the IgA antibody responses in contrast to the results in TABLE 3, in which the serum IgA response is of the same magnitude as the serum IgG response. Nevertheless, Svennerholm[36] did observe a significant correlation between the serum IgA titers and protection. The studies presented in FIGURE 1 and TABLE 3 support the previous reports that the CT-B is an effective mucosal immunogen. Our experiments, however, indicate a significant serum IgA response to cholera toxin B subunit. This serum IgA response to a mucosal immunogen may be important for the nursing mother, whose milk has the potential of providing protection for her offspring. Pierce[38,39] has shown the effectiveness of cholera toxin and its subunits as mucosal immunogens and has discussed some of the properties that appear to be important for the induction of a vigorous mucosal immune response. In TABLE 3 are shown some of our initial experiments with mucosal immunization that support his hypothesis that membrane binding is a significant factor. In these experiments, mucosal immunization with the high affinity membrane-binding protein, CT-B, resulted in a substantial serum IgA response, whereas immunization with dinitrophenylated (DNP)-ovalbumin failed to stimulate any serum IgA specific for DNP-ovalbumin. Mucosal immunization with DNP-peanut agglutinin, a protein that potentially could bind to membrane glycoproteins in the gut, stimulated a weak but significant serum IgA response.

ACKNOWLEDGMENTS

The authors would like to acknowledge the technical assistance of Robyn Meyer, John Cebra, and Sandra Halsey, as well as the helpful comments of Juliet Fuhrman and Chris Cordle.

REFERENCES

1. TOMASI, T. & J. BIENENSTOCK. 1968. Adv. Immunol 9: 1–96.
2. BRANDTZAEG, P. & E. SAVILAHTI. 1978. Adv. Exp. Med. Biol. 107: 219–226.
3. TOURVILLE, D., R. ADLER, J. BIENENSTOCK & R. TOMASI. 1969. J. Exp. Med. 129: 411–423.
4. CRAGO, S., R. KULHAVY, S. PRINCE & J. MESTECKY. 1978. J. Exp. Med. 147: 1832–1837.
5. O'DALY, J., S. CRAIG & J. CEBRA. 1971. J. Immunol. 106: 286–288.
6. CRABBÉ, P., A. CARBONARA & J. HEREMANS. 1965. Lab. Invest. 14: 235–248.
7. TOMASI, R., E. TAN, A. SOLOMON & R. PRENDERGAST. 1965. J. Exp. Med. 121: 101–124.
8. CRANDALL, R., J. CEBRA & C. CRANDALL. 1967. Immunol. 12: 147–158.
9. GOWANS, J. & E. KNIGHT. 1964. Proc. Royal Soc. Lond. B 159: 257–282.
10. GRISCELLI, C., P. VASSALLI & R. MCCLUSKY. 1969. J. Exp. Med. 130: 1427–1451.
11. ROUX, M., M. MCWILLIAMS, J. PHILLIPS-QUAGLIATA, P. WEISZ-CARRINGTON & M. LAMM. 1977. J. Exp. Med. 146: 1311–1322.
12. HUSBAND, A. & J. GOWANS. 1978. J. Exp. Med. 148: 1146–1160.
13. ORLANS, E., J. PEPPARD, J. REYNOLDS & J. HALL. 1978. J. Exp. Med. 147: 588–592.
14. JACKSON, G., I. LEMAITRE-COELHO, J. VAERMAN, H. BAZIN & A. BECKERS. 1978. Eur. J. Immunol. 8: 123–126.

15. BOURNE, F. & J. CURTIS. 1973. Immunol. **24:** 157–162.
16. HALSEY, J., B. JOHNSON & J. CEBRA. 1980. J. Exp. Med. **151:** 767–772.
17. MESTECKY, J., J. R. MCGHEE, R. ARNOLD, S. MICHALEK, S. PRINCE & J. BABB. 1978. J. Clin. Invest. **61:** 731–737.
18. MONTGOMERY, P., B. ROSNER & J. COHN. 1974. J. Immunol. Commun. **3:** 143–156.
19. CEBRA, J., P. GEARHART, J. F. HALSEY, J. HURWITZ & R. SHAHIN. 1980. J. Reticuloendothelial Soc. **28:** 61s–71s.
20. LAWRENCE, D. 1978. Invest. Cell Pathol. **1:** 5–22.
21. HANSON, L. 1961. Int. Arch. Allergy Appl. Immunol. **18:** 241–267.
22. BUTLER, J. 1979. Semin. in Perinatal. **3:** 255–270.
23. JACKSON, G. D., I. LEMAÏTRE-COELHO & J. P. VAERMAN. 1979. Protides Biol. Fluids Proc. Colloq. **25:** 919–922.
24. HALSEY, J. F., C. MITCHELL, R. MEYER & J. J. CEBRA. 1982. Eur. J. Immunol. **12:** 107–112.
25. COLWELL, M., R. MEYER, T. PAZDERNIK & J. F. HALSEY. 1980. Cell. Immunol. **52:** 229–238.
26. MCFARLANE, A. 1958. Nature (London). **182:** 53.
27. MCCOHANEY, P. & F. DIXON. 1966. Int. Arch. Allergy Appl. Immunol. **29:** 185–189.
28. KAARTINEN, M., T. IMIR, M. KLOCKARS, M. SANDHOLN & O. MAKELA. 1978. Scand. J. Immunol. **7:** 229–232.
29. STROBER, W., R. BLAESE & T. WALDMAN. 1970. J. Lab. Clin. Med. **75:** 856–862.
30. NEWBY, T. J. & J. BOURNE. 1977. J. Immunol. **118:** 461–465.
31. MONTGOMERY, P., S. KHALEL, J. GOUDSWAARD & G. VIRELLA. 1977. Immunol. Commun. **6:** 633–642.
32. DAHLGREN, U., S. AHLSTEDT, L. HEDMAN, C. WADSWORTH & L. HANSON. 1981. Scand J. Immunol. **14:** 95–98.
33. BOHL, E. N. & L. SAIF. 1975. Infect. Immun. **11:** 23–32.
34. BIENENSTOCK, J., M. MCDERMOTT & D. BEFUS. 1979. *In* Immunology of Breast Milk. P. Orga & D. Dayton, Eds.: 91–98. Raven Press. New York.
35. YARDLEY, J. H., D. KEREN, S. HAMILTON & G. D. BROWN. 1978. Infect. Immun. **19:** 589–597.
36. SVENNERHOLM, A., S. LANGE & J. HOLMGREN. 1978. Infect. Immun. **21:** 1–6.
37. FUHRMAN, J. & J. CEBRA. 1981. J. Exp. Med. **153:** 534–544.
38. PIERCE, N. F. & J. GOWENS. 1975. J. Exp. Med. **142:** 1550–1563.
39. PIERCE, N. F. 1978. J. Exp. Med. **148:** 195–206.

DISCUSSION OF THE PAPER

M. W. RUSSELL (*University of Alabama in Birmingham*): When you examined the molecular weight of the material you collected in milk, it eluted at high molecular weight on a Sepharose G-200 column. Can you elaborate on these findings further?

J. F. HALSEY (*University of Kansas, Kansas City*): The IgA elutes at void volume of a Sephadex G-200 column. When the material in milk is examined on an SDS polyacrylamide gel, it migrates as intact IgA.

RUSSELL: Our results are slightly different from yours. Although we would not deny there may be some transport of circulating polymeric IgA into milk, it is far less than what we find in bile. Dr. Challacombe and I injected IgA intravenously into monkeys and found radiolabeled material present in the saliva, a certain proportion of which did appear to be precipitable with anti-IgA. From analysis, however, on a sucrose density gradient, it was degraded. The IgA that transported into milk was 30% of what we had injected. I would worry if I were trying to analyze only a small amount going into the milk. The mouse is able to transfer a number of intact proteins into milk. Vaerman and others showed that MOPC-315 was very effectively transported into milk. We examined the transport of the MOPC-315 protein into milk and detected it by antibody titration. There was a small amount in milk, but not nearly as much as we found in bile.

HALSEY: Dr. Hanson and I have discussed species differences; rats and mice do appear to be different. Fifty percent of mouse serum IgA is polymeric, whereas virtually no polymeric IgA is found in rat serum. The rat is very efficient in removing polymeric IgA from its circulation.

J. P. VAERMAN (*Catholic University of Louvain, Brussels, Belgium*): I disagree with the statement that only monomeric IgA is found in rat serum. I think the reason for the difference is due to the technique used. Rocket electrophoresis was used to titrate IgA in gradient fractions. All immunodiffusion techniques are influenced by the molecular size of IgA. When we measured by Mancini's technique the IgA in successive fractions of eluates from molecular-sieve columns, we also found the largest rings with the monomeric fraction, but we found a large number of fractions that had small rings. If you add IgA concentration, however, and multiply the apparent concentrations of IgA by an appropriate correction factor, we obtain a higher proportion of polymeric IgA than of monomeric IgA.

I quite agree with the conclusion that the biliary transport system in mouse is less efficient than in the rat. Because of this difference you may observe milk transport of IgA in mice.

J. V. PEPPARD (*Chester Beatty Research Institute, Belmont, Surrey, England*): Intravenously, I injected radiolabeled rat IgA into lactating rats, and I found no transport of the IgA from the serum into the milk. You showed earlier that the IgM you injected is also transported. How do you account for this finding?

HALSEY: That has puzzled me from the beginning. In fact, human, as well as mouse, IgM are transferred.

DEFICIENT IgA SYNTHESIS VIEWED IN THE CONTEXT OF NORMAL DEVELOPMENT OF IgA B-CELLS

M. D. Cooper, P. Haber, W. E. Gathings, M. Mayumi, T. Kuritani, and D. E. Briles

The Cellular Immunobiology Unit of the Tumor Institute
Departments of Pediatrics and Microbiology
The Comprehensive Cancer Center
University of Alabama in Birmingham
Birmingham, Alabama 35294

IgA deficiency is the most frequently recognized type of immunoglobulin deficiency occurring in 1 or 2 per 1000 individuals of European ancestry.[1,2] Although IgA deficiency is usually considered as an isolated immunoglobulin deficit, this syndrome usually reflects the inability to produce both IgA_1 and IgA_2 antibodies.

In this report, we will compare the normal development of IgA B-cells and their plasma cell progeny with the development of this subpopulation of cells in individuals who have little or no serum IgA, but relatively normal overall levels of IgM and IgG.

Ontogeny of IgA B-Cells

The development of B-cells and plasma cells of all isotypes is inhibited when anti-μ antibodies are used to abort development of immature IgM B-cells.[3-6] The derivation of IgG and IgA B-cells from IgM-bearing B-cells is also reflected by the presence of surface IgM on immature IgG and IgA B-cells.[7,8] By contrast, most IgG and IgA B-cells in mature individuals lack detectable IgM on their surface. These results suggest that as B-cells switch from IgM to IgG or IgA, they pass through a transitional phase during which they continue to express IgM, and perhaps IgD as well.

Because IgG and IgA B-cells are acquired very early in development and are present in normal frequencies in athymic individuals, we have reasoned that heavy chain isotype switching does not require induction by antigens with T-cell help.[8] In the chicken, heavy chain isotype switching appears to occur exclusively within the bursa, the microenvironment in which B-cells are generated in birds.[3,6]

Heavy chain isotype switching has been observed as early as the pre-B-cell level in leukemias in mice and humans.[9-12] This switching appears to be a regular event in human pre-B-cell leukemias (Kubagawa, H., unpublished observations). On the other hand, heavy chains other than μ have not been observed in normal pre-B-cells.[13]

We have recently reexamined the roles of antigen and T-cells on the development of isotype diversity at the B-cell level. Germfree nu/nu and their nu/+ littermates acquired subpopulations of B-cells expressing μ, γ, and α isotypes at similar rates (Figure 1). This pattern of B-cell ontogeny did not differ

461

0077-8923/83/0409-0461 $1.75/0 © 1983, NYAS

from that previously observed for normal mice raised in a conventional environment.[8] This result is consonant with the idea that heavy chain isotype switching is an inherent feature of B-cell differentiation.

IgA B-cells could either be derived directly from IgM or by successive switches from IgM to IgG and from IgG to IgA. We initially proposed that the latter was the most likely developmental pattern, primarily because this pattern is the phylogenetic and ontogenetic order of heavy chain isotype development.[14] Treatment, however, with anti-γ antibodies consistently suppressed the development of murine IgG-plasma cells only; IgA-producing cells were not affected.[4,5] Immature IgA B-cells in mice and humans consistently express IgM, but not IgG

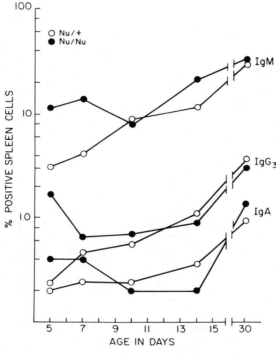

FIGURE 1.

as would have been expected if the successive isotype switching model were correct.[7,8] Moreover, the IgA$_1$ and IgA$_2$ B-cells belong to discrete subpopulations present in roughly equal numbers in newborn babies.[15] We have not found B-cells bearing both IgA$_1$ and IgA$_2$ at any time during development in the bone marrow, blood, or lymphoid tissues.

We have recently analyzed the immunoglobulin isotypes expressed by human B-cell precursors of plasma cells that can be induced by pokeweed mitogen (PWM). Monoclonal and affinity purified isotype specific antibodies have both been used in these studies.[16,17] Pokeweed mitogen induces B-cells from the blood of mature individuals to differentiate into plasma cells of all isotypes. The plasma cell induction is a T-cell dependent process that reaches its peak around the seventh day in lymphocyte cultures. Our results in these experiments can be summarized as follows. (1) Treatment of the PWM-stimulated lymphocytes with anti-μ antibodies inhibits most of the IgM-plasma cell precursors and approximately one-half of the B-cell precursors of IgG- and IgA-plasma cells. Selective removal of the IgM$^+$ B-cells before culture has the same effect. (2) Inhibition with anti-γ antibodies or selective depletion of IgG B-cells before culture with PWM suppressed only IgG-plasma cell development. (3) Inhibition with anti-α or depletion of IgA B-cells only impaired the development of IgA-producing cells. (4) Inhibition with monoclonal anti-α_1 antibody suppressed development of IgA$_1$- but not of IgA$_2$-plasma cells in the pokeweed model system.

These results infer that direct switches from IgM to each of the other heavy chain isotypes are the rule, and that successive isotype switches, although possible, are the exception. It would also appear that expression of a non-μ isotype on the B-cell surface indicates genetic commitment to the synthesis of that isotype; for example, IgA$_1$$^+$ B-cells with or without residual surface IgM will differentiate into IgA$_1$ plasma cells.

The molecular mechanism responsible for C$_h$ gene switching is still in debate. IgA-producing myeloma cells do so by joining a switch site 5' to the Cμ gene with a switch site 5' to the Cα gene with deletion of the intervening DNA.[18-20] If this arrangement were the sole mechanism for C$_h$ gene switching, the expression of IgM on IgA B-cells would presumably reflect residual mRNA and μ-chains made before the switch. Recently, however, an RNA splicing mechanism has been proposed for B-cells expressing two isotypes[12] (T. Honjo, personal communication). According to this hypothesis, DNA rearrangements would then be a secondary and final mechanism for isotype switching prior to terminal plasma cell differentiation.

IgA Deficiency

This immunodeficiency syndrome can have multiple causes, and few of the affected individuals appear to have structural abnormalities of the Cα genes. IgA deficiency can be inherited in a variety of transmission patterns, may be associated with congenital infections, and can be either acquired, or in some instances transient.[21-24]

More important, IgA B-cells can be found in virtually all IgA-deficient individuals,[25] but few of these B-cells differentiate either into IgA-plasma cells *in vivo*, or following stimulation by polyclonal mitogens *in vitro*.[26,27] We have examined the IgA B-cells in IgA-deficient individuals, and in 10 of 11 cases, more than 70% had both IgA and IgM on their surface.[28] This phenomenon is the phenotype of IgA B-cells in normal newborns.[7,15] By comparison, less than 20% of the IgA B-cells in mature individuals normally express surface IgM. Thus, IgA B-cells would appear to be arrested at an early stage in maturation in the IgA-deficient individuals.

Some IgA-deficient individuals produce anti-IgA antibodies of other isotypes.[22,29] Although these isotypes could suppress development of IgA B-cells, this finding would not appear to be a common basis for the deficiency, because antibodies to IgA are not found in all affected individuals, and anti-α antibodies are more likely to be found in the older IgA-deficient patients (our unpublished observations). Moreover, antibodies may be produced only against one α-isotype, although the deficiency is of both IgA_1 and IgA_2 antibodies.[22]

Although isolated IgA deficiency is classically diagnosed by the absence of serum IgA in the presence of normal or increased serum levels of IgM and IgG, the defect in antibody synthesis may extend to other immunoglobulin isotypes. In a recent study of 37 IgA-deficient individuals, 7 were found to be very deficient in IgG_2 as well.[30] In preliminary studies, we have examined the IgG subclasses of plasma cells induced by lipopolysaccharide (LPS). When blood mononuclear cells from normal individuals are cultured with LPS, IgG_2 plasma cells predominate in a T-cell dependent response.[31] This situation is not the case when blood cells from IgA-deficient individuals are stimulated by LPS (TABLE 1).

Most of the IgG antibodies that are made in response to polysaccharide antigens are of the IgG_2 isotype.[32] This finding led us to examine the response to the repeating phosphorylcholine (PC) determinants on pneumococcal polysaccharides. In approximately one-third of the IgA-deficient individuals, we could find virtually no IgM antibodies to phosphorycholine determinants (Briles, D. E.

TABLE 1

SUBCLASS DISTRIBUTION AMONG IgG-PLASMA CELLS INDUCED BY LPS*

	Percent IgG-Plasma Cells			
Blood MNC Donors	IgG_1	IgG_2	IgG_3	IgG_4
Healthy Controls:*				
(n = 6)	19 ± 12*	81 ± 13	<1	<1
IgA-Deficient Individuals:				
A	73	23	<3	<3
B	93	5	<1	<1

*One million blood mononuclear cells (MNC) were cultured with LPS (50 μg/ml) for seven days, and IgG-subclass distribution among IgG-plasma cells was determined by two-color immunofluorescence.
*Mean ± 1 S.D. of six experiments.

et al., unpublished observations). Among 50 healthy individuals, only 2 had low levels of IgM antibodies to phosphorylcholine. Thus, it would appear that IgA-deficient individuals may have a far more extensive abnormality in antibody responsiveness than the simple measurement of total IgM, IgG, and IgA levels might indicate.

Because T-cells exert control over B-cell proliferation and differentiation, it is logical to consider defective immunoregulation by T-cells as a possible cause for IgA deficiency. The demonstration that IgA-antibody responses are the most T-cell dependent[33,34] makes this hypothesis an especially attractive consideration. An embryonic thymus that is deficient in lymphopoietic activity is a consistent feature of the ataxia-telangiectasia syndrome that is often associated with IgA deficiency.[35] In addition to their IgM deficiency, individuals with ataxia-telangiectasia frequently have a severe deficiency of IgG_2 and less often of IgG_4.[36] In this volume are included three reports of T-cell lines that preferentially provide help for IgA responses (Michalek, Strober, and Tomasi). In a few individuals with IgA deficiency, T-cell suppressor activity, selective for IgA responses, has been demonstrated.[37-40] Whereas all of these clues point to the possibility that defective T-cell development and function could lead to a predominant deficiency of IgA responses, there is still no consistently demonstrable T-cell defect in IgA-deficient patients. The total number of T-cells appears to be normal in most IgA-deficient individuals, and the ratio of T4 helper:T5/T8 suppressor cells is usually normal.[41] Nevertheless, abnormalities of the interactions between T-cells and B-cells would still appear to be a fertile area for future research on the pathogenesis of IgA deficiency.

CONCLUSION

IgA B-cells are derived directly from IgM B-cells without an essential requirement for T-cell help. IgM is transiently expressed on immature IgA B-cells. T-cells are required for maturation of IgA B-cells into IgA-secreting plasma cells.

IgA-deficient individuals generate both IgA_1 and IgA_2 B-cells. These cells, however, are immature in phenotype, and like immature IgA B-cells in the normal newborn are not easily induced to become IgA-secreting plasma cells. In addition, these individuals frequently exhibit defective differentiation of IgG_2 B-cells and may also fail to make IgM antibodies to polysaccharide antigens. A combination of these antibody deficits may underlie the undue susceptibility to infections that is experienced by IgA-deficient individuals. Defective immunoregulatory interactions of T-cells with B-cells could prove to be a central lesion in this syndrome.

REFERENCES

1. BACHMANN, R. 1965. Studies on the serum γ-globulin level. III. The frequency of A-γ-A globulinemia. Scand. J. Clin. Lab. Invest. **17:** 316–320.
2. KOISTINEN, J. 1975. Selective IgA deficiency in blood donors. Vox Sang. **29:** 192–202.
3. KINCADE, P. W., A. R. LAWTON, D. E. BOCKMAN & M. D. COOPER. 1970. Suppression of immunoglobulin G synthesis as a result of antibody mediated suppression of immunoglobulin M synthesis in chickens. Proc. Natl. Acad. Sci. USA. **67:** 1918–1925.
4. LAWTON, A. R. & M. D. COOPER. 1974. Modification of B lymphocyte differentiation by anti-immunoglobulins. *In* Contemporary Topics in Immunobiology. M. D. Cooper and N. L. Warner, Eds.: Vol. 8: 193–225. Plenum Press. New York.
5. MANNING, D. D. 1975. Heavy chain isotype suppression: A review of the immunosuppressive effects of heterologous anti-Ig heavy chain antisera. J. Reticuloendothelial Soc. **18:** 63–86.
6. COOPER, M. D., J. F. KEARNEY, W. E. GATHINGS & A. R. LAWTON. 1980. Effects of anti-Ig antibodies on the development and differentiation of B cells. Immunol. Rev. **52:** 29–53.
7. GATHINGS, W. E., A. R. LAWTON & M. D. COOPER. 1977. Immunofluorescent studies of the development of pre-B cells, B lymphocytes and immunoglobulin isotype diversity in humans. Eur. J. Immunol. **7:** 804–810.
8. ABNEY, E. R., M. D. COOPER, J. F. KEARNEY, A. R. LAWTON & R. M. E. PARKHOUSE. 1978. Sequential expression of immunoglobulin on developing mouse B lymphocytes. A systematic survey which suggests a model for the generation of immunoglobulin isotype diversity. J. Immunol. **120:** 2041–2049.
9. VOGLER, L. B., J. L. PREUD'HOMME, M. SELIGMANN, W. E. GATHINGS, W. M. CRIST, M. D. COOPER & F. J. BOLLUM. 1981. Diversity of immunoglobulin expression in leukemic cells resembling B lymphocyte precursors. Nature (London) **290:** 339–341.

10. MAYUMI, M., H. KUBAGAWA, G. A. OMURA, W. E. GATHINGS, J. F. KEARNEY & M. D. COOPER. 1983. Studies on the clonal origin of human B cell leukemia using monoclonal anti-idiotype antibodies. J. Immunol. **130:** 671-677.

11. BURROWS, P. D., G. B. BECK & M. R. WABL. 1981. Expression of immunoglobulin heavy chains in different cells of a cloned mouse lymphoid cell line. Proc. Nat. Acad. Sci. USA. **78:** 564-568.

12. ALT, F. W., N. ROSENBERG, R. J. CASANOVA, E. THOMAS & D. BALTIMORE. 1982. Immunoglobulin heavy chain expression and class switching in a murine leukemia cell line. Nature (London) **296:** 325-331.

13. KUBAGAWA, H., W. E. GATHINGS, D. LEVITT, J. F. KEARNEY & M. D. COOPER. 1983. Immunoglobulin isotype expression of normal pre-B cells as determined by immuno-fluorescence. J. Clin. Immunol. **2:** 264-269.

14. COOPER, M.D., A. R. LAWTON & P. W. KINCADE. 1972. A two-stage model for development of antibody-producing cells. Clin. Exp. Immunol. **11:** 143-149.

15. CONLEY, M. E., J. F. KEARNEY, A. R. LAWTON & M. D. COOPER. 1980. Differentiation of human B cells expressing the IgA subclasses as demonstrated by monoclonal hybridoma antibodies. J. Immunol. **125:** 2311-2316.

16. LUCIVERO, G., A. R. LAWTON & M. D. COOPER. 1981. Pokeweed mitogen induced differentiation of human peripheral blood lymphocytes. II. Suppression of plasma cell differentiation by heavy chain specific antibodies and development of immuno-globulin class restriction. Hum. Lymph. Different. **1:** 27-36.

17. KURITANI, T. & M. D. COOPER. 1982. Human B cell differentiation. I. Analysis of immunoglobulin heavy chain switching using monoclonal anti-immunoglobulin M, G and A antibodies and pokeweed mitogen induced plasma cell differentiation. J. Exp. Med. **155:** 839-851.

18. HONJO, T. & T. KATAOKA. 1978. Organization of immunoglobulin heavy chain genes and allelic deletion model. Proc. Nat. Acad. Sci. USA. **75:** 2140-2144.

19. CORY, S. & J. ADAMS. 1980. Deletions are associated with somatic rearrangements of immunoglobulin heavy chain genes. Cell **19:** 37-51.

20. COLECLOUGH, C., D. COOPER & P. R. PERRY. 1980. Rearrangement of immunoglobulin heavy chain genes during B lymphocyte development as revealed by studies of mouse plasmacytoma cells. Proc. Nat. Acad. Sci. USA. **77:** 1422-1426.

21. GRUNDBACHER, F. J. 1972. Genetic aspects of selective immunoglobulin A deficiency. J. Med. Genet. **9:** 344-347.

22. VAN LOGHEM, E. 1974. Familial occurrence of isolated IgA deficiency associated with antibodies to IgA. Evidence against a structural gene defect. Eur. J. Immunol. **4:** 57-60.

23. PETTY, R. E., J. T. CASSIDY & D. B. SULLIVAN. 1973. Reversal of selective IgA deficiency in a child with juvenile rheumatoid arthritis after plasma transfusions. Pediatrics **51:** 44-48.

24. AMMAN, A. J. & R. HONG. 1971. Selective IgA deficiency. Presentation of 30 cases and a review of the literature. Medicine (Baltimore) **50:** 223-236.

25. LAWTON, A. R., S. A. ROYAL, K. S. SELF & M. D. COOPER. 1972. IgA determinants on B lymphocytes in patients with deficiency of circulating IgA. J. Lab. Clin. Med. **80:** 26-33.

26. DELEPASSE, G., P. GAUSSET, C. COUCHIE & A. GOVAERTS. 1976. Cellular aspects of selective IgA deficiency. Clin. Exp. Immunol. **35:** 296-305.

27. CASSIDY, J. T., G. OLDHAM & T. A. E. PLATT-MILLS. 1979. Functional assessment of a B cell defect in patients with selective IgA deficiency. Clin. Exp. Immunol. **35:** 296.

28. CONLEY, M. E. & M. D. COOPER. 1981. Immature IgA B cells in IgA deficient patients. N. Engl. J. Med. **305:** 495-497.

29. VYAS, G. N., L. HOLMDAHL, H. A. PERKINS & H. H. FUDENBERG. 1969. Serologic specificity of human anti-IgA and its significance in transfusion. Blood **34:** 573-581.

30. OXELIUS, V. A., A. B. LAURELL, B. LINDQUIST, H. GOLEBIOWSKA, U. AXELSSON, J. BJORKANDER & L. A. HANSON. 1981. IgG subclasses in selective IgA deficiency-Importance of IgG₂-IgA deficiency. N. Engl. J. Med. **304:** 1476-1477.

31. MAYUMI, M., H. KUBAGAWA & M. D. COOPER. 1983. IgG subclass expression by human B lymphocytes and plasma cells: B lymphocytes precommitted to IgG subclass can be

preferentially induced by polyclonal mitogens with T cell help. J. Immunol. In press.

32. RIESEN, W. F., F. SKVARIL & D. G. BROWN. 1976. Natural infection of man with group A streptococci. Levels, restriction in class, subclass, and type, and clonal appearance of polysaccharide grou-specific antibodies. Scand. J. Immunol. **5**: 383–390.

33. CLOUGH, J. D., L. H. MINES & W. STROBER. 1971. Deficient IgA antibody responses to arsanilic acid bovine serum albumin (BSA) in neonatally thymectomized rabbits. J. Immunol. **106**: 1624–1629.

34. CREWTHER, P. & N. L. WARNER. 1972. Serum immunoglobulins and antibodies in congenitally athymic (nude) mice. Aust. J. Exp. Biol. Med. Sci. **50**: 625–635.

35. PETERSON, R. D. A., M. D. COOPER & R. A. GOOD. 1965. The pathogenesis of immunologic deficiency diseases. Am. J. Med. **38**: 579–604.

36. OXELIUS, V. A. 1979. Quantitative and qualitiative investigations of serum IgG subclasses in immunodeficiency diseases. Clin. Exp. Immunol. **36**: 112–116.

37. WALDMANN, T. A., S. BRODER, R. KRAKAUER, M. DURM, B. MEADE & C. GOLDMAN. 1976. Defect in IgA secretion and in IgA specific suppressor cells in patients with selective IgA deficiency. Trans. Assoc. Am. Physicians **89**: 215–224.

38. ATWATER, J. S. & T. B. TOMASI. 1978. Suppressor cells and IgA deficiency. Clin. Immunol. Immunopathol. **9**: 379–384.

39. SCHWARTZ, S. 1980. Heavy chain specific suppression of immunoglobulin synthesis and secretion by lymphocytes from patients with selective IgA deficiency. J. Immunol. **124**: 2034–2041.

40. LEVITT, D. & M. D. COOPER. 1981. Immunoregulatory defects in a family with selective IgA deficiency. J. Pediatr. **98**: 52–58.

41. REINHERZ, E. L., M. D. COOPER, S. F. SCHLOSSMAN & F. S. ROSEN. 1981. Abnormalities of T cell maturation and regulation in human beings with immunodeficiency diseases. J. Clin. Invest. **68**: 699–705.

————————◆————————

DISCUSSION OF THE PAPER

R. M. E. PARKHOUSE (*National Institute for Medical Research, London, England*): Do you have any thoughts on the mechanism of anti-immunoglobulin inhibition of proliferation. Is it true that the signal is presumably from pokeweed mitogen and not from the immunoglobulin receptor?

M. D. COOPER (*University of Alabama in Birmingham*): I do not know the answer. There seems to be a signal overload during the stimulation, with both the T-cell helper factors that are generated in the pokeweed system together with the cross-linkage of the surface immunoglobulin receptors. At the late stage in B-cell differentiation, where the cells are preactivated, a signal from multiple surface receptors may result in the abortion of further differentiation.

PARKHOUSE: Anti-immunoglobulins stimulate B-cells. Have you tried Fab'$_2$ fragments for B-cell stimulation in the human system?

COOPER: The inhibition is effective with Fab'$_2$.

PARKHOUSE: Is there a difference then between human and mouse B-cells in that respect?

COOPER: No, because in mice you can inhibit LPS stimulation with Fab'$_2$ as well as with intact immunoglobulin.

PARKHOUSE: Can you get class specific stimulation of human B-cells with anti-immunoglobulin?

COOPER: Yes, Dr. Oppenheim reported several years ago that a proliferative, but not a differentiative, response is induced.

M. E. CONLEY (*University of Pennsylvania, Philadelphia*): Using exactly the same system with a monoclonal anti-alpha chain, we found that with high doses we saw a suppression. With very low doses, however, we saw a marked increase in the number of IgA_1 plasma cells without influencing the number of IgA_2 plasma cells in about half the individuals.

Z. OVARY (*New York University, New York, N.Y.*): In mice, on the first day, you had a respectable amount of surface immunoglobulins of all classes, but not IgE.

COOPER: The IgE B-cells are so infrequent that it is hard to enumerate them.

R.A. GOOD (*Oklahoma Medical Research Foundation, Oklahoma City*): I do not think the issue is a difference between the mouse and the human. Under appropriate conditions you can induce immunoglobulin production with anti-Fab'$_2$ reagents directed against immunoglobulins. One can induce both proliferation and terminal differentiation. The real question is whether Fab'$_2$ reagent will inhibit the development?

COOPER: Yes, it will.

GOOD: I think that the situation may depend on the conditions that concern the terminal differentiation, but you can get the terminal differentiation as well as proliferation with Fab'$_2$ reagents at least against IgM.

J.J. CEBRA (*University of Pennsylvania, Philadelphia*): All of us are convinced that switches can occur in single steps with consequent expression of downstream isotype such as G or A. They can also occur consecutively. You pointed out this fact in hybridoma and myeloma lines. The problem is what occurs naturally and physiologically. I think it is important to point out certain differences in the kinds of assays that different investigators use. In a short term pokeweed mitogen stimulation that endures for about four days, a couple of divisions occur, and one analyzes probable events that involve single switches followed by rapid maturation to plasma cells. In the clonal assay, as many as ten divisions can ensue over a 10 to 15 day period. So, in fact, one can see the downstream potential many generations later and the possibility of consecutive switches. What would happen *in vivo*? In acute immune responses, one sees more commonly what is seen from peripheral blood lymphocytes—a few divisions and rapid maturation. Perhaps in the Peyer's patches, where one might expect many divisions and few maturation signals, the likelihood of consecutive switches is greater. Therefore, both models would apply to different aspects in normal physiologic states. The question is: How selective is the subpopulation of B-cells that you are looking at with pokeweed mitogen? Are splenic and peripheral blood populations comparable? The latter contains a strong element of secondary, already primed cells.

COOPER: This topic is still an unsettled issue. We have examined splenic cells, and we find the same answer.

ISOLATION AND ANALYSIS OF ANTI-IDIOTYPIC ANTIBODIES FROM IgA-DEFICIENT SERA*

Charlotte Cunningham-Rundles

Memorial Sloan-Kettering Cancer Center
New York, N.Y. 10021

INTRODUCTION

More than half of IgA-deficient individuals have a marked excess of antibody to the common dietary antigens, bovine milk and serum proteins; this antibody presumably gains entrance into the systemic circulation because of a defective secretory mucosal barrier.[1,2] Because this excessive hyperpermeability is a chronic process, the serum of many IgA-deficient individuals contains large amounts of circulating immune complexes that we have previously shown to contain bovine protein antigens.[3,4] In animal studies, a very effective method for stimulating the production of anti-idiotypic antibodies is by the injection of antigen-antibody complexes, particularly if these complexes are formed in antibody excess.[5] For this reason, we studied the serum of two healthy IgA-deficient individuals in order to determine if a specific anti-antibovine protein antibody (anti-anticasein) could be isolated.

METHODS

Affinity Chromatography

Anticasein antibodies were isolated from 75 ml of serum from subject A and 85 ml from subject B by passage of a well-dialized, 50%-saturated $(NH_4)_2 SO_4$ precipitated IgG-containing fraction of serum on Sepharose 4B (Pharmacia Fine Chemicals) to which casein (ICN Nutritional Biochemicals, Cleveland, Ohio) had been coupled using cyanogen bromide (CNBr).[6] After removal of the nonadherent fractions by passage of 5 column volumes of phosphate-buffered saline (PBS), the adherent fractions were eluted by 0.1 M glycine HCl buffer, pH 2.7. These fractions, containing ~1.5 mg IgG/ml were passed over diethylaminoethyl (DEAE) cellulose equilibrated in 0.01 M Na phosphate buffer pH 7.1 to purify IgG and eliminate possible traces of casein that adhere to cellulose under these conditions. In some cases the anticasein fractions were also passed over Sephadex G-150 to collect fractions eluting the void volume. One mg of the resulting anticasein fractions of each subject were then coupled to 2 ml of CNBr-activated Sepharose 4B.[6] IgG fractions of serum A and B that had not adhered to casein-Sepharose, were passed on their respective anticasein columns and potential anti-anticasein antibodies were eluted by the glycine buffer. These anti-anticasein antibodies were further purified by passage over DEAE cellulose, and then G-150 Sephadex to collect fractions eluting in the void volume.

*This work was supported by grants AI-15809, CA-19267, and CA-29502 from the U.S. Public Health Service, grant ACS IM-245 from the American Cancer Society, grant HRC-1610 from the New York State Health Research Council, and the Zelda R. Weintraub Cancer Fund.

0077-8923/83/0409-0469 $1.75/0 © 1983, NYAS

Preparation Of Pepsin-Digested Alkaline Phosphatase-Labeled Anticasein

An aliquot of anticasein antibodies of each donor were pepsin digested,[7] and the Fab$'_2$ isolated by gel filtration on Sephadex G-150. Antigen-specific Fab$'_2$ of each aliquot were then isolated by repassage and elution from casein-Sepharose. Part of the pepsin-treated, affinity-repurified anticasein of serum A and B (containing about 150 μg IgG/ml) was then coupled to alkaline phosphatase (AP) at an enzyme/antibody ratio of 1:2.[3,8] The enzyme-antibody conjugates used were eluted in the void volume of a 6 × 0.2 cm column of Ultragel ACA-22 (LKB-Produkter Bromma, Sweden). The preparations were made 5% in chicken ovalbumin (three-times crystallized; Sigma Chemical Co., St. Louis, Mo.) to block residual glutaraldehyde and eliminate nonspecific reactions. Approximately 35% of the enzyme-antibody activity of these final preparations could be bound specifically to casein-Sepharose as determined in a separate elution study.

Assay for Anti-Anticasein

In separate tubes, increasing amounts (from 25 to 1,600 ng) of Fab$'_2$ anticasein of serum A or B were added to 600 ng of anti-anticasein of serum A or B, and 200 ng of AP labeled Fab$'_2$ anticasein were isolated from the same sera. In other tubes containing both anti-anticasein and AP-anticasein, possible inhibitors of the enzyme-labeled anticasein and anti-anticasein interaction were 10^{-3} M casein, 1 μg of the Fab$'_2$ of myeloma proteins HA and GU, or 1 μg of Fab$'_2$ of pooled human gamma globulin. In addition, 1 μg of pepsin-digested anticasein of subject B was tested with the anti-anticasein of subject A, and 1.6 μg of pepsin-digested anti-casein of subject A was tested with the anti-anticasein of subject B. In each tube, total volumes of 200 μl were achieved by additions of normal saline. After incubating these reactants overnight at 4° C, 100 μl of a 10% suspension of heat-killed, formalin-fixed *Staphylococcus aureus* (SA)[9] in PBS was added to each sample. After again incubating at 4° C for one hour, SA pellets were washed three times in PBS, containing 0.25% Tween-20 and 1 ml of a 1 mg/ml solution of *p*-nitrophenyl phosphate (Technicon Instruments Corp., Tarrytown, N.Y.).[3] After three hours at 25° C, SA pellets were removed by 10-minute centrifugation (730 g, GLC-2, Sorvall, Ivan Sorvall, Norwalk, Conn.), and the optical density (OD) 400 nm of the supernatant was read (Beckman Acta C iii spectrophotometer, Beckman Instruments, Inc., Fullerton, Ca.). Control samples contained no anticasein, no anti-anticasein, no enzyme-labeled anticasein, or SA alone.

Trace Iodination of Anti-Anticasein

An aliquot of anti-anticasein of subject B was trace iodinated by ^{125}[I] (New England Nuclear, Boston, Mass.) using chloramine T[10] and then extensively dialysed against PBS to remove unbound ^{125}[I]. The final specific activity was calculated to be 5.0 μCi/mg.

Sodium Dodecyl Sulfate Polyacrylamide Gel Electrophoresis

Aliquots of the anticasein antibodies of subjects A and B and the ^{125}[I] anti-anticasein of subject B were reduced and subjected to electrophoresis in

12-cm 5% polyacrylamide gels containing 0.1% sodium dodecyl sulfate (SDS).[11] The resulting gels were either stained with 0.05% Coomassie blue or sliced into 2-mm slices and counted in a Packard Autogamma Counter (Packard Instrument Co., Downers Grove, Ill.).

IgG Quantitation

Radial immunodiffusion[12] was used to determine IgG concentrations for levels ≥ 2 mg, and an ELISA method (to be described separately) for IgG concentrations falling between 10 ng/ml and 2 mg/ml.

In Vitro Production and Detection of IgG and κ-Casein Circulating Immune Complexes

Subject B was given 100 ml of bovine milk to drink after a 10 hour fast.[3] Serum samples drawn at 30 minute intervals for three hours were allowed to clot at room temperature for one hour, and the serum was removed after centrifugation. The amount of κ-casein containing immune complex was detected in a similar ELISA system using Raji cells that can identify as little as 0.11 ng κ-casein in immune complexes in human serum.[13]

Participation of Anti-Anticasein in Immune Complexes Formed In Vivo

For determining the amount of anti-anticasein binding to these naturally formed immune complexes, 25 μl aliquots of subject B's serum drawn at 30 minute intervals after milk ingestion, diluted 1:4 in normal saline, were incubated for 45 minutes with 1.0×10^6 Raji cells in 50 μl RPMI (Grand Island Biological Co., Grand Island, N.Y.). After washing 3 times in RPMI, Raji cell-bound complexes were again incubated in 50 μl RPMI containing ^{125}[I] anti-anticasein of subject B. After a six hour incubation at 4° C, the cell pellet was then washed three times in PBS and counted (Packard Autogamma Counter).

RESULTS

Subjects A and B were previously shown to form large amounts of IgG immune complex after milk challenge as shown in FIGURE 1, and both individuals were found to have large amounts of anticasein antibodies as determined in an ELISA.[3]

The anticasein antibody preparations isolated from the serum of these two individuals contained approximately 1.5 mg of IgG and the molecular weights of reduced samples analysed on SDS polyacrylamide gel electrophoresis were consistent with the molecular weight of H and L chains of IgG (53,000 and 23,000).

The anticasein antibodies of subjects A and B were used to prepare two second affinity columns for the isolation of anti-anticaseins. An iodinated, reduced further purified preparation of subject B's anti-anticasein was found to have a molecular weight profile of H and L chains of IgG on SDS polyacrylamide gel electrophoresis.

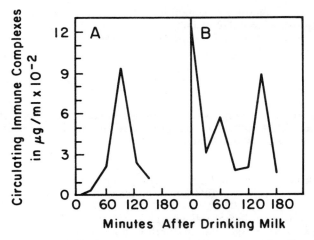

FIGURE 1. Two IgA-deficient subjects, A and B, were given 100 ml milk to drink. Serum samples drawn at 30 minute intervals were assayed for the presence of circulating immune complexes using the Raji cell ELISA assay.

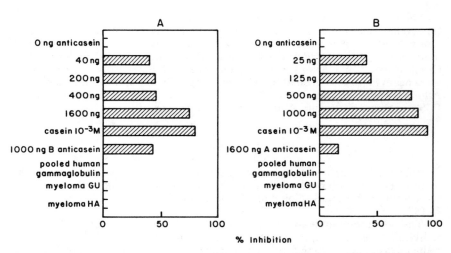

FIGURE 2. The ELISA *Staphylococcus aureus* assay shows that increasing amounts of anticaseins of subject A (panel A) or subject B (panel B) produce increasing inhibition of the binding of their respective anti-anticaseins to the alkaline phosphatase-labeled anticasein of each [the absorbance 400 nm (abscissa) indicates the relative binding of the enzyme-labeled anticasein]. Pooled human gamma globulin and two myeloma proteins produced no inhibition, but casein itself produced profound inhibition. Moderate inhibition appears to be present when the anticasein of subject A is tested with the anti-anticasein of subject B (panel B), or vice versa (panel A). The control, SA alone, is indicated.

To test the binding of the presumptive auto-idiotypic antibody to anticasein, a competition reaction using SA was devised. In these experiments, increasing amounts of nonlabeled anticasein were introduced to increasingly prevent a limited amount of enzyme-labeled anticasein from binding to anti-anticasein attached to S. aureus. FIGURE 2 shows that the binding of AP conjugated Fab$'_2$ anticasein of both IgA-deficient patients A and B (panel A and B) are progressively inhibited from binding to their respective anti-antibodies by increasing amounts of unlabeled Fab$'_2$ anticasein. Pepsin-treated pooled human gamma globulin or two IgG myeloma proteins did not inhibit the binding of anticasein to their respective anticasein antibodies. Casein (10^{-3} M) produced an 80% inhibition of idiotype binding for subject A and 95% inhibition for subject B, demonstrating that most, although not all, of the idiotypic antibodies, bind in or near, the antigen binding site. In addition, the anticasein of subject B inhibited by 43% the

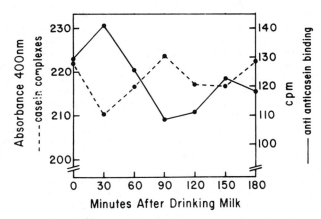

FIGURE 3. Subject B was given 100 ml of milk to drink. Kappa-casein containing immune complexes (----) were estimated by ELISA (Absorbance 400 nm) and the binding of anti-anticasein ^{125}[I] to the immune complexes present at each interval are given as cpm (.____.).

binding of subject A's anticasein to anti-anticasein; and the anticasein of subject A inhibited the same interaction of subject B by 34 percent.

In order to investigate the participation of anti-anticasein antibodies in in vivo immune complex formation as a possible function of serum casein concentrations, the serum of volunteer patient B was collected at 30 minute intervals for three hours after he had ingested 100 ml of milk. Using Raji cells to bind the immune complexes present in the serum at each interval, these complexes were then analysed for κ-casein and for the binding of his own ^{125}[I] anti-anticasein. FIGURE 3 shows that κ-casein-containing complexes first decreased after milk ingestion, slowly increased until the 90 minute interval, fell again at 120 and 150 minutes, and finally achieved a level somewhat below that originally present. The binding of anti-anticasein was found to be inverse: as the casein content diminished, anti-anticasein binding increased; as casein complexes increased, anti-idiotypic binding diminished. An alternating reciprocal binding of anti-

anticasein to these immune complexes, depending upon casein content, was thus observed.

These experiments show that a specific autologous anti-anticasein antibody can be isolated from the sera of IgA-deficient individuals. The antigenic individuality of the V_h region of human immunoglobulins, first described for humans by Kunkel et al.[14] and for rabbits by Oudin,[15] is the basis of the Jerne network hypothesis, which suggests that all in vivo antibody responses are normally balanced by the reciprocal production of idiotypes and autologous anti-idiotypes.[16] Current experimental evidence in murine models strongly favors cellular and humoral control by idiotype/anti-idiotype interactions,[17-19] but very few instances of autologous anti-idiotypes in human systems have yet been described. Possible exceptions include reports of a T-cell antibody with a specific suppressive action on the one-way mixed lymphocyte culture reaction identified in the serum of a long-surviving renal transplant patient,[20] immune complexes containing a tumor cytotoxin complex, and an antiglobulin detected in several normal sera.[21] (Because in this latter study, pooled human IgG also bound the tumor-antibody complex, nonspecific antibody interactions are difficult to exclude). Possible autologous anti-idiotypic activity has also been found in the IgM fractions of mixed cryoglobulins,[22] and in anti-DNA antibodies in the sera of patients with lupus erythematosus.[23]

In murine studies, anti-idiotypic antibodies induced by hyperimmunization with antibody can be nearly 100% inhibited from binding to idiotype by antigen, whereas similar antibodies raised by immunization with antigen antibody complexes can be 75% blocked by antigen,[5,23] indicating that the degree of saturation of antibody with antigen probably dictates the ultimate production of "site directed" versus "nonsite directed" anti-idiotype.[5,23] Because IgA-deficient humans have an intermittent saturation of anticasein antibody with ingested antigen,[3] it is most interesting that the degree of antigen inhibition found in subjects A and B (80, 95%) falls between the levels found in murine studies for immunization with antibody alone and immunization with antigen-antibody complexes.

These experiments suggest that the binding of a specific anti-idiotype into the circulating immune complexes of an IgA-deficient individual could depend upon the amount of antigen in these complexes. Because IgA-deficient individuals often have markedly increased antibody titers to bovine gamma globulin, α-lactalbumin, β-lactoglobulin, and ovalbumin, in addition to casein,[3,24] it is probable that anti-idiotypic antibodies corresponding to each of these antibodies are produced. One might expect that the circulating complexes so frequently present in the sera of these individuals could contain continuously fluctuating amounts of antigen and anti-idiotype, depending on diet.

The ultimate immunologic effect produced by the continuous production of idiotype and anti-idiotype is a critical issue. In murine studies, anti-idiotypes have been found to be capable of suppressing the expression of idiotypes[25,26] and may, in other systems, replace antigen as a trigger to idiotype production.[27] In addition, both idiotype[28] and anti-idiotype[29] have been found to generate T- suppressor cell activity in murine studies. It has, however, been uncertain to what degree murine experiments could be expected to elucidate human mechanisms. The experiments described here provide evidence of a naturally existing and unique model that may be used to explore these questions in human studies.

ACKNOWLEDGMENTS

The excellent assistance of Dr. D. Lawless, Mr. O. W. Gamble, Ms. Theodosia Zacharczuk, and the continued advice and supportive interest of Dr. R. A. Good are gratefully acknowledged.

REFERENCES

1. BUCKLEY, R. H. & S. C. DEES. 1969. Correlation of milk precipitins with IgA deficiency. New Engl. J. Med. **281:** 465–469.
2. CUNNINGHAM-RUNDLES, C., W. E. BRANDEIS, R. A. GOOD & N. K. DAY. 1978. Milk precipitins, circulating immune complexes and IgA deficiency. Proc. Nat. Acad. Sci. USA **75:** 3387–3389.
3. CUNNINGHAM-RUNDLES, C., W. E. BRANDEIS, R. A. GOOD & N. K. DAY. 1979. Bovine proteins and the formation of circulating immune complexes in selective IgA-deficiency. J. Clin. Inves. **64:** 272–297.
4. CUNNINGHAM-RUNDLES, C., W. E. BRANDEIS, B. SAFAI, R. O'REILLY, N. K. DAY & R. A. GOOD. 1979. Selective IgA deficiency and circulating immune complexes containing bovine proteins in a child with chronic graft vs. host disease. Am. Jour. Med. **67:** 883–890.
5. KLAUS, G. G. B. 1978. Antigen-antibody complexes elicit anti-idiotopes. Nature (London) **272:** 265–266.
6. MARCH, S. C., I. PARIKH & P. CUATRECASAS. 1975. Methods of affinity chromatography. Anal. Biochem. **60:** 149–155.
7. TURNER, M. W., H. H. BENNICH & J. F. NATVIG. 1970. Pepsin digestion of human G-myeloma proteins of different subclasses. I. The characteristic features of pepsin cleavage as a function of time. Clin. Exp. Immunol. **7:** 603–625.
8. ENGVALL, E. & P. PERLMANN. 1972. Enzyme-linked immunosorbant assay. J. Immunol. **109:** 129–135.
9. CUNNINGHAM-RUNDLES, C., F. P. SIEGAL & R. A. GOOD. 1978. Isolation and characterization of a human mononuclear cell Fc receptor. Immunochemistry **15:** 356–370.
10. HUNTER, W. M. & F. C. GREENWOOD. 1962. Preparation of iodine 131 labeled human growth hormone of high specific activity. Nature (London) **194:** 495–497.
11. LAEMMLI, U. K. 1970. Cleavage of structural proteins during the assembly of the head of bacteriophage T4. Nature (London) **227:** 680–685.
12. MANCINI, G., A. D. CARBONARA & J. F. HEREMANS. 1965. Immunochemical quantitation of antigen by single radial immunodiffusion. Int. J. Immunochem. **2:** 235–254.
13. CUNNINGHAM-RUNDLES, C. 1981. The identification of specific antigens in circulating immune complexes by an enzyme linked immunosorbant assay: detection of bovine κ-casein in IgG complexes in human sera. Eur. J. Immunol. **11:** 504–509.
14. KUNKEL, H. G., M. MANNIK & R. C. WILLIAMS. 1963. Individual antigenic specificity of isolated antibodies. Science **140:** 1218.
15. OUDIN, J. & M. MICHEL. 1963. A new form of allotypy of rabbit γ-globulins apparently correlated with antibody function and specificity. C.R. Acad. Sci. **257:** 805.
16. JERNE, N. K. 1974. The immune system; a web of v-domains. Ann. Immunol. Inst. Pasteur (Paris) **125c:** 375–389.
17. COSENZA, H. & H. KOHLER. 1972. Specific suppression of the antibody response by antibodies to receptors. Proc. Natl. Acad. Sci. USA **69:** 2701–2705.
18. HART, D. A., A. L. WANG, L. L. PAWLAK & A. NISONOFF. 1972. Suppression of idiotypic

specificities in adult mice by administration of anti-idiotypic antibody. J. Exp. Med. **135**: 1293-1300.

19. STRAYER, D. S., H. CONSENZA, W. M. F. LEE, D. A. ROWLEY & H. KOHLER. 1974. Neonatal tolerance induced by antibody against antigen-specific receptor. Science **186**: 640-643.

20. MIYAJIMA, T., R. HIGUCHI, H. A. KASHIWABARA, T. YOKOYAMA & S. FUJIMOTO. 1980. Anti-idiotype antibodies in a patient with functional renal graft. Nature (London) **283**: 306-307.

21. MORGAN, A. C., R. D. ROSSEN & J. J. TWOMEY. 1979. Naturally-occurring circulating immune complexes: normal human serum contains idiotype anti-idiotype complexes dissociable by certain IgG antiglobulins. J. Immunol. **122**: 1672-1680.

22. GELTNER, D., E. C. FRANKLIN & B. FRANGIONE. 1980. Anti-idiotypic activity with IgM fractions of mixed cryoglobulins. J. Immunol. **125**: 1530-1535.

23. JORGENSEN, T., G. GAUDERNACK & K. HANNESTAD. 1977. Production of BALB/c anti-idiotypic antibodies against the BALB/c myeloma protein 315 does not require an intact-ligand-binding site. Scand. J. Immunol. **6**: 311-318.

24. PUDIFIN, D. J., C. CUNNINGHAM-RUNDLES & R. A. GOOD. 1979. Circulating antibodies to chicken ovalbumin in IgA-deficient subjects. Fed. Proc. Fed. Am. Soc. Exp. Biol. **38**: 5263.

25. KOHLER, H. 1975. The response to phophorylcholine: Dissecting an immune response. Transplant Rev. **27**: 24-56.

26. NISONOFF, A. & S. A. BANGASSER. 1975. Immunological suppression of idiotypic specifities. Transplant Rev. **27**: 100-134.

27. TRENKER, E. & R. RIBLET. 1975. Induction of antiphosphorylcholine antibody formation by anti-idiotype antibodies. J. Exp. Med. **142**: 125.

28. JU, S. T., F. L. OWEN & A. NISONOFF. 1976. Structure of immunosuppression of a cross-reactive idiotype associated with anti-p-azophenylarsonate antibodies of strain-A mice. Spring Harbor Symp. Quant. Biol. **41**: 699-707.

29. EICHMAN, K., I. FALK & K. RAJEWSKY. 1978. Recognition of idiotypes in lymphocyte interactions. II. Antigen-independent cooperation between T and B lymphocytes that possess similar and complementary idiotypes. Eur. J. Immunol. **8**: 853-857.

DISCUSSION OF THE PAPER

L. Å. HANSON (*University of Göteborg, Göteborg, Sweden*): Do you have any notion as to the inflammatory capacity of the casein anti-casein complex compared to the anti-casein anti-anticasein complexes.

C. CUNNINGHAM-RUNDLES (*Memorial Sloan-Kettering Cancer Center, New York, N.Y.*): Rarely have we been able to demonstrate that the anti-casein casein complexes will fix complement. It happens in about one out of ten of the IgA-deficient individuals.

M. R. SZEWCZUK (*Queens University, Kingston, Ontario, Canada*): I just want to make a comment on some preliminary data from my laboratory. We presented TNP-bovine gamma globulin by gastric intubation and measured the hapten augmentable plaques. In young animals, we found that there was a high percentage of hapten augmentable plaques, as evidenced by autoanti-idiotypic antibody production. In older animals, this type of production was lost.

J. E. BUTLER (*University of Iowa, Iowa City*): Did you say why the major antigen in milk was the Fc portion of bovine IgM?

CUNNINGHAM-RUNDLES: I think it is unknown. I did not use it in my system as an antigen because it would have been difficult to exclude rheumatoid factors.

QUESTION: Do these patients experience any discomfort after they drink milk?

CUNNINGHAM-RUNDLES: Some of the patients have hives and joint pains, but we cannot make a close correlation.

M. W. RUSSELL (*University of Alabama in Birmingham*): Did you compare normal and IgA-deficient individuals, with respect to the isotype of other antibodies or immune complexes?

CUNNINGHAM-RUNDLES: I have not examined normal individuals at all. It is difficult to obtain enough anticasein with which to work. It appears that an anticasein antibody is almost always in the IgG_1 subclass.

J. MESTECKY (*University of Alabama in Birmingham*): I think this point is an interesting one, because Dr. Jackson worked with rabbit idiotypically cross-reactive antibodies to a large antigen such as human serum albumin. She observed a similar phenomenon. I think it is important to realize that this antigen has many antigenic determinants. This finding may be the reason why you are able to detect more cross-reactive antibodies than in usual systems that involve haptens. Do you know against what determinant on the casein molecule these antibodies are directed?

CUNNINGHAM-RUNDLES: I have done some cleavage experiments to see if I could detect what peptides are most antigenic. Caseins are remarkably heterogeneous, and the only preserved amino acid features are those that bind to calcium. The remainder of the sequence is quite diverse.

R. A. GOOD (*Oklahoma Medical Research Foundation, Oklahoma City*): It is fascinating that the antibodies produced against the milk proteins are IgG_1. What is the isotype of the anti-idiotypic antibodies?

CUNNINGHAM-RUNDLES: I do not know yet.

ALPHA-CHAIN DISEASE: AN IMMUNOPROLIFERATIVE DISEASE OF THE SECRETORY IMMUNE SYSTEM*

Maxime Seligmann† and J.C. Rambaud‡

†Laboratory of Immunochemistry and Immunopathology
INSERM U108, Research Institute on Blood Diseases
Laboratory of Oncology and Immunohematology of
The National Center for Scientific Research
Hôpital Saint Louis
Paris, France

‡Department of Gastroenterology
Research Unit on Physiopathology of Digestion, INSERM U54
Hôpital Saint Lazare
Paris, France

Alpha-chain disease, the most frequent of the heavy-chain diseases,[1] is a proliferative disorder of B-lymphoid cells affecting mainly young patients and involving primarily the secretory immune system. It is defined by the production of a population of immunoglobulin molecules consisting of incomplete alpha chains devoid of light chains.

The diagnosis of this condition can be suspected from clinical and pathological findings, but it relies entirely upon laboratory studies. The demonstration by immunochemical methods of the presence of this peculiar immunoglobulin molecule in the serum (and/or intestinal fluid or proliferating cells) is essential for establishing the diagnosis that may offer some difficulties in a routine laboratory. The diagnosis can easily be missed on the serum electrophoretic pattern, because the pathological protein is not detectable by this approach in more than half of the cases. Immunoelectrophoretic analysis of the patient's serum usually shows an abnormal component reacting with antisera to alpha chains, but not with antisera to kappa and lambda chains. The lack of precipitation of the anomalous component with antisera to light chains may be difficult to ascertain when the concentration of the heavy-chain disease protein is low. Moreover, it is by no means a sufficient criterion for the diagnosis, because some IgA-myeloma proteins with lambda chains fail to precipitate with most antisera to light chains.

The definite diagnosis of alpha-chain disease relies currently on the two following methods: 1) demonstration of the absence of conformational specificities of the Fab region that depends upon the presence of both heavy and light chains, by using highly selected antisera that contain precipitating antibodies to such configurational determinants;[2] and 2) demonstration of the absence of light-chain determinants by immunoselection (with highly selected antisera to kappa and lambda chains or to Fab alpha fragments) combined with immunoelectrophoresis.[3] These two methods have been compared by the criteria of sensitivity and suitability for testing in routine laboratories.[4] The latter has the advantage of slightly enhanced sensitivity, easier interpretation of the positive results and ability to detect the pathological protein when testing sera with very low levels of residual normal IgA. Radioimmunoassay using antisera or monoclonal antibodies

*This work was supported in part by DGRST Grant No. 82 L 0072.

478

0077–8923/83/0409–0478 $1.75/0 © 1983, NYAS

that would recognize unmasked Fc determinants unique to all naked alpha chains of a given subclass would represent an ideal approach. All attempts, however, to raise such antibodies have been unsuccessful thus far.

Alpha-chain disease is connected primarily with the IgA-secretory system. In three patients, with rather poorly documented pathological data, the disease was apparently confined to the respiratory tract. We believe that further cases of the respiratory form of the disease, as well as cases involving the salivary glands and other sites of secretory IgA production, will be described in the future.

All of the other patients presently reported were affected with the digestive form of alpha-chain disease that is localized mainly in the small intestine and the mesenteric lymph nodes.[5,6]

NATURAL HISTORY OF THE DIGESTIVE FORM OF ALPHA-CHAIN DISEASE

The natural history of alpha-chain disease is of utmost importance. It is well established that the lesions progress from an initial stage characterized by diffuse and extensive plasma-cell infiltration to an overt malignant lymphoma.[7] The early stage is usually featured by a diffuse infiltration of the lamina propria of the small intestine by mature plasma cells and sometimes "lymphoplasmacytoid" cells or small lymphocytes, without noticeable extension to the submucosa. Mesenteric lymph nodes are infiltrated by the same cells in follicular areas and medullary cords, without destruction of the nodal architecture nor invasion of the pericapsular fat. The late stage is characterized by the presence in the gut and/or mesenteric lymph nodes of a malignant lymphoma, usually of the large cell (immunoblastic) type and occasionally of the centroblastic-centrocytic type.[8] The evolution usually proceeds through an intermediate stage,[9] where the cellular infiltrate of the small intestine extends in some areas to the submucosa and even the muscularis propria, with the appearance of markedly dystrophic plasma cells and scattered immunoblasts. The same cellular infiltrate obliterates the lymph node architecture and invades pericapsular fat.

The extensive lymphoplasmacytic infiltration is mainly confined during the first stages to the enteromesenteric area. Infiltration of gastric, rectal, and colonic mucosae and of retroperitoneal lymph nodes is, however, not rare.[10] On the contrary, involvement of liver, spleen, mediastinal and peripheral lymph nodes, and of the bone marrow is a rare and late event, occurring at the stage of an overt malignant lymphoma. These data are in accordance with the well-known traffic of gut-associated B-cells.[11] In this respect, it is of interest to note that other sites of secretory IgA production are usually not involved in the digestive form of the disease. In a few cases of alpha-chain disease, the lymphoid proliferation does not involve the whole length of the small intestine: in one patient, it was located only to the ileum and the colon;[12] and in another case, the stomach and the colon were diffusely involved, whereas multilevel peroral biopsies of the small intestine were normal (J. Girodet, personal communication). These findings do not fit well with the present concepts of the IgA-secretory system of the digestive tract.

Apart from the tumoral symptoms and possible surgical abdominal complications at the latest lymphomatous stage, the clinical manifestations of alpha-chain disease are mainly those of a protein-losing enteropathy and of a severe malabsorption syndrome. The small intestine subtotal or total villous atrophy that is observed in most patients, plays a major role in the pathogenesis of malabsorption. At the initial stage, however, villous atrophy is inconstant, partial and patchy, and enterocyte morphology is normal. Oral antibiotics usually induce a prompt remission of the clinical and biological manifestations of malabsorption without any change in the intestinal mucosal lesions.[13] Thus, at this initial stage, colonization of the upper small bowel by bacteria and often by Giardia lamblia appears to be responsible for the occurrence of intestinal dysfunction. Bacteriological studies of the jejunal juice of several patients, however, showed a usually moderate bacterial overgrowth with nonsignificant concentrations of strict anaerobes.[14] These findings are different from those observed in the stagnant loop syndrome, and the possibility of enterotoxin production by intraluminal bacteria should be considered.

Some patients were present with the typical clinicopathological features of alpha-chain disease, whereas the presence of the characteristic heavy-chain disease protein could not be demonstrated in the serum. In one such patient, the alpha-chain disease protein was found in the jejunal juice, and in another patient it was demonstrated only in the proliferating cells.[15] The occurrence of such nonsecretory forms of alpha-chain disease should therefore be seriously considered, using immunofluorescence, immunoperoxidase, and biosynthesis studies, in patients with "immunoproliferative small intestinal disease"[6] and who are without detectable immunoglobulin abnormalities in serum and jejunal fluid.

Presently, we do not know whether the occurrence of an immunoblastic lymphoma, which may appear in any site of the lymphoplasmacytic infiltration featuring the initial stage, is a constant event in patients with alpha-chain disease who were not cured at an earlier stage. A purely plasmacytic infiltration of the small intestine was still found in a Tunisian patient 14 years after the clinical onset of the disease.[16] Conversely, a large cell lymphoma may be present as early as two months after the occurrence of the first symptoms. The mechanisms leading to the occurrence of the lymphoma remain unknown. An important point, however, is that there is good evidence that the large cells of the immunoblastic lymphoma arising in the late course of the disease are derived from the same B-cell clone as the initial plasma-cell proliferation. Alpha chains devoid of light chains were found on the surface of these large lymphomatous cells,[17] and studies of immunoglobulin biosynthesis have shown that these cells produce incomplete alpha chains that are incorporated into the plasma membrane, but not secreted.[18,19] These findings are analogous to those made in patients with chronic lymphocytic leukemia or Waldenström's macroglobulinemia and supervening immunoblastic lymphoma (Richter's syndrome).

That alpha-chain disease is not truly malignant in its initial stage is suggested by the occurrence of complete and prolonged remission achieved in a few patients treated with oral antibiotics alone.[13,20,21] Disappearance of the alpha-chain disease protein from the serum and intestinal fluid was noted in these patients, together with a normal histological appearance of multiple small bowel biopsies and negative immunofluorescence studies. It should be noted that these few patients with well-documented and lasting remissions had received tetracycline and that caryotypic studies of the proliferating plasma cells failed or were not performed.

Environmental factors providing a protracted antigenic stimulation in the gut may play an important role in the pathogenesis of alpha-chain disease. This possibility is suggested by the very peculiar geographic distribution[1] of the digestive form of the disease that appears to be extremely rare in Western developed countries. Although there is a wide spectrum of ethnic origin, most patients originated from, and had been living in, areas with a high degree of infestation by intestinal microorganisms and were exposed to conditions of poor hygiene. The postulated antigenic stimulation by specific or nonspecific intestinal microorganisms may have occurred many years before alpha-chain disease became clinically manifest. The environmental factors could have directly triggered the clonal proliferation or represented only predisposing factors. In either case, it is remarkable that the resulting plasma-cell proliferating appears to lead to the production of a heavy-chain disease protein rather than an entire myeloma globulin in the majority of patients.

Thus the natural history of alpha-chain disease raises a number of interesting problems and may constitute an important model for the understanding of the pathogenesis of human B-cell neoplasias.

Structural and Cellular Studies

Sequence data on alpha-chain disease proteins are scarce. This situation is partly due to great difficulties encountered in sequencing these proteins that often have heterogeneous terminal amino-sequences.[22] This heterogeneity is probably the consequence of a limited proteolysis occurring after the synthesis of an incomplete alpha-heavy chain. That the N-terminal residues found in seven such alpha-chain disease proteins were valine and/or isoleucine suggests that the degradation stopped at a given level for an unknown reason, such as enzyme specificity, steric hindrance, or the presence of a carbohydrate moiety. It should be noted, in fact, that the high carbohydrate content is an intriguing structural feature of most alpha-chain disease proteins and of many heavy-chain disease proteins, where unusual carbohydrate moieties, such as galactosamine in mu- or gamma-chain disease proteins, may be found at the aminoterminal end of the protein.[1]

The structural defect of most heavy-chain disease proteins is an internal deletion of the heavy chain.[1] Sequence data are available for only two alpha-chain disease proteins from our laboratory.[23,24] In both instances, the normal sequence of the alpha one chain constant region resumes at a valine residue in the hinge, just before the duplication of eight aminoacids.[23,25] This valine residue has a position similar to residue 216 of human gamma chains, which represents the site of resumption of normal sequence in many gamma-chain disease proteins. In a few other heavy-chain disease proteins, normal sequence resumes at other sites. For instance, in each of the three mu-chain disease proteins for which structural data are available,[1] the resumption of normal sequence occurs at the beginning of the constant domain C_{h1}, C_{h2}, or C_{h3}. In summary, an essential structural feature of heavy-chain disease proteins is that the gap, following an aminoterminal segment varying in length from 2 to about 100 residues, ends at an exon boundary and not at random.

The deletions in heavy-chain disease proteins usually affect two or even three heavy-chain domains, and the reason why they skip one or two potential joining regions is not yet fully understood. The study of DNA and RNA of proliferating cells producing these heavy-chain disease proteins should help us understand the nature of the recognition signals needed for splicing and elucidate the genomic defect responsible for the synthesis of these abnormal chains. Some data have recently become available for cells of murine myeloma mutants producing deleted heavy chains. The IF_2 gamma one variant, with a deletion of the entire C_{h1} domain, has a large genomic deletion, encompassing, in addition to the C_{h1} exon, part of the C_{h1} hinge-intervening sequence and at least 3 Kb to the 5' intron. At the 5' end of the reinitiation point, a $C\mu$ switch sequence was found.[26] These findings suggest that the production of the deleted protein could be related to an abnormal splicing. In two independently arising alpha mutants, both producing heavy chains with a C_{h1} deletion of approximately equal extent, different DNA patterns were found. One of these mutants has a genomic deletion encompassing all the C_{h1} exon plus portions of the intervening sequences. The other has a smaller deletion that does not remove the entire C_{h1} exon, suggesting that the remaining coding sequences are discarded during RNA processing.[27] This situation is somewhat analogous to that observed in the study of a kappa variant of MPC11, where the lack of the whole variable region results from aberrant splicing events due to a structural gene abnormality with absence of the J segment region and of the site for V-C_κ splicing.[28,29]

That the deletion of human-heavy chain disease proteins usually encompasses more than one domain could thus be due to abnormal splicing. A similar mechanism could explain another intriguing structural feature of several heavy-chain disease proteins. Whereas in many such proteins the aminoterminus can be identified as V_h, in some other proteins the aminoterminal stretch preceding the deletion represents sequences of unknown origin.[1] Such a strikingly abnormal aminoterminal sequence of about 40 residues has recently been established in a mu-chain disease protein. This finding could correspond to the translation of a persisting intervening sequence and abnormal splicing, although other hypotheses such as a missense repair fragment or even recombination with a viral genome cannot be excluded at present.

Another main feature of heavy-chain disease proteins is the lack of light chains. The failure of light chain synthesis is demonstrated in some,[30] but not all,[19] cases of heavy-chain disease. It is probably due to some regulatory rather than structural defect. A double defect of both light-chain and heavy-chain genes is difficult to visualize. A DNA defect responsible for the heavy-chain deletion could possibly encompass a site coding, for instance, for some crucial enzyme and could result in an error in light-chain RNA splicing and processing.

It seems likely that various genomic abnormalities can lead to the production of human alpha-chain disease proteins. The study of the proliferating cells producing such proteins will probably uncover various faulty mechanisms at the DNA or RNA levels and may help elucidate some important and presently unknown physiological mechanisms. It should be recalled that the clone producing the structurally abnormal heavy-chain disease proteins does not appear to be always malignant. Thus, the structural abnormality may not be directly linked to malignant transformation.

REFERENCES

1. SELIGMANN M., E. MIHAESCO, J. L. PREUD'HOMME, F. DANON & J. C. BROUET. 1979. Heavy Chain Diseases: Current Findings and Concepts. Immunol. Rev. **48:** 145–167.
2. SELIGMANN M., E. MIHAESCO, D. HUREZ, C. MIHAESCO, J. L. PREUD'HOMME & J. C. RAMBAUD. 1969. Immunochemical studies in four cases of alpha chain disease. J. Clin. Invest. **48:** 2374–2389.
3. DOE W. F., K. HENRY, J. R. HOBBS, F. AVERY JONES, C. E. DENT & C. C. BOOTH. 1972. Five cases of alpha chain disease. Gut **13:** 947–957.
4. DOE W. F., F. DANON & M. SELIGMANN. 1979. Immunodiagnosis of alpha chain disease. Clin. Exp. Immunol. **36:** 189–197.
5. RAMBAUD, J. C. & M. SELIGMANN. 1976. Alpha Chain Disease. Clin. Gastroenterol. **5:** 341–358.
6. WHO Meeting Report. 1976. Alpha chain disease and related small intestinal lymphoma. Arch. Fr. Mal. Appar. Dig. **65:** 591–607.

7. BOGNEL J. C., J. C. RAMBAUD, R. MODIGLIANI, C. MATUCHANSKY, C. BOGNEL, J. J. BERNIER, J. SCOTTO, P. HAUTEFEUILLE, E. MIHAESCO, D. HUREZ, J. L. PREUD'HOMME & M. SELIGMANN. 1972. Etude Clinique anatomo-pathologique et immunochimique d'un nouveau cas de maladie des chaines alpha suivi pendant cinq ans. Rev. Eur. Etud. Clin. Biol. **17**: 362-374.

8. NEMES Z., V. THOMAZY & G. SZEIFERT. 1981. Follicular centre cell lymphoma with alpha heavy chain disease. Virchows Arch. A **394**: 119-132.

9. GALIAN A., M. J. LECESTRE, J. SCOTTO, C. BOGNEL, C. MATUCHANSKY, J. C. RAMBAUD. 1977. Pathological study of alpha-chain disease, with special emphasis on evolution. Cancer (Brussels) **39**: 2081-2101.

10. RAMBAUD J. C. & A. GALIAN. 1981. La forme digestive de la maladie des chaines alpha. Ann. Gastroenterol. Hepatol. **17**: 37-43.

11. GUY-GRAND D., C. GRISCELLI & P. VASSALLI. 1974. The gut-associated lymphoid system: nature and properties of the large dividing cells. Eur. J. Immunol. **4**: 1661-1667.

12. SALIVANTI E., P. BRANDTZAEG & P. KUITUNEN. 1980. Atypical intestinal alpha chain disease evolving into selective immunoglobulin. A deficiency in a Finnish boy. Gastroenterology **79**: 1303-1310.

13. RAMBAUD J. C., J. L. PIEL, A. GALIAN, J. P. LECLERC, F. DANON, F. GIRARD-PIPAUD, R. MODIGLIANI & G. ILLOUL. 1978. Rémission complète clinique, histologique et immunologique d'un cas de maladie des chaînes alpha traité par antibiothérapie orale. Gastroenterologie Clin. Biol. **2**: 49-61.

14. GIRARD-PIPAUD F., M. HALPHEN, Y. PEROL, M. LARIVIERE & J. C. RAMBAUD. 1981. Etude bactériologique et parasitologique intestinale dans la maladie des chaînes alpha. Gastroenterologie Clin. Biol. **5**: 187A.

15. RAMBAUD J. C., A. GALIAN, F. DANON, J. L. PREUD'HOMME, M. WASSEF, M. LE CARRER, M. A. MEHAUT, O. VOINCHET & A. CHAPMAN. Alpha chain disease without qualitative serum IgA abnormality: report of two cases, including a "non-secretory" form. Cancer (Brussels) In press.

16. ABBANE S., F. TABBANE, M. CAMMOUN & N. MOURALI. 1976. Mediterranean lymphomas with heavy chain monoclonal gammopathy. Cancer (Brussels) **38**: 1989-1996.

17. BROUET J. C., D. Y. MASON, F. DANON, J. L. PREUD'HOMME, M. SELIGMANN, F. REYES, F. NAVAB, A. GALIAN, E. RENE & RAMBAUD J. C. 1977. Alpha chain disease: evidence for a common clonal-origin of intestinal immunoblastic lymphoma and plasmacytic proliferation. Lancet **1**: 861.

18. RAMOT B., M. LEVANON, Y. HAHN, N. LAHAT & C. MOROZ. 1977. The mutual clonal origin of the lymphoplasmocytic and lymphoma cell in alpha heavy chain disease. Clin. Exp. Immunol. **27**: 440-445.

19. PREUD'HOMME J. L., J. C. BROUET & M. SELIGMANN. 1979. Cellular immunoglobulins in human-γ and α-heavy chain diseases. Clin. Exp. Immunol. **37**: 283-291.

20. ROGE J., P. DRUET & C. MARCHE. 1970. Lymphome méditerranéen avec maladie des chaînes alpha: triple rémission clinique, anatomique et immunologique. Pathol. Biol. **18**: 851-858.

21. MONGES H., G. AUBER, A. CHAMLIAN, J. P. REMACLE, B. MATHIEU, A. COUGARD & H. ARROYO. 1975. Maladie des chaînes alpha a forme intestinale: présentation d'un cas traité par antibiothérapie avec rémission clinique, histologique et immunologique. Arch. Fr. Mal. Appar. Dig. **64**: 223-231.

22. SELIGMANN M., E. MIHAESCO & B. FRANGIONE. 1971. Studies on alpha chain disease. Ann. N.Y. Acad. Sci. **190**: 487-499.

23. WOLFENSTEIN-TODEL C., E. MIHAESCO & B. FRANGIONE. 1974. "Alpha chain disease" protein DEF: internal deletion of a human immunoglobulin A. heavy chain. Proc. Nat. Acad. Sci. USA. **71**: 974-978.

24. WOLFENSTEIN-TODEL C., E. MIHAESCO & B. FRANGIONE. 1975. Variant of a human immunoglobulin: Alpha chain disease protein AIT. Biochem. Biophys. Res. Commun. **65**: 47-53.

25. TUCKER P. W., J. L. SLIGHTOM & F. R. BLATTNER. 1981. Mouse IgA heavy chain gene sequence: Implications for evolution of immunoglobulin hinge exons. Proc. Natl. Acad. Sci. USA. **78**: 7684-7688.

26. DUNNICK W., T. H. RABBITTS & C. MILSTEIN. 1980. An immunoglobulin deletion mutant

with implications for the heavy-chain switch and RNA splicing. Nature (London) **286:** 669–675.

27. DACKOWSKI W. & S. L. MORRISON. 1981. Two heavy chain disease proteins with different genomic deletions demonstrate that nonexpressed heavy chain genes contain methylated bases. Proc. Natl. Acad. Sci. USA **78:** 7091–7095.

28. CHOI E., M. KUEHL & R. WALL. 1980. RNA splicing generates a variant light chain from an aberrantly rearranged gene. Nature (London) **286:** 776–779.

29. SEIDMANN J. G. & P. LEDER. 1980. A mutant immunoglobulin light chain is formed by aberrant DNA- and RNA- splicing events. Nature (London) **286:** 779–783.

30. BUXBAUM J. N. & J. L. PREUD'HOMME. 1972. Alpha and gamma heavy chain diseases in man: intracellular origin of the aberrant polypeptides. J. Immunol. **109:** 1131–1137.

DISCUSSION OF THE PAPER

W. STROBER (*National Institutes of Health, Bethesda, Md.*): Is it possible that the viral genome is present on the immunoglobulin portion of the genome? This may explain long N-terminal sequences.

M. SELIGMANN (*Hôpital Saint Louis, Paris, France*): I propose this explanation as a hypothesis to explain the long unknown N-terminal stretch found in some of the proteins but we have no experimental evidence.

M. BLAKE (*Rockefeller University, New York, N.Y.*): Are other mucosal surfaces involved?

SELIGMANN: In some of these patients there has been some pathology of other mucosal sites, but it has not been extensive. We have never found alpha-chain disease protein in the saliva of these patients.

J. MESTECKY (*University of Alabama in Birmingham*): Eight years ago, you published that the alpha-chain proteins present in the circulation were associated with J-chain. Is J-chain expressed at the cellular level when the cells are going through a transition toward lymphoma?

SELIGMANN: Dr. Preud'homme has found J-chain production in some of these cells. One of his patients that was studied was in the intermediate stage.

MESTECKY: Alpha-chain disease may be an excellent model for studying a possible mechanism for homing of IgA cells. Some investigators think that it is an antigen driven process, whereas others think that secretory component or other mechanisms may be involved. Have you examined salivary and lacrimal glands for the distribution of alpha-chain producing cells?

SELIGMANN: System pathologic studies of lacrimal and salivary glands are not available.

R. A. GOOD (*Oklahoma Medical Research Foundation, Oklahoma City*): There is an interesting point about the malignant transformation of the cells. Dr. Yunis has developed methods for identifying chromosomal abnormalities. Is there evidence for a chromosomal change during apparent malignant transformation of cells, or, do the cells have the chromosomal abnormality from the beginning?

SELIGMANN: In the few patients we have studied, we failed to detect chromosomal abnormalities at the various stages. We did not have any recent patients from which to obtain good evidence.

GOOD: Dr. Yunis claims that he can see chromosomal abnormalities in essentially all the malignant cells he has studied thus far. It would be an interesting approach to look at dividing cells at the different stages.

SELIGMANN: It will also be extremely important to determine whether there are caryotypic abnormalities in patients who are eventually in full remission after antibiotic treatment.

A. G. PLAUT (*Tufts-New England Medical Center, Boston, Mass.*): You screen for alpha-chain disease by immunoelectrophoresis. I think it is worthwhile emphasizing that the more facile screening techniques would be particularly valuable in diagnosing this disease. This is an illness that could be treated with antibiotics in its early stages; we can interrupt the progression of a relatively benign lesion to a lymphoma.

SELIGMANN: We thought it would be useful to have a good and sensitive screening method for systematic studies. We failed to find a better method than we described. Monoclonal antibodies that would be detecting heavy-chain disease proteins, and not the whole IgA molecules, might be useful in the near future.

P. BRANDTZAEG (*National Hospital, Oslo, Norway*): I looked at cells from several cases of alpha-chain disease and all of these were J-chain positive. With respect to the seeding of alpha-chain positive cells to other secretory sites, I studied a case from Finland in which the process was localized mainly to the large bowel and the distal small intestine. We never found the alpha-chain producing cells in the proximal small intestine, although this patient was studied over a period of six or seven years.

ABROGATION OF TOLERANCE TO FED ANTIGEN AND INDUCTION OF CELL-MEDIATED IMMUNITY IN THE GUT-ASSOCIATED LYMPHORETICULAR TISSUES*

Anne Ferguson, A. McI. Mowat,† and S. Strobel

*Gastrointestinal Unit
University of Edinburgh
Edinburgh, Scotland*

INTRODUCTION

There are many T-lymphocytes not only within the organized lymphoid tissues of the gastrointestinal tract, but also scattered within the mucosa as intraepithelial and lamina propria lymphocytes. Specific immunological responses to the feeding of protein antigen are multiple, and include a range of systemic humoral and cell-mediated immune responses, together with mucosal immunity (FIGURE 1). There is an increasing weight of evidence, from work in rodents, that the specific immunological responses to fed antigen are regulated by immunoregulatory T-cells in the organized lymphoid tissues of the gut. Until recently, our research program has concerned the effector limb of intestinal T-cell-mediated immunity (CMI). By using the animal models of allograft rejection of intestine, and graft-versus-host reaction, we have produced evidence that when a CMI reaction occurs in the small intestine mucosa, there is villous atrophy, crypt hyperplasia, and lymphocyte infiltrate—lesions associated with malabsorption.[1-5] Intestinal mucosal immune responses to food antigens are likely to be implicated in celiac disease and in other malabsorption syndromes with food protein intolerance.[6] Allergy to foods is an important component of atopic disease in infants.[7] In these and similar diseases, the primary pathology must be accepted as an abrogation of the normal, usually harmless immune response to dietary antigens, and so there is a need for the study of the mechanisms underlying induction of the various types of immune response to fed antigens, particularly induction of mucosal cell-mediated immunity.

Induction of systemic tolerance by feeding antigen is well documented,[8-11] although the mechanisms responsible remain controversial. There is, however, persuasive evidence that cellular suppressor mechanisms are related to systemic tolerance for CMI after the feeding of ovalbumin.[12-14] We therefore, empirically, decided to perform a series of experiments in which we would attempt to induce intestinal CMI to ovalbumin in mice that were orally immunized after pretreatment with cyclophosphamide (CY), because administration of CY in the dose 100 mg/kg enhances CMI reactions without an appreciable effect on antibody synthesis, by way of suppressor-cell inhibition.[15] These experiments also allowed us to develop an *in vitro* method for detection of CMI in the lymphoid tissues of

*This work has been supported by a grant from the Medical Research Council of the United Kingdom. Dr. A. Mowat was a recipient of the Allan Fellowship of the University of Edinburgh; Dr. S. Stobel was the recipient of a grant from the Deutsche Forschungsgemeinschaft, Str 210/2-3.

†Present address: Registrar in Bacteriology and Immunology, Department of Bacteriology and Immunology, Western Infirmary, Glasgow, Scotland.

0077-8923/83/0409-0486 $1.75/0 © 1983, NYAS

the gut. The experimental details and results have been published elsewhere in full.[16-18]

METHODS

Animals

BALB/c mice aged 6 to 10 weeks were used throughout. These mice were bred in the Animal Unit, Western General Hospital, Edinburgh, and maintained under conventional conditions on a pelleted diet that did not contain egg protein.

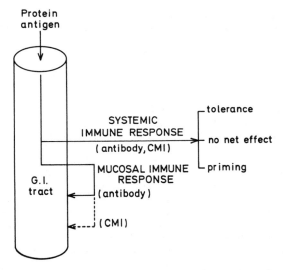

FIGURE 1. Diagrammatic representation of the range of systemic and mucosal immune responses to a fed protein antigen. On present evidence, there is a mucosal antibody response, but induction of mucosal CMI occurs only under experimental conditions or in disease.

Cyclophosphamide Treatment

Cyclophosphamide (Endoxana, WB Pharmaceuticals) was dissolved in saline and mice were given 100 mg/kg intraperitoneally two days before primary oral immunization with ovalbumin.

Oral Immunization

For primary immunization, mice were fed a single dose of either 2 mg or 25 mg ovalbumin (OVA) (Sigma Fraction V) in saline by intragastric tube. In some experiments a repeat feeding was performed in the following way. Twenty-eight days after the primary immunization, OVA, 2 mg/100 ml, was dissolved in the animals' drinking water so that each mouse ingested approximately 0.1 mg OVA daily. This feeding was continued for 10 days.

Skin Testing for Delayed Hypersensitivity

The presence of systemic delayed type hypersensitivity (DTH) was assessed in the various groups of immunized mice by intradermal skin tests using either flank or footpad skin. Mice were injected with 100 μg OVA in 0.05 ml saline intradermally on both shaven flanks, and double skinfold thickness was measured with calipers immediately before and 24 hours after injection, results being expressed as mean increment in skin thickness in millimetres at 24 hours. In other experiments, mice were tested by the increment in footpad thickness 24 hours after an intradermal injection of 100 μg OVA in 0.05 ml water. Control animals were injected with 0.05 ml saline only to assess the nonspecific response.

Lymphocyte Migration Inhibition Test

Mesenteric lymph nodes (MLN) from three to four mice were removed, washed in RPMI 1640 medium (Flow Laboratories) and trimmed of surrounding material before being gently cut up and passed through a fine wire mesh filter. After one passage through a 25 gauge needle, the cells were washed three times in RPMI 1640 and finally adjusted to 100×10^6 cells/ml in RPMI 1640. The cells were supplemented with 2 mmol/l glutamine, 100 μg/ml penicillin G, and 100 μg/ml streptomycin and buffered with 10 mmol/l hepes buffer. A standard migration inhibition test was then performed using 10 μl capacity glass capillary tubes in macrophage migration inhibition test plates (Sterilin Ltd.), the wells being filled either with 0.45 ml supplemented RPMI 1640 medium alone or medium containing 0.1 mg/ml ovalbumin. Six to eight wells were used for each antigen dose or for control cultures. After incubation at 37° C for 20 hours, migration areas were measured using a drawing tube attached to a dissecting microscope. The migration index was calculated as the mean area of migration in wells containing antigen divided by the mean area of migration in control wells.

Small Intestinal Epithelial Cell Kinetics

For measurements of intestinal mucosal architecture and mitotic activity of the crypts of Lieberkühn, villus length, crypt length, and crypt cell-production rate were examined in groups of animals by a technique first described by Clarke,[19] and previously used by our group in experiments on allograft rejection of gut.[3] Briefly, on the day of killing, all animals were given 7.5 mg/kg colchicine (BDH Pharmaceuticals Ltd.) intraperitoneally (i.p.), to arrest mitosis in metaphase. Individual animals were then killed at intervals from 20 to 100 minutes thereafter. Pieces of jejunum, 10 cm from the pylorus, were removed and fixed in 75% ethanol/25% acetic acid for six hours, then stained with a modified Feulgen stain. Villus length and crypt length were expressed in microns (μm) and the crypt cell-production rate (CCPR) expressed as net accumulation of metaphases/crypt/hour.

Intraepithelial Lymphocyte Counts

Pieces of jejunum were fixed in 10% buffered formal saline, paraffin embedded, 5 μm sections cut and stained with hematoxylin and eosin. A differential count was made of cell types within the epithelium covering the villi,[20] and the intraepithelial lymphocyte (IEL) count was expressed as the number of IEL/100 epithelial cells.

EXPERIMENTS AND RESULTS

Separate groups of animals were used for the measurements of lymph node cell migration, intestinal epithelial cell kinetics and IEL counts, studies of systemic immunization, and of systemic tolerance. Further groups of animals were used as positive controls having been systemically immunized with OVA in complete Freund's adjuvant; specificity controls were also performed using human serum albumin as an antigen.[17,21] Animals remained healthy throughout the experiments and the CY pretreated animals had no clinical side effects, weight gain being similar in all groups.

In general, four groups of animals were studied for each type of response. Untreated controls received water i.p. on day −2 and a water feed on day one. CY alone: animals received CY on day −2 and water or no further treatment thereafter. OVA alone: animals received water i.p. on day −2 and OVA feeding on day one. CY/OVA: animals received 100 mg/kg CY i.p. on day −2, and a feed of OVA on day one.

Systemic Immunity

The validity of intradermal skin testing as a measure of systemic DTH was confirmed by parenteral immunization of four mice that had received OVA in Freund's complete adjuvant and 21 days later were skin tested with 100 μg OVA (FIGURE 2). Similar skin testing was performed in orally immunized mice at 21 and 39 days after OVA feeding; no positive reactions were elicited in any of the orally immunized groups, including the CY/OVA treated animals (FIGURE 2).[18,21]

Systemic Tolerance

The presence or absence of tolerance induction was examined in the various experimental groups by immunizing all animals with 100 μg OVA in Freund's complete adjuvant intradermally, with DTH responses being measured 21 days later by a footpad swelling test. Results are summarized in FIGURE 3. Both doses of OVA used, 2 and 25 mg, suppressed a subsequent DTH response with 88% and 64% suppression ($p = 0.05$ in each case) in the fed mice when compared with water fed controls. The mice that were treated with CY before the feeding of 2 mg OVA had completely normal systemic DTH responses with no residual tolerance, and those mice CY pretreated, fed 25 mg OVA, had systemic DTH responses midway between control and tolerant animals, the value not being significantly different from either. Thus the tolerance for systemic DTH that was found after the feeding of OVA was abrogated by CY pretreatment.

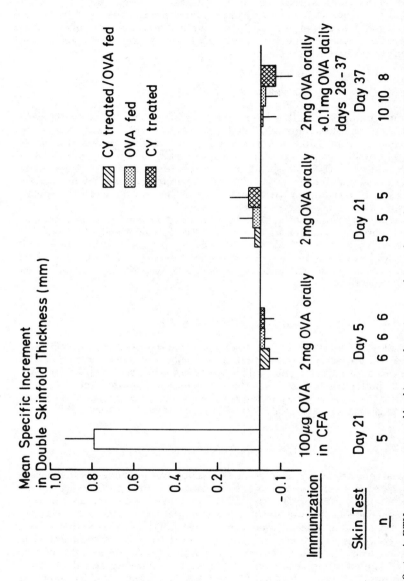

FIGURE 2. Systemic DTH responses, measured by skin test, after primary and secondary oral immunization with OVA in mice. A group of mice was also immunized with 100 μg OVA in complete Freund's adjuvant as positive controls. Results are expressed as mean specific increment in double skinfold thickness, 24 hours after 100 μg OVA in saline intradermally. Mean + 1 SD. Interval between immunization and skin test, and number of mice per group, are as shown.

Intestinal Cell Mediated Immunity—Migration Inhibition of Mesenteric Lymph Node Cells

Migration inhibition tests were performed with 0.1 mg/ml OVA and MLN cells taken at intervals from 1 to 22 days after oral immunization. Results are summarized in FIGURE 4. Animals fed OVA alone had no migration inhibition at any time, but animals given OVA preceded by CY had significant inhibition of migration at 24 hours after the OVA feed. A similar degree of migration inhibition persisted until 13 days after feeding. Two specificity controls were performed.[18] There was no migration inhibition of MLN in cells from OVA-immunized animals when the cells were incubated in the presence of human serum albumin, nor did OVA itself inhibit migration of MLN cells from unimmunized controls.

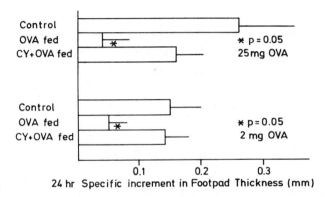

FIGURE 3. Effect of CY pretreatment on systemic tolerance induced by an OVA feed. Systemic DTH responses were measured by footpad swelling test three weeks after systemic immunization of all animals with 100 μg OVA in complete Freund's adjuvant. Bars represent mean specific increment in footpad thickness (millimetres) 24 hours after 100 μg OVA in saline, plus 1 SE. The three experimental groups are as shown. Prior OVA feeding, at both doses studied, induced systemic tolerance that was abrogated by CY pretreatment.

Intestinal Mucosal Architecture Changes after a Repeat Feed of Ovalbumin

Measurements of villus and crypt length, CCPR and IEL counts were made 10 days after OVA was fed again to the four experimental groups. Our previous work has shown that these two features can be used as indirect measures of the presence of a mucosal CMI reaction.[4,5] Although on conventional histology no abnormality of the mucosa was detected in any of the groups, objective measurements revealed minor but significant differences in the CY/OVA experimental mice. Results are illustrated in FIGURE 5. Villus length, crypt length, and CCPR were similar for the exclusively CY and OVA mice and untreated controls. CY/OVA animals, however, given a 10 day oral challenge with OVA, had significantly increased crypt length and CCPR compared with the other experimental groups. There were no significant differences between the groups with respect to villus length.

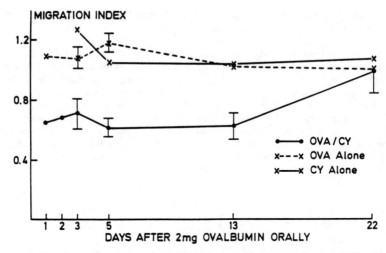

FIGURE 4. Development of migration inhibition in the MLN of mice fed OVA after CY pretreatment, and in mice fed exclusively OVA or given only CY. Where shown, bars represent mean ± 1 SD of three experiments (OVA/CY groups versus others, p < 0.01). Other results are for one experiment, and statistical analysis between groups was not possible.

Intraepithelial Lymphocyte Counts

As illustrated in FIGURE 6, IEL counts were significantly higher in the CY/OVA animals (mean 25.9) than in the other experimental and control groups (14.5, 15.9, and 14.1).

DISCUSSION

The experiments described in this paper have shown that under certain circumstances, oral immunization with the protein antigen OVA can induce a local CMI response in the gut-associated lymphoreticular tissues. Mice pretreated with 100 mg/kg CY before a feed of OVA had significant inhibition of migration in the presence of antigen and of MLN cells. They also had alterations in the structure of the intestinal mucosa after a repeat feeding of ovalbumin. These results suggest that CY pretreatment has induced intestinal cell-mediated immune responses.

The mechanism by which CY treatment has produced these effects in the gut is likely to be analogous to that which has been established in experiments on systemic immune responses—release of CMI reactions from suppressor control.[12-15] Thus we postulate that all of the effects observed in CY/OVA treated animals could be due to the effect of CY on T-suppressor cells. Two other possible actions of CY, however, should also be considered. The small intestine epithelium is one of the principal target organs for the cytotoxicity of many drugs, including CY, and so an increased permeability to proteins, or reduced enzyme content of cells of the intestinal mucosa may also be present. Alterations in the antigen handling properties of the gastrointestinal tract may influence CMI responses by leading to absorption of an unusually large amount of antigen, or alterations in the immunochemical nature of absorbed antigens. The maximal effect on the intestinal epithelium, however, of the dose of CY used occurs at 12–24 hours after drug administration,[22] and in our experiments OVA was fed at 48 hours. In addition to this potential alteration in the villus epithelium, an effect of CY on the lymphoid tissues of the gut, including Peyer's patches and surface epithelium overlying Peyer's patches, also deserves consideration; however, we have no information on this effect at the moment.

Support for the hypothesis that in these experiments we have reversed a background of homeostatic suppression of gut-associated CMI responses, comes from the considerable body of work on regulation of systemic delayed type hypersensitivity. The concept has arisen that there is normally a considerable

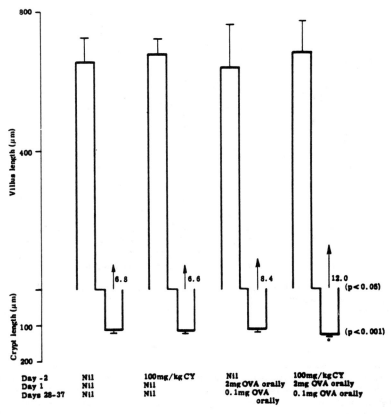

FIGURE 5. Mucosal architecture in jejunum of BALB/c mice treated as shown. Mucosal changes were measured after 10 days oral challenge with 0.1 mg OVA/day. Bars show means ± 1 SD for villus and crypt lengths, and arrows represent CCPR (six to eight mice per group).

degree of inhibitory control operating on the induction phase of DTH responses, and although we cannot draw any firm conclusions from the work described in this paper as to the nature of the postulated suppressor cells involved in regulating intestinal CMI, it is probably significant that T-suppressor cells for antibody production have been detected in Peyer's patches of orally immunized mice.[24,25] A similar system appears to exist for cell-mediated immune responses following oral immunization.[12] Future work on intestinal mucosal CMI responses and extension of this animal work into the clinical sphere, will require methods to detect and measure such responses. Our previous research on allograft rejection

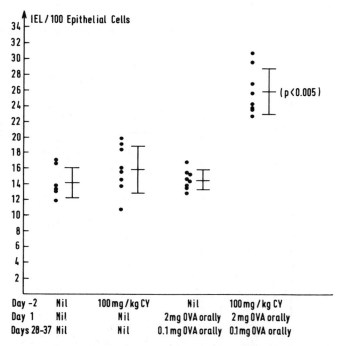

FIGURE 6. Intraepithelial lymphocyte counts in jejunum of BALB/c mice treated as shown. IEL counts measured after 10 days of oral challenge with 0.1 mg OVA/day. Results are expressed as mean ± 1 SD for each group of six to eight mice.

and graft-versus-host reaction identified the CCPR and IEL counts as reliable indices of mucosal CMI,[2-5] and these two parameters are sensitive, if not necessarily specific, indicators of a mucosal CMI reaction in experimental animals. These indices can now be supplemented by lymphocyte migration inhibition tests on MLN cells, and these tests should allow more detailed investigation of the effects on the intestinal mucosa and its lymphoid tissues of the manipulation of cell-mediated immune responses to fed antigens.

There is a growing body of evidence that says that mucosal T-cells represent a separate pool of lymphocytes from the systemic T-cell system, and have unique origins, routes of migration, and functions.[26] In theory, activation of the gut-associated lymphoreticular tissues with subsequent migration and differentiation of gut-associated lymphocytes need not involve activation of systemic-immune responses. Our findings of enhanced CMI responses in the gut in the absence of systemic DTH is further evidence supporting the segregation of mucosal and systemic T-cell populations.

ACKNOWLEDGMENT

We acknowledge the assistance of the staff of the Animal Unit, Western General Hospital, Edinburgh.

REFERENCES

1. FERGUSON, A. & D. M. V. PARROTT. 1973. Histopathology and time-course of rejection of allografts of mouse small intestine. Transplantation **15**: 546–554.
2. MACDONALD, T. T. & A. FERGUSON. 1976. Hypersensitivity reactions in the small intestine. 2. Effects of allograft rejection on mucosal architecture and lymphoid cell infiltrate. Gut **17**: 81–91.
3. MACDONALD. T. T. & A. FERGUSON. 1977. Hypersensitivity reactions in the small intestine. 3. The effects of allograft rejection and of graft-versus-host disease on epithelial cell kinetics. Cell Tissue Kinet. **10**: 301–312.
4. MOWAT, A. McI. & A. FERGUSON. 1981. Hypersensitivity reactions in the small intestine. 6. Pathogenesis of the graft-versus-host reaction in the small intestinal mucosa of the mouse. Transplantation **32**: 238–243.
5. MOWAT, A. McI. & A. FERGUSON. 1982. Intraepithelial lymphocyte count and crypt hyperplasia measure the mucosal component of the graft-versus-host reaction in mouse small intestine. Gastroenterology. **83**: 417–423.
6. FERGUSON, A. & A. McI. MOWAT. 1980. Immunological mechanisms in the small intestine. *In* Recent advances in gastrointestinal pathology. R. Wright, Ed.: 93–103. W. B. Saunders. Eastbourne, England.
7. BOCK, S. A., W. Y. LEE, K. K. REMIGIO & C. D. MAY. 1978. Studies of hypersensitivity reactions for foods in infants and children. J. Allergy Clin. Immunol. **62**: 327–334.
8. THOMAS, H. C. & D. M. V. PARROTT. 1974. The induction of tolerance to a soluble protein antigen by oral immunisation. Immunology **27**: 631–639.
9. ANDRE, C., J. F. HEREMANS, J. VAERMAN & C. L. CAMBIASO. 1975. A mechanism for the induction of immunological tolerance by antigen feeding: antigen-antibody complexes. J. Exp. Med. **142**: 1509–1519.
10. HANSON, D. G., N. M. VAZ, L. C. S. MAIA, M. M. HORNBROOK, J. M. LYNCH & C. A. ROY. 1977. Inhibition of specific immune responses by feeding protein antigens. Int. Arch. Allergy Appl. Immunol. **55**: 526–532.
11. SWARBRICK, E. T., C. R. STOKES & J. F. SOOTHILL. 1979. Absorption of antigens after oral immunisation and the simultaneous induction of specific systemic tolerance. Gut **20**: 121–125.
12. MILLER, S. D. & D. G. HANSON. 1979. Inhibition of specific immune responses by feeding protein antigens. IV. Evidence for tolerance and specific active suppression of cell mediated immune responses to ovalbumin. J. Immunol. **123**: 2344–2350.
13. CHALLACOMBE, S. J. & T. B. TOMASI. 1980. Systemic tolerance and secretory immunity after oral immunisation. J. Exp. Med. **152**: 1459–1472.
14. TITUS, R. G. & J. M. CHILLER. 1981. Orally induced tolerance: Definition at the cellular level. Int. Arch. Allergy Appl. Immunol. **65**: 323–328.
15. ASKENASE, P. W., B. J. HAYDEN & R. K. GERSHON. 1975. Augmentation of delayed-type hypersensitivity by doses of cyclophosphamide which do not affect antibody responses. J. Exp. Med. **141**: 697–702.

16. Mowat, A. McI. & A. Ferguson. 1981. Hypersensitivity reactions in the small intestine. 5. Induction of cell mediated immunity to a dietary antigen. Clin. Exp. Immunol. **43:** 574–582.
17. Mowat, A. McI., S. Strobel, H. E. Drummond & A. Ferguson. 1982. Immunological responses to fed protein antigens in mice 1. Reversal of oral tolerance to ovalbumin by cyclophosphamide. Immunology **45:** 105–113.
18. Mowat, A. McI., A. Ferguson. 1982. Migration inhibition of lymph node lymphocytes as an assay for regional cell mediated immunity in the intestinal lymphoid tissues of mice immunised orally with ovalbumin. Immunology. **47:** 365–370.
19. Clarke, R. M. 1970. Mucosal architecture and epithelial cell production in the small intestine of the albino rat. J. Anat. **107:** 519–529.
20. Ferguson, A. & D. Murray. 1971. Quantitation of intraepithelial lymphocytes in human jejunum. Gut **12:** 988–994.
21. Mowat, A. McI. 1981. Induction and expression of delayed hypersensitivity in the small intestine. PhD. Thesis, University of Edinburgh, Scotland.
22. Ecknauer, R. & U. Lohrs. 1976. The effect of a single dose of Cyclophosphamide on the jejunum of specified pathogen-free and germ-free rats. Digestion **14:** 269–280.
23. Schwartz, A., P. W. Askenase & R. K. Gershon. 1978. Regulation of delayed-type hypersensitivity by cyclophosphamide sensitive T-cells. J. Immunol. **121:** 1573–1577.
24. Ngan, J. & L. S. Kind. 1978. Suppressor T cells for IgE and IgG in Peyer's patches of mice made tolerant by the oral administration of ovalbumin. J. Immunol. **120:** 861–865.
25. Mattingly, J. A. & B. H. Waksman. 1978. Immunologic suppression after oral administration of antigen. I. Specific suppressor cells formed in rat Peyer's patches after oral administration of sheep erythrocytes, and their systemic migration. J. Immunol. **121:** 1878–1883.
26. Guy-Grand, D., C. Griscelli & P. Vassalli. 1978. The mouse gut T-lymphocyte, a novel type of T-cell: nature, origin and traffic in mice in normal and graft-versus-host conditions. J. Exp. Med. **148:** 1661–1677.

———————————◆———————————

DISCUSSION OF THE PAPER

J. R. McGhee (*University of Alabama in Birmingham*): How do you know that a suppressor cell is involved in systemic tolerance *in vivo*? Could you summarize the CMI test that you used?

A. Ferguson (*University of Edinburgh, Edinburgh, Scotland*): We transferred serum from animals fed with OVA, into the recipients, or sera from CY pretreated and OVA-fed donors. The abrogation of tolerance occurs if the recipients of the serum from OVA-fed animals are given cyclophosphamide. It is a CY-sensitive mechanism.

J. A. Mattingly (*Ohio State University, Columbus, Ohio*): Perhaps I have confirmed your results in an antibody system. Cyclophosphamide eliminated the suppressor cells from the spleen, but left the suppressor-inducer in the Peyer's patches. I was wondering whether the suppressor in the Peyer's patches can be a suppressor-effector for DTH rather than a suppressor-inducer for antibody.

J. M. Phillips-Quagliata (*New York University Medical Center, New York, N.Y.*): Have you tried to induce GVH reactions with peripheral node T-cells? If so, do they have the same effect on crypt length? Do mixed lymphocyte reaction (MLR) supernates have a similar effect?

FERGUSON: We have tried supernatants without any significant success. With regard to different cell types that induce GVH, we have used only spleen cells. Changes observed are really quite mild compared to those that have been reported by others.

DR. J. BIENENSTOCK (*McMaster University, Hamilton, Ontario, Canada*): What is the time scale of induction of mucosal CMI, and do you know whether your mesenteric lymph nodes contain functional suppressor cells? If so, when do they appear? Suppressor cells have been shown to appear first in Peyer's patches and then in mesenteric lymph nodes.

FERGUSON: Surprisingly, we found positive MIF tests from day 1 to day 21. When animals were refed, positive responses reappeared after 10 days. I am afraid we have no information on functional suppressor cells. Cells from Peyer's patches would be very difficult to use in the migration inhibition test.

SYNTHESIS AND SECRETION OF IgA, IgM, AND IgG BY PERIPHERAL BLOOD MONONUCLEAR CELLS IN HUMAN DISEASE STATES, BY ISOLATED HUMAN INTESTINAL MONONUCLEAR CELLS, AND BY HUMAN BONE MARROW MONONUCLEAR CELLS FROM RIBS*

Richard P. MacDermott, Mary G. Beale, Charles D. Alley,
Geoffrey S. Nash, Michael J. Bertovich, and M. Janice Bragdon

Division of Gastroenterology
Department of Medicine
Washington University School of Medicine
St. Louis, Missouri 63110

INTRODUCTION

Past studies on the synthesis and secretion of immunoglobulins by peripheral blood mononuclear cells (MNC) from patients with autoimmune diseases, by isolated intestinal MNC and by human bone marrow MNC, has resulted in conflicting results in each area. Therefore, we have examined the secretion of antibodies in general and IgA in particular by MNC from these tissues and disease states using long-term culture, in order to determine if alterations in cell migration from one compartment to another might occur.

Initially we examined the mitogenic and cytotoxic capabilities of isolated intestinal MNC from "normal" control specimens and resected intestinal specimens of patients with ulcerative colitis and Crohn's disease[1,2] and also the functional capabilities of human bone marrow MNC obtained by conventional aspirates and from ribs obtained at the time of thoracotomy.[3,4] Our studies revealed that isolated intestinal MNC from "normal" control specimens, as well as inflammatory bowel disease (IBD) specimens, are capable of lysing antibody-coated red blood cell targets, thus demonstrating classic killer-cell mediated cytotoxic capabilities, but are not capable of functioning as effector cells if antibody-coated cell line targets are used, or if cell line targets alone are used in a spontaneous cell-mediated cytotoxic cell assay.[1] Thus, isolated intestinal MNC contain a functional subclass of killer-cells effective against red blood cell targets but not cell line targets, and do not exhibit natural killer activity in the nonenhanced state. Furthermore, when allogeneic mixed leukocyte reactivity and cell-mediated lympholysis were examined, intestinal MNC from control and IBD specimens were capable of responding in the allogeneic mixed leukocyte reaction, but were not capable of lysing cells to which they had become sensitized in cell-mediated lympholysis.[2] Therefore, a functional subclass of T-cells naturally exists in the intestine that in other MNC populations, such as the peripheral blood, can only be observed after employing cell-separation techniques.

These observations point out the marked functional differences between MNC isolated from a solid organ, and those from peripheral blood, and indicate

*This work was supported in part by United States Public Health Service Grants AM21474 and AI15322.

0077-8923/83/0409-0498 $1.75/0 © 1983, NYAS

that theories on the etiology of autoimmune diseases based upon the functional capabilities of peripheral blood cells from humans or spleen cells from animals, do not necessarily hold when isolated MNC from solid organs are examined. In subsequent studies we have established that lectins and interferon will induce control intestinal MNC to become cytotoxic for cell line targets. Thus, exogenous agents or virally induced endogenous agents are capable of inducing cytotoxic effector function by isolated intestinal MNC, and may play a role in the immunopathogenesis of inflammatory bowel disease.

In studies of the cytotoxic capabilities of human bone marrow MNC, we observed that conventional aspirates resulted in cytotoxic effector function intermediate in level between that exhibited by pure human rib marrow MNC and pure peripheral blood mononuclear cells.[4] It therefore became apparent that much of the controversy in the literature with regard to immune function by marrow MNC was due to differences in aspiration techniques, resulting in various types of cells being examined by different laboratories. The variation in the volume of aspirates that have been utilized by different laboratories could have resulted in varying degrees of contamination by peripheral blood mononuclear cells. Thus we feel that in order to obtain a true picture of the functional capabilities of human bone marrow MNC, specimens obtained by curettage from human ribs at the time of thoracotomy should be utilized.[3,4]

In the present studies, we have examined the ability of MNC isolated from human intestine, human rib bone marrow, and the peripheral blood of patients with ulcerative colitis (UC), Crohn's disease (CD), systemic lupus erythematosus (SLE), and Henoch-Schönlein purpura (HSP), to synthesize and secrete IgA, IgM, and IgG. Our studies indicate that the human intestine is a major site of spontaneously synthesized dimeric IgA, and that human bone marrow is a major site of spontaneously synthesized monomeric IgA. Homing patterns and/or immunoregulation of B-cells capable of spontaneously developing into IgA, IgM, and IgG secretory cells appear altered in human disease states.

METHODS

Intestinal MNC were isolated and obtained as previously described[1,2,5] utilizing ethylenediaminetetraacetate (EDTA) washes to remove epithelial cells and overnight collagenase digestion followed by Ficoll-Hypaque and Percoll gradient purification. Human bone marrow MNC were obtained as previously described[3,4] from the ribs of patients undergoing thoracotomy and the MNC isolated from the marrow using centrifugation over Ficoll-Hypaque. Peripheral blood MNC were obtained from healthy, normal volunteers and from patients with CD, UC, SLE, and HSP as previously described.[5,6] Synthesis and secretion of IgA, IgM, and IgG was carried out using extensive washes of the cells followed by culture in microtiter plates at a concentration of 2×10^6 cells/ml in RPMI-1640 with 10% fetal calf serum (FCS) with or without a 1:100 dilution of pokeweed mitogen (PWN) for 7, 12, 14, 21, or 28 days.[5,6,7] A solid phase radioimmunoassay was carried out in order to measure the amounts of IgG, IgM, and IgA synthesized and secreted as described in detail in previous publications.[5,7] Cell-separation studies and surface-characteristic determinations were carried out using standard techniques as previously described.[8] Fractionation of IgA into monomeric and dimeric components was carried out using Sephacryl S-300 column chromatography.

TABLE 1

ANTIBODY SYNTHESIS AND SECRETION BY INTESTINAL
LAMINA PROPRIA MNC DURING 12-DAY CULTURE

		Immunoglobulin Concentration		
		IgA	IgM	IgG
"Normal" control	Media	19463 $\overset{\times}{\div}$ 1.30 (28)*	1808 $\overset{\times}{\div}$ 1.37 (28)	919 $\overset{\times}{\div}$ 1.34 (28)
	PWM	14427 $\overset{\times}{\div}$ 1.27 (28)	2792 $\overset{\times}{\div}$ 1.42 (28)	2216 $\overset{\times}{\div}$ 1.36 (28)
Ulcerative colitis	Media	11244 $\overset{\times}{\div}$ 1.49 (9)	630 $\overset{\times}{\div}$ 1.88 (9)	4867 $\overset{\times}{\div}$ 1.61 (9)
	PWM	3827 $\overset{\times}{\div}$ 1.41 (9)	509 $\overset{\times}{\div}$ 1.75 (5)	2169 $\overset{\times}{\div}$ 1.31 (9)
Crohn's disease	Media	3466 $\overset{\times}{\div}$ 1.66 (13)	465 $\overset{\times}{\div}$ 1.55 (13)	584 $\overset{\times}{\div}$ 1.71 (12)
	PWM	5985 $\overset{\times}{\div}$ 1.38 (13)	1955 $\overset{\times}{\div}$ 1.65 (13)	1286 $\overset{\times}{\div}$ 1.56 (12)

*Geometric mean $\overset{\times}{\div}$ SEM of ng/ml supernatant (number of specimens studied).

RESULTS

Examination of isolated intestinal MNC (TABLE 1) revealed that "normal" control intestinal cells exhibited high spontaneous synthesis and secretion of IgA, whereas cells obtained from the intestines of patients with CD and UC had reduced, though still significant, levels of spontaneous IgA secretion. As can be seen in TABLE 2, peripheral blood MNC from patients with CD, UC, SLE, HSP, exhibited markedly elevated synthesis and secretion of immunoglobulins in general, and IgA in particular. Addition of PWM to intestinal or peripheral blood

TABLE 2

ANTIBODY SYNTHESIS AND SECRETION BY PERIPHERAL BLOOD
MNC DURING 12-DAY CULTURE

		Immunoglobulin Concentration		
		IgA	IgM	IgG
Healthy Controls	Media	284 $\overset{\times}{\div}$ 1.68 (14)*	161 $\overset{\times}{\div}$ 1.60 (16)	280 $\overset{\times}{\div}$ 1.45 (17)
	PWM	1583 $\overset{\times}{\div}$ 1.62 (14)	1805 $\overset{\times}{\div}$ 1.62 (16)	2575 $\overset{\times}{\div}$ 1.66 (17)
UC Active†	Media	3500 $\overset{\times}{\div}$ 1.37 (8)	395 $\overset{\times}{\div}$ 2.31 (8)	1997 $\overset{\times}{\div}$ 1.55 (9)
	PWM	3258 $\overset{\times}{\div}$ 1.35 (7)	1190 $\overset{\times}{\div}$ 2.42 (7)	2505 $\overset{\times}{\div}$ 1.67 (8)
CD Active‡	Media	1325 $\overset{\times}{\div}$ 2.07 (4)	332 $\overset{\times}{\div}$ 2.31 (5)	307 $\overset{\times}{\div}$ 1.83 (5)
	PWM	2530 $\overset{\times}{\div}$ 1.45 (4)	821 $\overset{\times}{\div}$ 1.73 (5)	790 $\overset{\times}{\div}$ 1.61 (5)
SLE Active§	Media	2907 $\overset{\times}{\div}$ 1.21 (11)	477 $\overset{\times}{\div}$ 1.24 (11)	932 $\overset{\times}{\div}$ 1.42 (11)
	PWM	1020 $\overset{\times}{\div}$ 1.16 (11)	355 $\overset{\times}{\div}$ 1.43 (11)	662 $\overset{\times}{\div}$ 1.28 (11)
HSP Active¶	Media	2719 $\overset{\times}{\div}$ 1.35 (12)	898 $\overset{\times}{\div}$ 1.36 (12)	1317 $\overset{\times}{\div}$ 1.50 (12)
	PWM	684 $\overset{\times}{\div}$ 1.35 (12)	330 $\overset{\times}{\div}$ 1.66 (12)	598 $\overset{\times}{\div}$ 1.42 (12)

*Geometric mean $\overset{\times}{\div}$ SEM of ng/ml supernatant (number of individuals studied)
†Ulcerative colitis—7 untreated, 2 treated
‡Crohn's disease—all untreated
§Systemic lupus erythematosus—all untreated
¶Henoch-Schönlein purpura—all untreated

MNC of patients resulted in no enhancement of synthesis and secretions, and in many instances suppression of secretion was observed (TABLES 1 and 2). Coculture experiments (TABLE 3) demonstrated that peripheral blood MNC from patients with SLE and HSP exhibited a lack of normal T-suppressor cell capabilities in spontaneous antibody synthesis and the presence of T-suppressor cells under conditions of PWM stimulation. Follow-up studies of patients with HSP revealed elevated spontaneous synthesis and secretion of IgA with a return to normal levels of IgG and IgM secretion after patients had gone into disease remission.[6]

TABLE 3

COCULTURE EXPERIMENTS OF B-CELLS FROM CONTROLS, PATIENTS WITH HSP OR SLE WITH AUTOLOGOUS T-CELLS OR NORMAL ALLOGENEIC T-CELLS

Source	Cell Combinations	Stimulation	Immunoglobulin Concentration		
			IgA	IgM	IgG
Control (10)*	B	Media	115 $\overset{\times}{\div}$ 1.77†	201 $\overset{\times}{\div}$ 1.39	107 $\overset{\times}{\div}$ 1.40
		PWM	96 $\overset{\times}{\div}$ 1.66	198 $\overset{\times}{\div}$ 1.42	144 $\overset{\times}{\div}$ 1.38
	B + Auto T	Media	104 $\overset{\times}{\div}$ 1.42	170 $\overset{\times}{\div}$ 1.40	170 $\overset{\times}{\div}$ 1.43
		PWM	2092 $\overset{\times}{\div}$ 1.30	3271 $\overset{\times}{\div}$ 1.24	6614 $\overset{\times}{\div}$ 1.26
	B + Allo T	Media	70 $\overset{\times}{\div}$ 1.52	262 $\overset{\times}{\div}$ 1.42	98 $\overset{\times}{\div}$ 1.58
		PWM	1643 $\overset{\times}{\div}$ 1.34	1984 $\overset{\times}{\div}$ 1.61	3013 $\overset{\times}{\div}$ 1.37
HSP‡ (5)	B	Media	192 $\overset{\times}{\div}$ 1.57	160 $\overset{\times}{\div}$ 2.02	409 $\overset{\times}{\div}$ 1.71
		PWM	382 $\overset{\times}{\div}$ 1.35	145 $\overset{\times}{\div}$ 2.01	258 $\overset{\times}{\div}$ 1.54
	B + Auto T	Media	1143 $\overset{\times}{\div}$ 1.20	314 $\overset{\times}{\div}$ 2.18	586 $\overset{\times}{\div}$ 1.49
		PWM	345 $\overset{\times}{\div}$ 1.28	207 $\overset{\times}{\div}$ 1.68	419 $\overset{\times}{\div}$ 1.53
	B + Allo T	Media	293 $\overset{\times}{\div}$ 1.23	111 $\overset{\times}{\div}$ 1.82	154 $\overset{\times}{\div}$ 1.38
		PWM	2035 $\overset{\times}{\div}$ 1.21	2879 $\overset{\times}{\div}$ 1.45	6235 $\overset{\times}{\div}$ 1.47
SLE§ (5)	B	Media	806 $\overset{\times}{\div}$ 1.23	251 $\overset{\times}{\div}$ 1.79	845 $\overset{\times}{\div}$ 1.22
		PWM	367 $\overset{\times}{\div}$ 1.36	158 $\overset{\times}{\div}$ 1.56	324 $\overset{\times}{\div}$ 1.39
	B + Auto T	Media	1149 $\overset{\times}{\div}$ 1.17	288 $\overset{\times}{\div}$ 1.71	1373 $\overset{\times}{\div}$ 1.43
		PWM	154 $\overset{\times}{\div}$ 1.37	319 $\overset{\times}{\div}$ 1.59	316 $\overset{\times}{\div}$ 1.57
	B + Allo T	Media	279 $\overset{\times}{\div}$ 1.26	177 $\overset{\times}{\div}$ 1.79	447 $\overset{\times}{\div}$ 1.51
		PWM	1591 $\overset{\times}{\div}$ 1.40	1552 $\overset{\times}{\div}$ 1.22	4208 $\overset{\times}{\div}$ 1.14

*Number of individuals studied in parenthesis.
†Geometric mean $\overset{\times}{\div}$ SEM of ng/ml supernatant
‡Henoch-Schönlein purpura
§Systemic lupus erythematosus

TABLE 4

ANTIBODY SYNTHESIS AND SECRETION BY
HUMAN BONE MARROW MNC FROM RIBS

		Immunoglobulin Concentration		
		IgA	IgM	IgG
Total Bone Marrow	Media	3318 $\overset{\times}{\div}$ 1.39 (23)*	408 $\overset{\times}{\div}$ 1.43 (24)	1194 $\overset{\times}{\div}$ 1.51 (24)
	PWM	595 $\overset{\times}{\div}$ 1.34 (23)	164 $\overset{\times}{\div}$ 1.30 (24)	334 $\overset{\times}{\div}$ 1.35 (24)

*Geometric mean $\overset{\times}{\div}$ SEM of ng/ml supernatant (number of specimens studied)

Examination of antibody secretion by human bone marrow MNC (TABLE 4) revealed that high spontaneous synthesis and secretion of IgA was seen in most marrows examined, whereas a subset of marrows exhibited some IgG and, to a lesser degree, IgM secretion. IgA is the major immunoglobulin spontaneously synthesized and secreted by human bone marrow MNC *in vitro*. In the presence of PWM, human bone marrow synthesis and secretion of IgA was markedly inhibited (76.8 ± 3.2% in 23 specimens). The suppression of antibody synthesis by human marrow MNC in the presence of PWM was shown to be a cell-mediated event (TABLE 5) due to secretion of soluble suppressor factors (TABLE 6). Thus, human bone marrow MNC are not only capable of secreting large amounts of IgA, but also are capable of being stimulated to produce soluble suppressor factors that can inhibit antibody synthesis and secretion.

Finally, we have recently begun to study the characteristics of the IgA molecules synthesized and secreted by the various types of MNC that we have examined. Human bone marrow MNC primarily synthesized and secreted monomeric IgA, whereas intestinal MNC primarily secreted dimeric IgA (FIGURE 1), thus confirming the previous observations of Kutteh, Prince, and Mestecky.[9]

TABLE 5

SUPPRESSION OF HUMAN MARROW IgA SYNTHESIS BY PWM
PRETREATED AUTOLOGOUS MARROW MONONUCLEAR CELLS

Number of PWM Preincubated MNC* Added to 4 × 10⁵ MNC	Percent Suppression†
4.0×10^5	75 ± 6 (6)
2.0×10^5	78 ± 4 (6)
1.0×10^5	82 ± 3 (8)
5.0×10^4	78 ± 3 (3)
2.5×10^4	77 ± 6 (5)
1.3×10^4	67 ± 10 (3)
6.3×10^3	53 ± 15 (5)
1/100 dilution of PWM alone	85 + 3 (8)

*Cells incubated for one hour with a 1/100 dilution of PWM, washed three times to remove the PWM, then counted and added to cultures of autologous cells.

†Mean percent suppression ± SEM (number of samples) compared to simultaneous media controls. Geometric mean $\overset{\times}{\div}$ SEM for controls was 7376 $\overset{\times}{\div}$ 1.7 ng/ml IgA secreted for 10 samples.

Upon examination of intestinal MNC, it was observed that cells from patients with CD, cells from uninvolved intestine of patients with ulcerative colitis, and cells from control intestinal tissue gave similar patterns in which the majority of the secreted IgA molecules were dimeric (approximately 53 to 65%) (TABLE 7). By contrast, isolated intestinal MNC from involved portions of UC intestine showed a lower percentage of dimeric IgA (38.7 ± 12.5%) and an increased percentage of monomeric IgA (TABLE 7). Therefore, in the inflammatory infiltrate of intestinal MNC from UC patients, either B-cells capable of secreting monomeric IgA have migrated from extraintestinal sites, or the normal intestinal MNC that principally secrete dimeric IgA molecules have altered their secretion to include monomeric as well as dimeric IgA molecules.

TABLE 6

EFFECTS OF SUPERNATANTS FROM CULTURES OF PRETREATED
BONE MARROW MNC ON IGA SECRETION BY
ALLOGENEIC BONE MARROW CELLS

Culture Conditions	IgA Synthesis and Secretion (14 Days)	
	Concentration (ng/ml)*	Percent Suppression†
Media	9661 $\overset{\times}{\div}$ 2.69	—
PWM (1/100)	1841 $\overset{\times}{\div}$ 2.59	80.7 $\overset{\times}{\div}$ 2.3
Dilutions of supernatants from PWM pretreated cells‡		
1:1	1685 $\overset{\times}{\div}$ 2.73	82.0 $\overset{\times}{\div}$ 3.6
1:2	1906 $\overset{\times}{\div}$ 2.77	80.3 $\overset{\times}{\div}$ 1.2
1:4	2697 $\overset{\times}{\div}$ 3.62	69.3 $\overset{\times}{\div}$ 8.7
1:10	4857 $\overset{\times}{\div}$ 2.98	49.0 $\overset{\times}{\div}$ 5.8

*Geometric mean $\overset{\times}{\div}$ SEM for three separate experiments.
†Mean ± SEM of calculated percent suppression for three separate experiments.
‡Supernatant of seven day culture of bone marrow MNC after one hour pretreatment with 1/100 dilution of PWM.

DISCUSSION

Our studies to date have indicated that major alterations in antibody synthesis and secretion in general, and IgA secretion in particular, occur with intestinal MNC, human bone marrow MNC, and peripheral blood MNC isolated from patients with autoimmune disorders. The markedly heightened spontaneous IgA synthesis and secretion by control human intestinal MNC is not surprising, because the lamina propria is a rich source of B-cells that have the capability of developing into IgA-secreting plasma cells. In addition, the dimeric nature of the secreted IgA is also consistent with the ability of these cells to normally secrete dimeric IgA with J-chain that subsequently comes in contact with secretory component on the epithelial cell for secretion into the intestinal lumen. One possible explanation for our observed alterations of IgA secretion in IBD patients is that MNC in IBD patients are exhibiting an altered homing pattern, with intestinal cells capable of maturing into IgA-secreting cells, migrating to and remaining in the peripheral blood, rather than homing back to the intestine. This phenomenon would simultaneously account for both the decreased spontaneous IgA synthesis and secretion seen in IBD intestinal MNC populations as well as the increased spontaneous IgA synthesis and secretion observed by IBD peripheral blood mononuclear cells.

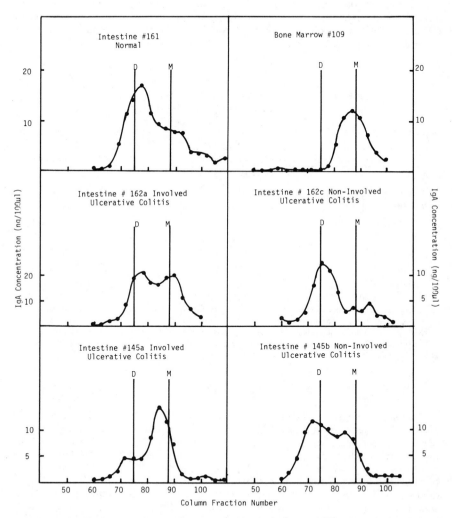

FIGURE 1. Column fractionation using Sephacryl S-300 of spontaneously secreted IgA by human rib bone marrow MNC, normal intestinal MNC, and MNC from involved or noninvolved bowel of UC patients. The column was standardized using monomeric IgA (M) from myeloma serum and dimeric IgA (D) from human colostrum.

TABLE 7

SYNTHESIS OF DIMERIC IgA BY INTESTINAL LAMINA
PROPRIA MNC DURING A 12-DAY CULTURE

	Percent Dimeric IgA*
"Normal" control	63 ± 3 (4)†
Crohn's disease	53 ± 1 (2)
Ulcerative colitis noninvolved bowel	65 ± 7 (2)
Ulcerative colitis involved bowel	39 ± 13 (5)

*Fractionation performed using Sephacryl S-300 column chromatography (see FIGURE 1).
†Mean ± SEM (number of specimens studied).

It should be noted that an alternative explanation for these results is that decreased IgA synthesis and secretion seen by intestinal MNC from IBD patients could represent a primary event, that is, a primary mucosal immunodeficiency could allow penetration of injurious agents and initiation of the inflammatory process. This situation would then suggest that the increased IgA synthesis and secretion by peripheral blood MNC from IBD patients is the result of a systemic immune response initiated by the penetrating agents. On the other hand, the similar alterations noted with peripheral blood MNC from both IBD and SLE patients raises the possibility that they both are either primary or secondary changes associated with autoimmune diseases.

It is important to consider the possible *in vivo* relevance of our present findings. Because major serum immunoglobulin abnormalities have not been previously noted in the types of patients studied in our present experiments, it is possible that the effects of our *in vitro* observations cannot be measured in the serum. It is important, however, to point out that the level of circulating immunoglobulin is a result of many different contributing factors, including synthesis, catabolism, and loss. Therefore, if IgA synthesis and secretion by IBD intestinal MNC is decreased and IgA synthesis and secretion by IBD peripheral blood MNC is increased, it is possible that the two alterations offset each other, resulting in normal circulating IgA levels. Another possibility is that increased IgA catabolism during the inflammatory reaction or increased gastrointestinal loss of IgA might offset increased IgA secretion by peripheral blood mononuclear cells. Furthermore, the increased IgA secretion by IBD peripheral blood MNC raises the distinct possibility that circulating IgA immune complexes may be seen *in vivo*. Thus, examination of sera from IBD patients for circulating IgA immune complexes is indicated. Moreover, the *in vivo* consequences of our *in vitro* observations may be manifested locally in the involved tissue rather than in the serum. Finally, normal hepatobiliary excretion of IgA may lead to clearance of the IgA that is synthesized in increased amounts.

After T-cell depletion, B-cell-enriched fractions from SLE patients maintained high levels of spontaneous IgG and IgA synthesis. Without identifying an inciting agent, these findings suggest that B-cells have been activated *in vivo* to mature into immunoglobulin-secreting plasma cells. When B-cells from either group of patients were cocultured with autologous T-cells, synthesis either remained the same or increased. More importantly, when T-cells from normal individuals were added to SLE or HSP B-cells, spontaneous immunoglobulin synthesis declined. This reduction was attributed to suppression rather than killing generated in an allogeneic mixed lymphocyte reaction, because patient

B-cells synthesized large amounts of immunoglobulin when cocultured with normal T-cells in the presence of pokeweed mitogen. By comparison, the failure of patient T-cells to inhibit autologous B-cell activity suggests a relative or absolute deficiency in T-suppressor cell function. Whether the defect in spontaneous T-suppressor cell function described here is a consequence of proportional changes in the numbers of T-helper and suppressor cells or whether it is secondary to other cellular disturbances such as defective T-cell stimulation by autologous non-T-cells is unknown. Nevertheless the present studies indicate that alterations in regulatory T-cell function are a critical component of the enhanced B-cell activity observed in patients with HSP and SLE. Clearly, further investigation into the nature of the T-cell population that is capable of spontaneously suppressing activated B-cells and is present in normal individuals is needed.

The marked synthesis and secretion of IgA by pure human bone marrow MNC is of importance because most previous investigators have concentrated primarily on the synthesis and secretion of IgG and IgM by human bone marrow. Furthermore, the observation that human bone marrow IgA is primarily monomeric confirms the recent characterization studies of Kutteh, Prince, and Mestecky.[9]

The enhanced spontaneous synthesis and secretion of immunoglobulins in general and IgA in particular, by peripheral blood MNC from patients with IBD as well as patients with SLE and HSP, is also consistent with altered patterns of migration due to inflammation or other stimuli. It should be noted that, in all of our studies, when markedly heightened spontaneous antibody synthesis and secretion has been observed, the addition of PWM results in a major suppression of the antibody synthesis and secretion. It is thus critical that the study of antibody secretion by human MNC consists not only of PWM stimulated antibody synthesis, but spontaneous antibody synthesis as well. It is possible to conclude from our studies that the description of PWM activable T-suppressor cells may be only part of the picture in disease states, and that a lack of suppressor cells that inhibit normal spontaneous antibody synthesis and secretion is also present in many instances.

We believe that further characterization of suppressor cell factors from tissues such as human bone marrow may be of importance in understanding normal regulatory mechanisms for antibody synthesis in the human. In particular, the presence of suppressor cells may not only play a role in antibody synthesis regulation, but could also be involved in the regulation of homing and recirculation patterns. Characterization of secreted IgA molecules in disease states by examining the subclasses of antibodies (IgA$_1$ and IgA$_2$) as well as the forms of IgA molecules secreted by peripheral blood MNC in patients with autoimmune disorders, may provide a better understanding of the types of alterations that can occur in the normal homing process.

SUMMARY

We have examined the secretion of IgA, IgM, and IgG by isolated human intestinal MNC, human bone marrow MNC from rib specimens, and peripheral blood MNC from patients with CD, UC, SLE, and HSP. "Normal" control intestinal MNC exhibited high spontaneous secretion of IgA, whereas intestinal MNC from UC and CD patients exhibited only modest increases in IgA secretion. Peripheral blood MNC from patients with CD, UC, SLE, and HSP exhibited markedly elevated spontaneous secretion of immunoglobulins in general and IgA in particular. Pure human bone marrow MNC exhibited high spontaneous secretion of IgA with modest amounts of IgG and normal IgM being secreted. The addition of PWM to cultures in which high spontaneous synthesis and secretion of immunoglobulins was seen, resulted in no further enhancement, and in some instances suppression, of antibody secretion. In patients with autoimmune disease, there appeared to be dual immunoregulatory defects, one involving a lack of normal T-suppressor cell functional capabilities for spontaneous antibody synthesis, and the other the presence of PWM activable T-suppressor cells. In human bone marrow, we have identified MNC that secrete suppressor factors in the presence of PWM and that are capable of inhibiting antibody synthesis and secretion.

Column separation using Sephacryl S-300 revealed that the IgA secreted by "normal" control intestinal MNC is predominantly dimeric, whereas the IgA secreted by human bone marrow MNC is predominantly monomeric. Furthermore, mucosal MNC from patients with CD and uninvolved intestine from patients with UC exhibited patterns similar to control intestinal MNC, being predominantly dimeric IgA with some monomeric IgA secreted. By contrast, intestinal MNC from patients with UC had a decreased proportion of dimeric IgA and increased proportion of monomeric IgA, thus indicating that IgA precursor B-cells may have migrated into the intestine from extraintestinal sites, or that the normal dimeric IgA-secreting cells in the intestine had begun secreting increased proportion of monomeric IgA as well. These studies indicate that homing patterns and/or immunoregulation of IgA-secreting cells are altered in human intestine, bone marrow, and autoimmune disease states.

REFERENCES

1. MacDermott, R. P., G. O. Franklin, K. M. Jenkins, I. J. Kodner, G. S. Nash & I. J. Weinrieb. 1980. Human intestinal mononuclear cells. I. Investigation of antibody-dependent, lectin-induced, and spontaneous cell-mediated cytotoxic capabilities. Gastroenterology **78:** 47–56.
2. MacDermott, R. P., M. J. Bragdon, K. M. Jenkins, G. O. Franklin, S. Shedlofsky & I. J. Kodner. 1981. Human intestinal mononuclear cells. II. Demonstration of a naturally occurring subclass of T-cells which respond in the allogeneic mixed leukocyte reaction but do not effect cell-mediated lympholysis. Gastroenterology **80:** 748–757.
3. Alley, C. D. & R. P. MacDermott. 1980. Investigation of the blastogenic and cytotoxic capabilities of human bone marrow: differences between aspirate and rib marrow. Blood **55:** 669–675.
4. Alley, C. D. & R. P. MacDermott. 1980. Separation and characterization of human bone marrow mononuclear cells from aspirates and ribs. J. Immunol. Methods **32:** 223–237.
5. MacDermott, R. P., G. S. Nash, M. J. Bertovich, M. V. Seiden, M. J. Bragdon & M. G. Beale. 1981. Alterations of IgM, IgG, and IgA synthesis and secretion by peripheral blood and intestinal mononuclear cells from patients with ulcerative colitis and Crohn's disease. Gastroenterology **81:** 844–852.
6. Beale, M. G., G. S. Nash, M. J. Bertovich & R. P. MacDermott. 1982. Similar disturbances in B cell activity and regulatory T cell function in Henoch-Schonlein purpura and systemic lupus erythematosus. J. Immunol. **128:** 486–491.
7. Nash, G. S., M. V. Seiden, M. G. Beale & R. P. MacDermott. 1982. A rapid miniaturized solid-phase radioimmunossay technique for secreted immunoglobulins, employing microtiter plates, antibody bound to polyacrylamide beads, and filter strip harvesting. J. Immunol. Methods **49:** 261–269.

8. MacDermott, R. P. & M. C. Stacey. 1981. Further characterization of the human autologous mixed leukocyte reaction (MLR). J. Immunol. **126:** 729–734.
9. Kutteh, W. H., S. J. Prince & J. Mestecky. 1982. Tissue origins of human polymeric and monomeric IgA. J. Immunol. **128:** 990–995.

DISCUSSION OF THE PAPER

J. Bienenstock (*McMaster University, Hamilton, Ontario, Canada*): Do you observe any differences in your results if bone marrow is obtained by aspiration or by curretage from ribs?

R. P. MacDermott (*Washington University, St. Louis, Mo.*): Dr. Good showed that if one aspirates more than 1 cc of bone marrow, the sample is significantly contaminated with peripheral blood.

R. A. Good (*Oklahoma Medical Research Foundation, Oklahoma City*): To obtain a sample of bone marrow that is functionally comparable to that obtained by a biopsy, you have to take aspirates as small as a tenth of a cubic centimeter. This situation is reflected in proliferative responses of the cells to phytohemagglutinin (PHA) and Con A. I do not think we can use aspiration of bone marrow, except as a crude approximation; we are mostly studying peripheral blood.

D. L. Delacroix (*Catholic University of Louvain, Brussels, Belgium*): Your studies of patients with Crohn's disease indicate that intestinal mononuclear cells from lamina propria secrete less IgA compared to normal individuals. You conclude that there might be some defect in homing of B-lymphocytes to gut mucosae in Crohn's disease that would explain lower IgA secretion. Did you determine the distribution of the Ig isotypes in cultured cells? In Crohn's disease, there is a marked change in the distribution of IgA and IgG cells in the lamina propria.

MacDermott: We have examined 13 specimens from patients with Crohn's disease for spontaneous secretion of immunoglobulins and we detect 3400 ng/ml IgA, 465 ng/ml IgM, and 584 ng/ml IgG. Therefore, IgA is secreted in greater quantities than in IgM or IgG in patients with Crohn's disease.

C. O. Elson (*Medical College of Virginia, Richmond, Va.*): It should be remembered that the yields of cells from the specimens of patients with Crohn's disease and also ulcerative colitis are three to four times larger then from a normal individual.

MacDermott: We have considered this factor. We have computed the results in terms of the numbers of cells, and we still see less IgA secreted per cell number or per gram of tissue than in the control specimens.

Elson: My question relates to the patients with lupus and Henoch-Schönlein purpura. If you take the patients' B-cells and mix them with normal T-cells, they no longer spontaneously synthesize immunoglobulins, but they stimulate with pokeweed mitogen. Have you mixed the patients' B-cells back with the patients' T-cells, and do they still show high spontaneous inhibition with pokeweed mitogen? In other words, did the cell separation affect the B-cells?

MacDermott: When you remove T-cells, you do not see spontaneous antibody synthesis by B-cells in normal controls. When, however, you remove the

T-cells from peripheral B-cells of these patients, you still see heightened spontaneous synthesis and secretion of antibodies. When you coculture B-cells with the patients' autologous T-cells, the altered pattern remains. When you coculture with normal allogeneic T-cells, then the pattern becomes reversed to normal.

ELSON: This situation may be a consequence of an acute phase reaction that we have never really realized before. Pneumonia and other diseases may exhibit a similar pattern of heightened synthesis of immunoglobulins. In other words, the B-cells, T-helper cells, and suppressors are all stimulated.

ORAL ROUTE AS METHOD FOR IMMUNIZING AGAINST MUCOSAL PATHOGENS

R. H. Waldman, Judy Stone, Valerie Lazzell, K.-Ch. Bergmann,
Rashida Khakoo, Arthur Jacknowitz, Steven Howard, and
Catherine Rose

School of Medicine
School of Pharmacy
West Virginia University
Morgantown, West Virginia 26506

The discipline of immunology developed in an attempt to prevent infectious diseases. Prevention has been extremely successful. The subdiscipline of secretory or mucosal immunology has not been nearly so successful in this regard, despite great progress in basic understanding of structure, cell traffic, and control. This aspect has been very disappointing, because soon after Hanson[1] and Tomasi[2] had demonstrated the presence and importance of secretory IgA, there was some hope for significant progress, recognizing that most infectious diseases enter the body through, or remain localized on, mucosal surfaces. It was generally assumed that local application of antigen was the best method for stimulation of a local antibody response, and several studies using different antigens and routes of administration supported this concept.[3-7]

Local immunization, however, by these various routes (nose drops, aerosol sprays, intravaginal applications) has many practical disadvantages. The concept of local immunization suggests that protection against respiratory pathogens would best result from aerosol delivery of vaccine. Local immunization against genital infections would certainly be inconvenient. Cooperative patients, highly trained personnel, and general acceptance is limited. Costly equipment is also required. In addition, there is the problem of attenuated versus inactivated viral vaccines. Trials suggest that live attenuated vaccines stimulate more solid immunity than do killed viral vaccines. This finding presents the problem that the virus must be attenuated sufficiently to cause few side effects, but still maintain immunogenicity. Additional concerns include the potential for reversion to virulence, and the problems of safety testing, storage, and stability.

The observation of Craig and Cebra[8] changed the thinking of many immunologists regarding the need to apply the antigen directly to the mucosal surface and supported the concept of a common mucosal defense system whereby an antigen that interacts with localized lymphoid tissue in the gut (gut-associated lymphoreticular tissue [GALT] or Peyer's patches) or in the respiratory tract (bronchial-associated lymphoreticular tissue [BALT]) will stimulate IgA-precursor cells that migrate to mucosal surfaces where they elaborate secretory IgA antibody specific for the initially sensitizing antigen. Such a concept, if confirmed in humans, could have a dramatic effect on immunization practices against many of the most important infectious diseases, including influenza and other respiratory viral pathogens, *Streptococcus pyogenes*, *S. mutans*, *Neisseria gonorrhea*, *Herpes simplex* virus, and *Chlamydia trachomatis*. Oral immunization to stimulate generally the secretory immune system might have many advantages, including effectiveness, safety, decreased side effects, cost, and potential for almost unlimited number and frequency of boosting.

510

0077-8923/83/0409-0510 $1.75/0 © 1983, NYAS

Despite the fact, however, that Craig and Cebra published their observation over ten years ago, very little in the way of application to infectious diseases protection has been attempted. Before this very modest amount of work is reviewed, it should be mentioned that general stimulation of mucosal antibodies has not been uniformly successful.

Oral immunization with live adenovirus vaccine in volunteers led to the development of sIgA coproantibodies and serum antibody, but no rise in nasal secretion sIgA antibody.[3,4] There are many hypothetical explanations for this "failure", but an explanation is beyond the scope of this paper, and one, or even a few, negative studies do not negate a theory.

There are also studies that suggest that local application of antigen is better at stimulating mucosal antibody. Ganguly *et al.*[5] demonstrated a significant rise in nasal antibody after intranasal application, but not after aerosol administration, of an attenuated rubella vaccine. This phenomenon has also been shown by Perkins *et al.*,[6] using a killed rhinovirus vaccine, and by Waldman *et al.*,[7] using a killed influenza virus vaccine. In the latter study, the vaccine was administered by nose

TABLE 1

ANTIBODY RESPONSE TO LIVE POLIO VACCINE ADMINISTERED ORALLY FOLLOWING PRIOR IMMUNIZATION OF DISTAL COLON[9]

Patient	Route of Immunization	Antibody Titer			
		Serum		Rectal	Pharyngeal
		IgG	IgA	IgA	IgA
No. 1	Baseline	32	0	0	0
	Colon	128	8	8	0
	Oral	256	8	8	8
No. 2	Baseline	0	0	0	0
	Colon	128	4	32	0
	Oral	256	8	16	8
No. 3	Baseline	8	0	0	0
	Colon	128	4	8	0
	Oral	256	4	16	4

drops or by aerosol, using particles of varying sizes. Small (1.5μ) particles elicited a strong sputum (lower respiratory) antibody response, whereas large particles $(40-100\mu)$ or nose drops, stimulated the best nasal antibody response. This finding suggested that local stimulation with antigen would only elicit antibody production in that limited area. That a more generalized secretory immune response was not seen may be attributable to limited amounts of lymphoid tissue present in the bronchi compared to that seen in the gut, that is, these findings may be a quantitative phenomenon.

Of particular interest is the study of Ogra *et al.*[9] in which 12 children with double-barrel colostomies were immunized in the distal colonic segment with live polio vaccine. Secretory IgA antibody was subsequently detected in the local segment of infected colon, but not in the other colonic limb or in nasal washings. Following closure of the colostomy, the polio vaccine was administered orally to three children. A significant sIgA response in the nasopharynx occurred (TABLE 1). The response of these three children could support the concept of a common mucosal defense system because nasal antibody followed oral administration. The lack of a nasal response following intracolonic immunization could again be

TABLE 2

SALIVARY IMMUNOGLOBULIN LEVELS, AGGLUTININ TITERS, AND EFFICACY OF ORAL IMMUNIZATION WITH S. MUTANS IN GNOTOBIOTIC RATS[10]

S. mutans Dose (CFU/gm)	Immunoglobulin Level (mg/ml)		Agglutinin Titer	Plaque Score
	IgG	IgA		
10^7	0.14	0.36	3.2	7.4
10^8	0.13	0.27	3.6	7.0
10^9	0.10	0.10	0.9	12.6
Infected only	0.08	0.08	0.3	15.1
Control	0.08	0.06	0	0

a quantitative phenomenon, that is, less GALT in the lower intestines as compared to the upper intestines.

Turning to the few promising studies relative to immunization against pathogens, Michalek et al.[10-11] have worked with Streptococcus mutans, the most important organism causing dental caries. In their rat model, they have shown that sIgA can be induced following ingestion of the killed organism and that, on subsequent rechallenge, these rats were protected against caries formation (TABLE 2). They also found that the magnitude of the response was dependent on antigen dose, and at least in gnotobiotic rats, high dose unresponsiveness was seen. In addition, protection was afforded against cross-reacting serotypes, and therefore, a lowly virulent strain could be used to elicit antibodies and protection against a highly virulent strain.

McGhee et al.[12] extended these observations to humans. A small group of volunteers were fed S. mutans, and within one week of ingestion, specific IgA antibodies were detected in both saliva and tears (TABLE 3). This observation has great potential in terms of caries prophylaxis.

Similar studies were recently conducted with a viral antigen. Mice were immunized against the influenza virus by various routes. An immunization schedule of three doses at fourteen day intervals was used. One week later the mice were exposed to an aerosol challenge of the live virus suspension. After two days the animals were sacrificed; bronchial lavage and blood samples were obtained. The cellularity of lavage fluid is a sensitive measure of intensity of infection, thus, lower cell counts correlate with protection. All of the nonparenteral routes showed significant, and almost identical protection against infection (TABLE 4). This finding correlated with the level of respiratory secretion antibody elicited by the immunization (TABLE 5), with respiratory antibody production being poorly stimulated by subcutaneous immunization, and being optimally

TABLE 3

AGGLUTININ TITERS IN HUMAN SALIVA FOLLOWING ORAL IMMUNIZATION WITH S. MUTANS

Period	Subject	1	2	3	4
Preimmunization		1	<1	1	1
Peak primary		5	4	3	6
Post primary		3	3	2	3
Peak secondary		10	7	8	9
Post secondary		5	3	5	5

TABLE 4

TOTAL CELL YIELD FROM LUNGS OF IMMUNIZED BALB/C MICE AND CONTROL ANIMALS
TWO DAYS AFTER INFECTION (AEROSOL CHALLENGE) WITH LIVE INFLUENZA VIRUS*

Group	Number	No. of Nucleated Cells × 10³		
		x̄†	S.E.‡	p
Controls				
no challenge	8	202	33	—
challenge	10	424	119	0.02
Nasal	10	213	39	N.S.
Oral	9	234	40	N.S.
Rectal	10	266	47	N.S.

*Mouse lungs lavaged with 4.5 ml phosphate buffered saline.
†x̄ = Mean
‡S.E. = Standard error

stimulated by intranasal immunization. There was no correlation between the titers of serum antibodies and hemagglutination inhibition titers in the lavage fluid.

With the encouraging results in the animal studies, we undertook a small pilot study with humans. Twenty-four young adult volunteers participated in a double-blind controlled study, in which they received either vaccine or placebo, administered orally or parenterally. The vaccine was the commercially available trivalent killed influenza vaccine consisting of 7 μg of hemagglutinin of each of A/Brazil/78 (H1N1), A/Bangkok/79 (H3N2), and B/Singapore-79. The vaccine was formulated in an enteric-coated capsule also containing D-xylose, which was used as a marker to ensure that the capsules dissolved in the small intestine. The dose of vaccine was ten capsules each morning for seven consecutive days, each capsule containing 7 μg of hemagglutinin of each antigen. Serum and nasal wash specimens were obtained as a baseline and at three weeks postvaccination. Antibody titers to A/Bangkok/79 (H3N2) were determined by hemagglutination inhibition in the serum and by the plaque reduction neutralization test in the nasal wash specimens. The pre- and postvaccination samples were simultaneously tested, in duplicate, by an investigator who was blinded with respect to the identity and immunization status of the volunteer whose specimens were being tested.

Oral immunization led to the production of nasal secretory antibody with a similar frequency and magnitude to that of the intramuscular vaccine group.

TABLE 5

RESULTS OF HEMAGGLUTINATION INHIBITION TESTS IN MICE AFTER DIFFERENT
IMMUNIZATION PROCEDURES WITH INFLUENZA VIRUS (A/PR/8/34)

Group	Number of animals	Mean Serum Antibody Titer	Lung Lavage Fluid* Percent With Detectable Antibody	Statistical Significance
Control	20	<1:10	5	—
Nasal	10	1:40	60	0.01
Oral	18	1:15	44	0.01
Rectal	20	1:20	40	0.05

*Lavage fluid after 20× concentration

TABLE 6

NASAL ANTIBODY RISE

Group	Mean Titer*		No. with Rise	
	pre-immunization	Three Week	≥2 fold	≥4 fold
Placebo	41	3	0	0
Intramuscular	105	373	6	4
Oral	59	116	5	4

*Reciprocal of arithmetic mean of 50% plaque reduction/IgA (mg/ml).

There was at least a four-fold rise in titer in 50% of both the oral and intramuscular vaccine recipients and at least a two-fold rise in titer in 75% of the volunteers in the parenteral vaccine group and in 63% of the volunteers in the oral vaccine group. The mean rise in titer was 2.0 in the oral group as compared to 3.6 for the intramuscular group (TABLE 6). Serum antibody, however, was not stimulated by oral vaccination, although it was stimulated in the intramuscular vaccine group, where a mean two-fold rise in titer was seen (TABLE 7). There were also no side effects following oral vaccination with influenza, compared to controls, in contrast to the experience with parenteral vaccination, where mild to moderate discomfort is common, and is a deterent to immunization.

A comparable antibody response was elicited after oral or parenteral immunization in nasal secretions, although a systemic antibody response was not stimulated by ingestion of the antigen. The lack of serum antibody response supports the concept of GALT, and suggests that there was local synthesis of secretory IgA in response to ingested antigen. This finding is significant, as a number of studies[13,14] have shown that secretory antibody correlates better with protection against viral infections of mucosal surfaces than does serum antibody. This finding may also be quite useful, as it would avoid potentially severe immune complex reactions, as occasionally occurs after parenteral respiratory syncytial virus vaccination, for example. On the other hand, if the secretory antibody failed as the body's "first line of defense", the lack of serum antibody could prove to be harmful.

Despite these concerns, oral vaccination has many advantages. A killed organism, as in the influenza study, could be used, eliminating the difficulties in developing an attenuated vaccine or concerns over possible reversion to virulence. Oral vaccines would not need to be highly purified, which would greatly simplify preparation. They would be easy and inexpensive to administer, and because of the relative absence of side effects, would be far more acceptable to

TABLE 7

SERUM ANTIBODY RESPONSE

Group	Mean Titer*		No. with >4 Fold Rise
	pre-immunization	Three Week	
Placebo	65	71	0
Intramuscular	54	93	3
Oral	59	49	0

*Reciprocal of arithmetic mean of hemagglutination inhibition titer

patients. This last point is especially important to consider when comparing oral immunization to other vaccination routes. The production of fever, diarrhea, runny nose, malaise, and sore arm associated with the parenteral vaccine are strong deterents, particularly when considering vaccination of chronically ill adults, children, and the elderly. Thus, oral immunization, by providing secretory antibody stimulation without the adverse effects associated with parenteral vaccination, may prove to be a far superior route of immunization.

SUMMARY

In the past three decades significant strides have been made in attempts at nonparenteral immunization. Appreciation of the importance of secretory immunity led to attempts to stimulate antibody production locally. The vaccines developed against respiratory pathogens as a result of this new knowledge have many practical limitations, such as the need for highly trained personnel, expensive equipment, very cooperative recipients for intranasal or aerosol administration, and a vaccine that is both adequately attenuated, immunogenic, and stable during storage. With recognition of the presence of a common mucosal defense system, new approaches to vaccine development have become possible. Oral immunization, by stimulating GALT, presents a promising approach for protecting many secretory surfaces against a variety of infectious agents. Recently, emphasis has been placed on developing an oral vaccine against *S. mutans*. McGhee *et al.* have demonstrated antibody to *S. mutans* in saliva and tears following oral ingestion of that antigen, without a rise in serum antibody, in both humans and rats. The rats were afforded protection from caries after rechallenge with both the original and cross-reacting serotypes of *S. mutans*. Similar results have recently been seen with viral antigens. Mice have been shown to have significant protection against influenza infection following oral immunization. And in a pilot study with human volunteers, the secretory antibody response in nasal washes was similar following either oral or parenteral vaccination.

Oral immunization may prove to be far superior to parenteral vaccination against a variety of pathogens, because of fewer side effects and greater ease in vaccine preparation and administration.

REFERENCES

1. HANSON, L. A. 1961. Comparative immunological studies of the immunoglobulins of human milk and blood serum. Arch. Allergy Appl. Immun. **18:** 241–267.
2. TOMASI, T. B., S. D. ZIGELBAUM. 1963. The selective occurrence of α A globulins in certain body fluids. J. Clin. Invest. **42:** 1552–1560.
3. SCOTT, R. H., B. A. DUDDING, S. V. ROMANO & P. H. RUSSELL. 1972. Enteric immunization with live adenovirus type 21 vaccine: II. Systemic and local immune responses following immunization. Infect. Immun. **5(3):** 300–304.
4. SCHWARTZ A. R., Y. TOYO & R. B. HORNICK. 1974. Clinical evaluation of live, oral types 1, 2, and 5 adenovirus vaccines. Amer. Rev. Respir. Dis. **109:** 233–238.
5. GANGULY, R., P. L. OGRA, S. REGAS & R. H. WALDMAN. 1973. Rubella immunization of volunteers via the respiratory tract. Infect. Immun. **8:** 497–502.
6. PERKINS, J. C., D. TUCKER, H. L. S. KNOPF, R. P. WENZEL, R. B. HORNICK, A. Z. KAPIKIAN & R. M. CHANOCK. 1969. Evidence for protective effect of an inactivated rhinovirus vaccine administered by the nasal route. Am. J. Epidemiol. **90(4):** 319–326.

7. WALDMAN, R. H., S. H. WOOD, E. J. TORRES & P. A. SMALL. 1970. Influenza antibody response following aerosol administration of inactivated virus. Am. J. Epidemiol. **91:** 575–584.

8. CRAIG, S. W. & J. J. CEBRA. 1971. Peyer's patches: an enriched source of precursors for IgA-producing immunocytes in the rabbit. J. Exp. Med. **134:** 188–200.

9. OGRA, P. & D. KARZON. 1969. Distribution of poliovirus antibody in serum, nasopharynx, and alimentary tract following sequential immunization of lower alimentary tract with polio vaccine. J. Immunol. **102**(6): 1423–1430.

10. MICHALEK, S. M., J. R. MCGHEE, & J. L. BABB. 1978. Effective immunity to dental caries: dose dependent studies of secretory immunity by oral administration of *Streptococcus mutans* to rats. Infect. Immun. **19**(1)217–224.

11. MICHALEK, S. M., J. R. MCGHEE, R. R. ARNOLD & J. MESTECKY. 1978. Effective immunity to dental caries: selective induction of secretory immunity by oral administration of *Streptococcus mutans* in rodents. Adv. Exp. Med. Biol. **107:** 261–269.

12. MCGHEE, J. R., J. MESTECKY, R. R. ARNOLD, S. H. MICHALEK, S. J. PRINCE & J. L. BABB. 1978. Induction of secretory antibody in humans following ingestion of *Streptococcus mutans*. Adv. Exp. Med. Biol. **107:** 177–184.

13. CATE, T. R., R. D. ROSSEN, R. G. DOUGLAS, W. T. BUTLER & R. B. COUCH. 1966. The role of nasal secretion and serum antibody in the rhinovirus common cold. Am. J. Epidemiol. **84:** 352–363.

14. SMITH, C. B., R. H. PURCELL, J. A. BELLANTI & R. M. CHANOCK. 1966. Protective effect of antibody to parainfluenza type 1 virus. N. Engl. J. Med. **275:** 1145–1152.

CELLULAR DETERMINANTS OF MAMMARY CELL-MEDIATED IMMUNITY IN THE RAT: KINETICS OF LYMPHOCYTE SUBSET ACCUMULATION IN THE RAT MAMMARY GLAND DURING PREGNANCY AND LACTATION*

Michael J. Parmely and Linda S. Manning

Department of Microbiology
University of Kansas Medical Center
Kansas City, Kansas 66103

INTRODUCTION

IgA-secreting plasma cells are a natural component of the mouse mammary gland and constitute the predominant immunoglobulin-secreting cell type present during the early postpartum period.[1-4] Two observations have provided strong evidence that a common pool of circulating mucosal B-cells provide the precursors for IgA-secreting plasma cells in the gland and that this pool is shared by the mouse mammary gland and small intestine. First, adoptive transfer studies indicate that the lactating gland is receptive to immigrating IgA⁺ B-lymphoblasts, especially those derived from gut-associated lymphoreticular tissues like the mesenteric lymph nodes (MLN).[2-4] Second, intestinal immunization in the mouse is an effective means of eliciting mammary secretory immunity[5,6] that again apparently depends on the migration of antigen-specific B-lymphoblasts along the entero-mammary axis.[6]

We have recently attempted to extend the concept of a shared pool of mucosae-seeking precursors to the study of mucosal T-cells and have chosen the rat mammary gland as a model. When labeled with ³H-thymidine (³H-TdR) and adoptively transferred to lactating syngeneic recipients, MLN and cervical lymph node (CLN) T-lymphoblasts demonstrated equal affinities for the mammary gland. We tentatively concluded from this observation that, in the rat, mammary gland T-cells were derived from peripheral as well as intestinal lymphoid tissues. An alternative interpretation would be that mucosal T-cells simply fail to migrate to the mammary gland in significant numbers and that the mammary gland lacks a significant T-cell component.

Studies of this nature emphasize the need for more information about the behavior of mucosal T-lymphocytes and their interactions with B-cells bearing cytoplasmic IgA (cIgA). Therefore the experiments performed earlier[7,8] and described herein were designed to answer the following general questions relating to this topic. Can significant numbers of cIgA⁺ B-cells, T-cells, and T-helper cells be found in the rat mammary gland, and how do their frequencies compare with those observed in the small intestine? What are the patterns of appearance of T- and B-cell subsets in the developing rat mammary gland during pregnancy and lactation and how do the two cell types differ in this regard? What evidence exists that mammary lymphocytes are derived from exogenous lym-

*This work was supported in part by National Institutes of Health Grants HD11787 and RR05373.

phoid tissues? Do gut-associated lymphoreticular tissues contain greater numbers of mammary lymphocyte precursors than peripheral lymphoreticular tissues? Is there a common mucosal immune system in the rat (as has been described for cIgA+ B-cells in the mouse) that serves as a source of mammary T- and B-cells?

We have taken a traditional experimental approach to these problems (immunofluorescence and adoptive transfer experiments) and have used a series of monoclonal antibodies to rat T-cells and the T-helper/inducer subset first described by Williams et al.[9,10] (so-called W3/13 and W3/25, respectively). Results of these studies indicate that the rat mammary gland collects T-, T-helper, and cIgA+ B-cells in quantities approximately one-fourth to one-third the levels seen in the small intestine (ileum). Adoptive transfer experiments suggest that many of the lymphocytes in the mammary gland are not directly derived from exogenous lymphoid sources, as appears to be the case with the small intestine. From this information, we are proposing that the rat lacks a common mucosal immune system of the type seen in the mouse, and instead, accumulates lymphocytes within the mammary gland by drawing on mucosal and peripheral circulating cell pools. We further hypothesize that mammary cIgA+ B-cells undergo extensive expansion in number within the local environment of the gland, and that this cellular proliferation is dependent on T-cells.

MATERIALS AND METHODS

Animals

Inbred female Fisher strain rats weighing 150–200g were obtained from Charles River (Wilmington, Mass.) or Microbiological Associates (Bethesda, Md.) and maintained at the University of Kansas Medical Center Animal Care Facilities. For studies requiring pregnant or lactating animals, Fisher females were mated with Dark Agouti (DA) males and were used as cell recipients during pregnancy, lactation, or weaning. Lactating recipients were left with their litters throughout the experiments. For the studies requiring postweaning recipients, the litters were removed at 20 days postpartum, and the females were used as cell recipients 5–9 days later.

Timed matings were performed for the studies requiring antepartum recipients. By this procedure, Fisher females were housed with DA males overnight and vaginal smears were checked the following morning for the presence of spermatozoa. If positive, the females were designated as day 21 antepartum and used as T-cell recipients during mid (5–9 days antepartum) or late (2–4 days antepartum) gestation.

Preparation and Labeling of Cell Suspensions

Mesenteric and cervical lymph node cells used in adoptive transfer experiments were prepared from syngeneic virgin female donors as previously described.[7] Mesenteric and cervical T-lymphocytes were prepared by our modification of the nylon wool adherence method of Julius et al.[11] Donor cells were labeled with ^{3}H-TdR (s.a. = 6 Ci/mmol; Schwartz-Mann, Orangeburg, N.Y.) by incubating them at a concentration of 5×10^7 cells/ml for 90 minutes at 37° C in Hanks Balanced Salt Solution (BSS) containing 10% calf serum and 25 μCi ^{3}H-TdR/ml.

In Vivo *Distribution of Adoptively Transferred Radiolabeled Cells*

Virgin, pregnant (5–9 day or 2–4 day antepartum), lactating (1–5 day or 9–12 day postpartum) or weaned (5–9 day post-weaning) female recipients were injected with 2–4 × 10^8 radiolabeled cells from syngeneic virgin female donors. The in vivo distribution of these donor cells was determined by two techniques: liquid scintillation counting (LSC) of solubilized recipient tissues[7] or autoradiography. For the latter technique, samples of tissues were quickly frozen in liquid nitrogen and sectioned to 4–7 μ thickness on a microtome (Cryostat II, American Optical, Buffalo, N.Y.), thaw-mounted on methanol-cleaned, gelatin-coated slides (1% gelatin, 1% chromium potassium sulfate) and stored for up to two weeks at $-20°$ C. The slides were dipped in photographic emulsion (NTB-2 or NTB-3, Eastman-Kodak, Rochester, N.Y.) that had been preheated to $40°$ C and diluted with an equal volume of 1% filtered detergent (Dreft) solution. After drying at room temperature, the slides were placed in light-tight slide boxes and stored at $4°$ C. After one to three days exposure, the slides were developed in Dektol (Eastman-Kodak). An entire experiment was dipped and developed at the same time. Slides were examined by light microscopy for the presence of labeled cells, and the data was expressed as the proportion of radiolabeled cells (cell smears), having counted at least one hundred cells, labeled cells/100 high powered field (HPF) (tissue sections), or percent injected labeled cells/10^3 HPF (×10^3). The last method allowed a correction for variations in the number of labeled cells injected based on differences in labeling indices of different cell populations. This approach also permitted a direct comparison of results in autoradiography to those obtained by liquid scintillation counting.

^{3}H-TdR-labeled cells were deposited on gelatin-coated microscope slides by cytocentrifugation, dipped in emulsion and developed together with tissue sections from the same experiments. These slides were then used to determine the percentage of radiolabeled lymphoblasts in a preparation and to determine T- and B-cell markers among radiolabeled cells (see *Combined immunofluorescence and autoradiography*). Cell inocula and tissue sections from paired animals receiving MLN or CLN cells were always assayed on the same day.

Antibodies

Rabbit anti-rat IgM, goat anti-rabbit IgG, rabbit anti-goat IgG, and rabbit anti-mouse IgG were obtained from Miles Laboratories (Elkhart, Ind.) or prepared in our laboratories. Rabbit anti-rat IgA was purchased from Nordic Immunological Laboratories (San Clemente, Calif.). Monoclonal W3/13 mouse anti-rat T-cell and W3/25 mouse anti-rat T-helper cell antibodies were obtained from Accurate Chemical and Scientific Corp. (Hicksville, N.Y.). Goat anti-rabbit IgG, rabbit anti-goat IgG, and an Fab$_2'$ fragment of rabbit anti-mouse IgG were conjugated with fluorescein isothiocyanate (FITC) according to the method of Beutner.[12] All antisera were heat inactivated ($56°$ C for 30 minutes) and centrifuged (135,000 × g for 60 minutes) before use. Aliquots were stored at $-70°$ C.

Indirect Immunofluorescence

The optimum concentration of each antiserum was determined by titration on control cells and tissues and varied depending on the lot used. For tissue immunofluorescence, cryostat sections of rat tissues were fixed in acetone for 10 minutes at room temperature and rinsed in phosphate-buffered saline (PBS). Twenty-five to 50 μl of an optimum concentration of the various antibodies (anti-IgM, anti-IgA, W3/13, or W3/25) was applied to each section and allowed to incubate for 30 minutes at room temperature in a moist chamber. The slides were then rinsed in PBS and washed twice for 15 minutes each at room temperature. The optimum concentration of the appropriate fluorescenated antibody was then applied and allowed to incubate an additional 30 minutes. Again the slides were washed and coverslips were applied with 80% glycerol in phosphate buffered saline. Control tissue sections were exposed to PBS and the fluorescenated antibodies alone. Sections were scored for the number of fluorescent cells/100 HPF at 400× magnification. Cytocentrifuge cell smears were similarly treated and scored as a percentage of total cells. Cell inocula and tissue sections from animals receiving MLN or CLN cells were always assayed on the same day.

Combined Immunofluorescence and Autoradiography

Frozen tissue sections and cell suspensions deposited on slides by cytocentrifugation were processed for indirect immunofluorescence as described. The slides were then fixed in acetone for 10 seconds and processed for autoradiography as described above. After exposure for one to four days, the slides were developed, coverslips were applied, and the sections were examined with a fluorescent microscope. Radiolabeled cells were located using the dark field optics, and the fluorescent nature of these cells was determined by changing to fluorescence optics. Five hundred to 2000 HPF (400× magnification) were scored for each tissue, and recipients of MLN or CLN were studied simultaneously.

Fluorescence Microscopy

Tissue sections and cell smears were examined for cells bearing surface or cytoplasmic antigens (IgM, IgA, W3/13, or W3/25) using appropriate fluorescein-conjugated reagents (see Antibodies) and a Zeiss fluorescence microscope equipped with an HBO 200 mercury light source. Routinely, 200–500 cells in cytocentrifuge smears or 500–2000 HPF (400× magnification) of each tissue were examined.

Statistical Analysis

Calculations of the means and standard deviations (S.D.) was performed and p values were determined by nonpaired, two-tailed Student's t-test. A significance level of $p < 0.01$ was used throughout.

RESULTS

The Natural Accumulation of Lymphocyte Subsets in the Rat Mammary Gland during Pregnancy, Lactation, and Weaning

Weisz-Carrington et al.[1] have reported that cIgA+ B-cells begin to appear in the mouse mammary gland during pregnancy and reach a maximum density late in lactation (20 days postpartum). To ascertain whether a similar pattern exists in the rat, cryostat sections of mammary glands and small intestines were prepared from Fisher rats at various stages of gestation or lactation and examined by indirect immunofluorescence with antibodies specific for IgA. A pattern of appearance of cIgA⁺ cells similar to that described for the mouse was observed in rat tissues (FIGURE 1).

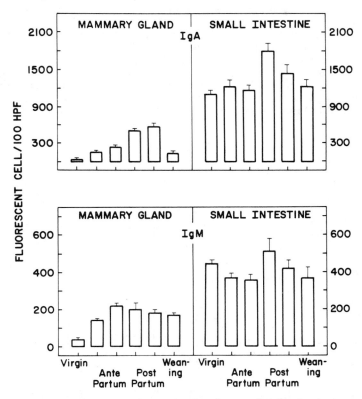

FIGURE 1. The natural accumulation of B-lymphocytes by the developing mammary gland. Mammary tissues were recovered from virgin, pregnant, lactating, or post-weaning Fisher strain female rats (see METHODS AND MATERIALS). Indirect immunofluorescence was performed on cryostat sections to enumerate cIgA⁺ or cIgM⁺ cells. Results are expressed as the means ±1 S.D. of the number of fluorescent cells/100 HPF (400× magnification). There were 5-6 animals tested in each group.

Cells bearing cytoplasmic IgA appeared in significant numbers by the thirteenth day of gestation and continued to increase in frequency throughout lactation to reach maximum levels by the second postpartum week. At this time, they were approximately one third as frequent as cIgA⁺ cells in the same animals' small intestines. Within a week after removing the sucklings, the frequency of cIgA⁺ cells in mammary tissues returned to levels comparable to those seen in virgin control animals.

Cells bearing cytoplasmic IgM were also present in the mammary glands and small intestines, albeit in lower numbers than cIgA+ cells. The appearance of cIgM+ cells in mammary tissues also paralleled glandular development, but preceded the expression of IgA among the lymphoid cells. Except for a transient increase during the first postpartum week, the density of B-cells in the small intestine bearing either IgM or IgA remained constant throughout the study period. Thus the development of the mammary gland leading to lactation was accompanied by an increase in the density of B-lymphocytes bearing IgM and/or IgA.

FIGURE 2 depicts the results of similar experiments performed to monitor stage-dependent changes in the frequencies of T-lymphocytes (W3/13+) or the T-helper (inducer) subset (W3/25+) in these two mucosal tissues. The density of T-cells remained constant within the intestine throughout this period at approximately seven W3/13+ cells per high powered field. This fact represents a frequency approximately half that of IgA+ cells in this organ in pregnant and lactating rats. The number of intestinal cells bearing membrane W3/25 antigens was also constant throughout this period, totalling approximately three cells per

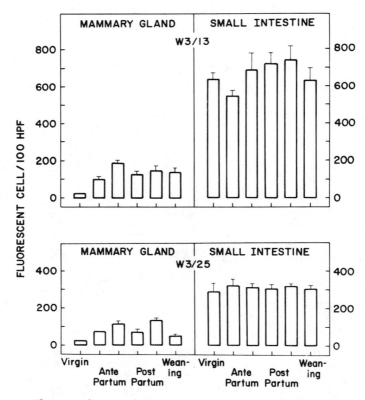

FIGURE 2. The natural accumulation of T-lymphocytes by the developing mammary gland. Indirect immunofluorescence was used to enumerate T-cells (W3/13) and T-helper cells (W3/25). See FIGURE 1.

TABLE 1

ANATOMICAL DISTRIBUTION OF T- AND B-LYMPHOCYTES WITHIN THE LACTATING RAT
MAMMARY GLAND*

Surface or Cytoplasmic Antigen	Tissue Distribution (Percent)			
	Intralobular Connective Tissue	Subepithelium	Epithelium	Alveolar Lumen
cIgA†	6 ± 4	84 ± 4	9 ± 5	1 ± 1
W3/13	3 ± 2	61 ± 8	32 ± 8	5 ± 2

*Mammary tissue was obtained from five lactating rats (6–10 days postpartum) and examined by indirect immunofluorescence for the location of IgA⁺ and W3/13⁺ cells.

†At this stage of lactation the densities of IgA⁺ and W3/13⁺ cells in the mammary gland were approximately 5 and 1.3 cells/HPF, respectively.

high powered field. In other words, approximately 40% of all T-cells in the intestines of these animals were W3/25⁺.

In the mammary gland, T-cells (W3/13⁺) reached maximum numbers late in gestation and then, unlike cIgA⁺ cells in the tissue, declined slightly with the onset of lactation. The T-inducer subset (W3/25⁺) showed a similar pattern, again declining in the early stages of lactation. By contrast to the small intestine, 70% of the T-cells in the mammary gland during gestation and early lactation and over 90% of T-cells during late lactation bore the W3/25 antigen (i.e., presumably belonged to the T-inducer subset[10]). Thus T-cells in the developing rat mammary gland reached maximum density by parturition when they were half as frequent as IgA⁺ cells and consisted primarily of the T-inducer subset.

Whereas over 80% of the IgA-containing B-cells were distributed within the subepithelium of the lactating mammary gland, 37% of the T-lymphocytes within this tissue were found either in the epithelial layer of alveoli or alveolar lumens. Intraepithelial as well as intraluminal T-cells showed membrane fluorescence typical of W3/13-binding cells in control tissues (periarteriolar lymphoid sheaths of the spleen, diffuse cortex of lymph nodes, intestinal mucosa, and Peyer's patches). Cells bearing cytoplasmic IgA were also seen in alveolar lumens, although they constituted a minor proportion (1%) of the total cIgA⁺ cells in the gland. Nonetheless, the number of intraluminal IgA-bearing cells was comparable to the number of W3/13⁺ cells found in alveolar lumens. Morphological assessment by fluorescence microscopy has not been sufficient to determine the nature of the intraluminal IgA⁺ cells, and for example, we cannot currently determine the contribution of milk macrophages[13] to these numbers (TABLE 1).

Mesenteric and Cervical Lymph Node Cells Have a Similar Affinity for the Lactating Mammary Gland

We have reported that, unlike the mouse,[2] rat MLN and CLN cells evidence equal potentials for migrating to the mammary gland throughout lactation.[7] Similar findings are reported in TABLE 2. Four pairs of lactating recipients (6–12 days post-partum) were injected intravenously with $2-4 \times 10^8$ ³H-TdR-labeled MLN or CLN cells. Twenty to twenty-four hours later, samples of tissues were recovered from the recipients and either quickly frozen in liquid nitrogen and sectioned on a cryostat or solubilized and prepared for liquid scintillation

TABLE 2

MIGRATION OF ³H-THYMIDINE-LABELED MLN AND CLN CELLS TO THE MAMMARY
GLANDS AND SMALL INTESTINES OF ADOPTIVE LACTATING RECIPIENTS: LIQUID
SCINTILLATION COUNTING VS. AUTORADIOGRAPHY

Technique	Radiolabeled Donor Cells	Recipient Tissue	
		Mammary Gland	Small Intestine
LSC†	MLN	0.26 ± 0.11*	7.00 ± 0.59
	CLN	0.27 ± 0.09	1.51 ± 0.44
	MLN:CLN‡	0.96	4.64
Autoradiography§	MLN	0.48 ± 0.13	7.52 ± 4.16
	CLN	0.30 ± 0.13	0.12 ± 0.04
	MLN:CLN	1.60	62.7

*Data represents $\overline{X}$ ± S.D.; n = 4

†LSC (liquid scintillation counting) data is expressed as percent injected radioactivity/g recipient tissue to adjust for differences in organ weights.

‡Ratio of activities in MLN recipient to CLN recipient tissues.

§Autoradiography data is expressed as percent injected labeled lymphoblasts/10^3 HPF ($\times 10^3$) so that comparisons could be made with LSC data, (see METHODS AND MATERIALS).

counting. The histological sections were subjected to autoradiography and analyzed for the frequency of radiolabeled donor cells.

The two techniques provided similar results. Radiolabeled MLN cells migrated to the small intestine of adoptive recipients in far greater numbers than did CLN cells. Nearly 5 times as much radioactivity and 60 times as many labeled cells were seen in the ileums of animals receiving MLN cells as compared to their CLN counterparts. This fact suggested that the principal source of lymphocytes in the small intestines of lactating rats was lymph nodes draining the intestine rather than peripheral lymphoid tissues.

By contrast, cells prepared from MLN or CLN had equal affinities for the mammary gland, regardless of the technique used to measure cell migration. Thus, substantial differences were seen between the cells localizing in the small intestines versus those found in the mammary glands. The former tended to favor donor gut-associated lymphoreticular cells, whereas the latter did not differentiate between the two populations. Moreover, these data suggest that a substandial proportion of mammary lymphocytes may be derived from exogenous sources.

The Migratory Patterns of Enriched T-Cell Populations Mimic the Natural Patterns of Accumulation of These Cells by Mucosal Tissues

We were next interested in determining whether a portion of the T-lymphocytes that appeared in the mammary gland during gestation and lactation (FIGURE 2) were potentially derived from exogenous sources. We reasoned that if this situation were the case, the patterns of CLN and MLN T-cell migration in adoptive pregnant or lactating recipients should parallel the natural course of appearance of T-cells in the organ during these periods.

Mesenteric and cervical lymph node T-lymphocytes were enriched by nylon wool adherence and contained >91% W3/13⁺, <1% IgA⁺, and <1% IgM⁺ cells.

Two to four hundred million ^{3}H-TdR-labeled T-enriched cells were then injected intravenously into syngeneic recipients. Recipients were either in midgestation (5–9 days antepartum), late gestation (2–4 days antepartum), early lactation (1–5 days postpartum), mid-lactation (9–12 days postpartum), or 5–9 days post-weaning. Tissue samples were recovered 20–24 hours after cell transfer, and radioactivity was determined by solubilization and liquid scintillation counting. The data, reported in FIGURES 3 and 4, is presented as a log of the ratio of radioactivity found in lactating recipients divided by that seen in virgin controls. This statistic has the advantage of depicting decreased cell migration to an organ with the same magnitude as increased cell accumulation.

It is apparent that the principal change in T-cell migration that accompanied

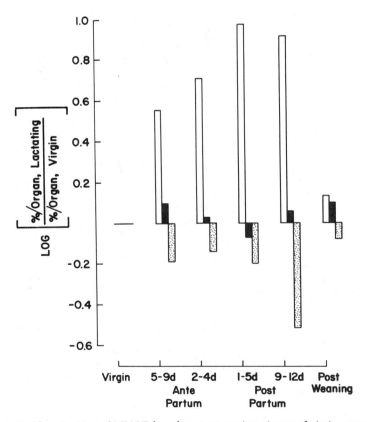

FIGURE 3. The migration of MLN T-lymphocytes to various tissues of virgin, pregnant, or lactating rats. Data is expressed as the log of the ratio of percent injected radioactivity/organ in pregnant or lactating recipients to that seen in virgin controls. Open bars = mammary glands; shaded bars = small intestines; stipled bars = lungs. T-cell migration to the mammary gland during gestation and lactation was significantly greater (p < 0.01) than that seen in virgin controls. The lungs accumulated significantly fewer cells (p < 0.01) at midlactation than did controls.

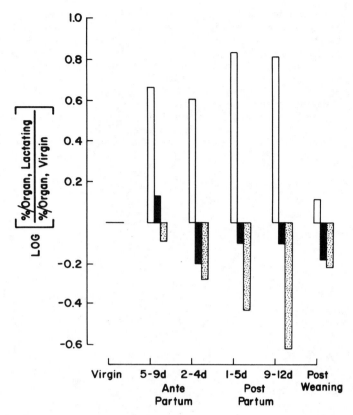

FIGURE 4. The migration of CLN T-lymphocytes to various tissues of virgin, pregnant, or lactating rats. See FIGURE 3. T-cell migration to the mammary gland during gestation and lactation was significantly greater (p < 0.01) than that seen in virgin controls. The lungs accumulated significantly fewer cells (p < 0.01) at midlactation than did controls.

gestation and lactation in these animals was a marked increase in accumulation by the mammary gland. Seven to ten times as many lymph node T-cells were retained by the gland during the first postpartum week than was seen in virgin animals. Moreover, the perinatal patterns, which essentially depict changes in receptivity of the mammary gland to migrating cells, were comparable for both T-cell sources (FIGURES 3 and 4) and were very similar in the prenatal period to the changes in host T-cell numbers (FIGURE 2).

Immediately following parturition, host W3/13+ cells declined somewhat in the gland (FIGURE 2), whereas migration studies (FIGURES 3 and 4) indicated that the mammary gland was, in fact, slightly more receptive to immigrating T-lymphoblasts. Overall these results suggest that mammary T-cells that appear in the gland in the perinatal period may be derived from exogenous tissue sites. If this is indeed the case, there is no reason to conclude that mucosal T-cells (such as those from MLN) have a selective affinity for the mammary gland.

The Mammary Gland and Small Intestine Derive Lymphoblasts from Different Circulating Pools

The T-cell-enriched populations prepared by nylon wool adherence and studied longitudinally throughout pregnancy and lactation (FIGURES 3 and 4) were >91% W3/13$^+$, <1% IgM$^+$, and <1% IgA$^+$. Since ^{3}H-TdR, however, labels a cycling lymphoblast subset within these MLN and CLN T-cell populations, we felt it was essential to determine the purity of the labeled subset. Contamination by a few radiolabeled cIgA$^+$ lymphoblasts might not be detected by immunofluorescence analysis of the entire cell population. To accomplish this analysis, ^{3}H-TdR-labeled MLN or CLN cells were deposited on microscope slides by cytocentrifugation, exposed to fluorescent antibodies (W3/13, W3/25, anti-IgM, and anti-IgA) and dipped in photographic emulsion. After three days exposure, the slides were developed and examined for the proportion of fluorescent cells, radiolabeled cells, and fluorescent/radiolabeled cells. Results are shown in TABLE 3 and demonstrate that nylon wool adherence efficiently depleted noncycling B-cells (IgM$^+$ or IgA$^+$), thereby enriching the T-cell population. An unexpected finding was the substantial number of IgA$^+$ and IgM$^+$ cells among the radiolabeled subset of nylon nonadherent cells. Thus IgA$^+$ B-lymphoblasts apparently were not adherent to nylon wool, and only partial depletion of IgM$^+$ lymphoblasts was realized. Because lymphoblasts bearing intracytoplasmic IgA

TABLE 3

T- AND B-CELL MARKERS DETECTED ON ^{3}H-THYMIDINE-LABELED LYMPHOBLASTS FROM MLN AND CLN AND T-LYMPHOCYTE PREPARATIONS FROM THESE NODES

Cell Preparation*	Percent Total Cells Bearing:†				Percent ^{3}H-TdR‡	Percent ^{3}H-TdR-Labeled Cells Bearing:§			
	W3/13	W3/25	cIgA	cIgM		W3/13	W3/25	cIgA	cIgM
MLN cells	64.0	45.0	4.8	14.3	4.8	49.5	40.0	19.5	34.5
	(3.5)	(2.8)	(0.4)	(3.2)	(0.8)	(2.1)	(2.8)	(0.7)	(2.1)
CLN cells	57.0	39.3	4.3	14.5	4.8	60.5	42.5	5.0	29.5
	(1.4)	(5.3)	(1.1)	(3.5)	(0.7)	(3.5)	(2.1)	(1.4)	(3.5)
MLN T-cells¶	92.5	51.3	1.3	1.5	4.1	75.3	42.0	14.5	12.5
	(0.7)	(6.0)	(0.4)	(0.0)	(1.3)	(6.8)	(4.2)	(2.1)	(0.7)
CLN T-cells	91.8	50.0	1.3	1.0	3.9	82.3	36.5	3.8	11.0
	(0.4)	(1.4)	(0.4)	(0.7)	(0.5)	(6.4)	(0.7)	(1.8)	(1.4)

*Cells were labeled with 25 μCi ^{3}H-TdR/5 $\times$ 10^7 cells/ml for 90 minutes at 37° C. After two washes in Hank's BSS containing 10% calf serum and two washes in PBS, the cells were deposited on methanol-cleaned, subbed slides by a cytocentrifuge and subjected to indirect immunofluorescence and autoradiography.

†Antibody specificities are described in METHODS AND MATERIALS. The results are presented as the means ± 1 S.D. for cell smears from three experiments.

‡Two hundred cells were counted per slide and the percent ^{3}H-TdR-labeled was determined. The results are presented as the means ± 1 S.D. (in parentheses) for cell smears from six experiments.

§At least one hundred ^{3}H-TdR-labeled cells were counted per preparation and the percent positive for each antiserum was determined. The results are presented as the means ± 1 S.D. (in parentheses) for cell smears from three experiments.

¶T-cells were prepared by nylon wool adherence according to Julius, et al.[11]

are known to have an affinity for mucosal tissues,[14-16] a reexamination of the adoptive transfer experiments was undertaken.

Rather than fractionating cells to prepare enriched subpopulations, we chose to utilize a technique employed most recently by Weisz-Carrington et al.[6] and McDermott and Bienenstock.[4] Radiolabeled unfractionated MLN and CLN cells were prepared and injected i.v. into lactating syngeneic recipients. Twenty to twenty-four hours later, mammary and intestinal tissues were recovered, and cryostat sections were prepared. The sections were then treated with fluorescen-ated antibodies to IgA, dipped in photographic emulsion and exposed for three to four days. After development, tissues were examined for the presence of donor (radiolabeled) cells and simultaneously scored by fluorescence microscopy for intracytoplasmic IgA. This approach allowed us to transfer unmanipulated MLN and CLN cells, and by scoring donor cells in recipient tissues for the presence of cIgA+ (B), we could derive information about the origins of cIgA+ (B) and cIgA- (T and other B) cells.

The predominant precursor source for cIgA+ B-cells capable of migrating to the ileum was the mesenteric lymph node. Over 100 times as many donor-derived

TABLE 4

PRESENCE OF CYTOPLASMIC IgA AMONG DONOR (RADIOLABELED) LYMPHOBLASTS LOCALIZING IN THE MAMMARY GLANDS AND SMALL INTESTINES OF ADOPTIVE RECIPIENTS

Recipient Tissue*	Donor Cells	^{3}H-TdR-labeled cells/100 HPF	Donor Cell Phenotype (Percent)	
			cIgA+	cIgA-
Small Intestine	MLN	68.1 ± 37.6	53	47
	CLN	1.2 ± 1.2	22	78
Mammary Gland	MLN	3.7 ± 0.8	43	57
	CLN	2.8 ± 2.7	25	75

*Three lactating (6–16 days postpartum) female rats received 2–4 × 10[8] ^{3}H-TdR-labeled CLN cells, and three matched recipients received the same number of MLN cells intravenously. Tissues were recovered 20–24 hours later and analyzed by autoradiography and indirect immunofluorescence for donor cells bearing cytoplasmic IgA.

cIgA+ cells appeared in the intestines of animals that received MLN cells than was seen in animals injected with CLN cells. The CLN-derived cells were predominantly cIgA-, suggesting that they bore other immunoglobulin isotypes or were T-lymphoblasts (TABLE 4).

Results with the mammary gland were remarkably different from those obtained with the small intestine, and suggested that this mucosal organ may derive many of its IgA-secreting plasma cells by a mechanism different from that described for the intestine. Thus the mammary gland did not accumulate as many IgA+-donor cells as did the small intestine, and the ratio of MLN-derived IgA+ cells to CLN-derived IgA+ cells did not approach the level seen in the intestine. Over one-half of the mammary-seeking MLN lymphoblasts and 75% of donor CLN lymphoblasts in this tissue were cIgA-. Again this fact suggested that the mammary gland may derive substantial numbers of its T-cells from both periph-eral and gut-associated lymphoreticular tissues. We are currently using this experimental approach to enumerate W3/13+ and W3/25+ cells among donor cells found in mammary tissues of adoptive recipients. This study should enable us to ascertain the tissue origins of mammary T-cells and the T-helper subset. Overall, the results in TABLE 4 confirm the hypothesis that the rat mammary gland and small intestine differ in the manner in which they collect cIgA⁺ B-lymphoblasts and suggest that the two tissues utilize different circulating precursor-cell pools.

DISCUSSION

Before an assessment of the origins of T- and B-lymphocytes in the rat mammary gland could be made, we needed to answer three questions. Do these cells exist in substantial numbers in the gland? Does a mucosae-seeking lymphocyte population exist in the rat? Do radiolabeled lymphocytes migrate to the mammary gland? The results of experiments reported here provided clear answers to the first two questions. Both cIgA⁺-plasma cells and W3/13⁺ or W3/25⁺ T-cells were found in the mammary gland during gestation and lactation, and their numbers were significant relative to the frequencies of the cells in the mucosa of the small intestine. Furthermore the ratio of T-cells to cIgA⁺ B-cells in the mammary gland during lactation (approximately 1:3) was comparable to the same ratio in the small intestine (approximately 1:2). One notable difference between the two organs was the predominance of W3/25⁺ (T-inducer) cells among T-cells of the mammary gland compared to a predominance of W3/25⁻ subsets in the small intestine. This fact may reflect the overall T-helper cell potential of these two organs (see below).

The results presented in TABLES 2 and 4 indicate that the MLN contains large numbers of cells capable of migrating to mucosal surfaces—in this case the small intestine. By autoradiographic analysis, 60 times more ³H-TdR-labeled MLN cells than radiolabeled CLN cells accumulated in the ileums of adoptive recipients. That these mucosae-seeking cells included both T- and B-lymphocytes was indicated by enumerating cIgA among the donor cells (TABLE 4), by transferring enriched T-cell populations from both lymph node sources[7] (FIGURES 3 and 4), and by results reported by a number of other investigators studying mucosal immunity in the rat.[14,16,17] Thus the rat mammary gland had a substantial endowment of cIgA⁺, W3/13⁺, and W3/25⁺ cells, and the animals possessed intestine-seeking B- and T-lymphoblast populations that we felt might serve as precursor sources for these cells.

Experiments designed to answer the third question—Do radiolabeled lymphocytes migrate to the mammary gland?—provided perplexing results. Because information regarding the densities of cIgA⁺ B-cells or T-cells in the mammary gland were unavailable at the time that we performed our initial cell migration studies,[7,8] we were not surprised to find that the gland accumulated far fewer donor lymphoblasts than did the small intestine. During the first postpartum week when cIgA⁺ cells in the small intestine outnumbered cIgA⁺ cells in the mammary gland by a factor of 3 (FIGURE 1), the number of ³H-TdR-labeled cIgA⁺ MLN B-lymphoblasts that migrated to the small intestine exceeded the number migrating to the mammary gland by a factor of 23 (TABLE 4). That is to say, far too few cIgA⁺ cells were collecting in the mammary gland to maintain the number of cells seen there if the kinetics of cell survival were similar in the two organs. In other words, based on the migration data alone, one would not have expected the density of cIgA⁺ B-cells that was observed in the lactating gland by immunofluorescence. Two explanations for this enigma might be offered. It is possible that most mammary IgA plasma-cell precursors are found in neither MLN nor CLN and reside instead in another lymphoid organ. Alternatively, the environmental conditions within the mammary gland and small intestine may differ, with the former favoring further clonal expansion of cIgA$^+$ B-cells and the latter limiting this capacity. We clearly favor the second hypothesis and reemphasize the temporal relationships between the arrival of cIgA$^+$ cells and T-cells in the gland and the predominance of cells of the T-inducer subset, especially in the postpartum period. This hypothesis would be compatible with low numbers of migrating cIgA$^+$ B-cells because subsequent cell division would greatly expand their numbers prior to terminal differentiation into IgA-secreting plasma cells. Furthermore, we would predict that this local amplification of B-cell clones is T-cell dependent.

Regarding the origins of T-cells in the mammary gland, the following observations have been made: (1) T-lymphoblasts prepared from MLN or CLN evidenced equal affinities for the mammary glands of adoptive lactating recipients; (2) both T-cell-enriched populations responded to developmental changes in the mammary gland (FIGURES 3 & 4) either induced by pregnancy or exogenously supplied lactogenic hormones.[8] Because these T-enriched populations were only 75–82% W3/13$^+$ and contained contaminating cIgA$^+$ cells (TABLE 3), we are currently unable to make a direct quantitative comparison between CLN and MLN T-cells. This information should be attainable by using combined immunofluorescence and autoradiography to enumerate W3/13$^+$ radiolabeled cells in the mammary tissues of adoptive recipients. Preliminary results using this approach indicate that CLN are a major source of mammary seeking T-cells in the rat (M. J. Parmely and L. S. Manning, unpublished data). Should these preliminary experiments be confirmed by further studies, they would suggest that optimum stimulation of specific mammary cell-mediated immunity (including, presumably, T-helper cell activity) would be accomplished by immunization regimens that include parenteral as well as oral challenge.

At the present time, we find no evidence for a common muscosal pool of T- or B-lymphocytes that preferentially provide large numbers of precursors for the mammary gland of the rat. Although ample evidence exists for a population of T- and B-lymphoblasts with affinity for the intestinal mucosa, these specific cells seem to ignore the mammary gland (TABLES 2 and 4) and in certain instances avoid accumulating in the lungs altogether[7] (FIGURES 3 & 4). We do not feel that these relationships reflect the "mucosal" nature of CLN,[18] chosen here as a control population. CLN cells did not migrate to the small intestine as efficiently as did MLN cells, and CLN cells have been a routine component of control "peripheral lymph node" cell populations studied in other laboratories.[14,2,4] Therefore the mammary gland appears to be distinguishable from the small intestine by the origins of its lymphocytes.

Cells-bearing W3/13 antigens were oftentimes located within the epithelia and alveolar lumens of the lactating mammary gland. We have not as yet studied the W3/25$^+$ subset in this regard, but would predict that it too would be present in substantial proportions within alveolar lumens. This prediction stems from the observation that human colostrum contains clones of T-cells capable of responding to soluble antigens and alloantigens in lymphoproliferative assays,[19,20] but appears to lack alloantigen-specific cytotoxic T-cell precursors.[21] Our data regarding the presence of IgA-bearing cells in rat milk (TABLE 1) is more difficult to interpret, because IgA-containing milk macrophages may contribute to these cell counts.

In summary, the present study documents the presence of substantial numbers of cIgA$^+$, W3/13$^+$, and W3/25$^+$ cells in the rat mammary gland. Adoptive transfer studies designed to determine their origin have confirmed the existence of mucosae-seeking T- and B-cell populations, but have failed to implicate them as the exclusive or even predominant source of mammary gland lymphocytes. Rather, we have interpreted the available data as suggesting that mammary $cIgA^+$ plasma cells arise from immigration of small numbers of precursors followed by their expansion within the gland by cell division. The pattern of appearance of T-cells in the mammary gland, the predominance of the T-helper cell subset, and the relative numbers of T-cell precursors in CLN and MLN compartments suggest that B-cell expansion is dependent on T-lymphocytes accumulated from both the mucosal and peripheral cell pools.

SUMMARY

The present study was undertaken to determine the pattern of T- and B-lymphocyte accumulation in the rat mammary gland during gestation, lactation, and weaning. Adoptive transfer experiments were then used to identify the likely source and extent of immigrating cells during this period. Our results indicate that the mammary gland accumulates levels of $cIgA^+$, $W3/13^+$, and $W3/25^+$ cells that are approximately one third their densities in the small intestine. Cell migration studies suggest that the input of immigrating B-cells is not sufficient to maintain these levels in the gland, and we have suggested that substantial clonal expansion must occur among $cIgA^+$ B-cells within the mammary tissue itself. The migratory behavior of T-cells, their pattern of appearance throughout gestation and lactation, and the predominance of the T-helper cell subset suggest that T-cells regulate B-cell development within the mammary gland.

ACKNOWLEDGMENTS

The authors wish to thank Linda Mauser, Sandra Kibalo, and Jennifer Lane for their expert technical assistance and Brenda Smith for preparing the manuscript.

REFERENCES

1. WEISZ-CARRINGTON, P., M. E. ROUX & M. E. LAMM. 1977. J. Immunol. **119:** 1306.
2. ROUX, M. E., M. MCWILLIAMS, J. M. PHILLIPS-QUAGLIATA, P. WEISZ-CARRINGTON & M. E. LAMM. 1977. J. Exp. Med. **146:** 1311.
3. BIENENSTOCK, J., M. MCDERMOTT & D. BEFUS. 1979. In Immunology of Breast Milk. P. L. Orga and D. Dayton, Eds.: 91–98. Raven Press. New York.
4. MCDERMOTT, M. R. & J. BIENENSTOCK. 1979. J. Immunol. **122:** 1892.
5. LAMM, M. E., P. WEISZ-CARRINGTON, M. E. ROUX, M. MCWILLIAMS & J. M. PHILLIPS-QUAGLIATA. 1979. In Immunology of Breast Milk. P. L. Orga and D. Dayton, Eds.: 105–109. Raven Press. New York.
6. WEISZ-CARRINGTON, P., M. E. ROUX, M. MCWILLIAMS, J. M. PHILLIPS-QUAGLIATA & M. E. LAMM. 1979. J. Immunol. **123:** 1705.
7. MANNING, L. S. & M. J. PARMELY. 1980. J. Immunol. **125:** 2508.
8. MANNING, L. S. & M. J. PARMELY. 1981. J. Reprod. Immunol. **3:** 522.
9. WILLIAMS, A. F., G. GALFRE & C. MILSTEIN. 1977. Cell **12:** 663.
10. WHITE, R. A. H., D. W. MASON, A. F. WILLIAMS, G. GALFRE & C. MILSTEIN. 1978. J. Exp. Med. **148:** 664.

11. JULIUS, M. H., E. SIMPSON & L. A. HERZENBERG. 1973. Europ. J. Immunol. **3:** 645.
12. BEUTNER, E. H., M. R. SEPULVEDA & E. V. BARNET. 1968. Bull. W.H.O. **39:** 587.
13. LAVEN, G. T., S. S. CRAGO, W. H. KUTTEH & J. MESTECKY. 1981. J. Immunol. **127:** 1967.
14. GRISCELLI, C., P. VASSALLI & R. T. McCLUSKEY. 1969. J. Exp. Med. **130:** 1427.
15. GUY-GRAND, D., C. GRISCELLI & P. VASSALLI. 1974. Europ. J. Immunol. **4:** 435.
16. PIERCE, N. F. & J. L. GOWANS. 1975. J. Exp. Med. **142:** 1550.
17. LOVE, R. J. & B. M. OGILVIE. 1977. Exp. Parasitol. **41:** 124.
18. TILNEY, N. L. 1971. J. Anat. **109:** 369.
19. PARMELY, M. J., A. E. BEER & R. E. BILLINGHAM. 1976. J. Exp. Med. **144:** 358.
20. PARMELY, M. J., D. B. REATH, A. E. BEER & R. E. BILLINGHAM. 1977. Transplant. Proc. **9:** 1477.
21. PARMELY, M. J. & S. B. WILLIAMS. 1979. *In* Immunology of Breast Milk. P. L. Orga and D. Dayton, Eds.: 173–180. Raven Press. New York.

DISCUSSION OF THE PAPER

J. R. McGHEE (*University of Alabama in Birmingham*): Your results obtained with monoclonal antibodies indicate that you deal with T-helper cells. Have you done any experiments either in antigen-specific systems with cells from orally immunized animals or in B-cell cultures to which you added these purified T-cells to determine whether they are indeed T-helper cells and will drive B-cells to divide and differentiate?

M. PARMELY (*University of Kansas, Kansas City*): The W325 antibody has been used by a number of groups, and they clearly detected the T-cell inducer subset, which is a Lyt-1 type cell in the rat. We have not done any direct experimentation on the functional activity of these cells, isolated either from the mammary gland or from other sources.

P. BRANDTZAEG (*National Hospital, Olso, Norway*): As far as I understand, you have not shown that there is a proliferation of IgA cells in the mammary glands.

PARMELY: That is correct.

BRANDTZAEG: I suggest on the basis of the isotype distribution of cells in lactating human mammary gland, that more than 10% of cells are not IgA cells. There is an intermediate proportion of IgD-producing cells compared to the lacrimal gland and gut mucosa. I suggest that perhaps there is a significant contribution from both tonsils and lymphoid tissues in the upper aero-digestive tract.

PARMELY: I suggested that the IgA-containing cells were not coming from either one of these lymph node populations. A great deal of the data presented at this conference, including your own, suggested that we need to examine lymphoid tissues as possible sources of IgA-precursor cells.

BRANDTZAEG: We agree that the common mucosal immune system may not be as common as some investigators have suggested.

A. O. ANDERSON (*University of Pennsylvania, Philadelphia*): A number of studies, including those of Dr. Cebra, indicate that the spleen is a substantial site of intermediary lodging of IgA-precursor cells. I notice you did not use the spleen for your IgA migrates. Have you done those studies?

PARMELY: No, we have not. We have examined the spleen and a variety of other lymphoid tissues and the migration of uridine-labeled cells.

N. F. PIERCE (*The Johns Hopkins University, Baltimore, Md.*): With respect to IgA B-cell blast homing, the basic idea is that they home selectively to mucosal rather than to nonmucosal surfaces. However, that does not mean that this homing may not be equal. We have shown that gut-derived IgA B-blasts may home with 20-30-fold greater selectivity to the gut as compared to the trachea. These IgA B-cell blasts home to the mammary gland in a pattern that is similar to the trachea. It seems to be important to show that they are not homing to spleen or to some nonmucosal site in a final way, because they could be homing selectively to mucosae, including the mammary gland, but in a relatively different degree, depending on which mucosal surface is examined.

PARMELY: Dr. Montgomery's data suggest that the cells may be derived from lymphoid tissues and be stimulated by immunizing events, occurring at the GI epithelium. Migration of IgA B-blasts is not sufficient to account for the number of cells there. There must be other contributing factors. We suggest that expansion in cell numbers is involved within the mammary gland itself.

M. LAMM (*Case Western Reserve University, Cleveland, Ohio*): I think there are important methodological differences between the studies performed in the mouse versus those studies in the rat. We have used pooled peripheral node cells, whereas Dr. Parmely has only used cells from the cervical lymph nodes. We cannot state how many IgA-producing plasma cells in the lactating mammary gland were the result of local proliferation. Nevertheless, when you take unseparated B- and T-donor cells from a mesenteric lymph node a day later, 90% of the cells are IgA producers. I think that these results alone would indicate that we are primarily discussing a B-cell phenomenon. I think it would be premature to start generalizing on the basis of studies in humans, where you cannot perform the same kind of experiment that can be done in the rodent.

PARMELY: The issue seems to be whether the cervical lymph node cells represent a peripheral source. There are several pieces of evidence to support this notion. The inability of these cells to home to mucosal surfaces and the work done by Griscelli and colleagues showing that rat peripheral and cervical nodes display the same homing pattern, indicate that these two sources of lymphocytes are comparable.

ESTROGEN-MEDIATED CONTROL OF THE SECRETORY IMMUNE SYSTEM IN THE UTERUS OF THE RAT*

Charles R. Wira, David A. Sullivan,† and Carola P. Sandoe

Department of Physiology
Dartmouth Medical School
Hanover, New Hampshire 03755

INTRODUCTION

From an endocrine standpoint, the uterus of the immature and ovariectomized adult rat has been the preferred organ for the study of the mechanism of estrogen action.[1,2] Estradiol has been known for a number of years to bind with high affinity to cytosol receptors present within the muscle, stromal, and epithelial cells of the uterus.[3-5] Following this initial interaction in the cytoplasm, the steroid-receptor complex moves into the nucleus to initiate alterations in DNA that, in turn, give rise to either new or increased messenger RNA synthesis.[6,7] These early biochemical changes occur rapidly and precede the wave of protein synthesis that is essential for uterine growth.[8]

As a part of this hormonally induced process, the uterus becomes prepared to receive the fertilized ovum. During the follicular or preovulatory phase of the reproductive cycle, the endometrium proliferates in response to estradiol.[9] This proliferation is accompanied by an increase in vascularization and blood flow as well as an increase in capillary permeability.[10,11] In the rat, this alteration in permeability results in fluid and protein accumulation in the uterus.[12] This permeability phenomenon has been termed water imbibition and occurs within hours of estradiol exposure.[13,14] During the luteal or postovulatory phase of the cycle, the glands of the endometrium become enlarged. This enlargement is accompanied by intraluminal secretions that serve as a nutritive source for the fertilized ovum from the time of ovulation through to implantation.[9]

In spite of the fact that much important information has been obtained about uterine secretions,[15] relatively little information exists on the role of these secretions in the defense against microbial organisms. Of particular interest is that, whereas the uterus is open to the external environment at certain stages of the reproductive cycle, it nevertheless is maintained as a sterile compartment.[16,17]

In considering the protective mechanisms that reside within the reproductive tract, several processes appear to be involved. Nonspecific anti-microbial factors such as peroxidase and lysozyme have been identified in uterine secretions and in amniotic fluid during pregnancy.[18-20] Also present within the uterus are several basic elements of the immune system. These include tissue plasma cells,[21] as well as IgA and IgG that are found in the uterus and uterine lumen.[22,23] By immunofluorescence analysis, diffuse noncellular staining of free immunoglobulins has been identified in the endometrial stroma, basement membrane, and epithelial cells that line the uterine lumen.[24-26] IgA and IgG cells are sometimes found, but

*This work was supported by Research Grant AI 13541 from the National Institutes of Health.

†Present address: Eye Research Institute of Retina Foundation, 20 Staniford Street, Boston, Mass. 02114.

0077-8923/83/0409-0534 $1.75/0 © 1983, NYAS

when present are sparsely distributed.[21,24-26] An additional constituent of the immune system is secretory component, which is present in uterine epithelial cells.[21,24-27] With regard to the secretions in the uterine lumen, IgA, IgG, and occasionally IgM have been identified.[23,28] Calculation of luminal IgA/IgG ratios indicate that unlike the serum, IgA is the predominant immunoglobulin.[29,30] When the size of IgA was examined, only polymeric IgA was found.[30,31] A particularly interesting finding has been that variations occur in the uterine immune system as a function of the estrous or menstrual cycle.[21,26,32] These variations suggested that sex hormones might regulate the immune system in the uterus.

In light of the valuable information available about both the mode of estradiol action as well as the presence of the immune system in the reproductive tract, we undertook to use the uterus of the rat as a model system to study the interactions of the female sex hormones with the secretory immune system. The results presented here demonstrate that the sex hormones have marked effects on various immunological parameters. In addition, these studies indicate that by hormonal manipulation of the reproductive tract, it has been possible to conclude that estrogens regulate several aspects of the immune system.

MATERIALS AND METHODS

General Procedures

Adult female virgin Sprague-Dawley-CD rats (Charles River Breeding Laboratories, Wilmington, Mass.) weighing between 150–250g were kept in constant temperature rooms with 12 hour intervals of light and dark. Animals at various stages of the estrous cycle were chosen after daily vaginal smears indicated that each rat had at least two normal four-day estrous cycles. Ovariectomies were carried out 6–15 days prior to each experiment.

Recovery of uterine luminal content was as previously described.[33] Briefly, immediately after decapitation, the uterine vascular bed was perfused by injecting saline through the descending aorta. After removing adherent material from the uterus by saline rinse, luminal content was collected by perfusing each horn with 0.1 ml of sterile saline. Recovered fluid was centrifuged (1,000 × g for four minutes) and supernatants were lyophilized and stored at $-20°C$ until assayed. At the time of assay, lyophilized samples were reconstituted with either distilled water or TKM buffer (50 mM Trizma (Sigma Chemical Co.), 25 mM KCl, 5 mM $MgCl_2$, pH 7.5). Tissue extracts were prepared from uteri as previousy described.[34,35] Briefly, uteri were homogenized in TKM buffer with a Polytron (Brinkmann) PT-10 at 3°C and then centrifuged at 10,000 × g for eight minutes to recover the supernatant fraction (cytosol). Plasma samples were obtained at the time of sacrifice by direct cardiac puncture of etherized rats with heparinized syringes. In order to measure circulating nucleated cells, blood (1.0 ml) was immediately mixed with 10 μl of sodium heparin (Calbiochem, B grade, USP/ml). Aliquots (10 μl) of blood were then diluted into 10 ml of saline. Nucleated cells were measured in a Coulter counter after cell suspensions were lysed by adding two drops of Zap-o-globin II (Coulter Diagnostics). Blood smears for differential counts were prepared at the time of blood collection.

Analysis of IgA, IgG, and Secretory Component

Immunoglobulin measurements were determined by radioimmunoassay (RIA) using either the solid phase[33] or double antibody precipitation technique.[35]

In the solid phase assay, rabbit anti-rat IgG (Miles Laboratory, Elkhart, Ind.) and goat anti-rat IgA (Dr. H. Bazin, Belgium) prepared against IgA-rich serum from rats with IR-22 immunocytomas were coupled either to cyanogen bromide activated microcrystalline cellulose or Sepharose 4B. Rat IgG and rat IgA obtained from immunocytoma serum (Bazin), the antigen components of the RIA, were radiolabeled with ^{125}I by using either the lactoperoxidase[33]or IODO-GEN[35] procedure. In the double antibody technique, rabbit anti-goat IgG and goat anti-rabbit IgG, purchased from Miles Laboratories, were used as second antibodies.

To detect the presence of secretory component in uterine secretions, Ouchterlony immunoprecipitation reactions were carried out in 1% agarose plates.[36] The end point of this assay was the formation of an immunoprecipitation band that resulted when uterine fluid (5 μl) containing secretory component was placed in one well and reacted with rabbit anti-rat secretory component (10 μl) (from Dr. B. Underdown, University of Toronto). Secretory component was also measured by RIA, using a double antibody precipitation technique.[36] Components of this assay included rat secretory component (Underdown) that was iodinated by the IODO-GEN procedure, rabbit anti-rat secretory component as the first antibody, and goat anti-rabbit IgG as the second antibody. As with the IgA and IgG RIAs described above, a standard curve was run with each set of unknown samples.

Immunofluorescence Analysis

Uteri to be examined by immunofluorescence microscopy were surgically removed and immediately frozen in liquid nitrogen. At the time of examination, specimens were transferred without thawing to a cryostat ($-20°$ C) and cut into eight μm sections. Immunofluorescent staining for IgA was carried out with the IgG fraction of goat anti-rat IgA that was conjugated to fluorescein isothiocyanate (FITC, Sigma Chemical Co., St. Louis, Mo.). Details of these procedures have been published previously.[37] FITC conjugates (initial concentration, 10 mg/ml) were used at a 1:28 dilution. Sections were evaluated with a Zeiss Photo III microscope illuminated by HB-200 mercury vapor labor. Zeiss excitation and barrier filters for fluorescein were used.

Hormone Preparation

Estradiol, progesterone, cortisol, estriol, and dihydrotestosterone, were purchased from Calbiochem (LaJolla, Calif.) and dissolved in ethanol. After the appropriate aliquots were evaporated to dryness, they were resuspended in either ethyl laurate or saline (0.9%) prior to subcutaneous injection (0.1 ml/rat/day). Controls received only solvent.

RESULTS

Effect of Estradiol on IgA and IgG in Uterine Secretions of the Ovariectomized Rat

FIGURE 1 shows the effect of estradiol and other steroids on the levels of IgA and IgG in uterine secretions following three days of hormone treatment. Of those hormones administered, only estradiol significantly increased IgA and IgG in the uterine lumen. By contrast, progesterone, cortisol, dihydrotestosterone, and estriol, when injected at doses that are known to elicit physiological effects in their respective target tissues, had no effect. We have observed in other studies,[33] that progesterone, when administered simultaneously with estradiol for three days, prevents the estradiol increase of both immunoglobulins. This antagonism exists irrespective of whether progesterone was given for all three days, for the last two days, or on the last day of a three-day estradiol treatment. No significant

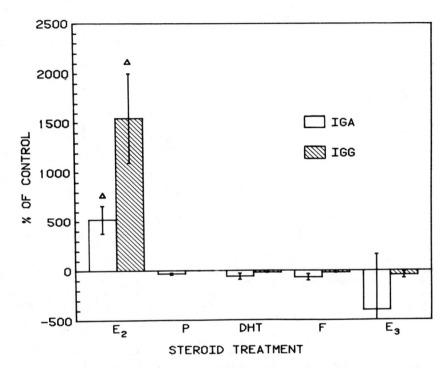

FIGURE 1. Influence of steroids on IgA and IgG in the rat uterus. Ovariectomized animals were injected daily with 0.1 ml of ethyl laurate or 0.1 ml of saline solution with either 1.0 µg of estradiol (E_2), or estriol (E_3), 2 mg of progesterone (P), 1.0 mg of cortisol (F), or dihydrotestosterone (DHT). Twenty four hours after the third injection, uterine luminal content was recovered and immunoglobulins measured. Results are expressed as percent of control $\pm$ SE (6 rats per group) that received only ethyl laurate or saline. Estimates of standard error were calculated as described in Meyer, S.L., Data Analysis for Scientists and Engineers. J. Wiley and Sons. New York. 1975, p. 40. $\triangle$, value differs from control values at $p < 0.01$. From Wira and Sandoe.[33]

variations were observed in serum IgA or IgG levels during the course of these experiments.

Gradual Accumulation of Immunoglobulins in Response to Estradiol

In light of the marked changes in IgA and IgG levels in the uterine lumen after multiple hormone treatments, we were interested in looking at the time course of

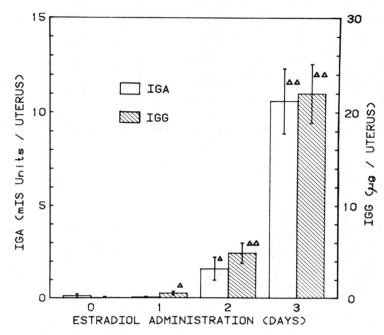

FIGURE 2. Time course of the effect of estradiol treatment on IgA and IgG recovered from the uterine lumen of ovariectomized rats. Estradiol (1.0 μg/0.1 ml) in ethyl laurate was given daily for one, two, or three days. Controls received only ethyl laurate. Animals were sacrificed 24 hours after the last injection. The bars represent the mean of five animals per group, and the vertical lines on the bars indicate the SE. IgA results are reported as immunocytoma serum (IS) units, where 1.0 IS unit is defined as the concentration of 1.0 mg of lyophilized immunocytoma serum per ml of distilled water. △, significantly (p < 0.01) greater than control. From Wira and Sandoe.[33]

immunoglobulin appearance in the uterus. As seen in FIGURE 2, when uterine secretions were collected at 24 hours after each of three daily estradiol injections, ovariectomized rats showed a gradual increase in IgA and IgG after two and three days of hormone treatment. In an earlier report,[33] we observed that after 6–14 days of daily hormone treatment, estradiol failed to maintain the increase in uterine IgA and IgG levels measured at three days. More recently, we have found that this drop is most likely due to the leakage of immunoglobulins from the uterus through the cervix into the vagina.[35] This conclusion is based on our observation that uterine IgA and IgG continued to accumulate in rats that were ligated at the uterine-cervical junction to prevent loss of uterine fluid.

Rapid Response of IgA and IgG to Estradiol

An observation that so far appears to have no parallel in other systems is that within the first hours after the administration of a single injection of hormone, there is a rapid accumulation of IgA and IgG in the uterus (tissue) and of IgG in the lumen. As shown in FIGURE 3, both IgA and IgG levels in the tissues increased markedly at three hours after hormone treatment. The increase in tissue IgG was also paralleled by a rapid rise in luminal IgG levels. By contrast, IgA levels in the uterine lumen did not change when compared to saline injected controls. In other experiments, we observed that the levels of IgA and IgG were highest at three and six hours after hormone treatment and then decreased to or approached control values at 25 hours.[35] The latter finding, of a decline at 25 hours, indicates why in our earlier studies, which had used 24 hours after estradiol injection as the time

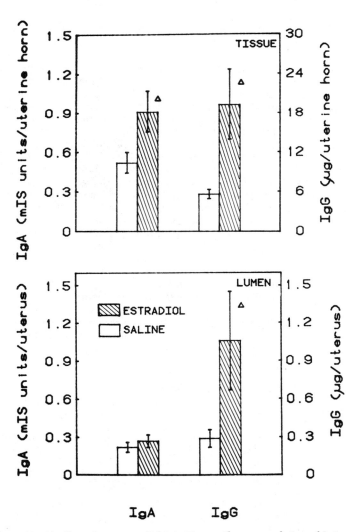

FIGURE 3. Rapid effect of one estradiol injection on the accumulation of IgA and IgG in the uterine tissue and the uterine lumina of ovariectomized rats. Animals were treated with estradiol (1 μg) in 0.9% saline three hours prior to sacrifice. △, significantly (p < 0.05) greater than control value. From Sullivan and Wira.[35]

interval for measuring uterine luminal accumulation, we failed to observe any signifcant increase in luminal IgA and IgG levels prior to two days of hormone treatment. By contrast to IgG, IgA in the uterine lumen increased initially at 18 hours after the second injection of estradiol and then continued to rise at all later time points measured.[38] We have also found that, whereas IgA in rat serum consists of monomers and polymers, it is completely polymeric and also bound to secretory component in the uterine lumen.[36,38]

Estradiol Stimulation of IgA and IgG Movement from the Uterus (Tissue) into the Uterine Lumen

The movement of IgA, but not IgG, from the uterus into the uterine lumen in response to estradiol goes against an apparent concentration gradient. As shown in TABLE 1, after three daily injections of estradiol, the concentration of IgA in the uterine lumen was significantly higher than that measured in the tissue. By contrast, IgG in the lumen was much lower than that measured in the tissue. These findings indicate that the mechanism(s) involved in the accumulation of IgA and IgG in the uterine lumen are distinctly different. In other studies, we have observed that coincident with the appearance of IgA in uterine secretions, there was a marked accumulation of IgA in the epithelial cells that line the uterine lumen.[39] In the absence of estradiol, very little IgA was found in these cells. Some, however, was present in the basement membrane region of the epithelial cells. Because IgA increased in these cells at a time that coincided with the maximal accumulation of IgA in the uterine lumen, we suggest that the epithelial cells in the uterus may play a central role in the luminal accumulation of IgA.

Effect of Estradiol on Lymphocytes in Rat Blood and on the Appearance of IgA-Positive Cells in the Uterine Tissues

To determine whether estradiol had any role in the migration of lymphocytes into the uterus of the rat, we measured the effect of estradiol on the number of

TABLE 1

THE CONCENTRATION OF IGA AND IGG IN THE UTERUS AND IN THE UTERINE SECRETIONS FOLLOWING THE TREATMENT OF OVARIECTOMIZED RATS WITH ESTRADIOL*

Immunoglobulin	Uterus	Uterine Fluid
IgA**	0.006 ± 0.0021†	0.130 ± 0.0150‡
	(4)‖	(4)
IgG	0.36 ± 0.0210§	0.016 ± 0.0054¶
	(4)	(4)

Data from Sullivan and Wira.[36]

*Rats were injected with estradiol (one μg/day for three days) in saline.

†IgA expressed as mIS units/mg tissue.

‡mIS units/μl uterine fluid.

§IgG expressed as μg/mg tissue.

¶μg/μl uterine fluid.

‖number of rats in each group.

**1.0 mIS unit is defined as the concentration of IgA in 1.0 μg of lyophilized immunocytoma serum per ml of distilled water.

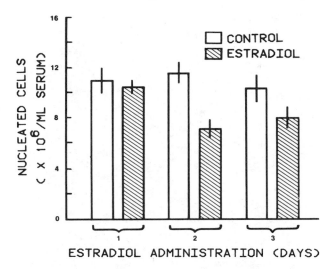

FIGURE 4. Time course of the effect of estradiol on circulating nucleated cells in blood from ovariectomized rats. Animals were injected daily for one, two, or three days with estradiol (1 μg/0.1 ml) in saline. Twenty-four hours after the last injection, animals (four to five per group) were anesthetized; blood was collected by direct cardiac puncture. See MATERIALS AND METHODS for details on cell counting. Bars and brackets indicate the mean ± SE for determinations. From Wira *et al.*[37]

circulating lymphocytes in the blood. As shown in FIGURE 4, when 1 μg of estradiol was administered daily to ovariectomized rats for three days, the number of circulating nucleated cells in blood gradually declined on days 2 and 3 by 25–30% of the control population. From differential smears on each of the blood samples, it was found that 80–90% of the nucleated cell population in both hormonally treated and control groups consisted of lymphocytes. In other experiments, the number of circulating lymphocytes was measured when progesterone was administered along with estradiol.[37] Under these conditions, the drop in lymphocytes was blocked by progesterone.

The reduction in circulating blood lymphocytes by estradiol coincides with the appearance of IgA-positive cells in the uteri of ovariectomized rats. By using fluoresceinated anti-rat IgA (FITC-anti IgA), IgA-positive cells were found in the uteri of ovariectomized rats treated daily with estradiol for three days. As seen in FIGURE 5A, no IgA-positive cells were found in the uteri of saline injected controls. With hormone treatment, IgA-positive cells (FIGURE 5B) appeared in the endometrium and myometrium in proportion to the length of hormone exposure. Time course studies indicated that a few cells were present at 24 hours after the first injection of estradiol (TABLE 2). As judged by representative sampling of sections cut from a number of different uteri at various stages of hormone exposure, greater numbers of IgA-positive cells were found in the uteri of rats treated with estradiol for two and three days. We also observed that progesterone blocked the hormonally induced accumulation of IgA-positive cells in the uterus. This block, however, appeared to be complete only when progesterone was administered along with estradiol for all three days, or for the last two days of hormone treatment. Of particular interest was our finding that IgA-positive cells appear to be present in the uteri of intact animals at all stages of the estrous cycle.

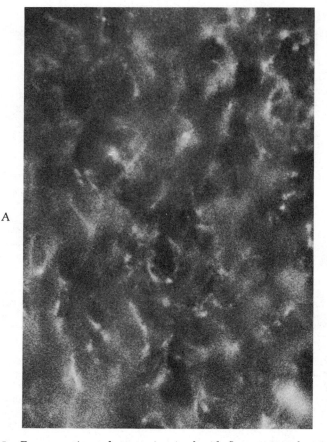

FIGURE 5. Frozen sections of rat uteri stained with fluoresceinated anti-rat IgA. A. Ovariectomized rat treated with saline for three days, no IgA-positive cells are present (160×); B. After three days of treatment with estradiol, 1 μg/day, IgA-positive cells are found both in the endometria and the myometria of ovariectomized rat uteri. From Wira et al.[37]

Because IgA levels are highest in the uterine lumen at proestrus and estrus,[33] when estrogens are known to be the dominant hormone present, it seems unlikely that the presence of these cells is the mechanism whereby estradiol exerts its cyclic influence on luminal IgA accumulation. Similar experiments with FITC anti-IgG have failed to demonstrate the presence of IgG-positive cells in the uterus irrespective of hormone treatment.

Regulation of Secretory Component by Estradiol in the Uteri of Ovariectomized Rats

The effect of estradiol on the appearance of secretory component in uterine secretions is shown in TABLE 3. When compared to controls, free secretory

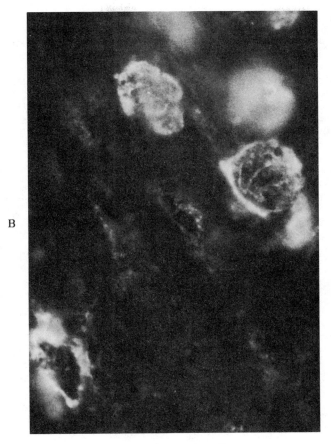

B

FIGURE 5 (continued)

component was initially detected in the uterine lumen 24 hours after the second injection of estradiol.[36] Also shown is our finding that free secretory component was present in all uterine secretions subsequent to day 2, irrespective of whether estradiol was administered daily for either three or eight days. Free secretory component was not detected in serum taken from either control or hormonally treated groups. In other studies, free secretory component was detected in the uterine secretions of intact female rats at the proestrus but not at the diestrus stage of the reproductive cycle.[36]

More recently, we have successfully developed an RIA to measure the amount of free secretory component in the uterine lumen. As seen in Table 4, initial experiments in which estradiol was administered to ovariectomized rats indicate that free secretory component in uterine secretions increases significantly when compared to ovariectomized controls. Also shown are the levels of IgA that increase markedly after three days of hormone treatment, as previously reported.

Estrogen Regulation of IgA in Neonatally Thymectomized Rats

In light of the marked effects of estradiol on IgA in the rat uterine lumen, we were interested in the possible role that T-cells might play in the expression of this hormone response. As seen in TABLE 5, when estradiol (1 μg/day for three days) is administered to neonatally thymectomized rats, the luminal accumulation of IgA is markedly reduced relative to both sham-operated and intact ovariectomized rats. IgA levels, while reduced, were nevertheless significantly higher than saline-injected controls. Uterine luminal IgG was also markedly reduced in the neonatally thymectomized rats.[31]

TABLE 2

THE PRESENCE OF IGA-POSITIVE CELLS IN THE UTERI OF INTACT RATS AT VARIOUS STAGES OF THE ESTROUS CYCLE, FOLLOWING OVARIECTOMY AND AFTER ESTRADIOL AND/OR PROGESTERONE TREATMENT OF OVARIECTOMIZED RATS

Endocrine State of Rats	Relative Number of IgA-Positive Cells in Endometrium and Myometrium*
Estrous cycle	+++
Ovariectomized	−
Ovariectomized and estradiol†	
a) day 1	+
b) day 2	+
c) day 3	++
Ovariectomized-progesterone‡	−
Ovariectomized-estradiol and progesterone§	
a) E$_2$-3P	−
b) E$_2$-2P	−
c) E$_2$-1P	++

Data from Wira et al.[37]
 *Number of IgA-positive cells; − nondetected; + few; ++ some; +++ many.
 †Estradiol = one μg/day
 ‡Progesterone = 2 mg/day
 §Estradiol administered daily for three days; E$_2$-3P, progesterone given with estradiol for all three days; E$_2$-2P, progesterone given with estradiol on last two days; E$_2$-1P, progesterone given on last day of three day estradiol treatment.

DISCUSSION

The results presented in this study indicate that estradiol has a marked stimulatory effect on several parameters of the immune system in the rat uterus. By ovariectomizing adult female rats to deplete them of endogenous estrogens, and then replacing estrogens with exogenous hormones, we were able to identify a temporal sequence of events that culminates in the accumulation of IgA and IgG in uterine secretions. Although at first IgA and IgG appeared to accumulate gradually over a period of days following estradiol treatment, it is now clear from our more recent studies that marked changes in uterine immunoglobulins occur within hours after hormone exposure. By measuring both tissue and luminal amounts of IgA and IgG, we found that, in parallel with the water imbibition step,

TABLE 3

TIME COURSE OF THE EFFECT OF ESTRADIOL TREATMENT ON THE PRESENCE OF FREE SECRETORY COMPONENT IN THE UTERINE LUMINA OF OVARIECTOMIZED RATS

Treatment*	Dose (μg)	Number	Percentage of Positive Responses
Saline†		13	0
One estradiol injection:			
3 hours	0.1	3	0
	1.0	3	0
	10.0	3	0
6 hours	1.0	4	0
12 hours	1.0	4	0
24 hours	1.0	4	0
Two estradiol injections:			
3 hours	1.0	4	0
6 hours	1.0	4	0
24 hours	5.0	2	100
Three estradiol injections:			
6 hours	5.0	2	100
24 hours	1.0	13	100
	5.0	2	100
Eight estradiol injections:‡			
24 hours	10.0	2	100

Data from Sullivan and Wira.[36]
*The number of hours after each injection at which samples were collected.
†Rats were randomly distributed so that some received saline (0.9%; 0.1 ml) for either one, two, or three days prior to sacrifice.
‡Rats had uteri ligated to prevent loss of uterine fluid through the cervix.

both immunoglobulins entered the tissue space three to six hours after estradiol administration and then declined towards control levels at 25 hours.[35] This pattern has been observed as well with multiple hormone injections and appears to be related to serum transudation (stromal edema) that occurs after each injection of estradiol.[31] By examining the luminal secretions in the hours immedi-

TABLE 4

IGA AND SECRETORY COMPONENT IN UTERINE SECRETIONS OF OVARIECTOMIZED RATS AFTER DAILY TREATMENT FOR THREE DAYS WITH ESTRADIOL (ONE μG/DAY) OR SALINE

	Number/Group	IgA (mIS units/uterus)*†	Secretory Component (μg/uterus)†
Control	12	0.07 ± 0.02	0.07 ± 0.02
Estradiol	7	3.06 ± 0.47‡	6.77 ± 0.81‡

Data from Sullivan and Wira.[36]
*IgA results are reported as immunocytoma serum (IS) units.
†Both IgA and secretory component were measured by radioimmunoassay. See METHODS section for details.
‡Significantly (p < 0.001) greater than ovariectomzied controls.
Each value represents the mean ± SE of the number of animals indicated.

ately after estradiol treatment, we found that the uterus handles IgG and IgA by distinctly different processes. At three hours and six hours, IgG levels were elevated in the uterine lumen, but IgA levels were not different from those of controls. By contrast, IgA accumulation in the uterine lumen did occur, but only after two to three days of hormone exposure.

One explanation for the rapid appearance of IgG, but not IgA or IgM in the uterine lumen after a single injection of estradiol, may be due to the size of the molecules involved. As we have discussed elsewhere,[35] because IgM and polymeric IgA are much larger than IgG, molecular weight restrictions may represent one possible means whereby IgA and IgM failed to move from tissue to lumen. This restriction, however, does not appear to exist from blood to tissue, because as a part of the phenomenon of water imbibition induced by estradiol, permeability changes in the vascular endothelium occur[40] that result in IgA, IgG, and IgM accumulation in the uterine tissues.[35]

Until recently, the presence of most, if not all, immunoglobulins in mucosal tissues was attributed to local synthesis by mucosal plasma cells.[41] Our finding

TABLE 5

THE EFFECT OF ESTRADIOL ON IGA LEVELS IN THE UTERINE LUMEN OF NEONATALLY THYMECTOMIZED RATS. ANIMALS WERE OVARIECTOMIZED 7–10 DAYS BEFORE BEING INJECTED WITH ESTRADIOL (ONE μG/DAY) FOR 3 DAYS. TWENTY-FOUR HOURS AFTER THE LAST INJECTION, RATS WERE SACRIFICED AND UTERINE SECRETIONS WERE COLLECTED.

| | | Estradiol Treated | | |
	Control*	Thymectomized	Sham	Intact
IgA*	0.16 ± 0.06	0.99 ± 0.51‡§	19.2 ± 5.9‡	12.6 ± 4.9‡
Number/group	10	5	8	8

Data from Sullivan and Wira.[31]

*Control group received 0.9% saline.

†mIS units/uterus.

‡Significantly ($p < 0.05$) greater than control.

§Significantly ($p < 0.05$) less than other estradiol-treated groups.

that no IgA-positive cells were present in the uterus at three hours[35] and that only few were present at 24 hours after a single estradiol treatment, suggests that very little of the tissue IgA is of local origin. Because we have found no IgG-positive cells in the uterus after hormone treatment,[34] but have demonstrated that [^{125}I]IgG equilibrates between blood and tissue,[35] we conclude that all of the IgG that accumulates in the tissue and uterine lumen after hormone treatment is of blood origin.

When IgA does accumulate in the uterine lumen after three days of estrogen treatment, several characteristics are prominent. First, IgA moves from tissue to lumen against an apparent concentration gradient. For example, IgA concentrations in uterine secretions have been found that are twenty-fold greater than those present in uterine tissue. Second, only polymeric IgA accumulates in the uterine lumen. By contrast, uterine tissue and blood have both polymeric and monomeric forms.[31] Third, IgA levels in uterine epithelial cells increase, as demonstrated by immunofluorescence analysis. In the absence of estradiol (control), very little IgA can be detected. These results suggest that estradiol, by an action on epithelial cells, may regulate IgA movement into the uterine lumen.

At other mucosal sites, IgA movement into luminal secretions appears controlled by secretory component.[42] This glycoprotein, which is synthesized by epithelial cells and hepatocytes,[43-45] both binds and transports specifically the polymeric form of IgA.[46-48] Given our findings that uterine IgA is associated with epithelial cells and that only polymeric IgA accumulates in the lumen, the possibility exists that estrogen action on uterine IgA movement may be mediated directly through secretory component.

This hypothesis is supported by our recent finding that estradiol plays an important role in the regulation of secretory component in the uterine lumen. Following estradiol treatment of ovariectomized rats, there was a time dependent accumulation of secretory component in the uterine lumen. This increase was specific for estradiol because other steroids such as cortisol and progesterone had no effect. For these reasons, estrogens are probably responsible for the increase in secretory component found during the reproductive cycle. As we report elsewhere in this Annal,[49] free secretory component was highest in the uterine lumen at proestrus when blood estrogen levels are known to be elevated,[50] and lowest at the diestrous stages of the cycle.

The presence of secretory component in the uterine lumen following estradiol treatment parallels the accumulation of IgA in uterine secretions.[38] Although our initial findings were qualitative, more recent quantitive results obtained by RIA[38] indicate that IgA and secretory component increased simultaneously at 18 hours after the second injection of estradiol. Because IgA in the uterine lumen is associated with secretory component,[36] the studies presented here support our working hypothesis that estradiol regulates IgA transport into the uterus by controlling the production of secretory component in uterine epithelial cells.

Whereas our finding that much of uterine tissue IgA is derived from serum, this fact does not preclude the possibility that some polymeric IgA may be synthesized locally. The results presented in this study indicate that in the absence of estradiol, no IgA-positive cells were present in the uteri of ovariectomized rats. With hormone exposure, IgA-positive cells appeared in the myometrium and endometrium in increasing numbers after one, two, and three days of estradiol treatment. Of particular interest was the finding that the appearance of IgA-positive cells in the uterus coincided with a drop in the number of circulating nucleated cells in blood, the majority of which were lymphocytes. The correlation between circulating lymphocytes and IgA-positive cells in the uterus was also found when progesterone was administered along with estradiol. Under these conditions, we observed that both the appearance of IgA-positive cells and the decline in circulating lymphocytes in blood were blocked when progesterone was administered along with estradiol. Several studies have indicated that mesenteric lymphocytes that migrate to mucosal sites such as the mammary gland,[51] cervix, and vagina,[52] are under endocrine control. Our findings suggest that under the appropriate hormonal balance, lymphocyte migration occurs to the uterus as well.

IgA-plasma cell infiltration and the secretion of IgA and IgG in the stroma of the uterus may be of particular importance at the time of blastocyst implantation into the uterus. Increasing numbers of IgA- and IgG-plasma cells have been found near the uterine glands during early pregnancy.[53-54] These studies suggested that locally synthesized immunoglobulins may play a role in either adoptive immunity or suppression of blastocyst rejection.

Regulation of the uterine immune system may, in part, be modulated through estradiol effects on the thymus. By measuring the uterine response to estradiol in neonatally thymectomized adult rats, we observed that the levels of IgA and IgG in the uterine lumen were markedly reduced. Others have shown as well that with the absence of an intact thymus, the secretory immune system, at a number of mucosal sites, is markedly altered.[55-57] In light of our observation that estradiol action in the uterus is diminished in the absence of the thymus, studies need to be undertaken to identify the mechanism(s) by which T-lymphocytes may alter the regulation of the uterine secretory immune system by estrogens.

In conclusion, our results suggest that estrogens regulate the secretory immune system in the reproductive tract at several levels. As shown in the schematic drawing (FIGURE 6), treatment with estrogen leads to a very rapid influx (three to six hours) from blood to tissue of polymeric and monomeric IgA, IgG, and IgM. This response is most likely due to changes in the uterine vasculature that result in increased uterine permeability within the first few hours after hormone exposure. Accompanying the flux of IgG into the uterus is its accumulation in the uterine lumen. This transfer of IgG is down a concentration gradient. When IgA begins to accumulate in uterine secretions (two to three days), it is moved from the tissue to the lumen against an apparent gradient. Secretory component also accumulates in the uterine lumen. This glycoprotein may bind and transport IgA from tissue

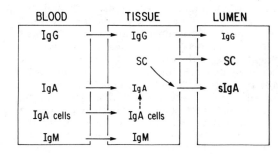

FIGURE 6. Schematic presentation of the possible sites at which estradiol may exert an influence on the immune system in the uterus of the rat.

into the uterine lumen. Also included is the estradiol-induced accumulation of IgA-positive cells in the uterus. The hatched line from tissue IgA-positive cells to IgA, though speculative, is included to suggest that in addition to serum transudation, local IgA synthesis may contribute to the pool of IgA that appears in the uterine tissue following hormone treatment.

ACKNOWLEDGMENTS

We are extremely indebted to Dr. Herve Bazin of the Catholic University of Louvain, Belgium, for his very generous gifts of goat anti-rat IgA and IgA-rich serum from rats with IR-22 immunocytomas. We also wish to express our appreciation to Dr. Brian Underdown of the University of Toronto, Toronto, Canada, for his kind gifts of rat secretory component and rabbit anti-rat secretory component.

REFERENCES

1. MUELLER, G. C., R. K. VONDERHAAR, U. H. KIM & U. LEMAHIEU. 1972. Estrogen action: An inroad to cell biology. Recent Prog. Horm. Res. **28:** 1–49.

2. JENSEN, E. V. & H. I. JACOBSON. 1962. Basic guides to the mechanism of estrogen action. Recent Prog. Horm. Res. **18:** 387–414.
3. GORSKI, J., D. TOFT, G. SHYAMALA, D. SMITH, & A. NOTIDES. 1968. Hormone receptors: Studies on the interaction of estrogen with the uterus. Recent Prog. Horm. Res. **24:** 45–80.
4. JENSEN, E. V., T. SUZUKI, T. KAWASHIMA, W. E. STUMPF, P. W. JUNGBLUT & E. R. DeSOMBRE. 1968. A two-step mechanism for the interaction of estradiol with rat uterus. Proc. Natl. Acad. Sci. U.S.A. **59:** 632–638.
5. McCORMACK, S. A. & S. R. GLASSER. 1980. Differential response of individual uterine cell types from immature rats treated with estradiol. Endocrinology **106:** 1634–1649.
6. MUELLER, G. C., J. GORSKI & Y. AIZAWA. 1961. The role of protein synthesis in early estrogen action. Proc. Natl. Acad. Sci. U.S.A. **47:** 164–169.
7. NOTEBOOM, W. D. & J. GORSKI. 1963. An early effect of estrogen on protein synthesis. Proc. Natl. Acad. Sci. U.S.A. **50:** 250–255.
8. REISS, N. A. & A. V. KAYE. 1981. Identification of the major component of the estrogen-induced protein of rat uterus as the BB isozyme of creatine kinase. J. Biol. Chem. **256:** 5741–5749.
9. WIRA, C. R. 1978. Physiology of reproduction. *In* Principles of Pediatrics, Health Care in the Young. McGraw-Hill Publishing Co. 305–310.
10. HECHTER, O., L. KROHN, & J. HARRIS. 1942. Effects of estrogens and other steroids on capillary permeability. Endocrinology **30:** 598–608.
11. KALMAN, S. M. 1955. Some studies on estrogens and uterine permeability. J. Pharmacol. Exp. Ther. **115:** 442–448.
12. KALMAN, S. M. & J. M. LOWENSTEIN. 1958. The effect of estrogens on the uptake of albumin and electrolytes by the rat uterus. J. Pharmacol. Exp. Ther. **122:** 163–167.
13. ASTWOOD, E. B. 1938. A six-hour assay for the quantitative determination of estrogen. Endocrinology **23:** 25–31.
14. TALBOT, N. B., O. H. LOWRY & E. B. ASTWOOD. 1940. Influence of estrogen on the electrolyte pattern of the immature rat uterus. J. Biol. Chem. **132:** 1–9.
15. SCHUMACHER, G. F. B. 1980. Humoral immune factors in the female reproductive tract and their changes during the cycle. In Immunological Aspects of Infertility, and Fertility Regulation. Dindsa, D. and G. Schumacher, Eds.: 93–141 Elsevier. North Holland.
16. SPARKS, R. A., B. G. A. Purrier & P. J. WATT. 1977. The bacteriology of the cervix and uterus. Brit. J. Obstet. Gynaecol. **84:** 701–704.
17. WIRA, C. R. & K. MERRITT. 1977. Effect of the estrous cycle, castration and pseudopregnancy on *E. coli* in the uterus and uterine secretions of the rat. Biol. Reprod. **17:** 519–522.
18. KLEBANOFF, S. J. & D. C. SMITH. 1970. Peroxidase-mediated antimicrobial activity of rat uterine fluid. Gynecol. Invest. **1:** 21–30.
19. GALASK, R. P. & I. S. SNYDER. 1970. Antimicrobial factors in amniotic fluid. Am. J. Obstet. Gynecol. **106:** 59–65.
20. BROWNLIE, J. & K. G. HIBBITT. 1972. Antimicrobial proteins isolated from bovine cervical mucus. J. Reprod. Fertil. **29:** 337–347.
21. TOURVILLE, D. R., S. S. OGRA, J. LIPPES & T. B. TOMASI, Jr. 1970. The human female reproductive tract: immunohistological localization of γA, γG, γM, "secretory piece," and lactoferrin. Am. J. Obstet. Gynecol. **108:** 1102–1108.
22. CINADER, B. & A. deWECK, Eds. 1976. Immunological Response of the Female Reproductive Tract. Scriptor. Copenhagen, Denmark.
23. WIRA, C. R. & C. P. SANDOE. 1977. Sex hormone regulation of IgA and IgG in rat uterine secretions. Nature (London) **268:** 534–536.
24. REBELLO, R., F. H. Y. GREEN & H. FOX. 1975. A study of the secretory immune system of the female genital tract. Brit. J. Obstet. Gynaecol. **82:** 812–816.
25. HURLIMAN, J., R. DAYAL & E. GLOOR. 1978. Immunoglobulins and secretory component in endometrium and cervix. Influence of inflammation and carcinoma. Virchows Arch. **377:** 211–223.
26. KELLY, J. K. & H. FOX. 1979. The local immunological defense system of the human endometrium. J. Reprod. Immunol. **1:** 39–47.

27. SYMONS, D. B. A. & J. HERBERT. 1971. Incidence of immunoglobulins in fluids of the rabbit genital tract and the distribution of IgG-globulin in the tissues of the female tract. J. Reprod. Fertil. **24**: 55-62.

28. CHANDRA, R. K., P. K. MALKANI & K. BHASIN. 1974. Levels of immunoglobulins in the serum and uterine fluid of women using an intra-uterine contraceptive device. J. Reprod. Fertil. **37**: 1-16.

29. VAERMAN, J. -P. & J. FERIN. 1974. Local immunological response in the vagina, cervix, and endometrium. Acta Endocrinologica [Suppl] (Kbh) **78**: 281-301.

30. MENGE, A. C. & M. E. LIEBERMAN. 1974. Antifertility effects of immunoglobulins from uterine fluids of semen-immunized rabbits. Biol. Reprod. **10**: 422-428.

31. SULLIVAN, D. A. & C. R. WIRA. 1983. Mechanisms involved in the hormonal regulation of immunoglobulins in the rat uterus. II. Uterine immunoglobulin response to multiple estradiol treatments. Submitted to Endocrinol.

32. WIRA, C. R. and C. P. SANDOE. 1978. Regulation by sex hormones of immunoglobulins in rat uterine and vaginal secretions. Adv. Exp. Med. Biol. **107**: 531-539.

33. WIRA, C. R. & C. P. SANDOE. 1980. Hormonal regulation of immunoglobulins: Influence of estradiol on immunoglobulins A and G in the rat uterus. Endocrinology **106**: 1020-1026.

34. WIRA, C. R. & D. A. SULLIVAN. 1981. Effect of estradiol and progesterone on the secretory immune system in the female genital tract. Adv. Exp. Med. Biol. **138**: 99-111.

35. SULLIVAN, D. A. & C. R. WIRA. 1983. Mechanisms involved in hormone regulation of immunoglobulins in the rat uterus. I. Uterine immunoglobulin response to a single estradiol treatment. Endocrinology **112**: 260-268.

36. SULLIVAN, D. A. & C. R. WIRA. 1981. Estradiol regulation of secretory component in the female reproductive tract. J. Steroid Biochem. **15**: 439-444.

37. WIRA, C. R., E. HYDE, C. P. SANDOE, D. SULLIVAN & S. SPENCER. 1980. Cellular aspects of the rat uterine IgA response to estradiol and progesterone. J. Steroid. Biochem. **12**: 451-459.

38. SULLIVAN, D. A. & C. R. WIRA. Unpublished observation.

39. WIRA, C. R., D. A. SULLIVAN & C. P. Sandoe. 1983. The role of estradiol in the accumulation of IgA and IgG in the rat uterine lumen. J. Steroid Biochem. In press.

40. TCHERNITCHIN, A. 1979. The role of eosinophil receptors in the non-genomic response to oestrogens in the uterus. J. Steroid Biochem. **11**: 417-424.

41. LAMM, M. E. 1976. Cellular aspects of immunoglobulin A. Adv. Immunol. **22**: 223-290.

42. GANGULY, R. & R. H. WALDMAN. 1980. Local immunity and local immune responses. Prog. Allergy **27**: 1-68.

43. CRAGO, S. S., R. KULHAVY, S. J. PRINCE & J. MESTECKY. 1978. Secretory component on epithelial cells is a surface receptor for polymeric immunoglobulins. J. Exp. Med. **147**: 1832-1837.

44. SOCKEN, D. J., K. N. JEEJEEBHOY, H. BAZIN & B. J. UNDERDOWN. 1979. Identification of secretory component as an IgA receptor on rat hepatocytes. J. Exp. Med. **50**: 1538-1548.

45. ZEVENBERGEN, J. L., C. MAY, J. C. WATSON & J. -P. VAERMAN. 1980. Synthesis of secretory component by rat hepatocytes in culture. Scand. J. Immunol. **11**: 93-97.

46. BRADTZAEG, P. 1974. Mucosal and glandular distribution of immunoglobulin components. Differential localization of free and bound SC in the secretory epithelial cells. J. Immunol. **112**: 1553-1559.

47. BROWN, W., K. ISOBE, P. K. NAKANE & B. PACINI. 1977. Studies on translocation of immunoglobulins across intestinal epithelium. IV. Evidence for binding of IgA and IgM to secretory component in intestinal epithelium. Gastroenterology **73**: 1333-1339.

48. NAGURE, H., P. K. NAKANE & W. R. BROWN. 1979. Translocation of dimeric IgA through neoplastic colon cells in vitro. J. Immunol. **123**: 2359-2368.

49. SULLIVAN, D. A. & C. R. WIRA. 1983. Estradiol regulation of secretory component in the rat uterus. Annals New York Acad. Sci. This volume.

50. NEQUIN, L. G., J. ALVAREZ & N. B. SCHWARTZ. 1979. Measurement of serum steroid and

gonadotropin levels and uterine and ovarian variables throughout 4 day and 5 day estrous cycles in the rat. Biol. Reprod. **20:** 659–670.

51. WEISZ-CARRINGTON, P., M. E. ROUX, M. MCWILLIAMS, J. M. PHILLIPS-QUAGLIATA & M. E. LAMM. 1978. Hormonal induction of the secretory immune system in the mammary gland. Proc. Natl. Acad. Sci. USA **75:** 2928–2932.

52. MCDERMOTT, M. R., D. A. CLARK & J. BIENENSTOCK. 1980. Evidence for a common mucosal immunologic system. II. Influence of the estrous cycle on B immunoblast migration into genital and intestinal tissues. J. Immunol. **124:** 2536–2539.

53. BERNARD, O., M-A. RIPOCHE & D. BENNETT. 1977. Distribution of maternal immunoglobulin in the mouse uterus and embryo in the days after implantation. J. Exp. Med. **145:** 58–75.

54. BERNARD, O., F. RACHMAN & D. BENNETT. 1981. Immunoglobulins in the mouse uterus before implantation. J. Reprod. Fertil. **63:** 237–240.

55. EBERSOLE, J. L., M. A. TAUBMAN & D. J. SMITH. 1979. The effect of neonatal thymectomy on the level of salivary and serum immunoglobulins in rats. Immunology **36:** 649–657.

56. EBERSOLE, J. L., M. A. TAUBMAN & D. J. SMITH. 1979. Thymic control of secretory antibody responses in the rat. J. Immunol. **123:** 19–24.

57. WEISZ-CARRINGTON, P., A. F. SCHRATER, M. E. LAMM & G. J. THORBECKE. 1979. Immunoglobulin isotypes in plasma cells of normal and athymic mice. Cell Immunol. **44:** 343–351.

DISCUSSION OF THE PAPER

J. BIENENSTOCK (*McMaster University, Hamilton, Ontario, Canada*): Do estradiol and perhaps other sex hormones induce secretory component in other tissues. Has anybody examined *in vitro* effects of such hormones or the expression of secretory component on hepatocytes?

WIRA (*Dartmouth Medical School, Hanover, N.H.*): In short term organ cultures of uterine segments taken from animals primed *in vivo* with estradiol, the secretory component accumulates in the incubation media. I am not aware of any published data that estradiol has a direct stimulatory effect.

BIENENSTOCK: I am aware of several papers, suggesting that estradiol causes changes in the endothelium of uterine capillaries and affects the post capillary venules as well as the numbers of cells that exit from the blood.

WIRA: This phenomenon has not been studied in the uterus, but does occur in peripheral lymph nodes. The number of high endothelial cells in post capillary vesicles increased after estradiol administration.

THE PROPERTIES AND ROLE OF RECEPTORS FOR IgA ON HUMAN LEUKOCYTES*

Michael W. Fanger, Steven N. Goldstine, and Li Shen

Departments of Microbiology and Medicine
Dartmouth Medical School
Hanover, New Hampshire 03755
Department of Oral Biology
School of Dentistry
Case Western Reserve University
Cleveland, Ohio 44106

INTRODUCTION

Receptors for the Fc portion of IgA (RFc_α) have been demonstrated on both the T- and non-T-lymphocytes of several species.[1-7] Although initially observed on only a small percentage of the lymphocyte population in the human,[1] recent studies indicate that a large percentage of human peripheral lymphocytes express RFc_α.[7] The vast majority of RFc_α bearing lymphocytes in the circulation are T-cells and overlap significantly with the T-lymphocyte population expressing receptors for the Fc portion of IgM (RFc_μ).[8] The association of RFc_α with the T-lymphocyte population suggests that these receptors may be involved in regulation of IgA responses. Moreover, studies with IgA myelomas in mice indicate that exposure to high concentrations of IgA alone can increase T-lymphocyte RFc_α expression[9,10] thus implying that the function(s) associated with RFc_α and RFc_α bearing lymphocytes can be modulated. Although some studies indicate that RFc_α bearing T-lymphocytes have no effect on IgA responses,[3] others[11] are more suggestive of an interrelationship, in that T-cells bearing RFc_α purified with a fluorescence-activated cell sorter were capable of specific enhancement of IgA production.

The demonstration of receptors for IgA on monocytes and polymorphonuclear cells (PMNs)[7] has suggested that on these cell populations RFc_α may have an effector function. In fact, it would appear that secretory IgA can synergize with IgG in promoting antibody-dependent cell cytotoxicity (ADCC) by human PMNs, monocytes, and lymphocytes.[12] The present paper considers the distribution and specificity of RFc_α among human leukocyte populations and the modulation of RFc_α on effector-cell subpopulations. Moreover, evidence is presented that indicates that RFc_α bearing leukocyte subpopulations from mucosal areas are able to phagocytose IgA-coated antigens.

*This work was supported by Research Grants AI-19053 from the Institute of Allergy and Infectious Disease, CA-31918 from the National Cancer Institute, and DE-05709 from the Institution for Dental Research of the United States Public Health Service. The Cytofluorograph was the generous gift of the Fannie Rippel Foundation and is partially supported by the core grant of the Norris Cotton Cancer Center (CA-23108).

0077-8923/83/0409-0552 $1.75/0 © 1983, NYAS

Methods and Materials

Cells

Human peripheral blood lymphocytes, monocytes, and PMNs were isolated from heparinized blood by gradient centrifugation on Ficoll Hypaque and by sedimentation in dextran.[7] Oral leukocytes were obtained from gingival crevices of healthy human volunteers.[13] Samples from 8 to 16 crevices per individual were collected and washed in Hanks Balanced Salt Solution. The oral leukocyte populations obtained were typically greater than 90% polymorphonuclear leukocytes of which at least 85% were viable.

Assays for Fc Receptors

Ox erythrocytes (ORBC) sensitized with rabbit IgG, mouse monoclonal IgM, or rabbit secretory IgA antibodies were used as indicator cells for the detection of

TABLE 1

Organ Distribution of Human Lymphocytes Bearing Receptors for Different Ig Classes

| | Lymphocytes Bearing Receptors for | | |
	IgG	IgM	IgA
Blood:			
Adult	22 ± 8	63 ± 8	51 ± 7
T	24 ± 8	68 ± 10	53 ± 8
non-T	75 ± 11	10 ± 5	7 ± 2
Neonatal	44 ± 5	42 ± 5	34 ± 4
Spleen	37 ± 7	30 ± 3	22 ± 4
Tonsils	11 ± 7	21 ± 16	38 ± 20
Bone Marrow	55 ± 11	13 ± 8	14 ± 11

cell populations expressing receptors for IgG (RFc_γ), IgM (RFc_μ), and IgA (RFc_α) respectively.[7,14] Secretory IgA antibody to ORBC was obtained from the milk of hyperimmunized rabbits and was purified as previously described.[7] The Orthocytofluorograph system 50H was used to quantitate binding of IgA immunoglobulin to these cell populations. Cells (2×10^6) were incubated with 50 μl fluorescein isothiocyanate (FITC) labeled human secretory IgA (0.5 mg/ml) for two hours at 4° C, washed in phosphate buffered saline, and analyzed by cytofluorography using a laser light at 480 nanameter wavelength maintained at constant light intensity with the Spectraphysics 265 exciter. The specificity of RFc_α was determined by studies on the inhibition of RFc_α rosette formation using various purified immunoglobulin preparations.[15,16] In particular, human secretory IgA, dimer IgA_2 and IgA_1 paraproteins, and their reduced and alkylated monomers, as well as a $C_{\alpha3}$ deficient IgA_1 paraprotein (Wal) were purified and utilized as previously described.[16]

Phagocytosis

Polymorphonuclear cells (5×10^6) in RPMI with 10% fetal calf serum were incubated with antibody-coated ORBC in a final volume of 0.5 ml for 10 minutes at 37° C. The cells were then centrifuged for five minutes at 1200 RPM and reincubated at 37° C for an additional 20 minutes. The supernatant was removed and 0.5 ml of ammonium chloride-TRIS-HCl buffer was added to the pellet to lyse extracellular ox erythrocytes. The cells were centrifuged onto slides at 500 rpm for five minutes, and the slides were fixed in methanol and stained with Wright's stain. Polymorphonuclear cells containing one or more ORBC were considered positive. The percentage of phagocytosis was determined by counting the number of positive PMNs per one hundred PMNs. In selected experiments the average number of ORBC phagocytosed per hundred PMNs was also determined.

RESULTS

Distribution and Specificity of RFc_α

Using ORBC sensitized with secretory IgA anti-ORBC antibody as an indicator system, we have found that large percentages of lymphocytes from the normal human tissues examined express RFc_α,[17] (TABLE 1). Although in organs such as tonsils, many of these RFc_α bearing cells are non-T-lymphocytes, the vast majority of RFc_α bearing lymphocytes in the peripheral blood are T-cells and are the same lymphocytes displaying RFc_μ.[17] As receptors associated with an apparent T-helper cell population, it is tempting to imagine that RFc_α on these cells have a regulatory role. The association of RFc_α with effector-cell populations,[7] including monocytes and both peripheral blood and oral PMNs (TABLE 2), suggests that RFc_α may facilitate protective interactions between the cells on which these receptors reside and IgA-coated antigen.

One approach to evaluating a potential effector function for these receptors has been to examine the nature of the interaction between RFc_α on these different cell populations and the various forms of IgA. Based on studies of the ability of different IgA preparations to block rosette formation between IgA-sensitized indicator cells and RFc_α bearing cells, it would appear that RFc_α can react with both the IgA_1 and IgA_2 subclasses, with secretory IgA, and with both monomer and dimer forms of IgA.[15,16] Thus, IgA preparations lacking secretory component and J-chain are effective blockers of RFc_α. Furthermore, the ability of an IgA paraprotein lacking a $C_{\alpha 3}$ domain and of $Fc_{2\alpha}$ fragments to block IgA-rosette

TABLE 2

RECEPTORS FOR IMMUNOGLOBULIN ON ORAL AND PERIPHERAL BLOOD
POLYMORPHONUCLEAR LEUKOCYTES

	Percent of PMNs Expressing Receptors for		
	IgA	IgM	IgG
Peripheral blood	35	0	82
Oral	62	0	46

TABLE 3

INDUCTION OF RFc_α ON PERIPHERAL BLOOD POLYMORPHONUCLEAR CELLS BY
INCUBATION WITH IGA

Experiment	Tube No.	Additions (µg)	Percent RFc_α	Bearing Cells*
A	1	None	—	42
	2	CLP-IgA	100	63
	3		30	54
B	1	None	—	38
	2	CLP-IgA	30	73
C	1	None	—	49
	2	CLP-IgA	30	68
	3	IgG	30	42
D	1	None	—	28
	2	CLP-IgA	30	57
	3	HsIgA	30	75

*PMNs were incubated with media alone or with various Ig preparations for 16 hours at 37° C in 5% CO_2 and then assayed for the percentage of cells forming rosettes with IgA-sensitized indicator cells.

formation indicate that RFc_α recognize structures in the C2 domain of the IgA α-chain.[15,16]

Modulation of RFc_a on Polymorphonuclear Cells

During studies on the specificity of RFc_α on human PMNs, it became clear that the degree of inhibition of IgA-rosette formation by certain IgA preparations was dependent on the way the blocking experiments were conducted. Additional studies demonstrated that under appropriate conditions IgA was, of itself, capable of enhancing the expression of RFc_α on human polymorphonuclear cells. In these experiments, PMNs were incubated at 37° C with a human myeloma IgA_1 paraprotein (CLP) or with human secretory IgA for 16 hours and then washed free of the IgA. A much larger percentage of PMNs incubated with IgA formed rosettes with IgA-sensitized ORBC than did untreated PMNs or PMNs treated under the same conditions with IgG (TABLE 3). Relatively low concentrations of IgA (30 µg/ml and 3 µg/ml) were capable, over a 16 hour period, of increasing the percentage of PMNs forming IgA rosettes. Moreover, the quality of the rosettes formed was much better than those formed by untreated PMNs; the rosettes were more stable and contained a larger number of red blood cells than IgA rosettes with untreated polymorphonuclear cells. Cells incubated with IgA did not form rosettes with unsensitized ORBC or with ORBC sensitized with IgM (TABLE 3).

In an attempt to develop a more quantitative appreciation for RFc_α expression and induction, cytofluorograph analysis of untreated and IgA-treated PMNs was carried out. As shown in FIGURE 1a, fluorescein conjugated human secretory IgA (FITC-HsIgA) stained a large percentage of human PMNs as compared with FITC-conjugated bovine serum albumin (FITC-BSA). After 16 hours of incubation with the CLP IgA paraprotein, PMNs had a considerably greater ability to react with FITC-HsIgA (FIGURE 1b) than did PMNs incubated in culture media

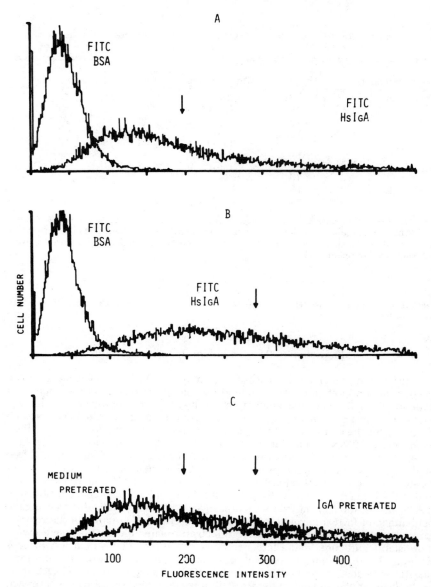

FIGURE 1. Cytofluorographic analysis of the binding of fluorescein conjugated BSA (FITC-BSA) or fluorescein conjugated human secretory IgA (FITC-HsIgA) to peripheral blood polymorphonuclear leukocytes. PMNs were pretreated for 16 hours at 37° C with medium alone (A), or medium containing 0.03 mg/ml of the CLP IgA paraprotein (B). A direct comparison of FITC-HsIgA binding to medium pretreated or CLP-IgA pretreated PMNs is shown in C. Arrows (↓) denote the mean fluorescence intensity of cells binding FITC-HsIgA. The mean is calculated as: $(1/N) \Sigma (N_x \cdot X)$ where N = total number of cells (10,000 in all samples), X = channel number, and N_x = number of cells in channel X.

alone (FIGURE 1a). A comparison of the cytofluorograph patterns of binding of FITC-HsIgA to PMNs before or after incubation with IgA (FIGURE 1c) demonstrates a shift in the mean fluorescence intensity from channel 199 to 285. Neither the binding of FITC-BSA, nor of FITC-conjugated human IgG (data not shown) to PMNs was enhanced by incubation of these cells with IgA. Furthermore, the interaction of FITC-HsIgA with PMNs could be blocked by HsIgA and by human IgA paraproteins. Incubation of PMNs with human IgG did not appear to enhance RFc_α expression, because no change in cytofluorograph pattern or mean fluorescence intensity of FITC-HsIgA staining was observed.

Phagocytosis

Our previous studies have indicated that IgA alone is unable to mediate ADCC by peripheral lymphocytes, monocytes, or PMNs.[12] Nonetheless, IgA is

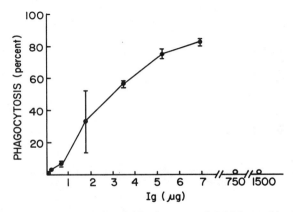

FIGURE 2. Phagocytosis by peripheral blood PMNs of ORBC sensitized with varying amounts of IgG (●) or IgA (○). Various quantities of immunoglobulin were used to sensitize 25 μl of a 2% suspension of ORBC. Results plotted are the mean and standard deviation of two replicate samples. Similar results were obtained in six other experiments.

able to synergize with IgG in mediating ADCC of ORBC, suggesting a role for RFc_α in this important effector function. In another series of experiments, we have examined the possible role of RFc_α in phagocytosis. Using optimal ratios of effector to target cells (1:10), we have found that ORBC sensitized with IgG antibody were readily phagocytosed by peripheral blood PMNs, whereas those ORBC sensitized with IgA antibody alone were not phagocytosed (Figure 2). These studies were done using concentrations of IgA that yielded IgA-sensitized indicator cells capable of optimal rosette formation with these same effector-cell populations. Thus, in spite of their ability to form rosettes with IgA-sensitized ORBC, these effector-cell populations were unable to phagocytose these targets.

In order to determine whether IgA antibody was capable of enhancing phagocytosis, ORBC were first coated with low concentrations of IgG anti-ORBC antibody. As illustrated in FIGURE 3, ORBC coated with IgG alone were phagocytosed by approximately 10% of the PMNs. In the presence of high concentrations of IgA antibody (1.2 mg), however, phagocytosis was increased by more than two-fold (FIGURE 3). These concentrations paralleled the amounts necessary for optimal IgA-rosette formation with this IgA preparation. Similar results were obtained in other studies and indicate that marked enhancement of phagocytosis by IgA antibody also occurred with various suboptimal quantities of IgG antibody (TABLE 4). In all cases, the addition of IgA to IgG-ORBC resulted in a two- to three-fold enhancement of phagocytosis. In no case was there phagocytosis of ORBC or IgA-ORBC.

Although it appeared as though IgA enhanced phagocytosis, it was important to evaluate the possibility that the increased phagocytosis was the result of very small amounts of IgG antibody in the IgA preparation. The level of contamination of the IgA preparations was examined by enzyme-linked immunoassay of the

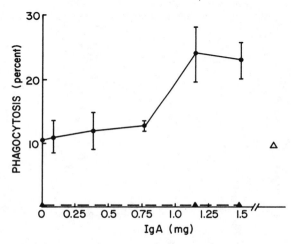

FIGURE 3. Phagocytosis by peripheral blood polymorphonuclear leukocytes of ORBC sensitized with IgG and IgA (●), IgM and IgA (▲), or IgM and IgG (△). The horizontal axis shows the quantity of IgA used to sensitize 25 μl of a 2% suspension of ORBC. Mouse hybridoma culture supernatant containing monoclonal IgM anti-ORBC was added to a 2% suspension of ORBC at a concentration that allowed optimal detection of RFc_{μ} bearing lymphocytes. IgG antibody was used at 1.0 μg to sensitize 25 μl of 2% ORBC targets.

concentrated antibody and found to be less than 0.1 μg IgG/mg IgA. Thus, in the experiment shown in TABLE 4 in which 600 μg of IgA significantly enhanced phagocytosis of IgG-coated ORBC, the contaminating IgG potentially added was less than 0.1 μg, a level below that causing minimal phagocytosis. Certainly the simple addition of the small amounts of IgG potentially present in the IgA preparation could not account for the increased levels of phagocytosis observed. Moreover, this phenomenon was specifically mediated by IgA, as enhanced phagocytosis was not observed on addition of IgM antibody to IgG-coated ORBC. In addition to increasing the percentage of PMNs that were phagocytic, the addition of IgA to IgG-ORBC also increased the number of ORBC phagocytosed per polymorphonuclear cell.

TABLE 4

SECRETORY IgA ANTIBODIES SYNERGIZE WITH IgG IN PROMOTING PHAGOCYTOSIS BY
HUMAN PERIPHERAL BLOOD POLYMORPHONUCLEAR CELLS*

Tube No.	Quanity of Ig (μg)† IgG	IgA	Percent Phagocytosis
1	—	—	0
2	—	600	0
3	1	—	2
4	1	600	10
5	2	—	11
6	2	600	29
7	6	—	39
8	6	600	80

*Similar results were obtained in eight other experiments.
†The quantity of immunoglobulin used to coat 25 μl of a 2% suspension of ORBC.

Because a larger percentage of oral PMNs express RFc_α than do their peripheral blood counterparts (TABLE 2), we examined the possibility that oral PMNs could phagocytose IgA-coated target cells. As shown in TABLE 5, in studies of oral PMNs from three different individuals, secretory IgA anti-ORBC antibody markedly enhanced the phagocytosis of IgG-coated ox erythrocytes. Perhaps more significantly, oral PMNs were capable of phagocytosing ORBC coated with IgA alone. Unsensitized ORBC were not phagocytosed by these cells. Again, the potential contaminating IgG in these IgA preparations was well below that necessary to account for the phagocytosis or synergy observed.

TABLE 5

SECRETORY IgA ANTIBODIES MEDIATE PHAGOCYTOSIS BY
ORAL POLYMORPHONUCLEAR CELLS*

Patients	Tube No.	Quantity of Ig (μg)† IgG	IgA	Phagocytosis Percent	ORBC/PMN
A	1	—	—	0	
	2	1.0	—	5	
	3	—	600	7	
	4	1.0	600	23	
B	1	—	—	0	
	2	4.0	—	40	
	3	—	600	6	
	4	4.0	600	64	
C	1	—	—	0	0
	2	4.0	—	80	2.3
	3	—	600	9	1.5
	4	4.0	600	89	3.6

*Oral leukocytes were collected from the gingival crevices of three different healthy adult volunteers. These results are representative of data obtained using oral leukocytes from 20 different patients.
†The quantity of immunoglobulin used to coat 25 μl of a 2% suspension of ORBC.

DISCUSSION

Receptors for the Fc portion of IgA are associated with a wide variety of leukocyte populations and subpopulations. Both peripheral blood T- and B-cells as well as lymphocytes from mucosal tissues express these receptors,[2,6,8] (Table 1). In the rabbit, a larger percentage of lymphocytes associated with mucosal tissues express RFc_α than do lymphocytes from systemic lymphoid organs.[4,18] That RFc_α in the human are primarily associated with the T-lymphocyte population expressing RFc_μ and categorized by some as a helper-cell population, suggests that RFc_α and RFc_α bearing T-cells play a role in regulation of secretory as well as systemic immune responses. This possibility is supported by the recent finding that RFc_α bearing T-lymphocytes purified by cell sorting were capable of specific enhancement of IgA production.[11]

In studies of mouse lymphocytes, other workers have found that incubation with high concentrations of IgA in vivo or in vitro results in a significant increase in the percentage of cells expressing RFc_α.[9,10] In this instance, these lymphocytes may represent suppressor-cell populations,[10] and a response of the immune system designed to dampen IgA production. In either case, it remains to be shown that the receptor itself is involved in either help or suppression. Moreover, considering the varied association of this receptor with different lymphocyte subpopulations, it is possible that RFc_α may be associated with both helper and suppressor populations. Were this the case, the function of RFc_α could be viewed as being dependent on the function of the subpopulation with which it was associated. Thus, on T-helper cells, RFc_α may facilitate manifestation of help, whereas on suppressor cells, the manifestation of suppression. One might view the function of RFc_α on lymphocytes, therefore, as secondary, but perhaps still important to the primary function of the cell population with which they are associated.

The association of RFc_α with effector-cell populations, including monocytes[7,16] and PMNs[7,16] (TABLE 2) implies that these receptors may be involved in facilitating interactions between phagocytic cells and IgA-coated targets. Our previous studies have shown that although human peripheral blood leukocytes are unable to manifest ADCC of ORBC coated with IgA alone, IgA anti-ORBC was capable of synergizing with suboptimal quantities of IgG anti-ORBC in ADCC of ORBC targets.[12]

Likewise, the present study of the properties of RFc_α in an erythrophagocytosis system suggests that, on blood PMNs, binding of these receptors alone does not trigger phagocytosis. Rather, RFc_α seem limited in their activity to enhancing phagocytosis mediated through RFc_γ, receptors already shown to be of major importance to this function.[19] The interpretation that there are cooperative interactions between these receptors is strengthened by the observation that challenge with IgA-ORBC and IgG-ORBC target cells, simultaneously, does not increase and occasionally decreases phagocytosis. Thus, to obtain IgA-mediated enhancement of phagocytosis of IgG-ORBC, the two antibody isotypes must be on the same target cell. These observations suggest that RFc_α on blood PMNs function to facilitate binding of IgG- and IgA-coated target cells.

The enhancement observed with the addition of IgA to IgG ORBC was most apparent under conditions that result in suboptimal IgG-mediated phagocytosis. As the amount of IgG antibody was increased and the percent of phagocytosis approached maximum levels for blood PMNs, the degree of enhancement by IgA was less marked. Similar trends were observed when the number of ORBC phagocytosed per PMN as monitored (TABLE 5).

If RFc$_\alpha$ and cells bearing these receptors play an active role in phagocytosis, it may be most clearly demonstrable on cells associated with mucosal surfaces. The data obtained by examining PMNs from the gingival crevices support this supposition. Not only does IgA enhance IgG-mediated phagocytosis, as with blood PMNs, but IgA itself appears to be capable of triggering phagocytosis by oral cells. The percentage of oral PMNs capable of phagocytosis of IgA-ORBC has consistently been between 5 and 10%. It seems unlikely that this phagocytosis is due to IgG contamination, because the level of IgG in the IgA preparations is far below that necessary for minimal phagocytosis. Moreover, blood PMNs have been consistently unable to phagocytose these targets.

It is possible that the unique phagocytic properties of oral cells may be nonspecific and the result of their exposure to oral fluids and bacteria. The role of RFc$_\alpha$ may, for example, parallel that of the complement receptors in phagocytosis, in that activated macrophages are capable of phagocytosis of C3b coated antigens, whereas normal, nonactivated macrophages are not capable of this activity.[20] Complement receptors mediate attachment of complement-coated antigens and enhancement of phagocytosis mediated by IgG antibody rather than having a more direct role in inducing the phagocytic event.[21] Although RFc$_\alpha$ on blood PMNs may function similarly, and although there is some evidence that oral PMNs have increased ability to reduce nitro blue tetrazolium dye relative to blood PMNs,[22] our studies of the phagocytic ability of oral and blood PMNs, using nonsensitized ORBC and IgG-ORBC, do not indicate enhanced phagocytic potential for oral polymorphonuclear cells.

An alternative possibility is that binding of IgA-sensitized targets to oral PMNs, through RFc$_\alpha$, triggers phagocytosis directly and that the apparent differences between blood and oral PMNs are a reflection of differences in the quality or quantity of RFc$_\alpha$ on these two cell populations. That there is a greater percent of detectable RFc$_\alpha$ bearing cells in the oral population (TABLE 2) may be a reflection of an overall increase in RFc$_\alpha$ density. We are presently exploring this possibility by a cytofluorographic comparison of these populations.

It may be of particular relevance in this context that the expression of RFc$_\alpha$ on lymphocytes[9,10] and, as shown in the present report, on PMNs is markedly enhanced by incubation with IgA. Incubation of PMNs with either human secretory IgA or an IgA paraprotein (CLP) resulted in increased numbers of RFc$_\alpha$ per cell (FIGURE 1) as well as an increase in the total number of PMNs bearing these receptors, whereas IgG at similar concentrations did not affect RFc$_\alpha$ expression. Induction by IgA was relatively specific for RFc$_\alpha$, because IgA-treated PMNs did not form rosettes with ORBC or IgM-ORBC, nor did these PMNs show increased uptake of FITC-BSA (or FITC-IgG) by cytofluorographic analysis.

A similar enhancement of Fc receptor expression has been reported on monocytes and a macrophage-like cell line U-937.[23] Two to ten-fold increases in binding of ^{125}I-labeled human IgG were observed after incubation of these cells with supernates from mixed lymphocyte cultures or lectin-stimulated mononuclear cells. This increased RFc$_\gamma$ expression appears concomitantly with an augmentation of the phagocytic and ADCC abilities of these cells.[24] Thus, modulation of Fc receptors on myeloid cells may be directly related to the manifestation of the lytic or phagocytic properties of these cells.

It seems significant that IgA-induced blood PMNs formed similar numbers of rosettes with IgA-ORBC as oral polymorphonuclear cells. This effect may be related to the presence of higher amounts of IgA and relatively lower amounts of other immunoglobulins in the gingival crevices, a situation similar to that in which increased RFc$_\alpha$ are induced *in vitro*. It is possible, for example, that PMNs migrating from the blood to the mucosal environment become exposed to greater levels of IgA, resulting in induction of higher numbers of IgA receptors per cell. This increased RFc_α expression may enhance the ability of the PMNs to participate in immune defense through IgA at the mucosal surface. This possibility is consistent with the observation that a larger percentage of oral PMNs than blood PMNs express RFc_α and may explain why oral PMNs can phagocytose through IgA alone, whereas blood PMNs require the additional presence of IgG antibodies for phagocytosis. In this regard, it would be important to evaluate the ability of IgA to induce increased RFc_α on oral PMNs and to examine the phagocytic ability of blood PMNs after induction of RFc_α with IgA. Overall, it is tempting to speculate that exposure to IgA or perhaps other constituents in the oral fluids could be a physiologic inducing signal that, by increasing RFc_α expression, could enhance the phagocytic or lytic potential of mucosal effector cells to lyse or phagocytose IgA-coated antigens.

REFERENCES

1. LUM, L. G., A. V. MUCHMORE, D. KEREN, J. DECKER, I. KOSKI, W. STROBER & R. M. BLAESE. 1979. J. Immunol. **122:** 65–69.
2. GUPTA, S., C. D. PLATSOUCAS, R. SCHULOF & R. A. GOOD. 1979. Cell. Immunol. **45:** 469.
3. LUM, L. G., E. BENVENISTE & R. M. BLAESE. 1980. J. Immunol. **124:** 702–707.
4. STAFFORD, H. A. & M. W. FANGER. 1980. J. Immunol. **125:** 2461–2466.
5. STROBER, W., N. E. HAGUE, L. G. LUM & P. A. HENKART. 1978. J. Immunol. **121:** 2440.
6. LUM, L. G., A. V. MUCHMORE, N. O'CONNOR, W. STROBER & R. M. BLAESE. 1979. J. Immunol. **123:** 714.
7. FANGER, M. W., L. SHEN, J. PUGH & G. M. BERNIER. 1980. Proc. Natl. Acad. Sci. USA **77:** 3640.
8. LYDYARD, P. M. & M. W. FANGER. 1981. Scand. J. Immunol. **14:** 509.
9. HOOVER, R. G. & R. G. LYNCH. 1980. J. Immunol. **125:** 1280.
10. HOOVER, R. G., B. K. DIECKGRAEFE & R. G. LYNCH. 1981. J. Immunol. **127:** 1560.
11. ENDOH, M., H. SAKAI, Y. NOMOTO, Y. TOMINO & H. KANESHIGE. 1981. J. Immunol. **127:** 2612.
12. SHEN, L. & M. W. FANGER. 1981. Cell. Immunol. **59:** 75–81.
13. SKAPSKI, H. & T. LEHNER. 1976. J. Periodontal Res. **11:** 19.
14. FANGER, M. W. & P. M. LYDYARD. 1979. J. Immunol. Methods **28:** 105.
15. FANGER, M. W. & P. M. LYDYARD. 1981. Mol. Immunol. **18:** 189.
16. FANGER, M. W., J. PUGH & G. M. BERNIER. 1981. Cell. Immunol. **60:** 324–334.
17. LYDYARD, P. M. & M. W. FANGER. 1981. Scand. J. Immunol. **14:** 509.
18. STAFFORD, H. A., K. L. KNIGHT & M. W. FANGER. 1982. J. Immunol. **128:** 2201–2205.
19. KLEBANOFF, J. J. & R. A. CLARK. 1978. The Neutrophil: Function and Clinical Disorders. 175–177. Elsevier. North Holland.
20. BIANCO, C., F. M. GRIFFIN & S. C. SILVERSTEIN. 1975. J. Exp. Med. **141:** 1278.
21. SCRIBNER, D. J. & D. FAHRNEY. 1976. J. Immunol. **116:** 892–897.
22. CHARON, J. A., Z. METZGAR, J. T. HOFFELD, J. I. GALLIN & S. E. MERGENHAGEN. 1982. J. Dent. Res. **61:** 333.
23. GUYRE, P. M., G. R. CRABTREE, J. E. BODWELL & A. MUNCK. 1981. J. Immunol. **126:** 666–668.
24. KOREN, H. S., S. J. ANDERSON & J. W. LARRICK. 1979. Nature (London) **279:** 328–330.

B. J. UNDERDOWN (*University of Toronto, Toronto, Ontario, Canada*): Did you show that the increased opsonization, mediated by IgA, was also inhibitable by free IgA in the medium?

M. W. FANGER (*Dartmouth Medical School, Hanover, N.H.*): Yes. Free IgA in the medium does inhibit IgA-mediated ADCC and opsonization mediated by macrophages.

J. M. SCHIFF (*University of Toronto, Toronto, Ontario, Canada*): Investigators usually do not check to see if a protein or a carbohydrate receptor is involved. Can you inhibit the binding and synergism with IgG?

FANGER: No, we cannot. The studies on specificity of binding have included pure immunoglobulins that should contain the similar sugars.

SHIFT: IgA has more carbohydrates, especially on the C2 domain.

FANGER: True. If RFc_α react with sugar moieties on IgA, however, they must be very characteristic sugars, because they are not on any of the other Ig classes we have examined.

R. J. GENCO (*State University of New York at Buffalo*): Do you have any evidence that this IgA receptor is involved in chemotaxis? The reason I ask is that Williams and van Epps have shown that IgA will inhibit chemotaxis.

FANGER: We have not performed any studies of chemotaxis. We have, however, used the same IgA protein (Wal) that lacks the C3 domain, as Drs. Williams and van Epps. This IgA molecule does not interfere with chemotaxis, but inhibits the binding to RFc_α significantly. These results indicate that if RFc_α are involved in chemotaxis, they cannot be triggered by an IgA half molecule.

GENCO: Do you know how the oral PMNs would express more IgA receptors?

FANGER: There may be some kind of inductive event that occurs in the oral tissues or environment that increases the expression of such receptors on oral polymorphonuclear cells.

NOVEL MUCOSAL ANTI-MICROBIAL FUNCTIONS INTERFERING WITH THE PLASMID-MEDIATED VIRULENCE DETERMINANTS OF ADHERENCE AND DRUG RESISTANCE

P. Porter and Margaret A. Linggood

Department of Immunology
Unilever Colworth Research Laboratory
Bedford MK44 1LQ England

INTRODUCTION

Enteropathogenicity of *E. coli* is intimately linked with host-specific adhesion factors, many of which are coded for by transmissible plasmids. Acquisition of such plasmids by strains of *E. coli* confers on the organism an ability to adhere to the anterior regions of the small intestine where the tissues are much more susceptible to the effects of enterotoxin. Over the years, a body of opinion has grown that emphasizes the importance of anti-adhesin antibodies in host protection against *E. coli* disease. Such a view has been put into extensive practice by employing K88 vaccines for maternal vaccination to prevent neonatal *E. coli* diarrhea in the pig. As a result, significant changes in the virulence determinants on porcine *E. coli* are emerging that suggest that the conventional anti-adhesin approach to vaccination may be too simplistic. The changes relate to the detection of new antigenic variants of K88 and the implication of the previously calf-specific adhesin K99 in pig strains.[1] Furthermore, where K88 was previously the reserve of the neonatal syndrome, it now complicates post-weaning disease that arises with greater virulence.[2]

There is no doubt that the anti-adhesin approach is a rational one even though the mode of vaccination and the effective immunoglobulin isotype may be questioned.[3] Effective immunization, however, must pay greater cognizance to the host-pathogen relationship in order to obviate major complications. It is in this respect that observations of *E. coli* infection in orally immunized pigs were of signal importance[4] in identifying a novel anti-microbial mechanism of the mucosal antibody system of the gut. In short, animals orally immunized with a heat inactivated *E. coli* vaccine showed a peculiar capacity to induce the loss of the K88 adhesin from a pathogen under test infection, whereas unimmunized littermates did not show this capacity. The infection was controlled in the vaccinated group, and after a short period an avirulent K88⁻ form of the administered pathogen was excreted. In the controls, however, the K88⁺ form was excreted for nearly two weeks with associated diarrhea.

This finding has led to a unique area of research concerning the role of the mucosal system in preserving a beneficial balance in the host-pathogen relationship by reducing the virulence of the pathogen in the environment. Subsequent *in vitro* studies have confirmed that antibodies produced by the oral immunization schedules have the capacity to induce the loss of K88ab and K88ac antigens in culture.[5] That the plasmid must be effectively eliminated has been confirmed indirectly by the failure of the organisms to reestablish the capacity to produce K88 antigens on subculture in the absence of antibody. Furthermore, in studies

0077-8923/83/0409-0564 $1.75/0 © 1983, NYAS

with an organism with a K88-linked plasmid function for raffinose fermentation, the antibodies induced the formation of raf⁻ strains at the same time.

Initial broad areas of interest concerning this phenomenon were the nature of the antigen or antigens involved, the mechanism by which the plasmid loss was affected, and the isotype efficiency in promoting the effect both *in vitro* and *in vivo*. Essential questions for the fullest application of this new principal in practice relate to the extent to which the mechanism covers other plasmid-mediated adhesion antigens in porcine enteropathogenic *E. coli* (EEC). Perhaps of greater importance is whether the same or a similar mucosal antibody function may ameliorate the epidemic spread of drug resistance. In this paper, we review our work on K88ab and K88ac, bring new data with regard to K88ad and K99 plasmids, extend the *in vivo* studies to examine the materno-neonatal link, and bring important new data on the effects of mucosal antibodies on the transmission of R factors. Such studies are supported with data from extensive experimentation with oral vaccination in sows and piglets; the composition and character of the vaccine has been previously described.[3]

IN VITRO STUDIES OF K88 PLASMID LOSS

The *in vitro* passaging of K88⁺ strains of *E. coli* in the presence of sera or milk wheys from immunized pigs can give rise to the loss of K88ab and K88ac plasmids from enteropathogenic strains.[5,6] FIGURE 1 shows the effect of passaging an O8:K87, K88ab strain in the presence of antibodies from a sow that had been immunized with heat-inactivated *E. coli* antigens. In this experiment, the bacteria were passaged five times, each passage for 12 hours, in nutrient broth containing 25% of the fraction under test. Under control conditions of culture there was no loss in ability to synthesize K88 antigens, but with antibodies in the culture, the O8 strain had become effectively K88⁻ after four to five passages. This loss of the ability to synthesize K88 was permanent and did not reemerge when the strain was grown in normal media. Investigation of Sephadex G-200 gel filtration fractions showed that the K88 plasmid "curing" activity of serum samples was predominantly located in the 7S IgG fractions. Both the IgG and the IgM/IgA fractions of milk wheys induced K88 loss, but the IgM/IgA fractions were more active (FIGURE 1).

A similar pattern of K88 plasmid loss was obtained when an O149:K91, K88ac strain was passaged through the immune fractions. In the strain used in this experiment, the genes for K88ac production and raffinose fermentation were on the same plasmid, and it was observed that the antibody induced loss of K88ac from the strain was always accompanied by the loss of the ability to ferment raffinose. On the other hand, any colonies that remained K88⁺ were also raf⁺, that is, the entire plasmid containing both the K88 and raf determinants was being eliminated.

There was no correlation between the ability of a serum or milk to induce K88 loss and its K88 antibody titer. When using the combined oral/parenteral schedule suitable for maternal immunization, K88 antibody levels in the serum and colostrum, samples from immunized pigs were generally low.[3] This finding was not unexpected. Although K88 antigen was present in the vaccine, K88 did not generate a secretory antibody response when priming by the oral route.[7] Oral immunization with heat-inactivated *E. coli* did, however, prime for parenterally boosted antibody responses to the serotype specific O-antigens, and in order to

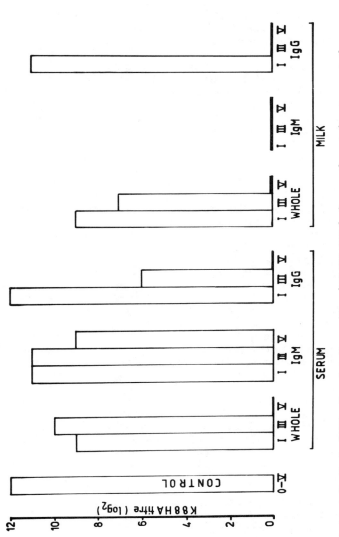

FIGURE 1. Synthesis of K88 antigen in cultures of *E. coli* 08:K87, K88ab after one, three, or five passages in the presence of antibodies from milk and serum fractions of an immunized (oral/parenteral) sow.

ascertain whether these specific antibodies were involved in the curing phenomenon, antisera were raised in pigs against heat-killed (121° C, 15 minutes) cells of a single serotype, 0149:K91, K88ac. These antisera had high titers of 0149 antibodies, but negligible levels of antibody to the O-antigens of the other enteropathogenic serotypes. K88$^+$ strains of the E. coli belonging to various O-serogroups were then passaged three times through broths containing 10% of the antisera or serum fractions under test. Each passage was for 24 hours. We found that factors present in the 0149 antisera could give rise to the elimination of K88 plasmids, not only from 0149 strains, but also from O8, O45, and O138 strains, that is, the "curing" activity of antisera was not O-serogroup specific. Absorption of the specific 0149 antibodies from the sera did not eliminate their "curing" activity (FIGURE 2). Similarly, it was possible to differentiate the "curing" activity from O-antibody by gel filtration as the 0149 antibodies were eluted in the IgM peak. The "curing" activity, however, was found in the IgG peak.[5]

Plasmid "curing" agents can give rise to the elimination of plasmids from a bacterial population basically by two different mechanisms. Some have a direct effect on the replication of the plasmid itself, whereas others select for any plasmid negative variants that have arisen spontaneously. Various experiments using the 0149 antisera described indicated that the plasmid eliminating antibodies belonged to the latter category of "curing" agent. K88$^+$ and K88$^-$ forms of the 0149 and O8 strains were grown in nutrient broth containing 10% of a "curing" or control serum, and bacterial counts were done at intervals over a period of 24 hours. The 0149 and O8 strains gave very similar growth curves, and those for the 0149 strain are shown in FIGURE 3. It will be seen that the K88$^+$ and K88$^-$ forms grew equally well in control serum, but growth of the K88$^+$ form was initially slower than that of the K88$^-$ form in the "curing" serum. The total viable counts of all the cultures were similar after 24 hours of growth, but at this stage the K88$^+$ form no longer constituted 100 percent of the bacteria present in the cultures initially inoculated with K88$^+$ organisms and grown in the presence of "curing" antibodies. In fact, K88$^-$ variants had begun to emerge after about 10 hours of growth in the presence of the antibodies.

So the presence of the K88 antigen, or factors associated with it, make K88$^+$ strains more susceptible to antibodies present in the sera and mammary secretions of immunized animals. Antibodies to the serotype specific O-antigens of the bacterial cell wall were clearly not important. Furthermore, K88 antibodies did not appear to be involved even though K88 "curing" antibodies are produced following immunization with K88$^+$, but not K88$^-$ strains. A possible explanation for this phenomenon is that the antigen involved is coded for by the K88 plasmid without necessarily being the K88 antigen itself.

ANTIBODY "CURING" EFFECTS ON OTHER ADHESION PLASMIDS IN PORCINE
ENTEROPATHOGENIC E. COLI

Recent studies[8] have suggested that a new variant of K88, identified serologically as K88ad, is emerging in porcine EEC due to selection pressure on the bacterial K88$^+$ population resulting from the widespread use of K88ab/ac vaccines. The intriguing possibility arose that here was a virulence factor that might evade the newly discovered plasmid elimination effect afforded by the antibodies so far investigated, particularly because the serotypes constituting the heat inactivated oral vaccine did not contain a K88ad plasmid.

In vitro studies of the plasmid "curing" effect were undertaken with milk

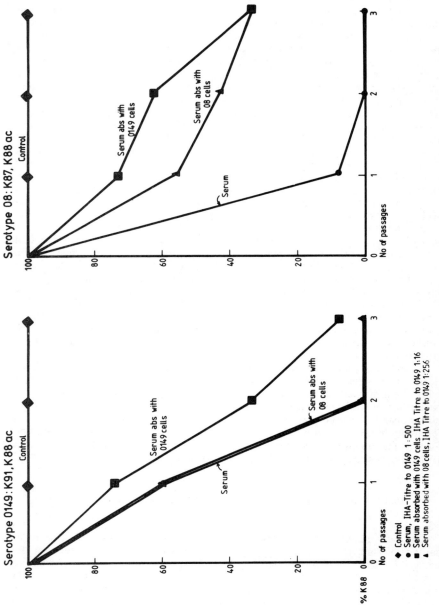

FIGURE 2. The effect of absorption of O-antibody on immune elimination of K88 antigen from porcine EEC.

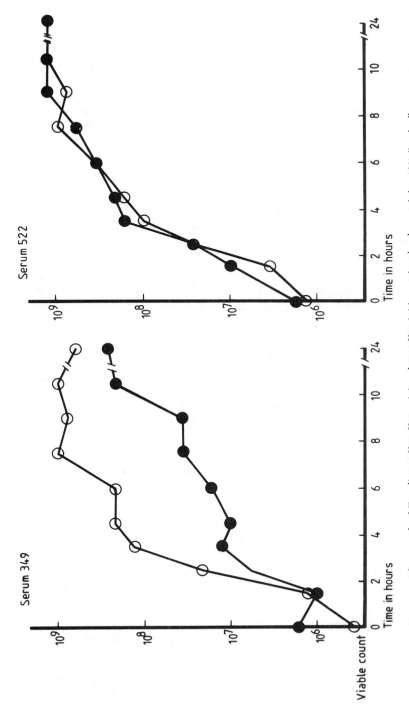

FIGURE 3. The growth of *E. coli* 0149:K91, K88ac (●) and 0149:K91 (○) in nutrient broth containing 10% "curing" serum (349) and 10% control serum (522).

whey from immunized sows. A direct comparison was made of the capacity of the milk antibodies in culture to "cure" K88ab, K88ac, and K88ad (FIGURE 4) from field strains of E. coli belonging to the O8 serogroup. No distinction emerged to suggest that the K88ad plasmid had a different stability. Furthermore, K88ac and K88ad were "cured" with equal facility from the different serogroups of E. coli O149 and O9 respectively. This finding further emphasizes the lack of association of the antibodies with the O-antigen because no pathogen of the O9 serogroup was incorporated in the vaccine.

The K99 plasmid must come into the same framework of examination for the consideration of the broad base of field efficiency of the E. coli vaccine. The K99 antigen was formerly considered to be an adhesion determinant specific for the calf; it is now, however, found frequently as the adhesin in porcine entero-pathogenic E. coli.[1]

The prospect that this antigen would also yield to antibody "curing" effects was examined with three field strains representing two different serogroups. Compared with the data for the K88 plasmids, the K99 "curing" effect of the sow milk antibodies was disappointingly negative (FIGURE 4). There was only limited evidence of a reduction in expression of K99 in the O8 serogroup and no evidence for the O101 serogroups. In view of the previous lack of serotype specificity for the K88 "curing" effect of antibodies, it was clear that the K99 plasmid was not subject to the same phenomenon; furthermore there was no marked difference between the abilities of K99$^+$ and K99$^-$ strains to grow in culture in the presence of the antibodies. Thus, selection pressure as one of the key factors in the phenomenon did not apply to the K99$^+$ strains. Again, because O8 antigen was a component of the vaccine and K88 "curing" had been achieved in the other O8 serogroups, it would appear that anti-O antibodies can be largely discounted as participating in the "curing" effect. Subsequent to these studies, we have detected that the K99 antigen does yield to "curing" with antibodies derived from vaccination with a live K12 K99$^+$ strain. Hence the phenomenon is open to investigation for the K99 plasmid with the eventual prospect for development of a suitable vaccine.

IN VIVO "CURING" OF K88 PLASMIDS IN THE IMMUNE SOW AND HER SUCKLING OFFSPRING

Under normal conditions of management, the sow is the major reservoir of infection for her offspring. The piglets, born without the benefits of transplacental transfer of immunity, meet the major infectious challenge of their new environment during the very act of seeking to suckle the colostrum that should sustain them with protective antibody. Using the combined oral/parenteral vaccination schedule for the maternal sow, we have observed plasmid "curing" in an E. coli infection induced in the sow some three days before parturition and the passive transfer of "curing" antibodies to her offspring.[9] As part of the trial of the maternal vaccination schedule, an immunized sow was dosed with large numbers of the E. coli O149: K91, K88ac pathogen during the three days prior to parturition so that the piglets would receive the infection naturally from the sow soon after birth. Loss of the K88 plasmid from the pathogen occurred rapidly in the gut of the immunized sow, and shortly after parturition, 70 percent of the O149 strain present in her feces was K88$^-$. The O149 strain was also isolated from the feces of the piglets. In 10 of the 11 piglets the K88$^+$/K88$^-$ proportions fluctuated, but followed a general trend of initially higher numbers of the K88$^+$ form, with the

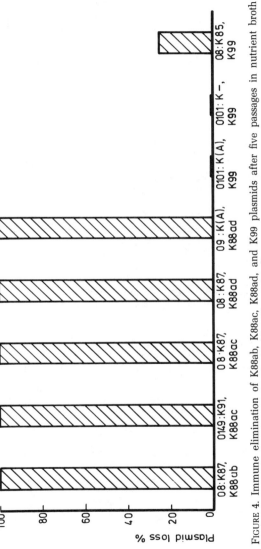

FIGURE 4. Immune elimination of K88ab, K88ac, K88ad, and K99 plasmids after five passages in nutrient broth containing 25% milk whey from an immunized (oral/parenteral) sow.

proporiton of the K88⁻ variant increasing until they formed practically 100 per-cent of the O149 population. In the 11th piglet, however, the reverse happened. Initially the K88⁺ variant formed only about 30 percent of the O149 strain present in the feces, but two days later, the K88⁺ form constituted 100 percent of the O149 population, and unlike its healthy, thriving littermates, the eleventh piglet developed severe diarrhea (TABLE 1).

An unimmunized sow was maintained in the same unit, and her litter was naturally infected with the K88⁺/K88⁻ mixture excreted by the immunized sow. In this unprotected litter, the K88⁺ type rapidly formed 100 percent of the O149 population in all the piglets, and half of them died from the infection during the first 48 hours.

The colostrum and milk from immunized sows contain a wide range of protecting antibodies, bactericidal and bacteriostatic antibodies, anti-adhesive antibodies, and antitoxins, but K88 "curing" antibodies are clearly also present as the process of plasmid elimination begun in the sow was continued in her offspring. In 10 of the 11 piglets from the immunized sow, the proportion of the K88⁻ form of the O149 strain continued to increase in spite of the advantage that the K88⁺ form would be expected to have because of its ability to adhere to intestinal epithelial cells. The rapid overgrowth of the K88⁺ form showed itself in the eleventh piglet in the litter, which may not have received sufficient colostral antibody from the sow, and in the unprotected litter in the adjacent pen that had received the same initial *E. coli* challenge.

Further evidence that a "curing" factor was present in the colostrum and milk of the immunized sow was obtained from *in vitro* culturing of the O149 strain in the presence of broth containing 10 percent of the immune fractions. After 72 hours of growth in the presence of immune whey from colostrum and first-day milk, the K88 plasmid had been eliminated from 100 and 63 percent, respectively, of the O149 colonies tested, whereas negligible plasmid loss had occurred from the strain when grown in the presence of wheys from the control sow (TABLE 1).

ORAL IMMUNIZATION AND DRUG RESISTANCE TRANSFER IN *E. COLI*

A notable feature of the extensive field trials undertaken with the oral/parenteral schedule vaccination for maternal sows in pig herds[10] was the dramatic reduction in need for therapeutic intervention with antibiotics. In trials involving more than 23,000 pigs, neonatal mortality was reduced by more than 50

TABLE 1

THE ELIMINATION OF K88AC FROM AN O149:K91, K88AC STRAIN OF
E. COLI IN VIVO AND *IN VITRO*

Sow	Piglet Mortality	Loss of K88 *in vivo*		Loss of K88 *in vitro* (72 hours)	
		In sow	In piglets (72 hours)	+10% colostrum	+10% milk
39 (immunized)	1/11	70%	65%*	100%	63%
			0%†		
42	9/13	0%	0%	6%	0%

*Average of 10 protected piglets.
†Piglet that developed diarrhea.

TABLE 2

EFFECT OF ORAL/PARENTERAL IMMUNIZATION OF SOWS WITH AN *E. COLI* VACCINE ON
ANTIBIOTIC THERAPY IN PIGLETS

Schedule	Number of Pigs	Pigs Treated per 100 Pigs Born		
		One day	Two days	Three days
Vaccinated	11566	21.1*	5.9*	1.3*
Control	9591	55.4	39.5	26.5

*p = <0.01

percent over the controls. This reduction was set against a background of medication in which the control litters had a need four times greater for treatment with antibiotics than did the litters from vaccinated sows. A further more important point emerged from the data that was a signal for the discovery of other antibody-mediated plasmid effects. The results were examined to determine the extent to which animals were subjected to medication, more particularly whether there was a beneficial response to one day's treatment or if there was a requirement for two, three, or more days' medication to overcome *E. coli* infection. The new data (TABLE 2) demonstrates the highly significant reduction in need for treatment of the progeny from the vaccinated sows, and moreover, demonstrates the significantly better response to treatment in the vaccinates compared with the controls.

The total reduction in need for therapeutic assistance in the vaccinated group was compounded from fewer animals needing treatment together with a superior responsiveness to therapy. Because the investigations were conducted simultaneously with paired litters in the same environment, the synergy of drug responsiveness with vaccination is a real phenomenon, not an artifact of different conditions, age, time or management.

In the light of the data derived from the studies of adhesion plasmids, we pursued, without success, the obvious inquiry as to whether sows' colostral antibodies could also induce the loss of R factors. Perhaps more pertinent, however, to the situation in young animals is the question of whether maternal antibodies might prevent the spread of drug resistance, that is, block the transfer of R factors. With this objective, we set up an *in vitro* model in which a high rate of transfer of the neomycin plasmid was achieved between a porcine EEC O149:K91,K88ac neo[+] and a nonpathogenic strain of *E. coli* P4, a streptomycin-resistant mutant. After 24 hours mixed culture, the numbers of transconjugants were counted on an agar medium containing streptomycin and neomycin.

In control media, the numbers of P4 neo[+] colony-forming units arising from a mixed culture of the pathogen and nonpathogen were more than 10^7 per milliliter. This exceedingly high rate of transfer provided a sensitive background against which to identify the effect of any antibody interfering with transfer. Studies were undertaken with wheys and sera from sows immunized late in gestation by natural infection with the live pathogen O149:K91, K88ac.[3] Significant reductions in the development of P4 neo[+] were recorded when the serum, colostrum, or milk samples of immunized sows or serum samples from their suckling piglets were added to the mating medium. Immune colostral wheys fractionated by gel filtration to achieve IgM, IgA, and IgG rich fractions were used to evaluate the specific activity of the antibody classes derived from the immunization schedule. All three classes of immunoglobulin participated in the neomycin plasmid transfer blocking effect (FIGURE 5), but IgG was much less effective than the mucosal immunoglobulins IgM and IgA.

The phenomenon of microbial adhesion is of considerable biological importance.[11] In the context of the host-pathogen interaction, antibodies at the site of

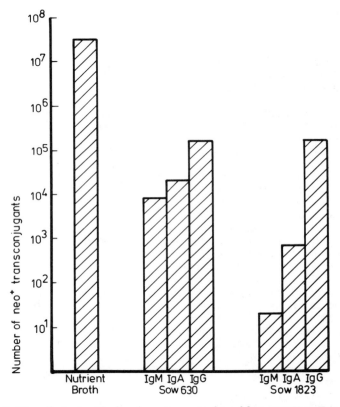

FIGURE 5. The effect of antibodies from immunized (oral live 0149:K91, K88ac *E. coli*)
sows on the rate of transfer of neomycin resistance plasmids between *E. coli* 0149:K91,
K88ac (donor) and 09:K36 (recipient).

bacterial adhesion will play an important defensive role in preventing microbial
colonization. This finding is readily demonstrated by studies employing host cell
membranes and antibodies against specific adhesion determinants.[12-14] The
protective value of anti-adhesins *in vivo* has been well demonstrated in mice with
experimental cholera[15] and with anti-K88 antibodies in porcine neonatal enteritis.[16]

There is probably no better model than the pig in which to study the influence of *E. coli* virulence determinants. Over the past decade specific adhesion determinants K88ab, K88ac, K88ad, K99, and 987P[17] have been identified. Vaccines have been developed with the primary objective of inducing sow milk antibodies that block intestinal adhesion in the neonate. Throughout such studies, great emphasis has been placed on the characteristics of the microbial antigens desirable for maternal immunization, but little attention has been paid to the passive antibody requirements of the neonate. Thus hyperimmunization of the sow leads to high levels of IgG antibodies that are transferred in the colostrum to the piglet, but are not designed specifically to act at mucosal surfaces, in particular, the intestinal tract.

In the study of enteric problems of the major domesticated animal species, we have maintained a consistent philosophy that in order to achieve successful immunization, one must mimic the consequences of natural infection. The immunization schedules used in the studies related here, are derived either from oral immunization with live pathogenic *E. coli* or from a safer oral/parenteral combination using heat inactivated *E. coli*.[3] The two schedules provide similar characteristics of antibody titer and immunoglobulin function dominated by IgM and IgA in sow colostrum and very comparable protective efficacy in the neonate. Using the same vaccine in a hyperimmunization schedule leading to colostral antibodies dominated by IgG, the protective efficacy in the neonate was substantially reduced in spite of *in vitro* determinations of antibody function being substantially the same or better in the case of anti-K88 activity.

Thus for passive protection, careful attention must be paid to the characteristics of the maternal response if the best protection for the neonate is to be attained. In the unimmunized herd situation, *E. coli* disease occurs as cyclical episodes, declining as the natural immune status of the herd increases and rising again as susceptibility returns with the throughput of new animals.

Apart from the best characteristics of the protective maternal immune response, one further significant factor has not been addressed in relation to herd immunity: the host is the controller of its own intestinal environment. The sow in particular is the source of pathogens that infect her offspring. Immunization must, therefore, take into account the long-term effects on the virulence of the pathogens that subsequently develop in the herd, and not just the immediate short-term protective effects. There is a tendency in pathogens for "masking" themselves to evade anti-microbial activities. In the natural cyclical circumstance of herd response to infection, there is no permanent antibody pressure, and virulence changes are slow to manifest themselves, particularly as the population of animals is also changing fairly rapidly. In a herd, however, hyperimmunized continuously to maintain a continuous high level of passive antibodies for the neonates against specific virulence determinants, complications might well be expected as a function of antibody pressure. This view is already being expressed in relation to the appearance of new adhesion determinants.[2,8]

It is in this respect that the finding of antibody-mediated plasmid "curing" represents more than an academic curiosity. The impact of the phenomenon in maintaining a safe environment in intensive agriculture is worthy of fullest investigation with attention to the characteristics of antigens involved and the most effective development of antibodies with reference to specific function as well as activity of immunoglobulins. On this basis the mucosal immunoglobulins must be most important, because EEC are not invasive, and the host is mainly in contact with the pathogen at its mucosal surface. Thus maternal antibodies must be of the IgM or IgA class and not IgG, which is much more easily induced and transferred in the colostrum of the sow.

The *in vitro* and *in vivo* loss of K88 function induced in the presence of antibodies is not just a feature of antigenic drift with easy potential for reversal. The studies with a K88-linked plasmid function for raffinose fermentation showed the combined and permanent loss of these functions following passage of the organisms in the presence of sows' milk antibodies. There was no recovery of the capacity to produce either activity once antibody pressure was removed, and passaging was continued in media without antibody. Selection pressure of antibody does play a role in the process, because it was established that K88$^+$ strains of *E. coli* grew with less facility than K88$^-$ strains of *E. coli* in the presence of "curing" antibodies. In the absence of antibody, the growth characteristics were substantially the same. Even if no other mechanism for induction of instability in the plasmid-bearing strain exists, then the selection pressure of the antibody will militate against successful establishment of the strain *in vivo*.

This phenomenon is unusual, however, because the plasmid is responsible for synthesizing a capsular antigen that assists in the resistance of the organism to bactericidal and bacteriostatic mechanisms. Furthermore, it is interesting that contrary to expectation, the antibody is not directed against the K88 antigen; in fact, specific anti-K88 antibodies were very poor at eliciting plasmid loss. A further intriguing point emerged when it was discovered that the antibody-mediated plasmid elimination effect proved to be not serotype specific, that is, unassociated with the O-antigen. The common antigen function does, however, appear to be limited to *E. coli* strains bearing the K88 plasmid, and "curing" antibody cannot be generated with strains without it. Therefore, it is probable that although the antigen may not be presented as a conventionally understood K88 determinant, it may well have some pilus association implicated with the K88 plasmid.

Plasmid-determined genes such as K88, Ent, and R factors can only be transferred if the donor strain of *E. coli* is also producing the sex pili necessary for conjugation. In some instances, the sex factors coding for the pili are covalently linked to their determinant genes. In others, several plasmids are present, and the determinants and sex factors are on separate pieces of genetic material. Some strains contain plasmids with determinant genes but no sex factors at all. These strains cannot act as plasmid donors unless sex factors are first transferred to them from other strains. For example, we have found that enterotoxin production in human pathogens is frequently nontransmissible in the sense that the strains contain Ent plasmids but no suitable sex factors. These pathogens, however, can acquire sex factors in matings with other strains that are donors of drug resistance plasmids. In this way the Ent plasmids of the pathogens can be mobilized and transferred to previously nonenterotoxigenic strains of *E. coli*. The widespread use of antibiotics in recent years has resulted in the rapid spread of R factors among intestinal bacteria, and this use may also induce the formation of new enterotoxigenic strains of *E. coli in vivo*.[18]

Plasmid transfer can be blocked using certain highly specific antisera prepared against the class of sex pilus coded for by the given sex factor.[19] Blocking, however, by specific anti-sex pilus antibodies and the "blocking" by milk wheys may not be due to the same mechanism. The apparent "blocking" by milk wheys may be a result of the presence of the sex pili making the piliated bacteria more susceptible to the antibodies present. This "blocking" would be particularly marked in bacteria that have just received sex factor plasmids and in which sex factor production is derepressed.

When strains of *E. coli* that contain derepressed sex factors are passaged in the presence of milk wheys, loss of the ability to produce sex pili can occur in a similar manner to the loss of the ability to produce K88 pili by K88$^+$ strains. Loss of sex factor activity can be demonstrated by the loss of the susceptibility of the strain to sex pilus-specific bacteriophages and the loss of the ability of the strain to act as a plasmid donor. In our experiments, we have not been able to "cure" R factor determinant genes from drug-resistant strains, but we have been able to eliminate their transmissibility. Antibody pressure appears to select for strains that have lost surface antigens such as sex pili or K88 antigens. Therefore, although the R determinant genes in our strains appear to be extremely stable, their associated sex factors can be lost on passaging the strains in the presence of immune milk wheys so that strains are no longer able to transfer their own R factors or mobilize Ent.

All these effects that arise out of oral immunization with antigens of porcine EEC are of great potential significance in intensive agriculture with high population densities of animals. The plasmid "curing" and "transfer blocking" phenomena attributable to the mucosal antibodies of the IgM and IgA classes in the intestinal tract will lead to a dramatic reduction in the concentration of virulence plasmids in the microbial population in the intestinal tracts of the animals and consequently the farm environment as a whole.

SUMMARY

Mucosal antibodies *in vivo* and *in vitro* interfere with the stability of plasmids coding for important virulence determinants in porcine enteropathogenic *E. coli* (EEC), such as the adhesion determinants K88ab and K88ac. The effector antibody is not directed against K88 antigens and is not serotype specific, but an antigen common to K88$^+$ strains is implicated. Further lack of pathogen specificity is exemplified by antibody elimination of the more recently discovered K88ad plasmid.

Antibodies that interfere with K88 plasmids do not affect K99, which now appears as an alternative adhesion factor in porcine enteropathogenic *E. coli*. This plasmid can be eliminated, however, by antibodies having K99 specificity.

In extending the studies to drug-resistance plasmids, further evidence has emerged that mucosal antibodies may assist in host control of the reservoir of R factors in the intestinal microflora. A major effector mechanism is that secretory IgA and IgM antibodies from orally immunized pigs can block the transfer of R factors between donor and recipient strains of *E. coli*.

REFERENCES

1. MOON, H. W., B. NAGY, R. E. ISAACSON & I. ØRSKOV. 1977. Occurence of K99 antigen on *Escherichia coli* isolated from pigs and colonisation of pig ileum by K99$^+$ enterotoxigenic *E. coli* from calves and pigs. Infect. Immun. **15:** 614–620.
2. SODERLIND, O., E. OLSSON C. J. SMITH & R. MOLLBY. 1982. The effect of parenteral vaccination of dams on the intestinal *Escherichia coli* flora in piglets with diarrhoea. Infect Immun. **36:** 900–906.
3. PORTER, P., M. A. LINGGOOD & J. W. CHIDLOW. 1978. Elimination of *Escherichia coli* K88 adhesion determinant by antibody in porcine gut and mammary secretions following oral immunisation. Adv. Exp. Med. Biol. **107:** 133–141.
4. PORTER, P., S. H. PARRY & W. D. ALLEN. 1977. Significance of immune mechanisms in relation to enteric infections of the gastrointestinal tract in animals. *In* Immunology of the Gut. **46:** 55–75. Ciba Foundation Symposium. Amsterdam: Excerpta Medica.

5. LINGGOOD, M. A., M. L. ELLIS & P. PORTER. 1979. An examination of the O and K specificity involved in the antibody-induced loss of the K88 plasmid from porcine enteropathogenic strains of *Escherichia coli*. Immunology **38**: 123–127.
6. LINGGOOD, M. A. & P. PORTER. 1978. Antibody induced elimination of the plasmid controlled K88 adhesion factor from a porcine enteropathogen. Immunology **35**: 125–127.
7. STOKES, C. R., T. J. NEWBY, J. H. HUNTLEY, D. PATEL & F. J. BOURNE. 1979. The immune response of mice to bacterial antigens given by mouth. Immunology **38**: 497–502.
8. GUINEE, P. A. M. & W. H. JANSEN. 1979. Behaviour of *Escherichia coli* K antigens K88ab, K88ac and K88ad in immunoelectrophoresis, double diffusion, and hemagglutination. Infect. Immun. **23**: 700–705.
9. LINGGOOD, M. A. & P. PORTER. 1980. The antibody mediated elimination of adhesion determinants from enteropathogenic strains of *Escherichia coli*. *In* Microbial Adhesion to Surfaces. R. C. W. Berkeley, J. M. Lynch, J. Melling, P. R. Rutter, and B. Vincent Ed.: 441–453. Ellis Horwood Ltd. Chichester.
10. CHIDLOW, J. W., J. A. BLADES & P. PORTER. 1979. Sow vaccination by combined oral and intramuscular antigen: a field study of maternal protection against neonatal *Escherichia coli* enteritis. Vet. Rec. **105**: 437–440.
11. GIBBONS, R. J. & J. VAN HOUTE. 1975. Bacterial adherence in oral microbial ecology. Annu. Rev. Microbiol. **29**: 19–44.
12. ELLEN, R. P. & R. J. GIBBONS. 1972. M Protein-associated adherence of *Streptococcus pyogenes* to epithelial surfaces: pre-requisite for virulence. Infect. Immun. **5**: 826–830.
13. WILSON, M. R. & A. W. HOHMANN. 1974. Immunity to *Escherichia coli* in pigs: adhesion of enteropathogenic *Escherichia coli* to isolated intestinal epithelial cells. Infect. Immun. **10**: 776–782.
14. PARRY, S. H. & P. PORTER. 1978. Immunological aspects of cell membrane adhesion demonstrated by porcine enteropathogenic *Escherichia coli*. Immunology **34**: 41–49.
15. FUBARA, E. S. & R. FRETER. 1973. Protection against enteric bacterial infection by secretory IgA antibodies. J. Immunol. **111**: 395–403.
16. RUTTER, J. M. & G. W. JONES. 1973. Protection against enteric disease caused by *Escherichia coli*—a model for vaccination with a virulence determinant. Nature (London) **242**: 531–533.
17. MOON, H. W., E. M. KOHLER, R. A. SCHNEIDER & S. C. WHIPP. 1980. Prevalence of pilus antigens, enterotoxin types, and enteropathogenicity among K88-negative, enterotoxigenic *Escherchia coli* from neonatal pigs. Infect. Immun. **27**: 222–230.
18. WACHSMUTH, I. K., S. FALKOW & R. W. RYDER. 1976. Plasmid-mediated properties of a heat-stable enterotoxin-producing *Escherichia coli* associated with infantile diarrhoea. Infect. Immun. **14**: 403–407.
19. HARDEN, V. & E. MEYNELL. 1972. Inhibition of gene transfer by antiserum and identification of serotypes of sex pili. J. Bacteriol. **109**: 1067–1074.

DISCUSSION OF THE PAPER

R. CURTISS III (*University of Alabama in Birmingham*): Is it really "curing" in the sense of loss of plasmid DNA, or could you have a phase variation with turn-on, turn-off of the gene?

P. PORTER (*Unilever Research, Sharnbrook, Bedford, England*): There is no evidence of a turn-on, turn-off mechanism. It is certainly an irreversible phenomenon and it is not a feature of antigenic modulation.

N. F. PIERCE (*The Johns Hopkins University, Baltimore, Md.*): Do you think there may be some aspects of the mechanism involved here that act specifically on the plasmid transfer process? Do you think what happens to plasmids is unique, or is it possible that there is a selection of serotype variants as in the gut of germfree mice that is chromosomally determined?

PORTER: No, because that is a reversible function. Sack and Miller observed that in the germfree mice, serum-sensitive forms were replaced by a smooth serum-resistant form, as the antibodies were formed. When this organism was taken into germfree mice, in the absence of antibodies, there was a reversal to the serum-sensitive form.

PIERCE: The chromosomal genetic material is not eliminated. Under antibody pressure, however, one has selection for variants, whether plasmid or chromosomally mediated, that seems to be similar.

PORTER: I think that is a part of the phenomenon. It is clear from the growth curves of the K88 strains that there is selection, but within it there is also some destabilization.

QUESTION: We have two chromosomal genes for other types of fimbriae, and in that instance, we see a selectiveness for phase variation. We see selection of phase-blocking mutants. The gene remains but the switch is blocked.

CURTISS: Fifteen years ago the idea of using immunological methods to intervene and block conjugation was considered when fimbriae, or sex pili, were first described. We now know, however, that there are some 25 incompatibile groups of conjugative plasmids in the enterics that specify at least 10 immunologically distinct conjugative pili. Synthesis of these pili by most of these plasmids is repressed. In terms of the magnitude of the problem are these phenomena really meaningful?

PORTER: The prevention of the epidemic spread of drug resistance is important as is reducing the reservoir of drug resistant bacteria. The host control of microflora may be one of the key factors of importance in public health.

RECEPTOR ANALOGUES AND ANTI-PILI ANTIBODIES AS INHIBITORS OF BACTERIAL ATTACHMENT *IN VIVO* AND *IN VITRO**

C. Svanborg Edén,[†] B. Andersson,[†] L. Hagberg,[†] L.Å.Hanson,[†]
H. Leffler, [‡] G. Magnusson,[§] G. Noori,[§] J. Dahmén,[§] and
T. Söderström[†]

[†]*Department of Clinical Microbiology*
[‡]*Department of Medical and Physiological Biochemistry*
University of Göteborg
Göteborg, Sweden
[§]*Swedish Sugar Company*
Arlöv, Sweden

INTRODUCTION

Mucous membranes form barriers between the surrounding outside and the tissues inside the body. The mucosal surfaces also constitute ecological niches for the bacterial populations that specialize in living under the local conditions.[1] The localization of bacteria in a certain site, their tissue tropism, depends in part on the capacity of the bacteria to bind to, and survive in association with, the mucosal surface.[2,3] Specific binding of bacteria to components of mucosal epithelial cells, that is, attachment, may be both a determinant of bacterial localization and a prerequisite for infection by way of mucous membranes.[4] As a consequence, treatments interfering with bacterial adhesion have a protective potential. Prevented from attaching, bacteria can be eliminated by mechanical and other unspecific defense mechanisms. Inhibition of adhesion may be accomplished by antibodies to the bacterial surface structures responsible for adhesion, or by any antibody that could agglutinate bacteria in the lumen, decreasing the concentration of bacteria available for interaction with the mucosa.[5] An alternative approach would be to interfere with bacterial adhesion by administration of soluble receptor analogues that competitively inhibit the interaction with epithelial cell receptors.[6] Both of these approaches require detailed information about the biochemical basis for the bacterial adhesion process. In this paper we focus on means for interfering with adherence of *Escherichia coli* that cause urinary tract infection, and draw parallels with recently obtained information on pneumococcal adherence.

The term urinary tract infection (UTI), defined as $\geq 10^5$ bacteria/ml urine, comprises several different disease entities. The severity of infection in the urinary tract free of obstructions and reflux, relates to the virulence factors of the infecting bacteria.[7] Strains causing acute pyelonephritis, often having a complete lipopolysaccharide and a capsular polysaccharide, are resistant to the bactericidal effect of serum. These strains produce hemolysin and attach to human uroepithelial cells. All of these properties are rarely found simultaneously in

*This study was supported by grants from the Swedish Medical Research Council (Project No. 215), the Swedish Board for Technical Development, the Volkswagon Foundation and the Ellen, Walter, and Lennart Hesselman Foundation for Scientific Research. T. Söderström was supported by the J. C. Kempe Memorial Foundation.

580

strains causing asymptomatic bacteriuria. We suggest that adhesive capacity is a factor that selects bacteria from the intestinal flora capable of reaching and infecting the urinary tract and a determinant of the localization of infection in the urinary tract. When obstructions, reflux, and possibly large volumes of residual urine are present, bacteria of low virulence may persist in the urinary tract, gain access to the kidney pelvis, and cause pyelonephritis.[8] The frequency of adhering bacteria in a group of patients with recurrent pyelonephritis and reflux was only about thirty per cent compared to about eighty per cent among the patient group free of reflux.

ADHESION MECHANISMS FOR BACTERIA IN THE URINARY TRACT

Bacterial attachment results from multiple interactions of bacterial surface ligands—adhesins—with epithelial cell receptors. Among urinary tract pathogens, different adhesion specificities are found for E. coli, Proteus mirabilis, Klebsiella, and Staphylococcus. Also within the group of uropathogenic E. coli, which cause about 80 percent of UTI in children, several adhesion specificities are known.[9] Binding to globoseries glycolipid receptors[10,11] explains the attachment to human uroepithelial cells of the majority of the pyelonephritic E. coli strains.[9,12] In addition, most strains bind to unidentified receptors probably containing mannose.[13] This binding type, found on most gram-negative bacteria, has not yet been directly related to virulence. One suggested function is binding bacteria to urinary tract slime.[14] Both binding to globoseries glycolipids and the mannose sensitive binding may be mediated by fimbriae (pili).[15,16]

IN VITRO INHIBITION OF ADHESION OF UROPATHOGENIC E. COLI

Receptor Sugars

The attachment of bacteria to human uroepithelial cells in vitro can be inhibited by glycolipids of the globoseries as well as the corresponding isolated oligosaccharides, including the simple disaccharide Galα1 → 4Galβ (TABLE 1). For the in vitro inhibition assay, bacteria harvested from tryptic soy agar plates and resuspended in phosphate buffered saline (PBS) were mixed with receptor glycolipid or saccharide. After incubation for 30 minutes at 37°C, allowing binding between bacteria and soluble receptor to take place, human uroepithelial cells from sedimented urine were added, and the adhesion was monitored as previously described.[9] As can be deduced from the table, the effeciency of the intact glycolipids on a molar basis, exceeded that of the isolated sugars. The tetrasaccharide globotetraose was a more efficient inhibitor than the Galα1 → 4Galβ disaccharide. The Galα1 → 4Galβ disaccharide is an integral part of the globoseries glycolipids either at a terminal or an internal position and can be a sufficient receptor site, although it does not give the best possible fit. Mannose or α-Methyl-mannoside did not affect the adhesion to human uroepithelial cells of strains tested.

Anti-Pili Antibodies

The exact structure of the adhesin on E. coli interacting with the glycolipid receptors is not known. Regardless of binding specificity, the pili thought to

TABLE 1

INHIBITION OF *IN VITRO* ADHESION BY GLOBOSERIES GLYCOLIPIDS AND ISOLATED
OLIGOSACCHARIDES*

Compound	Oligosaccharide Structure	Concentration† Required for 50% Inhibition of Adhesion of 10^9 Bacteria	
		(μg/ml)	(mM)
Globotetraosylceramide	GalNAcβ1→3Galα1→4Galβ1→ 4G1c-Cer	50	0.037
Globotetraose‡	GalNAcβ1→3Galα1→Galβ1→4 Glc	200	0.280
Digalactose	Galα1→4Gal	1300	3.800
α-Methyl-mannoside	CH$_3$O-Man	>10.000	

*E. coli 3669 was preincubated for 30 minutes at 37° C with decreasing amounts of soluble receptor analogue or PBS before addition of human uroepithelial cells. The number of adhering bacteria was determined by light microscopy.

†Mean of five experiments.

‡Globotetraose was obtained by ozonolysis of globotertaosylceramide; the structure was confirmed by nuclear magnetic resonance.[6]

interact with globoseries glycolipid receptors and those that bind mannosides, can be structurally similar in amino acid composition.[3,17] At least two groups of pili can be distinguished by their N-terminal amino acid sequence. One closely resembles that of mannose-binding pili except for the N-terminal; one retains that similarity at the very N-terminal but is different in the rest of the peptide chain.[17] The genes encoding the pili on uropathogenic *E. coli* have been found on the chromosome, as opposed to the plasmid encoded adhesions of enteropathogenic *E. coli*.[18] The structural relationship and the chromosomal localization of the genes suggest a common genetic origin of the pili on uropathogenic *E. coli*.

Among mannose-binding pili, a considerable degree of crossreactivity has been noticed.[19] Pili thought to bind to globoseries glycolipid receptors show a higher degree of serologic relationship within each OKH serotype than between different serotypes.[20] Anti-pili antibodies have previously been shown to inhibit attachment to human uroepithelial cells of the homologous strain.[21] Adhesion inhibition was also obtained with Fab' fragments. The inhibition by Fab' fragments indicates that the antigenic determinant(s) are adjacent enough to the receptor binding region on the pilus for the Fab' fragments binding to the antigenic determinant to block adhesion. On the other hand, the low degree of crossreactivity between pilus proteins with the same receptor specificity, suggests that the receptor binding region of the pilus is antigenically inactive. Hyperimmune serum prepared against whole pilus proteins are thus not expected to contain high levels of antibodies to the binding site. Antibodies to the immunogenic regions may still be active in blocking adherence if they cause steric hindrance or agglutination.

The access to monoclonal antibodies against pilus proteins has improved the possibilities for structure-function analysis. TABLE 2 shows the inhibitory effect on bacterial adhesion of pools of monoclonal antibodies to three pili thought to bind globoseries glycolipids and one mannose-binding pilus. The fusion and subcloning techniques for the hybridoma cell lines and the properties of the monoclonal antibodies have been described in part for the mannose-binding pili[22] and will be the topic of separate reports.

In Vivo Inhibition of Adhesion of Uropathogenic E. Coli

Animal Model

To evaluate the protective potential of anti-pili antibodies and soluble receptor sugars, an experimental model was developed. In contrast to the laboratory animals most commonly used for experimental UTI, rabbits, rats, and guinea pigs, the uroepithelial cells of mice were found to resemble those of the human in intensity and specificity of adhesion of pyelonephritogenic E. coli. Strains with Galα1 → 4Gal-binding capacity attached in high numbers, whereas strains with mannose-binding capacity only, attached in low numbers or not at all. To mimic the initial stages of urinary tract colonization by bacteria, the animals were sacrificed 16 hours after injection of bacteria into the urinary bladder. Kidneys and bladders were homogenized and the number of persisting bacteria were determined by viable counts and given as a percent of the inoculum concentration. To optimize the role of bacterial adhesion, no obstructive manipulations were used.[23]

Because of the variation in susceptibility to UTI among individual mice, a mixed infection protocol was chosen. Two bacterial strains, were used for infection, distinguishable from a mixture by resistance to different antibiotics. Their relative persistence in the urinary tract was compared. In this way the importance of a certain adhesive property could be evaluated in the individual animal, infected with bacterial strains that only differed with regard to their adhesins. Alternatively, a bacterial strain expected to be susceptible to a certain

TABLE 2

In Vitro Inhibition of E. coli Adhesion to Human Uroepithelial or Buccal Cells by Monoclonal Anti-Pili Antibodies*

E. coli Strains	Receptor Specificity of Pilus	Anti-Pilus Antibody	Adhesion (Bacteria/Cell)		
			Saline Control	Antibody (25 μl/0.5 ml)	Percent of Saline Control
O6:K13	mannose		99	0	0
Bam		pilus pool†	45	1	2
4283			85	0	0
3669	globoseries	pilus pool‡	48	1	2
1682	glycolipids		57	0	0

*Bacteria were preincubated with antibody for 30 minutes at 37° C before addition of epithelial cells.

†The anti-type 1 pilus pool contained hybridomas against E. coli H10407 and B9 pili, one of IgM and one of IgG isotype. A high degree of cross-reactivity between mannose-binding pili has previously been noticed.[22]

‡The pilus antibody pool was a mixture of hybridoma antibodies against pili from the three strains. The individual monoclonal antibodies reacted with the homologous pilus protein in ELISA at dilutions ≥10⁻⁵. All were of IgG isotype. The subclasses have not been identified. The degree of cross-reactivity and cross-inhibition has not yet been fully analyzed.

treatment could be mixed with a neutral strain. The effect of the treatment given could then be detected as a shift in the ratio of susceptible strain compared to the indicator strain. The role of different susceptibility of individual animals to infection could thus be neutralized.

Receptor Analogues

Of the available saccharides listed in TABLE 1, only globotetraose was tested for adhesion inhibition *in vivo* (TABLE 3). Two chemically induced mutants, *E. coli* HU824 and *E. coli* HU742, selected from a wild type pyelonephritogenic *E. coli* strain were used.[6,24] The mutants and parent were identical by the generotypic

TABLE 3

INHIBITION OF ASCENDING UTI IN MICE BY GLOBOETRAOSE*

Inoculum Mixture		No. Animals	Ratio of Recovery HU824 Str^R/HU742 Na1^R†			
				No. of Animals with Bacterial Recovery		
Mutants	Receptor Analogue		Common Median	Below Common Median	Above Common Median	Level of Signifi- cance
HU824 Str^R	Globotetraose	36		23	12	
+			0.352			p < 0.02
HU742 Na1^R	Saline control	49		19	30	

*The bacterial mixture injected intravesically consisted of *E. coli* HU824 Str^R and HU742 Nal^R, mutants of a wild-type pyelonephritogenic *E. coli* strain. The mutants were identical with regard to the genotypic and phenotypic traits available for testing, but retained either binding to globoseries glycolipids (HU824 Str^R) or to "mannosides" (HU742 Nal^R). The strains were distinguishable out of a mixture after induction of different antibiotic resistances. The bacterial mixture was preincubated with globotetraose.[6]

†Recovery = bacterial concentration in tissue/bacterial concentration in inoculum.

‡The mutants were constructed by R. and S. Hull in the laboratory of S. Falkow.[6,24] Significant differences were found both in kidneys and bladders.

and phenotypic characteristics available for testing, but differed in the receptor specificity of their adhesins. *E. coli* HU824 bound to globoseries glycolipid receptors, and the binding of *E. coli* HU742 was reversed by α-Methyl-mannoside. The difference in receptor specificity between the two mutants was characterized by adhesion inhibition by soluble receptor sugars as well as induction of binding to previously unreactive cells by receptor coating.[9,10] To allow separate detection from a mixed inoculum, *E. coli* HU742 was made resistant to nalidixic acid and HU824 to streptomycin. The bacterial mixtures were pretreated with globotetraose or α-Methyl-mannoside *in vitro* injection into the animals. The recovery of *E. coli* HU824 was reduced both in kidneys and bladders by globotetraose treatment. No significant effect was obtained with mannose treatment.

TABLE 4

PROTECTIVE EFFECT OF MONOCLONAL ANTI-TYPE 1 PILUS ANTIBODIES*

Experiment No.	Treatment Given	Kidney			Bladder		
		No. of Mice	Bacterial Recovery [Log 06K13/824]	Level of Significance	No. of Mice	Bacterial Recovery [Log 06K13/824]	Level of Significance†
1	anti-BSA	9	0.7	not significant	9	1.3	not significant
	PBS	9	0.1		9	1.7	
2	anti-type 1 pilus	8	−1.5	p < 0.05	10	−0.4	p < 0.05
	PBS	9	0.3		10	0.6	
3	anti-type 1 pilus	5	−0.4	not significant	8	0.5	p < 0.05
	PBS	8	0.1		10	1.4	

*A mixed inoculum of *E. coli* 06K13 and *E. coli* 824 was used. *E. coli* U6K13 carried pili reacting with the antibody given; *E. coli* 824 did not. The change in relative recovery of the two after intraperitoneal injection of antipili antibodies is shown.

†Paired Student's *t*-test.

Anti-Pili Antibodies

The protective effects of anti-pili antibodies against experimental UTI are shown in TABLES 4 and 5. Hyperimmune rabbit sera, induced against whole pili, were first chosen for passive protection. For these experiments the wild type strains used for pilus purification and mixed infections were used as infectious agents. Antibodies were added to the inoculum and incubated before infecting the animals. Little consistent protection was obtained (not shown).

The effect of monoclonal antibodies to a mannose-binding pilus is shown in TABLE 4. The antibodies were given intraperitoneally at a protein concentration of ~1 mg/ml (400 μg per mouse) three hours before the intravesical infection. Blood and urine samples for antibody determination were taken before intraperitoneal antibody injection, before intravesical infection, and at sacrifice. At the time of infection, significant circulating and urinary levels of the monoclonal antibodies were found by enzyme-linked immunosorbent assay (ELISA). A protective effect in the urinary bladder at a five percent level was seen in repeated experiments. No consistently significant protection was obtained in the kidneys. Monoclonal antibodies to bovine serum albumin (BSA) did not affect the infection. The low degree of protection by the anti-type 1 pilus antibodies might partly have been affected by the fact that E. coli O6:K13 possesses additional adhesive properties.

The effect of monoclonal antibodies to E. coli 1682 pili, binding to globoseries glycolipids, is shown in TABLE 5. The 7F5 clone produced IgG antibodies that inhibited attachment to mouse and human uroepithelial cells of E. coli 1682. The IgG antibodies produced by 6E6 did not block attachment. Both antibodies reacted strongly in ELISA with the isolated pilus protein as solid phase antigen (end point dilution $\geq 10^{-5}$). Neither antibody affected the adhesion of E. coli HU824, used as an indicator strain. Intraperitoneal injection of antibodies and intravesical challenge were performed as described above. A significant decrease in bacterial recovery was seen in kidneys and bladders of the animals injected with 7F5. The index strain was also affected. No significant decrease in infection rate with 1682 was seen after injection of the antibodies not inhibiting adhesion.

TABLE 5

PROTECTIVE EFFECT OF MONOCLONAL ANTIBODIES TO PILI BINDING TO GLOBOSERIES
GLYCOLIPIDS*

| Treatment Given | No. Animals | No. of Animals with Positive Cultures§ | | | |
| | | 1682 | | HU824 | |
		Kidney	Bladder	Kidney	Bladder
saline control anti-pilus antibody	10	10	7	9	10
7F5†	10	0	1	1	1
6E6‡	10	7	7	1	5

*A mixed inoculum of E. coli 1682, reacting with the anti-pili antibodies and E. coli HU824, not affected by the antibody in vivo, was given. The recovery in animals treated with antibodies or PBS is seen.

†Inhibitory for in vitro adhesion of 1682. No effect on the adhesion of HU824.

‡Noninhibitory for in vitro adhesion of 1682. No effect on the adhesion of HU824.

§>10 colonies in 0.1 ml of tissue homogenate.

TABLE 6

COMPARED INFECTIVITY OF E. COLI STRAINS WITH THE SAME ADHESINS, BUT DIFFERENT
VIRULENCE FACTORS*

Molecular Mixture	Serotype	Adhesion Specificity	Serum Resistance	Persistence in Kidney and Bladder
E. coli HU824	075 Kn.t.	globoseries glycolipids	resistant	
+				HU824 > 506 MR p < 0.05
E. coli 506 MR	Ont. K1	globoseries glycolipids	sensitive	

*E. coli HU824 was derived mutagenically from a wild-type pyelonephritogenic E. coli strain GR 12; E. coli 506 MR was constructed by cloning of the DNA coding for pilus formation into a fecal strain, E. coli 506, free of adhesive properties. The two strains were detected out of a mixture by presence (HU824) or absence (506 MR) of lactos fermentation, detected as yellow or blue colonies on a lactose-Bromthymol-Blue agar plate. The clones were constructed by R. and S. Hull in the laboratory of S. Falkow.[24]

In this case, however, the index strain was affected. The protective effect may, thus, depend on antibacterial mechanisms in addition to the blocking of adherence. Furthermore, the mechanism of transfer of antibodies from the circulation into the urine needs investigation.

ADHESION COMPARED TO OTHER BACTERIAL PROPERTIES

An attempt was made to compare adhesive capacity to other bacterial virulence factors regarding their importance for persistence in the mouse urinary tract. The E. coli strains chosen had the same receptor specificity of their pili, but differed in serotype, resistance to the bactericidal effect of serum, and probably other factors. E. coli HU824, retaining the virulence features of the wild-type parent, survived better in the mice than E. coli 506 MR—a normal fecal isolate into which pilus genes had been cloned (TABLE 6).

Pneumococcal Adherence

Recognition of oligosaccharide chains at epithelial cell surfaces seems to be a generalized mechanism of bacterial adherence. Pneumococci are frequent colonizers of the healthy nasopharynx as well as a cause of about 30 percent of bacterial otitis media.[23] Capacity to attach to human pharyngeal epithelial cells is higher for strains causing otitis media than for those associated with systemic disease.[24] Recently, it has been possible to identify saccharide receptor candidates for attaching pneumococci. The basis for this work was the progress regarding the mechanism of binding of Streptococcus pyogenes.[25] Fibronectin, a glycoprotein adsorbing onto epithelial cell surfaces, was recently found to bind S. pyogenes and pneumococci, although at different regions. In the collagen binding region of fibronectin, where the pneumococcal receptor was likely to be located, the saccharide sequence resembled that of E. coli lipopolysaccharide cores as well as the lactoneoseries of glycolipids. The latter compounds together with synthetic oligosaccharides, were tested (TABLE 7). Results obtained by adhesion inhibition

TABLE 7

INHIBITION OF ATTACHMENT TO HUMAN PHARYNGEAL EPITHELIAL CELLS OF *S. pneumoniae* 3114 BY RECEPTOR ANALOGUES

Compound	Chemical Structure of Characteristic Oligosaccharide Part	Adhesion	
		Concentration Inhibitor (μg/ml)	Percent Saline Control
Human fibronectin	NeuAcα2→4(6)Galβ1→4GlcNAc−	1	33
Lactoneotetraosylceramide	Galβ1→4GlcNAcβ1→3 Lac−	200	68
Sialyllactoneotetraosylceramide	NeuAcα2→3Galβ1→4GlcNAcβ1→3 Lac−	200	100
Lactoneotetraose	Galβ1→4GlcNAcβ1→3 Lac−	200	35
Lactosamine	Galβ1→4GlcNAc	1000	107

and induction of binding by receptor coating of unreactive target cells, suggest that glycoconjugates containing lacto-N-neotetraose (or part of this structure) act as receptors for attaching pneumococci.

DISCUSSION

Capacity to attach to the urinary tract mucosa has long been suggested to be essential for *E. coli* causing urinary tract infection. The evidence was derived mainly from *in vitro* work. With increased information on underlying host factors, more nuanced statements can be made. Adhesive capacity may be a prerequisite for bacteria infecting the healthy urinary tract. In patients with defects of urine flow, facilitating bacterial persistence in the urinary tract, attaching bacteria are, however, much less prevalent.

The *in vitro* work has led to the identification both of pili as one bacterial surface ligand involved in adhesion, and of the globoseries glycolipid receptors in the epithelial cell membrane, to which the majority of attaching pyelonephritogenic *E. coli* bind. Still, *in vitro* work never allows conclusions about the relative importance of different bacterial virulence factors. For this reason the ascending UTI mouse model was developed. The relevance of the information obtained from the mouse UTI model for the human situation may of course be debated. The model was designed to study the contribution of bacterial adhesion to virulence in the urinary tract. Its potential for the study of other pathogenetic mechanisms in human UTI remains to be investigated.

The evidence for a role of bacterial adhesion in ascending experimental UTI was three-fold. First, the expression of adhesins in the infecting bacteria affected their persistence in the mouse urinary tract. *E. coli* strains with genetically defined adhesins were used. Capacity to bind globoseries glycolipid receptors was sufficient for persistence in the kidney, whereas this property combined with "mannose" binding was optimal in the bladder. The functional equivalent of these binding patterns in the mouse is the capacity to associate with tissue that contains globoseries glycolipids and possibly "slime-binding" or association with mucus that contains "mannose." Second, bacterial persistence in kidneys and bladder were decreased by administration of soluble receptor analogues that specifically block the adhesion. Third, antibodies to pili, passively administered, protected against infection.

Only the passive administration of homologous anti-pili antibodies gave complete protection against infection. Increasing the amount of the receptor analogue or optimizing the antibody specificity may improve the chances for a broadly protective approach. Treatments interfering with bacterial adherence in humans will allow a more definite conclusion regarding the role of adhesion compared to other bacterial virulence factors. The ability to recognize and bind to oligosaccharides in epithelial cell surfaces seems to be a general mechanism of bacterial adhesion. Interference with adherence by administration of soluble receptor sugar may be useful also outside of the urinary tract. Indeed, it may already have been utilized by nature during breast-feeding (Hanson *et al.*, this volume), when the nasopharynx is flushed with free oligosaccharides, some of which serve as receptors for pneumococci and possibly other potential pathogens.

Our findings may have practical application for treatment and prophylaxis of UTI and other infections that occur in mucous membranes. In the delicate interaction between host and parasite, inhibition of one bacterial virulence factor like adhesion, may tilt the balance in favor of the host. Administration of receptor analogues or vaccination with pilus antigens may achieve this goal.

ACKNOWLEDGMENT

The monoclonal antibodies against the pili of *E. coli* 1682 were raised at the University of Michigan hybridoma facility by Ron Maciak, with the kind permission of Dr. J. L. Claflin.

REFERENCES

1. SAVAGE, D. C. L. 1972. Survival on mucosal epithelia, epithelial penetration and growth in tissues of pathogenic bacteria. Symp. Soc. Gen. Microbiol. **22:** 25–57.
2. GIBBONS, R. J. & J. VAN HOUTE. 1975. Bacterial adherence in oral microbial ecology. Am. Rev. Microbiol. **29:** 19–44.
3. LEFFLER, H., C. SVANBORG EDÉN, G. SCHOOLNIK & T. WADSTRÖM. 1982. Glycosphingo-lipids as receptors for bacterial adhesion. Host glycolipid diversity and other selected aspects. *In* Attachment of Microorganisms to the gastrointestinal mucosal surface. E. C. Boedeker, Ed. CRC Press. In press.
4. SMITH, H. W. & M. A. LINGOOD. 1971. Observations on the pathogenetic properties of K88, Hly and Ent plasmids of *Escherichia coli* with particular reference to porcine diarrhoea. J. Med. Microbiol. **4:** 467–485.
5. FUBARA, E. S. & R. FRETER. 1973. Protection against enteric bacterial infection by secretory IgA antibodies. J. Immunol. **111:** 395–403.
6. SVANBORG EDÉN, C., R. FRETER, L. HAGBERG, R. HULL, S. HULL, H. LEFFLER & G. SCHOOLNIK. 1982. Inhibition of experimental ascending urinary tract infection by receptor analogue. Nature. **298:** 560–562.
7. SVANBORG EDÉN, C., L. HAGBERG, L. Å. HANSON, T. K. KORHONEN, H. LEFFLER & S. OLLING. 1981. Adhesion of *E. coli* in urinary tract infection. *In* Adhesion and Microorganism Pathogenicity. 161–187. Ciba Symp. 80. Pittman Medical. Turnbridge Wells.
8. LOMBERG, H., L. Å. HANSON, U. JODAL, H. LEFFLER, S. JOHANSSON & C. SVANBORG EDÉN. P blood group phenotype, vesicoureteric reflux and susceptibility to recurrent pyelonephritis. Submitted for publication.
9. LEFFLER, H. & SVANBORG EDÉN, C. 1981. Glycolipid receptors for uropathogenic *E. coli* binding to human erythrocytes and uroepithelial cells. Infect. Immun. **34:** 920–929.
10. LEFFLER, H. & C. SVANBORG EDÉN. 1980. Glycolipid receptors for uropathogenic *E. coli* attaching to human urinary tract epithelial cells and agglutinating human erythrocytes. FEBS Lett. **8:** 127–134.
11. KÄLLENIUS, G., R. MÖLLBY, S. B. SVENSSON, J. WINBERG, A. LUNDBLAD, S. SVENSSON & B. CEDERGREN. 1980. The p^k antigen as receptor for the hemagglutinin of pyelonephritic *E. coli*. FEBS Lett. **7:** 297–302.
12. KÄLLENIUS, G., R. MÖLLBY, S. B. SVENSSON, I. HELIN, B. HULTBERG, B. CEDERGREN & J. WINBERG. 1981. Incidence of P-fimbriated *E. coli* in urinary tract infections. Lancet **2:** 1369–1372.
13. HAGBERG, L., U. JODAL, T. K. KORHONEN, G. LIDIN-JANSON, U. LINDBERG & C. SVANBORG EDÉN. 1981. Adhesion, hemagglutination and virulence of *E. coli* causing urinary tract infections. Infect. Immun. **31:** 564–579.
14. ØRSKOV, I., F. ØRSKOV & A. BIRCH-ANDERSEN. 1980. A fimbria *E. coli* antigen F7, determining uroepithelial adherence. Comparison with type 1 fimbriae which attach to urinary slime. Infect. Immun. **27:** 657–666.
15. SALIT, I. E. & E. C. GOTSCHLICH. 1977. Hemagglutination by purified type 1 *Escherichia coli* pili. J. Exp. Med. **146:** 1169–1181.

16. LEFFLER, H., H. LOMBERG, E. GOTSCHLICH, U. JODAL, T. K. KORHONEN, B. E. SAMUELSSON, G. SCHOOLNIK & C. SVANBORG EDÉN. 1982. Chemical and Clinical Studies on the Interaction of *E.coli* with host Glycolipid Receptors in Urinary Tract Infection. Scand. J. Infect. Dis. Suppl. **S33:** 26–32.
17. SVANBORG EDÉN, C., E. C. GOTSCHLICH, T. K. KORHONEN, H. LEFFLER & G. SCHOOLNIK. 1983. Aspects on structure and function of pili on uropathogenic *E. coli.* **S33:** 189–202.
18. ELWELL, L. P. & P. L. SHIPLEY. 1980. Plasmid-mediated factors associated with virulence of bacteria to animals. Am. Rev. Microbiol. **34:** 465–496.
19. BRINTON, C. C. Personal communication.
20. ØRSKOV, I., F. ØRSKOV, A. BIRCH-ANDERSEN, M. KANAMORI & C. SVANBORG EDÉN. 1982. O, K, H and fimbrial antigens in *E.coli* serotypes associated with pyelonephritis and cystitis. Scand. J. Infect. Dis. Suppl. **S33:** 18–26.
21. KORHONEN, T. K., H. LEFFLER & C. SVANBORG EDÉN. 1981. Binding specificity of piliated strains of *E. coli* and *S. typhimurium* to epithelial cells, saccharomyces cerevisiae cells and erythrocytes. Infect. Immun. **32:** 796–804.
22. SÖDERSTRÖM, T., C. C. BRINTON, C. BURCH, H. Å. HANSSON, L. A. HANSON, A. KARPAS, J. B. ROBBINS, R. SCHNEERSON, K. STEIN, A. SUTTON & W. VANN. 1983. Analysis of *E. coli* K antigens and type 1 pili with monoclonal antisera. Prog. Allergy. Suppl. **33:** 40–52.
23. HAGBERG, L., U. JODAL, T. K. KORHONEN, G. LIDIN-JANSON, U. LINDBERG & C. SVANBORG EDÉN. 1981. Adhesion, hemagglutination and virulence of *E.coli* causing urinary tract infection. Infect. Immun. **31:** 564–570.
24. SVANBORG EDÉN, C., R. HULL, S. HULL, S. FALKOW & H. LEFFLER. Target cell specificity of wild-type *E. coli* and mutants and clones with genetically defined adhesins. Nutr. Res. In press.
25. FINLAND, M. 1979. Pneumonia and pneumococcal infections. Am. Rev. Respir. Dist. **120:** 481–502.
26. ANDERSSON, B., B. ERIKSSON, A. FOGH, L. Å. HANSON, O. NYLÉN, H. PETERSON & C. SVANBORG EDÉN. 1981. Adhesion of Streptococcus pneumoniae to human pharyngeal epithelial cells *in vitro.* Infect. Immun. **32:** 311–317.
27. BEECHEY, E. H. 1981. Bacterial adherence. J. Infect. Dis. **143:** 325–345.
28. ANDERSSON, B., H. LEFFLER. G. MAGNUSSON & C. SVANBORG EDÉN. Glycoconjugate receptors for pneumococci attaching to human pharyngeal epithelial cells. Submitted for publication.

DISCUSSION OF THE PAPER

W. STROBER (*National Institutes of Health, Bethesda, Md.*): Has anybody used some of these sugars to try to suppress urinary tract infections?

C. SVANBORG EDÉN (*University of Göteborg, Göteborg, Sweden*): Not in humans.

QUESTION: Rhesus monkeys have the receptor, and it has been shown that a single dose of the β methyl-digalactose efficiently blocked the nephritis induced by such pressures and even blocked venous backflow.

M. BLAKE (*Rockefeller University, New York, N.Y.*): Because you are passively administering monoclonal antibodies in mice and then examining an effect on bacteria as you inject the bacteria into the urogenital tract, how does antibody reach the urine? What concentrations do you observe? Second, to which determinant is the monoclonal antibody directed?

SVANBORG EDÉN: We obtain significant levels of antibody by the ELISA assay in the urine of the animals at the time when the infection is given. I would not want to speculate about the mechanism of transfer. The specificity of the monoclonal antibodies is partially known. The type 1 monoclonals that we used are cross reactive with several type 1 pilus proteins. The monoclonals against *E. coli* 1682 pili have, so far, only reacted with the homologous pilus protein and with none other that we examined. We do not know yet which region of the pilus protein the monoclonals react with.

INTESTINAL UPTAKE OF MACROMOLECULES: *IN VITRO* AND *IN VIVO* STUDIES*

W. Allan Walker

Department of Pediatrics
Harvard Medical School
Pediatric Gastrointestinal and Nutrition Unit
Children's Service
Massachusetts General Hospital
Boston, Massachusetts 02114

Kurt J. Bloch

Department of Medicine
Harvard Medical School
Clinical Immunology and Allergy Units
Medical Services
Massachusetts General Hospital
Boston, Massachusetts 02114

At the International Symposium on the Immunoglobulin A System held at the University of Alabama in 1973, we reported on the role of immunization in controlling antigen uptake from the small intestine. In this report, we should like to summarize the results of subsequent *in vitro* studies and to report on the uptake of antigen from the intestinal lumen into the systemic circulation *in vivo*.

In the initial studies, germfree or conventionally raised rats were orally immunized with horseradish peroxidase (HRP) or bovine serum albumin (BSA), and the absorption of these antigens by everted gut sacs was tested *in vitro*. For these experiments, the jejunum and ileum were everted, and 5 cm long sacs were prepared and filled with Krebs-Ringer bicarbonate solution. Gut sacs were exposed to HRP or [^{125}I]BSA in this medium during 60 minutes incubation at 37° C in oscillating flasks. Thereafter the serosal contents were drained, and the content of antigen was determined by enzymatic methods (for HRP) or by crystal scintillation spectrometry of the trichlor acetic acid (TCA)-precipitable radioactivity (for BSA). In comparison with controls, a consistent decrease in peroxidase uptake was noted in both germfree and conventionally raised rats immunized with HRP; a similar decrease in BSA uptake was noted with gut sacs from rats immunized with bovine serum albumin. There was no difference in the uptake of an unrelated antigen.[2] The serum of orally immunized rats showed no antigen-binding activity detectable by radioimmunodiffusion; secretions and mucosal extracts showed antigen-binding activity attributable to IgG$_1$, but not to IgA antibodies.

Following intense parenteral immunization of conventionally raised rats with BSA or HRP emulsified in complete Freund's adjuvant, there was a significant and specific decrease in uptake of antigen by gut sacs from immunized compared to control rats.[3] The mechanism(s) whereby immunization interferes with the uptake of antigen was investigated.[4] In these studies, gut sacs from parenterally

*This work was supported by United States Public Health Service Grants AM-16269, AM-21505, and AM 23099.

0077-8923/0409-0593 $1.75/0 © 1983, NYAS

immunized and control rats were exposed to labeled antigen *in vitro*. The amount of antigen initially bound to the sacs, degraded by the sacs during incubation, and residually associated with the sacs after incubation was determined. To determine the breakdown of labeled antigen by the gut sacs, samples were removed from the incubation medium at intervals during the three hour incubation period. Total radioactivity in the samples was determined before and after precipitation with TCA (for BSA) or phosphotungstic acid (for HRP). It was shown that ^{125}I remaining in the supernate was present as free iodine or small peptides and that the radioactivity remaining in the supernate after precipitation of protein reflected breakdown of ^{125}I-labeled protein. By contrast to controls, gut sacs from immunized rats showed an increased initial adsorption of labeled antigen. Furthermore, gut sacs from immunized rats showed enhanced breakdown of labeled antigen on prolonged (three hour) incubation. Following incubation, gut sacs were rinsed, and the amount of protein-bound radioactivity eluted from the mucosal surface was determined. More radioactivity was present in the first rinse fluid of gut sacs from immunized compared to control rats. On density gradient ultracentrifugation of the former fluids, radioactivity was localized in the middle or bottom of the gradient, whereas radioactivity in the latter fluids was located at the top of the gradient. The rapidly sedimenting labeled antigen was coprecipitated in the reaction of rabbit anti-rat IgG_1 and rat IgG_1 protein, suggesting the presence of antigen-IgG_1 antibody complexes in the rinse fluid.[4]

These findings suggested that, *in vitro*, antigen became rapidly associated with antibodies present on the surface of the gut. Formation of antigen-antibody complexes seemed to prevent binding of antigen to, and subsequent pinocytosis by,[5] the intestinal epithelial cells. Antigen-antibody complexes retained in the mucous coat of the gut were degraded by local (in contrast to luminal) proteases.[14] Degradation of antigen may have further reduced the amount of antigen available for uptake.

In a subsequent study, we investigated the site of intestinal antibody activity. Weiser had previously shown that treatment with dithiothreitol can be used to remove the mucous coat from the intestine without interfering with the viability of the intestinal epithelial cells.[6] After establishing that the amount of dithiothreitol required did not interfere with the antigen-binding activity of conventional antibody molecules, we rinsed gut sacs prepared from the intestine of immunized and control rats with dithiothreitol. After treatment, there was no inhibition of antigen uptake by gut sacs from immunized compared to control rats, suggesting again that antibodies present in the mucous layer of the gut were responsible for inhibition of uptake.[7]

The source of proteases involved in enhanced degradation of antigen-antibody complexes present on the mucosal surface was studied.[8] For these experiments, gut sacs were prepared from BSA-immunized and control (saline)-injected rats. Intraperitoneal injections of antigen or saline emulsified in incomplete Freund's adjuvant were repeated several times. The rats were further modified by ligation of the pancreatic duct or by sham-operation 24 hours before the gut sacs were obtained for study. There was significantly less breakdown of [^{125}I]BSA by both jejunal and ileal gut sacs from BSA-immunized, pancreatic duct-ligated rats compared to gut sacs from BSA-immunized, sham-operated rats. One hour before sacrifice, it was possible to "reconstitute" the pancreatic duct-ligated rats by administration of pancreatic extracts. Subsequently, gut sacs were prepared for *in vitro* experiments. The magnitude of antigen breakdown by gut sacs from BSA-immunized, pancreatic duct-ligated rats treated with pancreatic extracts was similar to that observed previously with gut sacs from intact,

BSA-immunized rats. These experiments suggested that pancreatic enzymes adsorbed to the surface of the intestine contribute to the proteolysis of antigen and antigen-antibody complexes at this site.[8]

In a related *in vivo* experiment,[9] we examined the intraluminal events in the processing of a protein antigen, BSA, by the intestine of normal and orally

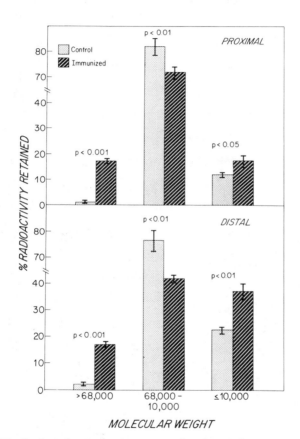

FIGURE 1. Distribution of radioactivity associated with BSA fragments in regions of an SDS-PAGE gel. The rinse fluid and mucosal extract obtained from the proximal (upper panel) and distal segment (lower panel) of the small intestine were separately applied to a 10% SDS-PAGE gel; the combined results of these analyses on rinse fluid and extracts from six immunized and six control rats are shown. (K. Y. Pang, W. A. Walker & K. J. Bloch.[9] With permission from *Gut*).

immunized rats. One hour after the administration of [^{125}I]BSA and labeled BSA by gavage, there was a difference in the distribution of radioactivity in the small intestine: control rats retained a significantly greater percentage of radioactivity in the proximal small intestine, whereas immunized rats retained a greater percentage of radioactivity in the distal small intestine (FIGURE 1). Radioactive

substances present in intestinal rinse fluids and mucosal extracts were characterized by sodium dodecyl sulfate-polyacrylamide gel electrophoresis (SDS-PAGE),
density gradient ultracentrifugation, and immunochemical methods. Rinse fluids
and mucosal extracts from immunized rats fed [^{125}I]BSA by gavage contained high
molecular weight components with characteristics of antigen-antibody complexes. Rinse fluids and extracts of normal rats contained more intact BSA and fewer
fragments than did fluids and extracts from immunized animals. These findings
suggested that oral immunization altered the distribution of antigen administered

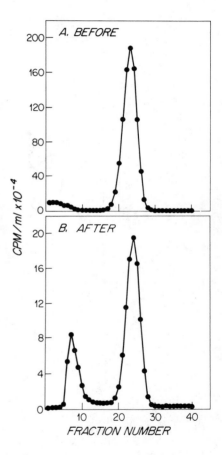

FIGURE 2. Bio-Gel P-60 chromatogram of
(A) ^{3}H-BSA dialysate, and (B) ^{3}H-BSA dialy-
sate incubated with normal rabbit serum. (J.
N. Udall et al.[10] With permission from
Immunology).

into the gut and that immunization enhanced the intraluminal degradation of
antigen.

UPTAKE OF PROTEIN ANTIGEN IN VIVO IN NORMAL RATS AND IN RATS WITH
PARTIAL VILLOUS ATROPHY, SYSTEMIC, OR LOCAL INTESTINAL ANAPHYLAXIS

Other investigators studying the transport of macromolecules across mucosal
surfaces have noted that techniques involving exogenously labeled macromole-

cules result in estimation of transport that exceeds estimates based on immuno-chemical methods. In preliminary experiments with either ^{125}I-, ^{14}C- or ^{3}H-labeled proteins, we encountered similar discrepancies. We therefore tested the possibility that radiolabeled fragments of macromolecules might bind to host proteins, resulting in an apparent increase in "size" of the fragments. Solutions of BSA labeled with tritium gas by the Wilzbach method were placed in cellulose dialysis bags with a molecular weight cut off of 12,000. After 30 minutes, radioactivity appearing outside the dialysis bag was measured and characterized. Appreciable radioactivity was detected and ascribed to the presence of ^{3}H-labeled amino acids, small peptides, and ^{3}H$_2$O. Incubation of the dialysate with whole serum led to binding of radioactivity to serum macromolecules, especially to albumin (FIGURE 2). In other experiments, dinitrophenylated (DNP) bovine gamma globulin was administered by gavage to adult rats. Dinitrophenylated-bearing fragments were identified in their serum by radioimmunoassay. These fragments were isolated by gel filtration and were labeled with ^{125}I. After radiolabeling, the fragments were mixed with normal rat serum and were also shown to bind to macromolecular constituents of rat serum. These findings suggested that different fragments may bind to native serum components. The observations may explain the overestimation of uptake of extrinsically labeled macromolecules from the gut, because following intestinal instillation of such labeled proteins, labeled amino acids, or small peptides generated by the digestive process, become absorbed and bound to serum macromolecules, thereby mimicking the uptake of macromolecules.[10]

In view of the problems posed by extrinsically labeled proteins, we chose to base our in vivo antigen (BSA) uptake studies on a radioimmunoassay for bovine serum albumin.[11] In these experiments, normal adult rats, weighing about 250 grams, were fed BSA and sodium bicarbonate by gavage. Serum was obtained at intervals after feeding and was tested for immunoreactive BSA (iBSA) by radioimmunoassay. Nanogram amounts of iBSA (mean peak value ~170 ng BSA per ml) were detected in serum of rats fed 1.0 gram BSA; peak serum values were observed at four to six hours after feeding. The molecular size of iBSA was approximately that of the administered BSA; no small fragments bearing BSA-antigenic determinants were detected.

The influence of intestinal inflammation on protein uptake was tested in two systems: infection of rats with Nippostrongylus brasiliensis and systemic and local intestinal anaphylaxis. Infection of rats with the nematode N. brasiliensis produces partial villous atrophy in segments of the small intestine harboring mature worms. The lesions are most intense between day 10 and day 17 of primary infection. Healing occurs after self-cure, which in our rat strain occurs by day seventeen. The uptake of BSA was tested in groups of rats throughout the course of a primary infection; enhanced uptake was observed in groups tested on day 12, 15, and 19, but not on day 29 or 39. A significant correlation was observed between the extent of morphologic alteration of the infected jejunum and the concentrations of iBSA detected in the blood of rats fed BSA[11] (FIGURE 3).

Mild systemic anaphylaxis was induced on day 40 of a primary infection with N. brasiliensis by the intravenous injection of worm extract or by the injection of egg albumin (EA) into rats immunized 14 days earlier with 100 μg EA and alum.[12] Mild systemic anaphylaxis led to the appearance of fluid separating the epithelium from the vascular core of the villi in the small intestine. Alteration of vascular and mucosal permeability was assessed semiquantitatively with the use of [^{125}I] rat serum albumin (RSA) immediately after challenge with antigen. Forty-five to sixty minutes later, rats were exsanguinated, and intestinal segments and their contents were removed. In comparison to controls, antigen-challenged rats showed enhanced retention of radioactivity in the wall of the duodenum and first and second halves of the small intestine. This measurement reflects the increased vascular permeability accompanying anaphylaxis. In addition, there were also increased amounts of TCA precipitable radioactivity present in the luminal contents of these segments of intestine, attesting to the leakage of intact [125I]RSA or large fragments from the interstitial spaces of the lamina propria into the intestinal lumen. This latter measurement reflects the increased mucosal permeability accompanying anaphylaxis.

Intestinal anaphylaxis also favored the reverse movement of protein from the

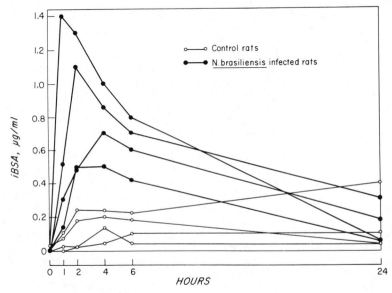

FIGURE 3. Amounts of iBSA detected in serum obtained from four uninfected and four *N. brasiliensis* infected rats at various intervals after feeding by gavage with 1000 mg BSA and 25 mg NaHCO₃. Feeding was performed on day 8 of a primary infection. (K. J. Bloch *et al*.[11] With permission from *Gastroenterology*).

lumen into the systemic circulation. For these experiments, immunized rats were gavaged with BSA, and one hour later, anaphylaxis was induced with either worm extract or egg albumin. Rats were bled and serum was examined for immunoreactive bovine serum albumin. In nearly all instances, greater amounts of iBSA were detected in the blood of rats subjected to mild systemic anaphylaxis than was found in saline-injected controls.

The effect of locally induced intestinal anaphylaxis on the uptake of a bystander antigen was also tested.[13] For these experiments, rats were immunized with small amounts of EA and alum so as to favor the production of IgE anti-EA antibodies. Local anaphylaxis was elicited by either intraduodenal or intragastric infusion of egg albumin. The occurrence of intestinal anaphylaxis under these circumstances was confirmed in some animals by measuring the extravasation of

[^{125}I]RSA into the walls of the intestine, as well as into the intestinal lumen. In other animals, intestinal anaphylaxis was elicited one hour after feeding by gavage with BSA: iBSA was sought in the blood of these animals at intervals after the induction of anaphylaxis. Again, a greater amount of iBSA as detected in the blood of rats subjected to local intestinal anaphylaxis than was found in the blood of control animals.[13]

The enhanced uptake of bystander protein that happens to be present in the intestine at the time of anaphylaxis might give rise to several immunological consequences. These include the possible induction of a local or systemic immune response to the bystander antigen; the induction of a local (gastrointestinal) immune response and systemic tolerance to the bystander antigen; or the induction of an IgE-antibody response to the bystander antigen. The latter might result in the broadening of anaphylactic sensitivity of the animal.

INTESTINAL GOBLET-CELL MUCUS RELEASE: THE ROLE OF IMMUNOLOGIC REACTIONS IN THE GUT

In the course of studies on intestinal uptake of macromolecules, as well as during intraluminal antigen challenge of immunized animals, we regularly observed the release of mucus from goblet cells. This phenomenon was first observed during studies on the *in vitro* uptake by rat small intestine of antigen-antibody complexes prepared in antibody excess. Response of gut sacs from normal rats to such complexes appeared to stimulate secretion of mucus, and complexes were associated with the mucus fraction. Based on these observations, it was suggested that mucus release stimulated by certain antigen-antibody complexes might rid the surface of the enterocyte of complexes that might otherwise be available for uptake into the lamina propria or other tissues of the host.[14]

In experiments performed with intact rats, the ability of antigen alone or of antigen-antibody complexes to stimulate goblet-cell mucus release was tested. Goblet-cell mucus release was assessed morphologically and by measuring ^{35}S-mucus release. The total number of goblet cells showing mucus release was significantly greater in rats exposed to complexes by intraduodenal instillation, than was observed in rats exposed to antigen. Considerably more radiolabeled mucus was released into the intestinal fluids of rats exposed to BSA-anti-BSA complexes than was observed in rats exposed to BSA alone.[15] Similar observations were made in orally immunized rats challenged by intraduodenal infusion of antigen. In these studies, mucus release was estimated from the amount of radioactivity present in the void volume (presumably as high molecular weight ^{35}S-labeled glycoprotein of goblet cell origin) of a Sepharose 4B gel filtration column to which intestinal washings from immunized, antigen-challenged rats had been applied.[16]

In rats immunized so as to favor the production of IgE antibodies to EA, infusion of antigen into the duodenum again stimulated the release of ^{35}S-labeled goblet-cell mucus. Goblet-cell mucus release was dependent on the dose of antigen infused, was antigen-specific, and was inhibited by pretreatment of rats with cyproheptadine. Enhanced release of goblet-cell mucus was transferred from immunized to normal rats with native, but not with heat-treated, antiserum—a finding consistent with the heat lability of IgE antibodies.[17] (FIGURE 4).

This series of experiments suggested that immunologically mediated release of mucus may provide the host with additional mechanisms for limiting uptake of intact antigen. Mucus released from goblet cells might increase the thickness of the mucous coat of the intestine, thereby increasing the mechanical barrier to penetration by macromolecules. Interaction between antigens, such as albumins, and mucous might increase the viscosity of mucous[18] thereby again enhancing its barrier function. In the animal that possesses a population of intestinal mast cells coated with IgE antibodies, an initial antigen-stimulated release of mucous might serve to limit further access of antigen to sensitized mast cells and might thereby ameliorate the severity of local intestinal anaphylaxis.

In summary, oral immunization and intense parenteral immunization with proteins led to the appearance of anti-protein antibodies in the mucous coat of the intestine. Studies performed with gut sacs from such animals showed that, *in vitro*, antigen could be bound to antibodies present in the mucous coat. The formation of antigen-antibody complexes at this site limited the access of antigen to the enterocyte surface from which systemic uptake might occur. Complexes

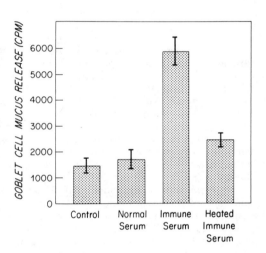

FIGURE 4. Release of goblet-cell mucus after duodenal infusion of 100 mg EA in rats passively prepared with normal serum, serum containing high titres of IgE anti-EA antibodies (immune serum), or the same serum previously heated at 56 for three hours (heated immune serum). Bars reflect the mean, and brackets reflect ± 1 SD of the release obtained in four rats. (K. J. Bloch et al.[17] With permission from the *Proceedings of the Eighty-First Ross Conference on Pediatric Research*).

retained in the mucous coat were susceptible to enhanced degradation by surface-associated enzymes that were at least partly pancreatic in origin. Antigen-antibody complexes did not necessarily remain associated with the surface of the intestine, because certain complexes were capable of stimulating goblet-cell mucous release and of being shed from the surface together with the mucous thus released.

In vivo studies disclosed that following gavage with large amounts of BSA, it was possible to detect nanogram quantities of immunoreactive BSA in the blood of rats. Intestinal inflammation produced by infection of rats with the nematode, *N. brasiliensis* or the induction of mild systemic or local intestinal anaphylaxis, enhanced the uptake of immunoreactive BSA serving as a bystander antigen. Some immunologic consequences of the enhanced uptake of a bystander antigen were considered.

In relation to the model of local intestinal anaphylaxis, it was demonstrated that the initial interaction of antigen with IgE antibodies on intestinal mast cells was capable of triggering goblet-cell mucous release. It was suggested that such mucous release might also have a protective function by limiting access of antigen to additional sensitized mast cells.

REFERENCES

1. WALKER, W. A., K. J. ISSELBACHER & K. J. BLOCH. 1974. Adv. Exp. Med. Biol. **45:** 295–303.
2. WALKER, W. A., K. J. ISSELBACHER & K. J. BLOCH. 1972. Science **177:** 608–610.
3. WALKER, W. A., K. J. ISSELBACHER & K. J. BLOCH. 1973. J. Immunol. **111:** 221–226.
4. WALKER, W. A., M. WU, K. J. ISSELBACHER & K. J. BLOCH. 1975. J. Immunol. **115:** 854–861.
5. CORNELL, R., W. A. WALKER & K. J. ISSELBACHER. 1971. Lab. Invest. **25:** 42–48.
6. WEISER, M. M. 1973. J. Biol. Chem. **248:** 2536–2541.
7. WALKER, W. A., K. J. ISSELBACHER & K. J. BLOCH. 1974. Am. J. Clin. Nutr. **27:** 1434–1440.
8. WALKER, W. A., M. WU, K. J. ISSELBACHER & K. J. BLOCH. 1975. Gastroenterology **69:** 1223–1229.
9. PANG, K. Y., W. A. WALKER & K. J. BLOCH. 1981. Gut **22:** 1018–1024.
10. UDALL, J. N., K. J. BLOCH, L. FRITZE & W. A. WALKER. 1981. Immunology **42:** 251–257.
11. BLOCH, K. J., D. B. BLOCH, M. STEARNS & W. A. WALKER. 1979. Gastroenterology **77:** 1039–1044.
12. BLOCH, K. J., A. M. LAKE, K. SINCLAIR & W. A. WALKER. 1981. In The Mucosal Immune System in Health and Disease. Proceedings of the Eighty-First Ross Conference on Pediatric Research. Ross Laboratories. Columbus, Ohio. 273–280.
13. BLOCH, K. J. & W. A. WALKER. 1981. J. Allergy Clin. Immunol. **67:** 312–316.
14. WALKER, W. A., S. N. ABEL, M. WU & K. J. BLOCH. 1976. J. Immunol. **117:** 1028–1032.
15. WALKER, W. A., M. WU & K. J. BLOCH. 1977. Science **197:** 370–372.
16. LAKE, A. M., K. J. BLOCH, M. R. NEUTRA & W. A. WALKER. 1979. J. Immunol. **122:** 834–837.
17. LAKE, A. M., K. J. BLOCH, K. J. SINCLAIR & W. A. WALKER. 1980. Immunology **39:** 173–178.
18. FORSTNER, J. F., I. JABBAT, B. P. FINDLAY & G. G. FORSTNER. 1977. Mod. Probl. Pediatr. **19:** 54–70.

DISCUSSION OF THE PAPER

M. LAMM (*Case Western Reserve University, Cleveland, Ohio*): Do you think that absorption in the intestinal lymph is unimportant, or were you not including this pathway of absorption of antigens in order to make the general point?

W. A. WALKER (*Harvard Medical School, Boston, Mass.*): I do not think there is enough information to say that the lymph drainage is not an additional important route.

J. V. PEPPARD (*Chester Beatty Research Institute, Sutton, Surrey, England*): Presumably, the immune complexes could be transported directly into the lumen of the gut by secretory component on the enterocytes before they reach the liver.

S. J. CHALLACOMBE (*Guy's Hospital, London, England*): Can you take any other secretory tissue, apply immune complexes or antigen, and induce release of mucous?

WALKER: We have not challenged other tissues except the intestine.

CHALLACOMBE: We have tried without any success.

P. BRANDTZAEG (*National Hospital, Oslo, Norway*): Have you examined in your experiments, which include a bystander antigen, the effect of specific antigen-antibody interaction on the absorption of bystander antigen?

WALKER: Yes. In our experiments, we used antibody directed against DNP BSA injected under two circumstances. Radiolabeled DNP BSA was injected simultaneously, and the elimination of immune complexes was measured. An additional antigen was injected as a bystander. Results obtained would suggest that a bystander antigen does not have any effect on the elimination of specific immune complexes. When an IgE antibody interacts with a specific allergen and produces a hypersensitivity reaction, the bystander antigen will be absorbed across the mucosal surface.

D. E. BOCKMAN: (*Medical College of Georgia, Augusta, Ga.*): There is a discrepancy between your suggestion that the presence of an antibody will exclude the antigens in the epithelial cell and your finding that suggests that complexes passing through the epithelial cell elicit expulsion of mucous from goblet cells. Do you have direct evidence that the antibody excludes the antigen from the epithelial cell.?

WALKER: I did not mean to imply that the complexes were formed on the surface. Antigens may pass through the surface, form complexes within the interstitium and interact with IgE attached to mast cells. This attachment, in turn, causes histamine release, and subsequent release of mucus from goblet cells. There may be a difference in the manner in which IgG or IgA complexes are handled by mucosal surfaces. Presumably, IgA acts as an exclusion complex-forming antibody, whereas IgG may actually cause an increased uptake.

R. A. GOOD: (*Oklahoma Medical Research Foundation, Oklahoma City*): There are some discrepancies with what we observe clinically. When Dr. Cunningham-Rundles was studying the adsorption of antigens in patients with selective absence of IgA, I discussed this problem with Dr. Levinsky, and he told me that in patients with atopic allergy, IgE allergy, there was a marked increased uptake of antigen, comparable to our patients with selective absence of IgA. Subsequently, we observed that patients with Bruton's agammaglobulinemia, who lacked the total immunity system, had not absorbed as much of the antigen as the patients with selective absence of IgA. These observations suggest that allergic reaction or antigen-antibody complex reactions may, under certain circumstances, enhance the uptake of antigen, as well as be a barrier to its uptake.

T- AND B-CELL MEMORY ON MUCOSAL SURFACES

R. Ganguly and R. H. Waldman

University of South Florida
Veterans Administration Medical Center
Tampa, Florida 33612
West Virginia University School of Medicine
Morgantown, West Virginia 26506

Secretory IgA is the predominant immunoglobulin in external secretions.[1-3] Amoss and Taylor, in 1917,[4] found that poliomyelitis activity could be neutralized by substances obtained from nasal washings. Besredka, in 1927,[5] proposed the presence of a local immune system resident on mucosal surfaces. Bull and McKee, in 1929,[6] showed that intranasal instillation of pneumococci resulted in resistance to infection with the same organism in the absence of demonstrable serum antibodies in patients. Using viral antigens, much of the data were obtained that support the concept of local mucosal immunity.[7]

Cell-mediated immunity (CMI) on secretory surfaces is less clearly understood, however. During the past decade, studies conducted in this area suggested that the local induction of CMI on mucosal surfaces is feasible.[8-12] The appearance of sensitized lymphocytes in the respiratory tract was compared with those in the spleens of guinea pigs after administration of dinitrophenylated human gamma globulin (DNP-HGG) either locally (nose drops) or by injection.[13] The results indicated that CMI, as evidenced by inhibition of macrophage migration in the presence of antigen, was associated with lymphocytes obtained from the respiratory tracts of guinea pigs immunized by DNP-HGG in nose drops, but not from those immunized parenterally. Splenic lymphocytes from parenterally immunized animals inhibited macrophage migration, whereas those from locally immunized animals did not. Thus, this type of immunity is now accepted as a part of the secretory immune system, which previously has been described only in terms of humoral immunity, with secretory IgA antibody as its predominant component.

Minimal information, however, is available regarding the existence of and mechanisms involved in eliciting mucosal memory responses.[14,15] Earlier investigations did not demonstrate the existence of a strong anamnestic humoral response following oral administration of antigen.[16,17] More recent studies analyzed and detected a local memory response with IgA-containing cells in mesenteric lymph nodes, spleen,[19,20] and in the lamina propria of the gut.[21-23]

Using live attenuated rubella vaccine, we assessed the effects of booster immunization by way of the nasopharyngeal tract in human volunteers.[24] The subjects in four groups received the primary sensitization by various routes, that is, subcutaneously, by aerosol, spray, or nose drops. It was found that following primary exposure to the vaccine, nose drops and spray groups developed higher nasal antibody levels compared to the levels in the aerosol and subcutaneous groups (TABLE 1). Upon secondary challenge with the vaccine by the intranasal route, local secretory antibody was found to be enhanced in groups where preexisting antibody levels were low. Individuals in the nose drops and spray groups showed neither viral shedding nor changes in the local antibody levels (TABLE 2). None of the volunteers in any group developed viremia; however, local colonization of the virus was frequently encountered (as detected in the nasal

603

0077-8923/83/0409-0603 $1.75/0 © 1983, NYAS

TABLE 1

NASAL SECRETION ANTIBODY IN VOLUNTEERS
IMMUNIZED WITH RUBELLA VACCINE BY VARIOUS ROUTES[24]

Vaccine Groups	No. With Antibody Rise/No. Tested	Geometric Mean Titer*
Aerosol	9/11	1:3
Spray	5/6	1:4
Nose Drops	9/9	1:7
Subcutaneous	4/8	1:2

*Includes entire group, both those who had significant antibody rise and those who did not.

wash specimens) in subcutaneous and aerosol groups. They also had lower levels of nasal antibodies. When individual volunteers were evaluated, we saw that virus shedding and a rise in secretory antibody occurred in volunteers who had nasal antibody at the time of challenge (TABLE 3). It is possible that the quality of secretory antibody, depending upon the route of primary exposure, was different in those who were protected as compared to those who were not. Furthermore, local cellular immunity might have played a significant role in protection because such mechanisms of cellular immunity are known to exist in connection with viral antigens on secretory surfaces.[25]

McGhee and coworkers demonstrated that ingestion of S. mutans antigen by human volunteers induces the selective appearance of sIgA antibody at distant sites in salivary and lacrimal secretions in the absence of a detectable serum response.[26] They also studied the dynamics of antibody production observed after a second series of antigen ingestion. Their data strongly imply that a secondary response, associated with the IgA class, can be induced in external secretions following reexposure to the antigen (TABLE 4).

In a recent report, Keren, et al.[27] have also directly demonstrated in intestinal secretions an IgA-memory response to orally administered bacteria, that is, Shigella flexneri antigens. These investigators outlined the use of the chronically isolated ileal loop model in rabbits[28] to follow the kinetics of the mucosal IgA-memory response in intestinal secretions after oral immunization and challenge with Shigella antigen. The animals received three weekly peroral doses of

TABLE 2

RESPONSE TO BOOSTER IMMUNIZATION IN VOLUNTEERS
COMPARED TO SERONEGATIVE CONTROLS[24]

Group (No.)	Symptoms*	Antibody Response†	
		Serum	Secretory
Vaccines:			
Subcutaneous (8)	0	0	3
Nose Drops (13)	0	0	0
Aerosol (13)	0	0	2
Spray (12)	0	0	0
Control (9)	4	9	9

*Pharyngitis, rhinitis, rash, low-grade fever, adenopathy, or rash.
†Number with fourfold or greater rise.

10^{10} live *S. flexneri* strain X 16 and then were allowed to rest for 60 days after the third oral immunization. At this point, chronically isolated loops were created, and a single oral challenge with 10^{10} live *S. flexneri* strain X 16 was given. A striking IgA-memory response was found in secretions from this group of rabbits (TABLE 5). No such memory response was seen when killed *Shigella* were used to prime and challenge the rabbits. These studies provide conclusive data that peroral immunization will produce a local IgA-anamnestic response in the intestinal tract.

Studies from our laboratory have indicated earlier that local CMI exhibits memory.[29] In previously sensitized animals, reexposure to influenza antigen elicited an earlier local CMI response compared to the primary response, although there was no difference in the magnitude or duration of this activity (TABLE 6). This anamnestic response on respiratory mucosal surfaces may be important from the standpoint of protection, because the period of a few days between the onset of local CMI in sensitized and nonsensitized individuals may

TABLE 3

VOLUNTEERS SHOWING RESPONSE TO SECONDARY EXPOSURE
TO LIVE ATTENUATED RUBELLA VACCINE[24]

Volunteers	Group Primary Sensitization	Serum Ig Antibody Prior to Challenge	Secretory Antibody Titers*		Virus Shedding*
			Pre-challenge	Post-challenge	
JC	SQ†	1:64	1:2	1:2	+
LB	SQ	1:64	1:8	1:2	+
BJ	SQ	1:64	1:4	1:16	−
JL	SQ	1:64	<1:1	1:8	−
MV	SQ	1:128	1:8	1:32	−
CF	Aerosol	1:64	1:4	1:4	+
DS	Aerosol	1:32	1:2	1:2	+
TM	Aerosol	1:64	<1:1	<1:1	+
BS	Aerosol	1:128	1:4	1:16	−
SR	Aerosol	1:64	1:4	1:16	−

*nasal wash specimens
†SQ = subcutaneous group

determine the outcome of infection. Conceivably, protection from local CMI is a result, not of enduring immunity, but of the rapid activation of immune lymphocytes following reintroduction of the organism.

In another study in guinea pigs, we compared the development of local humoral and cellular immunities following booster immunization. Using bivalent influenza virus vaccine, the animals were primed either intranasally or by footpad route. To determine the memory response, approximately 45 days after the primary dose, the animals received the vaccine either by the same route as primary sensitization or by the cross immunization route. Development of the humoral and cellular immunities was then tested as described previously.[29,30] Hemadsorption inhibition neutralization technique was employed for specific antibody determination in the lung lavage fluids of the animals against influenza virus. Production of migration inhibitory factor by the pulmonary cells was assessed using normal guinea pig peritoneal macrophages as indicator cells.

TABLE 4

PRIMARY AND SECONDARY IMMUNE RESPONSES OF AGGLUTININ TITERS OF SELECTED SAMPLES OF PAROTID SALIVA AND TEARS OF VOLUNTEERS INGESTING S. mutans OMZ-176[25]

Period	Subject 1		Subject 2		Subject 3		Subject 4	
	Parotid	Tears	Parotid	Tears	Parotid	Tears	Parotid	Tears
Preimmunization	1 [2]*	<1 [1]	<1 [1]	<1 [1]	1 [1]	1 [1]	1 [2]	1 [2]
Peak primary	5 [8]	5 [9]	4 [7]	6 [8]	3 [8]	6 [8]	6 [9]	7 [8]
Peak secondary	10 [12]	9 [12]	7 [9]	11 [12]	8 [11]	9 [11]	9 [12]	10 [>12]

*Log_2 agglutinin titer determined by microtitrations with 2×10^8 colony forming units (CFU)/ml of formalin-killed *Streptococcus mutans* OMZ-176. Numbers in parentheses represent the log_2 agglutinin titers after washing and reacting with anti-α specific antiserum. No enhancement of titers occurred with anti-μ or anti-γ serum.

TABLE 5

LOCAL IgA-MEMORY RESPONSE IN RABBIT ILEAL LOOP SECRETIONS
AFTER ORAL PRIMING WITH LIVE SHIGELLA × 16[27]

Day After Challenge*	Not Primed†	Live Shigella × 16‡	Significance§
0	0.047 ± 0.006¶	0.234 ± 0.086	0.0026
1	0.041 ± 0.012	0.213 ± 0.066	0.0029
2	0.062 ± 0.013	0.499 ± 0.134	0.0001
3	0.047 ± 0.014	0.567 ± 0.133	0.0001
4	0.136 ± 0.042	1.778 ± 0.438	0.0001
5	0.218 ± 0.103	1.626 ± 0.387	0.0001
6	0.435 ± 0.149	1.610 ± 0.298	0.0007
7	0.519 ± 0.513	1.833 ± 0.350	0.0014
8	0.591 ± 0.306	1.363 ± 0.248	0.0151
10	0.532 ± 0.210	.979 ± 0.249	N.S.‖

*Day 0 = day of final antigen challenge.
†Animals given 10^{10} live shigella × 16 orally on day 0 (number = 19).
‡Animals given 10^{10} live shigella × 16 orally on days −75, −68, and −61 before oral challenge on day 0 (number = 10).
§As determined by F-test.
¶Results expressed as mean OD 405 nm/100 min ± SEM of IgA antibodies specific for shigella antigen as determined by ELISA.
‖N.S. = not significant (>0.02 by F-test).

The results are shown in FIGURES 1 and 2. As evident from the data, local primary humoral, and cellular immunities were better elicited by local immunization (FIGURES 1 & 2, Section A versus D). This fact was evident, considering the time of first appearance of the activity as well as in their magnitudes compared to the parenteral group. Following booster immunization by the same route, the nasal immunization group showed a heightened and earlier response in nasal-antibody production (FIGURE 1, Section B). Migration inhibitory factor production appeared earlier compared to the primary response (FIGURE 2, Section B).

Clearly then, local booster sensitization elicits memory responses in both cellular and humoral immunities. The group receiving the vaccine both times by the footpad route also responded earlier with heightened reactivity compared to the primary response (FIGURES 1 & 2, Sections E). This response, however,

TABLE 6

IMMUNOLOGIC MEMORY IN ALVEOLAR LYMPHOCYTES AFTER
SECONDARY ANTIGENIC STIMULATION WITH INFLUENZA VACCINES[29]

Route of Vaccination	Source of Lymphocytes	Percent Inhibition of Macrophage Migration							
		Primary				Secondary			
		2 Days	4 Days	14 Days	28 Days	2 Days	4 Days	14 Days	28 Days
Nasal	Lung	3	20	35	10	24	20	28	40
	Spleen	2.5	10	2	13	20	5	42	12
Footpad	Lung	2	3	30	10	15	12	15	10
	Spleen	2	18	54	30	23	28	25	26

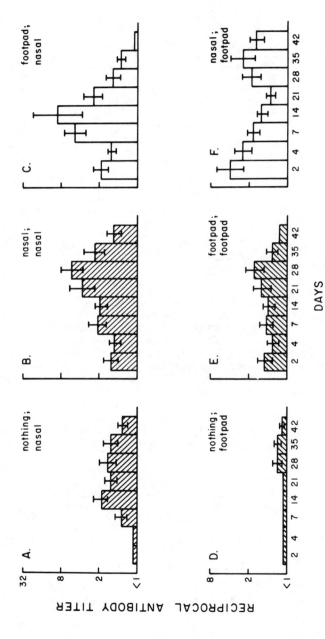

FIGURE 1. Bronchial antibody response to influenza vaccine in guinea pigs following primary and secondary immunizations.

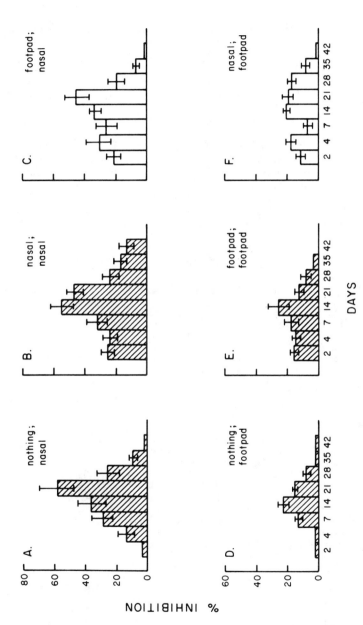

FIGURE 2. Migration inhibitory factor production by lung lavage cells in guinea pigs following primary and secondary immunizations with influenza vaccine.

appeared rather attenuated when compared to the counterpart sensitized both times intranasally (FIGURES 1 & 2, Sections B). As may be seen from the data (FIGURES 1 & 2, Sections C and F), the local and systemic dichotomy of the immune system, with regard to the requirements for local and systemic sites of antigen application, could be overcome, at least partially, by administering cross-immunization route boosters. The lower levels of local immune response were largely compensated for in the parenterally primed animals when they received the booster by intranasal route (FIGURES 1 & 2, Sections C).

SUMMARY AND CONCLUSIONS

The secretory immune system exhibits memory responses in both B- and T-cell systems. Booster immunization mediates rapid activation of immune lymphocytes that may be important for host protection. Local memory responses may be generated following application of the antigen systemically or at other distant mucosal sites. The dichotomy between the systemic and local immune systems could be overcome, at least partially, in memory responses, depending upon the route and amount of antigen employed for the booster immunization.

REFERENCES

1. TOMASI, T. B., E. M. TAM, A. SOLOMON & R. A. PENDERGAST. 1965. J. Exp. Med. 121: 101.
2. CRABBE, P. A., A. O. CARBONARA & J. F. HEREMANS. 1965. Lab. Invest. 14: 135.
3. GANGULY, R. & R. H. WALDMAN. 1980. Prog. Allergy 27: 1.
4. AMOSS, H. L. & E. TAYLOR. 1917. J. Exp. med. 25: 507.
5. BESREDKA, A. 1927. Local Immunization. Williams and Wilkins. Baltimore. p. 181.
6. BULL, C. G. & C. M. McKEE. 1929. Am. J. Hyg. 9: 490.
7. WALDMAN, R. H. & R. GANGULY. 1974. J. Infect Dis. 130: 419.
8. GALINDO, B. & O. N. MYRVIK. 1970. J. Immunol. 105: 227.
9. KABE, J., Y. AOKI & T. MITAMOTO. 1971. J. Allergy 47: 59.
10. MIYAMOTO, J., J. KABE, M. NODA, N. KOBAYASHI & K. MIURA. 1971. Am. Rev. Resp. Dis. 103: 509.
11. PERNIS, V. 1965. Arch Environ Health 10: 289.
12. YAMAMOTO, K., R. L. ANACHER & E. RIBI. 1970. Infect. Immun. 1: 595.
13. HENNEY, C. S. & R. H. WALDMAN. 1970. Science 169: 696.
14. NASH, D. R. & B. HOLLE. 1973. Clin. Exp. Immunol. 13: 573.
15. KAWATA, H., Q. N. MYRVIK & E. S. LEAKE. 1964. J. Immunol 93: 433.
16. ANDRE, C., H. BAZIN & J. F. HEREMANS. 1973. Digestion 9: 166.
17. OGRA, P. L. 1969. In The Secretory Immunologic System. D. H. Dayton, Jr., P. A. Small, Jr., R. M. Chanock, H. E. Kauffman and T. B. Tomasi, Eds.: 259. Proceedings. Conference at Vero Beach. National Institute of Child Health and Human Development. Bethesda, Md.
18. OGRA, P. L. & D. T. KARZON. 1969. J. Immunol. 102: 15.
19. BAZIN, H., G. LEVI & G. DORIA. 1970. J. Immunol. 105: 1049.
20. HURME, M. & S. KONTIAINEN. 1976. Scand. J. Immunol. 5: 339.
21. PIERCE, N. F. 1978. J. Exp. Med. 148: 196.
22. ROBERTSON, P. W. & G. N. COOPER. 1973. Aust. J. Exp. Biol. Med. Sci. 51: 575.
23. HUSBAND, A. M. & J. L. GOWANS. 1978. J. Exp. Med. 148: 1146.
24. GANGULY, R., P. L. OGRA, S. REGAS & R. H. WALDMAN. 1973. Infect. Immun. 8: 497.
25. WALDMAN, R. H., C. S. SPENCER & J. E. JOHNSON III. 1972. Cell Immunol. 3: 294.
26. McGHEE, J. R., J. MESTECKY, R. R. ARNOLD, S. M. MICHALEK, S. J. PRINCE & J. L. BABB. 1978. Adv. Exp. Med. Biol. 107: 177.

27. KAREN, D. F., S. E. KERN, D. H. BAUER, P. J. SCOTT & P. PORTER. 1982. J. Immunol. **128:** 475.
28. KAREN, C. F., H. COLLINS, P. GEMSKI, P. S. HOLT & S. B. FORMAL. 1981. Infect. Immun. **31:** 1193.
29. GADOL, N., J. E. JOHNSON & R. H. WALDMAN. 1974. Infect. Immun. **9:** 858.
30. WALDMAN, R. H., S. H. WOOD, E. J. TORRES & P. A. SMALL, JR. 1970. Am. J. Epidemiol. **91:** 575.

DISCUSSION OF THE PAPER

T. LEHNER (*Guy's Hospital, London, England*): The actual increase in T-cell and antibody titers were very convincing data, but when one thinks about secondary responses, there are four criteria to consider: titers appear faster, the higher titer is observed, they last a longer time, and have a higher affinity. Could you tell us what the interval was between the two immunization periods, and whether you are convinced these titers are actual secondary responses.

R. GANGULY (*West Virginia University, Morgantown, W.Va.*): There are several studies that have showed a secondary humoral response. We observed an increased response; it appeared earlier, but variations were seen in the duration, especially in the secretory antibody response. The interval was 45 days in the last study.

M. W. RUSSELL (*University of Alabama in Birmingham*): How significant do you regard a one to eight titer that seemed to be the best response you elicited in external secretions even on a second priming?

GANGULY: A systemic response is not heightened, but local antibody response would be significant. This fact must be considered when an animal is challenged with a small quantity of antigen.

E. M. ANDREW (*National Institute for Medical Research, London, England*): On the subject of the duration of the secondary response, I found that the secondary IgA response to particulate antigens, such as sheep red blood cells or bacteria, lasts up to one year after injecting antigen directly into the Peyer's patches and examining rat bile for specific antibodies. This response is transferable by cells from the thoracic duct.

LEHNER: Can you induce such a long-lasting secretory immune response by oral immunization?

ANDREW: No, we found that oral immunization produces variable responses.

A. O. ANDERSON (*University of Pennsylvania, Philadelphia*): I just wanted to address a comment to Dr. Russell. There are situations where antibody titers of one to eight or less of these lethal viruses, for which we have no vaccines, are totally protective, whereas titers of one to one million do not protect at all.

LEHNER: I should like to support this notion; it is not a question of titer. The avidity of the antibody might be at least as important as the titer itself.

OCCURRENCE AND NATURE OF BACTERIAL IgA PROTEASES*

M. Kilian,[†] B. Thomsen,[†] T.E. Petersen,[‡]
and H.S. Bleeg[†]

[†]Department of Oral Biology
Royal Dental College
DK-8000 Aarhus, Denmark
[‡]Department of Molecular Biology
University of Aarhus
Aarhus, Denmark

INTRODUCTION

Secretory immunoglobulin A (sIgA) is the principal mediator of specific immunity on human mucosal surfaces. Although the exact mechanisms are partly unclear, it is generally accepted that sIgA antibodies maintain the integrity of the mucous membranes by reducing their colonization by microorganisms, by neutralizing toxins and viruses, and by preventing the penetration of microbial and other antigens and allergens through the surfaces.[1] IgA in serum appears to play an important role in the regulation of inflammatory responses particularly in submucosal tissues.[1] Recent studies in rodents have suggested, furthermore, that serum IgA is involved in the disposal of antigens from the circulation.[2]

For sIgA to successfully protect mucosal surfaces it must resist proteolytic attack from digestive and microbial enzymes that occur in these environments. Changes in the structure of IgA induced by bacteria was first demonstrated *in vitro* by Müller in 1971.[3] He reported that strains of *Neisseria meningitidis* and *N. gonorrhoeae* possess proteolytic activity that invariably induce selective changes in the electrophoretic mobility of human IgA. Although the exact nature of these changes were not identified, Müller suggested that bacterium-induced alterations of IgA is a possible factor in the pathogenesis of infections caused by *N. meningitidis* and *N. gonorrhoeae*. Strains of a number of other bacterial species, including *Pseudomonas aeruginosa*, *Bacteroides melaninogenicus*, and *Proteus vulgaris*, were shown to have a strong proteolytic activity capable of causing progressive degradation of IgA. In addition, several human-pathogenic organisms induced changes in the electrophoretic mobility of IgA and various other human serum glycoproteins by attacking their carbohydrate moieties.

The existence of a bacterial proteolytic enzyme with the capacity to induce specific cleavage of IgA in the hinge region, yielding intact Fab_α and Fc_α fragments was first reported by Metha and coworkers in 1973.[4] The enzyme was demonstrated in human feces of six normal subjects examined. The intestinal bacterium responsible for this cleavage has never been identified. Subsequent studies by Plaut, Genco, and Tomasi revealed that a similar enzymatic activity is present in human saliva, and that an organism indigenous to the oral cavity, *Streptococcus sanguis*, produces an enzyme with this characteristic activity.[5]

*This work was supported by The Danish Medical Research Council, Grants No. 12-1790 and 12-3239, and by Ingeborg og Leo Dannins Legat for Videnskabelig Forskning.

Studies of partially purified enzyme (IgA protease) from *S. sanguis* revealed a remarkable substrate specificity for human IgA_1 that is the predominant subclass in serum (90–95% of IgA) and amounts to 50–75% of IgA in secretions.[1] The IgA_2. IgG, IgM, IgD, and IgE isotypes of human immunoglobulin, and IgA from a variety of animal species were not susceptible to the streptococcal enzyme.[5,6] Because subsequent studies have identified bacteria with the capacity to cleave IgA_2, we will refer to the originally described IgA proteases as IgA_1 protease.

OCCURRENCE OF IgA PROTEASES

Since the original detection of IgA_1 proteases in strains of *Streptococcus sanguis*, a comprehensive survey of bacteria, mycoplasma, fungi, and viruses has been carried out in order to identify microorganisms that share this property.[7-9] TABLES 1 and 2 list the species affiliation of more than 800 microbial strains that have been examined in our laboratory. These screenings revealed the occurrence of IgA_1 cleaving enzymes in a small number of bacterial species, whereas none of the examined species of mycoplasma (*M. pneumoniae*), fungi (*Candida albicans*), or viruses (*Herpes simplex*, poliovirus) had IgA_1 protease activity.

Interest in the IgA_1 proteases was greatly stimulated by the finding that the species of bacteria that possess this activity are not mutually related by taxonomic criteria, but by their association with a few distinct groups of infectious diseases (TABLE 2). Thus they include the three principal etiologic agents in bacterial meningitis, the cause of gonorrhoea, the suspected etiologic agents in periodontal disease, and the two streptococcal species responsible for the initiation of plaque formation on teeth.

Bacterial Meningitis

It is of particular interest that the three principal causes of bacterial meningitis in humans, *Haemophilus influenzae*, *Neisseria meningitidis*, and *Streptococcus pneumoniae*, all produce enzymes capable of cleaving human IgA_1.[10-12] In addition to meningeal infections, these bacteria are frequent causes of acute and chronic infections of the human respiratory tract, its sinuses, and the middle ear. Members of these species may also constitute a minor part of the microflora of the upper respiratory tract without causing detectable disturbances. Thus, *H. influenzae* can be isolated from the nasopharynx of 75% of children below the age of seven years, and from about 35% of healthy adults. In healthy individuals, however, *H. influenzae* constitutes less than 1% (range, 0–5%) of the total cultivable flora of the nasopharynx.[13] Significantly increased proportions of both *H. influenzae* and *S. pneumoniae* have been demonstrated in nasopharynx of children with recurrent secretory otitis media.[14]

Within the species *H. influenzae*, strains causing invasive diseases as meningitis and epiglottitis can be clearly differentiated by serological and biochemical means from strains isolated from chronic respiratory infections or from healthy carriers.[15] It is important to emphasize that all sero- and biotypes of *H. influenzae*, as is the case with *N. meningitidis* and *S. pneumoniae*, produce IgA_1 protease.[11,12,16] As will be discussed below, however, the enzymes produced by the various types are not identical.

Only rare strains of *N. meningitidis* and *H. influenzae* have been found to lack

TABLE 1

SPECIES OF BACTERIA, MYCOPLASMA, AND YEAST THAT ARE UNABLE TO CAUSE
PROTEOLYTIC DEGRADATION OF HUMAN IgA*

Actinomyces	israelii, naeslundii, odontolyticus, viscosus
Actinobacillus	actinomycetemcomitans
Bacteroides	gracilis, fragilis, levii, oralis, vulgatus
Bordetella	bronchiseptica, parapertussis, pertussis
Branhamella	catarrhalis
Candida	albicans
Clostridium	tetani, welchii
Corynebacterium	diphteriae, haemolyticum, pyogenes
Eikenella	corrodens
Escherichia	coli (serotypes O1:K1:H7,O2:K1:H5,O2:K2ac:H1,O4:K12:H5, O6:K13:H1,O18:K1:H7,O18ac:K1,O83:K1,O112ac:H46)
Flavobacterium	meningosepticum
Fusobacterium	nucleatum
Gardnerella	vaginalis
Haemophilus	aphrophilus, ducreyi, haemolyticus, parainfluenzae, segnis
Kingella	kingae
Klebsiella	aerogenes, oxytoca, pneumoniae
Lactobacillus	acidophilus, casei, salivarius
Legionella	pneumophila
Leptotrichia	buccalis, dentium
Listeria	monocytogenes
Moraxella	osloensis, pnenylpyruvica
Mycobacterium	tuberculosis
Mycoplasma	pneumoniae
Neisseria	flavescens, lactamica, sicca
Nocardia	asteroides, braciliensis
Propionibacterium	acnes
Rothia	dentocariosa
Salmonella	typhi, typhimurium
Shigella	boydii, dysenteriae, flexneri, sonnei
Staphylococcus	aureus, epidermidis
Streptococcus	acidominimus, agalactiae, anginosus, faecalis, faecium, milleri, mutans, uberis (Lancefield serogroups A,B,C,D,E,F,G,M,N)
Veillonella	alcalescens, parvula
Vibrio	alginolyticus, cholerae, parahaemolyticus
Yersinia	enterocolitica, pestis

*A detailed list of examined strains can be obtained from the authors.

IgA$_1$ proteases. Among 100 typable and nontypable strains of N. meningitidis,
Mulks et al. found only two strains that lacked the property.[16] Seven out of 105
strains of H. influenzae examined in our laboratory did not have IgA$_1$ protease.
These negative strains included two strains of H. influenzae serotype b, which
had been isolated from cases of meningitis in the 1940s, and five recent
noncapsulated isolates from normal respiratory tracts. If a suitable animal model
was found, it would be of considerable interest to compare the pathogenicity of
such negative strains with strains possessing IgA$_1$ protease activity. No strain of
S. pneumoniae so far examined lacked IgA$_1$ proteases.[11,12]

    An organism referred to as H. aegyptius, which is closely related to
H. influenzae, but causes a special acute form of conjunctivitis, particularly under

hot climates, also produces IgA$_1$ protease.[11] This organism appears to be able to colonize human conjunctivae without preceding viral or chlamydial infection.

In contrast to the mentioned species, nonpathogenic members of the genera *Haemophilus* and *Neisseria* lack IgA$_1$ protease activity (TABLE 1).[11,12,17] There is one exception, *H. parahaemolyticus*, which will be discussed below.

Gonorrhoea

IgA$_1$ protease activity has been demonstrated in all examined strains of *N. gonorrhoeae* isolated from gonorrhoea as well as from disseminated gonococcal infection. Both strains of the piliated, infectious forms (colony types T1 and T2) and the noninfectious forms (colony types T3 and T4) excrete the enzyme.[10]

TABLE 2

BACTERIAL SPECIES THAT PRODUCE PROTEASES ATTACKING IgA$_1$ OR IgA$_2$ AND THEIR PRINCIPAL ASSOCIATION WITH INFECTIOUS DISEASES

Disease	Species	Cleavage of*	
		IgA$_1$	IgA$_2$
Meningitis, respiratory tract infections			
	Haemophilus influenzae	Fab/Fc	—
	Neisseria meningitidis	Fab/Fc	—
	Streptococcus pneumoniae	Fab/Fc	—
Gonorrhea			
	Neisseria gonorrhoeae	Fab/Fc	—
Destructive periodontal disease			
	Bacteroides asaccharolyticus	Fc remaining	—
	Bacteroides buccae	Fab/Fc ·	—
	Bacteroides gingivalis	Fab/Fc, or complete	—, or complete
	Bacteroides intermedius	complete	complete
	Bacteroides loescheii	Fab/Fc	—
	Bacteroides melaninogenicus	Fab/Fc	—
	Bacteroides oris	Fab/Fc	—
	Bacteroides denticola	Fab/Fc	—
	Capnocytophaga ochracea	Fab/Fc	—
	Capnocytophaga gingivalis	Fab/Fc	—
	Capnocytophaga sputigena	Fab/Fc	—
Initial dental plaque formation, gingivitis (?)			
	Streptococcus mitior†	Fab/Fc	—
	Streptococcus sanguis†	Fab/Fc	—
Miscellaneous			
	Haemophilus parahaemolyticus†	Fab/Fc	—
	Haemophilus aegyptius	Fab/Fc	—
	Gemella haemolysans	Fab/Fc	—
	Pseudomonas aeruginosa†	Fab/Fc?	?

*Fc remaining = Fc part of immunoglobulin remained intact, whereas Fab part was completely degraded; complete = complete degradation of immunoglobulin into small-molecular-weight fragments; Fab/Fc = cleavage of immunoglobulin in hinge region to yield intact Fab and Fc fragments.

†Only some strains of these species produce IgA$_1$ protease.

Periodontal Disease

Peridontal disease is an inflammatory response in the supporting tissues of teeth to penetrating products of the bacteria that accumulate in the gingival crevice. It has been calculated that periodontal disease is the most frequent infectious disease affecting humans. Numerous recent studies of the microbial communities associated with destructive periodontal disease in humans have implicated a group of gram-negative, anaerobic, and capnophilic rods as the principal etiologic agents. We recently reported that most of these suspected pathogens, namely *Bacteroides melaninogenicus* (subspecies *melaninogenicus* and *intermedius*), *B. asaccharolyticus*, and the three *Capnocytophaga* species, are capable of inducing proteolytic degradation of IgA_1. In addition to IgA_1, some of these species were found to induce complete degradation of IgA_2, sIgA, and polyclonal IgG.[18]

The taxonomy of the genus *Bacteroides* has been the subject of comprehensive studies during the past few years. As a result, extensive reclassifications and the establishment of several new species are currently being proposed. Motivated by these changes, we examined an additional collection of representative strains including type strains of newly proposed species for their ability to cleave IgA_1 and IgA_2. TABLE 2 shows the results of these studies.

As shown in TABLE 2 *Bacteroides buccae*, *B. loescheii*, *B. melaninogenicus*, *B. oris*, *B. denticola*, *Capnocytophaga ochracea*, *C. gingivalis*, *C. sputigena*, and some of the strains of *B. gingivalis* cleaved IgA_1 in the hinge region of the alpha-chain in a manner resembling that seen with, for example, *S. sanguis*. Most strains, however, of *B. gingivalis* and all strains of *B. intermedius* and *B. asaccharolyticus* showed a more pronounced proteolytic activity. *B. asaccharolyticus* strains induced complete degradation of the Fab part of IgA_1, leaving the Fc part intact.[18] Strains of the two other species digested the whole IgA_1 molecule into small peptides that were undetectable by immunochemical means. In addition, strains of these two species caused complete degradation of IgA_2 and sIgA.[18]

Besides colonizing pathologic periodontal pockets around teeth, several of the *Bacteroides* species may be isolated from the human vagina and intestinal canal.[19,20] Bacteria of these species may be responsible for the cleaved IgA originally observed in gut secretions by Metha et al.[4]

Dental Plaque Formation

The two streptococcal species *S. sanguis* and *S. mitior* have been found responsible for the initiation of plaque formation on tooth surfaces. Within four hours after cleaning, tooth surfaces are covered with a monolayer of bacteria of the two species. Both species have also been implicated in the etiology of recurrent ulcers of the oral mucosa.[21] *Streptococcus mitior*, particularly, forms part of the normal flora of the oral and pharyngeal mucosa.

Strains of both *S. sanguis* and *S. mitior* produce IgA_1 protease.[5,7,22] In contrast to the above-mentioned bacteria, however, only some strains of these two streptococcal species are protease positive. On human cheek mucosa, approximately 68% of isolates of *S. mitior* produce IgA_1 protease, whereas among otherwise identical isolates from pharyngeal mucosa less than 6% cleave IgA_1.[22] The reasons for these differences are unclear, but the different proportions may be a reflection of the degree of selection pressure exerted by sIgA on the two mucosal surfaces.

Miscellaneous

Male was the first to demonstrate IgA$_1$ protease activity in a strain of *H. parahaemolyticus*.[12] Among 14 strains of that species examined in our laboratory, three strains, including the type strain (NCTC 8479), cleaved IgA$_1$. As discussed below, however, the IgA$_1$ proteases produced by at least two of these strains differ in important ways from IgA$_1$ proteases from other bacteria.

Haemophilus parahaemolyticus can be detected in bacteriological samples from the oral cavity and pharynx of most healthy individuals.[13] The organism is by most clinical bacteriologists considered nonpathogenic, but there are occasional reports of severe infections caused by *H. parahaemolyticus*.[15] Furthermore, Sims has reported that *H. parahaemolyticus* is one of the most common isolates from purulent infections in the oral cavity.[23]

During a study of the biochemical characteristics of streptococci and related bacteria, we unexpectedly detected IgA$_1$ protease activity in two strains of *Gemella haemolysans*. Although there have been doubts, this organism is considered a Gram-positive coccus. Facklam demonstrated that it closely resembles *Streptococcus morbillorum* and questions the validity of its status as a separate taxonomic entity.[24] Two strains of *S. morbillorum* examined by us, however, did not have IgA$_1$ protease activity.

Gemella haemolysans has been demonstrated in significant proportions in dental plaque from Tanzanian children,[25] and has been isolated from bronchial secretions and slime from the respiratory tract.[26] Its pathogenic potential is unclear.

Recently, Döring and coworkers demonstrated that two extracellular enzymes isolated from a strain of *Pseudomonas aeruginosa* were capable of attacking immunoglobulins.[27] One of these enzymes, an elastase, induced breakdown of the heavy chains of IgA$_1$ and IgG$_1$ myeloma proteins. Given that sIgA was cleaved by this enzyme to a degree where no intact heavy chains could be observed, indicates that IgA$_2$ is also susceptible to cleavage. The other pseudomonas enzyme, an alkaline protease, was considerably less active. It cleaved only IgA$_1$, and only after incubation for several days.[27] Further studies are required to determine where these enzymes attack the heavy chains of IgA$_1$, IgA$_2$, and IgG$_1$.

The natural habitat of *P. aeruginosa* appears to be soil and water, and the virulence of this organism is considered low in humans. It is a common cause, however, of wound and respiratory infection in severely debilitated patients. Like *H. influenzae*, *P. aeruginosa* is often isolated during acute exacerbations from the lower respiratory tract of children with cystic fibrosis.

The incidence of IgA-cleaving activity in strains of *P. aeruginosa* is not clear. None of 15 clinical isolates of *P. aeruginosa* examined by us showed IgA$_1$ protease activity under standard conditions.[11]

CHARACTERISTICS OF IgA$_1$ PROTEASES

All the IgA$_1$ proteases that have been examined in any detail can be described as extracellular, metal-chelator sensitive endopeptidases. Enzymes from *S. san-*

guis, *S. mitior*, *S. pneumoniae*, and *C. ochracea* are inhibited by 5mM ethylenediaminetetraacetate (EDTA), whereas an EDTA concentration higher than 125 mM is required for the inactivation of IgA_1 proteases from *N. meningitidis*, *N. gonorrhoeae*, *H. influenzae*, and *B. melaninogenicus*. This significant difference in EDTA sensitivity may mean that the two mentioned groups of enzymes belong to separate types of metal-dependent proteases, that is, neutral proteases and alkaline proteases, respectively.[28] We have found that another metal-chelating compound, bathocuproine disulfonate (Sigma), invariably inhibits the IgA_1 proteases from all of the above-mentioned bacteria at a concentration of 10 mM. Traditional inhibitors of serine proteases, such as phenylmethylsulfonyl-

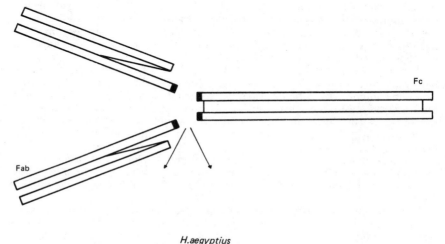

FIGURE 1. Primary structure of the hinge region of human IgA_1 and the sites susceptible to cleavage by bacterial IgA_1 proteases.[6,10,29,30]

fluoride, diisopropylfluorophosphate, and aprotinin, have no effect on the activity of the IgA_1 proteases.

Although by such properties, the IgA_1 proteases conform with well-known groups of bacterial proteases,[28] they appear to be unique with regard to specific activity. Thus, all the IgA_1 proteases, for which the specific activity has been identified, attack either prolyl-seryl or prolyl-threonyl peptide bonds. The susceptible bonds are all located in the hinge region of the heavy chain of IgA_1,[6,10,16,29,30] within a 13-amino acid sequence, which is lacking in the $alpha_2$ chain (FIGURE 1).

As shown in FIGURE 1, IgA_1 proteases from *S. sanguis* and *S. pneumoniae* cleave a prolyl-threonyl bond between residues 227-228. Protease from *N. gonorrhoeae* cleave a different prolyl-threonyl bond at position 235-236, and protease of *H. aegyptius* cleave a prolyl-seryl peptide bond at position 231-232. Recently, Mulks *et al.* reported that strains of *N. meningitidis* possess either a protease cleaving, a prolyl-threonyl bond, or a prolyl-seryl bond (FIGURE 1).[16] Each meningococcal isolate yielded only one of these enzymatic specificities. Furthermore, a certain correlation between the serogroup of the isolates and type of protease produced was demonstrated.[16] A similar heterogeneity within both *H. influenzae* and *N. gonorrhoeae* was suggested by Insel *et al.* who observed differences in molecular weights of IgA$_1$ fragments produced by different isolates of the two species.[31]

For the genus *Haemophilus*, we have confirmed the heterogeniety with regard to IgA$_1$ proteases by demonstrating that clinical isolates of *H. influenzae* produce either proteases attacking the prolyl-seryl bond at position 231-232, or proteases attacking the prolyl-threonyl bond at position 235-236 (FIGURE 1), or both types of enzyme simultaneously.[30] As will be discussed below, however, analysis of IgA$_1$ proteases released by a large number of clinical isolates of *H. influenzae* with enzyme-neutralizing antibodies have revealed an additional, and unexpected, complexity.

The specific activity of the IgA proteases produced by the *Bacteroides* and *Capnocytophaga* species listed in TABLE 2 has not yet been determined. The pattern of cleavage and the selective cleavage of IgA$_1$ by most of these species suggest that they produce IgA$_1$ proteases of the traditional type.[18] Whether this finding is the case for *B. asaccharolyticus, B. gingivalis,* and *B. intermedius*, which induce extensive degradation of IgA, remains to be elucidated. Sequential studies of the degradation of both IgA$_1$ and IgA$_2$ by these organisms suggest an initial cleavage of the IgA molecule in the hinge region (perhaps by a specific IgA endopeptidase) followed by extensive degradation of the Fab and Fc fragments.[18] Further studies are required to identify the responsible enzymes. Such studies may reveal a specific IgA$_2$ protease.

EXAMINATION OF IGA$_1$ PROTEASES WITH
ENZYME-NEUTRALIZING ANTIBODIES

Immunization of rabbits to IgA$_1$ protease preparations results in antibodies with enzyme-neutralizing activity. We have applied such antibodies to the study of the relationships between IgA$_1$ proteases produced by different species and proteases produced by different isolates of the same species.

IgA$_1$ proteases were isolated from two strains of *N. meningitidis* (serogroups Y and V135), one strain each of *S. sanguis* (ATCC 10556), *S. mitior* (NCTC 7864), *S. pneumoniae* (VK6), *N. gonorrhoeae* (VK17), *H. aegyptius* (NCTC 8502), and nine strains of *H. influenzae* (HK393, 368, HK224, HK295, HK38, HK284, HK221, HK390, HK277). White rabbits were immunized by subcutaneous injection of 0.5 ml of protease preparation mixed with 0.5 ml of Freund's incomplete adjuvant at intervals of two weeks. Seven to 10 days after the fourth injection of antigen the animals were bled by heart puncture and the immunoglobulin fraction of the sera was isolated and redissolved in Tris/HCl buffer to about one fourth of the original volume.

Each of the antisera were tested against all enzyme preparations in enzyme inhibition experiments. For these experiments, the protease preparations were adjusted to a standard activity. Quantitation of IgA$_1$ protease activity and titration of enzyme-neutralizing antibodies were carried out by a rocket immunoelectro-phoresis assay. The principle of the assay is illustrated in FIGURE 2.

Two rabbits immunized with protease from the strain of *S. mitior* consistently failed to produce inhibiting antibodies against the homologous IgA$_1$ protease. All other antisera caused complete inhibition of the homologous IgA$_1$ proteases in dilutions up to 1:192-768. Cross-inhibition experiments using unabsorbed antisera and antisera absorbed with inactivated enzyme preparations revealed that 1) the pneumococcus IgA$_1$ protease is unrelated to proteases produced by *S. sanguis* and *S. mitior*, in spite of the fact that their specific activity is identical; 2) each of the two strains of *N. meningitidis* produced at least two IgA$_1$ proteases, one of which is antigenically related to the protease produced by the strain of *N. gonorrhoeae*; 3) apart from the latter relationship, IgA$_1$ proteases produced by the strains of *S. pneumoniae*, *N. meningitidis*, *N. gonorrhoeae*, and *H. influenzae* are mutually different.

The 9 antisera produced against the *Haemophilus* strains were applied in a study of IgA$_1$ proteases produced by 98 strains of *H. influenzae*, 9 strains of *H. aegyptius*, and 3 strains of *H. parahaemolyticus*.[30] As noted above, molecular weight determinations and partial amino acid sequencing of fragments of IgA$_1$ cleaved by strains of *H. influenzae* revealed only two types of IgA$_1$ proteases (FIGURE 1) that could be present alone or in combination in different strains. Studies using enzyme-neutralizing antisera, however, disclosed a remarkable degree of complexity. Within 107 strains of *H. influenzae* and *H. aegyptius*, 15 different patterns of enzyme inhibition could be demonstrated with the use of the 9 antisera. Cross-inhibition experiments and the use of absorbed antisera revealed that strains belonging to 8 of these 15 patterns produced 1 or 2 proteases, each cleaving the prolyl-seryl bond at position 231-232. Strains assigned to four of

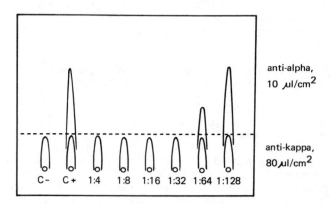

FIGURE 2. Rocket immunoelectrophoresis technique used for quantitation of IgA$_1$ protease activity and titration of enzyme-neutralizing antibodies. One volume of IgA$_1$ protease preparation was mixed with one volume of two-fold dilutions of antiserum. After incubation for two hours at 37° C 1 volume of a solution of IgA$_1$ myeloma protein (Fri) was added to give a final concentration of 0.5 mg/ml. The reaction mixture was incubated for two hours at 37° C followed by immediate electrophoresis at 2V/cm for 24 hours. The wells contained 5 μl of reaction mixture. The primary gel, which contains antiserum against light chain (Dakopatts, Copenhagen, A 192), holds back uncleaved IgA and Fab fragments. The secondary gel, which contains antiserum against alpha-chain (Dakopatts, Copenhagen, A 092), allows quantitation of Fc fragments.

TABLE 3

IgA$_1$ Protease Pattern of 54 Encapsulated Strains of *H. Influenzae*

Serotype	Total No. of Strains	IgA$_1$ Protease Pattern*					
		1	4	5	7	8	9
a	3	0	0	0	0	3	0
b	35	35	0	0	0	0	0
c	2	0	2	0	0	0	0
d	4	0	0	0	4	0	0
e	5	1	0	4	0	0	0
f	5	0	3	0	0	0	2

*Based on patterns of inhibition by antisera against nine prototypes of *H. influenzae* IgA$_1$ proteases.[30]

the patterns produced one or two proteases that cleaved the prolyl-threonyl bond at position 235-236, and strains of the two remaining patterns produced both types of enzymes simultaneously. Furthermore, the results of these studies indicated that within the species *H. influenzae* and *H. aegyptius*, at least three IgA$_1$ proteases attacking the prolyl-seryl bond (231-232) and at least three proteases attacking the prolyl-threonyl bond (235-236) were produced by different strains. The above-mentioned 15 different inhibition patterns are a result of different permutations of these different proteases.

In view of this unexpected complexity, it is reassuring that a correlation between the "IgA$_1$ protease pattern" and other characteristics of the strains was demonstrated. Thus, among encapsulated strains of *H. influenzae*, a distinct correlation between capsular serotype and the "IgA$_1$ protease pattern" was observed (TABLE 3). It is of particular interest that all 35 strains of serotype b, the serotype that is responsible for virtually all cases of *H. influenzae* meningitis and epiglottitis, were assigned to one particular "IgA$_1$ protease pattern" (pattern 1 (TABLE 3).[30]

Two of the strains of *H. parahaemolyticus* were different from all other strains because they were inhibited by human and nonimmune rabbit sera. The inhibiting factor was unrelated to the immunoglobulin fraction. The remaining strain of *H. parahaemolyticus* was not inhibited by nonimmune sera and could not be assigned to any of the above-mentioned 15 patterns.

CONCLUSIONS

IgA$_1$ proteases have been demonstrated in the principal etiologic agents of bacterial meningitis, gonorrhoea, and periodontal disease and in two streptococcal species responsible for the initiation of dental plaque formation. In addition, some strains of the species *H. parahaemolyticus*, *Gemella haemolysans*, and *Pseudomonas aeruginosa* release proteases capable of cleaving IgA$_1$. Strains of the two *Bacteroides* species *B. gingivalis* and *B. intermedius* are also capable of inducing extensive degradation of IgA$_2$.

The IgA$_1$ proteases are all metal-chelator sensitive, extracellular endopeptidases and are highly unusual with regard to specific activity. All enzymes that have been examined in detail cleave one of several prolyl-seryl or prolyl-threonyl peptide bonds present in the hinge region of the heavy chain of IgA$_1$.

IgA$_1$ proteases of two distinct specificities have been demonstrated within both N. meningitidis and H. influenzae, and preliminary observations suggest a similar pattern in N. gonorrhoeae. The application of enzyme-neutralizing antibodies to the study of IgA$_1$ proteases from strains of H. influenzae and H. aegyptius revealed at least 15 different patterns of IgA$_1$ protease activities that showed a correlation to capsular serotype. A similar complexity may exist within other species of IgA$_1$ protease-producing bacteria.

ACKNOWLEDGMENT

Some of the work reported herein was initiated in Dr. J. Mestecky's laboratory. We thank Dr. Mestecky for continuous stimulation and for providing some of the immunoglobulin preparations used in the study.

REFERENCES

1. HANSON, L. Å., and P. BRANDTZAEG. 1980. The mucosal defense system, In Immunologic disorders in infants and children. E. R. Stiehm and V. A. Fulginiti, Eds.: 137–164. The W.B. Saunders Co., Philadelphia.
2. RUSSELL, M. W., T. A. BROWN & J. MESTECKY. 1981. Role of serum IgA. Hepatobiliary transport of circulating antigen. J. Exp. Med. 153: 968–976.
3. MÜLLER, H. E. 1971. Immunoelectrophoretische Untersuchen zur Einwirkung bakterieller Enzyme auf menschliche Plasmaprotein. Zbl. Bakteriol. Hyg. I. Abt. Orig. A. 217: 254–274.
4. METHA, S. K., A. G. PLAUT, N. J. CALVANICO & T. B. TOMASI, JR. 1973. Human immunoglobulin A: production of an Fc fragment by an enteric microbial proteolytic enzyme. J. Immunol. 111: 1274–1276.
5. PLAUT, A. G., R. J. GENCO & T. B. TOMASI, JR. 1974. Isolation of an enzyme from Streptococcus sanguis which specifically cleaves IgA. J. Immunol. 113: 289–291.
6. PLAUT, A. G., R. WISTAR, JR & J. D. CAPRA. 1974. Differential susceptibility of human IgA immunoglobulins to streptococcal IgA protease. J. Clin. Invest. 54: 1295–1300.
7. GENCO, R. J., A. G. PLAUT & R. C. MOELLERING, JR. 1975. Evaluation of human oral organisms and pathogenic Streptococcus for production of IgA protease. J. Infect. Dis. 131 (Suppl.): S17–S21.
8. KORNFELD, S. J. & A. G. PLAUT. 1981. Secretory immunity and the bacterial IgA proteases. Rev. Infect. Dis. 3: 521–534.
9. KILIAN, M. 1982. Bacterial enzymes degrading human IgA$_1$. In Seminars in infectious disease. L. Weinstein and B. N. Fields Eds.: Vol. 4: 213–224. Thieme-Stratton Inc. New York.
10. PLAUT, A. G., J. V. GILBERT, M. S. ARTENSETEIN & J. D. CAPRA. 1975. Neisseria gonorrhoeae and Neisseria meningitidis: extracellular enzyme cleaves human immunoglobulin A. Science 190: 1103–1105.
11. KILIAN, M., J. MESTECKY & R. E. SCHROHENLOHER. 1979. Pathogenic species of the genus Haemophilus and Streptococcus pneumoniae produce immunoglobulin A1 protease. Infect. Immun. 26: 143–149.
12. MALE, C. J. 1979. Immunoglobulin A1 protease production by Haemophilus influenzae and Streptococcus pneumoniae. Infect. Immun. 26: 254–261.
13. KILIAN, M. & W. FREDERIKSEN. 1981. Ecology of Haemophilus, Pasteurella and Actinobaccilus. In Haemophilus, Pasteurella and Actinobacillus M. Kilian, W. Frederiksen, and E. L. Biberstein Eds.: 11–38. Academic Press. London.
14. RUOKONEN, J., K. SANDELIN & J. MÄKINEN. 1979. Adenoids and otitis media with effusion. Ann. Otol. Rhinol. Laryngol. 88: 166–171.

15. FREDERIKSEN, W. & M. KILIAN. 1981. *Haemophilus-Pasteurella-Actinobacillus:* Their significance in human medicine. *In Haemophilus, Pasteurella* and *Actinobacillus.* M. Kilian, W. Frederiksen, and E. L. Biberstein Eds.: 39–55. Academic Press. London.

16. MULKS, M. H., A. G. PLAUT, H. A. FELDMAN & B. FRANGIONE. 1980. IgA proteases of two distinct specificities are released by *Neisseria meningitidis.* J. Exp. Med. **152:** 1442–1447.

17. MULKS, M. H. & A. G. PLAUT. 1978. IgA protease production as a characteristic distinguishing pathogenic from harmless *Neisseriaceae.* N. Engl. J. Med. **299:** 973–976.

18. KILIAN, M. 1981. Degradation of immunoglobulins A1, A2, and G by suspected principal periodontal pathogens. Infect. Immun. **34:** 757–765.

19. DUERDEN, B. I. 1979. The isolation and identification of bacteroides spp. from the normal human vaginal flora. J. Med. Microbiol. **13:** 79–87.

20. DUERDEN, B. I. 1979. The isolation and identification of bacteroides spp. from the normal human faecal flora. J. Med. Microbiol. **13:** 69–78.

21. DONATSKY, O. 1976. A leucocyte migration study on the cell-mediated immunity against adult human oral mucosa and streptococcal antigens in patients with recurrent aphtrous stomatitis. Acta Pathol. Microbiol. Scand. Sect. C. **84:** 227–234.

22. KILIAN, M. & K. HOLMGREN. 1980. Ecology and nature of immunoglobulin A1 protease-producing streptococci in the human oral cavity and pharynx. Infect. Immun. **31:** 868–873.

23. SIMS, W. & M. R. PATH. 1974. The clinical bacteriology of purulent oral infections. Br. J. Oral Surg. **12:** 1–2.

24. FACKLAM, R. R. 1977. Physiological differentiation of viridans streptocci. J. Clin. Microbiol. **5:** 184–201.

25. KILIAN, M., A. THYLSTRUP & O. FEJERSKOV. 1979. Predominant plaque flora of Tanzanian children exposed to high and low water fluoride concentrations. Caries Res **13:** 330–343.

26. REYN, A. 1974. Gemella Berger 1960, *In* Bergey's Manual of Determinative Bacteriology. R. E. Buchanan and N. E. Gibbons Eds.: **253:** 516–517. The Williams & Wilkins Co. Baltimore.

27. DÖRING, G., H.-J. OBERNESSER & K. BOTZENHART. 1981. Extracellular toxins of *Pseudomonoas aeruginosa* II. Effect of two proteases on human immunoglobulins IgG, IgA and secretory IgA. Zbl. Bakt. Hyg., 1. Abt. Orig. A **249:** 89–98.

28. MORIHARA, K. 1974. Comparative specificity of microbial proteinases. Adv. Enzymol. Relat. Areas Mol. Biol. **41:** 179–243.

29. KILIAN, M., J. MESTECKY, R. KULHAVY, M. TOMANA & W. T. BUTLER. 1980. IgA1 proteases from *Haemophilus influenzae, Streptococcus pneumoniae, Neisseria meningitidis,* and *Streptoccocus sanguis:* comparative immunochemical studies. J. Immunol. **124:** 2596–2600.

30. KILIAN, M., B. THOMSEN, T. E. PETERSEN & H. S. BLEEG. 1983. Molecular biology of *Haemophilus influenzae* IgA proteases. Mol. Immunol. In press.

31. INSEL, R. A., P. Z. ALLEN & I. D. BERKOWITZ. 1982. Types and frequency of *Haemophilus influenzae* IgA1 proteases. *In* Seminars in infectious disease. L. Weinstein and B. N. Fields, Eds.: Vol 4: 225–231. Thieme-Stratton Inc., New York.

DISCUSSION OF THE PAPER

R. J. GENCO (*State University of New York at Buffalo*): Does the treatment with enzymes from *B. melaninogenicus, gingivalis,* and *intermedius* result in a complete destruction of the IgA molecule, comparable to pronase digestion? Was the

IgA reductively cleaved under dissociating conditions to show this complete digestion? Under certain conditions trypsin, for example, cleaves but only within the domain that is held by a disulfide. If you reduce disulfide bonds in the presence of dissociating solvents, the molecule will fall apart.

M. KILIAN (*Royal Dental College, Aarhus, Denmark*): It appears that the strains of B. *melaninogenicus* cleave only one peptide bond, in the hinge region. The strains of B. *gingivalis* and *intermedius* cause the complete degradation of the IgA. You do not have to pretreat the IgA in order to observe this cleavage. The sequential studies of the cleavage seem to indicate that these organisms produce a specific endopeptidase capable of cleaving the IgA in the hinge region like the other bacteria. Once the IgA molecule is opened, exopeptidases and perhaps other endopeptidases complete digestion.

GENCO: It is a fascinating observation that the B. *gingivalis* and *intermedius* are unique among these oral gram-negative organisms in producing a large number of amino peptidases.

T. LEHNER (*Guy's Hospital, London, England*): The site of predilection is the hinge region. Is there anything particularly significant about a hinge region that so many organisms act in that particular site?

KILIAN: Structural models of the hinge region suggest that this region is the most susceptible site of the IgA molecule.

W. STROBER (*National Institute of Health, Bethesda, Md.*): If the bacteria can elaborate so many different kinds of enzymes, why do bacteria not also elaborate enzymes that cleave IgA_2?

KILIAN: I think we have to know more about the functions of IgA_1 and IgA_2. Perhaps bacteria do not have to cleave IgA_2 in order to produce disease.

G. ACOSTA (*Instituto Mexicano del Seguro Social, Mexico D.F., Mexico*): Is it possible to induce antibodies of the IgA class against IgA_1 protease?

KILIAN: It is possible to raise antibodies against the IgA_1 proteases. We have raised them in rabbits, but we have also demonstrated that highly purified preparations of colostral sIgA exhibit antibody activity against the IgA_1 proteases.

J. E. BUTLER (*University of Iowa, Iowa City*): Are these enzymes secreted into the media, or are they present on the membrane? Do differences exist in their secretion during different phases of bacterial growth?

KILIAN: They seem to be true extracellular enzymes.

GENCO: Can you induce the production of these enzymes? It is known that B. *gingivalis* produces collagenase only if grown in ascitic fluid.

KILIAN: No, these seem to be constituative enzymes.

INHIBITION OF BACTERIAL IgA PROTEASES BY HUMAN SECRETORY IgA AND SERUM*

Joanne V. Gilbert, Andrew G. Plaut,† and Brook Longmaid

Gastroenterology Unit
Department of Medicine
Tufts-New England Medical Center Hospital
Boston, Massachusetts 02111

Michael E. Lamm‡

Department of Pathology
New York University School of Medicine
New York, New York 10016

Introduction

IgA proteases are extracellular proteolytic enzymes of bacterial pathogens including *Neisseria gonorrhoeae*, *Neisseria meningitidis*, *Hemophilus influenzae*, *Streptococcus pneumoniae*, and *Streptococcus sanguis*.[1] These proteases each exhibit highly selective substrate specificity, cleaving one of the peptide bonds in the replicated hinge region of the human IgA_1 heavy polypeptide chain. In the course of our studies on these enzymes, it was observed that a pool of normal human colostral secretory IgA was resistant to hydrolysis, an unexpected finding because at least half of this IgA preparation was composed of protease-susceptible IgA_1 protein. Moreover, in the presence of low levels of this secretory IgA, the IgA proteases were unable to hydrolyze serum IgA substrates, indicating that the secretory protein was a direct inhibitor of enzyme activity. Also, human serum and plasma inhibited the enzymes, and this anti-protease activity was localized to the IgG fraction of serum. Because these data indicated that IgA-protease inhibition is widespread in secretions and plasma and is exclusively found among immunoglobulin molecules, we predicted that inhibition was through an anti-enzyme antibody mechanism.[2] Our initial findings, reported here, indicate that this hypothesis is probably correct.

Methods

All bacteria used were clinical isolates from patients at the New England Medical Center Hospital, with the exception of *Streptococcus sanguis*, which was purchased from the American Type Culture Collection (ATCC catalogue #10556). *Neisseria gonorrhoeae* types T1 and T4 were identified by examining colonies on nutrient agar under a dissecting microscope.[3] The *Neisseria meningitidis* strain

*This research was supported by Grants AI-14648, AI-15071, and CA-23885 from the National Institutes of Health, Bethesda, Md. 20205.

†Address all correspondence to Andrew G. Plaut, New England Medical Center Hospital, 171 Harrison Avenue, Boston, Mass. 02111.

‡Present address: Institute of Pathology, Case-Western Reserve University, Cleveland, Ohio 44106.

0077-8923/83/0409-0625 $1.75/0 © 1983, NYAS

used in these studies yielded type 1 IgA protease specificity, as defined earlier from this laboratory.[4]

IgA proteases were obtained from the extracellular medium of bacterial liquid cultures grown at 37° C for 18 hours. Neisseria species were inoculated into two liters Brain Heart Infusion broth (Difco Laboratories, Detroit, Mich.) supplemented with IsoVitalex (BBL, Cockeysville, Md.) and grown with gentle swirling, in an atmosphere of 5% CO_2 in air. *S. sanguis* was grown in stationary one liter Todd-Hewitt broth cultures. Enzyme was partially purified from bacteria-free spent media by precipitation in 60% ammonium sulfate followed by sequential chromatography of the dissolved enzyme on Biogel P100 and Sephadex G150, where enzyme eluted just after the void volume peak. Throughout purification, enzyme was monitored by qualitative assay of IgA hydrolysis on cellulose acetate membranes.[5] The final enzyme preparations used in our studies contained less than 2% of the protein in the starting material, and specific activity was increased approximately 800-fold during the purification procedure.

Secretory IgA was purified[6] from individual colostrum of three women and also from a colostrum pool from ten additional donors. Human monoclonal IgA and IgG were purified from plasma of patients with multiple myeloma. Purified proteins made radioactive were labeled with ^{125}I by the chloramine-T method of Hunter and Greenwood.[7] Human serum Cohn Fraction II, a polyclonal IgG preparation, was obtained from Sigma Corporation, St. Louis, Mo., and used without further purification.

Quantitative enzyme assay was in Tris-HCl buffer 0.05 M, pH 8.1, the substrate being a mixture of [^{125}I]serum IgA and the same protein, unlabeled, at a ratio of 1:25 by weight. In principle, the assay measures release of IgA Fab fragments per unit time. For assay of neisserial enzymes, sialic acid was removed from the substrate by *Clostridium perfringens* neuraminidase (Sigma Corp., St. Louis, Mo.); this was required because gonococcal Fc_α and Fab_α hydrolysis products overlap during cellulose acetate electrophoresis, a technical problem lessened by preliminary removal of charged sialic acid residues from the Fab_α.[8] The neuraminidase preparation used had no demonstrable proteolytic activity against human IgA_1 or IgG.

In a typical enzyme assay, 5 μl enzyme was mixed with 20 μl substrate, the final incubation mixture containing 8.8 μg IgA (352 $\mu g/ml$) having approximately 10^6 cpm. During a 45-minute incubation at 37° C, samples were removed at intervals and the enzyme activity stopped by adding an equal volume of 450 mM ethylenediaminetetraacetic acid (EDTA) held in solution in buffer at 37° C. Following electrophoresis on cellulose acetate membranes, the radioactivity in newly released Fab_α fragments was determined by counting the appropriate region on the cut membrane. As previously reported,[5] the hydrolysis of human serum IgA by microbial IgA proteases is linear using this method. One unit of IgA protease activity has been defined[5] as that enzyme activity cleaving one microgram human serum IgA per minute at 37° C.

To study IgA-protease inhibition, 10 μl aliquots of inhibitory sera or dilutions of secretory IgA were mixed with 5 μl enzyme solution containing approximately 0.03 units of activity. After this mixture had incubated 30 minutes at 37° C, an assay of remaining enzyme activity was conducted as outlined above. An enzyme control tube received bovine serum albumin (5.0 mgm/ml) instead of inhibitor and was assigned 100% activity, allowing inhibition to be expressed on a percentage basis. The contribution of added secretory or serum IgA to the substrate pool was not considered in calculations of protease activity.

For assays of IgA-protease hydrolysis of secretory IgA, separation of hydrolytic products was by polyacrylamide gel electrophoresis (PAGE) in 9% slab gels containing 0.1% sodium dodecyl sulfate (SDS) after disulfide reduction of samples in 0.125% β-mercaptoethanol and 1.25% SDS.[9] After fixing and staining of gels, autoradiography was used to locate the [^{125}I]Fd (heavy chain portion of the Fab fragment) hydrolysis product of IgA, and these bands were removed for counting by cutting the dried gel.

Trypsin assay to measure anti-tryptic activity of normal serum and serum Ryd used *p*-tosyl-*l*-arginine methyl ester (TAME, Worthington Biochemical Corp., Freehold, N.J.) as substrate in Tris HCl buffer, pH 8.1, containing 0.0115 M CaCl$_2$.

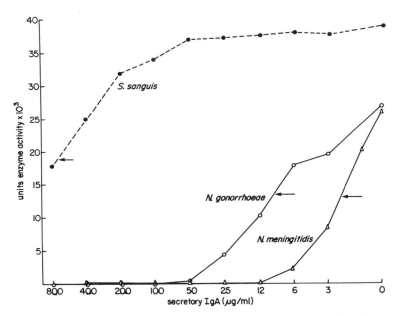

FIGURE 1. Inhibition of three IgA proteases by varying concentrations of purified, pooled human colostral secretory IgA. The arrows indicate the amount of IgA required for 50% inhibition of each enzyme. Neisserial enzymes were inhibited at 10 μg/ml secretory IgA or less; inhibition of *S. sanguis* protease required much higher concentrations.

Trypsin cleavage of the TAME substrate was followed spectrophotometrically at 247 nm.[10]

RESULTS

Inhibition of IgA Proteases by Colostral Secretory IgA

Gonococcal, meningococcal, and *S. sanguis* IgA proteases were all inhibited by exposure to secretory IgA, the degree of inhibition determined by the amount of colostral IgA added (FIGURE 1). For purposes of uniformity, the level of inhibitor

TABLE 1A

INHIBITION OF TWO IgA PROTEASE ENZYMES BY
PURIFIED HUMAN COLOSTRAL SECRETORY IgA

Colostral IgA Donor	N. gonorrhoeae Protease (0.030 Units)	S. sanguis Protease (0.035 Units)
1.	75.0*	240*
2.	25.2	182
3.	45.0	155
Secretory IgA	9.2	700

*μg/ml secretory IgA required for 50% inhibition

that reduced activity by 50% was recorded (TABLE 1A). Using the pooled colostral IgA, meningococcal protease activity was 50% inhibited at levels of 2.4 μg secretory IgA/ml, gonococcal enzyme at 9.2 μg/ml, and S. sanguis at 700 μg/ml. Because this was a pooled secretory IgA preparation to which one woman may have contributed, by chance, all inhibiting IgA, we verified the findings by

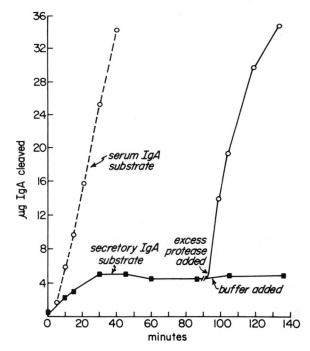

FIGURE 2. SDS-PAGE of serum and secretory IgA substrates separately exposed to gonococcal IgA protease. Serum IgA was readily hydrolyzed, but the same amount of enzyme cleaved only minor amounts of secretory IgA. Hydrolysis stopped after 30 minutes. Subsequent addition of large amounts of enzyme overcame the inhibiting activity of the secretory IgA protein, and it rapidly hydrolyzed. Buffer added as control to an aliquot of this digest yielded no additional hydrolysis.

examining IgA preparations that were individually purified from colostrum of three donors. These gave 50% inhibition of gonococcal protease at 75.0, 25.2, and 45.0 μg secretory IgA/ml, and 50% inhibition of S. sanguis protease at 240, 182, and 155 μg/ml, respectively (TABLE 1A).

Because these experiments examined secretory IgA inhibitor that was itself a potential substrate, it was necessary to determine if inhibition of serum IgA hydrolysis in the presence of secretory IgA was through substrate competition. Accordingly, we did an experiment to directly determine if the secretory IgA protein was cleaved when acting as an enzyme inhibitor. [^{125}I]secretory IgA was mixed with unlabeled secretory IgA (weight ratio 1:25); this mixture was then used as the only substrate for 0.64 units of N. gonorrhoeae protease under conditions otherwise identical with our inhibition assays. The final secretory IgA-substrate concentration was 350 μg/ml. A control tube containing no secretory IgA was used to measure the activity of the same enzyme preparation on serum IgA substrate. The large amount of enzyme (0.64 units) used in this study maximized the opportunity for secretory IgA hydrolysis to occur; the level of enzyme used was based on preliminary studies showing that 350 μg/ml secretory IgA still inhibited this amount of protease activity. In this experiment Fab and Fc hydrolysis products were resolved on SDS-PAGE, and the results are shown in FIGURE 2. The control N. gonorrheae IgA protease rapidly cleaved serum IgA substrate, but comparable amounts of the same enzyme preparations gave sluggish and progressively diminishing hydrolysis of secretory IgA that stopped entirely after 30 minutes. Upon addition of fresh enzyme (1.0 units) to half of this dormant digestion mixture, the residual secretory IgA was cleaved because enough enzyme was added to overcome inhibition. In the other half of the digest, to which control buffer had been added, we observed no additional secretory IgA cleavage up to 140 minutes of incubation. This experiment revealed that in the course of inhibiting gonococcal IgA protease, colostral IgA is not itself appreciably hydrolyzed, allowing the conclusion that inhibition is not the result of expansion of the substrate pool by the added IgA.

Inhibition of IgA Proteases by Human Serum

Gonococcal and meningococcal IgA proteases were inhibited by all normal human sera examined. Among normal sera obtained from ten healthy adult men and women the titers giving 50% inhibition of gonococcal and meningococcal protease ranged from 1:10 to 1:250. Inhibition levels were found higher in patients with gonorrhea; for example, serum from a typical patient on the first day of symptomatic acute gonococcal urethritis showed 50% inhibition of gonococcal protease at a dilution of 1:560, and 50% inhibition of meningococcal protease at a titer of 1:650, levels not seen in healthy normal subjects (FIGURE 3). In sharp contrast, S. sanguis IgA protease activity was unaffected by human serum, retaining full activity at all dilutions greater than 1:10. This phenomenon was true of normal serum and serum from patients with high titer gonococcal protease inhibition. The inhibitory data from serum specimens is summarized in TABLE 1B.

In order to characterize the serum inhibitor, a specimen from a patient having an anti-gonococcal protease titer (50% inhibition) of 1:1100 was chromatographed on Sepharose 6B. Alternate fractions were assayed for their capacity to inhibit N. gonorrhoeae enzyme (FIGURE 4). The inhibitor was found to cochromatograph with IgG and IgA, but not with IgM-containing fractions, and those eluted

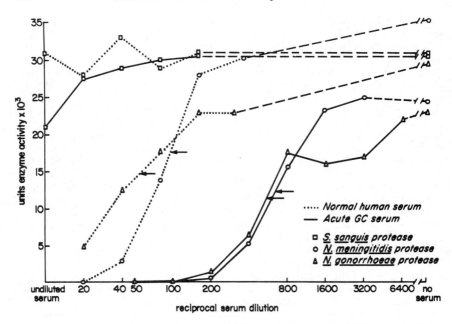

FIGURE 3. Inhibition of *S. sanguis, N. gonorrhoeae,* and *N. meningitidis* IgA proteases by normal human serum and serum from a patient with gonococcal urethritis (acute GC). The heavy dashed line carries each curve to a point showing enzyme activity in the absence of serum; arrows indicate 50% inhibition. Patient serum had titers to both meningococcal and gonococcal enzyme that were higher than those in normal serum. Notably, neither serum significantly inhibited *S. sanguis* enzyme.

TABLE 1B

INHIBITION OF TWO IGA PROTEASE ENZYMES BY NORMAL AND PATIENT SERUM

Serum Donor	*N. gonorrhoeae* Protease (0.030 Units)	*S. sanguis* Protease (0.035 Units)
Ten healthy adults	10–250*	0
Acute serum, gonococcal		
urethritis (6 patients)	560	0
	1100	0
	150	N.D.†
	200	N.D.
	320	N.D.
	1700	N.D.
Human umbilical cord serum	250	0
Patient Ost (IgA deficient)	175	0
Patient Ryd		
(agammaglobulinemia)	0	0

*Reciprocal of serum titer causing 50% inhibition.
†N.D. = Not determined.

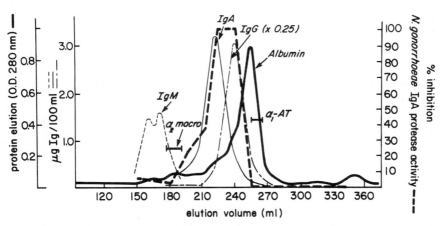

FIGURE 4. Molecular sieve fractionation (Sepharose 6B) of serum from a patient with acute gonococcal urethritis. Inhibitor (heavy dashed line) cochromatographed with IgG and IgA immunoglobulin. Eluates containing IgM, α-1-anti-trypsin (α_1-AT) and α-2-macroglobulin (α_2-macro) were not inhibitory.

fractions that contained the two major plasma protein inhibitors, α-1-anti-trypsin and α-2-macroglobulin, were not inhibitory beyond minor levels that could be explained by chromatographic overlap of small amounts of IgG and IgA. As shown in TABLE 2, polyclonal serum IgG in the form of Cohn Fraction II showed nearly 50% inhibition of *N. gonorrhoeae* protease at levels of 40 μg/ml, whereas a monoclonal human serum IgG protein gave no inhibition up to levels of 320 μg/ml, a result showing that inhibition by IgG could not be attributed to a nonspecific property of the immunoglobulin protein itself.

To verify that plasma immunoglobulins alone, principally IgG, inhibited IgA protease, we examined three sera whose content of immunoglobulin was deficient. Serum Ryd was that of a 59-year old woman with adult onset immunodeficiency that contained undetectable (less than 1% normal) levels of IgG, IgA, and IgM. The two other sera studied were those of a healthy 33-year old man (Ost) with isolated, complete absence of serum IgA, and normal umbilical cord serum containing IgG, but no IgA. The cord and Ost serum devoid of IgA showed 50% inhibition of gonococcal enzyme at dilutions of 1:250 and 1:175, values that fell within the normal range. Cord and Ost specimens also did not

TABLE 2

PERCENT INHIBITION OF *N. GONORRHOEAE* IgA PROTEASE BY
NORMAL HUMAN SERUM IgG (COHN FRACTION II) AND
MONOCLONAL HUMAN SERUM IgG

	Concentration of IgG (μg/ml)				
Type of IgG	320	160	80	40	20
Human Cohn Fraction II	100	100	77	47	25
Human myeloma IgG (monoclonal)	0	0	0	N.D.	N.D.*

*N.D. = Not determined.

inhibit *S. sanguis* enzyme. Serum Ryd failed to inhibit all IgA proteases, those of *N. gonorrhoeae*, *N. meningitidis*, and *S. sanguis* and has been the only serum we have studied to date that totally lacks any inhibitory activity. These data (TABLE 1b) confirmed that the presence of IgA is unnecessary for human sera to inhibit IgA protease, but more importantly, they showed that the absence of all immunoglobulin as exemplified by the agammaglobulinemic Ryd specimen renders serum noninhibiting. To confirm that the anti-tryptic activity of serum Ryd was otherwise normal, it was examined for its content of the two major nonantibody serum protease inhibitors, α-1-anti-trypsin and α-2-macroglobulin. Both proteins were detected by Ouchterlony analysis, using specific rabbit antisera (Atlantic Antibodies, Scarborough, Maine), and the capacity of Ryd serum to inhibit bovine trypsin was indistinguishable from normal human serum, as seen in FIGURE 5.

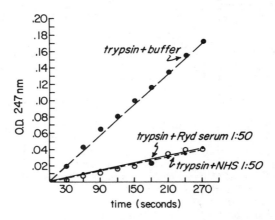

FIGURE 5. Inhibition of bovine trypsin by normal and Ryd (agammaglobulinemic) serum was the same, indicating that the nonimmunoglobulin protease inhibitor activity in Ryd was quantitatively normal. Substrate is TAME, assay at pH 8.1.

DISCUSSION

The principal findings in this study are that purified human colostral secretory IgA at unexpectedly low concentrations inhibits microbial IgA protease by a mechanism that does not result in its own hydrolysis, and that human serum also inhibits microbial IgA protease, with most of the inhibitor being present in IgG fractions. Several lines of evidence indicate that the process by which this inhibition occurs is through an antibody mechanism. First, human myeloma (monoclonal) IgA and IgG paraproteins do not inhibit IgA protease, indicating that structural features of these immunoglobulins in themselves do not have the capacity to bind or otherwise interrupt activity of IgA proteases. Second, although results are presently preliminary, patients recovering from infections by IgA protease-positive bacteria have inhibitory titers in serum that are higher than normal. Although bacterial infections may lead to increases of the multiple nonimmunoglobulin plasma proteinase inhibitors as acute phase reactants, we have shown that the two major proteins of this kind, α-1-anti-trypsin and α-2-macroglobulin do not participate in the reduction of IgA-protease activity brought about by the serum of patients with gonococcal infection. In such sera fractionated by ion exchange and molecular sieving techniques, IgG was found to have the most pronounced inhibitory activity; IgA-containing fractions were also inhibiting, but titers were lower than those of IgG. Third, human serum (patient Ryd) that is devoid of immunoglobulin has no demonstrable anti-IgA protease activity, whereas sera lacking IgA, but having otherwise normal content IgG are indistinguishable as inhibitors from normal human serum. Fourth, equal amounts of secretory IgA purified from colostrum of individual women show variation in IgA-protease inhibitory activity, indicating that inhibition is a property of a subfraction of these isolated proteins. We do not as yet know whether IgA_1, IgA_2, or both isotypes present in our pooled secretory IgA preparations are inhibitory, but we are continuing our efforts to isolate the inhibitory subpopulations from the preparation. Our preliminary experiments have shown that monomeric secretory IgA Fab_α fragments will reduce gonococcal enzyme activity, whereas Fc_α fragments do not reduce activity. Regardless of the actual mechanism involved, it is clear that secretory IgA is directly inhibitory to the microbial IgA proteases, a finding that has been confirmed by Kilian and coworkers.[11]

A puzzling but nonetheless consistent finding in our experiments has been the resistance of *S. sanguis* IgA protease to serum inhibition. Although this inhibition could be explained by the streptococcal enzymes being less antigenic than those of the neisserial species, the anti-protease could also be directed toward regions of the enzyme that are sufficiently distant from the active site so that even when the enzyme is complexed, IgA cleaving activity remains intact. In preliminary experiments not reported here, insoluble staphylococcal protein A that binds IgG-immune complexes will not absorb soluble streptococcal protease activity in the presence of serum, suggesting that a noninhibitory complex of IgG and enzyme is unlikely. Interpretation of these studies, however, must await the determination of which isotype of IgG carries anti-protease activity. Because we do not know the amount of protein per unit activity for each IgA protease, resistance of the streptococcal enzyme to inhibition may reflect differences in specific activity, and it is possible that serum inhibitor is insufficient, on a molar basis, to inactivate the enzyme from this species. This possibility can only be confirmed when the enzymes are purified to homogeneity, allowing the actual content of enzyme antigen in our reaction mixtures to be determined with certainty.

Because the IgA proteases from different species show differences in IgA_1 substrate specificity and susceptibility to EDTA inhibition, natural or experimentally produced antibody may eventually prove valuable as a probe to examine the structural feature of these enzymes. The discordance of streptococcal and neisserial protease inhibition by the same serum specimens may be the first indication that such studies would be fruitful. It should be noted, however, that the serum of a patient with gonococcal infection (FIGURE 1) had high levels of inhibition to both the gonococcal and meningococcal enzyme, indicating that cross-reactivity of IgA proteases of closely related species is to be expected. This cross-reactivity would limit the value of anti-protease activity as a test for infection by these organisms, unless species-specific enzyme epitopes can be identified and isolated for use in serology.

In summary, inhibition of proteases by human serum IgG and secretory IgA adds a new and complicating aspect to the study of these unique enzymes. Although it is not unexpected that antibody responses to these enzymes would occur, considering the frequency with which protease-positive bacteria enter the circulation at mucosal surfaces, the presence of such inhibitors could be a factor in determining the outcome of colonization or early mucosal penetration by these pathogens. The biological importance of serum IgA-protease inhibition is less clear, because the defensive role of circulating IgA in human beings is not well defined, and there is even data indicating that circulating anti-bacterial IgA may enhance virulence.[12] At present, we can predict that if IgA proteases have a role in bacterial virulence, then the balance between enzymatic activity and inhibitory levels, in secretions and serum, may be decisive in the control of pathogenic events.

ACKNOWLEDGMENTS

We would like to thank Dr. Nelia Murkofsky, Dr. William McCormack, and Dr. Fred Rosen for providing valuable specimens used in this study.

REFERENCES

1. KORNFELD, S. J. & A. G. PLAUT. 1981. Secretory immunity and the bacterial IgA proteases. Rev. Infect. Dis. **3:** 521–534.
2. PLAUT, A. G., J. V. GILBERT, M. E. LAMM, H. E. LONGMAID & N. A. MURKOFSKY. 1979. Inhibition of microbial IgA protease activity by human secretory IgA and human serum. Fed. Proc. Fed. Am. Soc. Exp. Biol. **38:** 1224 (abstract no. 5275).
3. KELLOGG, D. S., JR., W. L. PEACOCK, JR., L. DEACON & C. I. PIRKLE. 1963. Neisseria gonorrhoeae I. Virulence genetically linked to clonal variation. J. Bacteriol. **85:** 1274–1279.
4. MULKS, M. H., A. G. PLAUT, H. A. FELDMAN & B. FRANGIONE. 1980. IgA proteases of two distinct specificities are released by Neisseria meningitidis. J. Exp. Med. **152:** 1442–1447.
5. PLAUT, A. G., J. V. GILBERT & I. HELLER. 1978. Assay and properties of IgA protease of Streptococcus sanguis. Adv. Exp. Med. Biol. **107:** 489–495.
6. LAMM, M. E. & J. GREENBERG. 1972. Human secretory component. Comparison of the form occurring in exocrine immunoglobulin A to the free form. Biochemistry **11:** 2744–2750.
7. HUNTER, W. M. & F. C. GREENWOOD. 1962. Preparation of iodine-131-labelled human growth hormone of high specific activity. Nature (London) **194:** 495–496.
8. PLAUT, A. G., J. V. GILBERT & A. H. RULE. 1978. Isolation and properties of the immunoglobulin A proteases of Neisseria gonorrhoeae and Streptococcus sanguis. In Immunobiology of Neisseria gonorrhoeae. G. F. Brooks, E. C. Gotschlich, K. K. Holmes, W. D. Sawyer and F. E. Young, Eds.: 279–284. American Society of Microbiology. Washington, D.C.
9. LAEMMLI, U. K. 1970. Cleavage of structural proteins during the assembly of the head of bacteriophage T4. Nature (London) **227:** 680–685.
10. HUMMEL, B. C. W. 1959. A modified spectrophotometric determination of chymotrypsin, trypsin and thrombin. Can. J. Biochem. Physiol. **37:** 1393.
11. KILIAN, M., J. MESTECKY, R. KULHAVY, M. TOMANA & W. T. BUTLER. 1980. IgA1 proteases from Haemophilus influenzae, Streptococcus pneumoniae, Neisseriae meningitidis and Streptococcus sanguis: comparative immunochemical studies. J. Immunol. **124:** 2596–2600.
12. GRIFFISS, J. McL. 1982. Epidemic meningococcal disease: synthesis of a hypothetical immunoepidemiologic model. Rev. Inf. Dis. **4:** 159–172.

DISCUSSION OF THE PAPER

N. J. CALVANICO (*Veterans Administration Medical Center, Wood, Wis.*): In view of the exclusive specificity of the enzyme even on similar types of linear sequences that have a proline-threoxine 3*d* bond, it is surprising that you do not observe cleavage with IgA protease. Have you considered the possibility that the enzyme may be specific for tertiary structure on the IgA molecule?

A. G. PLAUT (*Tufts-New England Medical Center, Boston, Mass.*): There is no question that the tertiary configuration could be important in enzyme specificity. In collaboration with Dr. Burton, we have designed peptide inhibitors and substrates for these proteases. It is difficult to add the carbohydrates on the peptides. In addition, the susceptible bonds are not in the milieu of the rest of the molecule with the Fc and Fab on flanking sides. At this time our data are difficult to understand.

M. KILIAN (*The Royal Dental College, Aarhus, Denmark*): You mentioned that you do not see inhibition of *Streptococcus sanguis* IgA protease enzyme activity by normal human serum. We have raised neutralizing or inhibiting antibodies against proteases from the *Hemophilus, Meningococcus,* and *Gonococcus* and repeatedly tried to raise inhibiting antibodies against proteases from *Streptococcus sanguis* and *Streptococcus mitior*. Antibodies against these proteases are never inhibitory to the enzyme activity. It is possible that the active site of the enzyme is hidden and, therefore, is not antigenic.

PLAUT: We have tried to find whether the antibody to *S. sanguis* derived from IgA protease could be directed against a site other than the active site. We need positive evidence for this possibility.

J. R. McGHEE (*The University of Alabama in Birmingham*): Have you considered monoclonal antibodies to different determinants on these IgA proteases?

PLAUT: Yes, but we do not have them yet.

L. Å. HANSON (*University of Göteborg, Göteborg, Sweden*): Our previous findings indicate that there is an enzyme reductase isolated from the liver that splits secretory IgA, releases SC, and digests the IgA molecule. The hypothesis that similar enzymes may be produced by *E. coli* could relate to your findings.

S. J. CHALLACOMBE (*Guy's Hospital, London, England*): I was interested in your observation of the inhibition by secretory IgA. There have been a number of reports in the literature of modulation of enzyme activity by purified colostral or salivary IgA. Few of these studies actually make the distinction between a nonspecific effect of IgA and a specific effect of IgA antibody. Do you know whether the inhibitory effect is actually due to antibody or some other binding effect?

PLAUT: If antibody is responsible for the enzyme inhibition, then the IgA proteases represent a major antigenic stimulus to the secretory immune system. Dr. Kilian has shown that antiserum could be raised in animals. The inhibitor is in the Fab region of the molecule and has nothing to do with the Fc fragment or secretory component. These data suggest that the inhibitor is antibody until proven otherwise.

K. MOSTOV (*The Rockefeller University, New York, N.Y.*): Does the secretory component stabilize and protect the IgA molecule from degradation?

PLAUT: Our data indicate that the secretory component and the Fc region are not involved in the protection of the secretory IgA molecule from these enzymes. The data originally published by other investigators suggests that secretory IgA is resistant to proteolytic cleavage. Generalized proteases, such as trypsin and chymotrypsin were used. I believe that the secretory component does not protect the IgA molecule against IgA$_1$ proteases.

M. LAMM (*Case Western Reserve University, Cleveland, Ohio*): Variations of the titers of neutralizing antibodies from person to person indicate specificity rather than nonspecificity.

PLAUT: That is right. We examined individual women's colostrum for neutralizing antibodies per microgram of IgA. In normal women the titers varied considerably, and the same amount of IgA inhibited the enzyme differently.

ADJUVANTS FOR SECRETORY IMMUNE RESPONSES*

Martin A. Taubman, Jeffrey L. Ebersole, Daniel J. Smith, and
Wendy Stack

Department of Immunology
Forsyth Dental Center
Boston, Massachusetts 02115

INTRODUCTION

Experiments suggest that Peyer's patch cells are precursors that home to distant secretory sites,[1] including the salivary glands.[2] There is direct evidence that oral administration of antigen can result in the induction of salivary antibody.[3-5] It has also recently been demonstrated that the salivary immune response can be modulated by prior procedures such as priming[6] or by immunization by combined routes.[7] These combined procedures give rise to enhanced immune responses and can select for IgA precursor clones expressing various affinities.[8] These phenomena are influenced by the nature of the antigen (soluble vs. particulate)[9] and also by the route and mode of immunization.

Induction of Secretory Antibody: Use of Adjuvants

Early studies indicated that secretory IgA antibodies could be induced in colostrum[10,11] and saliva[12] by immunization in the glandular vicinity with antigen incorporated in complete Freund's adjuvant (CFA). Although adjuvants are not required for a secretory antibody response,[13] certain adjuvants may demonstrate selective effects on the secretory immune system. Adjuvants may also be used as molecular probes to investigate events occurring during a secretory immune response.

Muramyl Dipeptide (MDP)

The synthetic muramyl dipeptide N-acetylmuramyl-L-alanyl-D-iso-glutamine (MDP) has been found to be the minimal essential structure that duplicates the activity of the mycobacteria of complete Freund's adjuvant.[14,15] These water-soluble compounds show adjuvanticity by various routes, including oral administration.[16,17] It has been suggested that stimulation of macrophages[18,19] and/or enhanced stimulation of T-helper cell function[20,21] by MDP is responsible for its adjuvant activity. The ability of MDP to enhance an immune response when administered by the oral route, the demonstrated effectiveness of the oral route in stimulating a secretory immune response,[3-5] coupled with the highly thymus-dependent nature of secretory immune responses[22,23] suggested that MDP, administered orally, might be effective as an adjuvant for the secretory immune response. In a continuing series of experiments, we have investigated the effects

*This work was supported by Grant DE-04733 from the National Institute of Dental Research and by Public Health Service Career Development Award DE-00075 (to Jeffrey L. Ebersole).

0077-8923/83/0409-0637 $1.75/0 © 1983, NYAS

of this adjuvant substance on the secretory (salivary) immune response. Parameters examined in these studies included the effect of oral administration of MDP and antigen (Streptococcus mutans or glucosyltransferase),[24,38] the effect of route of administration of adjuvant and antigen, the effect of covalent bonding of MDP to antigen, and the effect of antigen ovalbumin (OVA) administration in incomplete Freund's adjuvant (IFA). Secretory and systemic immune responses were evaluated by an enzyme-linked immunosorbent assay (ELISA).[23,25]

RESULTS

Effect of Oral Administration of Muramyl Dipeptide

The effects of oral administration of MDP on the immune response to orally administered bacterial antigen and to a subsequent infection with bacteria bearing this surface antigen are shown in FIGURE 1. In this experiment, animals were (A) immunized orally (p.o.) with glucosyltransferase (GTF) after either administration of MDP orally or after injection subcutaneously (s.c.) with MDP. The immune responses in serum (IgG) and saliva (IgA) were also monitored at several intervals after infection with S. mutans (B). The salivary IgA responses were elevated only in the group receiving oral MDP. Serum responses were not detected after the oral administration of GTF, but were present after the infection (FIGURE 1). Serum IgG levels directed to GTF were only elevated after S. mutans infection of animals that received either subcutaneous MDP or oral MDP. The data indicate that oral MDP can enhance a secretory immune response to oral antigen, whereas either mode of administration (p.o. or s.c.) enhanced the serum antibody response following infection with GTF bearing S. mutans. The mechanism of the enhanced secretory immune response may be by way of stimulation of gut-associated lymphoreticular tissue. These data indicate that the secretory response can be controlled by varying the route of administration of adjuvant and antigen. This prospect was studied further in a second series of experiments.

Effect of Route of Administration of Adjuvant and Antigen

In these experiments, the effect of route of MDP administration on the secretory immune response to gastrically intubated GTF antigen was investigated (FIGURE 2). Groups received intragastric (i.g.) MDP, or MDP injected subcutaneously in the scruff of the neck before i.g. administration of GTF (A). Also shown are responses in the same group of animals after a second i.g. administration of GTF (B). Antibody to GTF was determined by the ELISA procedure using isotype specific antiserums.[25] Intragastric MDP administered on day 0 resulted in an enhanced salivary IgA immune response after each of two courses of intragastric administration of GTF. No such enhancement of the IgA response was seen when MDP was injected subcutaneously followed by intragastric GTF, except during a second administration of antigen. No serum response was detected. Thus, the route of adjuvant administration can selectively enhance secretory immune responses.

An additional experiment was performed to examine the effect of route of adjuvant administration on secretory immune responses to local injection of antigen in the salivary gland vicinity (s.g.v.; FIGURE 3). The antigen, GTF, was injected two separate times in the vicinity of the four major salivary glands as

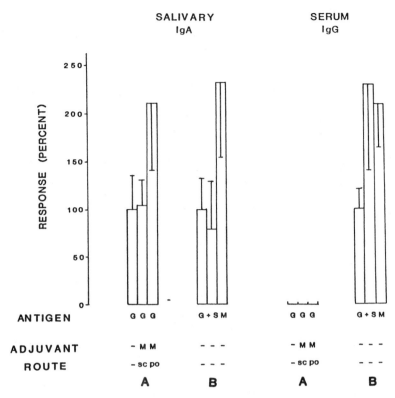

FIGURE 1. Effect of oral or s.c. administration of MDP on the immune response to oral administration of GTF or infection with *S. mutans* bearing surface GTF. Groups of Sprague Dawley rats (5–6) were first administered GTF orally (p.o.) (Stage A). These same animals were subsequently infected with *S. mutans* 29–31 days later (B). Salivary IgA and serum IgG responses are shown after oral administration (p.o.) of GTF[38] (G) (15 μg for 5 consecutive days in each 7 day period for 26 days) and (B) after *S. mutans* infection (G + SM). Antibody responses were determined by ELISA[23,25] as greater than the mean values (plus 2 standard deviations) recorded for the negative control group. This assay seems to be independent of antibody affinity as shown by the similarity in slope of dilution profiles of numerous different antisera to the same antigen.[39] Responses are expressed as the percent of the antibody activity after administration of antigen without adjuvant. Treatments for the individual groups after p.o. administration (A) and after infection (B) are indicated beneath the bars showing the group mean response. Bracket indicates standard error. The first group shown received no adjuvant, the next group received adjuvant (MDP) subcutaneously (s.c., 100 μg in scruff of neck), and another received MDP (M) p.o. (1 mg) on the first day of the experiment less than one hour before GTF was administered. IgA bars (day 8; day 65) represent peak responses observed after oral GTF and after *S. mutans* strain 6715 (G + SM) infection. The mean level of salivary IgA antibody of the group receiving p.o. MDP was significantly elevated (two-way analysis of variance of response points; all time points not shown) when compared to the group not receiving antigen after p.o. antigen ($p < 0.03$) and after infection ($p < 0.02$). IgG bars (day 8; day 38) show no response after GTF administration, but show antibody response after *S. mutans* infection. The mean serum IgG antibody level of the group receiving p.o. MDP was significantly elevated when compared with the no adjuvant group ($p < 0.01$).

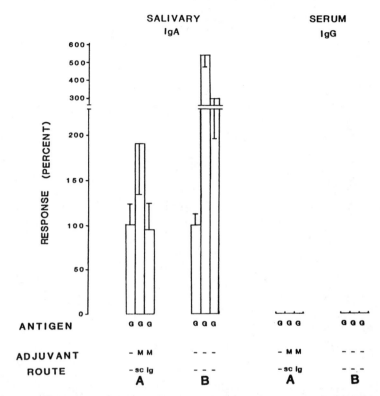

FIGURE 2. Effect of intragastric (i.g.) or subcutaneous (s.c.) administration of MDP on the immune response to i.g. administration of GTF. Salivary IgA and serum IgG responses are shown (A) after i.g. administration of GTF (15 μg, 23 times in a 26 day period), or (B) after a second i.g. GTF administration for eight consecutive days on days 85 to 92. There were six to nine Sprague Dawley rats per group. Treatments for the individual groups are indicated beneath the bars showing the group mean response. The first group received no adjuvant. On the first day of the experiment, one group received MDP (M) subcutaneously (s.c., 200 μg in scruff of neck), and the other received MDP (M; 1 mg) i.g. GTF was also administered on the same day within one hour. Responses are expressed as the percent of response after administration of antigen without adjuvant. IgA bars (day 41; day 118) represent the peak response observed after the i.g. GTF administration (A) and after second i.g. GTF administration (B). The absence of IgG bars (day 41; day 118) indicates that no response was seen from any group after either GTF administration. Antibody responses were determined from ELISA data as greater than the values recorded for the negative control group plus 2 standard deviations. The bracket indicates the standard error of relative mean response of the group described below the appropriate column. After the first GTF administration, animals receiving i.g. MDP showed a significant elevation when compared to the group receiving GTF alone (p < 0.04; two-way analysis of variance of response points; all time points not shown). After the second GTF administration, both i.g. (p < 0.001) and s.c. (p < 0.02) groups, responses were elevated (day 118).

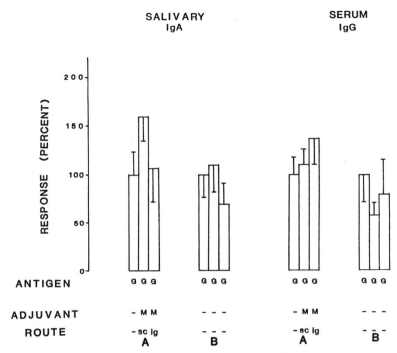

FIGURE 3. Effect of i.g. or s.c. administration of MDP on the immune response to injection of GTF in the salivary gland vicinity. There were five to six Sprague Dawley rats per group. Treatments for the individual groups are indicated beneath the bars showing the group mean response. The first group received no adjuvant. One group received MDP (M) subcutaneously (s.c., 200 μg in the scruff of neck), and the other received MDP (M; 1 mg) i.g. the first day of the experiment. GTF (15 μg) was injected in the vicinity of the four major salivary glands (s.g.v.) on day 1 and day 61. Responses are expressed as the percent of response after administration of antigen without adjuvant. IgA bars (day 17; day 68) represent the peak response observed after the first salivary gland administration of GTF (A) and also after the second GTF administration (B). IgG bars (day 17; day 68) also show the mean response levels at the times of peak response after each GTF injection. Antibody responses were determined, from ELISA data, as greater than the values recorded for negative controls plus 2 standard deviations of that value. Bracket indicates standard error of the mean relative response of the group described below the appropriate bar. After the first GTF injection only the animals receiving s.c. MDP showed significant elevation when compared to the group receiving GTF without MDP (p < 0.02; two-way analysis of variance of response curves).

described previously.[13,26] The salivary IgA and serum IgG responses were measured after the first (A) and after the second (B) injections. Subcutaneous administration of MDP (day 0) gave rise to an enhanced salivary IgA response after the primary administration of antigen, compared to animals that did not receive the adjuvant. There were no apparent differences between groups after a second immunization in the salivary gland vicinity. On the other hand GTF-immunized groups given i.g. MDP or given no MDP showed no difference in antibody responses. Therefore s.c. immunization with MDP followed by salivary gland vicinity injection of antigen gave rise to an enhanced primary secretory imune response; however, no such enhancement was seen when the MDP was administered intragastrically.

Effects of Conjugation of Muramyl Dipeptide to Antigen

It has been shown that covalent conjugation with MDP to antigen can increase antibody production to the antigen[27] and can also give rise to antibody to the MDP.[28] Still others have shown that MDP conjugation to antigen can result in the induction of isotype specific (IgE) T-suppressor cells. Other isotypes (IgG) are unaffected.[29,30] In the experiments described here, the effects of conjugation of MDP to GTF on the serum and secretory immune response were studied (FIGURE 4). The presence of MDP with the antigen enhanced the serum IgG response to primary injection only at the high dose of MDP and GTF. None of the doses of MDP and GTF tested, either conjugated or mixed with GTF, enhanced or suppressed salivary IgA antibody to GTF. Doses of MDP that may enhance systemic response may not enhance secretory response. This may also be dependent, however, on the antigen dose. Injection of MDP conjugated to GTF does not appear to enhance the serum response beyond the effect of mixing MDP and antigen. Likewise, conjugated MDP does not preferentially enhance or suppress secretory immune responses to GTF at least at the conjugation level obtained in this study. It is possible that in addition to the nature of the antigen, the substitution ratio may influence the ability of the MDP conjugate to affect immune responses.

Effects of MDP on Secretory Responses to Antigen (Ovalbumin) Administered in Incomplete Freund's Adjuvant

We also studied the effects of MDP on the secretory antibody response to OVA administration. In this experiment, varying doses of MDP were administered with ovalbumin. In the data shown (FIGURE 5), injection of 200 micrograms of MDP was necessary to enhance the salivary immune response to ovalbumin. Also, the effect of administering OVA in IFA in conjunction with injection of MDP at a different site (scruff of the neck) was studied. In these experiments, animals receiving MDP showed elevated levels of salivary antibody, but the major effect was seen in the animals receiving OVA in incomplete Freund's adjuvant. The serum response in these animals was also vastly increased. In this particular experiment, however, no serum IgG response was noted in the animals receiving a single OVA injection without incomplete Freund's adjuvant. The responses were also examined at day 28 at which time the IgA response of the groups receiving injection of OVA without IFA were diminishing (not shown). The salivary IgA and serum IgG responses of animals that had received OVA plus IFA continued to increase at this time (data not shown). The administration of antigen with IFA gives rise to a considerably enhanced response that manifests different kinetics than the administration of antigen alone. MDP combined with IFA may or may not have a synergistic effect in enhancing immune responses.

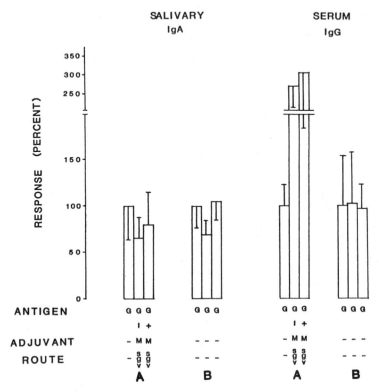

FIGURE 4. Effect of conjugation of MDP to antigen on the immune response to injected GTF. MDP(M) was conjugated to GTF(G) using the carbodiimide procedure.[27] Salivary IgA and serum IgG responses are shown after s.g.v. administration of GTF (146 μg) without MDP or MDP(M) conjugated to GTF (G; 50 μg MDP; 146 μg GTF) or an admixture of MDP plus
$$\text{GTF (G; 50 μg MDP} \underset{M}{\overset{|}{+}} \text{146 μg GTF).}$$
There were six to eight animals per group. Responses are expressed as the percent of response after administration of antigen without adjuvant. IgA bars (day 7/10; day 133/136) represent peak response observed after the s.g.v. injection (A) or after the second injection of GTF (146 μg) without MDP (B). IgG bars (day 7/10; day 133/136) show the mean response levels at the times of peak response after each GTF injection. Antibody responses were determined from ELISA data, as greater than the values recorded for negative controls +2 standard deviations of that value. Bracket indicates standard error of the mean response of the group described below the appropriate column. After the first GTF injection, only the groups of animals receiving MDP conjugate showed elevated serum IgG responses when compared to the group receiving GTF without MDP (conjugate p < 0.03; admixture p < 0.05). Lower doses were not effective.

DISCUSSION

Peyer's patches can serve as an enriched source of precursor cells, giving rise to mesenteric lymph node (MLN) blasts that selectively home to secretory tissues. It has recently been shown that dividing MLN cells bearing IgA demonstrate selective localization in salivary glands.[2] Presumably, this type of event is

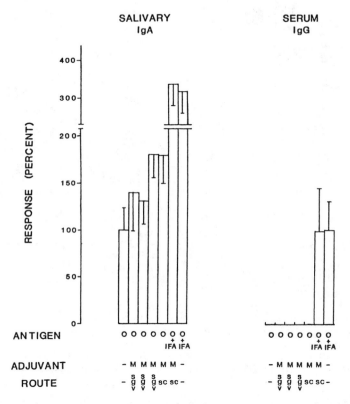

FIGURE 5. Effect of injection of MDP on immune response of rats to OVA or OVA (0) plus incomplete Freund's adjuvant (IFA). Salivary IgA and serum IgG responses are shown after s.g.v. injection of OVA without MDP(M) or with varying amounts of MDP (5 μg-second bar, 50 μg-third bar, 200 μg-fourth bar). OVA was also injected in IFA, and MDP (200 μg) was injected s.c. (in the scruff of the neck). There were 8–10 animals per group. Responses are expressed as the percent of response after administration of antigen without adjuvant. IgA bars (day 21) represent mean response after the s.g.v. injection. IgG bars show the mean response levels 21 days after OVA injection. Antibody responses were determined from ELISA data as greater than the values recorded for negative controls plus 2 standard deviations of that value. Bracket indicates standard error of the mean response of the group described below the appropriate column. After the OVA injection, the two groups receiving 200 μg MDP demonstrated elevated salivary IgA antibody (MDP s.g.v.—$p < 0.04$; MDP s.c.—$p < 0.05$), and both groups receiving IFA were highly elevated ($p < 0.005$ one-way analysis of variance). Only the serum response of the groups receiving IFA were significantly elevated, and these did not differ from one another.

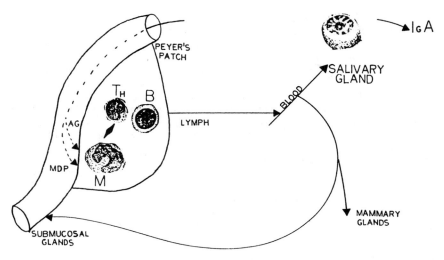

FIGURE 6. Interactions that may be involved in generating a salivary response to intragastric administration of adjuvant (MDP) and antigen (AG). The Peyer's patch macrophage or M-cell is represented by (M); also shown are T-helper cells (TH) and antigen-sensitive precursor B-cells (B).

initiated when specialized microfold M-epithelial cells covering the Peyer's patch follicle are exposed to antigen in the intestinal lumen.[31] These cells are actively engaged in internalization functions and apparently serve to sample the luminal antigen contents.[32] Numerous studies have shown that in addition to these M-cells, both T- and B-cells and macrophages are present in Peyer's patches. These T- and B-cells are antigen sensitive and can respond by synthesizing antibody in culture.[33] It has also been demonstrated that MDP can stimulate macrophages to produce interleukin I[34] and that MDP can act as a T-cell replacing factor for B-cells.[35]

Recent studies have also shown that MDP has an effect on Peyer's patch macrophages.[36] MDP promoted enhanced *in vitro* immune responses in Peyer's patch cultures derived from either normal or orally primed C3H/HeN (lipopolysaccharide (LPS) responder) mice, but not in Peyer's patch cultures from C3H/HeJ (LPS nonresponder) mice.[36] Cultures of Peyer's patch cells (containing macrophages) from LPS responder mice demonstrated enhanced plaque-forming cell responses to MDP that could be further enhanced after addition of splenic macrophages. No enhancement in LPS nonresponder mice Peyer's patch cells was seen after MDP unless spleen cells from responder mice were added. Thus, some evidence has accumulated indicating that MDP may affect Peyer's patch macrophages. It is our contention that, not only can MDP affect Peyer's patch macrophages, but that M-cells may also be target cells for MDP. Recently, we have developed a technique for enriching single cell suspensions of rat Peyer's patches for M-cells.[37] These putative M-cells appear to be Ia positive.[37]

If the assumption is made that the effect of MDP in Peyer's patch is on M-cells and/or on macrophages, the following potential interactions could occur to generate the responses seen in the current investigations. FIGURE 6 shows schematically the interactions that might be involved in generating the response to intragastric administration of adjuvant and antigen. The macrophage (or M-cell) and associated antigen can interact by generating T-helper cells in such a way as to increase migration of antigen-sensitive precursor B-cells by way of the lymph and blood to the salivary gland (and possibly to other remote secretory organs). These cells then differentiate into plasma cells producing IgA. The result is the production of salivary antibody. In the situation where MDP was injected, no enhanced sIgA antibody synthesis was observed; however, the MDP may have stimulated cellular interaction in certain peripheral locations, resulting in enhanced salivary antibody synthesis if antigen was also available at the peripheral location. Data support the concept of the route of administration of adjuvant and antigen as critical in selectively stimulating a secretory immune response. We have shown that MDP is an effective adjuvant for secretory immune responses. It should be pointed out, however, that the effect of MDP was limited when compared with the adjuvanticity of IFA (FIGURE 5). The knowledge of combinations of route of adjuvant and antigen administration are potentially quite attractive in selectively enhancing a secretory immune response.

SUMMARY

Salivary IgA responses of rats receiving MDP were elevated after oral GTF administration and after infection with S. mutans bearing surface GTF. Intragastric administration (but not injection) of MDP enhanced salivary IgA responses to i.g. GTF. Subcutaneous injection (but not i.g. administration) of MDP enhanced IgA responses to GTF injected in the salivary gland vicinity. Conjugation of MDP to GTF did not enhance the secretory response to the antigen. Nevertheless, s.g.v. administration of OVA in IFA dramatically enhanced the secretory and serum responses. Injection of MDP may further enhance the secretory response. The combination of routes of adjuvant and antigen administration were critical in selectively enhancing a secretory immune response.

ACKNOWLEDGMENTS

The authors thank Dr. Ralph Kent for statistical advice, Dr. H. Kiyono, Dr. J. McGhee, Dr. J. Kearney, and Dr. S. Michalek for the opportunity to read their manuscript prior to publication. We also appreciate the expert technical assistance of Ronald Reger and the secretarial assistance of Rhonda Falk.

REFERENCES

1. CRAIG, S. W. & J. J. CEBRA. 1971. Peyer's patches: An enriched source of precursors for IgA-producing immunocytes in the rabbit. J. Exp. Med. 134: 188–200.
2. JACKSON, D. E., E. T. LALLY, M. C. NAKAMURA & P. C. MONTGOMERY. 1981. Migration of IgA bearing lymphocytes into salivary glands. Cell. Immunol. 63: 203–209.
3. MICHALEK, S. M., J. R. MCGHEE, J. MESTECKY, R. R. ARNOLD & L. BOZZO. 1976. Ingestion of Streptococcus mutans induces secretory immunoglobulin A and caries immunity. Science 192: 1238–1240.
4. MESTECKY, J., J. R. MCGHEE, R. R. ARNOLD, S. M. MICHALEK, S. J. PRINCE & J. L. BABB. 1978. Selective induction of an immune response in human external secretions by ingestion of bacterial antigen. J. Clin. Invest. 61: 731–737.
5. SMITH, D. M., M. A. TAUBMAN & J. L. EBERSOLE. 1979. Effect of oral administration of glucosyltransferase antigens on experimental dental caries. Infect. Immun. 26: 83–89.

6. COX, D. S. & M. A. TAUBMAN. 1982. Salivary antibody response and priming stimulated by soluble or particulate antigens injected at a remote secretory site. Mol. Immunol. **19:** 171–718.
7. COX, D. S. & M. A. TAUBMAN. 1982. Systemic priming of the secretory antibody response with soluble and particulate antigens and carriers. J. Immunol. **128:** 1844–1848.
8. COX, D. S., M. A. TAUBMAN, D. J. SMITH & L. CARTELLI. 1982. Antibody affinity in milk and serum produced after gastric intubation and local injection of soluble or particulate antigen. Fed. Proc. Fed. Am. Soc. Exp. Biol. **41:** 293.
9. COX, D. S., M. A. TAUBMAN, J. L. EBERSOLE & D. J. SMITH. 1980. Secretory antibody response to local injection of soluble or particulate antigens in rats. Mol. Immunol. **17:** 1105–1115.
10. GENCO, R. J. & M. A. TAUBMAN. 1969. Secretory γ A antibodies induced by local immunization. Nature (London) **221:** 679–681.
11. TAUBMAN, M. A. & R. J. GENCO. 1971. Induction and properties of rabbit secretory γ A antibody directed to group A streptococcal carbohydrates. Immunochemistry **8:** 1137–1155.
12. TAUBMAN, M. A. 1973. Role of immunization in dental disease. *In* Comparative Immunology of the Oral Cavity. S. Mergenhagen and H. Scherp, Eds.: 138–158. U.S. Government Printing Office. Washington, DC.
13. TAUBMAN, M. A., D. J. SMITH & J. L. EBERSOLE. 1981. Conventional and specialized rodent models for studies of immune mechanisms and dental caries. Proceedings 'Symposium on Animal Models in Cariology.' J. M. Tanzer, Ed.: 439–450. Sp. Supp. Microbiology Abstracts. Washington, D.C.
14. ELLOUZ, F., A. ADAM, F. CIORBARU & E. LEDERER. 1974. Minimal structural requirements for adjuvant activity of bacterial peptidoglycan derivatives. Biochem. Biophys. Res. Commun. **59:** 1317–1325.
15. KOTANI, S., Y. WATANABE, T. KINOSHITA, T. SHIMONO, T. MORISAKI, T. SHIBA, S. KUDUMOTO, Y. TARUMI & K. IKENAKA. 1975. Immunoadjuvant activities of cell walls and their water-soluble fractions prepared from various gram-positive bacteria. Biken J. **18:** 105–111.
16. CHEDID, L., F. AUDIBERT, P. LEFRANCIER, J. CHOAY & E. LEDERER. 1976. Modulation of the immune response by a synthetic adjuvant and analogs. Proc. Nat. Acad. Sci. USA **73:** 1472–1475.
17. CHEDID, L. & F. AUDIBERT. 1977. Chemically-defined bacterial products with immuno-potentiating activity. J. Infect. Dis. **136** (Suppl): 246–251.
18. NAGAO, S., A. TANAKA, Y. YAMAMOTO, T. KOGA, K. ONOUE, T. SHIBA, K. KUSUMOTO & S. KOTANI. 1979. Inhibition of macrophage migration by muramyl peptides. Infect. Immun. **24:** 308–312.
19. FEVRIER, M., J. L. BIRRIEN, C. LECLERC, L. CHEDID & P. LIACOPOULOS. 1978. The macrophage, target cells of the synthetic adjuvant muramyl dipeptides. Eur. J. Immunol. **8:** 558–562.
20. SUGIMOTO, M., R. N. GERMAIN, L. CHEDID & B. BENACERRAF. 1978. Enhancement of carrier-specific helper T cell function by the synthetic adjuvant, N-acetyl-muramyl-L-alanyl-D-isoglutamine (MDP). J. Immunol. **120:** 980–982.
21. LOWY, I., J. THEZE & L. CHEDID. 1980. Stimulation of the *in vivo* dinitrophenyl antibody response to the DNP conjugate of L-glutamic acid-L alanine-L-tyrosine (GAT) polymer by a synthetic adjuvant, muramyl dipeptide (MDP): Target Cells for adjuvant activity and isotypic pattern of MDP-stimulated response. J. Immunol. **124:** 100–104.
22. EBERSOLE, J. L., M. A. TAUBMAN & D. J. SMITH. 1979. The effect of neonatal thymectomy on the level of salivary and serum immunoglobulins in rats. Immunology **36:** 649–657.
23. EBERSOLE, J. L., M. A. TAUBMAN & D. J. SMITH. 1979. Thymic control of secretory antibody responses. J. Immunol. **123:** 19–24.
24. TAUBMAN, M. A. & D. J. SMITH. 1977. Effects of local immunization with glucosyltransferase on experimental dental caries in rats and hamsters. J. Immunol. **118:** 710–720.
25. TAUBMAN, M. A., D. J. SMITH & J. L. EBERSOLE. 1978. Antibody binding of glucosyltrans-

ferase enzyme preparations from homologous and heterologous serotypes of *S. mutans*. Adv. Exp. Med. Biol. **107:** 317–327.

26. TAUBMAN, M. A. & D. J. SMITH. 1974. Effects of local immunization with *Streptococcus mutans* on induction of salivary immunoglobulin A antibody and experimental dental caries in rats. Infect. Immun. **9:** 1079–1091.

27. LANGBEHEIM, H., R. ARNON & M. SELA. 1978. Adjuvant effect of a peptidoglycan attached covalently to a synthetic antigen provoking anti-phage antibodies. Immunology **35:** 573–579.

28. REICHERT, C. M., C. CARELLI, M. JOLIVET, F. AUDIBERT, P. LEFRANCIER & L. CHEDID. 1980. Synthesis of conjugates containing N-acetylmuramyl-L-alanyl-D-isoglutaminyl (MDP). Their use as hapten-carrier systems. Mol. Immunol. **17:** 357–363.

29. KISHIMOTO, T., Y. HIRAI, K. NAKANISHI, I. AZUMA, A. NAGAMATSU & Y. YAMAMURA. 1979. Regulation of antibody response in different immunoglobulin classes. VI. Selective suppression of IgE response by administration of antigen-conjugated muramylpeptides. J. Immunol. **123:** 2709–2715.

30. LECLERC, C., E. BOURGEOIS & L. CHEDID. 1982. Demonstration of muramyl dipeptide (MDP)-induced T suppressor cells responsible for MDP immunosuppressive activity. Eur. J. Immunol. **12:** 249–252.

31. OWEN, R. L. & A. J. JONES. 1974. Epithelial cell specialization within human Peyer's patches: An ultrastructural study of intestinal lymphoid follicles. Gastroenterology **66:** 189–203.

32. BOCKMAN, D. E. & M. D. COOPER. 1973. Pinocytosis by epithelium associated with lymphoid follicles in the Bursa of Fabricus, Appendix, and Peyer's patches. An electron microscopic study. Amer. J. Anat. **136:** 455–477.

33. KAGNOFF, M. F. & S. CAMPBELL. 1974. Functional characteristics of Peyer's patch lymphoid cells. I. Induction of humoral antibody and cell-mediated allograft reactions. J. Exp. Med. **139:** 398–406.

34. BYERS, N. 1982. Effects of muramyl dipeptides on the *in vitro* synthesis of interleukin I by guinea pig adherent peritoneal cells. Fed. Proc. Fed. Am. Soc. Exp. Biol. **41:** 564. Abstract 1720.

35. WATSON, J. & C. WHITLOCK. 1978. Effect of a synthetic adjuvant on the induction of primary immune responses in T cell-depleted spleen cultures. J. Immunol. **121:** 383–389.

36. KIYONO, H., J. R. MCGHEE, J. F. KEARNEY & S. M. MICHALEK. 1982. Enhancement of *in vitro* immune responses of murine Peyer's patch cultures by concanavalin A, muramyl dipeptide and lipopolysaccharide. Scand. J. Immunol. **15:** 329–339.

37. PAPPO, J., J. L. EBERSOLE, M. A. TAUBMAN & D. J. SMITH. 1982. Isolation and characterization of M cells and macrophages in rat Peyer's patches. Fed. Proc. Fed. Am. Soc. Exp. Biol. **41:** 434.

38. SMITH, D. J., M. A. TAUBMAN & J. L. EBERSOLE. 1979. Preparation of glucosyltransferase from *Streptococcus mutans* by elution from water-insoluble polysaccharide with a dissociating solvent. Infect. Immun. **23:** 446–452.

39. EBERSOLE, J. L., D. E. FREY, M. A. TAUBMAN & D. J. SMITH. 1980. An ELISA for measuring serum antibodies to *Actinobacillus actinomycetemcomitans*. J. Periodontal Res. **15:** 621–632.

DISCUSSION OF THE PAPER

J. R. McGHEE (*University of Alabama in Birmingham*): All of your experiments have been done *in vivo*. Have you performed any experiments in nude rats?

M. A. TAUBMAN (*Forsyth Dental Center, Boston, Mass.*): We are currently establishing some experiments in nude rats and in neonatally thymectomized animals.

T. LEHNER (*Guy's Hospital, London, England*): Did you look for helper suppressor cells? Did you see any increase in the antibody titers without reimmunization around 14 days after primary immunization? Was it a bimodal distribution of your antibodies? As described by several investigators one can elicit a secondary response without injecting additional antigens.

TAUBMAN: We have not observed any increase in antibodies without reimmunization.

QUESTION: Investigators tend to use the carbodiimide coupling procedure without the realization that this is an effective way to destroy proteins. It was shown, for instance, that about 99% of the native determinants of diphtheria toxin are destroyed. Moreover, you crosslink proteins, and the antibody raised against such antigen will not react well with native proteins. A number of new antigenic determinants are created by carbodiimide coupling.

TAUBMAN: Several investigators have shown that MDP conjugated to antigen becomes immunogenic. We are currently examining antibodies in both the saliva and the serum for the presence of anti-MDP using an ELISA assay with MDP conjugated to BSA.

N. F. PIERCE (*The Johns Hopkins University, Baltimore, Md.*): One of the major advantages of an adjuvant would be to simplify the immunizing regimen. You have to give so many doses of GTF because it is poorly immunogenic. Have you done any studies with MDP with simpler immunizing regimens to show that you can induce higher antibody titers by a mucosal route of immunization?

TAUBMAN: We are studying an immunization regimen with single doses of antigen. The problem is that it is difficult to purify GTF in large quantities. Single administration with higher doses of GTF may be less feasible.

S. J. CHALLACOMBE (*Guy's Hospital, London, England*): I was surprised by your statement that you did not find tolerance after this long-term oral immunization with MDP and GTF. One would expect to find systemic tolerance when challenged. Did the GTF linked with the MDP induce systemic tolerance?

TAUBMAN: No. We observed a higher serum response in those animals; this indicated that they were primed.

MCGHEE: Dr. Michael has found that ovalbumin orally administered with MDP in some cases accelerates tolerance induction.

TAUBMAN: In our experiments, ovalbumin was injected and there was a serum response.

CHALLACOMBE: Did you induce tolerance to the GTF alone, without the MDP?

TAUBMAN: Definitely not.

EFFECT OF ADJUVANTS ON ORALLY ADMINISTERED ANTIGENS

R.J. Genco, R. Linzer, and R.T. Evans

Department of Oral Biology
State University of New York at Buffalo
School of Dentistry
Buffalo, New York 14214

Oral immunization with live organisms that colonize the gastrointestinal tract has proven to be remarkably effective against mucosal infections. A well-known example is the attenuated oral polio vaccine described by Saban that provides protection against paralytic polio as well as the carrier state, and induces mucosal antibodies of the IgA class as well as serum antibodies. Recently, a new oral vaccine against typhoid fever was described by Wahdan and coworkers.[1] These authors showed striking protection against the disease after ingestion of three doses of an attenuated mutant strain of *Salmonella typhi*, each containing about 10^9 live bacteria. After three years of observation of over 16,000 children given the attenuated strain, the attack rate was 0.2 cases per 10,000 children in contrast to five cases per 10,000 children in the control group of over 15,000 children. This remarkable protection rate of 95% afforded by the vaccine is encouraging for those working with diseases where the infectious agent can be inhibited by immunity induced at mucosal surfaces. Unfortunately, however, limited success has been obtained in stimulating immunity to infectious agents by oral administration of inactivated or killed organisms. In general, ingestion of nonviable microbial antigens, or of characterized protein or carbohydrate antigens, does not result in significant induction of immune response except under unique circumstances, and may result in oral tolerance. It appears that massive amounts of fed antigen are required to stimulate an immune response. For example, from a report by Clancy and Pucci,[2] it can be estimated that from 300–900 mg of bovine serum albumin (BSA) are required to induce an immune response in rabbits by feeding the antigen, whereas only 2 mg injected in the foot pad will induce a comparable immune response. Similarly, Smith and coworkers,[3] Mestecky, et al.,[4] and Michalek, et al.[5] found that large doses of antigen were required to induce a secretory immune response when administered orally. Furthermore, Michalek and coworkers[5] found that only a very narrow dose range of killed bacterial cells administered in the drinking water or food was effective in inducing a salivary antibody response.

The mucous membranes are in constant contact with a large amount and variety of antigenic materials, and other immunostimulatory molecules. In this environment the lymphoid tissue without effective regulation might undergo excessive stimulation. It is reasonable, then, that mucosal immunosuppressant mechanisms minimize immune responses to fed antigens. To overcome these suppressive regulatory mechanisms, specific conditions such as large amounts of fed antigens in the proper immunogenic form are necessary. Such regulation of mucosal immunity may be important for survival of the organism, otherwise responses by potentially pathogenic organisms would be preempted or suppressed by responses to less important immunostimulatory substances that exist in large quantities on mucosal surfaces. In this study, we attempt to potentiate the

650

0077–8923/83/0409–0650 $1.75/0 © 1983, NYAS

immunogenicity of antigen given orally by administering these antigens in adjuvants, and by this, to stimulate immunity, particularly in the secretory immune system.

MUCOSAL IMMUNE SYSTEM REGULATORY MECHANISMS

The regulatory mechanisms operative in the mucosal immune system can be considered in three main categories: those that are responsible for tolerance or oral unresponsiveness; those that result in oral immunization as evidenced by priming for an immune response or by induction of an immune response by oral presentation of antigen; and that immunoglobulin class-specific regulation of the mucosal immune response that results in induction of IgA antibodies and at the same time, suppression of IgG, IgM, and IgE antibodies. (For recent reviews see Bienenstock, *et al.*[6] and Strober *et al.*[7])

Present concepts on the mechanisms operative in mucosal immunity can explain in bold strokes how the feeding of antigen results in the production of secretory antibodies and at the same time can induce systemic unresponsiveness or hyporesponsiveness. Much of the antibody found in exocrine secretions is of the IgA class and is synthesized by plasma cells in the respiratory/gastrointestinal lamina propria and in the interstitial areas of exocrine glands from which secretions arise.[8,9] A central finding in the explanation of the mechanism by which antigen initiates the expression of IgA antibodies in mucosal or exocrine sites was made by Craig and Cebra[10] who showed that the B-follicles in Peyer's patches were enriched sources of precursors for IgA-plasma cells. Studies of the homing of immunoblasts to the gut, and recirculation of lymphocytes from the lymphatics to the blood and tissues,[11,12] showed that precommitted IgA immunoblasts appear to arise from Peyer's patches, pass through the mesenteric lymph nodes into the intestinal lymphatics and into the circulation by way of the thoracic duct. From the circulation, the IgA immunoblasts selectively lodge in the gut lamina propria and to the exocrine glands. These findings help to explain why a mucosal antigenic challenge is more efficient than parenteral stimulation in eliciting secretory antibodies. This phenomena was clearly demonstrated by the studies of Montgomery and coworkers[13] who showed that rabbits immunized orally with dinitrophenylated-pneumococci (DNP-PN) produced high levels of colostral IgA antibodies directed to DNP in the absence of detectable serum antibodies using a technique that could detect as little as 0.01 μg of antibody. These investigators also showed[14] that high titers of serum antibody were produced to DNP-PN in systemically immunized animals in the absence of a detectable IgA. Furthermore, the mammary response to oral immunization with DNP was not affected by high titers of systemic antibodies to DNP. Hence, it did not appear that antigen was absorbed from the gastrointestinal tract and directly stimulating cells in the mammary gland, but rather that precursors of antibody-forming cells were initially sensitized in the intestine and seeded to a distal exocrine secretory site such as the mammary gland. The appearance of IgA antibodies in secretions such as saliva, induced by feeding antigen has been described in man[4] and in rodents;[3,5,17] however, efforts to stimulate salivary antibodies by feeding killed bacteria to monkeys has been unsuccessful.[18,55,56] The most plausible explanation for the occurrence of secretory IgA antibodies in exocrine secretions remote from the stimulus by way of the gut is that there is a selective seeding of the precursors of the IgA-producing cells to interstitial tissues of exocrine glands. Presumably antigenic stimulation of IgA precursors occurs in the mucosal lymphoid accumulations, mainly the Peyer's patches. Thereafter, cell division and eventual migration, homing and seeding to distal sites, and maturation then leads to the appearance of IgA-plasma cells producing specific antibody to fed antigens in the lamina propria of the gut and in the interstitial tissues of the exocrine glands.

It appears that secretory IgA responses are governed by regulatory mechanisms that act to enhance the secretory IgA response, while other regulatory mechanisms are set into motion that suppress serum antibody responses. Using a mitogen-activated indicator system, Elson and coworkers[15] found in vitro, that concanavalin A pulsed spleen T-cells suppressed immunoglobulin synthesis of all immunoglobulin classes including IgA, whereas similarly, Con A pulsed Peyer's patch T-cells added to Peyer's patch cultures, which also contained LPS, caused suppression of IgM and IgG synthesis, while enhancing IgA synthesis. Apparently then, Con A pulsed cells from Peyer's patches, but not from spleen, have a differential effect on immunoglobulin synthesis with a net helper effect for IgA, and a suppressor effect for IgM and IgG. A similar conclusion was reached in the studies of Richman and coworkers[16] who showed that feeding of the dietary protein antigen ovalbumin, induced differential isotype-specific regulation of gut-associated lymphoreticular tissue resulting in antigen-specific IgA T-helper cell production. At a later time in the same experiments, they demonstrated IgG-suppressor cell function. Cells mediating antigen-specific IgG suppression and IgA help were clearly shown to be T-cells in their study. The simultaneous induction of T-helper cells for IgA, and T-suppressor cells for systemic immunoglobulins such as IgG, IgM, and possibly IgE, may in part explain the repeated observation of induction of secretory IgA antibodies by feeding of antigen in man,[4] and in rodents.[3,5,17] These results also explain, in part, induction of oral tolerance or unresponsiveness following feeding as described by Chase,[19] Mattingly, and Waksman.[20]

Briefly then, it appears that fed antigens stimulate precursor B-lymphocytes in the Peyer's patches to become antigen-stimulated IgA-precursor lymphoblasts. In addition, T-helper cells for IgA and T-suppressor cells for IgG, IgM, and IgE are stimulated by antigens or mitogens that gain access to the Peyer's patches. The IgA-precursor cells then migrate through the intestinal lymphatics to the mesenteric lymph nodes that are enriched for IgA-plasma cells. From there, they enter the thoracic duct and circulation. The lymphoblasts in the circulation then home to the lamina propria of the gut and to the interstitial tissue of exocrine glands such as the lacrimal glands, salivary glands, mammary glands and to the respiratory, intestinal, and genital-urinary tracts. It appears that homing from the blood vessels to the exocrine interstitial tissues and the lamina propria is a random process; however, antigen also appears to play a role. The large lymphocytes in the thoracic duct that home to the lamina propria are the precursors of the IgA-synthesizing cells of the gut as established by experiments of Guy-Grand and coworkers,[21] and Pierce and Gowans.[22] Factors that effect the migration of these large lymphocytes into the lamina propria and the interstitial tissue are not clearly elucidated; however, it does appear that antigen may play an important role in their localization based upon the original work of Gowans and Knight.[23] It has been proposed[24] that there is random migration of the large lymphocytes in the thoracic duct; however, this is tempered by an intrinsic property of the small intestine that favors the emigration of these large lymphocytes into the lamina propria. Furthermore, once the cells have homed, antigen-dependent immobilization of these cells occurs that keeps them there. It is also likely that antigen-drive proliferation can occur at local secretory sites once the IgA-precursor cells have homed to the region. Husband and Gowans[25] showed that large lymphocytes migrate to secretory sites independently of antigen and are responsible for the early secretory antibody seen at sites distant from antigenic stimulus. They propose that these cells probably die *in situ*; however, if antigen remains or antigen is reintroduced into the site, there is an increase in antigen-driven proliferation of cells that produce the specific antibody. Evidence for local antigen-stimulation in the salivary glands comes from the studies of Emmings, Evans, and Genco,[26] in which intraductal immunization of monkey parotid glands resulted in stimulation of IgA-specific antibodies from the immunized glands with no detectable antibody in the nonimmunized contralateral glands.

THE IMPORTANCE OF IgA ANTIBODIES IN SECRETIONS

IgA is the major immunoglobulin in most secretions[71] and as such may provide protection against infections of mucous membranes and other structures bathed by these secretions. IgA, however, is inefficient in acting as a bacteriocidal or opsonic antibody or in other complement-dependent reactions. Functions such as viral neutralization and inhibition of bacterial adherence to surfaces were proposed to account for its biologic effects.[72] Specific IgA antibody mediated inhibition of bacterial adherence to oral epithelium,[73] intestinal mucosa,[74] urinary tract,[75] and genital epithelium[76] have been described. IgA can also exert protective effects by neutralizing toxins or destructive enzymes, an activity that does not require accessory cells or complement.[77] It has been proposed that IgA antibodies work in concert with factors in secretions such as lactoferrin to inhibit bacterial growth.[78]

Studies of immunity to dental caries caused by *Streptococcus mutans* have provided a fertile area for investigation of the function of secretory IgA antibodies. A series of studies have shown that feeding of *Streptococcus mutans* or its antigens induces secretory IgA antibody found in saliva. Reduced *Streptococcus mutans*-induced caries in rodents often is correlated with the appearance of salivary IgA anti-*S. mutans* antibodies.[3,5] Although these studies provide evidence for the role of salivary IgA in protection against caries, varying amounts of salivary IgG antibody are often found in rat saliva, and its role, as well as the role of cellular immunity, has not been fully evaluated. Parenteral immunization of subhuman primates with *Streptococcus mutans* has also been found to reduce dental caries.[79-81] High titers of serum antibody were induced in the studies. The salivary immune response, however, was low or not evaluated. It was not clear whether serum antibodies entering the saliva through the gingival crevice, or low levels of salivary antibodies, or other forms of protective immunity resulted in the caries reduction reported. Evans, *et al.*[82] report a marked reduction in *S. mutans* colonization of the monkey dentition in animals with elevated salivary IgA antibodies, suggesting that IgA anti-*S. mutans* activity could reduce *S. mutans* levels, and hence, caries in this model. From the caries vaccine studies, it is reasonable that salivary IgA antibodies are responsible for the caries reduction seen; however, the role of serum derived antibodies remains to be clarified.

THE ROLE OF ANTIGEN

Antigen may function at several levels in mucosal immunity. First, antigenic stimulation of gut-associated lymphoreticular tissue (GALT) such as Peyer's patches may occur from the intestinal lumen after oral administration of antigen. Second, parenteral immunization from the blood stream may immunize the

GALT, including the Peyer's patches. This immunization apparently occurs when animals are hyperimmunized parenterally, and exhibit a secretory immune response, but it is probably not a major mechanism for inducing secretory immunity. Third, local antigen application would provide the final antigen-induced proliferation leading to maturation and persistence or immobilization of IgA-producing lymphoblasts in the distal exocrine and lamina propria sites.

It is clear then that an important encounter of antigens with immunocompetent cells occurs in the intestine and leads to a secretory immune reaction. Antigen uptake, processing, and presentation by macrophages, which are thought to be early events in induction of most immune responses, are of concern as they function in the intestine, particularly in the Peyer's patches. The epithelium covering the dome of the Peyer's patches is specialized[27] and appears to function in antigen sampling.[28] These dome epithelial cells are not typically columnar. They lack microvilli, have many cytoplasmic vacuoles, and have been called M-cells because of the presence of microfolds. Similar epithelial cells have been found in bronchial-associated lymphoreticular tissues that are considered to be the respiratory tract equivalent of gut-associated lymphoreticular tissue.[29] Bockman and Cooper[30] showed pinocytosis of ferritin particles by the epithelium over the Peyer's patches. Hence, it appears that antigen can gain access to the lymphoid tissues of Peyer's patches through the specialized epithelium separating the lymphoid elements of the patches from the intestinal lumen.

Evidence has been presented that suggests that a defect exists in the ability of macrophages of the Peyer's patches to process antigen,[31,32] and it is clear that local antibody production does not occur in gut-associated lymphoreticular tissues.[33,34] This lack of in vivo local antibody synthesizing capability in Peyer's patches is further complicated by the findings of Kiyono[35] who showed that murine Peyer's patches possess macrophages capable of accessory functions for in vitro immune responses, as well as the precursor T- and B-cell populations necessary for an in vitro IgA response. Because these components are found in enzymatically disassociated Peyer's patch cells, the authors suggest that the in vivo architecture of Peyer's patches prevents the complex interactions necessary for this response.[35] It is possible that the initial inductive events of antibody synthesis take place in the Peyer's patches in situ, but that important additional cell interactions that lead to final differentiation of IgA-synthesizing plasma cells occur at distal mucosal sites under the influence of local antigen or polyclonal stimulants.

Although chronic mucosal exposure to organisms that colonize and replicate within the gastrointestinal tract is an effective means of stimulating secretory antibody, less consistent stimulation has been observed with nonliving antigens. An effective mehtod of increasing the immunogenicity of weak immunogens has been through the use of adjuvants. It is with this objective in mind, that is, to increase the secretory immune response to well-defined, nonliving antigens, that we embarked on a course of investigation of the effect of adjuvants on orally administered antigens. Rationale for use of two such adjuvants, 6-O-stearoyl-N-acetylmuramyl-L-alanyl-D-isoglutamine (S-MDP) and liposomes, will be discussed below.

LIPOSOMES AS ADJUVANTS

Liposomes are microscopic structures consisting of one of more concentric lipid bilayers, enclosing aqueous compartments. Studies with liposomes over the last decade have provided considerable insight into the physicochemical and chemical nature of cell membranes. Liposomes have also been studied clinically as pharmacological capsules for delivery of therapeutic agents. More recently, their use as immunological adjuvants has been explored. Liposomes can be formed from synthetic and natural phospholipids, often with added cholesterol. Their major constituent is usually phosphatidylcholine, but other phospholipids can be added to confer positive or negative charges. Liposomes have been divided into three classes based upon their size and unilamellar or multilamellar nature. Multilamellar vesicles are very heterogeneous and can be extremely large, ranging in size up to fractions of a millimeter. Unilamellar vesicles consist of a single lipid bilayer surrounding an aqueous compartment. The small unilamellar vesicles, are are those vesicles that range in size from 200–500 angstroms and are generally prepared by ultrasonic dispersion. Large unilamellar vesicles range in diameter from 600 angstroms to several microns, and are bound by one, or at most a few, lipid bilayers. Liposomes in the one micron range have little reported toxicity,[36] and they have been safely administered to humans in doses of approximately 50 mg.[37,38]

Allison and Gregoriadis[39] found that diphtheria toxoid administered intravenously in negatively charged liposomes elicited formation of higher concentrations of antibody than are elicited by antigen alone. Since then, liposomes have been shown to augment the immune response to a number of antigens including purified proteins such as albumin and immunoglobulins,[40] cell surface antigens,[41] parasitic antigens,[42] and viral antigens including the hepatitis B-surface antigen.[43,44] In vivo[45] and in vitro[46] studies show that liposomes behave as T-cell independent immunogens. Tadakuma and coworkers[47] found that hapten epitope density plays a critical role in induction of in vitro immune responses to immunogens using liposome model membranes sensitized with haptenic groups. The use of liposomes with well-defined antigens clearly has had tremendous value in the elucidation of mechanisms by which B-cells are activated by antigens. Liposome-associated immunogens may offer decided advantages in systems that are highly T-dependent such as the IgA system, because the T-dependency can apparently be minimized or reduced with the use of liposome-associated antigen.[48]

Liposomes have low intrinsic immunogenicity, apparently due to the poor immunogenecity of phosphatidylcholine, a major constituent of most liposomes. Other phospholipids, however, such as cardiolipin, phosphatidylinositol, phosphatidylglycerol, and phosphatidic acid are immunogenic, particularly when incorporated into liposomes.[49] Shuster and coworkers[50] found the liposomes containing lipid A augment immune responses to the lipid A and induce antibodies against the liposomal contents including phosphocholine, phosphatidylcholine, and sphingomyelin. Whether or not this is a general phenomenon of induction of immunogenicity to liposomes or lipids by adjuvants incorporated into liposomes requires further investigation. The significance of the induced antibodies to lipid also is unknown; however, these antibodies may have biological activity, because these lipids are major cell constituents.

Liposomes had been given with antigens by various routes, including intravenous, intraperitoneal, subcutaneous, and intramuscular, and have been found to act as adjuvants with varying success depending upon the route of immunization. Oral use of liposomes as adjuvants has not been reported, and it is the purpose of the present study to investigate this potential. Liposomes, however, have been administered orally for other purposes, and early findings suggest that part of the orally administered phospholipids can be absorbed intact. For example, there is general agreement that orally administered insulin entrapped in liposomes can cause a decrease in blood glucose in diabetic rats.[51] There is some uncertainty, however, as to the extent to which liposomes remain intact in the gastrointestinal tract *in vivo*. (For review of these considerations see Ryman, *et al.*[38])

Insight into a partial explanation for the uncertainty over the fate of *in vivo* orally administered liposomes comes from the study of Rowland and Woodley[52] who found that stable liposomes comprised of distearoylphosphatidylcholine/ cholesterol can penetrate that rat gut wall *in vitro* and reach the serosal fluid in relatively intact form. A possible explanation for this is the stability of both dipalmitoylphosphatidylcholine and distearoylphosphatidylcholine, which *in vivo* at 37° C are below their transition temperatures of 41° C and 58° C respectively.[53] Also, the possibility of absorption through the oral mucous membranes, and not through the gastrointestinal mucous membranes, could explain some of the variability in the absorption of *per os* administered liposomes. Hence, there is an indication that at least some of the intragastrically or orally administered liposomes, especially those that are "stable", can resist extremes of pH and the presence of bile salts and pancreatic lipase, and can be absorbed intact from the human intestinal lumen.[54]

In summary, the selection of liposomes for use as oral adjuvants is based upon their demonstrated adjuvanticity, the possibility that stable liposomes may be absorbed from intestinal contents, the fact that they are not intrinsically immunogenic, and their conversion of T-dependent immunogens to T-independent immunogens. These properties suggest that liposomes may be effective adjuvants for stimulating the mucosal immune system when administered by the oral route.

MURAMYL DIPEPTIDE AS AN ADJUVANT

The minimal adjuvant active structure of bacterial peptidoglycans was determined to be N-acetylmuramyl-L-alanyl-D-isoglutamine, referred to as muramyl dipeptide or MDP.[57-59] MDP appears to be comparable to complete Freund's adjuvant; however, it has certain advantages. For example, it is not in itself immunogenic, and moreover, it is devoid of acute toxicity in mice and does not produce the side effects associated with complete Freund's adjuvant such as lymphoid hyperplasia, increased susceptibility to endotoxins, and adjuvant polyarthritis.[60] Although MDP is shown to be devoid of several of the secondary effects inherent to bacterial adjuvants, it is capable of inducing changes in body temperature.[61] Recently, a new synthetic muramyl dipeptide adjuvant devoid of pyrogenicity was described by Chedid and coworkers.[62] The relationship between well-defined synthetic molecules, such as MDP, and immunoregulatory activities is summarized by Chedid and Lederer.[63] The mechanism of action of MDP has been studied in various systems, and it appears to induce both a humoral immune response as well as cellular immunity. Leclerc and coworkers[64] have shown that MDP enhances *in vivo* and *in vitro* immune respones to T-dependent antigens as well as *in vitro* responses of nude mice to T-independent antigens such as trinitrophenolpolyacrylamide. The authors suggest that their data support the contention that muramyl dipeptide exerts a direct effect on B-cells and that it also can mimic the function of T-helper cells. Watson and Whitlock[65] found that MDP stimulated an *in vitro* primary immune response to sheep red cells in T-depleted nude mouse spleen cultures. They conclude that T-cell replacing activity of muramyl dipeptide is most likely explained by the MDP interacting directly with B-cells to mimic the T-helper cell function in the induction of an antibody response.

In an investigation of the influence of various routes of administration of MDP, Chedid and coworkers[66] showed that MDP did not have to be administered with the antigen by the same route to exert its adjuvant effect. The compound was found to be active even when administered *per os* and when the antigen BSA was given subcutaneously. Various chemical conjugations of muramyl dipeptides have been attempted, and offer promise for production of immunologic adjuvants with desirable properties. For example, Kotani and coworkers[67] showed that replacement of the primary hydroxyl group at the C-6 position of the *N*-acetylmuramyl moiety of MDP by a lauroyl, stearoyl, or docosanoyl group produced MDP derivatives with adjuvant activities. Siddiqui and coworkers[42] showed that 6-O-stearoyl-*N*-acetylmuramyl-L-alanyl-D-isoglutamine (S-MDP) can replace complete Freund's adjuvant in vaccination of owl monkeys against infection with the human malarial parasite *Plasmodium falciparum*. In these studies, S-MDP was used with carrier liposomes, and the crude *Plasmodium* vaccine was incorporated into the adjuvant-liposome complex. This vaccine induced protection from parasitic challenge by the parasite. In addition, serum from the monkey significantly inhibited parasite multiplication, and antibodies were detected by immunofluorescence techniques in the monkeys after the second vaccination.

In summary then, based upon the extensive literature showing marked adjuvant activity of muramyl dipeptides and their stearoyl derivative, we set out to test the effectiveness of S-MDP used with carrier liposomes in the induction of an immune response with gastrically administered antigen.

Experiments to Assess the Role of Adjuvants Administered with Oral Antigen

To determine the effects of adjuvants administered with oral antigens, Osborne-Mendel rats were immunized with the soluble protein BSA in the adjuvants. The Osborne-Mendel rats were derived from a pathogen-free strain obtained from Dr. Rachel Larson at the National Institute of Dental Research and were bred and barrier maintained in our animal facilities. They have been extensively used for caries immunization studies, and we and others have shown that feeding this strain of rats with cells of *Streptococcus mutans* will induce a salivary antibody response that correlates with the protection conferred against *Streptococcus mutans*-induced caries. The rats were weaned when 21 days old, and put on the Charles River RMH 1000 diet and water *ad libitum*. Within one or two days after weaning, female litter mates were assigned to various experimental groups, and initial immunization was begun. The rats were also given a booster immunizaiton 21 days later (See FIGURE 1). They were bled, and pilocarpin-stimulated whole saliva was collected at days 21, 35, and 49.

The antigen used was crystalline BSA (Sigma Chemical Co., St. Louis, Mo.). Liposomes were prepared by a modification of the procedure of Inoue.[68] Briefly, equimolar amounts of lecithin (dipalmitoyl-DL-α-phosphatidylcholine, Grade I, approximately 99%; Sigma), and cholesterol (Sigma grade 99+%, Sigma) were dissolved in 1 ml chloroform in a conical glass tube. The chloroform was evaporated by a stream of N_2 gas. Bovine serum albumin at the desired concentration in phosphate buffered saline at pH 7.4 was added to the lipid-coated tube, and liposomes were produced by sonication for 20 seconds at room temperature using a Branson 350 Sonicator at a pulse setting of 50% and power setting of one. The S-MDP incrorrated liposomes were prepared by recovering the liposomes by centrifugation at 3,000 RPM for 10 minutes, and by incubating the liposomes with S-MDP at 37° C for 15 minutes. The original antigen-containing supernate was then added to return the liposome suspension to the appropriate concentration.

Liposomes containing 40 μM cholesterol and 40 μM of lecithin prepared with varying amounts of BSA were recovered by centrifugation. They were then washed and dissolved in chloroform/water to determine the incorporated protein as measured by the Lowry procedure.[69] When 200, 20, and 2 mg/ml BSA were used, 5.6, 6.0, and 8.1% respectively of the BSA was recovered from the liposomes. Antibodies were measured by a microtiter modification of the enzyme-linked immunosorbent assay (ELISA) as described by Engvall and Perlman,[70] using 10 μg/ml BSA to coat wells of Dynatech microtiter plates (Cooke, Arlington, Va.).

The immunoglobulin class of BSA reactive antibodies was determined with rabbit or goat antisera specific to rat IgA, IgG, or IgM. The reaction was developed by incubating the anti-immunoglobulin reagents specifically bound to the ELISA plates with alkaline phosphatase-labeled antibodies to rabbit Ig or goat IgG. Specificity was assessed with purified rat Ig bound to the plates as well as by immunoelectrohporesis of the anti-immunoglobulin reagents.

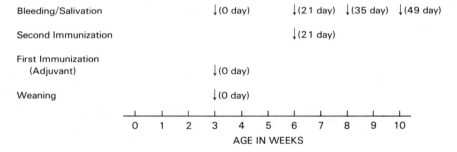

FIGURE 1. Typical experimental design.

In the first experiment, the effect of complete Freund's adjuvant is compared to liposomes and liposomes plus S-MDP on rats when immunized subcutaneously in the salivary gland region. Bovine serum albumin, at a dose of 500 μg, which is suboptimal in inducing a serum immune response, was used. The liposomes contained 2 μM each of cholesterol and lecithin and the S-MDP at 50 μg per animal, per dose. The serum response of these parenterally immunized rats is summarized in FIGURE 2. Complete Freund's adjuvant provided a strong adjuvant effect resulting in high titers of IgG antibody appearing earlier (21 days) as compared to no adjuvant where some of the rats had only low titers of IgG antibodies at 35 and 49 days. IgM and IgA antibodies were not demonstrable at any time during the immunization in the animals subcutaneously immunized with 500 μg BSA in the absence of adjuvant. Liposomes and S-MDP-liposomes also potentiated the antibody response as evidenced by a strong IgG response at 21, 35, and 49 days. In addition, an early IgM response was seen at 21 days in the liposome and S-MDP-liposome immunized animals. Complete Freund's adjuvant stimulated a serum IgA response at all time intervals. In contrast, in the

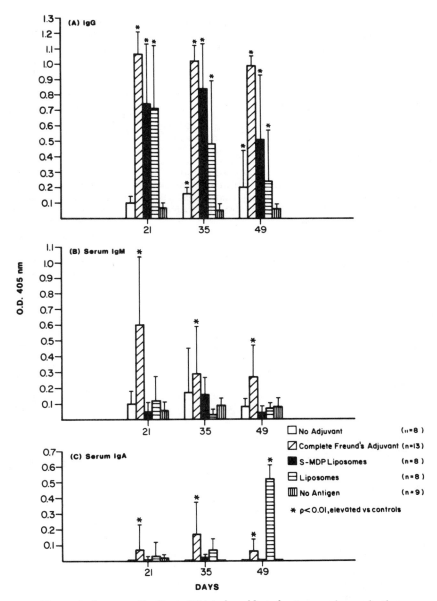

FIGURE 2. Serum antibodies to BSA induced by subcutaneous immunization.

TABLE 1

SALIVARY ANTIBODY RESPONSE TO BSA
SUBCUTANEOUSLY ADMINISTERED WITH ADJUVANTS

Immunization (Subcutaneous)	n	Salivary Antibody on Day 49	
		IgG	IgA
Antigen, No Adjuvant	6	0.17 ± 0.33*	0.02 ± 0.02*
Complete Freund's Adjuvant	7	0.66 ± 0.04†	0.05 ± 0.02†
6-O-stearoyl-MDP-Liposomes	8	0.16 ± 0.12†	0.02 ± 0.03
Liposomes	8	0.09 ± 0.03	0.02 ± 0.02
No Antigen, No Adjuvant	9	0.07 ± 0.04	0.01 ± 0.03

*$\bar{x}$ ± S.D.; optical density (O.D.) 405 nm, 1/20 dilution (dil.).
†p < 0.01, significantly elevated as compared to controls.

S-MDP-liposome group, no detectable serum IgA-antibody production was seen, whereas in the liposome group, serum IgA production was seen at the latest interval. This experiment shows that liposomes and S-MDP-liposomes can act as adjuvants for parenterally administered BSA resulting in induction of IgG and IgM anti-BSA antibodies. Neither of these adjuvants appears, under the conditions tested, to give as potent or prolonged a serum reponse as that obtained with complete Freund's adjuvant.

The salivary antibody response to BSA administered subcutaneously in these same animals is given in TABLE 1. Salivary IgG or IgA antibodies were not

TABLE 2

SERUM ANTIBODY RESPONSE TO BSA
ORALLY ADMINISTERED WITH 6-O-STEAROYL-MDP-LIPOSOMES

Immunization (Oral)	n	Antibody Isotype	Serum Antibody on		
			Day 21	Day 35	Day 49
Controls					
5 mg BSA,		IgG	0.10 ± 0.02*	0.08 ± 0.06*	0.04 ± 0.03*
No Adjuvant,	7	IgM	0.04 ± 0.03	0.08 ± 0.04	0.08 ± 0.04
1 mg BSA Boost		IgA	—	0	0.01 ± 0.03
25 mg BSA,		IgG	—	0.04 ± 0.03	0.04 ± 0.06
No Adjuvant,	6	IgM	—	0.03 ± 0.08	0.08 ± 0.06
5 mg BSA Boost		IgA	—	0	0
6-O-stearoyl-MDP-Liposomes					
5 mg BSA,		IgG	0.07 ± 0.07	0.02 ± 0.02	0.06 ± 0.03
S-MDP-Liposomes,	9	IgM	0.06 ± 0.02	0.03 ± 0.03	0.08 ± 0.03
1 mg BSA Boost		IgA	0	0.01 ± 0.02	0.02 ± 0.04
25 mg BSA,		IgG	0.06 ± 0.05	0.07 ± 0.04	0.10 ± 0.06
S-MDP-Liposomes,	9	IgM	0.02 ± 0.02	0.07 ± 0.03	0.08 ± 0.41
5 mg BSA Boost		IgA	0.06 ± 0.02	0.02 ± 0.02	0.30 ± 0.09†
100 mg BSA,		IgG	0.07 ± 0.02	0.02 ± 0.08	0.03
S-MDP-Liposomes	6	IgM	0.06 ± 0.04	0.07 ±	0
20 mg BSA Boost		IgA	0.16 ± 0.11†	0.05 ± 0.05	0.01 ± 0.01

*$\bar{x}$ ± S.D.; O.D. 405 nm, 1/50 dil.
†Significant at p < 0.01.

detected when BSA was administered subcutaneously in the absence of adjuvants or with liposomes; however, complete Freund's adjuvant and S-MDP liposomes resulted in a detectable IgG response in the saliva at 49 days. Only the complete Freund's adjuvant immunized group induced a salivary IgA response, and this was a weak, although statistically significant, response seen at 49 days. It can be concluded from the responses of the subcutaneously immunized animals that the liposomes and S-MDP-liposomes are effective adjuvants for a serum antibody response; however, neither appears to induce a salivary IgA response when administered subcutaneously.

The next experiment was designed to test the effects of these adjuvants on the response to orally administered bovine serum albumin. In TABLE 2, the serum

TABLE 3

SERUM ANTIBODY RESPONSE TO BSA
ORALLY ADMINISTERED IN LIPOSOMES

Immunization (Oral)	n	Isotype	Serum Antibody on		
			Day 21	Day 35	Day 49
Controls					
5 mg BSA,		IgG	0.10 ± 0.02*	0.08 ± 0.06*	0.04 ± 0.03*
No Adjuvant,	7	IgM	0.04 ± 0.03	0.08 ± 0.04	0.08 ± 0.04
1 mg BSA Boost		IgA	—	0	0.01 ± 0.03
No Antigen,		IgG	0.07 ± 0.03	0.05 ± 0.04	0.06 ± 0.03
No Adjuvant,	9	IgM	0.06 ± 0.05	0.09 ± 0.04	0.08 ± 0.05
No Boost		IgA	0.02 ± 0.02	0	0
Liposomes					
5 mg BSA,		IgG	0.03 ± 0.02	0.07 ± 0.03	0.11 ± 0.03†
Liposomes	9	IgM	0.06 ± 0.02	0.10 ± 0.04	0.07 ± 0.05
1 mg BSA Boost		IgA	0.02 ± 0.01	0.03 ± 0.01	0.34 ± 0.15†
25 mg BSA,		IgG	0.05 ± 0.04	0.13 ± 0.12	0.22 ± 0.32†
Liposomes,	8	IgM	0.07 ± 0.02	0.08 ± 0.02	0.08 ± 0.04
5 mg BSA Boost		IgA	0.03 ± 0.02	0.04 ± 0.02	0.13 ± 0.12†
100 mg BSA,		IgG	0.02 ± 0.04	0.03 ± 0.02	0.11 ± 0.17†
Liposomes,	9	IgM	0	0.08 ± 0.01	0.07 ± 0.03
5 mg BSA Boost		IgA	0.06 ± 0.02	0.01 ± 0.01	0.14 ± 0.10†

*$\bar{x} \pm$ S.D.; O.D. 405 nm, 1/50 dil.
†Significant at $p < 0.01$.

antibody response is tabulated, and it can be seen that using two concentrations, 5 and 25 milligrams of BSA in the absence of adjuvants, no serum response was seen in any of the immunoglobulin classes tested from 21 to 49 days. When S-MDP-liposomes were used as adjuvants with BSA (20 μM each of cholesterol and lecithin, and 500 μg S-MDP per dose) the only specific serum antibodies seen were in the IgA class late in immunization (49 days). When BSA-liposomes were used with the same three concentrations of BSA, somewhat greater serum responses were seen (TABLE 3). For example, IgG and IgA responses were seen at all three doses at day 49; however, an IgM response was not seen at any interval or any dose.

Because feeding has been reported to induce a salivary IgA-antibody response with low or no serum response, it was of interest to study the salivary antibody response in these same animals. The salivary IgA responses are tabulated in TABLE 4. As can be seen, the S-MDP-liposome immunized animals had salivary antibodies in IgA class at the highest dose of BSA used (100 mg). Salivary IgG and IgA antibody at the other doses were negative. Similarly, the group administered the antigen in liposomes (without S-MDP) also showed salivary antibodies in the IgA class at the highest dose, that is, 100 mg of BSA used to prepare the liposomes. In another experiment, rats immunized orally with BSA in S-MDP-liposomes were found to have IgA anti-BSA antibodies in their saliva at 21 and 35, as well as 49 days, suggesting that the first immunization with oral adjuvant was effectively stimulating the salivary immune response (FIGURE 3).

These results show that a salivary IgA response is reproducibly stimulated in rats by feeding liposome antigen and S-MDP-liposome antigen combinations. The amount of antigen associated with the liposomes when the concentration of 100 milligrams per ml of BSA is used to prepare the vesicles, is approximately 5–8 percent of the total antigen present. Hence, the liposomes contain 5–8 milligrams of antigen. Because even 5–25 milligrams of antigen administered without adjuvant failed to induce either a serum or a secretory immune response under the conditions tested, it is reasonable that the antigen-containing liposomes are quite effective in augmenting an IgA response with little or no serum response.

TABLE 4

SALIVARY ANTIBODY RESPONSE TO BSA
ADMINISTERED ORALLY WITH 6-O-STEAROYL-MDP-LIPOSOMES AND IN LIPOSOMES

Immunization (Oral)	n	Antibody Isotype	Salivary Antibodies on Day 49
Controls			
5 mg BSA, No Adjuvant	6	IgG	0.01 ± 0.02*
1 mg BSA Boost		IgA	0
No Antigen, No Adjuvant	9	IgG	0.07 ± 0.04
No Boost		IgA	0.01 ± 0.03
6-O-stearoyl-MDP-Liposomes			
5 mg BSA, S-MDP-Liposomes		IgG	0.07 ± 0.02
1 mg BSA Boost	7	IgA	0.01 ± 0.01
25 mg BSA, S-MDP-Liposomes		IgG	0.03 ± 0.02
5 mg BSA Boost	9	IgA	0.09 ± 0.04
100 mg BSA, S-MDP-Liposomes		IgG	0
20 mg BSA Boost	6	IgA	0.15 ± 0.02†
Liposomes			
5 mg BSA, Liposomes		IgG	0.09 ± 0.05
1 mg BSA Boost	7	IgA	0.02 ± 0.02
25 mg BSA, Liposomes		IgG	0.04 ± 0.07
5 mg BSA Boost	7	IgA	0.08 ± 0.05
100 mg BSA, Liposomes		IgG	0
20 mg BSA Boost	8	IgA	0.21 ± 0.07†

*$\overline{x}$ ± S.D.; O.D. 405 nm, 1/20 dil.　†Significant at $p < 0.01$.

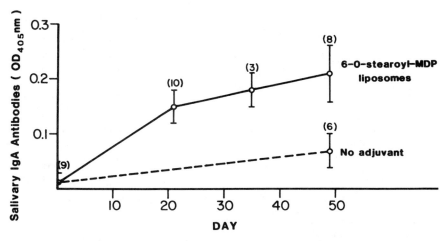

FIGURE 3. Salivary IgA antibodies resulting from feeding BSA.

These experiments provide a convenient method for immunizing animals to induce a salivary IgA-antibody response to a protein antigen in the absence of an appreciable serum IgG or IgM response. The kinetics of the response and the effect on antibodies of other classes and cellular immunity also can be assessed using this system. This method of stimulating the mucosal immune system by incorporation of antigen into liposomes that then can be taken orally may be useful in providing protective immunity to infectious agents using purified antigens of the virulent organisms incorporated into liposomes.

The mechanism of action of these adjuvants in stimulating a mucosal immune response by oral feeding is not clear; however, it is possible that binding of antigen by its hydrophobic regions to the liposome surface decreases the thymic dependency of the BSA by providing a critical epitope density on the surface. The liposome antigen complex may attach to gut epithelial cells, particularly the dome epithelial cells, and be taken up in a more immunogenic fashion. It is also possible that the liposomes may decrease the need to stimulate macrophages, or for macrophage processing, which appears to be important in the induction of IgA antibodies. The role of liposome antigen complexes in suppression of systemic antibody production may also result from similar properties that stimulate suppressor cells or factors efficiently.

REFERENCES

1. WAHDAN, N. H., C. SERIE, Y. CERISIER, S. SALLAM & R. GERMANIER. 1982. A controlled field trial of live *Salmonella typhi* strain Ty 21a oral vaccine against typhoid: three year results. J. Infect. Dis. **145:** 292–295.
2. CLANCY, R. & A. PUCCI. 1978. Sensitization of gut-associated lymphoid tissue during oral stimulation. Aust. J. Exp. Biol. Med. Sci (Part 3): 337–340.
3. SMITH, D. J., M. A. TAUBMAN & J. EBERSOLE. 1979. Effect of oral administration of glucosyltransferase antigens on experimental dental caries. Infect. Immun. **26:** 82–89.
4. MESTECKY, J., J. R. McGHEE, R. R. ARNOLD, S. M. MICHALEK, S. J. PRINCE & J. L. BABB.

1978. Selective induction of an immune response in human external secretions by ingestion of bacterial antigen. J. Clin. Invest. **61:** 731–737.

5. MICHALEK, S. M., J. R. McGHEE & J. C. BABB. 1978. Effective immunity to dental caries: dose-dependent studies of secretory immunity by oral administration with *Streptococcus mutans* in rats. Infect. Immun. **19:** 217–224.

6. BIENENSTOCK, J., A. D. BEFUS & M. McDERMOTT. 1980. Mucosal Immunity. *In* Monographs in Allergy. **16:** 1–18. Karger. Basel.

7. STROBER, W., L. K. RICHMAN & C. O. ELSON. 1981. The regulation of gastrointestinal immune responses. *In* Immunology Today. 156–162. Elsevier. North Holland Biomedical Press.

8. CRABBE, P. A., A. O. CARBONARA & J. F. HEREMANS. 1965. The normal human intestinal mucosa as a major source of plasma cells containing λ-a-immunoglobulin. Lab Invest. **14:** 235–248.

9. TOMASI, T. B. JR., E. M. TAN, A. SOLOMON & R. A. PRENDERGAST. 1965. Characteristics of an immune system common to a certain external secretion. J. Exp. Med. **121:** 104–124.

10. CRAIG, S. W. & J. J. CEBRA. 1971. Peyer's patches: An enriched source of precursors for IgA-producing immunosites in the rabbit. J. Exp. Med. **134:** 188–200.

11. HALL, J. G. & M. E. SMITH. 1970. Homing of lymph born immunoblasts to the guts. Nature (London) **226:** 252–262.

12. GOWANS, J. L. & E. J. KNIGHT. 1964. The route of recirculation of lymphocytes in the rat. Proc. R. Soc. London Ser. B. **159:** 257–282.

13. MONTGOMERY, P. C., J. COHN & E. T. LALLY. 1974. The induction and characterization of secretory IgA antibodies. *In* The Immunoglobulin A System, J. Mestecky and A. R. Lawton, Eds.: Adv. Exp. Med. Biol. **45:** 453–462, Plenum Press. New York.

14. MONTGOMERY, P. C., I. LEMAITRE-COELHO & E. T. LALLY. 1976. Effects of circulating antibodies on secretory IgA antibody induction following oral immunization with DNP-PN. Ric. Clin. Lab 6 Suppl. 3:93–99.

15. ELSON, C. O., J. A. HECK & W. STROBER. 1974. T-cell regulation of murine IgA synthesis of the polyclonal stimulation of IgA production *in vitro* by LPS is likely under the control of an IgA specific T-helper cell. J. Exp. Med. **149:** 632–643.

16. RICHMAN, L. K., A. S. GRAEFF, R. YARCHOAN & W. STROBERG. 1981. Simultaneous induction of antigen-specific IgA helper T-cells and IgG suppressor T-cells in the murine Peyer's patch after protein feeding. J. Immunol. **126:** 2079–2083.

17. MATTSBY-BALTZER, I., L. A. HANSON, S. OLLING & B. KAIJSER. 1982. Experimental *Escherichia coli* ascending pyelonephritis in rats: active peroral immunization with live *Excherichia coli*. Infect. Immun. **35:** 647–653.

18. CHALLACOMBE, S. J. & T. LEHNER. 1979. Salivary antibody reponses in rhesus monkeys immunized with *Streptococcus Mutans* by the oral, submucosal, or subcutaneous routes. Arch. Oral. Biol **24:** 917–925.

19. CHASE, M. W. 1946. Inhibition of experimental drug allergy by prior feeding of a sensitizing agent. Proc. Soc. Exp. Biol. Med. **61:** 257–259.

20. MATTINGLY, J. A. & B. H. WAKSMAN. 1978. Immunologic suppression after oral administration of antigen. I. Specific suppressor cells found in rat Peyer's patches after oral administration of sheep erythrocytes and their systemic migration. J. Immunol. **121:** 1878–1883.

21. GUY-GRAND, D., C. GRISCELLI & P. VASSALLI. 1974. The gut-associated lymphoid system: major improperties of the large dividing cells. Eur. J. Immunol. **4:** 435–443.

22. PIERCE, N. F. & J. L. GOWANS. 1975. Cellular kinetics of the intestinal immune response to cholera toxoid in rats. J. Exp. Med. **142:** 1550–1563.

23. GOWANS, J. L. & E. J. KNIGHT. 1964. The route of recirculation of lymphocytes in the rat. Proc. R. Soc. London Ser. B. **159:** 257–282.

24. HUSBAND, A. J., H. J. MONIÉ & J. L. GOWANS. 1976. The natural history of the cells producing IgA in the Gut. *In* Immunology of the Gut. Ciba Foundation. **46:** 29–54.

25. HUSBAND, A. J. & J. L. GOWANS. 1978. The origin and antigen-dependent distribution of IgA-containing cells in the intestine. J. Exp. Med. **148:** 1146–1160.

26. EMMINGS, F. G., R. T. EVANS & R. J. GENCO. 1975. Antibody response in the parotid fluid

and serum of irus monkeys (*Macaca fascicularis*) after local immunization with *Streptococcus mutans*. Infect. Immun. **12**: 281–292.

27. OWEN, R. L. & A. L. JONES, 1974. Epithelial cell specialization within human Peyer's patches: An ultrastructural study of intestinal lymphoid follicles. Gastroenterology **66**: 189–190.

28. OWEN, R. L. 1977. Sequential uptake of horseradish peroxidase by lymphoid follicle epithelium of Peyer's patches in normal, unobstructed mouse intestine: An Ultrastructural Study. Gastroenterology **72**: 440–451.

29. BIENENSTOCK, J., N. JOHNSTON & D. Y. E. PEREY. 1973. Bronchial lymphoid tissue. I. Morphologic characteristics. Lab. Invest. **28**: 686–692.

30. BOCKMAN, E. & M. D. COOPER. 1973. Pinocytosis by epithelium associated with lymphoid follicles in the bursa of fabricius, appendix and Peyer's patches. An electron microscopic study. Am. J. Anat. **136**: 455–478.

31. HUNTER, R. L. 1972. Antigen trapping in the lamina propria and production of IgA antibody. J. Reticuloendothelial Soc. **11**: 245–252.

32. KAGNOFF, M. F. & S. CAMPBELL. 1974. Functional characteristics of Peyer's patch lymphoid cells. I. Induction of humoral antibody and cell-mediated allograft reactions. J. Exp. Med. **139**: 398–406.

33. BIENENSTOCK, J. & J. DOLEZEL. 1971. Peyer's patches: lack of specific antibody-containing cells after oral and parenteral immunization. J. Immunol **106**: 938–945.

34. HENRY, C., W. P. FAULK, L. KUHN, J. M. YOFFEY & H. H. FUDENBERG. 1970. Peyer's patches; immunologic studies. J. Exp. Med. **131**: 1200–1210.

35. KIYONO, H., J. R. McGHEE, M. J. WANNEMUEHLER, M. V. FRANGAKIS, D. M. SPALDING, S. M. MICHALEK & W. J. KOOPMAN. 1982. *In vitro* Immune response to a T-cell dependent antigen by cultures of disassociated Murine Peyer's patch. Proc. Nat'l. Acad. Sci. USA **79**: 596–600.

36. KIMELBERG, H. K. & E. G. MAYHEW. 1978. Properties and biological effects of liposomes and their uses in pharmacology and toxicology. CRC Crit. Rev. Toxicol. **6**: 25–79.

37. GREGORIADIS, G., C. P. SWAIN, E. J. WILLS & A. S. TAVILL. 1974. Drug-carrier potential of liposomes in cancer chemotherapy. Lancet **1**: 1313–1316.

38. RYMAN, B. E., R. F. JEWKES, K. JEYASINGH, M. P. OSBOURNE, H. M. PATEL, V. J. RICHARDSON, M. H. N. TATTERSALL & D. A. TYRELL. 1978. Potential applications of liposomes to therapy. Ann. N.Y. Acad. Sci. **308**: 281–307.

39. ALLISON, A. C. & G. GREGORIADIS. 1974. Liposomes as immunological adjuvants. Nature (London) **252**: 252.

40. VAN ROOIJEN, N. & R. VAN NIUWMEGAN. 1980. Liposomes in immunology: Evidence that their adjuvant effects results from surface exposition of the antigens. Cell. Immunol. **49**: 402–407.

41. GERLIER, D., F. SAKAI & J. F. DORE. 1980. Induction of antibody response to liposome-associated gross virus cell-surface antigen. Br. J. Cancer **41**: 236–242.

42. SIDDIQUI, W. A., D. W. TAYLOR, S. C. KAN, K. KRAMER, S. M. RICHMOND-CRUM, S. KOTANI, T. SHIBA & S. KUSUMOTO. 1978. Vaccination of experimental monkeys against *Plasmodium falciparum*: a possible safe adjuvant. Science **201**: 1237–1238.

43. GREGORIADIS, G. & E. K. MANEIUS. 1980. Liposomes as immunologic adjuvants for hepatitis B surface antigens. *In* Liposomes in Immunobiology. B. H. Tom and H. R. Six, Ed.: 271–283. Elsevier. North Holland Inc. New York.

44. MANEIUS, E. K., C. CAMERON & G. GREGORIADIS. 1979. Hepatitis B surface antigen containing liposomes enhance humoral and cell-mediated immunity of the antigen. FEBS Lett. **102**: 107–111.

45. YASUDA, T., G. F. DANCEY & S. C. KINSKY. 1977. Immunogenic properties of liposomal model membranes in mice. J. Immunol. **119**: 1863–1867.

46. YASUDA, T., T. TADAKUMA, C. W. PIERCE & S. C. KINSKY. 1979. Primary *in vitro* immunogenicity of liposome model membranes in mouse spleen cultures. J. Immunol. **123**: 1535–1539.

47. TADAKUMA, T., T. YASUDA, S. C. KINSKY & C. W. PIERCE. 1980. The effect of epitope dentisty on the *in vitro* immunogenicity of hapten-sensitized liposomal model membranes. J. Immunol. **124**: 2175–2179.

48. VAN HOUTE, A. J., H. SNIPPE & J. M. N. WILLERS. 1979. Characterization of immunologic

properties of haptenated liposomal model membranes in mice. I. Thymus independence of the antigen. Immunology **37**: 505-514.

49. ALVING, C. R. 1977. Immune reactions of lipids in lipid model membranes. In The Antigens M. Seila, Ed., Vol. 4: 1-72. Academic Press. New York.

50. SHUSTER, B. G., M. NEIDIG, B. M. ALVING & C. R. ALVING. 1979. Production of antibodies against phosphocholine, phosphatidylcholine, spinghomyelin, and lipid A by injection of liposomes containing lipid A. J. Immunol. **122**: 900-905.

51. DAPERGOLAS, G. & G. GREGORIADIS. 1976. Hypoglycemic effect of liposome-entrapped insulin administered intragastrically into rats. Lancet **2**: 824-827.

52. ROWLAND, R. & J. F. WOODLEY. 1981. The uptake of distearoylphosphatidylcholine/cholesterol liposomes by rat intestinal sacs in vitro. Biochim. Biophys. Acta **673**: 217-223.

53. LADBROOKE, B. D. & D. CHAPMAN. 1969. Thermal analysis of lipids, proteins and biological membranes. A review and summary of some recent studies. Chem. Phys. Lipids **3**: 304-356.

54. ROWLAND, R. N. & J. F. WOODLEY. 1980. The stability of liposomes in vitro to pH, bile salts, and pancreatic lipase. Biochim. Biophys. Acta **620**: 400-409.

55. WALKER, W. A. & K. J. ISSELBACHER. 1976. Intestinal antibodies. Physiol. Med. **297**: 767-773.

56. LINZER, R., R. T. EVANS, F. G. EMMINGS & R. J. GENCO. 1981. Use of combined immunication routes in induction of a salivary immunoglobulin A response to Streptococcus mutans in Macaca fasicularis monkeys. Infect. Immun. **31**: 345-351.

57. ELLOUZ, F., A. ADAM, R. CIORBARU & E. LEDERER. 1974. Minimal structural requirements for adjuvant activity of bacterial peptidoglycan derivatives. Biochem. Biophys. Res. Comm. **59**: 1317-1325.

58. MERSER, C., P. SINAY & A. ADAM. 1975. Total synthesis adjuvant activity of bacterial peptidoglycan derivatives. Biochem. Biophys. Res. Comm. **66**: 1316-1322.

59. KOTANI, S., Y. WATANABE, F. KINOSHITA, T. SHIMONO, I. MORISAKI, T. SHIBA, S. KUSUMOTO, Y. TARUMI & K. IKENAKA. 1975. Immunoadjuvant activities of synthetic N-acetyl-muramyl-peptides or -amino acids. Biken. J. **18**: 105-111.

60. CHEDID, L. & T. AUDIBERT. 1977. Recent advances in the use of the synthetic immunoadjuvants muramyl dipeptide and analogues. In Microbiology. D. Schlessinger, Ed.: 388-394. American Society of Microbiology. Washington, D.C.

61. KOTANI, S., Y. WATANABE, T. SHIMONO, K. HARADA, T. SHIBA, S. KUSUMOTO, K. YOKOGAWA & M. TANIGUCHI. 1976. Correlation between the immunoadjuvant activities and pyrogenicities of synthetic N-acetyl-muramyl-peptides or alpha amino acids. Biken. J. **19**: 9-13.

62. CHEDID, L. A., M. A. PARANT, F. M. AUDIBERT, G. J. RIVEAU, F. J. PARANT, E. LEDERER, J. P. CHOAY & P. L. LEFRANCIER. 1982. Biological activity of a new synthetic muramyl peptide adjuvant devoid of pyrogenicity. Infect. Immun. **35**: 417-424.

63. CHEDID, L. & E. LEDERER. 1978. Past, present and future of the synthetic immunoadjuvant MDP and its analogs. Biochem. Pharmacol. **27**: 2183-2186.

64. LECLERC, C., BOURGEOIS, E. & L. CHEDID. Enhancement by muramyl-dipeptide of in vitro nude mice responses to a T-dependent antigen.

65. WATSON, J. & C. WHITLOCK. 1978. Effect of a synthetic adjuvant on the induction of primary immune responses in T Cell-depleted spleen cultures. J. Immunol. **121**: 383-389.

66. CHEDID, L., F. AUDIBERT, P. LEFRANCIER, J. CHOAY & E. LEDERER. 1976. Modulation of the immune response by a synthetic adjuvant and analogs. Proc. Natl. Acad. Sci. USA **73**: 2472-2475.

67. KOTANI, S., F. KINOSHITA, I. MORISAKI, T. SHIMONO, T. OKUNAGA, H. TAKADA, M. TSUJIMOTO, Y. WATANABE, K. KATO, T. SHIBA, S. KUSUMOTO & S. OKADA. 1977. Immunoadjuvant activities of synthetic 6-O-acyl-N-acetylmuramyl-L-alanyl-D-isoglutamine with special reference to the effect of its administration with liposomes. Biken. J. **20**: 95-103.

68. INOUE, K. 1974. Permeability properties of liposomes prepared from dipalmitoyllecithin, dimyristoyllecithin, egg lecithin, rat liver lecithin, and beef brain sphingomyelin. Biochim. Biophys. Acta **339**: 390-402.

69. LOWRY, O. H., N. J. ROSEBROUGH, A. L. FARR & R. J. RANDALL. 1951. Protein measurement with the folin phenol reagent. J. Biol. Chem. **193:** 265–275.
70. ENGVALL, E. & P. PERLMANN. 1972. Enzyme-linked immunosorbent assay, ELISA. III. Quantitation of specific antibodies by enzyme-labeled anti-immunoglobulin in antigen-coated tubes. J. Immunol. **109:** 129–135.
71. TOMASI, T. B. & S. ZIGELBAUM. 1963. The selective occurrence of gamma-1-a-globulin in certain body fluids. J. Clin. Invest. **42:** 1552–1560.
72. GENCO, R. J. 1969. *In* The secretory immunologic system. D. H. Dayton, P. A. Small, R. M. Chanock, H. E. Kaufman and T. B. Tomasi, Eds.: 253–255. U.S. Department of Health, Education, and Welfare, Public Health Service, National Institutes of Health. Bethesda, Md.
73. WILLIAMS, R. C. & R. GIBBONS. 1972. Inhibition of bacterial adherence by secretory immunoglobulin A: A mechanism of antigen disposal. Science **177:** 697–699.
74. FUBARA, E. S. & FRETER, R. 1973. Protection against enteric bacterial infection by secretary IgA antibodies. J. Immunol. **111:** 395–403.
75. SVANBORG-EDEN, C. & A. M. SVENNERHOLM. 1978. Secretory immunoglobulin A and G antibodies prevent adhesion of *Escherichia coli* to human urinary tract epithelial cells. Infect. Immun. **22:** 790–797.
76. TRAMONT, E. C. 1977. Inhibition of adherence of *Neisseria gonorrhoreae* by human genital secretions. J. Clin. Invest. **59:** 117–124.
77. FUKUI, Y., K. FUKUI & T. MORIYAMA. 1973. Inhibition of enzymes by human salivary immunoglobulin A. Infect. Immun **8:** 335–340.
78. ROGERS, H. J. & C. SYNGE. 1978. Bacteriostatic effect of human milk on *Escherichia coli:* The role of IgA. Immunology **34:** 19–28.
79. BOWEN, W. H., B. COHEN, M. COLE & G. COLEMAN. 1975. Immunisation against caries. Brit. Dent. J. **139:** 45–58.
80. LEHNER, T., S. CHALLACOMBE AND J. CALDWELL. 1975. Immunological and bacteriological basis for vaccination against dental caries in rhesus monkeys. Nature (London) **254:** 517–520.
81. LEHNER, T., M. W. RUSSELL, J. CALDWELL & R. SMITH. 1981. Immunization with purified protein antigens from *Streptococcus mutans* against dental caries in rhesus monkeys. Infect. Immun. **34:** 407–415.
82. EVANS, R. T., F. G. EMMINGS & R. J. GENCO. 1975. Prevention of *Streptococcus mutans* infection of tooth surfaces by salivary antibody in irus monkeys (*Macaca fascicularis*). Infec. Immun. **12:** 293–302.

DISCUSSION OF THE PAPER

J. R. McGHEE (*University of Alabama in Birmingham*): Do you know whether orally administered liposomes are taken up in the Peyer's patches?

R. J. GENCO (*State University of New York at Buffalo*): We have not yet examined this possibility. We initiated experiments to follow the fate of the liposome with various antigens, including viruses.

T. LEHNER (*Guy's Hospital, London, England*): Are you suggesting that the MDP preferentially induces an enhanced IgA but not IgG response?

GENCO: Yes. The liposomes with or without MDP preferentially induce a salivary IgA response in the absence of a salivary IgG and serum IgG, IgA, or IgM responses. Certain groups of animals, however, showed an IgA response in the serum. Therefore, liposome antigen mixtures presented orally appear as a fairly effective way to induce a salivary IgA response in the absence of a serum response. One could manipulate the timing, the dose, and the type of liposome to elicit salivary response, and possibly tear and milk IgA responses.

A. O. ANDERSON (*University of Pennsylvania, Philadelphia*): Did you ever induce a response with the sterile MDP that was higher than with the liposomes alone?

GENCO: We did not. The ELISA assay does not really allow you to quantitate antibody. ELISA titers are a function both of amount of antibody and affinity. We did not think that it was appropriate to use a standard amount of antibody. Therefore, I have no good basis for comparison.

ANDERSON: I agree with your work, because I observe the same type of results when I use MDP. I do not observe much potentiation at all.

THE INFLUENCE OF MURAMYL DIPEPTIDE ON THE
SECRETORY IMMUNE RESPONSE

J. E. Butler, H. B. Richerson, P. A. Swanson, W. C. Kopp,
and M. T. Suelzer

Departments of Microbiology and Internal Medicine
The University of Iowa Medical School
Iowa City, Iowa 52242

INTRODUCTION

Most pathogens enter their mammalian hosts through the respiratory or gastrointestinal systems; both are regarded as part of the secretory immune system. These systems are also exposed to nonliving antigenic substances. Emphasis in our laboratory is focused on the immune response to inhaled antigens and the relevance of this response to acute and chronic lung diseases.

The mucosal surfaces of the gut and upper respiratory tract are intricately associated with IgA-producing plasma cells[1-3] and believed to be responsible for transport of dimeric IgA (as sIgA) to the lumenal surfaces.[4-6] Cell populations of alveoli consist largely of macrophages (>90% in normal mammals[7-9]), and alveolar fluids contain a proportionately larger amount of IgG than is found in the bronchial region.[10-14] The immune system functioning at these mucosal and alveolar surfaces is presumably equipped to defend against infective mechanisms of the respiratory and intestinal pathogens such as adhesion and subsequent colonization of epithelial surfaces and invasion of cells and tissues. Exposure of mucosal surfaces to bacteria, viruses, or their products is effective in stimulating local immune responses.[15-20] In fact microbial flora might be responsible for stimulating the development of the mucosal immune system.[21,22] The stimulatory effect of microbial agents may result from their ability to colonize or adhere to surface epithelia, selectively stimulate gut-associated lymphorecticular tissue (GALT),[23] or stimulate phagocytosis through their particulate nature. Whereas microbial antigens may be more effective in stimulating local IgA responses,[24] such responses can also be stimulated with nonmicrobial antigens.[24-26]

The effectiveness of microbial agents in stimulating local IgA could also result from the stimulatory effect of nonantigenic bacterial components; the B-cell mitogenic action of bacterial endotoxin and adjuvant properties of bacterial cell walls and cell-wall products are well known.[27] Recently, N-acetylmuramyl-L-alanyl-D-isoglutamine (muramyl dipeptide or MDP) has been described as being the minimal adjuvant-active structure of mycobacteria constituting complete Freund's adjuvant.[28,29] As MDP is derived from peptidoglycan cell components (and these are common to gram-positive and gram-negative bacteria as well as other procaryotes[29]), the possibility that the local immune system is exposed to MDP or MDP-like agents during bacterial infection is likely.

Muramyl dipeptide has been shown to be nonimmunogenic in mice,[30] and we have shown that it is nonmitogenic in the rabbit.[31] Studies in other species do not agree on the mechanism of action of MDP *in vivo* or *in vitro*. Some studies indicate that MDP acts directly to stimulate macrophages,[32] whereas others conclude that the initial target cell is a lymphocyte.[33] Unpublished data from our laboratory suggest that both macrophages and T-cells are targets. Lymphocytes

669

0077-8923/83/0409-0669 $1.75/0 © 1983, NYAS

binding MDP appear to be T-cells as determined by double-label immunofluorescence. (Antiserum to rabbit T-cells was kindly provided by Dr. Katherine Knight, University of Illinois.) Muramyl dipeptide, like the parent mycobacterium, promotes increased humoral immune responses, and in mice has been shown to preferentially stimulate IgG_1 responses to dinitrophenyl (DNP).[34] Selective suppression of IgE responses has also been reported.[35]

We have previously shown that inhaled soluble protein antigens provoke local and systemic immunologic responses in the lung and gut.[36] The initial inhalation of antigen by animals parenterally primed with complete Freund's adjuvant and antigen results in inflammatory alveolitis that wanes over time during repeated antigen inhalation. If MDP is inhaled with antigen, alveolitis fails to wane, and chronic disease results.[31] Therefore, we wondered whether MDP was acting as a polyclonal or selective stimulator of some facet of the immune system, which might explain the development of chronic disease.

Data presented here show that when MDP is administered with a soluble antigen by chronic aerosol, serum IgA antibody levels are increased three times above that of non-MDP treated controls, such that the serum IgG to IgA antibody ratio is significantly reduced. The IgG:IgA ratio in lung lavage fluids of those MDP-treated animals not developing alveolitis is also reduced when compared to controls. This effect requires parenteral priming with antigen to be observed. Immunohistochemical studies fail to identify an increase in the relative proportion of IgA-antibody containing cells in the lower lung, mediastinal lymph nodes, or small bowel. Nearly 100% of the antibody-containing cells in the gut of MDP-treated rabbits are of the IgG class. The biliary levels or ratio of IgA and IgG antibodies in bile are, however, unaffected by the addition of MDP to inhaled antigen. The influence, if any, of this enhanced IgA response in explaining the maintenance of chronic disease in repeatedly aerosolized rabbits has not been determined.

MATERIALS AND METHODS

Experimental Design

Random bred New Zealand white rabbits were used in all chronic inhalational experiments. Each treatment group contained four rabbits (FIGURE 1). Each animal was immunized in the toe pads with 0.2 ml of a mixture of ovalbumin (OVA) (1 mg) and MDP (100 μg) emulsified in incomplete Freund's adjuvant (IFA). This dosage was distributed among eight toe pads of the four feet. Control groups received either MDP in IFA or OVA in IFA.

Animals were chronically administered OVA and MDP twice weekly for four to six weeks by placing them in a chamber connected to a deVilbis ultrasonic nebulizer. A total chamber dose of 10 ml saline containing 100 mg of OVA and 1 mg of MDP was used. Control group animals for the effect of aerosol MDP received only OVA. Controls for the effect of parenteral priming received OVA and MDP, but were given only MDP and saline in IFA at immunization (FIGURE 1).

Animals were sacrificed 48–96 hours after the final challenge, and blood, bronchoalveolar lavage washings (BAW), and various tissues were collected. In one experiment, saline intestinal wash fluid and bile were also collected. Bronchoalveolar lavage wash, bile, and intestinal wash fluid were immediately mixed with an equal volume of a protease inhibitor mixture containing 20 mM

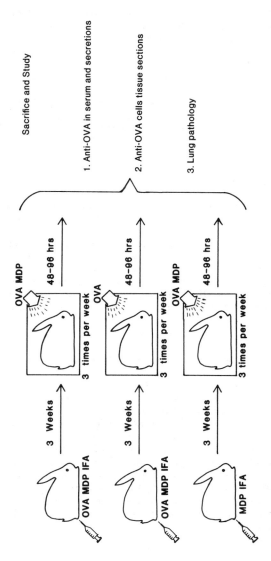

FIGURE 1. Experimental design of experiments including immunization and chronic inhalational challenge. Animals were immunized with 1 mg of ovalbumin (OVA) and 100 µg of muramyl dipeptide (MDP). Aerosol challenges consisted of 100 mg of OVA and 1 mg of MDP. IFA = incomplete Freund's adjuvant.

ethylenediametetraacetate (EDTA), 20 mM parachloromercuribenzoic acid, and 3.4 mM phenylmethylsulfonylfluoride. In certain cases BAW and intestinal wash fluids were concentrated prior to analyses.

Source of Antigen and Muramyl Dipeptide

Ovalbumin was purchased as 3× crystalline protein from Miles Laboratories, Elkhart, Ind., and MDP was either purchased from GIRPI, Paris, France or synthesized by C. Barfkneckt and C. H. Hubert of the School of Pharmacy, University of Iowa.

Antibody and Albumin Measurement

IgG and IgA antibodies were measured in serum, BAW, bile, and intestinal washings using the amplified enzyme-linked immunosorbent assay (a-ELISA).[37,38] Initial studies were performed in conventional polystyrene tubes, whereas more recent studies were performed in microtiter wells using Immulon II plastic from Dynatech. Antibody activities in rabbits were expressed in absolute units using either the "direct ELISA" method in tubes[39] or by comparison to a reference standard when microtiter wells were used. The preparation of antisera to rabbit immunoglobulin for use in the a-ELISA has been described previously.[36,37] Albumin was measured in serum and BAW by radial diffusion as previously described.[36]

Density Gradient Ultracentrifugation

Characterization of the IgG immune response as monomeric or dimeric was performed using a micromethod of sucrose density ultracentrifugation developed by T. K. Koertge.[40] Briefly, 200 μl of 20% sucrose was placed in the bottom of a cellulose nitrate tube designed for the Beckman SW Ti60 rotor. This was overlaid with 1.0 ml of 8.0% sucrose, and the remainder of the tube was filled with water. The sample to be assayed (100 μl) was layered under the water and the chilled tubes centrifuged for three hours at 45,000 rpm. Tubes were fractionated into 100 μl fractions using a conventional paraffin oil fractionator. Antibody distribution was assayed by the a-ELISA as described elsewhere.[38] MOPC (mineral oil induced plasmacytoma) 315 monomeric and dimeric IgA were used as reference proteins. These were kindly provided by Dr. Richard Lynch, Department of Pathology, University of Iowa.

Immunohistochemistry and Histopathology

IgA and IgG anti-OVA-containing plasma cells were enumerated as described previously.[36] Briefly, tissues were prepared using the cold-ethanol fixation method of Sainte-Marie,[41] deparaffinated and treated with OVA conjugated to tetrarhodamine isothiocyanate (TRITC) according to the method of Goldstein and Cebra.[42] After washing in cold phosphate buffered saline (PBS), sections were treated either with DTAF (ditriazinoaminofluorescein)-conjugated guinea pig anti-rabbit γ- or α-chain antisera. DTAF was conjugated to the 33% ammonium sulfate insoluble fraction of the respective guinea pig antisera using the method of Blakeslee[43] except that a 10-fold molar excess of DTAF to protein was used. The fluorescein/protein ratios of the conjugates was 2.9 and 2.56 for anti-γ and anti-α respectively. Specificity and interference were tested by reagent reversal and blocking experiments. The most brilliant rhodamine positive cells in all fields were polymorphonuclear leukocytes, and these were not enumerated. The cell numbers reported here are those regarded as plasma cells by the criteria of their morphology and uniform intracellular staining with both rhodamine (antigen-binding) and fluorescein (immunoglobulin).

RESULTS

TABLE 1 presents the mean concentration of serum IgG and IgA anti-OVA in 16 parenterally primed rabbits receiving chronic aerosol challenge of MDP and OVA and in 12 parenterally primed controls that received only ovalbumin. Chronic MDP aerosol challenge tended to cause an elevation of serum antibody responses that is significant only for IgA.

TABLE 1

THE INFLUENCE OF INHALED MDP ON SERUM IgG
AND IgA ANTI-OVA IN PARENTERALLY PRIMED RABBITS

Nature of Chronic Challenge	n	Anti-OVA (μg/ml ± S.D.)		Antibody Ratio IgG:IgA
		IgG	IgA	
MDP + OVA	16	1,286 ± 1,005	33.9 ± 19.1†	38
		331 − 4,300*	9.2 − 85.1	
OVA	12	1,197 ± 468	9.4 ± 3.5	127
		488 − 1,860*	2.1 − 16.2	

*Range observed
†Significantly greater than the mean of all 28 rabbits, p < 0.05.

Chronic inhalational challenge with MDP and antigen leads to chronic hypersensitivity pneumonitis.[31] The degree of alveolitis was graded histopathologically from 0–4 in 0.5 unit intervals by examination of lung sections prepared from formalized tissue collected at sacrifice. The validity of this grading system could also be secondarily confirmed by the measurement of albumin levels in the BAW collected at sacrifice. The correlation between these two systems is shown in FIGURE 2. By grading the degree of alveolitis resulting from chronic challenge, the MDP-treated animals described in TABLE 1 can be subdivided into those with severe alveolitis and those with little or no alveolitis (pathology score ≤ 0.5). Data on these subdivided groups are presented in TABLE 2. Rabbits with chronic disease show a two-fold increase in their serum IgA anti-OVA levels compared to their healthy, MDP-treated counterparts. A similar increase is, however, also seen for IgG antibody in serum. Healthy MDP-treated rabbits have a mean IgA anti-OVA level in their BAW that exceeds the mean level of IgG anti-OVA, whereas this situation is reversed in chronically diseased rabbits. Hence, by separating animals into healthy and diseased groups the same phenomenon of selective elevation of IgA anti-OVA that was observed in the sera of MDP-treated rabbits can also be seen in bronchoalveolar lavage washings. It should be noted in TABLE 2 that the major effect of chronic disease on humoral immunity is the elevation of IgG antibody in bronchoalveolar lavage washings. The elevation of IgG anti-OVA in the BAW of rabbits with chronic disease can also be expected to occur as a result of transudation from serum resulting from the alveolitis. When the levels of IgG antibody in BAW are corrected, however, for the effect of transudation (TABLE 3), the increased IgG:IgA antibody ratio in the BAW of diseased animals when compared to healthy rabbits, cannot be explained by this transudation. Rather, an increase in the number of IgG-producing cells in the lung proper or associated lymph nodes must be occurring.

To determine the effect of chronic inhalation of MDP and antigen without initial parenteral immunization, rabbits were immunized with MDP and saline in IFA prior to chronic aerosol challenge. TABLE 4 shows that without parenteral

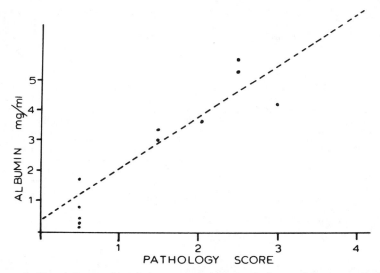

FIGURE 2. Correlation analyses between graded lung pathology and the concentration of albumin in lung lavage fluids.

antigen priming, the selective influence of MDP on the IgA-antibody response is not observed.

In an experiment using eight parenterally primed rabbits, four were given MDP and OVA by aerosol, whereas the remainder received only ovalbumin. Bile and intestinal wash as well as serum and BAW were collected at sacrifice. TABLE 5 shows that whereas preferential elevation of IgA antibody was seen in serum and BAW, no effect was observed on biliary IgG or IgA levels, or the IgA:IgG ratio in this body fluid. The principal antibody in intestinal washings was IgG by a factor of 1000-fold. In fact, IgA anti-OVA could not be detected in the intestinal wash fluids of some rabbits even after concentration. This fact resulted in our inability to properly compare the IgG:IgA antibody activity in the washings in terms of the influence of muramyl dipeptide.

TABLE 2

IgG and IgA Anti-OVA in Sera and BAW of Rabbits with and without Chronic Alveolitis

Treatment and Condition	n	Serum Anti-OVA*			BAW Anti-OVA*		
		IgG	IgA	IgG/IgA	IgG	IgA	IgG/IgA
MDP No Disease	6	623 ± 229	18.9 ± 4.8	33	98 ± 138	297† ± 155	0.32‡
MDP Alveolitis	10	1,683 ± 1,089	42.9 ± 18.7	39‡	529 ± 540	384 ± 373	1.37
No MDP	12	1,197 ± 468	9.4 ± 3.5	127	121 ± 113	138 ± 60	0.87

* Antibody concentrations are given in $\mu g/ml$
† Not significantly different than IgA anti-OVA in the BAW of other groups, p > 0.1
‡ Significantly lower than non-MDP treated rabbits, p < 0.05

TABLE 3

CORRECTION OF LOCAL ANTI-OVA CONCENTRATIONS FOR TRANSUDATION FROM SERUM*

Animal No.	Pathology Score	Serum Anti-OVA & Albumin			BAW Anti-OVA and Albumin			Corrected Anti-OVA in BAW	
		IgG µg/ml	IgA µg/ml	Albumin (mg/ml)	IgG µg/ml	IgA µg/ml	Albumin (mg/ml)	IgG µg/ml	IgA µg/ml
#4	3.0	8,680	85.1	25.3	2,590	980	4.35	1,670	974
#2	0.5	2,790	22.2	24.1	370	230	0.8	336	230
#3	2.5	2,940	59.7	21.1	5,190	2,220	5.75	4,684	2,213
#11	0.0	1,210	1.3	24.1	330	180	0.35	330	180

*The formula used to correct for transudation is given below. $\overline{X}$ is albumin concentration of nine control rabbits = 0.353 ± 0.16 mg/ml; Ab = antibody and Alb = albumin.

$$\text{Corrected BAW } [Ab] = \text{Observed BAW } [Ab] - \frac{[\text{serum Ab}]}{[\text{serum Alb}]} \times \text{increase in } [\text{BAW Alb}] \times \frac{D^{Ab}}{D^{Alb}},$$

where D is the diffusion coefficient:

$$\frac{D^{IgG}}{D^{Alb}} = 0.72; \frac{D^{IgA}}{D^{Alb}} = 0.59.$$

TABLE 4

INFLUENCE OF PARENTERAL PRIMING ON SERUM AND BAW LEVELS OF ANTI-OVA IN CHRONICALLY MDP AEROSALIZED RABBITS

Animal No. & Experiment§	Pathology Score	Serum Anti-OVA*			BAW Anti-OVA		
		IgG	IgA	IgG/IgA	IgG	IgA	IgG/IgA
#10 07-02	0.0	430	0.73	589	3.9	3.3	1.2
#11 07-02	0.0	490	1.55	316	18.9	27.9	0.67
#9 08-29	0.5	1,590	1.4	1,136	340	130	2.61
#10 08-29	0.0	2,300	2.4	958	320	300	1.07
#11 08-29	0.0	1,210	1.3	930	330	180	1.83
#12 08-29	0.0	520	0.3	1,733	130	30	4.33
$\overline{X}$ values	0.08	1,090 ± 755	1.28† ± 0.7	944	190 ± 159	108 ± 127	1.95‡
$\overline{X}$ of healthy, parenterally primed animals	≤0.5	623 ± 229	18.9 ± 4.8	32	98 ± 138	297 ± 155	0.32

*Antibody concentrations in $\mu g/ml$.
†Significantly lower than $\overline{X}$ of healthy, parenterally primed animals, $p < 0.001$.
‡Significantly greater than for healthy, parenterally primed animals, $p < 0.05$.
§Individual animals listed were not parenterally primed.

TABLE 5

IgG and IgA Anti-OVA in Bile and Intestinal Washings of Parenterally Primed, Chronically MDP-Treated Rabbits

Chronic Challenge	n	X̄ Pathology Score	anti-OVA (µg/ml) X̄ ± S.D.						IgG/IgA in	
			Bile			Intestinal Wash†				
			IgG	IgA	IgG/IgA	IgG	IgA	IgG/IgA	Serum	BAW
MDP + OVA	4	1.0	3.2 ± 1.1	320 ± 263	0.010	115 ± 200	0.063‡	1,825	47	0.038
OVA	4	0.37	2.8 ± 0.7	277 ± 159	0.010	93 ± 156	0.047‡ ± 0.013	1,978	117	0.59

*Bile was collected from the gall bladder with a syringe and diluted 1 + 1 with a protease inhibitor solution. See MATERIALS AND METHODS.
†Approximately 20–25 cm of the ileum was removed and filled with ≈50 cc of physiological saline. After 15–30 minutes of gentle massage, the bowel was emptied and the contents centrifuged for 15 minutes at 10,000 rpm. An aliquot of the supernatant was diluted 1 + 1 with the protease inhibitor solution. See MATERIALS AND METHODS for further details.
‡IgA anti-OVA was only detected in one animal of the MDP-OVA group and three animals of the non-MDP group.

Studies in our laboratory[38,44] have indicated, at least for DNP, a pronounced bias of ELISA assays for antibodies of high affinity or multivalency.[40] We have also observed the general absence of a prozone phenomenon when measuring IgM antibodies even in the presence of very high levels of IgG.[45] Recently we have shown a four-fold greater binding of MOPC 315 dimer over MOPC 315 monomer to DNP-gelatin or *o*-dinitrocarboxylphenol in extreme antigen excess.[40] These observations collectively caused us to be concerned that the increases in serum IgA antibody that we report here in MDP-treated rabbits could result from bias in the ELISA for the selective appearance of IgA in the sera of MDP-treated animals that was of higher valency and could therefore exhibit higher avidity and

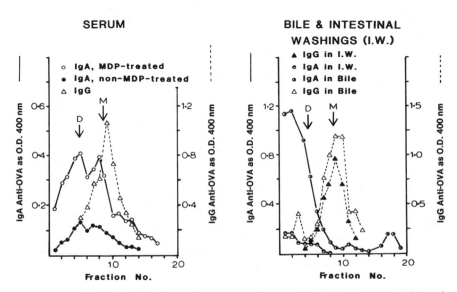

FIGURE 3. The sedimentation behavior of IgA and IgG anti-OVA in serum, bile, and intestinal wash fluids of selected animals. The two sera tested for IgA anti-OVA were used at the same dilution, otherwise sera and secretions were tested at dilutions that optimized detection of the respective antibodies. The bottom of the centrifuge tube is at the left. D = sedimentation position of radiolabeled MOPC 315 dimer. M = sedimentation position of radiolabeled MOPC 315 monomer.

consequently greater detectability at low serum dilutions. To test this possibility, representative sera were fractionated by a modified sucrose density ultracentrifugation method. The results of this study are shown in FIGURE 3. These data show that there is no difference in the sedimentation characteristics of serum IgA anti-OVA in MDP-treated versus non-MDP-treated rabbits, but rather only a difference in activity. The data presented in FIGURE 3 also show that the IgG anti-OVA in bile, intestinal wash, and serum behaves as a monomeric antibody. We have previously shown this to be true for the IgG in bronchoalveolar lavage washings.[36]

The data presented in the previous tables and figures leave the issue of the origin of the increased IgA anti-OVA in serum and some BAWs unresolved.

Initial attempts to investigate this issue were undertaken using double-label immunofluorescence and cold ethanol-fixed tissue. The most striking observation from both MDP and non-MDP treated rabbits was the presence of large numbers of neutrophils that bound the labeled antigen, but not the anti-globulins, to give a granular appearance. In some high power fields (40 × 8), more than 100 of these brightly labeled cells were present. In the small intestine, the IgG anti-OVA plasma cells were found in the same regions. In the lung parenchyma, both plasma cells and neutrophils were most abundant near blood vessels and bronchioles. In animals with chronic lung disease, antibody-containing cells were also seen in the granulomas present. IgA-positive cells were most often seen in thin alveolar septa. Macrophages were abundant in the alveoli, and as reported previously,[36] were often positively labeled with anti-α, even though they did not bind rhodamine ovalbumin. Cells that were smaller than typical alveolar macrophages, but distinctly not plasma-cell like were also observed. These stained with anti-α and anti-γ, but not with rhodamine ovalbumin. They may have been lymphoblasts.

The number of fluorescein and rhodamine cells were enumerated, and the data for three tissues are presented in TABLE 6. "Anti-OVA Cells Containing IgG or IgA" refer to those cells that were double-labeled, that is, were IgG or IgA containing anti-OVA cells. Immunization by aerosol caused an increase in both IgG and IgA cells in the mediastinal lymph node and lung, but not in the small intestine. Parenteral priming versus aerosol alone caused an increase in the number of anti-OVA cells in the lung, but not the mediastinal lymph node or intestine. The major class of anti-OVA containing cells in all three tissues was IgG; from 75–100 percent of these cells were IgG positive. In neither the lung nor mediastinal lymph node was there evidence for an increase proportion of IgA anti-OVA cells in chronic-MDP-treated rabbits. In fact, there was a trend for MDP treatment to increase the proportion of IgG anti-OVA cells (TABLE 6). Of the differences observed, the tendency for nearly all anti-OVA cells in the small intestine to be of the IgG class in MDP-treated rabbits was most obvious. The abundance of IgG anti-OVA cells in the gut is consistent with the prominence of IgG anti-OVA in intestinal washings.

Discussion

The data presented in this report currently describe only a phenomenon of the humoral response to inhaled antigen without providing evidence for the mechanisms responsible. The principal phenomenon observed is the elevation of serum IgA-antibody levels in animals receiving MDP by inhalational challenge compared to controls receiving only antigen. The molecular size profile of the IgA in serum of MDP-treated animals does not differ from that of the IgA anti-OVA in non-MDP treated animals, ruling out the possibility of bias in the measurement system, resulting from the accumulation of, for example, sIgA in serum that could originate in the respiratory tract. sIgA in bile and intestinal washings sediments to a different position than the typical monomeric and dimeric IgA in serum (FIGURE 3). Whereas it may be argued that MDP accelerates affinity maturation of the IgA response, such that the results are biased by increases in affinity rather than concentration, the serum IgA anti-OVA in both MDP and non-MDP treated rabbits exhibits the same "hook" or prozone affect in the ELISA when tested in the presence of high levels of IgG anti-OVA (data not presented). Hence, substantial affinity or avidity differences are unlikely. It is our belief, therefore,

TABLE 6

The Isotypic Distribution of Anti-OVA Containing Cells*

Tissue Examined	Experimental Treatment	Total Cells		Total Anti-OVA Cells	Anti-OVA Cells Containing		Percent of Anti-OVA Cells Labeled With	
		IgG	IgA		IgG	IgA	Anti-γ	Anti-α
Lung Parenchyma	Untreated Controls	5.5 ± 1.3	4.0 ± 1.2	0.0	0.0	0.0	0.0	0.0
	Nonprimed, non-MDP	26 ± 5.4	9.3 ± 4.8	10.6 ± 5.1	8.0 ± 4.2	1.4 ± 0.7	75.3	13.2
	Parenterally primed non-MDP, 1978†	33 ± 10	19 ± 8	20.0 ± 3.7	16.3 ± 1.5	4 ± 2	81.5	20
	1982	N.D.‡	N.D.	55.4 ± 22	51.3 ± 15	6.5 ± 7.0	92.6	11.7
	Parenterally primed, MDP, 1982	N.D.	N.D.	39.7 ± 15	31 ± 16	6.2 ± 2.2	78.1	15.6
Mediastinal Lymph Node	Untreated Controls	24.9 ± 2.5	7.8 ± 3.8	0.0	0.0	0.0	0.0	0.0
	Nonprimed, non-MDP	127 ± 27	19 ± 70	31.9 ± 13.8	30 ± 11	3.3 ± 2.5	93.8	10.3
	Parenterally primed non-MDP, 1978	71 ± 26	16 ± 11	23.5 ± 8.6	26 ± 11	2.6 ± 2.1	89.6	8.9
	1982	N.D.	N.D.	130 ± 60	115.7 ± 56	10 ± 0.8	89.0	7.7
	Parenterally primed MDP, 1982	N.D.	N.D.	65 ± 24	71 ± 23	0.8 ± 0.9	106	1.2
Small Bowel	Untreated Controls	40.6 ± 18	265 ± 72	0.0	0.0	0.0	0.0	0.0
	Nonprimed, non-MDP	50 ± 64	176 ± 42	2.3 ± 1.4	2.0 ± 0.8	0.25 ± 0.5	91	11.4
	Parenterally primed, non-MDP, 1978	31.5 ± 18	205 ± 33	6.6 ± 3.0	5.3 ± 4.0	1.2 ± 1.3	78.7	17.8
	1982	N.D.	N.D.	24.7 ± 7.1	22.5 ± 7.5	4.3 ± 2.0	91.1	17.4
	Parenterally primed MDP, 1982	N.D.	N.D.	39.3 ± 12	40.6 ± 8.5§	2.7 ± 1.5	103	6.8

*Data presented is $\bar{X}$ ± S.D. of the sum of cells seen in 10 high power (40 × 8) microscope fields.

†All data shown for normal controls, nonprimed MDP animals and primed rabbits labeled 1978 were obtained from different groups of rabbits than used in the 1982 studies. Furthermore, animals were challenged only twice weekly in the 1982 study.

‡N.D. = Not done.

§The greater number of double-labeled cells than anti-OVA cells is due to random counting errors when only ten field are counted.

that the quantitative data on IgA antibodies presented here reflects true differences in the concentration of these antibodies in serum and secretions.

Whereas chronic inhalation of antigen and MDP typically results in chronic hypersensitivity pneumonitis,[31] our findings that some rabbits fail to develop such disease has been of use in revealing the phenomenon we describe. Typically the BAW of animals with chronic alveolitis contains considerable amounts of IgG antibodies to the inhaled antigen[31] (TABLE 2). The tendency for the BAW of healthy MDP-treated rabbits to contain a greater proportion of IgA antibodies than their healthy, non-MDP treated controls suggests that the increased IgA anti-OVA seen in serum probably originates in the respiratory tract. In sheep, lymphatic drainage from the lung is known to contribute sizeable amounts of IgA and IgM to the blood vascular system.[46] The data on antibody-containing cells fail to indicate an increase in the proportion of IgA anti-OVA cells in the lower lung or draining lymph nodes. Therefore either this technique is insensitive to such differences, or the IgA antibody originates elsewhere in the pulmonary tract, presumably in the upper bronchi or upper respiratory mucosae. It is well established that the upper and lower pulmonary system differ markedly in the proportion of immunoglobulin of different classes that are present;[10-14] IgA predominates in the upper tract and IgG in the lower.

The exact fate of inhaled antigen or MDP has not been determined in our system. It is known that >80% of inhaled antigen is swallowed and appears in the stomach of the rabbit,[47] (H. B. Richerson, unpublished data). Antigen that remains in the lungs is taken up by alveolar macrophages,[48] may enter the bronchial-associated lymphoreticular tissue (BALT) across specialized epithelial covering,[49] or can be absorbed into the circulation by alveolar epithelia.[50] In the immunization model described here the latter mechanism is likely to play a more important role than usual, because when parenterally primed rabbits are exposed to inhaled antigen, they develop acute hypersensitivity pneumonitis even in the absence of muramyl dipeptide.[51] This is characterized by serum transudation in much the same manner as for rabbits with chronic disease (TABLE 3), except that minimal, if any, locally produced antibody is present prior to challenge.[36] In any case, these inflammatory conditions could presumably make it easier for inhaled antigen to be systemically absorbed by the lungs of animals with disease than by those without, although this possibility has not been studied in our model.

Muramyl dipeptide has been shown to bind to both macrophages and lymphocytes,[32,33] although its fate in our rabbits after inhalation challenge is unknown. If stimulation of a particular cell type (or suppression of others) by inhaled, MDP is responsible for the phenomenon we report here; its fate after inhalation could be instructive in elucidating the mechanism involved.

Selective stimulation of certain antibody isotypes or subisotypes by certain antigens or adjuvants has been reported. For example, use of water-in-oil emulsions of ϕX174 enhanced the IgG_2 response of guinea pigs to the phage, compared to ϕX174 given in saline alone.[52] Lowy et al. (1980) have reported a selective stimulation of IgG_1 responses in mice to DNP given MDP,[34] and Kishimoto et al.[35] report that MDP selectively suppressed IgE-antibody responses. Enhancement or suppression by MDP may be dose dependent.[53] A pronounced and atypical IgG_1 response of cattle to Brucella abortus infections is known to occur,[54,55] and lipopolysaccharide from this organism behaves differently than E. coli lipopolysaccharide in terms of the isotypic expression of antibodies stimulated from mouse lymphocytes.[56] Hence, bacterial components appear to possess the capacity to influence isotype selection by precursor or B-lymphocytes; this phenomenon has special significance for the secretory immune system because of its constant exposure to such agents.

The nature of the antigen may also influence the isotype of the antibody response. This is documented for human IgG_2 subclass antibodies, some of which constitute the principle response to carbohydrate antigen.[57] We have currently switched antigens from ovalbumin (used here) to flourescyl proteins. Whereas data on IgA and IgG antibodies to both hapten and carrier have been measured in animals undergoing acute hypersensitivity pneumonitis,[48] more data from chronic studies will be needed before we can say for certain that MDP produces the same selective increase in IgA antibody to either hapten, carrier, or both as reported here for ovalbumin.

Despite the fact that rabbits chronically challenged with aerosolized antigen ingested a high percentage of the inhaled dose, we found only rare IgA antibody-containing cells in the intestine of rabbits whether or not they were given MDP (TABLE 6). Initial parenteral priming appears to affect only modestly the results, but not in terms of the isotype of the antibody-containing cells in the gut. In all chronically treated animals, IgG-containing cells constitute >80% of the total number of antibody-containing cells (TABLE 6). This observation suggests that ingested antigen is very likely not responsible for the stimulation of the antibody production in the gut, and that homing to the gut of IgA-precursor cells stimulated in the respiratory tract does not occur to any significant extent. The high proportion of IgG-containing cells in the gut is consistent with the predominance of IgG anti-OVA in intestinal wash fluids. This high proportion of IgG antibodies is atypical for antibody responses stimulated by controlled immunization of the gut,[16,58] although parenteral challenge of primed animals can result mainly in an IgG response in the gut.[59] The failure to detect significant numbers of IgA antibody-containing cells in the gut is in agreement with the studies of McDermott and Bienenstock,[60] who showed that most blast cells from BALT return to the respiratory mucosa. Our results suggest that major trafficking of IgA-producing cells stimulated in the lung to the gut does not occur in our model, but could mean that such trafficking does occur for IgG cells primed by inhaled antigen.

REFERENCES

1. TOMASI, T. B. JR. & J. BIENENSTOCK. 1968. Secretory Immunoglobulins. Adv. Immunol. **9:** 1–96.
2. CRABBÉ, P. A., A. O. CARBONARA & J. F. HEREMANS. 1965. The normal human intestinal mucosa as a major source of plasma cells containing γA immunoglobulin. Lab. Invest. **14:** 235–248.
3. MARTINEZ-TELLO, F. J., D. G. BRAUN & W. A. BLANC. 1968. The immunoglobulin production in the bronchial mucosa and bronchial lymph nodes in chronic bronchopulmonary disease, particularly in cystic fibrosis of the pancreas. J. Immunol. **101:** 989–1003.
4. TOURVILLE, D. R., R. H. ADLER & J. BIENENSTOCK. 1969. The human secretory immunoglobulin system: Immunohistological localization of γA, secretory "Piece," and lactoferrin in normal human tissues. J. Exp. Med. **129**(2): 411–429.
5. POGER, M. E. & M. E. LAMM. 1974. Localization of free and bound secretory component in human intestinal epithelial cells. J. Exp. Med. **139:** 629–642.
6. BRANDTZAEG, P. 1974. Mucosal and glandular distribution of immunoglobulin components: differential localization of free and bound SC in secretory epithelial cells. J. Immunol. **112**(4): 1553–1559.
7. KALTREIDER, H. B. & S. E. SALMON. 1973. Immunology of the lower respiratory tract: Functional properties of bronchoalveolar lymphocytes obtained from the normal canine lung. J. Clin. Invest. **52:** 2211–2217.
8. FORD, R. J. & C. KUHN. 1973. Immunologic competence of alveolar cells. I. The

plaque-forming response to particulate and soluble antigens. Am. Rev. Resp. Dis. **107:** 763–770.

9. REYNOLDS, H. Y. & H. H. NEWBALL. 1974. Analysis of protein and respiratory cells obtained from human lungs by bronchial lavage. J. Lab. Clin. Med. **84:** 559–573.

10. KALTREIDER, H. B. & M. K. L. CHAN. 1976. The class-specific immunoglobulin composition of fluids obtained from various levels of the canine respiratory tract. J. Immunol. **116**(2): 423–429.

11. WALDMAN, R. H., P. F. JURGENSEN, G. N. OLSEN, R. GANGULY & J. E. JOHNSON, III. 1973. Immune response of the human respiratory tract. I. Immunoglobulin levels and influenza vaccine antibody response. J. Immunol. **111:** 38–41.

12. REYNOLDS, H. Y., W. M. MERRILL, E. P. AMENTO & G. P. NAEGEL. 1977. Immunoglobulin A in secretions from the lower human respiratory tract. Adv. Exp. Med. Biol. **107:** 553–5564.

13. MORGAN, K. L., A. M. HUSSEIN, T. J. NEWBY & F. J. BOURNE. 1980. Quantification and origin of the immunoglobulins in porcine respiratory tract secretions. Immunology **41:** 729–736.

14. HAND, W. L. & J. R. CANTEY. 1974. Antibacterial mechanisms of the lower respiratory tract. I. Immunoglobulin synthesis and secretion. J. Clin. Invest. **53:** 354–362.

15. OGRA, P. L. 1969. The secretory immunoglobulin system of the gastrointestinal tract. In The Secretory Immunologic System. D. H. Dayton, Jr., P. A. Small, Jr., R. M. Chanock, H. E. Kaufman and T. B. Tomasi, Jr., Eds.: 259–279. USPHS Publ.

16. PORTER, P., R. KENWORTHY, D. E. NOAKES & W. D. ALLEN. 1974. Intestinal antibody secretion in the young pig in response to oral immunization with *Escherichia coli.* Immunology **27:** 841–853.

17. BELLANTI, J. A., M. S. ARTENSTEIN & E. L. BUESCHER. 1965. Characterization of virus neutralizing antibodies in human serum and nasal secretions. J. Immunol. **94**(3): 344–351.

18. PIERCE, N. F. & J. L. GOWANS. 1975. Cellular kinetics of the intestinal immune response to cholera toxoid in rats. J. Exp. Med. **142:** 1550–1563.

19. FAZEKAS DE ST. GROTH, S., M. DONNELLEY & D. M. GRAHAM. 1951. Studies in experimental immunology of influenza. VIII. Pathotopic adjuvants. Aust. J. Exp. Biol. Med. Sci. **29:** 323–337.

20. FUHRMAN, J. A. & J. J. CEBRA. 1981. Special features of the priming process for a secretory IgA response. B cell priming with cholera toxin. J. Exp. Med. **153:** 534–544.

21. CRABBÉ, P. A., H. BAZIN, H. EYSSEN & J. F. HEREMANS. 1968. The normal microbial flora as a major stimulus for proliferation of plasma cells synthesizing IgA in the gut. Int. Arch. Allergy Appl. Immunol. **34:** 362–375.

22. BENVENISTE, J., G. LESPINATS & J. C. SALOMON. 1971. Serum and secretory IgA in axenic and holoxenic mice. J. Immunol. **108:** 1656–1662.

23. CARTER, P. B. & F. M. COLLINS. 1975. Peyer's patch responsiveness to *Salmonella* in mice. J. Reticuloendothelial Soc. **17**(1): 38–46.

24. COX, D. S., M. A. TAUBMAN, J. L. EBERSOLE & D. J. SMITH. 1980. Secretory antibody response to local injection of soluble or particulate antigens in rats. Mol. Immunol. **17**(9): 1105–1115.

25. CRABBÉ, P. A., D. R. NASH, H. BAZIN, H. EYSSEN & J. F. HEREMANS. 1969. Antibodies of the IgA type in intestinal plasma cells of germfree mice after oral or parenteral immunization with ferritin. J. Exp. Med. **130**(4): 723–738.

26. HEREMANS, J. F. & H. BAZIN. 1971. Antibodies induced by local antigenic stimulation of mucosal surfaces. Annals. N.Y. Acad. Sci. **190:** 268–275.

27. WHITEHOUSE, M. W. 1977. The chemical nature of adjuvants. In Immunochemistry: An Advanced Textbook L. E. Glynn and M. M. Steward, Eds. J. Wiley. New York.

28. ELLOUZ, F., A. ADAM, R. CIORBARU & E. LEDERER. 1974. Minimal structure requirements for adjuvant activity of bacterial peptidoglycan derivatives. Biochem. Biophys. Res. Commun. **59:** 1317–1325.

29. CHEDID, L., F. AUDIBERT & A. G. JOHNSON. 1978. Biological activities of muramyl dipeptide, a synthetic glycopeptide analogous to bacterial immunoregulating agents. Prog. Allergy **25:** 63–105.

30. LOWY, I., C. LECLERC, E. BOURGEOSIS & L. CHEDID. 1980. Inhibition of mitogen-induced

polyclonal activation by a synthetic adjuvant, muramyl dipeptide (MDP). J. Immunol. **124**(1): 320–325.

31. RICHERSON, H. B., M. T. SUELZER, P. A. SWANSON, J. E. BUTLER, W. C. KOPP & E. F. ROSE. 1982. Chronic hypersensitivity pneumonitis produced in the rabbit by the adjuvant effect of inhaled muramyl dipeptide (MDP). Am. J. Pathol. **106**(3):409–420.

32. TANAKA, A., S. NAGAO, K. IMAI & R. MORI. 1980. Macrophage activation by muramyl dipeptide as measured by macrophage spreading and attachment. Microbiol. Immunol. **24**: 547–557.

33. SUZIMURA, K., M. UEMIYA, I. SAIKI, I. AZUMA & Y. YAMAMURA. 1979. The adjuvant activity of synthetic N-acetylmuramyl dipeptide: Evidence of initial target cells for the adjuvant activity. Cell. Immunol. **43**: 137–149.

34. LOWY, I., J. THEZE & L. CHEDID. 1980. Stimulation of the *in vivo* dinitrophenyl antibody response to the DNP conjugate of L-glutamic acid^{60}-L-alanine^{30}-L-tyrosine^{10} (GAT) polymer by a synthetic adjuvant, muramyl dipeptide (MDP): target cells for adjuvant activity and isotypic pattern of MDP-stimulated response. J. Immunol. **124**(1): 100–104.

35. KISHIMOTO, T., Y. HIRAI, K. NAKANISHI, I. AZUMA, A. NAGAMATSU & Y. YAMAMURA. 1979. Regulation of antibody response in different immunoglobulin classes. VI. Selective suppression of IgE response by administration of antigen-conjugated muramyl peptides. J. Immunol. **123**(6): 2709–2715.

36. BUTLER, J. E., P. A. SWANSON, H. B. RICHERSON, H. V. RATAJCZAK, D. W. RICHARDS & M. T. SUELZER. 1982. The local and systemic IgA and IgG antibody responses of rabbits to a soluble inhaled antigen. Measurement of responses in a model of acute hypersensitivity pneumonitis. Am. Rev. Resp. Dis. **126**: 80–85.

37. BUTLER, J. E., P. L. McGIVERN & P. SWANSON. 1978. Amplification of the enzyme-linked immunosorbent assay (ELISA) in the detection of class-specific antibodies. J. Immunol. Methods **20**: 365–383.

38. BUTLER, J. E. 1981. The amplified ELISA: Principles and applications for the comparative quantitation of class and subclass antibodies and the distribution of antibodies and antigens in biochemical separates. Methods Enzymol. J. J. Langone and H. Vunakis, Eds.: **73B**: 482–523.

39. BUTLER, J. E., L. A. CANTARERO & P. L. McGIVERN. 1980. Measurement of bovine subclass antibodies (IgG1 and IgG2) using the amplified enzyme-linked immunosorbent assay. Mol. Immunol. **17**: 645–653.

40. KOERTGE, T. E. 1983. Immunochemical studies on the enzyme-linked immunoadsorbent assay (ELISA) and its application to studies on the transport of monomeric and polymeric antibodies. Ph.D. Thesis. University of Iowa.

41. SAINTE-MARIE, G. 1961. A paraffin embedding technique for studies employing immunofluorescence. J. Histochem. Cytochem. **10**: 250–256.

42. CEBRA, J. J. & G. GOLDSTEIN. 1965. Chromatographic purification of tetramethylrhodamine-immune globulin conjugates and their use in the cellular localization of rabbit γ-globulin polypeptide chains. J. Immunol. **95**: 230–245.

43. BLAKESLEE, D. & M. G. BAINES. 1976. Immunofluorescense using DTAF. I. Preparation and fractionation of labelled IgG. J. Immunol. Methods. **13**: 305–320.

44. BUTLER, J. E., T. L. FELDBUSH, P. L. McGIVERN & N. STEWART. 1978. The enzyme-linked immunosorbent assay (ELISA): A measurement of antibody concentration or affinity? Immunochemistry **15**: 131–136.

45. BUTLER, J. E., P. L. McGIVERN, L. A. CANTARERO & L. PETERSON. 1980. Application of the amplified enzyme-linked immunosorbent assay: Comparative quantitation of bovine serum IgG1, IgG2, IgA and IgM antibodies. Am. J. Vet. Res. **41**: 1479–1491.

46. GORIN, A. B. & J. GOULD. 1979. Immunoglobulin synthesis in the lungs and caudal mediastinal lymph node of sheep. J. Immunol. **123**: 1339–1342.

47. WILLOUGHBY, J. B. & W. F. WILLOUGHBY. 1977. *In vivo* responses to inhaled proteins I. Quantitative analysis of antigen uptake, fate and immunogenicity in a rabbit model system. J. Immunol. **119**(6): 2137–2146.

48. BUTLER, J. E., H. B. RICHERSON, P. A. SWANSON, M. T. SUELZER & W. C. KOPP. 1983. The carrier requirement for development of acute hypersensitivity pneumonitis in a rabbit model. Int. Arch. Allergy Appl. Immunol. **70**. In press.

49. TENNER-RACZ, K., P. RACZ, Q. N. MYRVIK, J. R. OCKERS & R. GEISTER. 1979. Uptake and transport of horseradish peroxidase by lymphoepithelium of the bronchus-associated lymphoid tissue in normal and Bacillus Calmette-Guerin-immunized and challenged rabbits. Lab. Invest. 41(2): 106–115.

50. BRALEY, J. F., L. B. PETERSON, C. A. DAWSON & V. L. MOORE. 1979. Effect of hypersensitivity on protein uptake across the air-blood barrier of isolated rabbit lungs. J. Clin. Invest. 63: 1103–1109.

51. RICHERSON, H. B., F. H. F. CHENG & S. C. BAUSERMAN. 1971. Acute experimental hypersensitivity pneumonitis in rabbits. Am. Rev. Respir. Dis. 104: 568–575.

52. WILKINSON, P. C., W. A. FLEMING & R. G. WHITE. 1967. The effect of adjuvants on biosynthesis of 19S and 7S antibody against bacteriophage ϕX174 in the guinea pig. Immunology 13: 603–611.

53. LECLERC, C., D. JUY, E. BOURGEOIS & L. CHEDID. 1979. In vivo regulation of humoral and cellular immune responses of mice by a synthetic adjuvant, N-acetyl-muramyl-L-alanyl-D-isoglutamine, muramyl dipeptide or MDP. Cell. Immunol. 45: 199–206.

54. LAMB, V. L., L. M. JONES, G. G. SCHURIG & D. T. BERMAN. 1979. Enzyme-linked immunosorbent assay for bovine immunoglobulin subclass specific responses to lipopolysaccharides of Brucella abortus. Infect. Immun. 26(1): 240–247.

55. BUTLER, J. E., G. I. SEAWRIGHT, P. L. MCGIVERN & M. GILSDORF. 1981. Class and subclass antibody response of B. abortus strain 19-vaccinated and field-strain-challenged cattle: Evidence for a predominant IgG1 response in infected animals. In The Ruminant Immune System J. E. Butler, Ed.: 790–791. Plenum Press. New York.

56. KURTS, R. & D. BERMAN. Personal communications.

57. KUNKEL, H. G. & W. J. YOUNT. 1970. Heavy-chain subgroups of γG and γA globulins. In Immunoglobulins E. Merler, Ed.: 137–145. Nat'l Acad. Sci. Washington, D.C.

58. YARDLEY, J. H., D. F. KEREN, S. R. HAMILTON & G. D. BROWN. 1978. Local (immunoglobulin A) immune response by the intestine to cholera toxin and its partial suppression with combined systemic and intraintestinal immunization. Infect. Immun. 19(2): 589–597.

59. SVENNERHOLM, A. M., S. LANGE & J. HOLMGREN. 1980. Intestinal immune response to cholera toxin: Dependence on route and dosage of antigen for priming and boosting. Infect. Immun. 30: 337–341.

60. MCDERMOTT, M. R. & J. BIENENSTOCK. 1979. Evidence for a common mucosal immunologic system. I. Migration of B immunoblasts into intestinal, respiratory and genital tissues. J. Immunol. 122: 1892–1898.

DISCUSSION OF THE PAPER

QUESTION: It has been claimed that MDP stimulates IgA secretion. Does it do anything at all?

J. E. BUTLER (The University of Iowa, Iowa City): We have examined the mitogenic effects of MDP in vitro and its ability to stimulate polyclonal responses in vivo. MDP has none of these effects.

QUESTION: So, it does not stimulate the IgA responses without the antigen?

BUTLER: No. MDP preparations that were purchased from France as well as those we synthesized ourselves are not stimulating by themselves.

S. J. CHALLACOMBE (Guy's Hospital, London, England): These adjuvants would be particularly useful if they not only helped to induce the response, but made such a response longer lasting. Do you have any information concerning the duration of immune response in the MDP-treated animals?

BUTLER: Because these animals are sacrificed for histologic purposes shortly after the last exposure, we have not done these experiments. The purpose of these experiments was not to study the effect of MDP on the IgA response, but to examine the effect on the development of chronic disease.

J. R. McGHEE (*University of Alabama in Birmingham*): How do you know that you are not inducing with MDP an accelerated form of tolerance, or lack of responsiveness in terms of numbers of responding cells?

BUTLER: We followed the serum antibody response, not the cells. We do not know whether there is a selective suppression of IgG response; we observe a heightened IgA response after MDP administration.

T. LEHNER (*Guy's Hospital, London, England*): Is MDP pyrogenic or cytotoxic?

BUTLER: According to the literature, MDP is pyrogenic and toxic at high doses. At levels of 100 μg, MDP may have some rather negative effects in rat ileal loops.

ESCHERICHIA COLI STRAINS PRODUCING STREPTOCOCCUS MUTANS PROTEINS RESPONSIBLE FOR COLONIZATION AND VIRULENCE*

Roy Curtiss III,† Robert G. Holt, Raúl G. Barletta
James P. Robeson,‡ and Shigeno Saito

Institute of Dental Research
and
Department of Microbiology
University of Alabama in Birmingham
Birmingham, Alabama 35294

INTRODUCTION

Streptococcus mutans is a principal etiologic agent of dental caries and is likely one of the most ubiquitous bacterial infectious disease agents worldwide.[1-3] The ability of S. mutans to colonize the oral cavity is due to sucrose-independent and sucrose-dependent adherence to the pellicle-coated tooth surface with glucan facilitated aggregation between cells to result in plaque. Cariogenicity is then caused by the ability of S. mutans in plaque to metabolize free sugars and both extra and intracellular complex carbohydrates to yield predominantly lactic acid.[1-3] The S. mutans gene products that contribute to colonizing ability and thus virulence include glucosyltransferases, glucan-binding proteins, and a diversity of less well-characterized cell-surface proteins and carbohydrate antigens that may also promote adherence or aggregation.

Until recently, S. mutans was unable to be analyzed genetically by classical methods of mutagenesis and gene transfer for mapping and complementation. We thus chose to use gene cloning technologies to introduce S. mutans genes into suitable strains of Escherichia coli K-12. S. mutans plasmid[4] and chromosomal[5-7] genes are expressed very well in E. coli. For example, the S. mutans gene for aspartic acid semialdehyde dehydrogenase possesses a very unique promoter sequence region that results in 7% of the total E. coli protein being the product of this one S. mutans gene.[5,7] Furthermore, S. mutans gene products can substitute for E. coli gene products that are missing because of the presence of gene mutations or deletions in the E. coli recipient strain.[5,7] In that regard, Perry and Kuramitsu[8] have developed a method for transformation of S. mutans strain GS-5 (serotype c), making it possible to mutate S. mutans genes cloned in E. coli, to return them to S. mutans and then to examine the effect of a known mutation altering a well-characterized gene product on S. mutans virulence. Similarly, we have been able to use antibodies against S. mutans gene products made by

*Research was supported by Public Health Service Grant DE-02670 from the National Institute of Dental Research and by a Public Health Service Postdoctoral Traineeship, T32 DE 07026, from the National Institute of Dental Research to Robert G. Holt.

†To whom correspondence should be addressed.

‡Present Address: Laboratorio de Microbiología, Universidad Católica de Valparaíso, Casilla 4059, Valparaíso, Chile.

0077-8923/83/0409-0688 $1.75/0 © 1983, NYAS

recombinant *E. coli* strains to select *S. mutans* mutants lacking that gene product.

We have begun systematically to clone *S. mutans* genes encoding cell-surface proteins and then to determine the contribution of these gene products to the ability of *S. mutans* to colonize the tooth surface. An associated objective is to use some of the *S. mutans* gene products synthesized by recombinant *E. coli* clones for the analysis of the immune response to *S. mutans* and for the development of an effective anti-caries vaccine.

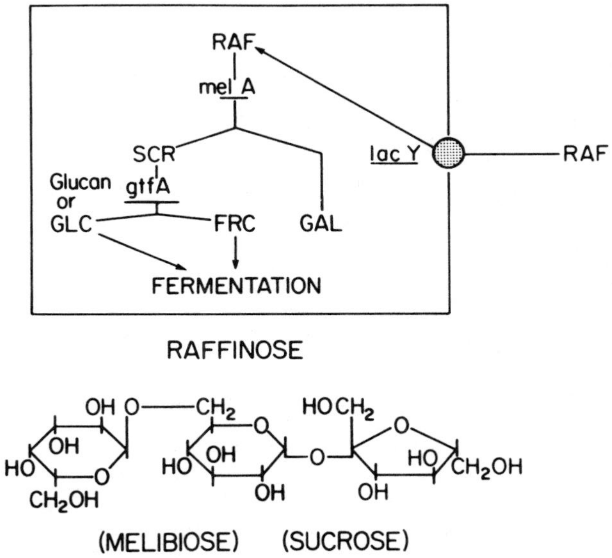

FIGURE 1. Strategy for successful cloning of *S. mutans* genes specifying enzymes for hydrolysis of sucrose into strains of *E. coli* K-12 (see text).

RESULTS

Cloning of S. mutans *Genes with Sucrose Hydrolyzing Activity*

E. coli is unable to metabolize sucrose because of the absence of enzymes with invertase-like activity and furthermore is unable to transport sucrose efficiently across the cytoplasmic membrane. Because we were uncertain whether *S. mutans* gene products with sucrose hydrolyzing activity would leave the cytoplasm, it was necessary to devise a means to present sucrose to such enzymes in the *E. coli* cytoplasm. FIGURE 1 depicts the strategy for accomplishing this. The trisaccharide raffinose is an α-galactoside containing galactose and glucose in an $\alpha-1\rightarrow6$ linkage; thus raffinose can be transported across the *E. coli* cytoplasmic membrane by way of the galactoside permease that is the product of the *lacY* gene. Raffinose can then induce expression of the genes in the *mel* operon with the *melA* gene specifying an α-galactosidase that cleaves raffinose to yield galactose and sucrose. We thus shotgun cloned *S. mutans* PS14 (serotype *c*) DNA using

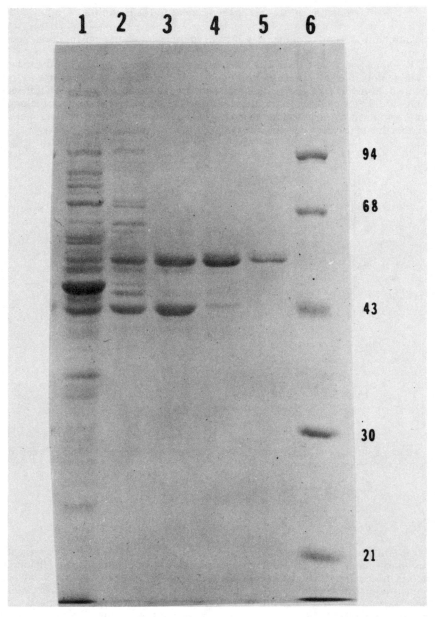

FIGURE 2. SDS-polyacrylamide gel electrophoresis of proteins in fractions containing *gtfA* enzyme activity at different stages of purification. Activity was measured by generation of reducing sugars from sucrose.[9] Lane 1: crude extract of *E. coli* K-12 containing pYA601 obtained by sonication followed by sedimentation of cell debris. Lane 2: fractions after chromatography on a DE-52 column. Lane 3: fractions after chromatography on an Ultrogel AcA54 column. Lane 4: fractions after chromatography on an Ultrogel AcA44 column. Lane 5: purified *gtfA* enzyme following precipitation with 33% ammonium sulfate. Lane 6: molecular mass markers (kdal).

the pBR322 plasmid cloning vector into an *E. coli* strain possessing a deletion of the *gal* operon and selected recombinant clones able to grow on raffinose as the sole carbon source.[6,9] Treatment of *E. coli* cells able to grow on raffinose with toluene led to a linear increase in the amount of reducing sugar generated over time when sucrose was used as a substrate. One of the recombinant *E. coli* clones with sucrose hydrolyzing activity contained a recombinant plasmid designated pYA601. Analysis of proteins specified by the recombinant plasmid, pYA601, using purified minicells containing the plasmid, revealed the presence of a 55,000 molecular weight protein encoded by 1730 base-pair fragment of *S. mutans* DNA. Based on the molecular weight of this protein, a strategy was devised for its purification to homogeneity (FIGURE 2). This purified protein could then be used

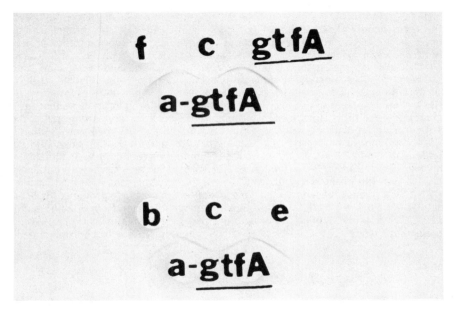

FIGURE 3. Immunodiffusion analysis employing antibodies against purified *gtfA* protein produced by *E. coli* (a-*gtfA*) and extracts of cell-surface proteins obtained from *S. mutans* strains in serotypes *b*, *c*, *e*, and *f* and the purified *gtfA* protein from the serotype *c* *S. mutans* strain, PS14.

to prepare monospecific and monoclonal antibodies against the protein as well as to characterize the protein for its enzyme activity.

The protein encoded by pYA601 is a glucosyltransferase[6,9] that hydrolyzes sucrose to synthesize a glucan polymer and an equivalent amount of fructose. Antibody against the product of this gene that we have designated *gtfA* reacts with immunologically identical proteins from serotypes *c*, *e*, and *f* *S. mutans* strains and cross-reacts with a protein from serotype *b* *S. mutans* (FIGURE 3). No reaction was detected with proteins produced by *S. mutans* serotypes *a*, *d*, or *g*.

The purified glucosyltransferase has a K_m of 1.2 *mM* for sucrose, a pH optimum of about 6.5 and hydrolyzes sucrose to a water-soluble glucan of low molecular weight and fructose. This glucosyltransferase does not require a primer, and the protein is transported across the E. coli cytoplasmic membrane into the periplasm without processing or modification. Thus, E. coli containing the pYA601 plasmid can grow on sucrose because sucrose is transported across the outer membrane into the E. coli periplasm. E. coli recombinants containing pYA601 synthesize about 100,000 molecules of the gtfA enzyme per cell. This fact accounts for about 3 to 4% of the total E. coli soluble protein.

Cloning of S. mutans Genes Specifying Cell-Surface Proteins Lacking Enzyme Activity

DNA from S. mutans strain 6715 (serotype g) was shotgun cloned into the cosmid vector, pJC74,[10] so as to reduce the size of the clone bank that would need to be screened for expression of S. mutans cell-surface protein antigens. The cosmids packaged in vitro into infectious λ-phage particles were introduced into an E. coli strain lysogenic for the λcI857 thermo-inducible prophage and plated at 30°C. Colonies were patched onto an agarose medium containing high titer antisera raised against S. mutans cell-surface proteins, and after overnight incubation at 30°C, the plates were shifted to 42°C to cause thermo-induction of the λ-prophage leading to lysis of cells and release of protein antigens that they contain.[11] Precipitin rings formed around those colonies expressing a protein antigen reacting with the antibodies in the minimal agarose medium.[6,12] One of the recombinant clones produced a strong precipitin band and has been studied most extensively. This clone contained the recombinant cosmid, pYA721, that had an 8.3 kilobase insert of S. mutans 6715 DNA. This insert was subsequently cloned into the plasmid vector, pACYC184, to yield the recombinant plasmid, pYA726.[12] We have designated the gene specifying this surface protein antigen as spaA and have purified the spaA protein to homogeneity both from S. mutans and from E. coli recombinants. The protein purified from S. mutans has an apparent molecular weight of 210,000 by SDS-polyacrylamide gel electrophoresis and of

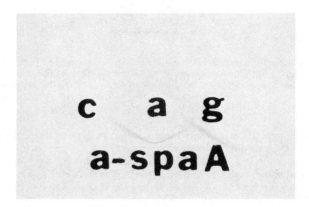

FIGURE 4. Immunodiffusion analysis of cell-surface proteins produced by S. mutans serotypes a, c, and g against antisera raised to purified spaA protein (a-spaA). It should be noted that proteins from serotypes c, e, and f are all identical in regard to response to a-spaA serum as are the proteins produced by serotypes d and g S. mutans strains.

TABLE 1

PRESENCE OF ANTIGENS CROSS-REACTING WITH 6715 *SPAA* PROTEIN AMONG THE
VARIOUS SEROTYPES OF *S. MUTANS*

Strain	Serotype	Supernatant Fluid*	Cell Surface†
HS6	*a*	Yes	Yes
BHT	*b*	No	No
Ingbritt	*c*	Yes	Yes
OMZ176	*d*	Yes	Yes
LM7	*e*	Yes	Yes
OMZ175	*f*	Yes	Yes
6715	*g*	Yes	Yes

*Extracellular protein fractions of the various *S. mutans* serotypes grown in defined media[12] were prepared from cell-free culture supernatant fluids and were examined for antigens cross-reacting with the *spaA* protein of *S. mutans* 6715 by immunodiffusion analysis.

†*S. mutans* cells of the various serotypes were grown in defined media[12] and washed with 5 *M* NaCl. The presence of cell-surface antigens cross-reacting with the *spaA* protein of *S. mutans* 6715 was determined by direct immunofluoresence using rhodamine-conjugated a-*spaA* as a probe.

180,000 when produced by *E. coli*. *E. coli* cells with the *spaA* gene produce 7% of their total soluble protein as the *spaA* protein and translocate 60% of this protein to the periplasmic space.[12] The *spaA* protein reacts with antibody against the *spaA* protein as well as with antibody against the antigen I/II, purified and characterized from serotype *c* *S. mutans* strains by Russell, *et al.*[13] In addition, antibody purified against the *spaA* protein reacts with antigen I/II from serotype *c* and also with antigens produced by serotypes *a, d, e, f,* and *g,* but not by *b* strains of *S. mutans* (FIGURE 4, TABLE 1). The *spaA* protein produced by *S. mutans* contains an antigenic determinant not present on the *spaA* protein produced by *E. coli* recombinants. This phenomenon is possibly due to the absence of carbohydrate antigenic determinants on the *E. coli*-produced gene product. This hypothesis is currently under test. The *spaA* protein is found free in the supernatant fluid of *S. mutans* strains grown in FMC medium[12] (TABLE 1), but is also found to be tightly bound to the cell surface even after washing in 5 *M* NaCl. By using antibodies directed against the *spaA* protein, it has been shown that these antibodies will inhibit sucrose-induced aggregation between *S. mutans* cells. Furthermore, *S. mutans* mutants lacking the *spaA* protein as selected by using antiserum against the *spaA* protein are also defective in aggregation.

DISCUSSION

We have found that a diversity of *S. mutans* genes for cell-surface protein antigens from both serotype *c* and serotype *g* strains are expressed very well in strains of *E. coli* K-12. Furthermore, most of these *S. mutans* cell-surface proteins are able to be translocated across the *E. coli* cytoplasmic membrane into the *E. coli* periplasm. Because of this fact, we are continuing to identify and characterize other *S. mutans* cell-surface protein antigens produced by recombinant *E. coli* strains. Analysis of these proteins is facilitated by the fact that there are few, if any, *E. coli* proteins that cross-react with *S. mutans* proteins or vice versa. Monoclonal antibodies against the *spaA* and *gtfA* proteins have been produced from hybridomas,[14] and these monoclonal antibodies are being used to facilitate purification of the spaA and gtfA proteins by immunoabsorbent chromatography. It should be pointed out that relatively satisfactory methods for the purification of these proteins from E. coli, as well as S. mutans, have been worked out.

Other workers have used purified glucosyltransferases[15-17] and the antigen I/II protein,[13] also termed B,[18,19] from serotype c and g S. mutans strains to immunize rats, hamsters, and Rhesus monkeys to evaluate induction of immunity to S. mutans-induced dental caries. Some,[15,19] but not all,[16,17] of these studies gave promising results.

Because of these previous studies, the purified S. mutans cell-surface proteins are being used in several interrelated investigations. Dr. Michalek, Dr. McGhee, and their colleagues are using these proteins, as well as lipoteichoic acid and type-specific carbohydrate antigens, to screen humans as a function of age for titers of various Ig isotypes in saliva and serum. Both enzyme-linked immunosorbent assays (ELISA) and radioimmunoassays (RIA) have been developed for most of these S. mutans cell-surface proteins. These individuals are also being evaluated for caries incidence, and for titers and serotypes of S. mutans in plaque. High titers of antibodies, especially secretory IgA, against one or more of these antigens in conjunction with low titers of S. mutans in plaque and/or low incidence of dental caries would be suggestive of protein antigens that should be explored for their ability to induce protective immunity against S. mutans-induced dental caries.

In this last regard, we are collaborating with Dr. Mestecky, Dr. Michalek, Dr. McGhee, and their colleagues to use purified protein antigens for oral (by gastric intubation) and systemic immunization of mice and gnotobiotic rats to analyze the immune response and evaluate effective immunity to S. mutans-induced dental caries. We have also devised a new approach for oral immunization so as to stimulate cells of the Peyer's patches to result in a strong secretory IgA response. Specifically, we are starting with enteric pathogens that are able to attach to and invade cells of the gut-associated lymphoreticular tissue (GALT) and then rendering them avirulent by genetic manipulation as used in our development of the safer E. coli host, χ1776, for recombinant DNA research.[20] These avirulent pathogens can then be endowed with genetic information to permit high-level production of S. mutans cell-surface protein antigens, and because of their ability to attach to and invade cells of the GALT, we anticipate that a secretory immune response against these S. mutans protein antigens will be induced. If so, a safe effective vaccine against S. mutans-induced dental caries should become a reality. In addition, this method would also be applicable to vaccine construction and immunization to preclude infection by any viral, bacterial, mycotic, or parasitic agent that invades a mucosal surface.

ACKNOWLEDGMENTS

We thank Sylvia Larrimore and Hettie Murchison for technical assistance and Pat Pierce for help in preparation of this manuscript.

REFERENCES

1. NEWBRUN, E. 1973. Cariology. The Williams & Wilkins Co., Baltimore.
2. GIBBONS, R. J. & J. VAN HOUTE. 1975. Dental caries. Annu. Rev. Med. 26: 121–136.

3. HAMADA, S. & H. D. SLADE. 1980. Biology, immunology, and cariogenicity of *Streptococcus mutans*. Microbiology Rev. **44:** 331–384.

4. HANSEN, J. B., Y. ABIKO & R. CURTISS III. 1981. Characterization of the *Streptococcus mutans* plasmid pVA318 cloned into *Escherichia coli*. Infect. Immun. **31:** 1034–1043.

5. CURTISS, R. III, E. K. JAGUSZTYN-KRYNICKA, J. B. HANSEN, M. SMORAWINSKA, Y. ABIKO & G. CARDINEAU. 1982. Expression of *Streptococcus mutans* plasmid and chromosomal genes in *Escherichia coli* K-12. In *Microbial Drug Resistance*. S. Mitsuhashi, Ed.: Vol. *3:* 15–25. University Park Press, Baltimore.

6. CURTISS, R. III, J. P. ROBESON, Y. ABIKO, R. BARLETTA & M. SMORAWINSKA. 1982. Synthesis and function of *Streptococcus mutans* cell surface proteins in *Escherichia coli*. In *Microbiology-1982*. D. Schlessinger, Ed.: 253–257. ASM Publications, Washington, D.C.

7. JAGUSZTYN-KRYNICKA, E. K., M. SMORAWINSKA & R. CURTISS III. 1982. Expression of *Streptococcus mutans* asparate semialdehyde dehydrogenase gene cloned into plasmid pBR322. J. Gen. Microbiol. **128:** 1135–1145.

8. PERRY, D. & H. K. KURAMITSU. 1981. Genetic transformation of *Streptococcus mutans*. Infect. Immun. **32:** 1295–1297.

9. ROBESON, J. P., R. G. BARLETTA & R. CURTISS III. 1983. Expression of a *Streptococcus mutans* glucosyltransferase in *Escherichia coli*. J. Bacteriol. **153:** 211–221.

10. COLLINS, J. 1979. *Escherichia coli* plasmids packageable *in vitro* in λ bacteriophage particles. Methods Enzymol. **68:** 309–326.

11. SKALKA, A. & L. SHAPIRO. 1976. *In situ* immunoassays for gene translation products in phage plaques and bacterial colonies. Gene **1:** 65–79.

12. HOLT, R. G., Y. ABIKO, S. SAITO, M. SMORAWINSKA, J. B. HANSEN & R. CURTISS III. 1982. *Streptococcus mutans* genes that code for extracellular proteins in *Escherichia coli* K-12. Infect. Immun. **38:** 147–156.

13. RUSSELL, M. W., L. A. BERGMEIER, E. D. ZANDERS & T. LEHNER. 1980. Protein antigens of *Streptococcus mutans*: purification and properties of a double antigen and its protease-resistant component. Infect. Immun. **28:** 486–493.

14. DAUGHERTY, D. F., D. E. COLWELL, R. G. HOLT, R. CURTISS III, J. R. McGHEE & S. M. MICHALEK. 1982. Fed. Proc. Fed Am. Soc. Exp. Biol. **41:** 596.

15. TAUBMAN, M. A. & D. J. SMITH. 1977. Effects of local immunization with glucosyltransferase fractions from *Streptococcus mutans* on dental caries in rats and hamsters. J. Immunol. **118:** 710–720.

16. RUSSELL, R. R. B. & G. COLMAN. 1981. Immunization of monkeys (*Macaca fascicularis*) with purified *Streptococcus mutans* glucosyltransferase. Arch. Oral Biol. **26:** 23–28.

17. COHEN, B., G. COLMAN & R. R. B. RUSSELL. 1979. Immunization against dental caries: further studies. Br. Dent. J. **147:** 9–14.

18. RUSSELL, R. R. B. 1979. Wall-associated protein antigens of *Streptococcus mutans*. J. Gen. Microbiol. **114:** 109–115.

19. LEHNER, T., M. W. RUSSELL, J. CALDWELL & R. SMITH. 1981. Immunization with purified protein antigens from *Streptococcus mutans* against dental caries in Rhesus monkeys. Infect. Immun. **34:** 407–415.

20. CURTISS, R. III, D. A. PEREIRA, J. C. HSU, S. C. HULL, J. E. CLARK, L. J. MATURIN, Sr., R. GOLDSCHMIDT, R. MOODY, M. INOUE & L. ALEXANDER. 1976. Biological containment: the subordination of *Escherichia coli* K-12. In *Recombinant Molecules: Impact on Science and Society*. R. F. Beers, Jr. and E. G. Bassett, Eds.: 45–56. Raven Press. New York.

DISCUSSION OF THE PAPER

T. LEHNER (*Guy's Hospital, London, England*): I am impressed by the cross-reactivity between serotypes, except for serotype *b*, which is a rat strain. Can you tell us whether there is complete or partial cross reactivity, because you have not shown us all the data on this situation?

R. CURTISS (*University of Alabama in Birmingham*): Only partial cross-reactivity occurs here. Hopefully by using the cloned genes from serotypes c, a, and g, we will be able to determine what particular domains in this very large protein are shared and those that are dissimilar.

LEHNER: It also appears that this protein has the two antigen determinants that we called antigens I and II. Have you tried to digest away the antigen I component of this antigen I/II complex to leave the antigen II behind?

CURTISS: Dr. Russell and Dr. Holt in our laboratory have shown that most of the similarity between the *spa* A proteins from serotypes c and g seem to be in the antigen I component.

LEHNER: I was going to ask about the considerable ease with which you have identified the antigen I/II. What about the antigen III/IV? Have you found any other synthesized by *E. coli* that you could use?

CURTISS: We have quite a diversity of recombinant clones that produce at least 10 different *S. mutans* cell-surface proteins, and we just have not characterized all of these. They do not have glucosyltransferase activity. One of the problems is that we have not used the antibodies against antigen III or IV to analyze any of our clones. This method might be the simplest way, assuming that they will also be cross-reactive.

L. J. SAIF (*Ohio Agricultural Research and Development Center*): For your future studies, if you used avirulent enteric strains, do you think that they, indeed, would be able to attach and colonize?

CURTISS: Yes. We are currently using derivatives of *Salmonella* and *Salmonella-Escherichia* hybrids. Others have used a *Salmonella* derivative that lacks the ability to produce enterochelin, and although it is avirulent, this strain still invades. The real problem with their mutant is that it ends up in the spleen, where it persists for several months. We are developing strains that will not get that far, but hopefully, will just hang up in the Peyer's patches.

M. BLAKE (*Rockefeller University, New York, N.Y.*): Do you have evidence that your *E. coli* regulates the genes that you are introducing?

CURTISS: Yes.

BLAKE: Do you have any difficulty with a posttranslational modification problem? Do you think that will be a problem in the future?

CURTISS: The answer to the first question is yes. We do get genes regulated in some cases. Ordinarily, they are constitutively expressed in *E. coli*, in fact, at a very high level. But, a cluster of three or four genes for galactose metabolism are coordinately regulated in *E. coli* in the same manner as they are in *S. mutans*. Although we thought we had an operon, we did not. There are at least three transcriptional units, and one of the gene products actually is a positive regulator acting to cause increased synthesis of the other enzymes in the pathway.

In terms of posttranslation modification, we now have antibodies that are directed at the unique antigenic determinants on some of these proteins made in *S. mutans* that are not present on the proteins made in *E. coli*. These antibodies are now being used to screen for cloning of the genes that would cause the proteins in *E. coli* to be modified. So, by using sequential cloning, we assume that we will be able to demonstrate the synthesis of glycoproteins by recombinant techniques, where we have to introduce genes for several enzymes from the donor—in this case *S. mutans*. This technique should then allow one to look at the different antigens with and without the modifications, in terms of their ability to induce a protective response.

BIOLOGIC FUNCTION OF THE SERUM IgA SYSTEM: MODULATION OF COMPLEMENT-MEDIATED EFFECTOR MECHANISMS AND CONSERVATION OF ANTIGENIC MASS*

J. McLeod Griffiss

Channing Laboratory
Department Of Medicine
Brigham And Women's Hospital
Harvard Medical School
Boston, Massachusetts 02115

INTRODUCTION

The physiologic function of serum IgA remains largely obscure despite a rapid increase in understanding of the secretory IgA immune system.[1] Because the first component of complement does not bind to glycosyl receptors in the alpha-chain hinge region, IgA does not activate complement under biologic conditions. More importantly, it blocks activation of complement, whether initiated directly by binding of complement components or indirectly through binding by IgM or IgG, and regardless of the pathway of activation.[2-4] Thus, serum IgA blocks all complement-mediated immune effector mechanisms, as well as some complement independent mechanisms (TABLE 1). Because unrestricted complement activation would be deleterious, it has been suggested that serum IgA functions as a modulator of complement activation, that is, as an anti-inflammatory Ig.[9]

Studies of the role of serum IgA in the induction of epidemic susceptibility to disseminated meningococcal disease provide data that not only support the hypothesis that serum IgA functions as a regulatory immunoglobulin, but also that serum IgA acts to preserve antigenic mass by shunting small antigenic loads into immune processing cells and away from polymorphonuclear leukocytes (PMN). These data also provide a focus for generalization to other bacteria and other disease states and for the development of a schematic model of the mucosal immune response that incorporates serum IgA.

SERUM IgA AND DISSEMINATED MENINGOCOCCAL DISEASE

It is well established that immune lysis, a complement-mediated effector mechanism initiated by circulating antibody, provides man with a barrier to dissemination of *Neisseria meningitidis* from the upper respiratory mucosa.[10-12] Such bactericidal antibody contributes to maintenance of the normal commensal relationship.[12]

Initially, the absence of bactericidal activity in the serum of individuals at risk of disseminated meningococcal disease was thought to reflect an absence of meningococcal antibody.[13] This interpretation did not take into account differ-

*This work was supported in part by Grant No. AI 15241 and Research Career Development Award No. AI 00328 from the National Institutes of Health, Bethesda, Maryland.

0077-8923/83/0409-0697 $1.75/0 © 1983, NYAS

TABLE 1

IMMUNE EFFECTOR MECHANISMS KNOWN TO BE INHIBITED BY SERUM IGA

Complement-dependent Immune lysis[2] PMN chemotaxis[4-6] PMN phagocytosis[7,8] Cutaneous anaphylaxis[4] Arthus reaction[4]
Complement-independent PMN chemotaxis[9] PMN phagocytosis[7]

ences in initiation of effector functions among Ig isotypes that were not then known. The major circulating Ig isotypes vary greatly in their ability to initiate immune lysis. IgM is invariably bactericidal; the bactericidal capacity of IgG is at best only one-half that of IgM.[14,15] IgG isotypes that activate complement poorly (IgG_2 and IgG_4) may not initiate immune lysis at all, and IgA blocks its initiation by both IgM and IgG.[2] This latter inhibition is antigen specific, that is, both the blocking IgA and the lytic antibody compete for the same antigenic sites.[2]

Blocking of lysis by IgA accounted for the absence of lytic activity in the serum of susceptible military recruits, during an outbreak of groups B, C, and Y disease,[16] and Finnish children during an epidemic of group A disease.[17] For most individuals during epidemics, susceptibility is a function of the presence of meningococcal IgA.[12,16,17]

CONTROL OF CIRCULATING IGA LEVELS

It is one thing to modulate complement activation and quite another to abrogate a major bacterial defense mechanism, thereby exposing the host to sure death. Evolutionary conservation of down-regulation of complement by serum IgA would require that its level be tightly controlled. In FIGURE 1, the concentration of IgA in the serum of a single individual over a period of one month, and at several points over the subsequent six years, is depicted. Except for a single three-day period, day to day variations are within the measurement error of the assay itself, despite continuous antigen processing at mucosal surfaces. Although some variation did occur over the following six years, it is remarkable that five years later, the IgA level was unchanged. This consistency indicates that turnover of serum IgA must be very rapid.[18]

Hepatic clearance now appears to be the primary mechanism by which this consistency is effected.[1] In addition, it has recently been shown that high levels of circulating IgG act to block antigen uptake by Peyer's patches following enteral immunization, thereby suppressing induction of IgA.[19] This suppression is a form of negative feedback control that requires passive diffusion of IgG from serum to gut lumen.

FUNCTIONAL CONTROL OF IGA BLOCKADE

Studies of IgA blockade of immune lysis of N. meningitidis provide evidence of two, more subtle, control mechanisms. In my initial studies, IgA blocking of

IgG-initiated lysis was found to be a function of the ratio of IgA to IgG, suggesting competition by the Ig isotypes for the same binding sites.[2] This competition was subsequently confirmed using dinitrophenyl (DNP)-sensitized erythrocytes and an IgA-myeloma protein.[3] Strain-specific IgG, however, is absent from the sera of susceptibles at the time of bacterial dissemination, although strain-specific IgM is present.[16,20] This fact suggests that IgA blocking of IgM-initiated lysis involves a separate mechanism more sensitive to quantitative changes. To explore this possibility, studies were designed to analyze, qualitatively and quantitatively, the interactions of target cells (organisms), effector molecules (lytic Ig), and inhibitor molecules (IgA).[15]

Blocking by IgA of IgG-initiated immune lysis was again found to be a sigmoidal function of the ratio of lytic to blocking antibody and independent of the concentration of IgG or IgA alone, or of target cells. Complete inhibition occurred at an IgA:IgG ratio of 0.5; that is, an amount of IgA that bound one-half as much antigen as did the IgG completely blocked the latter's initiation of lysis. Activation of complement by IgG requires doublet formation: two molecules of IgG must bind closely enough apposed for a single molecule of complement to bridge their Fc regions.[11] At saturation of antibody-binding sites, one molecule of IgA effectively blocks two molecules of IgG by preventing doublet formation. As a consequence of its competitive nature, IgA blocking of IgG is not affected by changes in inoculum size, does not produce a prozone effect, and is relatively insensitive to changes in IgA concentration within the normal range.[21] Thus, IgG exerts a subtle, functional control over IgA blocking of complement activation, and individuals with strain-specific IgG are not susceptible to the blocking effect of IgA concentrations within the physiologic range.[16,20]

By contrast, IgA blocking of IgM-initiated lysis is a noncompetitive, linear function of the ratio of IgA to antibody binding sites (organisms) and independent of the concentration of IgM. At concentrations of IgA sufficient to saturate antibody binding sites, IgM is an impotent bystander.[15] By virtue of its noncompetitive nature, IgA blocking of IgM is extremely sensitive to changes in IgA

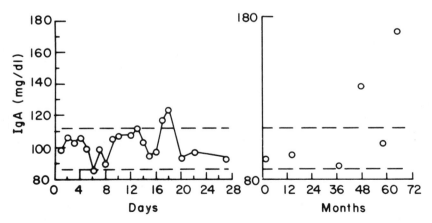

FIGURE 1. Concentration of IgA within the serum of a single individual over a period of one month and at several points over the subsequent six years, as measured by radial immunodiffusion (Behring Werke). The 95% confidence interval of the assay, determined for nine replicate measurements of a control serum, are projected around the initial value (boundary limits).

TABLE 2

CHARACTERISTICS OF IGA BLOCKING OF IMMUNE LYSIS INITIATED BY IGM AND IGG

Characteristic	IgM	IgG
Inhibition	Noncompetitive	Competitive
Ratio	IgA:organisms	IgA:IgG
Complete block	Saturation of antibody binding sites	1 IgA:2 IgG
Inoculum effect	yes	no
Prozone	yes	no
Sensitivity to IgA concentration	high	low
Binding affinity	IgM $\geqslant$ IgA	IgG = IgA

concentration and to inoculum size; a given concentration of IgA will effectively block IgM-initiated lysis of a small inoculum, but have no effect on lysis of a much larger inoculum,[21] provided that IgM concentration is sufficient to saturate the additional binding sites. This inoculum effect provides an additional fail-safe control mechanism. Whereas concentrations of IgA sufficient to completely inhibit lysis of biologically realistic inocula ($<10^3$ organisms/ml) are quite common in human serum, the increase in binding sites on larger and more ominous inocula dilutes their blocking effect, permitting binding by IgM and initiation of complement-mediated defenses. Although only of serologic interest, it should be noted that IgA produces a prozone with IgM, an indication that complete block would result if smaller inocula were tested.[21]

Neither of the two mechanisms described above is dependent upon differences in Ig-binding affinity—at least as measured by disassociation constants.[15] The molecular basis for IgA blocking of IgG and IgM remains totally unknown. The two blocking mechanisms are summarized in TABLE 2; IgA control mechanisms are summarized in TABLE 3.

ANTIBACTERIAL EFFECT OF IGA

If serum IgA provides a generalized, and precisely and redundantly controlled, mechanism for the prevention of complement activation by insignificant inocula, it must also provide for their clearance. Although IgA does not opsonize for PMN phagocytosis, it does opsonize for a complement-independent bactericidal activity of monocytes.[22,23] Presumably, this anti-bacterial mechanism involves phagocytosis, since IgA does not appear to initiate antibody-dependent cellular cytotoxicity,[24] and intrinsic radiolabel was not released during cell death (unpublished observation). Regardless of its nature, monocyte-macrophage anti-bacterial activity would provide for clearance of modest inocula of IgA-opsonized

TABLE 3

CONTROL OF BLOCKING EFFECTS OF SERUM IGA

Inoculum effect limitation (IgM)
Rapid hepatic clearance
Competitive damping by IgG

Suppression of IgA induction at Peyer's patch level (IgG)

organisms. In turn, phagocytosis by monocyte-macrophages would facilitate presentation of bacterial antigens to other limbs of the immune system, enhancing subsequent immune response and leading to a reversal of IgA blockade. In effect, opsonization by IgA would effectively shunt small inocula away from phagocytosis by PMN—an immunological dead end—and into monocyte-macrophages—an immunological beginning, thus preserving antigenic mass for optimal immune processing. Enhancement of the immune response to soluble antigens by complexing with specific IgA has been demonstrated in mice.[25]

INDUCTION OF SERUM IgA

An understanding of the kinetics of induction of serum IgA is necessary for understanding both its physiologic role and its relationship to the epidemiology of meningococcal disease. Induction requires priming of either the gut-associated lymphorecticular tissue (Peyer's patches or GALT) or its analog along the bronchial tree, bronchial-associated lymphoreticular tissue, (BALT). Certainly the meningococcus is an unlikely colonizer of the gastrointestinal tract, but colonization of deep bronchial surfaces would result in pneumonia. The most obvious assumption, that nasopharyngeal colonization augments serum IgA, is not a satisfactory explanation, because established carriers never develop disseminated disease.[12] The time between exposure and dissemination is extremely short in noncolonized individuals who do develop disease,[26] and the route of priming is not explained by nasopharyngeal colonization.

The parsimony of antigenic expression among microorganisms of diverse genera[27] provides an alternative hypothesis.[12] The normal enteric flora contain several bacteria that elaborate surface antigens that are immunochemically identical to those of N. meningitidis. Unapparent colonization by these bacteria might be the stimulus for meningococcal IgA antibody.[12] Immunologically, it is the chemical structure of antigens, rather than the biochemical attributes of the elaborating microorganism, that is important.

To test this hypothesis, I colonized myself with a strain of Streptococcus faecalis isolated from the rectal culture of an alcoholic habitué of the skid row community of Seattle, Washington, during an epidemic of disseminated group A meningococcal disease among the skid row populations of the U.S. Pacific Northwest.[28] This S. faecalis strain elaborates a surface polymer of mannosamine phosphate that is immunologically indistinguishable from the capsular polysaccharide of group A N. meningitidis.

Colonization was accomplished by drinking 50 ml of an overnight culture (Todd-Hewitt broth) suspended in one-half pint of milk. Rectal, nasopharyngeal cultures, and serum samples were obtained daily. Cultures were performed on "halo plates" containing equine antiserum raised to viable group A N. meningitidis. This technique provided rapid identification of aerobic bacteria elaborating the group A capsular polysaccharide.

IgA, IgG, and IgM specific for the group A capsular polysaccharide were each quantified in each of the serum samples by the method of Käyhty.[29] Briefly, the total group A polysaccharide binding capacity and the concentration of antigen that would be around 20% bound were determined by $(NH_4)_2SO_4$ precipitation[30] for each sample. Each sample was then reassayed using this antigen concentration and immune precipitation. Goat anti-human IgM, IgG, and IgA (heavy chain specific) were each added to separate tubes at a concentration previously determined to maximally precipitate antibody of their respective isotypes.[29] In addition, serum was processed so as to preserve intrinsic complement and its lytic activity determined for the strain of group A *N. meningitidis* responsible for the outbreak in Seattle.

In FIGURE 2, certain preliminary data are depicted. Colonization with the study strain of *S. faecalis* was apparent for two periods during the first two weeks after ingestion. The break in stool recovery may represent insensitivity of the recovery technique or "curing" of colonization, followed by recolonization from the newly contaminated environment. Over the first 12 days of colonization, IgA concentration declined by 25%, but increased sharply on day 13 and continued to rise over the next five days. By contrast, IgM concentration remained stable for

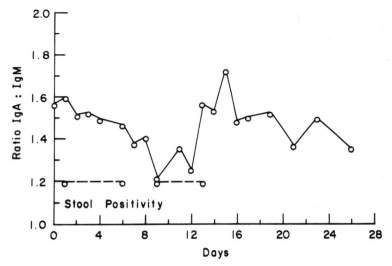

FIGURE 2. Ratio of group A meningococcal capsular polysaccharide IgA to IgM in the serum of a single individual following intentional enteric colonization. The test strain was a group A *Neisseria meningitidis*; the colonizing strain was a *Streptococcus faecalis* that elaborates a surface antigenic structure that is identical to the Group A meningococcal capsule. Days during which the *S. faecalis* strain was recovered on stool culture are indicated (Positive stool, O---O). Specific IgA and IgM were determined by radioimmunoprecipitin, utilizing intrinsically labeled group A capsular polysaccharide. Pertubations in the observed ratio reflect, primarily, alterations in specific IgA.

the first nine days and then dropped by 12% over days eleven to fifteen. IgG concentration remained stable throughout the period of observation; total binding capacity reflected changes in IgA concentration. The observed changes in IgA concentration did not reflect changes in total serum IgA (FIGURE 1). Fluctuations in specific IgA and IgM are depicted as the ratio in FIGURE 2. The marked increase in the ratio of IgA to IgM following curing of colonization coincided with a sharp decrease in lytic capacity for the study strain of group A *N. meningitidis*.[11] The significance of these changes cannot be tested statistically, because each serum sample is dependent, in a statistical sense, on the previous sample. A time-series statistical model for application to these data is currently being developed.

These data clearly demonstrate pertubations in specific Ig isotypes within stable overall concentrations attendant upon neocolonization and the limited duration of such changes. The sharp rise in specific IgA, coincidental with a decline in specific IgM and in total lytic capacity, are quite consistent with those reported for the serum IgA response to *Vibrio cholerae* colonization.[31] They also demonstrate the difficulty of studying the question epidemiologically: if the maximum serum IgA reponse occurs after "curing" of colonization, then individuals who have sickened because of high IgA levels would no longer be carriers of the inducting enteric organism.

These data are quite preliminary, and the kinetics of IgA induction during epidemics of meningococcal disease remain unclear. For example, nasopharyngeal presentation of the cross-reacting antigen by the meningococcus may also be required for induction of high levels of serum IgA.[17] Regardless of the exact details, the scenario proposed here and in reference 12 remains logical and feasible and is supported by what little data are available.

RELATIONSHIP OF SERUM IgA TO MUCOSAL IMMUNITY

FIGURE 3 depicts a schematic model of the IgA-immune system that combines aspects of the serum response presented above with what is known of the secretory reponse. Critical to this synthesis is the observation of Cantey, *et al.*, that bacterial binding to Peyer's patches precedes binding to villus epithelium for a strain of encapsulated *Escherichia coli*.[32,33] Assuming that binding to Peyer's patches induces antigen specific IgA-precursor cells, IgA would be produced prior to the possible transit of the bacteria through the villus epithelium. Upon entrance into lymph channels or circulation, such bacteria would be immediately opsonized with IgA, preventing complement activation and facilitating uptake by monocytes-macrophage, particularly Kupffer cells. Excess IgA would be removed by hepatic cells, whereas IgM would remain constant or increase modestly as a result of immune processing of phagocytosed bacteria. Meanwhile, antigen specific IgA-plasma cells would have seeded distal mucosal sites, arming the host against bacteria presenting this antigen. In the absence of further stimulation, IgA-plasma cells would die and serum IgA and IgM levels decline, making room for the products of newly stimulated immunocyte clones. Alternatively, if the same antigen were to be presented to mucosal surfaces, a brisk secretory IgA response would ensue; if presented parenterally, IgM, followed by IgG, would be produced, influenced by activated macrophages. IgG would damp IgA blockade, opsonize bacteria for PMN clearance, and suppress IgA induction at the gut level by competing for antigen intraluminally. This sequence of events would follow enteral presentation of each new antigen, as well as stimulation of BALT. In this way, the gut- and bronchial-associated lymphoreticular tissues would act as immune sentinels, sampling environmental antigens, encountered in the food we eat and the air we breathe, respectively.

CLINICAL IMPLICATIONS

Despite the redundancy of controls, the system remains delicately balanced. Pathologic states that interfere with hepatic clearance of serum IgA, such as severe cirrhosis, result in the accumulation of oligoclonal serum IgA that inhibits chemotaxis[5,6] and prevents complement-mediated bacterial clearance, resulting

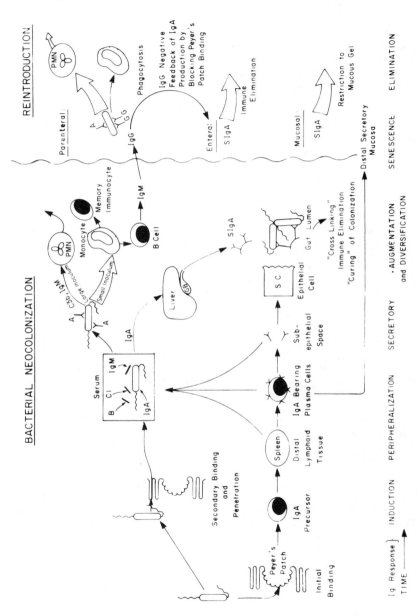

FIGURE 3. Schematic representation of the relationship of the serum IgA response to other components of mucosal immunity. See text for details. Cl = complement.

in sepsis.[20] Significantly, when cirrhotic patients become septic, specific IgG is absent from their serum.[20]

Because the phagocytic capacity of the monocyte-macrophage compartment is finite, if unmeasured in man, it could be exceeded by IgA-opsonized bacteria. This situation would seem more likely in infants, in whom the absolute capacity would be reduced. In addition, clinical states that decrease the monocyte-macrophage compartment (siderosis, chemotherapy) might create conditions in which a normal IgA response might be deleterious.

Finally, it is clear that the epidemic induction of aberrantly high specific IgA levels accounts for outbreaks of meningococcal meningitis, although the inducing events remain uncertain.

CONCLUSION

Clearly, IgA possesses ideal properties for a regulatory molecule: the effects of IgA are highly specific (antigen-binding) and subject to the same regulation as other components of the immune system; IgA has a short half-life (rapid turnover); IgA's regulatory effects are redundantly controlled; and IgA initiates an alternative defense mechanism. The induction of IgA following mucosal colonization insures its presence in the circulation when its regulatory effect is needed and provides an additional dimension to overall mucosal immunity. As with all physiologic regulatory mechanisms, disturbances and imbalances may have pathologic consequences.

ACKNOWLEDGMENT

I would like to thank Barbara Chamberlain for assistance in the preparation of this manuscript.

REFERENCES

1. RUSSELL, M. W., T. A. BROWN & J. MESTECKY. 1981. Role of serum IgA. Hepatobiliary transport of circulating antigen. J. Exp. Med. **153:** 968–976.
2. GRIFFISS, J. McL. 1975. Bactericidal activity of meningococcal antiserum. Blocking by IgA of lytic antibody in human convalescent sera. J. Immunol. **114:** 1779–1784.
3. RUSSELL-JONES, G. J., P. L. EY & B. L. REYNOLDS. 1980. The ability of IgA to inhibit complement-mediated lysis of target red blood cells sensitized with IgG antibody. Mol. Immunol. **17:** 1173–1180.
4. RUSSELL-JONES, G. J. 1980. The inhibition of complement-mediated phenomena by IgA. (Thesis). Univer. of Adelaide, Adelaide, South Australia.
5. VAN EPPS, D. E. & R. C. WILLIAMS, JR. 1976. Suppression of leukocyte chemotaxis by human IgA myeloma components. J. Exp. Med. **144:** 1227–1242.
6. MADERAZO, E. G., P. A. WARD & R. QUINTILIANI. 1975. Defective regulation of chemotaxis in cirrhosis. J. Lab. Clin. Med. **85:** 621–630.
7. VAN EPPS, D. E., K. REED & R. C. WILLIAMS, JR. 1978. Suppression of human PMN bactericidal activity by human IgA paraproteins. Cell. Immunol. **36:** 363–376.
8. WILTON, J. M. A. 1978. Suppression by IgA of IgG mediated phagocytosis by human polymorphonuclear leukocytes. Clin. Exp. Immunol. **34:** 423–428.
9. VAN EPPS, D. E. & S. L. BROWN. 1981. Inhibition of formylmethionyl-leucyl-phenylalanine-stimulated neutrophil chemiluminescence by human immunoglobulin A paraproteins. Infect. Immun. **34:** 864–870.

10. GRIFFISS, J. McL. 1982. Human serum IgA and susceptibility to disseminated meningococcal disease. *In* Bacterial Vaccines. Seminars in Infectious Diseases. L. Weinstein and B. N. Fields, Eds.: Vol. **4**: 13–18. Theime-Stratton. New York.
11. GRIFFISS, J. McL. 1982. Serum IgA: Modulation of complement activation and induction of susceptibility to bacterial dissemination. Infection. **10**: 246–251.
12. GRIFFISS, J. McL. 1982. Epidemic meningococcal disease: Synthesis of a hypothetical immunoepidemiologic model. Rev. Infect. Dis. **4**: 159–172.
13. GOLDSCHNEIDER, I., E. C. GOTSCHLICH & M. S. ARTENSTEIN. 1969. Human immunity to the meningococcus. I. The role of humoral antibodies. J. Exp. Med. **129**: 1307–1326.
14. FRANK, M. M. 1979. Complement system in host defense and inflammation. Rev. Infect. Dis. **1**: 483–501.
15. GRIFFISS, J. McL. & D. K. GOROFF. 1983. IgA blocks IgM and IgG initiated immune lysis by separate molecular mechanisms. J. Immunol. **130**. In press.
16. GRIFFISS, J. McL. & M. A. BERTRAM. 1977. Immunoepidemiology of meningococcal disease in military recruits. II. Blocking of serum bactericidal activity by circulating IgA early in the course of invasive disease. J. Infect. Dis. **136**: 733–739.
17. KÄYHTY H., H. JOUSIMIES-SOMER, H. PELTOLA & H. MÄKELÄ. 1981. Antibody response to capsular polysaccharides of A and C *Neisseria meningitidis* and *Haemophilus influenzae* type b during bacteremic disease. J. Infect. Dis. **143**: 32–41.
18. TOMASI, T. B., JR. 1968. Human immunoglobulin A. N. Engl. J. Med. **279**: 1327–1330.
19. PIERCE, N. F. 1980. Suppression of the intestinal immune response to cholera toxin by specific serum antibody. Infect. Immun. **30**: 62–68.
20. FIERER, J. & F. FINLEY. 1979. Deficient serum bactericidal activity against *Escherichia coli* in patients with cirrhosis of the liver. J. Clin. Invest. **63**: 912–921.
21. GRIFFISS, J. McL. & D. K. GOROFF. Inoculum sensitivity of IgA blockade of immune lysis of *Neisseria meningitidis*. Submitted.
22. LOWELL, G. H., L. S. SMITH, J. McL. GRIFFISS, B. L. BRANDT & R. P. MACDERMOTT. 1980. Antibody-dependent mononuclear cell-mediated anti-meningococcal activity. Comparison of the lytic effects of convalescent and post-immunization immunoglobulins G, M, and A. J. Clin. Invest. **66**: 260–267.
23. LOWELL, G. H., L. S. SMITH, J. McL. GRIFFISS & B. L. BRANDT. 1980. IgA-dependent monocyte-mediated antibacterial activity. J. Exp. Med. **152**: 452–457.
24. FANGER, M. W., L. SHEN, J. PUGH & G. M. BERNIER. 1980. Subpopulations of human peripheral granulocytes and monocytes express receptors for IgA. Proc. Natl. Acad. Sci. USA **77**: 3640–3644.
25. STOKES, C. R., E. T. SWARBRICK & J. R. SOOTHILL. 1980. Immune elimination and enhanced antibody responses: functions of circulating IgA. Immunology **40**: 455–458.
26. EDWARDS, E. A., L. F. DEVINE, C. H. SINGBUSCH & H. W. WARD. 1977. Immunological investigations of meningococcal disease. III. Brevity of group C acquisitions prior to disease occurrence. Scand. J. Infect. Dis. **9**: 105–110.
27. GRIFFISS, J. McL. & GOROFF, D.K. 1981. Immunological cross-reaction between a naturally occurring galactan, agarose, and an LPS locus for immune lysis of *Neisseria meningitidis* by human sera. Clin. Exp. Immunol. **43**: 20–27.
28. GRIFFISS, J. McL., B. L. BRANDT, D. GREGORY, G. A. FILICE & G. W. COUNTS. 1977. Epidemic group A meningococcal disease in the Pacific Northwest—an immunologic paradox. Clin. Res. **25**: 376 A.
29. KÄYHTY, H. 1980. Comparison of passive hemagglutination, bactericidal activity and radioimmunological methods in measuring antibody responses to *Neisseria meningitidis* group A capsular polysaccharide vaccine. J. Clin. Microbiol. **12**: 256–263.
30. BRANDT, B. L., M. S. ARTENSTEIN & C. D. SMITH. 1973. Antibody responses to meningococcal polysaccharides. Infect. Immun. **8**: 590–596.
31. WALDMAN, R. H., Z. BENCIC, R. SAKAZAKI, R. SINHA, R. GANGULY, B. C. DEB & S. MUKERJEE. 1971. Cholera Immunology. I. Immunoglobulin levels in serum, fluid from the small intestine, and feces from patients with cholera and noncholerraic diarrhea during illness and convalescence. J. Infect. Dis. **123**: 579–586.

32. CANTEY, J. R., W. B. LUSHBAUGH & L. R. INMAN. 1981. Attachment of bacteria to intestinal epithelial cells in diarrhea caused by *Escherichia coli* strain RDEC-1 in the rabbit: stages and role of capsule. J. Infect. Dis. **143:** 219–230.
33. CANTEY, J. R. & L. R. INMAN. 1981. Diarrhea due to *Escherichia coli* strain RDEC-1 in the rabbit. The Peyer's patch as the initial site of attachment in colonization. J. Infect. Dis. **143:** 440–446.

———————◆———————

DISCUSSION OF THE PAPER

D. F. KEREN (*The University of Michigan, Ann Arbor, Mich.*): I have a question about the functional significance of IgA. The most common type of isolated antibody in the kidney is IgA; it is usually found with complement and not with other immunoglobulin classes. Do you think what you have described is a general phenomenon, and that IgA blocks all these complement pathways? Alternatively, is IgA peculiar to bacteria, perhaps to meningococcus?

J. M. GRIFFISS (*Harvard Medical School, Boston, Mass.*): This question is one of aggregation. Aggregated IgA will activate complement, both through the alternative pathway and the classical pathway. The antigenic array of epitopes on the surface of bacteria is such that aggregation cannot occur. In the kidney, where clumps of IgA are brought into the mesangium, complement activation could occur. This question is simply a matter of a steric array of antigens on the surface of the bacteria, against which is the natural situation that we have to defend ourselves.

PASSIVE IMMUNITY TO TRANSMISSIBLE GASTROENTERITIS VIRUS: INTRAMAMMARY VIRAL INOCULATION OF SOWS*

Linda J. Saif and E. H. Bohl

Ohio Agricultural Research and Development Center
Department of Veterinary Science
Wooster, Ohio 44691

INTRODUCTION

Transmissible gastroenteritis (TGE) is a highly contagious enteric coronaviral disease of swine with a high mortality rate in pigs under two weeks of age. The TGE virus primarily infects the small intestinal villous epithelium causing villous atrophy and severe diarrhea.[1] Our previous reports have indicated that optimal passive immunity to TGE is related to frequent ingestion of milk containing high titers of sIgA neutralizing antibody.[2-7] Additional studies have focused upon methods to stimulate these IgA antibodies in swine mammary secretions.[2-7]

Although evidence supports the concept that the mammary gland is part of the mucosal immune system characterized by a predominance of locally synthesized sIgA in external secretions[8-10] and a preponderance of IgA plasmacytes adjacent to the secretory epithelia,[8,11,12] the origin of these cells was obscure until recently. It is well documented from early studies with TGE virus and *Escherichia coli* in swine,[2-7,13] and subsequent studies using a variety of antigens in many other species including man,[14-18] that specificities of milk sIgA reflect prior antigen encounters in the intestinal tract. We initially reported evidence for a gut-mammary immunologic link after observing that TGE viral antibodies of the sIgA type occurred in milk of swine only as a result of previous viral infection of the gut.[2-7] Based on this finding, we originally proposed that IgA TGE-sensitized immunocytes may migrate from the gut to the mammary gland.[2,3] Direct proof of this entero-mammary-immunologic axis came from recent cell migration investigations that have shown that lymphoblasts, most of which are committed to IgA synthesis, migrate from gut-associated lymphoreticular tissue (GALT) to the lamina propria of the intestine[19] and also to the mammary gland during late pregnancy and lactation.[20,21]

Whereas antigen administered orally generally elicits sIgA antibodies in milk, contradictory results exist concerning stimulation of sIgA milk antibodies in monogastric animals by direct mammary gland inoculation with various antigens. Previous studies of intramammary inoculation of pregnant swine with TGE virus[2-4] or *Escherichia coli*[13] have shown that only IgG antibodies are elicited in mammary secretions. Other studies have reported either an IgG-[22] or an IgA-antibody response in milk after direct injection of the mammary glands of pregnant swine, rabbits, guinea pigs, or rats with various antigens.[23-27]

This study addresses the question of the lacteal entrance of an enteric virus in

*This investigation was supported in part by Public Health Service Research Grant AI-10735 from the National Institute of Allergy and Infectious Diseases and by special grant 59-2392-0-2-068-0 from the Science and Education Administration, U.S. Department of Agriculture.

lactating animals either artificially by way of injection or naturally through infected piglets as a possible means of priming or boosting the sIgA antibody response in milk. In the present report, the immune response of the nonlactating or lactating mammary gland is examined after direct injection of a live viral antigen (TGE virus). Specific antibody titers and the immunoglobulin isotypes of these antibodies in mammary secretions from intramammarily injected seronegative and seropositive (orally primed) sows are compared.

MATERIALS AND METHODS

Experimental Animals

Four pregnant swine were obtained from the Ohio Agricultural Research and Development Center swine herds. All swine except one (sow #3683) were serologically negative for TGE antibodies by the plaque reduction virus neutralization test prior to viral inoculation. Sow #3683 had previously been naturally infected with TGE virus and had serum and milk TGE antibodies at the time of inoculation. Two animals had farrowed previously (#19-2 & #3683), whereas the other two were first litter gilts (#3634 & #1452).

Viruses

The TGE viruses used in this study were described in detail previously.[2] A live-attenuated high passaged Purdue strain of TGE virus was serially passaged 116 times in primary porcine kidney cell cultures and is referred to as the P-116 strain. The virus titer was 7.5×10^6 plaque-forming units (PFU)/ml. A commercial live-modified TGE virus, Porsivac (Fort Dodge Laboratories, Fort Dodge, Iowa) was used in one animal (gilt #3634). Virulent TGE virus of gut origin, referred to as the Miller #4 strain was used for challenge of suckling pigs. All piglets of a litter except one contact control were orally challenged with two ml of a 1:100 dilution of the Miller #4 virus at three to four weeks postfarrowing. Piglets from gilt #3634 were orally challenged a second time at 37 days postfarrowing (DPF) with undiluted virulent TGE virus.

Intramammary Vaccination

Prior to inoculation, mammary glands were sprayed with a local topical anesthetic spray (benzocaine). All animals were intramammarily injected (IMm) into each of three glands on the left side of the udder using a 20-gauge one-inch needle. Two ml of virus were injected into the mammary tissue at the base of each teat. Sows were injected and litters challenged as outlined in TABLE 1.

Immunofluorescent (IF) Staining

A cell-culture immunofluorescent test was used for detection of TGE virus from milk and rectal swab fluid (one swab in four ml of tissue culture fluid). This test was performed on centrifuged (800 × g for 30 minutes) milk and rectal swab fluid in swine testes cells as described previously.[28] A few milk samples were also

INTRAMAMMARY VACCINATION OF SOWS WITH TGE VIRUS: EXPERIMENTAL PROTOCOL

Sow	TGE Antibody Status	Time of Vaccination DPF	Virus Strain	Challenge of Piglets/DPF
1452	Seronegative	22 and 8 days prefarrowing	Purdue (P-116) TGE	—
3634	Seronegative	3 DPF	Porsivac TGE (Ft Dodge)	+/24,37
19-2	Seronegative	4 DPF	Purdue (P-116) TGE	+/26
3683	Naturally infected (seropositive)	3 DPF	Purdue (P-116) TGE	+/23

titrated for infectious virus by a plaque test in swine testes cells. A direct IF staining procedure was used on small intestinal mucosal smears from euthanatized piglets to confirm TGE infection.[29]

Collection of Specimens and Antibody Titrations

Methods used for collection and processing of serum and milk from sows were the same as described previously.[3] Milk was always collected from the three injected glands (inj. glds.) and pooled. It was also collected from at least three noninjected glands on the noninjected side (NI glds-NI side) of the udder. These samples were also pooled. In two animals (#3634 & #3681) milk was also collected and pooled from the noninjected glands on the injected side (NI glds-inj. side) of the udder. A plaque reduction test was used for detection of TGE virus and OSU (Ohio State University) porcine rotavirus virus neutralizing antibodies,[2,30] and titers were expressed as the reciprocal of the sample dilution, resulting in an 80% reduction in plaques.

Gel Filtration

Gel filtration using Biogel A-1.5m (BioRad Laboratories, Richmond, Calif.) and 0.1 M Tris-0.2 M NaCl buffer, pH 8 was conducted as described previously.[3] The optical density (O.D.) of the collected fractions (4 ml) was determined at 280 nanometers. Selected fractions were tested for porcine IgM, IgA, and IgG by the micromodification of Ouchterlony's double immunodiffusion test, using monospecific rabbit anti-porcine IgM, sIgA, and IgG antisera prepared as described earlier.[3] These fractions were also tested for TGE antibodies by the plaque reduction virus neutralization test.

RESULTS

Intramammary Inoculation of a Seronegative Pregnant Gilt

The antibody titers in serum and milk of gilt #1452 are summarized in TABLE 2. Also shown are the immunoglobulin isotypes of TGE antibodies in milk. Milk antibody titers from injected glands were consistently higher than titers in milk from noninjected glands (1.5–2.5 times higher). Gel filtration studies of 3 and 34

DPF milk indicated TGE antibodies were primarily associated with IgG fractions (third peak) and with lower titers in the sIgA fractions (second peak), especially at 3 DPF (TABLE 2). Piglets in this litter were not challenged and the sow's serum and milk antibody titers decreased greatly throughout the lactation period.

Intramammary Inoculation of Seronegative Lactating Swine

Virus Shedding

Following IMm vaccination of gilt #3634, shedding of TGE virus was detected in high titers in milk from injected glands only, at one and three days postvaccination (DPV, TABLE 3). All nine nursing piglets developed mild diarrhea and six of the nine piglets shed TGE virus in feces at three to nine DPV of this gilt (TABLE 3). One diarrheic piglet was euthanatized at five DPV and small intestinal mucosal smears were positive for TGE viral antigen in intestinal epithelial cells as determined by IF staining.

After oral challenge of eight piglets with virulent TGE virus at 24 DPF, only one piglet developed mild diarrhea at two days postexposure (DPE, TABLE 3). This piglet was euthanatized at three DPE, and small intestinal smears were IF negative for TGE viral antigen. After a second oral challenge with undiluted virulent TGE virus at 37 DPF, all nursing piglets remained clinically normal, and shedding of TGE virus was not detected by the cell-culture immunofluorescent test on rectal specimens collected at one to seven DPE. No virus was detected in rectal swabs collected from gilt #3634 throughout this experiment (TABLE 3), nor was this gilt observed sick or with diarrhea, either after IMm vaccination or after the challenge of her suckling piglets.

Similar TGE virus shedding patterns were detected for sow 19-2 and her piglets after IMm vaccination of this sow (TABLE 4). Virus was shed in high titers

TABLE 2

TGE ANTIBODY TITERS IN SERUM AND MILK AND IN THE IgA AND IgG FRACTIONS OF MILK FROM INTRAMAMMARILY VACCINATED GILT 1452. PIGLETS WERE NOT CHALLENGED.

			TGE Antibody Titer*					
				Milk				
Days Pre- or Postfarrowing (DPF)	Days Postvaccination (DPV)	Serum	Inj. Glds.†			NI Glds.–NI Side		
			Whey	IgA‡	IgG‡	Whey	IgA	IgG
−22	0	<1						
−8	14	40						
3	25	390	1,700	20	170	700	2.4	80
13	35		>1,024			550		
20	42	320	130			90		
34	55	28	160	3.5	9.2	87	2.6	5.3

*Reciprocal of dilution giving an 80% plaque reduction of TGE virus.

†Mammary glands 1, 3, and 6 on the left side of the udder were injected with Purdue (P-116) strain of live-attenuated TGE virus at 22 and 8 days prefarrowing. This gilt was seronegative for TGE antibodies at the time of the first injection. NI = noninjected.

‡Milk whey was fractionated on Biogel A-1.5m columns and peak fractions tested for immunoglobulins and TGE antibodies.

TABLE 3

DETECTION OF TGE VIRUS IN MILK FROM INTRAMAMMARILY VACCINATED SOW 3634 AND RECTAL SWABS FROM HER PIGLETS USING A CELL CULTURE-IF TEST

Days Postfarrowing →	3	4	6	10	11	12	13	24	25	26	27	28	30
Pig No. / Days Postexposure	0*	1	3	7	8	9	10	0†	1	2	3	4	6
1	—	—	−2	−2	−1	—	—	—	—	—	—	—	—
2	—	—	+1	−1	—	—	—	—	—	—	—	—	—
3	—	—	+2	+3	+1	—	—	—	—	—	—	—	—
4	—	—	+3	+2	−1	—	—	—	—	−1	−1¶	—	—
5	—	—	+3	+2§									
6	—	—	−2	−3	−1	—	—	—	—	—	—	—	—
7	—	−1‡	−2	+1	−1	—	—	—	—	—	—	—	—
8	—	—	−2	−2	−1	—	—	—	—	—	—	—	—
9	—	+1	−1	−1	−1	—	—	—	—	—	—	—	—
Sow 3634	—	—	—	—	—	—	—	—	—	—	—	—	—

Milk

	3	4	6	10
Inj. glds.‖	—	+	+	—
NI glds.-inj. side**	—	—	—	—
NI glds.-NI side††	—	—	—	—

*Days postintramammary vaccination of the sow.
†Days postoral challenge of pigs with virulent TGE virus.
‡Subscript indicates diarrhea: 1 = pasty stool; 2 = semiliquid stool; 3 = liquid stool.
§Pig no. 5 was euthanatized at 11 days of age, and enterocytes were IF positive for TGE.
¶Pig no. 4 was euthanatized at 27 days of age and enterocytes were IF negative for TGE.
‖Mammary glands 1, 3, and 4 on the left side of the udder were injected with live attenuated Porsivac TGE virus (Ft. Dodge Laboratories, Iowa).
**NI glds.-inj. side = Noninjected glands on the injected side (left).
††NI glds.-NI side = Noninjected glands on the noninjected side (right).

TABLE 4

DETECTION OF TGE VIRUS IN MILK FROM INTRAMAMMARILY VACCINATED SOW 19-2 AND RECTAL SWABS FROM HER PIGLETS USING A CELL CULTURE-IF TEST

Days Postfarrowing →	4	5	6	9	10	11	12	18	26	27	30	31	32
Pig No. / Days Postexposure	0*	1	2	5	6	7	8	14	0†	1	4	5	6
1	—		+	+	−1	−2	−2						
2	—		+	—	—			−3¶					
3	—			—	+3§								
4	—		−	+	+2	−2	—	−3			—	−1	−2
5	—			—	−2	−1	—	−1	—	−1	+1	−1	—
6	—			—	−1	−2	−2	−3	—	—	+2	+2	−1
7	—			+2‡	−2	+3	−2	—	—	—	—	−1	—
Sow 19-2	—	—	—	—	—	—	—	—	—	—	—	—	—

Milk

	4	5	6	9	10	11	12	18	26	27	30	31	32
Inj. glds.‖	—	+	+	+				—					
NI glds.-NI side**	—	—	—	—									

*Days postintramammary vaccination of the sow.
†Days postoral challenge of pigs with virulent TGE virus.
‡Subscript indicates diarrhea: 1 = pasty stool; 2 = semiliquid stool; 3 = liquid stool.
§Pig no. 3 was euthanatized at 10 days of age; enterocytes were IF positive for TGE.
¶Pig no. 2 was euthanatized at 18 days of age; enterocytes were IF negative for TGE.
‖Mammary glands 1, 3, and 4 on the left side of the udder were injected with Purdue (P-116) strain of live-attenuated TGE virus at four DPF.
**Noninjected glands on the noninjected side (right).

(1.5 × 10⁵ PFU/ml) in milk from injected glands only at one, two, and five DPV. Six of seven nursing piglets developed mild diarrhea and five of the seven piglets shed TGE virus in feces at five to seven DPV of the sow. A diarrheic piglet euthanatized at six DPV was IF positive for TGE viral antigen in small intestinal mucosal smears. After oral challenge of four piglets with virulent TGE virus at 26 DPF, all four developed mild diarrhea, and two piglets shed virus in their feces at four to five DPE (TABLE 4). No virus was detected in rectal swabs from sow 19-2, nor was this sow sick either after IMm vaccination or challenge of her suckling piglets.

Antibody Response

TGE antibody titers in serum and milk and immunoglobulin isotypes of these milk antibodies from gilt #3634 are summarized in TABLE 5. Also shown are the rotavirus antibody titers in milk from this animal. TGE antibody titers in milk from injected glands were greater than titers in milk from noninjected glands. There was an increase in milk TGE antibody titers after challenge of the piglets with virulent virus (24 DPF) even though virus shedding by the sow or piglets was not observed at this time. Rotavirus milk antibody titers (presumably due to previous natural infection of this sow with rotavirus) were not consistently higher in milk from injected versus noninjected glands. Milk TGE antibodies from both injected and noninjected glands were associated with only IgM (first peak) and sIgA (second peak) fractions at 17 DPF (FIGURE 1) and only sIgA and IgG fractions at 45 DPF (TABLE 5).

Summarized in TABLE 6 are the TGE serum antibody titers and both TGE and rotavirus milk antibody titers from sow 19-2. Also shown are the immunoglobulin isotypes of milk TGE antibodies as indicated by gel filtration studies. Similar to the previous animal, TGE antibody titers in milk from injected glands were consistently greater (about 1.5–4 times greater) than titers from noninjected glands and greater or equal to serum titers except for the 44 DPF sample. In comparison, rotavirus milk antibody titers (presumably due to previous natural infection) were not consistently higher in milk from injected versus noninjected glands (TABLE 6). Serum and milk TGE antibody titers of this sow increased greatly (3.5–20 times) following oral challenge of her nursing piglets, two of which shed virus after challenge. As in gilt #3634, TGE antibodies in milk at 23 DPF from both injected and noninjected glands of this sow were present in both IgM and sIgA Biogel fractions with only very low titers in IgG fractions. At 45 DPF, TGE antibody activity was mainly detected in the sIgA and IgG fractions of milk.

Intramammary Inoculation of a Naturally Infected Lactating Sow

TGE antibody titers in serum and milk of sow #3683 are summarized in TABLE 7 as are the immunoglobulin isotypes of milk TGE antibodies. After IMm vaccination, both serum and milk antibody titers increased greatly with milk titers greater than those in serum (except at 35 DPF). Milk antibody titers were always greatest in milk from the injected glands followed by lower milk titers from noninjected glands on the injected side and usually lowest in milk from glands on the noninjected side. After challenge of nursing piglets at 23 DPF with virulent TGE virus, both serum and milk antibody titers increased slightly. Biogel column chromatography of milk indicated that TGE antibodies were primarily associated

TABLE 5

ANTIBODY TITERS IN SERUM AND MILK AND IN THE IgM, IgA, AND IgG FRACTIONS OF MILK FROM INTRAMAMMARILY VACCINATED GILT 3634. PIGLETS WERE CHALLENGED WITH VIRULENT TGE VIRUS AT 24 DPF.

Days Postfarrowing (DPF)	Days Postvaccination (DPV)	TGE Antibody Titer*										Rotavirus Antibody Titer[a]	
		Serum	Milk									Milk	
			TGE Inj. Glds.†				NI Glds.-Inj. Side	NI Glds.-NI Side				TGE Inj. Glds.	NI Glds.
			Whey	IgM‡	IgA‡	IgG‡	Whey	Whey	IgM	IgA	IgG		
3	0	<1	<1				<1	<1				280	230
10	7	67	98				21	34					
17	14	1300	460	31	4.5	<1	100	140	1.7	2.2	<1	320	200
31	28		390				70	92				240	330
45	42	>1024	760	<1	24	125	>256	>256	<1	28	105	420	540

*Reciprocal of dilution giving an 80% plaque reduction of TGE virus or OSU porcine rotavirus.
†Mammary glands 1, 3, and 4 on the left side of the udder were injected with Porsivac TGE virus (Fort Dodge Laboratories, Iowa) at three DPF. This gilt was seronegative for TGE antibodies at the time of injection, but had been naturally infected with rotavirus.
‡Milk whey was fractionated on Biogel A-1.5m columns, and peak fractions were tested for immunoglobulins and TGE antibodies.

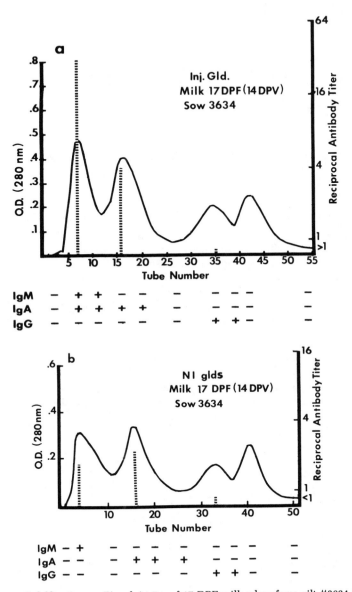

FIGURE 1. Gel filtration on Biogel A1.5m of 17 DPF milk whey from gilt #3634 that was intramammarily vaccinated with live attenuated TGE virus at three DPF. (a) Milk from injected glands; (b) Milk from noninjected glands. Vertical bars represent TGE virus neutralizing antibody titers detected in the unconcentrated fractions. Presence of the Igs in the various fractions is indicated by a +.

TABLE 6

ANTIBODY TITERS IN SERUM AND MILK AND IN THE IgM, IgA, AND IgG FRACTIONS OF MILK FROM INTRAMAMMARILY VACCINATED SOW 19-2. PIGLETS WERE CHALLENGED WITH VIRULENT TGE VIRUS AT 26 DPF.

Days Postfarrowing (DPF)	Days Postvaccination (DPV)	TGE Antibody Titers*									Rotavirus Antibody Titers*	
			Milk								Milk	
			TGE Inj. Glds.†				NI Glds.-NI Side					
		Serum	Whey	IgM‡	IgA‡	IgG‡	Whey	IgM	IgA	IgG	TGE Inj. Glds.	NI Glds.
4	0	<1	<1				<1				280	230
9	5	1.5	5				3					
12	8	27	33				8					
16	12	78	78				28					
23	19	180	320	2.6	7.6	1.6	170	4.2	3.7	1.4	850	1,550
30	26	380	370				86				1,700	1,300
44	39	5,600	1,300	2.5	18	28	1,700	2.7	21	42	420	600

*Reciprocal of dilution giving an 80% plaque reduction of TGE virus or OSU porcine rotavirus.

†Mammary glands 1, 3, and 4 on the left side of the udder were injected with Purdue (P-116) strain of live-attenuated TGE virus at four DPF. This sow was seronegative for TGE antibodies at the time of injection, but had been naturally infected with rotavirus.

‡Milk whey was fractionated on Biogel A-1.5m columns, and peak fractions were tested for immunoglobulins and TGE antibodies.

TABLE 7

TGE Antibody Titers in Serum and Milk and in the IgM, IgA, and IgG Fractions of Milk from Intramammarily Vaccinated Sow 3683. Piglets were Challenged with Virulent TGE Virus at 23 DPF.

Days Postfarrowing (DPF)	Days Postvaccination (DPV)	Serum	TGE Antibody Titer* Milk								
			Whey	Inj. Glds.†			NI Glds.-Inj. Side	Whey	NI Glds.-NI Side		
				IgM‡	IgA‡	IgG‡			IgM	IgA	IgG
3	0	60	500	4.0	68	10		420	3.5	95	5.0
9	6	1,500	4,096	12	370	21	2,100	1,600	NT§	280	3.0
16	13	3,100	8,600				7,600	4,096			
23	20	820	1,300	3.6	280	3.0	1,100	910			
35	32	1,100	1,024				520	600			
48	45	200	1,300				1,100	1,000			

*Reciprocal of dilution giving an 80% plaque reduction of TGE virus.
†Mammary glands 1, 3, and 5 on the left side of the udder were injected with Purdue (P-116) strain of live-attenuated TGE virus at three DPF. This sow had been previously naturally infected with TGE virus.
‡Milk whey was fractionated on Biogel A-1.5m columns, and peak fractions were tested for immunoglobulins and TGE antibodies.
§NT = not tested.

with sIgA fractions. These titers increased several fold as early as six DPV in milk from both injected and noninjected glands.

Diarrhea was not detected in the sow and piglets after IMm vaccination of the sow; however, after oral challenge of the piglets with virulent virus, two of the eight developed mild transient diarrhea at four DPE. Rectal swabs and milk samples were not collected for virus detection.

DISCUSSION

Studies of the mammary glands of swine and other monogastric species have shown a preponderance of IgA-plasma cells in the connective tissue adjacent to the ducts and alveoli.[8,11,12] The number of these cells increases in the mammary gland very late in gestation (one to two weeks prefarrowing) and during lactation.[11,12] These observations correlate with cell migration studies in mice that have shown the migration of IgA-bearing immunoblasts from the GALT to mammary glands late in pregnancy and during lactation under the influence of pregnancy-associated hormones.[20,21]

Investigators have further reported that few IgA-plasma cells are present in the mammary gland in a resting state or throughout most of the gestation period.[11,12] These findings may explain our current observations that IMm inoculation of a seronegative animal with live-attenuated TGE virus during pregnancy results in primarily IgG TGE antibodies in milk, whereas IMm injection during lactation elicits sIgA and IgM TGE antibodies in milk. These results concur with our previous reports that IMm or intramuscular inoculation of pregnant swine with live-attenuated TGE virus stimulates only IgG TGE milk antibodies.[2,3]

One factor that may have influenced stimulation of a sIgA milk antibody response after IMm inoculation might be that TGE virus replicates in the injected lactating, but not in the nonlactating mammary gland. Evidence for this phenomenon was the shedding of the virus in high titers in milk from injected glands only (one to five DPV) and the subsequent viral infection of the nursing piglets. This observation was further supported by IF studies that showed the presence of TGE virus-fluorescing cells lining the alveoli in an injected mammary gland (but not in the noninjected gland) collected by biopsy from one animal at two DPV (L. J. Saif, A. Brunner, E. H. Bohl, and D. R. Redman, unpublished observations). Similar studies by Kemeny and Woods[31] have shown that IMm injection of TGE antibody seronegative lactating sows with live virulent TGE virus also results in virus shedding in milk. In their report, all sows shed virus in high titers in milk from injected glands at one to six DPV, and two of the three sows also shed virus in very low titers in milk from noninjected glands at one to three DPV. In contrast to our studies using attenuated virus, all virulent virus-injected sows in their study became clinically ill and shed TGE virus in low titers in their feces. Moreover, mortality was 100% among their nursing piglets, whereas no piglets died in our study.

Lactogenesis may provide a highly susceptible population of rapidly proliferating mammary epithelial cells similar to villous epithelial cells in the small intestine. It is these rapidly developing intestinal enterocytes that are the target cell of TGE virus infection.[1] Replication of TGE virus in lactating mammary gland tissue may provide a mass antigenic stimulus to underlying IgA immunocytes leading to secretion of IgA antibodies in milk. Studies that have reported IgA antibodies in milk from rabbits or swine following IMm injection have usually employed adjuvants that would presumably also localize the antigen in mammary tissue providing prolonged antigenic stimulation.[23,25,27]

An alternative explanation might be that the IMm injected attenuated virus reached the intestine of the sow by way of the circulation or orally through fecal shedding by the infected piglets, subsequently leading to secretion of IgA antibodies in milk. Intestinal exposure by way of the circulation cannot be excluded in the present study, but this probably did not occur in previous studies of IMm inoculation of pregnant animals, because only IgG antibodies were detected in milk.[2-4] Several observations also make intestinal infection of the sow through the oral route unlikely. These include the reported difficulty in orally infecting the gut of adult swine with live-attenuated TGE virus. In our studies, even repeated oral dosing of pregnant sows with attenuated virus resulted in primarily IgG TGE antibodies in milk with lesser amounts of sIgA, and we believe this paucity of milk IgA antibody to be indicative of failure to infect the gut of the sow with the virus.[4-6] In the present study, neither fecal shedding of TGE virus nor diarrhea was evident in the two sows, even after exposure to infected piglets.

In a recent experiment in one sow, older seropositive TGE actively immune foster piglets (about two weeks after oral exposure to virulent TGE virus) were substituted for her natural piglets prior to IMm injection. These piglets did not develop diarrhea, nor was virus shedding detected after IMm injection of the sow. An IgA and IgM TGE antibody response, however, was still evident in this sow's milk (L. J. Saif and E. H. Bohl, unpublished observations).

A further question this study raises is the source of IgA TGE antibodies in milk from noninjected glands. Others have also reported that vaccination of one mammary gland gives rise to antibody activity in the other glands that was not due to passive transfer from serum.[26,27] TGE virus was not detected in milk from noninjected glands, although this fact does not preclude possible low levels of virus or viral antigen. Other possibilities might be transfer of IgA antibodies or IgA immunocytes derived from the injected glands to noninjected glands by way of the circulation. Alternatively, if disseminated antigen reached and was processed by GALT, IgA immunoblasts may migrate to both injected and noninjected glands with increased titers in the injected glands due to the presence of the antigen. Increased milk antibody titers in injected glands were probably not due to an inflammatory response with transudation of serum antibodies, because milk antibody titers to the unrelated virus, porcine rotavirus (due to previous natural infection of the animals) were not generally greater in milk from TGE virus-injected versus noninjected glands (TABLES 5 and 6).

Finally, this study has shown a rapid high increase in sIgA TGE antibody titers in milk after IMm immunization of a TGE naturally infected (orally primed) lactating sow. These findings for the mammary gland are similar to observations made by Pierce and Gowans[32] and Husband and Gowans[33] for the intestine. Their studies suggested that although initial migration of immunocytes is antigen independent, presence of an antigen results in a higher and prolonged response in the gut. Explanations suggested by Husband and Gowans may also be extrapolated to the mammary gland, where local presentation of antigen may result in enhanced recruitment of recirculating TGE-sensitized IgA-precursor cells, or antigen-driven clonal expansion of mammary gland IgA-precursor cells that originated in the GALT.

These findings raise the question of whether a natural lacteal entrance of enteric viruses may occur in lactating sows through exposure to infected piglets that may shed these viruses in their saliva. The biologic significance of this route of exposure would be to increase rapidly the secretion of sIgA milk antibodies, particularly against enteric organisms for which the dam has been orally primed, thereby providing rapid enhanced passive immunity to the gut of the neonate.

SUMMARY

Sows were injected intramammarily with live-attenuated TGE virus, an enteric coronavirus—one sow during pregnancy and three sows during lactation. All sows were TGE antibody seronegative prior to inoculation except for one naturally infected sow inoculated during lactation. The animal injected during pregnancy had primarily IgG TGE antibodies in milk from all glands. By contrast, sows injected during lactation had IgA and IgM initially, and later IgA and IgG TGE antibodies in milk from injected and noninjected glands. The seropositive sow had elevated IgA TGE antibody titers in milk after IMm injection. Both seronegative sows inoculated intramammarily during lactation shed TGE virus in milk from injected glands, and their nursing piglets developed mild diarrhea and shed virus in their feces at three to nine DPE of the sows. Milk from IMm injected glands generally had higher TGE antibody titers than milk from noninjected glands. These results suggest that TGE virus replicates in lactating mammary gland tissue, thereby stimulating IgA immunocytes, leading to secretion of IgA antibodies in milk. Whether the intramammary route presents a natural route of enteric virus exposure in lactating animals (by way of infected nursing piglets), leading to IgA-antibody secretion in milk, requires further investigation.

ACKNOWLEDGMENTS

We thank Ms. Sandy Dutton, Ms. Kathy Miller, Ms. Peggy Weilnau, and Ms. Bonnie Landmeier for their skilled technical assistance.

REFERENCES

1. HOOPER, B. E. & E. O. HAELTERMAN. 1966. Concepts of pathogenesis and passive immunity in transmissible gastroenteritis in swine. J. Am. Vet. Med. Assoc. **149:** 1580–1586.
2. BOHL, E. H., R. P. K. GUPTA, F. M. W. OLQUIN & L. J. SAIF. 1972. Antibody responses in serum, colostrum and milk of swine after infection or vaccination with transmissible gastroenteritis virus. Infect. Immun. **6:** 289–301.
3. SAIF, L. J., E. H. BOHL & K. P. GUPTA. 1972. Isolation of porcine immunoglobulins and determination of the immunoglobulin classes of transmissible gastroenteritis viral antibodies. Infect. Immun. **6:** 289–301.
4. BOHL, E. H. & L. J. SAIF. 1975. Passive immunity in transmissible gastroenteritis of swine: Immunoglobulin characteristics of antibodies in milk after inoculating virus by different routes. Infect. Immun. **11:** 23-32.
5. SAIF, L. J. & E. H. BOHL. 1979. Passive immunity in transmissible gastroenteritis of swine: Immunoglobulin classes of milk antibodies after oral/intranasal inoculation of sows with a live low cell culture-passaged virus. Am. J. Vet. Res. **40:** 115-117.
6. SAIF, L. J. & E. H. BOHL. 1979. Role of secretory IgA in passive immunity of swine to enteric viral infections. In Immunology of Breast Milk. P. L. Ogra and D. Dayton, Eds.: 237-248. Raven Press. New York.
7. SAIF, L. J. & E. H. BOHL. 1981. Passive immunity against enteric viral infections. In Proceedings of the Third International Symposium on Neonatal Diarrhea. S. D.

Acres, A. J. Forman and H. Fast, Eds.: 83-101. University of Saskatchewan. Saskatoon, Canada.

8. PORTER, P., D. E. NOAKES & W. D. ALLEN. 1970. Secretory IgA and antibodies to *E. coli* in porcine colostrum and milk and their significance in the alimentary tract of the young pig. Immunology **18:** 245-257.

9. BOURNE, F. J. & J. CURTIS. 1973. The transfer of immunoglobulins IgG, IgA and IgM from serum to colostrum and milk in the sow. Immunology **24:** 157-161.

10. TOMASI, T. B. 1976. The immune system of secretions. Foundations of Immunology Series. Prentice-Hall. New York.

11. BROWN, P. J., F. J. BOURNE & H. R. DENNY. 1975. Immunoglobulin-containing cells in pig mammary gland. J. Anat. **120:** 329-335.

12. WEISZ-CARRINGTON, P., M. E. ROUX & M. E. LAMM. 1977. Plasma cells and epithelial immunoglobulins in the mouse mammary gland during pregnancy and lactation. J. Immunol. **119:** 1306-1309.

13. PORTER, P. & W. D. ALLEN. 1972. Classes of immunoglobulins related to immunity in the pig: A review. J. Am. Vet. Med. Assoc. **160:** 511-518.

14. MONTGOMERY, P. C., J. COHN & E. T. LALLY. 1974. The induction and characterization of secretory IgA antibodies. *In* The Immunoglobulin A System. J. Mestecky and A. R. Lawton, Eds.: 453-462. Plenum Press. New York.

15. ALLARDYCE, R. A., D. J. C. SHERMAN, D. B. L. MC CLELLAND, K. MARWICK, A. J. SIMPSON & R. B. LAIDLOW. 1974. Appearance of specific colostrum antibodies after clinical infection with *Salmonella typhimurim*. Brit. Med. J. **3:** 307.

16. GOLDBLUM, R. M., S. AHLSTEDT, B. CARLSSON, L. A. HANSON, U. JODAL, G. LIDINJANSON & A. SOHL-AKERLUND. 1975. Antibody-forming cells in human colostrum after oral immunization. Nature (London) **257:** 797-799.

17. MICHALEK, S. M., J. R. MC GHEE, J. MESTECKY, R. R. ARNOLD & L. BOZZO. 1976. Ingestion of *Streptococcus mutans* induces secretory immunoglobulin A and caries immunity. Science **192:** 1238-1240.

18. AHLSTEDT, S., B. CARLSON, S. P. FALLSTROM, L. A. HANSON, J. HOLMGREN, G. LIDINJANSON, B. S. LINDBLAND, U. JODAL, J. KAISER, A. SOHL-AKERKINO, & C. WADSWORTH. 1977. Antibodies in human milk and serum induced by enterobacteria and food proteins. *In* Immunology of the Gut. 115-129. Elsevier. Amsterdam.

19. CRAIG, S. W. & J. J. CEBRA. 1971. Peyer's patches: An enriched source for IgA-producing immunocytes in the rabbit. J. Exp. Med. **132:** 18.

20. ROUX, M. E., M. MC WILLIAMS, J. M. PHILLIPS-QUAGLIATA, P. WEISZ-CARRINGTON & M. E. LAMM. 1977. Origin of IgA-secreting cells in the mammary gland. J. Exp. Med. **146:** 1311-1322.

21. WEISZ-CARRINGTON, P., M. E. ROUX, M. MC WILLIAMS, J. M. PHILLIPS-QUALIATA & M. E. LAMM. 1978. Hormonal induction of the secretory immune system in the mammary gland. Proc. Natl. Acad. Sci. USA **75:** 2928-2932.

22. HURLIMANN, J. & M. LICHAA. 1976. Local immunization in the mammary glands of the rabbits. J. Immunol. **116:** 1295-1301.

23. GENCO R. J. & M. A. TAUBMAN. 1969. Secretory IgA antibodies induced by local immunization. Nature (London) **221:** 679-681.

24. STEWARD, N. W. 1971. Resistance of rabbit secretory IgA to proteolysis. Biochem. Biophysics Acta. **236:** 440-449.

25. EDDIE, D. S., M. L. SCHULKIND & J. B. ROBBINS. 1971. The isolation and biologic activities of purified secretory IgA and IgG anti-*Salmonella typhimurium* "0" antibodies from rabbit intestinal fluid and colostrum. J. Immunol. **106:** 181.

26. MC DOWELL, G. H. 1973. Local antigenic stimulation of guinea-pig mammary gland. Aust. J. Exp. Biol. Med. Sci. **51:** 237-245.

27. BOURNE, F. J., T. J. NEWBY & J. W. CHIDLOW. 1975. The influence of the route of vaccination on the systemic and local immune response in the pig. Res. Vet. Sci. **18:** 244-248.

28. BOHL, E. H. 1979. Diagnosis of diarrhea in pigs due to transmissible gastroenteritis virus or rotavirus. *In* Viral Enteritis in Humans and Animals. R. Scherrer and F. Bricout, Eds.: Vol. 90: 341-343. Inserm. Paris, France.

29. FREDERICK, G. T., E. H. BOHL & R. F. CROSS. 1976. Pathogenicity of attenuated strains of TGE for newborn pigs. Am. J. Vet. Res. **37:** 165–169.
30. MATSUNO, S., S. INOUYE, & R. KONO. 1977. Plaque assay of neonatal calf diarrhea virus and the neutralizing antibody in human sera. J. Clin. Microbiol. **5:** 1–4.
31. KEMENY, L. J. & R. D. WOODS. 1977. Quantitative transmissible gastroenteritis virus shedding patterns in lactating sows. Am. J. Vet. Res. **38:** 307–310.
32. PIERCE, N. F. & J. L. GOWANS. Cellular kinetics of the intestinal immune response to cholera toxoid in rats. J. Exp. Med. **142:** 1550–1563.
33. HUSBAND, A. J. AND J. L. GOWANS. 1978. The origin and antigen-dependent distribution of IgA-containing cells in the intestine. J. Exp. Med. **148:** 1146–1152.

DISCUSSION OF THE PAPER

P. PORTER (*Unilever Research, Shambrook, Bedford, England*): Would you comment on the different protective efficiency of IgA versus IgG? You showed a schedule, that was intramammary that gave a high level of IgG, and in the challenge situation in the piglets, it seemed to have a high protective efficiency. Is there any basis for producing IgA that necessitates intramammary injection as opposed to parenteral administration?

L. J. SAIF (*Ohio Agriculture Research and Development Center*): We have found that if IgG is present in high enough titer in the milk or colostrum, it can be protective when the piglets are challenged. We have not been able to maintain, however, this high IgG level in the colostrum. In fact, if we took the same piglets that had been challenged at three days postfarrowing from sows that have been vaccinated intramammarily, and rechallenged them at two weeks, they would then be susceptible to infection. So the problem has been that the IgG titers drop very dramatically in the milk and, therefore, do not remain consistently elevated, as do the IgA anti-TGE antibody titers.

R. A. GOOD (*Oklahoma Medical Research Foundation, Oklahoma City*): Can you accomplish the same goal by intraepithelial immunization, as you can by injecting directly into the mammary gland tissue? Did you find virus in the noninjected portions of mammary tissue?

SAIF: We have not tried to inject the virus by way of the teat canal. As to the question of whether we found any TGE virus in the noninjected glands, we did not find any evidence of TGE virus shedding. Furthermore, when we looked at the noninjected glands by immunofluorescence, no evidence of fluorescent positive cells were seen. Antibody was present in milk from the noninjected glands. I think the best explanation for this phenomenon might be that the antigen did, indeed, get carried by the circulation to the GALT, which then seeded both the injected and noninjected glands. The titers would be consistently higher in the injected gland because of the presence of the antigen.

GOOD: Do you have any direct evidence of this in terms of shedding of virus from the GI tract?

SAIF: No.

C. R. WIRA (*Dartmouth Medical School, Hanover, N.H.*): Did you carry your sows through a second pregnancy to see if there was any mammary memory in terms of antibody titers in the milk?

SAIF: Regarding this topic, we have been interested in trying to confirm when the mammary-gut axis might be established. We have taken the nursing neonate that has been orally challenged with the TGE virus, while it was nursing the sow, and then allowed this animal to grow up and breed. The animal was kept confined so that it was not exposed to TGE virus, and then we looked at its milk and serum antibodies. There were very low titers, so apparently we have not established this type of gut-mammary axis in a very young animal.

PORTER: I can also comment on this point. We had the same objective that has been described here with the *E. coli* schedules. We have no evidence of mammary memory, and we have taken them through three or four farrowings.

B. PERI (*The University of Chicago, Chicago, Ill.*): Have you any explanation for the rise in titers you saw in the absence of virus?

SAIF: The only explanation we would propose would be that the nursing piglets probably did become subclinically infected with the virus. They then probably shed the virus. We would then postulate that the sow was reexposed by either the oral route or possibly even by the lacteal route.

ORAL IMMUNIZATION AGAINST EXPERIMENTAL CHOLERA: THE ROLE OF ANTIGEN FORM AND ANTIGEN COMBINATIONS IN EVOKING PROTECTION*

Nathaniel F. Pierce, William C. Cray, Jr., and John B. Sacci, Jr.

Department of Medicine
Johns Hopkins University School of Medicine
and
Baltimore City Hospitals
Baltimore, Maryland 21224

John P. Craig

Department of Microbiology
State University of New York
Downstate Medical Center
Brooklyn, New York 11203

René Germanier and Emil Fürer

Swiss Serum and Vaccine Institute
Berne, Switzerland

INTRODUCTION

Two lines of evidence strongly suggest that immunization for cholera should be given orally, aiming to evoke a protective sIgA response in the small intestine. First, the infection is superficial. Ingested *Vibrio cholerae* adhere to the small bowel mucosa, multiply, and release a protein enterotoxin that acts directly on mucosal cells to cause fluid secretion. Secretory antibody (mostly sIgA) is the only immunologic effector known to act at the mucosal surface or within the gut lumen, where these events can be interrupted. Second, an enteric mucosal sIgA response is probably best stimulated by locally applied antigen. Immature B-cells precommitted to synthesis of IgA are especially numerous in gut-associated lymphoreticular tissue[1] and are efficiently exposed to luminal antigens by a specialized mucosal antigen sampling mechanism.[2] By contrast, parenteral immunization is usually inefficient at evoking mucosal sIgA responses, and may actually suppress them.[3]

Some progress toward a practical oral cholera vaccine has been made using live avirulent mutants of *V. cholerae* or nonliving antigens, but a product combining safety, efficiency, and efficacy has not been achieved. Among the antigens produced by *V. cholerae*, cholera toxin (CT), or its derivatives, have been most extensively studied as immunizing materials. Cholera toxin is a potent mucosal immunogen; small amounts applied to intestinal mucosa cause vigorous local sIgA-antitoxin responses and protect experimental animals against oral

*This work was supported by Research Grant AI-14480 and Research Contract AI-92601, both from the National Institute of Allergy and Infectious Diseases, National Institutes of Health. Research facilities were provided by the Gerontology Research Center, National Institute of Aging, under its Guest Scientist Program.

724

challenge with virulent *V. cholerae*.[4,5] The doses required, however, to achieve protection also cause transient diarrhea, which is an unacceptable side effect for a practical vaccine. This situation has prompted us to seek alternate methods by which antitoxic immunity, alone or in combination with anti-bacterial immunity, might be achieved. In specific, we have sought to determine whether antitoxic protection can be induced by minimally toxic derivatives of CT, and whether other antigens of *V. cholerae* combined with CT can evoke synergistically protective mucosal immune responses and thus avoid the need to immunize with large, potentially toxic doses of cholera toxin.

The results of our recent studies are summarized here. Although they focus on the practical problem of oral immunization against cholera, it is hoped that they will also add understanding on how variations in antigen form, or the use of antigen combinations, affect the induction of protective mucosal sIgA responses in general.

MATERIALS AND METHODS

Animals

Rats were inbred Lewis females from Charles River Breeding Laboratories, Wilmington, Mass; they weighed 125–150g when first studied. Dogs were healthy mongrels weighing 6.5 to 15 kilograms.

Antigens

Purified CT and B subunit were prepared by Dr. R. A. Finkelstein. B subunit was derived from a *V. cholerae* mutant that produces B subunit, but not the A subunit, of cholera toxin.[6] Crude cholera toxin (CrT) was a lyophilized culture filtrate of *V. cholerae*, Ogawa, B1307. CrT from which CT had been selectively removed by passage through an antitoxin affinity column (termed toxin-depleted CrT) was provided by Dr. R. O. Thomson, Wellcome Research Laboratories, Beckenham, Kent, England. Glutaraldehyde-inactivated toxoid, made by treating purified CT with glutaraldehyde,[7] was provided by Wyeth Laboratories, Radnor, Penn. Heat-aggregated cholera toxin (HACT) was prepared by heating purified CT at 60° C for 20 minutes in Tris-ethylenediamino tetra acetate (EDTA) buffer. This caused formation of stable, minimally toxic aggregates of CT with molecular weights ranging to 2.5×10^6. HACT also contained a small amount of B subunit.[8]

Assays

The toxicity of CT and related materials was determined in rabbits by the skin vascular permeability assay.[9] The toxicities of B subunit, HACT, and glutaraldehyde toxoid, relative to purified CT, are shown in TABLE 1. Antitoxin responses in biopsies of intestinal mucosa were determined by a fluorescent antibody technique that revealed antitoxin-containing plasma cells (ACC) in the lamina propria.[10] ACC were enumerated and results expressed as ACC/mm^3. Results in groups of animals are reported as geometric means ± SE; for each immunization group, biopsies were obtained from five to seven animals.

TABLE 1

RELATIVE TOXICITY OF PURIFIED ANTIGENS DERIVED FROM CHOLERA TOXIN

Antigen	Relative Toxicity (Percent)*
Cholera toxin	100
Heat-aggregated toxin	1.2
Glutaraldehyde toxoid	.0002
B subunit	none

*Determined by rabbit skin vascular permeability assay.[9]

Immunization

Rats were immunized by direct intraduodenal inoculation of antigen.[10] Dogs were immunized orally as described elsewhere;[5] each immunization group contained 14–23 dogs.

Challenge of Dogs

Dogs were challenged orally with 10^{11} V. cholerae, Ogawa 395, or Inaba B36237, three weeks after immunization as previously described.[5] Equal numbers of immune and nonimmune animals were challenged together. About 50 percent of nonimmune dogs developed severe or lethal diarrhea with either challenge strain, usually within 24 hours after challenge. Results are expressed as the percent protection against severe or lethal diarrhea in immunized animals compared to concurrently challenged nonimmune controls. Statistical analysis is by Student's t-test.

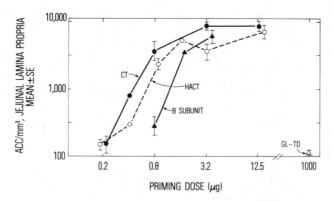

FIGURE 1. Compared priming efficiency of CT and related antigens. Rats were primed intraduodenally with varying doses of CT, HACT, B subunit, or glutaraldehyde toxoid (GL-TD). On day 14 all rats were challenged with 12.5 µg CT intraduodenally; jejunal biopsies were obtained on day 19 and scored for ACC. Results are expressed as geometric means; n = five to eight rats per data point.

RESULTS

Mucosal Priming with CT and Its Derivatives

Purified CT and three purified derivatives (HACT, B subunit, and glutaraldehyde toxoid) were compared for their ability to prime for a mucosal antitoxin response in rat jejunum. The results (FIGURE 1) show that HACT was nearly as effective as CT, and B subunit was only slightly less effective; glutaraldehyde toxoid, however, was ineffective. The calculated ED_{50} dose (i.e. the amount required to prime for a secondary ACC response of $1000/mm^3$) for priming by

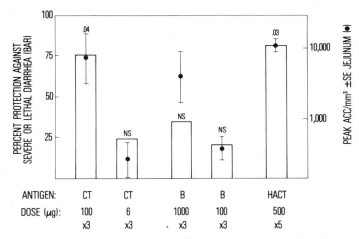

FIGURE 2. Protection of dogs immunized orally with CT or related antigens. Dogs were immunized orally with varying doses of CT, B subunit, or HACT. The first 3 doses were at 21 day intervals; any additional doses were at 7 day intervals. Each immunization group contained 14–23 dogs. Seven days after immunization, jejunal biopsies were taken from five to seven animals in each group and scored for ACC, results being expressed as geometric means. Three weeks after immunization, immunized dogs and an equal number of nonimmune controls were challenged orally with 10^{11} viable V. *cholerae*, Ogawa 395. Challenge outcome is expressed as percent protection against severe or lethal diarrhea when compared with concurrently challenged controls. P values above bars refer to statistical significance of protection; NS = not statistically significant (p > 0.05).

each antigen was (in µg): CT—0.4, HACT—0.6, B subunit—1.1, and glutaraldehyde toxoid—>1000.

Protection of Dogs Immunized Orally with CT or Its Derivatives

Dogs were immunized orally with purified CT, B subunit, or HACT, and challenged three weeks later with virulent V. *cholerae*. Transient diarrhea followed oral immunization in 69% of dogs given 100 µg CT (it was severe in

13%), and in 6% given 6 µg CT; diarrhea did not occur in dogs given B subunit or HACT.

The magnitude of antitoxic responses in jejunal mucosa, taken six to seven days after immunization, and the degree of protection against challenge for dogs immunized with each antigen, are shown in FIGURE 2. Oral immunization with three 100 µg doses of CT evoked vigorous mucosal ACC responses and protected significantly against severe or lethal cholera-like diarrhea; a 16-fold lower dose, however, caused much smaller ACC responses and was nonprotective. Immunization with B subunit was less effective than CT in two respects: comparable doses caused much smaller mucosal ACC responses, and large doses, which caused substantial ACC responses, were not significantly protective. Similar ACC responses produced by CT immunization, however, were protective. By contrast, oral immunization with HACT caused large mucosal ACC responses and was

TABLE 2

MUCOSAL ANTITOXIN RESPONSES AND PROTECTION OF DOGS IMMUNIZED WITH
CRT OR TOXIN-DEPLETED CRT

Dose (mg)	No. of Doses	Equivalent Dose of CT (µg)*	ACC/mm³, jejunum†	Percent Protection‡	P
CrT					
1,000	3	37	12,400	100	0.002
1,000	2	37	1,600	78	0.03
63	3	2.3	750	81	0.008
63	2	2.3	280	90	0.003
63	3	2.3	210	44§	NS
16	3	0.6	230	31	NS
Toxin-depleted CrT					
1,000	3	—	140	44	NS

*Based upon measured toxic activity of CrT.

†Geometric mean ACC response in jejunal biopsies taken six to seven days after immunization, when the response was greatest.

‡Protection against severe or lethal disease when compared with concurrently challenged nonimmune controls.

§Challenge was with V. cholerae, Inaba B36237; in all other groups, challenge was with V. cholerae, Ogawa 395.

highly protective; however, more doses were given than in the preceding studies, so strict comparison of these results is not possible.

Efficacy of CrT and Toxin-Depleted CrT as Oral Immunogens

In further studies, dogs were immunized orally with CrT and then challenged with virulent V. cholerae, Ogawa 395, the same serotype used to prepare CrT. Several schedules proved highly protective (TABLE 2), the simplest being a two-dose regimen in which each dose of CrT contained 2.3 µg CT; this evoked barely detectable jejunal ACC responses and caused slight diarrhea in only 21% of dogs. This regimen did not protect, however, when challenge was with V. cholerae of the Inaba serotype.

By contrast to CrT, toxin-depleted CrT was ineffective as an oral immunogen

TABLE 3

COMPARED PROTECTIVE EFFICACY OF CT, B SUBUNIT, CRT, AND TOXIN-DEPLETED CRT

	Protective Dose 50*	
Antigen	Whole Material	As CT or B Subunit
Crude toxin	26 mg	1µg
Pure toxin	—	25 µg
B subunit	—	>1000 µg
Toxin-depleted crude toxin	>1000 mg	—

*Based on studies using three-dose immunization schedules.

even though large doses, each equivalent to 1000 mg of CrT, were given (TABLE 2).

Compared Efficacy of CT, B Subunit, CrT, and Toxin-depleted CrT as Oral Immunogens

The relative efficacy of each antigen used in these studies was determined by calculating the dose required, in a three-dose schedule, to confer 50% protection (protective dose$_{50}$; PD$_{50}$) against severe or lethal diarrhea (TABLE 3). Expressed in terms of CT or B subunit content, the relative efficacy was CrT > CT > B subunit, whereas the relative efficacy was CrT> toxin-depleted CrT when total doses of crude materials were compared. The peak mucosal ACC responses associated with 50% protection also varied markedly depending upon the antigen used for oral immunization (TABLE 4).

COMMENTS

These studies show that antigen form and antigen combinations are important determinants of the efficacy of oral immunization for cholera in experimental animals.

We have shown previously that mucosally applied CT readily evokes IgA

TABLE 4

RELATION OF PROTECTION TO MUCOSAL ACC RESPONSE IN DOGS IMMUNIZED WITH CT, B SUBUNIT, OR CRT

Antigen	Peak Mucosal ACC Response Associated with 50 Percent Protection*
Crude toxin	200
Pure toxin	1,600
B subunit	>4,500†

*Based upon curves defined when the mean ACC response for each immunization regimen was plotted against protection induced by that regimen. Protection was against severe or lethal disease; ACC responses are per mm^3 in jejunal lamina propria.

†By linear extrapolation of the curve defined by the two studies with B subunit, 50,000 ACC/mm^3 would be required for 50 percent protection.

ACC in the enteric lamina propria of rats,[4,10] and that lamina propria ACC are the source of secreted antitoxin that protects dogs against enteric challenge with cholera toxin.[11] The present study, and another study recently published,[5] show that oral CT also evokes protection against challenge with virulent V. cholerae, that protection correlates with the magnitude of the peak mucosal ACC response, and that protective doses of CT cause transient diarrhea in a majority of dogs.

The striking effectiveness of CT as a mucosal immunogen has been attributed to its ability to bind to ganglioside receptors on intestinal epithelium and/or submucosal lymphoid cells, and to its activation of adenylate cyclase in lymphoid cells;[4] the latter property may have an adjuvant effect[4] and may favor production of a predominantly IgA response.[12] The failure of priming by glutaraldehyde toxoid, which is immunogenic when given parenterally, may be largely because it lacks these features. The explanation for the poorer performance of B subunit is speculative. Its poorer ability to evoke mucosal ACC responses may reflect its lack of an adenylate cyclase stimulating effect (which requires the A subunit of CT), whereas the failure of protection by ACC responses, nearly equal to those produced by protective doses of CT, could reflect a protective role for antibody to the A subunit that is usually considered a much inferior antigen, or could occur if anti-B subunit were less avid than anti-cholera toxin. An alternate possibility is that the predominant ACC isotype evoked by B subunit might not be IgA. Others have shown that enteric priming of mice with B subunit provokes sensitized Peyer's patch B-cells that are mostly of non-IgA isotypes, whereas CT priming evokes mostly IgA priming.[12] Although B subunit may prove effective as a booster antigen for responses primed by CT, these studies suggest it may be substantially inferior to CT for use as an oral vaccine component in nonprimed individuals.

HACT was the only toxin-derived antigen that caused vigorous mucosal ACC responses and protection without causing diarrhea during immunization; this situation suggests that HACT may have practical value as a safe and effective component of an oral vaccine for cholera. The mucosal immunogenicity of HACT is unexplained, but has also been observed by others.[13] The immunogenicity seems greater than would be expected from its residual toxic activity (equivalent to 6 μg CT/500 μg HACT), but could reflect enhancement of the ACC response to inactivated "toxoid" by residual active toxin trapped in the heat-induced aggregate. An alternate possibility is that aggregation per se may enhance the mucosal immunogenicity of this soluble protein, thus "making up" for the loss of immunogenicity that would be expected to accompany a reduction in toxicity. Whether aggregation might enhance the mucosal immunogenicity of other proteins is unknown.

The marked efficacy of CrT as an oral immunogen appeared to be due to synergistic protection evoked by antitoxic and anti-bacterial antibodies, although only the mucosal antitoxic response was measured directly. Evidence for such synergy was the much smaller PD_{50} for CrT than for its components (CT and toxin-depleted CrT) when each was used separately. This interpretation accords with prior reports of synergistic protection in rabbits immunized parenterally with cholera toxoid or CT plus killed V. cholerae or its lipopolysaccharide (LPS).[14,15] Protection in those studies was probably due to serum-derived IgG antibodies, whereas protection in the present study was likely caused by locally elaborated IgA antibodies.

Another possible explanation for the protective efficacy of CrT is that it evoked greater immune responses to bacterial antigens than did toxin-depleted CrT. This might occur if CT in CrT had an adjuvant effect upon the immune responses to coadministered bacterial antigens. Although this possibility is not excluded in the present study, a prior study has failed to show any enhancing effect of CT upon the mucosal immune response to a "bystander" antigen.[4]

A variety of nontoxin antigens of V. cholerae may have contributed to the protection evoked by crude cholera toxin. These might include LPS, flagellar antigen, outer membrane proteins, hemagglutinins, proteases, and neuraminidase. In this study, indirect evidence suggests that protection was partly due to the serotype-specific O antigen associated with lipopolysaccharide. This conclusion is based on failure of a "threshold" protective dose of CrT (63 mg given three times) derived from an Ogawa serotype of V. cholerae to protect against challenge by an Inaba serotype. Confirmation of this observation and determination of the protective roles of other bacterial antigens of V. cholerae require further study.

The synergistic protection noted in these studies has important practical implications for the development of effective oral vaccines for cholera and related enterotoxin-mediated bacterial diarrheas. It suggests that specific antigen combinations, or even crude antigen mixtures, may be especially effective. In the case of cholera vaccine, the combination of HACT with other bacterial antigens, including LPS, appears especially attractive because it appears to be safe (i.e. not causing diarrhea during immunization) and probably evokes synergistic protection. Whether similar synergy can be shown for protection against mucosal pathogens such as Neisseria gonorrheae, Hemophilus influenzae, Streptococcus mutans, or other enteric pathogens is uncertain; however, it is an attractive possibility.

REFERENCES

1. GEARHART, P. J. & J. J. CEBRA. 1979. Differentiated B lymphocytes potential to express particular antibody variable and constant regions depends on site of lymphoid tissue and antigen load. J. Exp. Med. 149: 216–227.

2. OWEN, R. L. 1977. Sequential uptake of horseradish peroxidase by lymphoid follicle epithelium of peyer's patches in the normal unobstructed mouse intestine: an ultrastructural study. Gastroenterology 72 (3): 440–451.

3. PIERCE, N. F. & F. T. KOSTER. 1980. Priming and suppression of the intestinal immune response to cholera toxoid/toxin by parenteral toxoid in rats. J. Immunol. 124: 307–311.

4. PIERCE, N. F. 1978. The role of antigen form and function in the primary and secondary intestinal immune responses to cholera toxin and toxoid in rats. J. Exp. Med. 148: 195–206.

5. PIERCE, N. F., W. C. CRAY, JR., & P. F. ENGEL. 1980. Antitoxic immunity to cholera in dogs immunized orally with cholera toxin. Infect. Immun. 27: 632–637.

6. HONDA, T. & R. A. FINKELSTEIN. 1979. Selection and characteristics of Vibrio cholerae mutant lacking the A (ADP-ribosylating) portion of the cholera enterotoxin. Proc. Natl. Acad. Sci. USA 76: 2052–2056.

7. RAPPAPORT, R. S., G. BONDE, T. MCCANN, B. A. RUBIN & H. TINT. 1974. Development of a purified cholera toxoid. II. Preparation of a stable, antigenic toxoid by reaction of purified toxin with glutaraldehyde. Infect. Immun. 9 (2): 304–317.

8. GERMANIER, R., E. FURER, S. VARALLYAY & T. M. INDERBITZEN. 1976. Preparation of a purified antigenic cholera toxoid. Infect. Immun. 13 (6): 1692–1698.

9. CRAIG, J. P. 1971. Cholera toxins. In Microbial Toxins. S. Kadis, T. C. Montie, and S. J. Ajl, Eds.: Vol. 2A: 189–254. Academic Press. New York.

10. PIERCE, N. F. & J. L. GOWANS. 1975. Cellular kinetics of the intestinal immune response to cholera toxoid in rats. J. Exp. Med. 142: 1550–1563.

11. PIERCE, N. F., W. C. CRAY, JR. & B. K. SIRCAR. 1978. Induction of a mucosal antitoxin response and its role in immunity to experimental canine cholera. Infect. Immun. 21: 185–193.

12. FUHRMAN, J. A. & J. J. CEBRA. Personal Communication.
13. FUJITA, K. & R. A. FINKELSTEIN. 1972. Antitoxic immunity in experimental cholera: comparison of immunity induced perorally and parenterally in mice. J. Infect. Dis. **125** (6): 647–655.
14. PETERSON, J. W. 1979. Synergistic protection against experimental cholera by immunization with cholera toxoid and vaccine. Infect. Immun. **26**: 594–598.
15. SEVENNERHOLM, A.-M. & J. HOLMGREN. 1976. Synergistic protective effect in rabbits of immunization with *Vibrio cholerae* lipopolysaccharide and toxin/toxoid. Infect. Immun. **13**: 735–750.

———————◆———————

DISCUSSION OF THE PAPER

P. PORTER (*Unilever Research, Shambrook, Bedford, England*): Work by one of my colleagues, Dr. Lingood, demonstrated a heat stable enterotoxin that was related to heat labile enterotoxin of *E. coli*. After oral immunization, it induced antitoxin immunity in the ligated gut test, which was quite contrary to our expectations. I notice that in your work you are carefully doing your heat aggregation at 60 degrees. I presume this is based on concern for the biofunction of the enterotoxin as opposed to its antigenicity. Is this the case?

N. F. PIERCE (*The Johns Hopkins University, Baltimore, Md.*): It is really based upon the concern that with higher heating, we would denature the protein. We have not, however, done studies with higher temperatures.

J. A. MATTINGLY (*Ohio State University, Columbus, Ohio*): Does the glutaraldehyde toxoid subunit contain the O somatic antigen?

PIERCE: No, the toxoid is highly purified.

MATTINGLY: Do you think the toxin must be biologically active to induce an immune response?

PIERCE: It depends perhaps on how the immune response is measured; certainly the B subunit does generate an immune response, and it is not toxic. It is, however, not very efficient in generating an immune response, and the immune response, when generated, does not appear to be very protective. There is the possibility that the B subunit may not be evoking primarily an IgA response. The toxin provokes almost entirely an IgA response, but we have not evaluated the isotype response to the B subunit. Dr. Furhman has some evidence, based upon clonal precursor analysis, that Peyer's patches immunized with B subunit contain a different array of clonal precursors, with less commitment to IgA than obtained with cholera toxin. I tend to believe that a small amount of toxic activity may be advantageous.

QUESTION: Did you ever try to combine the lipopolysaccharide in the pure form with the B subunit and see whether you could make a good immunogen?

PIERCE: We plan to do studies of this nature. In the present work, we decided to load the situation in our favor and not presume which antigen may be contributing from the crude material.

S. J. CHALLACOMBE (*Guy's Hospital, London, England*): In previous work, you have shown that you can get a longer lasting secretory response if you give a prior intraperitoneal immunization in your system. Because you have large numbers of antibody-containing cells after these three intragastric immunizations, how long does this protection last?

PIERCE: The work with intraperitoneally immunized animals does not provoke a longer response, but instead, a shorter response. We suspect that may be due to some suppressor mechanisms that are concurrently generated by the intraperitoneal antigen. The duration of the response in rats immunizied entirely orally reaches its peak five or six days after immunization and declines steadily, so that by two weeks it has declined by about 75 to 80 percent. One can still detect, however, small numbers of antitoxin-containing cells in animals biopsied three months later. The numbers are two or three percent, maybe even only one percent, of the peak levels. How important that 1 percent level is, I cannot say.

M. F. KAGNOFF (*University of California at San Diego, La Jolla*): Have you looked at the binding to the cell membrane of this heat inactivated material?

PIERCE: No; however, we know that it has some ability to bind GM-1 ganglioside, and so I presume it has some ability to bind to receptors; however, I cannot give quantitative data on this point.

LOCAL IgA-MEMORY RESPONSE
TO BACTERIAL ANTIGENS*

David F. Keren, Patricia J. Scott, Roderick A. McDonald,
and Scott E. Kern

Department of Pathology
The University of Michigan Medical Center
Ann Arbor, Michigan 48109

INTRODUCTION

For over 100 years, it has been known that oral immunization can protect against challenge by certain enteropathogenic bacteria.[1-3] The mechanism of this protection was unclear as most individuals did not demonstrate strong serum agglutinins to the orally administered vaccine. Work by Davies in 1922 provided evidence that agglutinating antibodies in stool specimens from patients with dysentery correlated better with the disease activity than serum antibody levels.[4] Following the demonstration by Tomasi et al. in 1965 that IgA was the main antibody on mucosal surfaces, a new area of investigation was opened that led to the elucidation of the mechanism of protection by oral vaccination.[5]

In order to follow the development of the local IgA-immune response, we developed a chronically isolated ileal loop model in rabbits.[6] This model allowed us to sample ileal loop secretions daily. In other studies, we immunized the isolated segment directly with bacteria, toxins, or other macromolecules.

In the present study, we have used this model to demonstrate that a mucosal IgA-memory response can be elicited following oral immunization with *Shigella flexneri* antigen.

MATERIALS AND METHODS

Preparation of Chronically Isolated Ileal Loops

The surgical creation of ileal, Thiry-Vella loops in rabbits has been described in detail previously.[6] In brief, while three to four kg New Zealand White rabbits are anesthetized with xylazine and ketamine, a midline abdominal incision is made and the terminal ileum is identified. A 20 cm segment of ileum containing a grossly identifiable Peyer's patch is isolated with its vascular supply intact. Silastic tubing (Dow-Corning) is sewn into each end of the isolated segment. This tubing is then brought out through the midline incision and tunneled subcutaneously to the nape of the neck where it is exteriorized and secured. Intestinal continuity is restored by an end-to-end anastomosis, and the midline incision is closed in two layers.

Each day approximately two to four ml of secretions and mucous that collect in the isolated loops are expelled by injecting 20 ml of air into one of the silastic tubes. The slightly opaque, colorless fluid and mucous expelled from the tubing is

*This work was supported in part by the U.S. Army Medical Research and Development Command Contract DAMD 1/-80-C-0113.

studied for specific immunoglobulin content. A subsequent flush with 20 ml of sterile saline helps to remove adherent mucous. This saline is then removed by repeated gentle flushes of air. With proper daily care, 80%–90% of rabbits can complete experiments lasting one to two months.

Enzyme-Linked Immunosorbent Assay (ELISA)

The ELISA procedure has been described in detail previously.[7,8] Briefly, microtiter wells are coated with a solution containing *Shigella flexneri* lipopolysaccharide (Westphal preparation). Immediately prior to testing serum samples or loop secretions, the antigen solution is removed, and wells are washed with a phosphate buffer containing Tween 20 (PT). The fluid to be assayed is diluted in the PT buffer and incubated in the coated wells and in uncoated wells (to control for nonspecific adsorption) for four hours on horizontal rotary shaker. The plates are washed with PT and incubated with either alkaline phosphatase-conjugated goat anti-rabbit IgA or staphylococcal protein A overnight on the shaker. Following another PT wash, substrate reaction is carried out with nitrophenyl phosphate in carbonate buffer. The OD 405 nm of the substrate reaction is determined using a Titer Tek microELISA reader. Kinetics of the enzyme-substrate reaction are extrapolated to 100 minutes. The OD 405 nm of uncoated wells is subtracted from the OD 405 nm of coated wells. Specific IgG and IgA standards prepared as described previously[7] are processed daily with the unknown fluids.

Bacterial Preparations

Three live *Shigella* strains, one acetone-killed strain, and one Westphal lipopolysaccharide preparation containing *Shigella flexneri 2a* somatic antigens were used in these studies. *Shigella flexneri* strain M4243 was shown to invade the surface epithelium and to persist with ulcer formation.[9] *Shigella* X16 is a hybrid of *S. flexneri-Escherichia coli* that invades surface epithelium, may form ulcers, but does not thrive (persist) in guinea pig intestine.[10] *S. flexneri* strain 2457-0 does not form ulcers and does not invade surface epithelium.[11] The preparations of acetone-killed strain M4243 (AK-M4243) and the *Shigella* lipopolysaccharide preparations have been described previously.[11-13]

Shedding of Live Shigella

The presence of live bacteria in the stool and in loop secretions was assessed by culturing both stool samples and loop secretions on MacConkey agar plates as previously described.[14]

Statistical Analysis

Statistical analysis of the data was performed in the Midas computer of the Statistical Research Laboratory at The University of Michigan. The F-test result and significance were determined for each group.

RESULTS

In earlier studies, we immunized the chronically isolated ileal loops directly with various antigen preparations. This immunization was done by injecting live or killed antigen preparations in 4 ml of phosphate-buffered saline directly into the isolated loops. This material was left in the loops overnight and flushed out the next morning. Data from some of these earlier studies are summarized in FIGURE 1. In these studies, we found that chronically isolated ileal loops stimulated by various preparations of *Shigella* antigen contain considerable secretory IgA activity, but at most, trivial IgG activity against these antigens.[13,14] Virtually no IgA and usually no or trivial IgG directed against *Shigella flexneri* antigens were found in sera from these rabbits.

When the isolated ileal loops were immunized directly with 10^8 live bacteria, in doses given on days 0, 7, and 14 (day of surgery = day -1), there was no significant difference in the local IgA response for the three live antigen forms used (invasive M4243, invasive *Shigella* X16, noninvasive 2457-0).[15] As shown in FIGURE 1, however, acetone-killed *Shigella flexneri* achieved a weaker local IgA response in the isolated ileal loop secretions. The lipopolysaccharide preparation

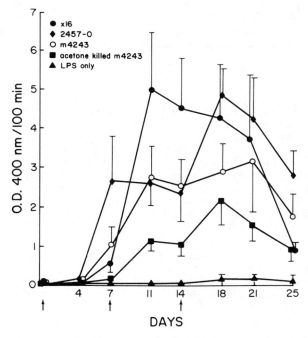

FIGURE 1. Mean IgA anti-shigella responses in ileal loop secretions from groups of rabbits immunized directly in the isolated loop with 10^8 live M4243, X16, 2457-0, 2.5 mg of acetone-killed M4243 per ml, or 100 ug of hot phenol-water prepared *Shigella* LPS. The vertical axis expresses the net optical density (O.D.) and the horizontal axis indicates days after first intraloop stimulation. Standard errors of mean (SEM) indicated. (D.F. Keren et al.[15] With permission from *Infection and Immunity*).

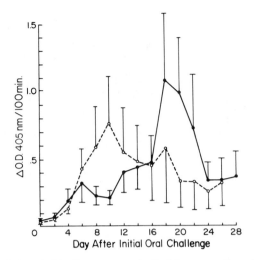

FIGURE 2. Mean IgA anti-shigella responses in ileal loop secretions from rabbits immunized orally with a single dose of 10^{10} live *Shigella* X16 on day 0 (○) or from rabbits given 10^{10} live *Shigella* X16 on days 0, 7, and 14 (●). SEM indicated. (D.F. Keren.[8] With permission from the *Journal of Immunology*.)

(given in a dose equivalent to the amount of lipopolysaccharide in 10^8 bacteria) was ineffective in achieving a significant mucosal immune response.[5]

Whereas our chronically isolated ileal loop model in rabbits has been useful for following the kinetics of the local immune response to initial antigen stimulation, it has been difficult to use this model for studying the local IgA-anamnestic response of the bowel. First, it is difficult to maintain these isolated ileal loops for periods longer than one month. Animals that do survive for long periods of time (some have been kept alive with isolated ileal loops for as long as 10 months), usually require several subsequent surgical procedures to drain abscesses and correct abdominal problems. Further, some animals require antibiotic therapy for various related and unrelated infections. It is obvious that these are undesirable events in an experimental model to follow the immune response against infectious diseases. Second, by directly immunizing the isolated ileal loops, we are creating an extremely artificial situation. That is, if one were immunizing a population, or if an infection were occurring naturally, the vaccine or pathogen would pass through gastric acid, bile, pancreatic digestive enzymes, and normal intestinal flora and food products. Any or all of the aforementioned might alter the ability of the orally administered antigen to stimulate the mucosal immune response.

Therefore, in order to make our model system more relevant to both the natural infection and to a potential vaccine program for humans, we immunized the animals orally, rather than stimulating the isolated ileal loops directly. The local IgA response was followed by studying the secretions from the isolated ileal loops for specific IgA activity at various times following oral immunization. The isolated ileal loops are separated from the intestinal contents and, therefore, are never directly exposed to the antigen.

This approach evolves from the theory that a common mucosal immune system exists. That such a system exists has been demonstrated by several laboratories.[16-18] If this common mucosal immune system exists, it should be possible to create the isolated ileal loop, give an oral dose of antigen to that animal and follow the intestinal responses in the local secretions.

Indeed, following a single oral dose of 10^{10} live *Shigella* X16, the kinetics of the local IgA response in the chronically isolated ileal loop secretions paralleled the response seen when the loops were directly immunized with the same live antigen (FIGURE 2).[8] No enhancement of this response was seen following three doses of live oral *Shigella* X16. When 10^{10} heat-killed *Shigella* X16 were given orally, similar, albeit weaker, local IgA responses were seen (FIGURE 3).[8] In

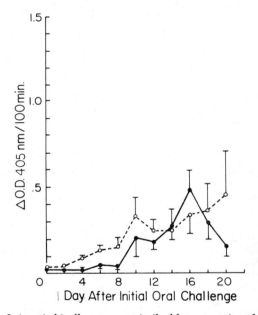

FIGURE 3. Mean IgA anti-shigella responses in ileal loop secretions from rabbits immunized orally with a single dose of 10^{10} heat-killed *Shigella* X16 on day 0 (o) or from rabbits given 10^{10} heat-killed *Shigella* X16 on days 0, 7, and 14 (●). SEM indicated. (D.F. Keren.[8] With permission from the *Journal of Immunology*.)

neither situation were there significant local IgG or serum IgG or IgA responses directed against these bacteria.

To determine whether a local IgA-memory response could be elicited by oral priming, a group of ten rabbits that did not have chronically isolated ileal loops was primed by giving three weekly, oral doses of 10^{10} live *Shigella* X16 to each rabbit. The animals were rested for two months after the third dose. Then, a chronically isolated ileal loop was surgically created in each animal and the animals were challenged with a single oral dose of 10^{10} live *Shigella* X16 on the day after surgery.

TABLE 1

LOCAL IGA-MEMORY RESPONSE IN RABBIT ILEAL LOOP SECRETIONS AFTER ORAL PRIMING WITH LIVE *SHIGELLA* X16[8]

Day After Challenge*	Not Primed†	Live *Shigella* X16‡	Significance§	F-STAT**
0	.047 ± .006¶	.234 ± .086	.0026	10.077
1	.041 ± .012	.213 ± .066	.0029	9.825
2	.062 ± .013	.499 ± .134	.0001	19.205
3	.047 ± .014	.567 ± .133	.0001	19.086
4	.136 ± .042	1.778 ± .438	.0001	27.790
5	.218 ± .103	1.626 ± .387	.0001	23.568
6	.435 ± .149	1.610 ± .298	.0007	13.173
7	.519 ± .513	1.833 ± .350	.0014	11.358
8	.591 ± .306	1.363 ± .248	.0151	6,322
10	.532 ± .210	.979 ± .249	N.S.‖	—

*Day 0 = Day of final antigen challenge
†Animals given 10^{10} live *Shigella* X16 orally on day 0 (n = 19)
‡Animals given 10^{10} live *Shigella* X16 orally on days −75, −68, −61 prior to oral challenge on day 0 (n = 10)
§As determined by F-test
¶Results expressed as mean optical density (O.D.) 405 nm/100 minutes ± standard error of mean (S.E.M.) of IgA antibodies specific for *Shigella* antigen as determined by ELISA
‖ N.S. = not significant (>.02 by F-test)
**F-STAT = F-test value

A striking local IgA-memory response was seen in these animals as compared to the nonprimed animals (TABLE 1).[8] By contrast, the animals that received this same dosage schedule with killed *Shigella* X16 followed by a challenge with a single dose of killed *Shigella*, showed no evidence of a local IgA-memory response (TABLE 2).[8]

TABLE 2

LACK OF IGA-MEMORY RESPONSE AFTER ORAL PRIMING WITH KILLED *SHIEGELLA* X16[8]

Day After Challenge*	Not Primed†	Primed With Killed *Shigella* X16‡	Significance
0	.040 ± .008¶	.057 ± .02	N.S.‖
2	.046 ± .011	.040 ± .14	N.S.
4	.089 ± .016	.108 ± .05	N.S.
6	.140 ± .031	.173 ± .063	N.S.
8	.161 ± .049	.120 ± .041	N.S.

*Day 0 = day of final antigen challenge
†Unprimed animals given 10^{10} killed *Shigella* X16 orally on day 0 (n = 12)
‡Animals orally primed with 10^{10} killed *Shigella* X16 on days −75, −68, −61 prior to oral challenge on Day 0 (n = 11)
§Significance assessed by F-test
¶Results expressed as mean optical density (O.D.) 405nm/100 minutes ± S.E.M. for *Shigella* antigen as determined by ELISA
‖ N.S. = Not significant (>.02 by F-test)

During these studies, some rabbits were given erythromycin for pulmonary infections. All of the rabbits given the erythromycin developed poor local IgA-memory responses (FIGURE 4). To see if this erythromycin effect could be repeated, a second group of rabbits was given the regimen for the memory studies with live *Shigella* X16 and then given erythromycin concurrently with the challenge. As shown in FIGURE 4, a significantly lower IgA-memory response was seen in the erythromycin-treated rabbits.

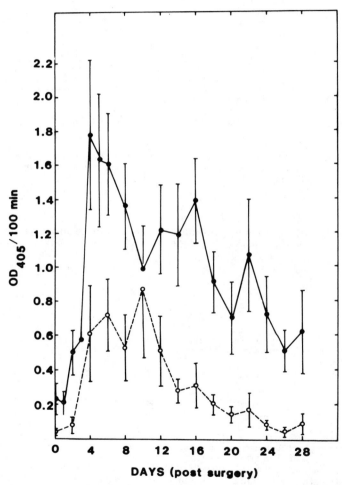

FIGURE 4. Mean IgA anti-shigella response in secretions from isolated ileal loops of rabbits primed with three oral doses of 10^{10} live shigella on days -74, -67, and -60 and challenged with a single oral dose on day 0 (one day after surgical creation of the isolated ileal loop.) One group of rabbits had no exposure to erythromycin (●); the other was given erythromycin for several days before and after the challenge dose of live *Shigella* X16 (○). SEM indicated.

DISCUSSION

In the present studies, we have used our chronically isolated ileal loop model in rabbits as a probe to follow the local IgA-memory response of the intestine after either oral or parenteral priming.

In our previous studies, we have shown that the intestinal secretions from chronically isolated ileal loops directly stimulated with various Shigella preparations will contain considerable secretory IgA but no, or only little, IgG directed against the Shigella.[6-8, 13-15] The lack of locally produced IgG is not due to rapid degradation of IgG as the isolated loops are separated from the proteolytic effects of gastric acid, bile, and the enzymes trypsin, pepsin, and chymotrypsin.[19] Also, direct stimulation of the isolated loops by Shigella antigens has resulted in little or no systemic (serum) IgG against Shigella, unless the systemic immune response was previously primed by a subcutaneous or intravenous dose of Shigella.[15]

Although direct immunization of the chronically isolated ileal loop was useful for studying the kinetics of the local IgA response to Shigella antigens, it had major drawbacks. First, the effects of gastric acid, bile, and pancreatic digestive enzymes on either a natural infection or a potential oral vaccine were artifically bypassed by directly stimulating the chronically isolated ileal loops. Second, for studying the mucosal memory response, it was difficult to maintain chronically isolated loops for periods lasting longer than one to two months. Therefore, in the present study, rather than directly stimulating the isolated loops, we used the chronically isolated loops as a probe for following the local immune response. Because we were interested in studying the intestinal response, we chose an oral route of immunization. Pierce has demonstrated that the site of mucosal stimulation influences where the locally stimulated B-cells will lodge.[20]

These studies show that the kinetics of the IgA response to Shigella in our isolated ileal loops after a single oral immunization follow the same sequence as when the isolated loops were stimulated directly; this finding is further evidence for the common mucosal immune system. Further, it establishes this model system as a valid probe for events occurring locally in the intestine. We have then taken advantage of this system to determine whether a mucosal memory response to Shigella can be elicited by oral priming.

It is clear that we were able to achieve a mucosal memory response when live, but not killed, Shigella X16 were used to prime and challenge the rabbits orally.

The difference between the orally administered killed Shigella and live Shigella may be due to several factors. First, the live Shigella are able to multiply in the intestine. We found that stool from rabbits given oral Shigella would contain Shigella for as long as 10 days after each oral dose. No loop fluids were found to contain Shigella. This pattern of shedding is similar to that described for Shigella flexneri when they were administered orally to monkeys.[11] Therefore, the actual dose of Shigella X16 for animals that received live oral Shigella was considerably greater than those that received killed Shigella. Second, Shigella X16 is a locally invasive strain. Actual invasion of the epithelium may be necessary for achieving or for enhancing the mucosal IgA-memory response. We do not think that the latter is the case, because preliminary studies in our laboratory using the noninvasive Shigella flexneri strain 2457-0 have shown a mucosal IgA-memory response similar to that of the invasive Shigella X16. Last, the challenge antigen may be of importance. The challenge antigen for the rabbits primed with killed Shigella was heat-killed. It may be important to have a live bacteria for an effective challenge. This situation may be a dose-related phenomenon.

Our studies using parenteral priming have shown no mucosal IgA-memory response in spite of the presence of systemic IgG against *Shigella* antigen.

Last, we record a peculiar effect of the antibiotic erythromycin on the local IgA-memory response of orally primed rabbits. When rabbits were treated with erythromycin at the time of their challenge dose, no local IgA-memory response could be demonstrated in most of the rabbits. Only two of the ten rabbits studied showed evidence of an IgA-memory response. The mechanism of action of this effect is unclear at the present time. This effect could be of importance, however, in any vaccine program using live, attenuated bacteria.

In summary, the present studies offer our chronically isolated ileal loop model as a probe to follow the mucosal primary and memory responses to orally or parenterally administered *Shigella* antigens. We have shown that a significant local memory response is achievable by oral priming with live invasive, but not with heat-killed *Shigella* X16. Concurrent antibiotic administration may be able to alter the ability of animals to elicit such a mucosal memory response.

ACKNOWLEDGMENT

The authors thank Mrs. Mary Ann Byrnes for her excellent assistance in preparing this manuscript.

REFERENCES

1. PASTEUR, L. 1880. Cited by Calmette, A. 1923. Les vaccinations microbiennes par voie buccale. Ann. Inst. Pasteur. **37:** 900–920.
2. FERRAN, J. 1885. Cited by A. P. Fernandez. Vae Inventoribus Magnis! El doctor Ferran y el colera morbo asiatico en la guerra europea. Barcelona. Imp. La Renaixenza-Xucla 13. 133–151. 1921.
3. BESREDKA, A. 1927. De la vaccination par voie buccale contre la dysenterie, la fievre typhoide et le cholera. Rev. d'Hyg. et de Med. Prev. **49:** 445–463.
4. DAVIES, A. 1922. An investigation into the serological properties of dysenteric stool. Lancet. **2:** 1009–1012.
5. TOMASI, T. B., E. M. TAN, A. SOLOMON & R. A. PRENDERGAST. 1965. Characteristics of an immune system common to certain external secretions. J. Exp. Med. **121:** 101–124.
6. KEREN, D. F., H. L. ELLIOTT, G. D. BROWN & J. H. YARDLEY, 1975. Atrophy of villi with hypertrophy and hyperplasia of Paneth cells in isolated (Thiry-Vella) ileal loops in rabbits. Gastroenterology **68:** 83–93.
7. KEREN, D. F. 1979. Enzyme-linked immunosorbent assay for immunoglobulin G and immunoglobulin A antibodies to *Shigella flexneri* antigens. Infect. Immun. **24:** 441–448.
8. KEREN, D. F., S. E. KERN D. H. BAUER, P. J. SCOTT & P. PORTER. 1982. Direct demonstrtation in intestinal secretions of an IgA memory response to orally administered *Shigella flexneri* antigens. J. Immunol. **128:** 475–479.
9. FORMAL, S. B., T. H. KENT, S. AUSTIN & E. H. LABREC. 1966. Fluorescent antibody and histological study of vaccinated and control monkeys challenged with *Shigella flexneri*. J. Bacteriol. **19:** 2368–2376.
10. FORMAL, S. B., E. H. LABREC, T. H. KENT & S. FALKOW. 1965. Abortive intestinal infection with an *Escherichia coli—Shigella flexneri* hydrid strain. J. Bacteriol. **89:** 1374–1382.
11. FORMAL, S. B., E. H. LABREC, A. PALMER & S. FALKOW. 1965. Protection of monkeys against experimental shigellosis with attenuated vaccines. J. Bacteriol. **90:** 63–68.
12. FORMAL, S. B., R. M. MAENZA, S. AUSTIN, & E. H. LABREC. 1967. Failure of parenteral

vaccines to protect monkeys against experimental shigellosis. Proc. Soc. Exp. Biol. Med. **125:** 347–349.

13. KEREN, D. F., P. S. HOLT, H. H. COLLINS, P. GEMSKI & S. B. FORMAL. 1978. The role of Peyer's patches in the local immune response of rabbit ileum to live bacteria. J. Immunol. **120:** 1892–1896.

14. KEREN, D. F., P. S. HOLT, H. H. COLLINS, P. GEMSKI & S. B. FORMAL. 1980. Variables affecting the local immune response in Thiry-Vella loops. I. Role of immunization schedule, bacterial flora, and postsurgical inflammation. Infect. Immun. **28:** 950–956.

15. KEREN, D. F., H. H. COLLINS, P. GEMSKI, P. S. HOLT & S. B. FORMAL. 1981. Role of antigen form in development of mucosal IgA response to *Shigella flexneri* antigens. Infect. Immun. **31:** 1193–1202.

16. CEBRA, J. J., R. KAMAT, P. GEARHART, S. M. ROBERTSON & J. TSENG. 1977. The secretory IgA system of the gut. *In* Immunology of the gut. CIBA Foundation Symposium **46:** 5–28.

17. MCWILLIAMS, M., J. M. PHILLIPS-QUAGLIATA & M. E. LAMM. 1977. Mesenteric lymph node B lymphoblasts which home to the small intestine are precommitted to IgA synthesis. J. Exp. Med. **145:** 866–875.

18. MCDERMOTT, M. R. & J. BIENENSTOCK. 1979. Evidence for a common mucosal immunologic system. I. Migration of B immunoblasts into intestinal, respiratory, and genital tissues. J. Immunol. **122:** 1892–1897.

19. KEREN, D. F., P. J. SCOTT & D. BAUER, 1981. Variables affecting the local immune response in Thiry-Vella loops. II. Stability of antigen-specific IgG and secretory IgA in acute and chronic Thiry-Vella loops. J. Immunol. **124:** 2620–2624.

20. PIERCE, N. F. & W. C. CRAY, JR. 1982. Determinants of the localization, magnitude, and duration of a specific mucosal IgA plasma cell response in enterically immunized rats. J. Immunol. **128:** 1311–1315.

DISCUSSION OF THE PAPER

A. J. HUSBAND (*The University of Newcastle, Newcastle, Australia*): We know that IgA is intimately bound up with intestinal mucus. Did you handle your samples in any special way to accommodate for the mucus production that changes in isolated loops?

D. F. KEREN (*The University of Michigan, Ann Arbor, Mich.*): We handle all our specimens in the same way. We immediately centrifuge them and remove the mucus that might have some IgA bound to it. We assay the overlying clear supernatants that we obtain from these.

HUSBAND: You showed that you had IgA antibody produced in isolated, nonimmunized loops when you immunized the intact intestine.

KEREN: That is correct.

HUSBAND: And do you propose that this is a counterpart of the common mucosal immune system?

KEREN: Yes.

HUSBAND: I would suggest that the cells that are migrating to those loops are in transit. In the absence of antigen in those loops, they would not be induced to proliferate and persist. Does your data support my explanation of that result, that the IgA-antibody levels in these loops are more transient or lower in magnitude than a loop that is directly immunized?

KEREN: It seems improbable, because the antibody that we see does seem to persist for at least three to four weeks, albeit, at relatively lower levels. One would think that if antibody were just passing through the loops, that it would not persist quite that long.

HUSBAND: Does that antibody level, however, compare favorably with antibody levels in directly immunized loops?

KEREN: No. The antibody in the directly immunized loops was much higher.

RESTRICTIONS ON MUCOSAL B-LYMPHOCYTE FUNCTION IN MAN*

Robert Clancy,† Allan W. Cripps, Alan J. Husband,
and Maree Gleeson

Department of Pathology
Faculty of Medicine
University of Newcastle
Hunter Immunology Unit
Newcastle, Australia

Our interest in the development and control of the local immune response in man relates to the establishment of oral immunization strategies that are dependent on the responsiveness of mucosal B-cells to locally presented antigen, and on a lymphocyte traffic that enables antibody secretion to occur at distant mucosal sites. We report results from three studies that examine different aspects of the capacity of mucosal B-cells to respond to stimulation.

OSCILLATORY PATTERN OF IGA SECRETION IN SALIVA OF INFANTS (FIGURE 1)

Saliva was collected from 63 normal infants, at 13 time intervals in the first year of life. Saliva was clarified by centrifugation and immunoglobulins measured by electroimmunodiffusion.[1] Milk contamination was excluded by immunoelectrophoresis using a rabbit antiserum to human colostral whey. Anti-E. coli antibodies were detected by hemagglutination of cells sensitized with a pooled "0" antigen.[2]

Albumin and IgG were present in high concentrations at birth (5.7 ± 0.6 and 3.6 ± 0.8 mg/dl respectively), but decreased in parallel to low values at two months of age, representing a transient "leaky" membrane. IgA was detected by three weeks of age, increasing to peak at six weeks (1.8 ± 0.8 mg/dl) at levels within the adult range (0.2–8.8 mg/dl). Subsequently, levels oscillated with a trough at three months (0.6 ± 0.2 mg/dl) rising again to adult levels by eight months (1.4 ± 0.3 mg/dl). The difference between IgA levels at 6 and 12 weeks was significant ($p < 0.01$). No E. coli antibody was detected in saliva samples tested in the first six months of life (compared to detection of E. coli antibody in the saliva of 63% of normal adults).

SALIVARY ANTIBODY RESPONSE TO AN ORAL BACTERIAL VACCINE DEPENDS ON THE PREIMMUNIZATION ANTIBODY LEVEL

An orally killed polyvalent bacterial vaccine (Buccaline Berna, Swiss Serum, Switzerland) was given to healthy volunteers at birth, one, and two months. Each course contained 3.5×10^{10} H. influenzae organisms. Antibody was detected by a

*We thank NH and MRC and Ciba-Geigy (Australia) for support.
†Address for correspondence: Professor R. Clancy, Department of Pathology, Faculty of Medicine, University of Newcastle, Newcastle, NSW Australia.

745

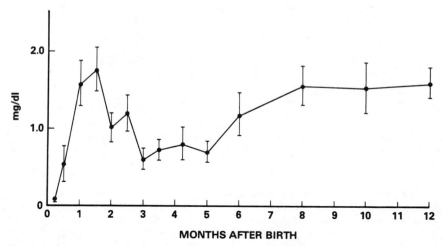

FIGURE 1. Graph to demonstrate oscillatory pattern of development of secretory IgA levels in 63 infants through the first year of life (mean ± SE).

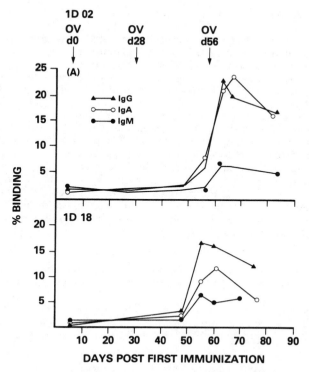

FIGURE 2. Salivary antibody response in two subjects taking three courses of an oral polyvalent killed bacterial vaccine containing *H. influenzae*.

TABLE 1

SALIVARY IgA SPECIFIC ANTI-*H. INFLUENZAE* ANTIBODY LEVELS FOLLOWING ORAL
BACTERIAL VACCINE

Responder* (7)		Nonresponder (10)	
Pre-Birth	Post (Day 62)	Pre-Birth	Post (Day 62)
1.7†	12.00	4.99	3.49
±	±	±	±
0.24	2.90	0.89	0.59

*Increase in binding by >1%
†Mean ± SE

class specific solid phase radioimmunoassay using rabbit anti-human immuno-beads (Bio-Rad Lab, USA) and *H. influenzae* specific antigen.[3] The time course of salivary IgA antibody in "responders" is indicated in FIGURE 2. Analysis of the antibody response at day 62 (TABLE 1) indicates those subjects that developed increased levels of antibody binding after immunization (i.e. ≥1%) when compared with "nonresponders." Similar observations were made, though at lower levels, for IgG and IgM antibody. No increase in serum antibody was detected in any patient.

HUMAN GUT MUCOSA CONTAINS REGULATORY T-LYMPHOCYTES AND B-LYMPHOCYTES CAPABLE OF RESPONDING TO THESE T-CELLS

T- and B-lymphocyte enriched cell populations were prepared from histologically normal human gut mucosa[4] and cocultured in various ratios to examine the effect of low and high proportions of T-cells on immunoglobulin secretion from a fixed number of B-cells[5] maintained at 50,000/0.2 ml culture. IgA, IgG, and IgM concentrations were determined on seven day culture supernatants.[6] Cocultures contained pokeweed mitogen at a 1:200 concentration. From dose-response curves, B:T-cell ratios of 2:1 and 2:10 were chosen to determine T-cell help and suppression respectively. T-cell mediated help (arbitrarily defined as an increase

TABLE 2

HELP PROVIDED BY GUT MUCOSAL T-LYMPHOCYTES

Source	IgG		IgA		IgM	
	B-cells*	Percent Help†	B-cells	Percent Help	B-cells	Percent Help
Stomach	53 (3)‡	40	540 (5)	30	130 (2)	28
Ileum	38 (2)	520	40 (3)	200	45 (5)	4000
Colon	34 (1)	90	350 (2)	33	85 (1)	200
Blood	140 (10)	210	44 (10)	220	170 (10)	180

*Ig secretion in ng/ml
†Percent increase in Ig secretion at B:T = 2:1 (see text)
‡( ) = Number of experiments

TABLE 3

SUPPRESSION OF MUCOSAL B-CELLS BY MUCOSAL T-CELLS

Source	Percent Inhibition of Ig Secretion (At B:T = 2:10)*		
	IgG	IgA	IgM
Stomach	22 (4)†	25 (4)	48 (4)
Ileum	94 (2)	76 (3)	72 (5)
Blood	43 (10)	66 (10)	34 (10)

*Expressed as a percent of Ig secretion at B:T = 2:1
†( ) = Number of experiments

of immunoglobulin concentration of ≥50 ng/ml) was demonstrated for IgG in five of six experiments, IgA in eight of ten experiments, and IgM in eight of eight experiments. T-cell mediated suppression (arbitrarily defined as a reduction of ≥20% of immunoglobulin concentration with a B:T = 2:10 when compared with a B:T = 2:1) was demonstrated for IgG in four of six experiments, IgA in six of seven experiments, and IgM in seven of nine experiments (TABLES 2 and 3).

DISCUSSION

Components of three studies on the development and control of local immunity in man are presented as they relate to B-cell responsiveness.

First, the ontogeny of secretory immunity was studied by measuring immunoglobulin and *E. coli* antibody in saliva through the first year of life. After a transient period of "mucosal leakiness," characterized by high levels of IgG and albumin in saliva, IgA appears in an oscillatory pattern, before it stabilizes at adult levels, at about eight months. The failure to detect *E. coli* antibody in saliva in the first six months despite colonization by *E. coli* is most consistent with a polyclonal activation of IgA B-cells by products from colonizing bacteria. Only IgM was detected in short duration "bursts" that appeared to correlate in individuals with dietetic changes. The oscillatory pattern of IgA secretion and the

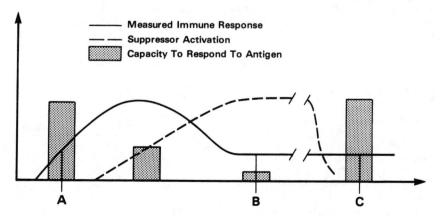

FIGURE 3. Graph to demonstrate hypothesis that B-cell responsiveness is determined by balance struck between intrinsic capacity of B-cells to respond and suppressor influences.

limited "bursts" of IgM appearing in saliva best fit a model of a stimulus-activated succession of waves of activation and feedback suppression.

Second, both T-suppressor and helper cells capable of regulating mucosal B-cell function were demonstrated within human gut mucosa using a method of coculture that had demonstrated defects in human autoimmune disease.[5] This observation complements previous studies that demonstrated that human gut T-cells can inhibit antigen- or mitogen-initiated lymphocyte proliferation.[4]

Third, the ability of an orally administered killed bacterial vaccine to stimulate antibody secretion in saliva was influenced by the preimmunization antibody level. This finding suggests that either local antibody at a low level may interfere with antigen handling, or that low levels of antibody reflect a sensitization of both B-cells and suppressor mechanisms that limit subsequent responsiveness.

Two of the above studies have used events in saliva to monitor the effects of stimuli acting at the level of the gut. Local stimulation, antigen transfer, or an IgA pump mechanism cannot be rigidly excluded, but the most likely link between gut and salivary mucosal surfaces is a selective cell traffic.[7] The data obtained in these studies collectively support the hypothesis that the capacity of primed mucosal B-lymphocytes to respond to antigen, or mitogen, is determined by the degree of suppressor-cell influence at that time; activation and suppression follow a stimulus in successive but overlapping waves of variable duration. Thus, the capacity to secrete antibody at any time in response to an antigenic stimulus depends on the balance struck between antigen reactive cells, their intrinsic capacity to respond to stimulus, and the degree of extrinsic suppression (FIGURE 3).

REFERENCES

1. LAURELL, C. B. 1972. Scand. J. Clin. Lab. Invest. (Suppl. 124) **29**.
2. SUZUKI, T., E. GORZYNSKI & E. NETER. 1964. J. Bacteriol. **88**: 1240.
3. DAVIES, J. L., C. R. LAUGHTON & J. R. MAY. 1974. J. Clin. Pathol. **27**: 265.
4. PUCCI, A. & R. CLANCY. 1979. Ric. Clin. Lab. **9**: 237.
5. TRENT, R., R. CLANCY, V. DAVIS & A. BASTEN. 1981. Clin. Exp. Immunol. **45**: 9.
6. CLANCY, R., A. CRIPPS & H. CHIPCASE. Submitted for publication.
7. RUDZIK, O., R. CLANCY, D. PEREY & J. BIENENSTOCK. 1975. J. Immunol. **114**: 1599.

DISCUSSION OF THE PAPER

J. R. McGHEE (*University of Alabama in Birmingham*): I am concerned about your separated cells, in the last part of your talk, with regard to your criteria for T- and B-cells. How did you determine this criteria?

R. CLANCY (*University of Newcastle, Newcastle, Australia*): Our criteria for these particular studies were that the T-cells were E-rosette positive, whereas, B-lymphocytes have membrane immunoglobulin fluorescence.

P. BRANDTZAEG (*National Hospital, Oslo, Norway*): How did you collect your saliva? My question is related to the effect of flow rate on the concentrations of

IgA that are quite dramatic. I wonder if there is an age dependence on the flow rate of the saliva that could cause this drop in levels of IgA in the babies.

CLANCY: We have used unstimulated saliva, which is easy to get from babies. The only time we required stimulation with a drop of lemon was in the first week of life. We have had some difficulty in getting significant amounts of saliva. We have not done flow rates in these children. We are trying to use an epidemiological approach. All I can say is that the albumin levels remain constant in these samples. I suppose one could not strictly say that there is not some specific variable on flow rates at the second month.

MONOCLONAL ANTIBODIES RECOGNIZING THE SECRETED AND MEMBRANE DOMAINS OF THE IgA DIMER RECEPTOR*

Lukas C. Kühn† and Jean-Pierre Kraehenbuhl

Institute of Biochemistry
University of Lausanne
CH-1066 Epalinges, Switzerland

INTRODUCTION

Polymeric immunoglobulins, assembled and secreted by mature plasma cells, are unidirectionally translocated across epithelial cells of exocrine glands and mucous surfaces.[1-4] The transport mechanism involves binding to specific basolateral cell-surface receptors, adsorbtive endocytosis, intracellular vesicular transport, and release into external fluids.[5-11]

The predominant secretory immunoglobulin in most exosecretions consists of a J-chain-containing dimer of immunoglobulin A (IgA dimer), associated with secretory component (SC), a hydrophilic glycoprotein of epithelial origin.[12] Early investigators observed that the formation of IgA dimer-SC complexes occurs during transepithelial transport.[13] This finding led them to the idea that SC might mediate IgA-dimer translocation.[14] In support for such a proposal, immunocytochemical localization with anti-SC antibodies displayed SC-antigenic determinants not only in the rough endoplasmic reticulum, the Golgi complex, and intracellular vesicles,[6,7,9-11] but also at the basolateral plasma membrane of epithelial cells.[7,9,15] Direct binding of IgA dimer to intact epithelial cells or enriched plasma membrane fractions have shown specific and high affinity interaction with membrane-associated SC, confirming its role as a surface receptor.[15,16]

Recent experiments, in a cell-free translation system with heterologous microsomal membranes, indicate that SC is synthesized exclusively as a transmembrane protein with a cytoplasmic extension of 15 kilodaltons.[17] The *in vitro* translated SC has been shown to bind specifically to IgA dimer.[17] Affinity-purified IgA dimer receptor from rabbit liver and mammary gland is identical with affinity-purified membrane SC, revealing a group of amphiphilic proteins with apparent molecular weights of 120, 116, 95, and 91 kilodaltons.[18] In one-dimensional peptide maps, the liver membrane SC shares extensive structural homology with SC from rabbit milk.[18] Milk SC is equally heterogenous with molecular weights of 83, 80, 58 and 55 kilodaltons. The membrane receptors for IgA dimer appear, therefore, to be precursor molecules of the mature secretory forms of secretory component.[17,18] Release of SC from membranes must involve proteolytic cleavage of the membrane precursor, leaving behind a 35 kilodalton membrane peptide.

To gain further insight into the receptor-mediated endocytosis and transport of

*This work was supported by Grant No. 672-0-80 from the Swiss National Science Foundation.
Address for correspondence: Dr. Lukas C. Kühn, Department of Biology, Yale University, Kline Biology Tower, P. O. Box 6666, New Haven, Conn. 06511.

0077-8923/83/0409-0751 $1.75/0 © 1983, NYAS

IgA dimers, we have prepared monoclonal antibodies[19] against the purified rabbit liver IgA dimer receptor (membrane secretory component). Both antibodies described in the current paper efficiently immunoprecipitate membrane SC; however, only one of them is capable of interacting with free SC from milk. Thus they are directed against antigenic determinants on two distinct domains of the IgA dimer receptor, the membrane anchorage peptide and the ectoplasmic domain that gives rise to secreted secretory component.

MATERIALS AND METHODS

Reagents and Animals

Protein A-Sepharose-CL-4B was obtained from Pharmacia Fine Chemicals, polyethylene glycol 1500 from Schwarz/Mann, rabbit IgG-anti-mouse Ig from Nordic Immunology, and goat anti-mouse heavy chain class- and subclass-specific antisera from Cappel. Other chemicals were purchased as reported.[18] The mouse myeloma cell line SP2/0 was kindly provided by Dr. M. Nabholz. Cells and hybrids were grown in Dulbecco's modified Eagle's medium (DMEM) with high glucose (4.5 g/l) supplemented with 10% fetal calf serum from Gibco, 10 mM Hepes (N-2 hydroxyethylpiperazine-N-2 ethane sulfonic acid), folic acid (12 mg/l), arginine (200 mg/l), asparagine (36 mg/l), 50 μM 2-mercaptoethanol, penicillin 100 (IU/ml), and streptomycin (100 μg/ml). Selective HAT (hypoxathine, aminopterine, thymidine)-medium contained in addition 0.1 mM hypoxanthine, 0.4 μM aminopterin, and 16 μM thymidine.[20] Eight-week-old female BALB/c mice and four-month-old DBA mice were from the breeding colony at the Swiss Cancer Institute in Lausanne.

Immunization

Rabbit liver IgA dimer receptor used for immunization was purified as described[18] by anti-SC affinity chromatography followed by preparative polyacrylamide gel electrophoresis in sodium dodecylsulfate (SDS-PAGE). BALB/c mice were immunized twice, with an interval of three weeks, by intraperitoneal injections of 50 μg receptor in complete and incomplete Freund's adjuvant. Three days after the second injection, the spleen was removed under sterile conditions.

Cell Fusion

Hybridization was performed according to a standard method.[21] 10^8 viable spleen cells were mixed with 10^7 SP2/0 myeloma cells and pelleted in serum-free DMEM. Cells were loosened by tapping, and 0.4 ml of a 50% solution of polythelene glycol was added dropwise over a period of one minute under constant gentle mixing at 37° C. After one additional minute, and within the following five minutes, the cell suspension was diluted dropwise with serum-free HAT-medium to 5 ml, and 15 minutes later to 100 ml in complete HAT-medium. Aliquots with 10^5 or 10^4 spleen cells were immediately pipetted into 96 well Falcon plates on top of feeder layers. Feeder layers had been plated two days earlier with 2×10^4 peritoneal macrophages from DBA mice. Fresh HAT-medium was added seven days after fusion. Culture supernatants of growing hybrid colonies were screened on days 10 to 17.

Monoclonal Antibody Production

The presence of specific monoclonal antibodies in culture supernatants was tested by immunoprecipitation of radiolabeled IgA dimer receptor. Triplicates with 50 μl culture supernatant and 50,000 cpm of antigen, iodinated by the chloramine-T method,[18,22] were incubated overnight at 4° C in a final volume of 100 μl buffer containing 50 mM Tris-HCl, pH 8.3, 0.5% bovine serum albumin, 0.05% SDS, and 0.5% Triton X-100. A second overnight incubation after addition of 1 μg rabbit IgG anti-mouse Ig in 50 μl buffer was followed by incubation for four hours at 4° C with a 100 μl suspension of 1 μl packed protein A-Sepharose and 9 μl Sepharose 4B. The radioactivity adsorbed on Sepharose was counted after one wash with 3 ml 0.1 M Tris-HCl pH 8.3. Positive supernatants precipitated up to 3000 cpm, whereas background levels ranged at 500 cpm.

Positive hybrid colonies were cloned by limiting dilution. Ascites fluids with titers up to 10 mg/ml were obtained by intraperitoneal injection of 10^7 cloned hybridoma cells into pristane-primed DBA mice.

Immunoprecipitations and Sodium Dodecylsulfate Polyacrylamide Gel Electrophoresis

Iodinated IgA dimer receptor (0.4 × 10^6 cpm) or affinity purified[18] milk sIgA (1.7 × 10^6 cpm) were immunoprecipitated with 2 μl ascites fluid and 10 μl protein A-Sepharose according to the above protocol. The step including rabbit IgG anti-mouse Ig was omitted. Sepharose beads were washed three times and analyzed on a 5–13% polyacrylamide gel.[23] For autoradiography, dried gels were exposed to Kodak XS-5 films.

RESULTS

The screening of 330 culture wells containing hybrid cells revealed two hybridoma colonies whose supernatants were consistently anti-receptor antibody positive. The monoclonal antibodies have been designated anti-SC 166 and anti-SC 303. In Ouchterlony double diffusion, both antibodies exhibited heavy chains of the IgG$_1$ subclass. Upon immunoprecipitation of iodinated liver IgA dimer receptor (membrane SC), both higher ($M_r \sim$ 120 and 116 kilodaltons) and lower ($M_r \sim$ 95 and 91 kilodaltons) molecular weight forms were precipitated with either one of the monoclonal antibodies (FIGURE 1, lanes 2 and 3). The amount of antigen precipitated by a mixture of both antibodies, corresponded to the sum of each separate precipitation (FIGURE 1, lane 5). Free SC from milk competed the precipitation with anti-SC 303, but not with anti-SC 166 (FIGURE 1, lanes 6 and 7). Likewise, only anti-SC 303 could precipitate iodinated free SC present in an affinity-purified milk sIgA-preparation (FIGURE 1, lanes 8 and 9). This result was confirmed in samples with mixed IgA dimer receptor and sIgA (FIGURE 1, lanes 14 and 15). Nonspecific adsorption to protein A-Sepharose was not observed. Interestingly, anti-SC 303 did not precipitate covalent sIgA (FIGURE 1, lane 9).

Additional experiments performed on deoxycholate-solubilized proteins of rabbit liver microsomal membrane fractions showed that both monoclonal antibodies exclusively immunoprecipitated the IgA dimer receptor (results not shown). The antigenic site, however, recognized by anti-SC 303 was destroyed upon reduction and alkylation of the receptor.

DISCUSSION

Since its discovery more than 15 years ago,[13] the secretory component (SC) has been considered a possible mediator in the transport of polymeric immunoglobu-

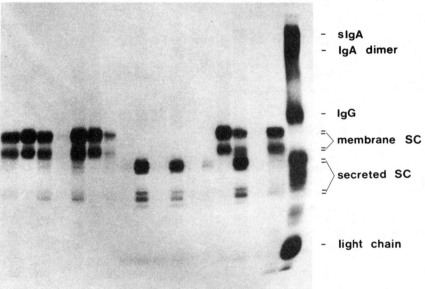

FIGURE 1. Immunoprecipitates with mouse monoclonal antibodies and protein A-Sepharose of radioiodinated rabbit liver IgA dimer receptor (lanes 1 to 7 and 14 to 17) or a mixture of rabbit milk free SC and covalently bound SC (sIgA) (lanes 8 to 15 and 18) were analyzed by SDS-PAGE on a 5–13% gel. Lanes 1, 17, and 18 show the antigens prior to precipitation as a reference. Immunoprecipitations were performed as described in MATE-RIALS AND METHODS with the following antibodies: lanes 2, 8, and 14—anti-SC 166; lanes 3, 9, and 15—anti-SC 303; lanes 4 and 10—no antibody; lanes 5 and 11—mixture of anti-SC 166 and 303; lanes 6 and 12—anti-SC 166 preincubated for one hour at 37° C with 100 μg unlabeled rabbit milk free SC; lanes 7 and 13—anti-SC 303 preincubated with SC.

lins.[14] Several transport models have been proposed.[4] With the accumulation and refinement of immunocytochemical data,[5–11] and more recently by *in vitro* binding studies with radiolabeled IgA dimer,[15,16] it has become clear that SC-like antigens with IgA-dimer binding properties are expressed at the basolateral surface of epithelial cells in both glandular and mucosal tissues. *In vivo* studies on the perfused rat liver confirmed the role of SC-like binding sites in the IgA dimer translocation process from serum into bile.[3,24,25]

The relationship between the hydrophilic SC and membrane associated SC-like antigens have recently been examined at the molecular level.[17,18] It is now well established that SC is exclusively synthesized as a transmembrane protein and that membrane SC functions as the IgA dimer receptor both in rabbit liver and mammary gland.[17,18,26] Solubilized rabbit membrane and secreted SC show striking homologies in their molecular weight heterogeneity,[18] peptide maps,[18] high affinity interaction with IgA dimer (affinity constant $\sim 10^8$ M^{-1}),[18,27] and the presence of antigenic sites recognized by xenogeneic,[18] allogeneic[28] (unpublished results), and monoclonal anti-SC 303 antibodies. All these features are shared by the higher and lower molecular weight forms of rabbit SC, suggesting no functional difference despite the heterogeneity. These results, in conjunction with fucose-labeling experiments showing that the label appeared first on the sinusoidal membrane of rat hepatocytes and later in bile,[29] lead to the conclusion that the IgA dimer receptor is the precursor of secreted secretory component.

In order to release mature SC, or receptor-bound IgA dimer (sIgA) into exosecretion, a proteolytic cleavage of receptors must occur at an as yet unknown location along the IgA dimer transport pathway. The enzyme involved is not known, nor has it been shown that the cleavage is sufficient to ensure rapid release into exosecretion. Considering our experimental evidence of an epithelial SC-receptor,[15] it is conceivable that mature SC, once generated by the cleavage, retains some affinity to its counterpart, the membrane anchorage peptide. IgA dimer might influence such an affinity.

The concept of a precursor relationship between IgA dimer receptor and mature secreted SC explains several important features of IgA dimer transport through epithelial cells: the expression of SC-antigenic determinants at the basolateral cell surface, the vectorial nature of the transport process, the formation of sIgA, and its release into secretion upon exocytosis. The unique properties of a receptor that is cleaved to give rise to a secreted protein implies that each IgA dimer receptor can operate only once. From the amount of receptor present in rabbit liver[18] and the daily output of SC into bile, we estimate that all the receptors are replaced about 10 times per day. In the lactating mammary gland the estimate is even higher. This rapid turnover implies an extraordinary high rate of membrane receptor synthesis and a receptor half life that compares to the time required for its basolateral expression and intracellular transport.[29] This phenomenon suggests a continuous flow of SC from the Golgi complex, by way of the basolateral surface to the apical surface. It has been observed that this flow is independent of ligand-receptor interactions.[30]

In order to gain further insight into the fate of the rabbit IgA dimer receptor during endocytosis and intracellular transport, we have prepared monoclonal antibodies. One of our antibodies, the anti-SC 303, clearly is directed against the receptor domain that is secreted. Its poor interaction with sIgA suggests that it recognizes an SC-antigenic determinant that is hidden in the SC-IgA dimer complex. Hidden determinants have been described in the human species and their use has provided immunocytochemical evidence that covalent interaction of SC with IgA dimer occurs during the transepithelial transport.[5] The other monoclonal antibody, anti-SC 166, distinguishes between membrane and secreted SC, and is therefore directed against the membrane domain of the IgA dimer receptor. As a consequence of receptor cleavage, this domain can be expected to accumulate as a 35 kilodalton peptide on the apical membrane. We have recently investigated the localization of this peptide on thin frozen sections from rabbit liver and found strong immunofluorescence with anti-SC 166, but not with anti-SC 303, on the canalicular hepatocyte membrane (unpublished results). Experiments to determine whether anti-SC 166 is directed to the cytoplasmic extension are in progress. It has been proposed that this domain might contain information needed for membrane protein sorting.[17] The clustering and uptake of receptors into endocytotic vesicles and the intracellular vectorial translocation of these vesicles[9,25] may involve interactions between cytoplasmic sites on the receptor and cytoskeletal proteins. Monoclonal antibodies to these sites could provide a tool to study such interactions and to isolate the transport vesicles.

SUMMARY

The receptor that mediates the specific uptake and intracellular transport of dimeric immunoglobulin A (IgA dimer) in mucosal and glandular epithelia is identical with a transmembrane precursor of secreted secretory component. During transport, the IgA dimer receptor (membrane SC) is cleaved into two domains, a membrane anchorage peptide and secreted secretory component. We have produced monoclonal antibodies with distinct specificity against both domains of the rabbit IgA dimer receptor. Two mouse hybridoma lines were obtained by fusion of SP2/0 myeloma cells with spleen cells from mice immunized with purified receptor from rabbit liver and by screening of culture supernatants in an immunoprecipitation assay with radiolabeled receptor. One antibody, designated anti-SC 303, reacts both with membrane and secreted SC and is therefore directed to a determinant on the secreted domain of the IgA dimer receptor. The other antibody, anti-SC 166, unable to interact with secreted SC, recognizes the membrane domain of the receptor. We discussed the unique precursor relationship between a cell-surface receptor and a secreted protein and its implications in the IgA dimer transport system.

ACKNOWLEDGMENTS

We wish to thank Ms. Maya Günthert for technical assistance, Dr. Michael Kamarck for his critical reading of the manuscript, and Ms. Marie Siniscalchi for secretarial assistance.

REFERENCES

1. LAMM, M. E. 1976. Adv. Immunol. **22**: 223–290.
2. KRAEHENBUHL, J. P. & L. C. KÜHN. 1978. In Transport of Macromolecules in Cellular Systems, Life Science Research Report. S. Silverstein, Ed.: 213–218. Dahlem Konferenzen Berlin.
3. VAERMAN, J. P. & I. LEMAÎTRE-COELHO. 1979. In Protein Transmission through Living Membranes, W. A. Hemmings, Ed.: 383–398. Elsevier. North Holland.
4. BRANDTZAEG, P. 1981. Clin. Exp. Immunol. **44**: 221–232.
5. BRANDTZAEG, P. 1974. J. Immunol. **112**: 1553–1559.
6. KRAEHENBUHL, J. P., L. RACINE & R. E. GALARDY. 1975. Ann. N.Y. Acad. Sci. **254**: 190–202.
7. BROWN, W. R., Y. ISOBE, & P. K. NAKANE. 1976. Gastroenterology **71**: 985–995.
8. CRAGO, S. S., R. KULHAVY, S. J. PRINCE & J. MESTECKY. 1978. J. Exp. Med. **147**: 1832–1837.
9. NAGURA, H., P. K. NAKANE & W. R. BROWN. 1979. J. Immunol. **123**: 2359–2368.
10. BIRBECK, M. S. C., P. CARTWRIGHT, J. G. HALL, E. ORLANS & J. PEPPARD. 1979. Immunology **37**: 477–484.

11. RENSTON, R. H., A. L. JONES, W. D. CHRISTIANSEN, G. T. HRADEK & B. J. UNDERDOWN. 1980. Science **208:** 1276–1278.
12. TOMASI, T. B. & H. M. GREY. 1972. Prog. Allergy **16:** 81–213.
13. TOMASI, T. B., E. M. TAN, A. SOLOMON & R. A. PRENDERGAST. 1965. J. Exp. Med. **121:** 101–124.
14. SOUTH, M. A., M. D. COOPER, F. A. WOLLHEIM, R. HONG & R. A. GOOD. 1966. J. Exp. Med. **123:** 615—627.
15. KÜHN, L. C. & J. P. KRAEHENBUHL. 1979. J. Biol. Chem. **254:** 11072–11081.
16. SOCKEN, D. J., K. N. JEEJEEBHOY, H. BAZIN & B. J. UNDERDOWN. 1979. J. Exp. Med. **50:** 1538–1548.
17. MOSTOV, K. E., J. P. KRAEHENBUHL & G. BLOBEL. 1980. Proc. Natl. Acad. Sci. USA **77:** 7257–7261.
18. KÜHN, L. C. & J. P. KRAEHENBUHL. 1981. J. Biol. Chem. **256:** 12490–12495.
19. KÖHLER, G. & C. MILSTEIN. 1975. Nature (London) **256:** 495–497.
20. LITTLEFIELD, J. W. 1964. Science **145:** 709–710.
21. GALFRÉ, G., S. C. HOWE, C. MILSTEIN, G. W. BUTCHER & J. C. HOWARD. 1977. Nature (London) **266:** 550–552.
22. GREENWOOD, F. C., W. M. HUNTER & J. S. GLOVER. 1963. Biochem. J. **89:** 114–123.
23. MAIZEL, J. V. 1971. Methods Virol. **5:** 179–246.
24. FISHER, M. M., B. NAGY, H. BAZIN & B. J. UNDERDOWN. 1979. Proc. Natl. Acad. Sci. USA **76:** 2008–2012.
25. MULLOCK, B. M. & R. H. HINTON. 1981. Trends Biochem. Sci. **6:** 188–191.
26. KÜHN, L. C. & J. P. KRAEHENBUHL. 1982. Trends Biochem. Sci. **7:** 299–302.
27. KÜHN, L. C. & J. P. KRAEHENBUHL. 1979. J. Biol. Chem. **254:** 11066–11071.
28. KNIGHT, K. L., M. ROSENZWEIG, E. A. LICHTER & W. C. HANLY. 1974. J. Immunol. **112:** 877–882.
29. MULLOCK, B. M., R. H. HINTON, M. DOBROTA, J. PEPPARD & E. ORLANS. 1980. Biochem. J. **190:** 819–826.
30. MULLOCK, B. M., R. S. JONES & R. H. HINTON. 1980. FEBS Lett. **113:** 201–205.

DISCUSSION OF THE PAPER

B. J. UNDERDOWN (*University of Toronto, Ontario, Canada*): Have you any data related to the point raised by others that there may be a receptor for polymeric IgA other than secretory component? When you isolate the receptor on an IgA column, do you ever see any other components, or does your monoclonal antibody to the ectoplasmic domain of SC inhibit the IgA transport?

L. C. KÜHN (*University of Lausanne, Epalinges, Switzerland*): We have not yet done any transport studies *in vivo.* Using IgA-Sepharose for adsorbtion, we could not see any additional components adsorbed when compared to anti-secretory component-Sepharose. All bands that we could see were identical in both affinity columns; these results indicate that there is no additional IgA receptor, at least not with sufficiently high affinity in order to be detected by this kind of technique.

J. M. SCHIFF (*University of Toronto, Toronto, Ontario, Canada*): I was interested in the heterogeneity of secretory component. I noticed that in your peptide map, you separated SC-derived peptides so that they could be classified into two groups. The question is: Are they not splitting into large sizes and small sizes?

KÜHN: Large size molecules from the membrane have peptides in common with the large size of the secreted form of SC, and the small size membrane molecules have peptides in common with the small size of the secreted form. If you calculate the molecular weight of each of the peptides and try to make an aligning peptide map, you come up with the model I have shown. The large and small size forms of SC actually have a common domain.

SCHIFF: Are they allotypes?

KÜHN: No. But in secretion, we can distinguish four proteins, that is, two doublets, an upper and lower, for each allotype. We obtained antibodies from Drs. Hanly and Knight who performed extensive studies on these allotypes. Both upper and lower molecular forms have the allotypic determinant. On SDS polyacrylamide gels, crosslinked by diallyltartardiamide instead of bisacrylamide, one can distinguish the two allotypes. There are four bands for each homozygous animal. In addition, we usually find three degradation products that are derived from one of the two allotypes.

SCHIFF: Is there one gene for secretory component, or two?

KÜHN: We cannot answer this question before having done the analysis at the DNA level. I think that we can expect to find either a gene duplication, or some kind of transposition where we have a smaller gene, in common for both forms, that would be linked or not to extragenous DNA. The third possibility would be that we have one gene and differential splicing.

T. B. TOMASI (*University of New Mexico, Albuquerque, N.M.*): Would you clarify for me what you think is going on with the transport across the cell? You have here an unusual type of situation compared to the coated pit and coated vesicle type of mechanism. The material being transported goes through to the other side of the cell. The only other similar situation I know of is in the placenta. One possibility would be that the receptor, in this case secretory component, stays attached to IgA all the way through and comes out on the other side together with the IgA molecule. If that is the case, then the SC attached to the IgA would be larger by the size of your transmembrane C terminal portion that has a molecular weight of 30,000. The other possibility would be that the receptor is proteolyzed, and in this case, IgA would acquire another secretory component. This secretory component would be the same secretory component that was created by differential RNA splicing to generate the secretory form rather than the transmembrane form. If the latter is the case, then the free secretory component should have the same C terminal structure as the secretory component attached to the IgA molecule. If the former is the case, then the C terminal part of the molecule might be different. If the receptor is removed from IgA, is it completely proteolyzed or is it reinserted into the membrane?

KÜHN: I believe that IgA remains attached to the receptor all the way through the cell and that proteolytic cleavage of the receptor allows the release of sIgA. No mRNA coding for the secreted forms have been found, indicating that all secreted SC derive from cleaved membrane SC. I have the feeling that one secretory component molecule is used as a receptor only once in its lifetime. The reason I believe this, is that one finds an excess of secretory component in secretions of all species. There is always an excess of free SC over IgA. I think the transport, and indeed, the route of transport is taking place whether there is IgA or not. The splitting of the receptor is also taking place whether there is IgA or not.

TOMASI: Do you know whether the C terminal is free, or is it bound?

KÜHN: Dr. Mostov examined the N-terminus. Given that N-terminus is the same, I would think that the C terminal end is different in secreted and membrane SC. There is no difference in secreted SC bound to IgA and free secretory component. They are exactly the same molecules.

M. LAMM (*Case Western Reserve University, Cleveland, Ohio*): Dr. Good, do you think we should stop calling this molecule secretory component and go back to transport piece?

R. A. GOOD (*Oklahoma Medical Research Foundation, Oklahoma City*): I have insisted on this name for a long time. The question I had goes back to initial observations in the agammaglobulinemic patient, or in the patient with selective absence of IgA. In secretions of such patients, one finds large amounts of the secretory component. How do you visualize the initiation of this transport motion within the cell? Is it constantly going on or is it generated by the combination with the immunoglobulin? I would think that the observation in the immunodeficient patient would suggest that the process is related to the receptor and not related to the combination.

KÜHN: The results that Dr. Mostov presented favor the former possibility. He detected a mature form of SC without the addition of IgA to epithelial cells.

SECRETORY IgA ANTIBODIES FROM BILE OF IMMUNIZED RATS REACTIVE WITH TROPHOZOITES OF ENTAMOEBA HISTOLYTICA

G. Acosta, R. Campos, C. Barranco, A. Isibasi, and J. Kumate

División Inmunoquímica
Unidad de Investigación Biomédica
Instituto Mexicano del Seguro Social
03020 Mexico D.F., México

INTRODUCTION

Amoebiasis is an infection produced by the ingestion of cysts of *Entamoeba histolytica*. Once the cyst undergoes a transformation into trophozoites, it attaches itself to intestinal epithelial cells, causing dysentery and colon ulceration. Taking into account that the predominant antibodies in intestinal secretions are of the IgA class, it is possible that the presence of trophozoites of *Entamoeba histolytica* in the large intestine induces the production of specific IgA antibodies against the parasite. Because of the problems of inducing experimental intestinal amoebiasis, it is difficult to obtain antibodies against the parasite from the intestine. Under normal circumstances, a large amount of secretory IgA is secreted daily in the duodenum by way of the bile.[1] In previous work using this model, we assayed the induction of specific IgA antiamoeba antibodies, immunizing rats through different routes. We obtained positive results immunizing the rats intraperitoneally and challenging them intracaecally with trophozoites.[2] The aim of the present work is to investigate any possible reactions of secretory IgA immunoglobulin, purified from bile of immunized rats, with trophozoites of *Entamoeba histolytica*.

MATERIALS AND METHODS

Entamoeba histolytica *Cultures*

Trophozoites of *Entamoeba histolytica*, strain HK 9, were grown axenically for 72 hours, in a medium containing trypticase, yeast extract, iron, and bovine serum as described by Diamond,[3] and before use, washed six times with saline.

Immunization Protocol

A group of 32 rats (150–200 g) were injected four times intraperitoneally with 2×10^6 trophozoites. Two weeks later, the group was given a boostered injection intracaecally with the same number of trophozoites. The control group was not

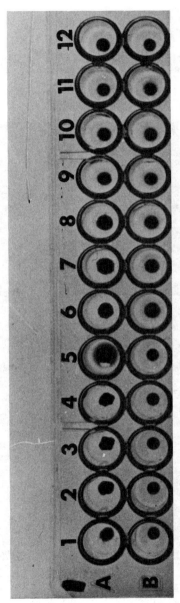

FIGURE 1. Indirect hemagglutination, sheep erythrocytes sensitized with lipopeptidephosphoglycan extracted from trophozoites of *E. histolytica* by a phenol-water method. Upper wells (A): Secretory IgA obtained from the bile of rats immunized with trophozoites of *E. histolytica* agglutinates and sensitized red blood cells in a titer of 1:128. Lower wells (B): Iga obtained from control rats.

immunized. After cannulation of the common bile duct on the day of the boosters, bile was collected 5–7 days thereafter.

Purification of sIgA from Rat Bile

The bile of immunized rats and controls was pooled separately, concentrated by vacuum ultrafiltration, and filtered on Ultrogel AcA 22 column as previously reported.[4]

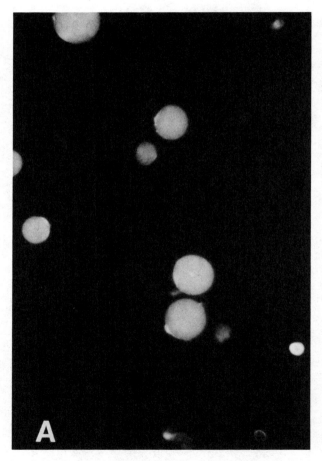

FIGURE 2. Capping in *E. histolytica* induced by antibodies. On picture A, trophozoites were incubated with anti-*E. histolytica* secretory IgA (1 mg/ml) and then exposed to FITC-rabbit IgG antirat IgA for 15 minutes at 4° C, washed thoroughly, and incubated for an extra 15 minutes at 37° C. On picture B: Trophozoites were incubated with secretory IgA from control rats under the same conditions.

Antisera

Rabbit specific antisera against rat IgA used in all experiments was provided by J.P. Vaerman (Unit of Experimental Medicine, Catholic University of Louvain, Brussels, Belgium). Rabbit antisera against whole serum was prepared in our laboratory.

Indirect Hemagglutination

Sheep red blood cells were washed three times in PBS. A pellet of 250 μl of cells was mixed with 0.75 mg of lipopeptidephosphoglycan, extracted from the same strain of trophozoites by a phenol-water method,[5] and incubated at 37°C for

FIGURE 2 (continued)

30 minutes with agitation. They were centrifugated and washed twice; the supernatant fluid was removed. The cells were suspended at 1.5% in PBS containing 1% normal rabbit serum. Two hundred microliters of secretory IgA obtained from immunized and control rats were diluted separately in PBS, containing 1% normal rabbit serum, using a Cooke microtiter plate. Finally, 25 μl of the 1.5% of sensitized red cells suspension were added to all the wells.

Indirect Immunofluorescent Studies

Two hundred microliters of secretory IgA, obtained from immunized and control rats were incubated with 3×10^5 trophozoites for 15 minutes at 4°C, washed twice with saline, and incubated at 37°C for 10, 30, and 45 minutes. The cells were fixed with 1% paraformaldehyde, washed, and incubated with 100 μl of rabbit IgG antirat IgA and conjugated with fluorescein isothiocyanate (FITC) as reported by Johnson et al.[6] They were then incubated for 30 minutes at room temperature, washed, and examined with an epifluorescence microscope (UnivaR, Reichert, Austria).

RESULTS

Hemagglutination Titers

The IgA purified fraction of the bile from the rats immunized with trophozoites was compared by hemagglutination to the same fraction of control bile, after adjusting both to 1 mg/ml. The control bile IgA-fraction did not agglutinate sensitized red blood cells, whereas the IgA fraction from the immunized rats agglutinated sensitized red blood cells in a titer of 1:128 (FIGURE 1).

Indirect Immunofluorescent Studies

The two samples of purified IgA fractions obtained from control and immunized rats were used at 1 mg/ml. Incubating at 4°C for 10 minutes, only the sIgA obtained from immunized rats bound to the surface of Entamoeba histolytica. After the trophozoites were washed and incubated for the same period of time at 37°C, it was observed that secretory IgA anti-amoeba was concentrated in a typical cap (FIGURE 2). Thirty minutes later, all trophozoites had released their caps into medium.

DISCUSSION

It has been reported that sera of patients with invasive amoebiasis contain antibodies of IgG class against amoeba. When the antibodies are bound to the trophozoites, they induce surface redistribution of membrane components, and the formed caps are released. This evasive mechanism helps trophozoites overcome the effect of antibodies to amoeba.[7]

It is feasible that under normal circumstances IgA antibodies act in intestinal amoebiasis. Our results demonstrated that rats, challenged intracaecally with trophozoites, synthesize IgA antibodies found in bile. These antibodies react with material extracted from the same strain of trophozoites and also bind to the surface of the amoeba. The amoebas form fewer caps compared to those formed with IgG. This formation might be explained by low titers of antibodies or special properties of secretory IgA (higher molecular weight, dimeric structure). It is possible, but no proved, that this class of immunoglobulin plays an important role in intestinal immunity and protection against the parasite.

ACKNOWLEDGMENTS

We wish to thank A. Ramirez for technical assistance.

REFERENCES

1. LEMAITRE-COELHO, I., G. D. F. JACKSON & J. P. VAERMAN. 1977. Rat bile as a convenient source of secretory IgA and free secretory component. Eur. J. Immunol. **7:** 588.
2. ACOSTA, G., C. BARRANCO, R. CAMPOS, A. RAMIREZ, A. ISIBASI & J. KUMATE. 1981. Induction of antibodies of secretory IgA class in the bile of rats immunized with trophozoites of *Entamoeba histolytica*. Arch. Invest. Med. (Mex.) (Supl. 2) **12**(4): 64.
3. DIAMOND, L. S. 1968. Technique of axenic cultivation of *Entamoeba histolytica* like amoeba. J. Parasit. **54:** 1047.
4. ACOSTA, G., C. BARRANCO-ACOSTA, E. VAN ROOST & J. P. VAERMAN. 1980. Isolation and characterization of secretory IgA (sIgA) and free secretory component (FSC) from rat bile. Mol. Immunol. **17:** 1525.
5. ISIBASI, A., M. S. CRUZ, A. RAMIREZ & J. KUMATE. 1981. Immunochemistry of an antigen; lipopeptidephosphoglycan. A phenol-water extraction from trophozoites of *E. histolytica* cultured axenically. Arch Inv. Med. (Mex.) Supl. 2 **12**(4) suppl. 2: 63.
6. JOHNSON, G. D. E., J. MOLBOROW & J. DORLING. 1978. Immunofluorescence and Immunoenzyme techniques. *In* Handbook of Experimental Immunology. P. M. Weir, Eds.: 15: 11–13 Blackwell Scientific Publications Ltd. Oxford.
7. CALDERON, J., MA. L. MUÑOZ & H. M. ACOSTA. 1980. Surface Redistribution and Release of antibody induced caps in Entamoeba. J. Exp. Med. **151:** 185.

IgA ANTIBODY LEVELS IN HUMAN TEARS, SALIVA, AND SERUM*

Mathea R. Allansmith, Jeffrey L. Ebersole, and
Christine A. Burns

Department of Ophthalmology
Harvard Medical School
Eye Research Institute of Retina Foundation
Boston, Massachusetts 02114

The predominance of secretory IgA (sIgA) in secretions suggests that sIgA has a role in protecting mucosal surfaces.[1] IgA prevents bacteria from adhering to the mucosa[2,3] and also disposes of bacteria.[4] Although sIgA is the predominant immunoglobulin in tears,[5] it has not been demonstrated to prevent or reduce bacterial colonization of the ocular surface.[6]

Natural agglutinins to the oral Streptococcus, *Streptococcus mutans* (*S. mutans*), are present in tears,[7] although the bacterium found is a nonocular antigen.[8] In humans, ingestion of *S. mutans* causes the simultaneous appearance of anti-*S. mutans* sIgA antibodies in tears and saliva.[9,10] sIgA has also been found at peripheral sites such as the mammary and salivary mucosal surfaces after oral administration of antigen.[9,11-13] Arnold, Mestecky, and McGhee[14] found naturally occurring antibodies to five serotypes of *S. mutans* in saliva, colostrum, and serum. The relatively low antibody levels in serum compared with those in colostrum and saliva suggest that stimulation by *S. mutans* occurred remote from the site of bacterial growth, the oral mucosa.

It was of interest to determine whether remote site stimulation by the oral antigen *S. mutans* occurred in the ocular system. The presence of *S. mutans* antibodies in tears would suggest that the ocular immune system is involved in a common mucosal system.[15,16]

The presence and level of IgA antibodies to the oral microorganism *S. mutans* were determined in human tears, parotid saliva, and serum by a modified, indirect enzyme-linked immunosorbent assay. IgA antibodies were found in the tears of all 15 subjects (TABLE 1). The IgA-antibody levels in tears and saliva were not significantly different. This finding suggests that the level of IgA-antibody activity per volume is independent of the naturally occurring site of the antigen, and that local stimulation does not cause a significant difference in the antibody level per volume of secretion between exocrine sites. Much higher levels of IgA antibody were present in serum, suggesting that after oral ingestion of antigen, both the systemic and exocrine systems are stimulated. IgG antibodies to *S. mutans* were also found in human tears, saliva, and serum (TABLE 2). No relationship between serum levels, and tear and saliva levels was found for either IgA or IgG antibodies. Thus the antibodies in tears and saliva did not appear to have leaked from serum.

We conclude that there may be remote regulation of both the ocular and the parotid IgA- and IgG-antibody systems.

*This work was supported in part by Grant no. EY 02882 from the National Eye Institute.

TABLE 1

ANTI-*STREPTOCOCCUS MUTANS* IGA-ANTIBODY LEVELS IN INDIVIDUAL TEARS, PAROTID
SALIVA, AND SERUM

Subject	Level of anti-*S. mutans* IgA antibody (ELISA units)		
	Tears	Saliva	Serum
1	294	81	2,028
2	252	300	6,552
3	708	279	3,016
4	102	291	6,656
5	216	110	27,872
6	240	108	8,528
7	450	53	4,784
8	168	720	7,176
9	255	120	9,048
10	330	45	15,080
11	216	126	4,784
12	300	36	22,464
13	180	136	20,800
14	240	168	14,560
15	159	273	4,320
Median	216	110	6,552
Range	(102–708)	(36–720)	(2,028–27,872)
Mean	274.0	189.7	10,511.2
SEM	37.6	44.7	2,032.1

TABLE 2

ANTI-*STREPTOCOCCUS MUTANS* IGA-ANTIBODY LEVELS IN INDIVIDUAL TEARS, PAROTID
SALIVA, AND SERUM

Subject	Level of anti-*S. mutans* IgG antibody (ELISA units)		
	Tears	Saliva	Serum
1	135	234	48,100
2	354	122	33,800
3	7584	258	40,040
4	348	147	35,360
5	4368	204	197,600
6	4992	177	36,920
7	468	147	27,560
8	348	462	49,920
9	564	171	99,840
10	636	273	53,040
11	204	255	34,320
12	246	255	107,520
13	7680	267	242,688
14	9216	156	196,608
15	366	243	230,400
Median	354	177	40,040
Range	(135–9216)	(122–462)	(27,560–242,688)
Mean	2500.6	224.7	95,581.1
SEM	854.1	21.57	20,597.0

REFERENCES

1. TOMASI, T. B., JR & J. BIENENSTOCK. 1968. Secretory immunoglobulins. Adv. Immunol. **9:** 1–96.
2. FUBARA, E. S. & R. FRETER. 1973. Protection against enteric bacterial infection by secretory IgA antibodies. J. Immunol. **111:** 395–403.
3. SVANBORG-EDEN, C. & A. M. SVENNERHOLM. 1978. Secretory immunoglobulin A and G antibodies prevent adhesion of *Escherichia coli* to human urinary tract epithelial cells. Infect. Immun. **22:** 790–791.
4. WILLIAMS, R. C. & R. J. GIBBONS. 1972. Inhibition of bacterial adherence by secretory immunoglobulin A: A mechanism of antigen disposal. Science **177:** 697–699.
5. KNOPF, H. L. S., D. M. BERTRAN & A. Z. KAPIKIAN. 1970. Demonstration and characterization of antibody in tears following intranasal vaccination with inactivated type 13 rhinovirus: A preliminary report. Invest. Ophthalmol. **9:** 727–734.
6. MCKAY, E. & H. THOM. 1969. Observations on neonatal tears. J. Pediatr. **75:** 1245–1256.
7. ALLANSMITH, M. R., C. A. BURNS & R. R. ARNOLD. 1982. Comparison of agglutinin titers to *Streptococcus mutans* in tears, saliva, and serum. Infect. Immun. **35:** 202–205.
8. ALLANSMITH, M. R., H. B. OSTLER & M. BUTTERWORTH. 1969. Concomitance of bacteria in various areas of the eye. Arch. Ophthalmol. **82:** 37–42.
9. MCGHEE, J. R., J. MESTECKY, R. R. ARNOLD, S. M. MICHALEK, S. J. PRINCE & J. L. BABB. 1978. Induction of secretory antibodies in humans following ingestion of *Streptococcus mutans*. Adv. Exp. Med. Biol. **107:** 177–184.
10. MESTECKY, J., J. R. MCGHEE, R. R. ARNOLD, S. M. MICHALEK, S. J. PRINCE & J. L. BABB. 1978. Selective induction of an immune response in human external secretions by ingestion of bacterial antigen. J. Clin. Invest. **61:** 731–737.
11. AHLSTEDT, S., B. CARLSSON, L. A. HANSON, & R. M. GOLDBLUM. 1975. Antibody production by human colostral cells. Immunoglobulin class, specificity and quantity. Scand. J. Immunol. **4:** 535–539.
12. MICHALEK, S. M., J. R. MCGHEE, J. MESTECKY, R. R. ARNOLD & L. BOZZO. 1976. Ingestion of *Streptococcus mutans* induces secretory immunoglobulin A and caries immunity. Science **192:** 1238–1240.
13. MONTGOMERY, P. C., K. M. CONNELLY, J. COHN & C. A. SKENDERA. 1978. Remote-site stimulation of secretory IgA antibodies following bronchial and gastric stimulation. Adv. Exp. Med. Biol. **107:** 113–122.
14. ARNOLD, R. R., J. MESTECKY & J. R. MCGHEE. 1976. Naturally occurring secretory immunoglobulin A antibodies to *Streptococcus mutans* in human colostrum and saliva. Infect. Immun. **14:** 355–362.
15. BIENENSTOCK, J. M., M. MCDERMOTT & D. BEFUS. 1979. A common mucosal immune system. *In* Immunology of breast milk. P. L. Ogra and D. Dayton, Eds.: 91–98. Raven Press. New York.
16. MCDERMOTT, M. R. & J. BIENENSTOCK. 1979. Evidence for a common mucosal immunologic system. I. Migration of B immunoblasts into intestinal, respiratory and genital tissues. J. Immunol. **122:** 1892–1898.

EFFECT OF ENTERIC PRIMING WITH REOVIRUS AND LIPOIDAL AMINE ADJUVANT ON MUCOSAL LYMPHATIC TISSUE AND ANTI-VIRAL IgA SECRETION*

Arthur O. Anderson, Alan Plotner, and Donald H. Rubin

University of Pennsylvania
Philadelphia, Pennsylvania 19104

Priming by a mucosal route has been shown to be superior to parenteral inoculation in eliciting a protective secretory IgA response.[1] Indeed, parenteral priming often depresses subsequent IgA responses elicited by mucosal challenge and vice versa.[2] In addition, inactivated, attenuated, or toxoided antigens often fail to retain the essential immunogenic properties needed for an IgA response, and unmodified pathogens carry with them unacceptable toxicity. We explored the feasibility of using a mucosal adjuvant to potentiate the intestinal secretory IgA response to Reovirus serotype 1/Lang. The lipoidal amine N, N-dioctadecyl-N', N'-bis(2-hydroxyethyl) propanediamine (CP 20,961) (FIGURE 1) was used, because previous studies documented its effectiveness in potentiating an antiviral IgG response when used for parenteral priming.[3] CP 20,961 also appeared to spontaneously form antigen-bearing liposomes when mixed with nonpolar soybean oil lipids (FIGURE 2). The reovirus system has been utilized as a model for viral gastrointestinal disease.[4,5] Reovirus serotype 1/Lang binds specifically to membraneous (M)[6] cells, and it can be recovered in high titers from Peyers patches and intestinal secretions in adult mice (D. Rubin, unpublished results). Fifty-one BALB/c mice were given a single intraduodenal (ID) priming dose of live or partially UV inactivated reovirus (10^{10} particles), reovirus plus CP 20,961 (0.3mg) in soybean lipid, or adjuvant alone. Virus-specific IgA levels in intestinal secretions were measured by ELISA from 1–14 days following priming. In addition, mucosal-associated lymphatic tissues were excised, weighed, and examined histologically. The use of CP 20,961 increased reovirus specific IgA in secretions threefold on day 7 and nearly fourfold (TABLE 1) on day 14 after a single ID dose compared to mice inoculated with reovirus alone. The lymphoid compartments of the spleen and Peyer's patches (PP) were markedly enlarged at all time points after use of combinations of antigen and adjuvant (TABLES 2 & 3 and FIGURE 3a to e). In the absence of antigen, CP 20,961 appeared to increase extramedullary hematopoiesis (EMH) in the splenic red pulp without affecting follicle formation, whereas adjuvant plus virus was not associated with significant EMH stimulation. In PP, the antigen and [^{3}H]CP 20,961 accumulated as multilamellar liposome-like bodies within macrophages under the dome epithelium (FIGURE 2). There was an initial increase in small B-cells in the corona that was followed by expansion of the follicles up to twice their size (FIGURES 3d and e). Reovirus in the presence of CP 20,961 mimicked chronic antigen exposure by inducing the development of additional PP between day 7 and 14. Studies of the biological effects of parenterally administered immunological adjuvants indi-

*This work was supported by BRSG 5 SO7 RR 05415 20, Pfizer Central Research, and a National Institutes of Health Grant to D.H. Rubin, No. 1 R22 A1 1855-01.

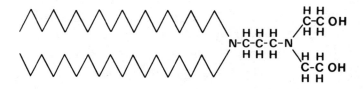

N,N-dioctadecyl-N',N'-bis(2-hydroxyethyl) propanediamine [CP20961]

+

Soybean lipid emulsion and Antigen =

  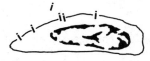

FIGURE 1. The structure of the lipoidal amine adjuvant resembles polar molecules that form lipid components of cell membranes. This might contribute to its affinity of membranes and its capacity to generate liposomes on aggitation with nonpolar lipids.

cated that they enhance lymphoid cell migration into regional lymphatic tissues,[3] increase the burst size of expanding clones of primed lymphocytes, and increase the output of accessory cell types (macrophages and dendritic cells) in thoracic duct lymph.[7,8] The local and systemic effects of CP 20,961 suggest that it might enhance mucosal immunity by producing similar effects on populations of lymphoid cells in the spleen and PP that are responsible for IgA-committed responses.[1] Localization of the adjuvant and antigen by macrophages in the dome

TABLE 1

LEVELS OF REOVIRUS-SPECIFIC ANTIBODY IN INTESTINAL SECRETIONS AFTER PRIMARY IMMUNIZATION

| | Antibody Levels by Elisa Units* | | | | | |
| | IgA | | | IgG | | |
Experimental Group	Day 3	Day 7	Day 14	Day 3	Day 7	Day 14
Reovirus 10^{10} p† (1/Lang)	529	588	234	60	0	15
Reovirus 10^{10} p + CP 20,961 0.3 mg	63	1,352	849	55	78	0
Reovirus 10^{10} p, 10^4 PFU‡ (UV inac)	0	0	867	0	0	0
Reovirus (as above) + CP 20,961	345	160	220	0	0	100
Cholera toxin 10 mcg	0	0	0	0	0	0
CP 20,961 alone	ND	0	0	0	0	0

*As determined by ELISA using monospecific heavy chain antisera. Values expressed as the mean optical density reading at 405nm ($\times 10^{-3}$) of duplicate tests per sample (1/20 dilution of original) per group after two hours of incubation with substrate.
†p = particles
‡PFU = plaque-forming units

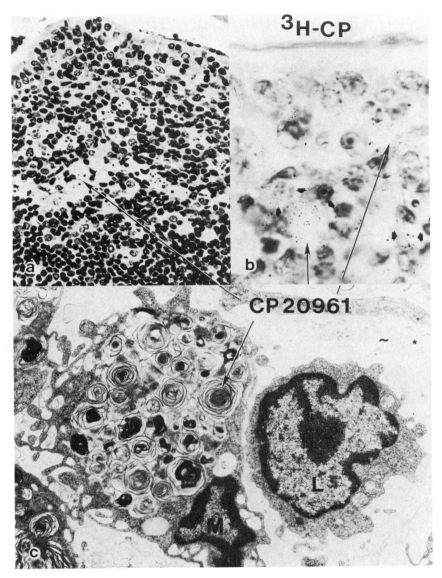

FIGURE 2. Tritiated CP 20,961 was administered enterically as described and radioautography showed that the label accumulated in swollen macrophage-like cells under the Peyers patch dome epithelium. This figure shows this histologically (a), radioautographically (b), and ultrastructurally (c).

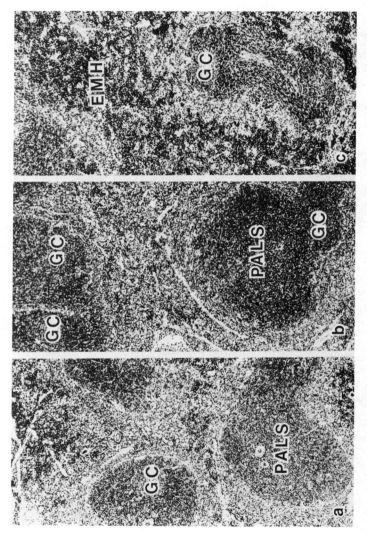

FIGURE 3.   Reovirus infection following enteric inoculation appears to cause sequestration of small lymphoid cells in the periarteriolar lymphatic sheath (PALS) of the spleen (a) and the corona of Peyer's patches.[2] Use of adjuvant with reovirus results in early enlargement of the PALS followed by increased germinal center formation in the spleen (b) and PP (e) by the seventh day after priming. Adjuvant alone causes some increase in follicles, but most of the spleen enlargement is due to increased extramedullary hematopoeisis (c).

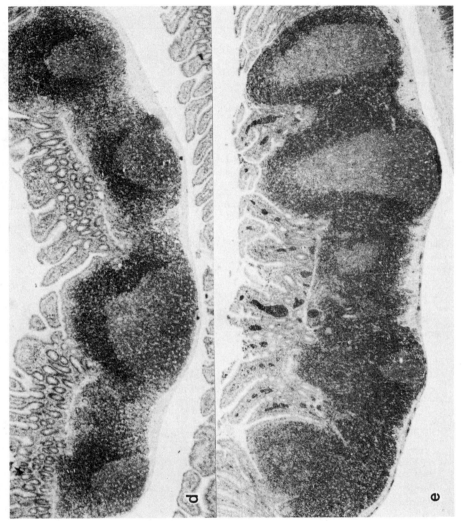

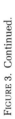

FIGURE 3. Continued.

TABLE 2

RESPONSE OF LYMPHATIC TISSUES TO ENTERIC IMMUNIZATION WITH REOVIRUS 10^{10} P
PLUS 0.3MG CP 20,961 (PFIZER)*

Treatment ID†		Wet weight in mg ± 1 SD			
		Spleen	Mesenteric L.N.	Peyers Patches	Number PP
Untreated		97.30 ± 9	53.73 ± 13	43.68 ± 12	7.33 ± 1
Reovirus + CP 20,961	day 1	110.95 ± 16	60.15 ± 3	68.52 ± 8	8.00 ± 1
Reovirus + CP 20,961	day 3	164.12 ± 35	57.98 ± 11	68.33 ± 6	8.67 ± 1
Reovirus + CP 20,961	day 7	126.73 ± 12	61.12 ± 9	74.25 ± 21	9.67 ± 1
Reovirus + CP 20,961	day 14	130.05 ± 21	60.00 ± 7	67.84 ± 4	12.33 ± 1
Reovirus alone	day 1	N.D.	N.D.	N.D.	N.D.
Reovirus alone	day 3	148.60 ± 30	53.94 ± 3	58.13 ± 5	8.00 ± 2
Reovirus alone	day 7	123.56 ± 56	55.90 ± 17	53.87 ± 6	8.33 ± 1
Reovirus alone	day 14	113.86 ± 9	50.06 ± 5	75.83 ± 9	11.33 ± 1
CP 20,961 alone	day 1	N.D.	N.D.	N.D.	N.D.
CP 20,961 alone	day 3	112.32 ± 9	63.12 ± 3	61.44 ± 7	7.54 ± 1
CP 20,961 alone	day 7	126.65 ± 8	61.93 ± 6	54.64 ± 10	6.30 ± 1
CP 20,961 alone	day 14	120.84 ± 5	79.96 ± 8	52.73 ± 9	6.88 ± 1

*All tissues were maintained at uniform hydration by fixation in 10% buffered formalin.
†Three mice per group were immunized by direct ID inoculation of the respective agents; the control was sham incised. All mice were of identical age at the time of sacrifice.

region of PP may be responsible for the restricted stimulation of mucosal-associated lymphatic tissues.

ACKNOWLEDGMENTS

We are grateful to Dr. J. J. Cebra and Dr. J. A. Fuhrman for advice and encouragement.

TABLE 3

ALTERATION OF SPLENIC LYMPHOID COMPARTMENTS INDUCED
BY ENTERIC IMMUNIZATION

Experimental Group	Mass of Lymphatic Tissue (mg)*			
	Germinal Center	PALS†	Marginal Zone	Extramedullary Hematopoiesis
Untreated control	1.94	14.69	14.68	6.81
Reovirus + CP 20,961 day 1	2.09	58.47	24.74	2.50
Reovirus + CP 20,961 day 3	4.43	86.49	37.25	4.10
Reovirus + CP 20,961 day 7	8.87	39.53	28.76	10.13
Reovirus + CP 20,961 day 14	8.71	42.78	27.44	9.90
Reovirus alone day 7	3.58	35.46	35.95	10.37
CP 20,961 alone day 7	3.67	21.02	19.25	31.66

*The mass of lymphocytes constituting each anatomic compartment was calculated by measuring the percent volume (by planimetry) and multiplying it by the wet weight. Because the lymphoid mass is directly proportional to the number of lymphocytes present (i.e. a 20 mg lymph node contains 10^9 cells), it is clear to see that substantial redistribution and/or proliferation of lymphocytes occurred.
†PALS = periarteriolar lymphatic sheath.

REFERENCES

1. FUHRMAN, J. A. & J. J. CEBRA. 1981. J. Exp. Med. **153:** 534–544.
2. PIERCE, N. F. & F. T. KOSTER. 1980. J. Immunol. **124:** 307–311.
3. ANDERSON, A. O. & J. A. REYNOLDS. 1979. J. Reticuloendothelial Soc. **26:** 667–680.
4. JOKLIK, W. K. 1981. Microbiology Rev. **45:** 483–501.
5. FLEWETT, T. H. & G. N. WOODE. 1978. Arch. Virol. **57:** 1–21.
6. WOLF, J. L., D. H. RUBIN, R. FINBERG, R. S. KAUFFMAN, A. H. SHARPE, J. S. TRIER & B. N. FIELDS. 1981. Science **212:** 471–472.
7. ANDERSON, A. O., J. T. WARREN & D. L. GASSER. 1981. Transplant. Proc. **13:** 1460–1468.
8. ANDERSON, A. O. & J. T. WARREN. 1982. Adv. Exp. Med. Biol. **149:** 791–799.

T-CELL HELP FOR THE IgA RESPONSE IN CAF$_1$ MICE

Margaret Arny, Patricia Kelly-Hatfield, Michael E. Lamm, and
Julia M. Phillips-Quagliata

New York University Medical Center
New York, New York 10016

Plasma cells in the lamina propria of the intestine are predominantly IgA-producing cells. This phenomenon contrasts with plasma cells in most lymphoid tissues that are primarily IgG- and IgM-producing cells. It has been suggested that regulatory T-cells in Peyer's patches (PP) and mesenteric nodes (MN) encourage the development of IgA-committed cells that home to the lamina propria and differentiate into plasma cells. Our interest has been to determine if there is more T-cell help for the IgA response in PP and MN than in other lymphoid organs.

Our approach has been to compare carrier-primed, nylon wool-purified, Lyt-2.2 plus C-depleted T-cells from PP, MN, and peripheral nodes (PN) in their ability to help a secondary IgA anti-TNP response *in vitro*. CAF$_1$ male mice were used in all experiments. Donors of PP and MN T-cells were primed intraduoden-ally with 2×10^8 sheep red blood cells (SRBC) or 0.2–2 mg keyhole limpet hemocyanin (KLH). Peripheral node T-cells were taken from mice primed subcutaneously with either 2×10^8 SRBC or 200 μg KLH in CFA. The source of primed B-cells was anti-Thy-1.2 plus C-treated spleen cells of mice immunized at least 30 days earlier with 100 μg dinitrophenylated (DNP)-KLH and 2×10^9. *B. pertussis* in alum. Primed T-cells were titrated into 1 cc MiniMarbrook cultures containing 6–8×10^6 DNP-primed B-cells and either 1×10^6 TNP-SRBC or 0.1 μg DNP-KLH or TNP-KLH. After a four-day culture, IgM, IgA, and IgG plaque-forming cells (PFC) were enumerated with the Jerne plaque assay.

In an initial series of experiments, the helping ability of SRBC-primed PP, MN, and PN T-cells were compared on days 3, 7, and 11 after priming. Mesenteric node and PP T-cells helped equivalent ratios of IgM, IgA, and IgG PFC on each day after priming. Peripheral node T-cells helped slightly more IgA and IgG compared to IgM PFC than did MN or PP T-cells. Although help for all isotypes appeared somewhat later in MN than in PP or PN, there was no indication within any organ that help for IgM, IgA, and IgG appeared at different rates. These results indicate that SRBC-primed T-cells from PP and MN do not provide any more help than PN T-cells for a secondary IgA response.

It is possible that the nonspecific helper factors known to act in these cultures obscure differences in IgA help provided in a cognate manner. To determine if this is in fact the case, we attempted to repeat the experiments by comparing the help provided by KLH-primed T-cells in the presence of DNP-keyhole limpet hemocyanin. In this system antigen nonspecific factors play less of a role. To date, we have been unable to prime PP and MN with keyhole limpet hemocyanin. PN T-cells, however, were primed very well with keyhole limpet hemocyanin.

On comparing the helping ability of KLH- and SRBC-primed PN T-cells for the same population of DNP-primed B-cells, we noted that KLH-primed T-cells helped a much lower ratio of IgA:IgM plaque-forming cells. This was a very consistent finding and was not due to the particular concentration of antigen we initially chose to use. Addition of supernatants from Concanavalin (Con A)-stimulated spleen cells to cultures with KLH-primed T-cells and DNP-KLH did not lead to an increase in the IgA:IgM ratio. When help was provided by Con A supernatants in the presence of TNP-SRBC the IgA:IgM ratio of PFC was similar to that in cultures where help was provided by SRBC-primed T-cells, suggesting that nonspecific helper factors acting in the latter cultures stimulate the high IgA response. These results are consistent with the idea that there are two populations of B-cells that can differentiate into IgA-producing cells; one that responds to cognate T-cell help and another that responds only to nonspecific factors in the presence of TNP-sheep red blood cells.

IMMUNOLOGY OF THE MUCOSAL RESPONSE TO ANTIGENS OF DIETARY AND MICROBIAL ORIGIN AFFECTING INTESTINAL FUNCTION AND NUTRITIONAL PERFORMANCE

M. E. J. Barratt, W. D. Allen, and P. Porter

Immunology Department
Unilever Research Laboratory
Sharnbrook, Bedfordshire, England

In the young animal the main antigenic problems affecting immune function and related integrity of the gut surface are of microbial or dietary origin. In the young preruminant calf, we have characterized two distinctly different immune responses to antigens presented orally, one detrimental and the other beneficial.

The young calf responds to certain soya proteins in its diet by developing high levels of serum antibody associated with an IgG_1 precipitin that fixes complement.[1] This antibody response relates to the type of soya protein fed, physiological disturbances in the intestine, and the degree of lowered nutritional performance obtained.[2,3] The response was greater in younger animals and was enhanced by passive acquisition of maternal antibody to soya protein from colostrum.[4] Biopsy studies showed that there was partial atrophy of the villi and intensive mononuclear-cell infiltration of the lamina in these animals.[1] Significant improvements in performance, together with a lack of antibody response could be obtained by feeding soya proteins lacking in the antigenic components responsible for the observed morphological disturbances.

Studies in calves in which Thiry-Vella intestinal loops had been established showed that there was no noticeable secretion of intestinal antibody in response to perfusion of soya protein. This phenomenon is in contrast to the response of young calves to bacterial polysaccharide antigens administered orally. Here, a marked secretory antibody response occurs that is predominantly associated with IgA and IgM. There was no detectable serum antibody response to these antigens. Oral immunization of young calves with milk replacer diets containing enteropathogenic *E. coli* antigens resulted in significant improvements in health and performance when compared to animals not immunized.[5]

In conclusion, two contrasting immune responses to antigens presented by way of the intestinal mucosa have been identified in the young preruminant calf. Both responses exert a significant effect on the health and nutritional performance of the animal, the one beneficial and the other detrimental.

REFERENCES

1. BARRATT, M. E. J., P. J. STRACHAN & P. PORTER. 1978. Antibody mechanisms implicated in digestive disturbances following ingestion of soya protein in calves and piglets. Clin. Exp. Immunol. **31:** 305–312.
2. VAN LEEUWEN, J. M., H. J. WIEDE & C. C. BRAAS. 1969. The nutritive value of soya bean oil meal in comparison with dried skimmed milk. Versl. Landbouwkd. Onderz. **732:** 12.
3. SMITH, R. H. & J. W. SISSONS. 1975. The effect of different feeds, including those

containing soya bean products, on the passage of digesta from the abomasum of the pre-ruminant calf. Br. J. Nutr. **33:** 329–349.

4. BARRATT, M. E. J. & P. PORTER. 1979. Immunoglobulin classes implicated in intestinal disturbances of calves associated with soya protein antigens. J. Immunol. **123:** 676–680.

5. PORTER, P., M. E. J. BARRATT & W. D. ALLEN. 1981. Intestinal response to dietary and bacterial antigens affecting health and performance in the calf. *In* The Ruminant Immune System. J. E. Butler, Ed.: 649. Plenum Publishing Corporation. New York.

GUT-ASSOCIATED PRECURSOR IMMUNOCOMPETENCE IN RELATION TO BACTERIAL POLYSACCHARIDE DEXTRAN B-1355 SUBSISTS IN ABSENCE OF SYSTEMIC RESPONSE*

Clara G. Bell

Department of Microbiology and Immunology
University of Illinois at the Medical Center
Chicago, Illinois 60680

The systemic immune response to bacterial polysaccharides, which have determinants cross-reactive with gut-microflora antigens, is marked by a triple anomaly: delay in onset, restriction in specificity, and decline in expression with age.[1,2,3] To understand the manner in which the murine immune response to polysaccharide, a paradigm of the human anti-polysaccharide response, is activated and maintained within the constraints of its micro-environment, a dissection was made of the BALB/c Ig_h-1^{al} (al) allogroup response to *Leuconostoc mesenteroides* dextran B-1355 S [carrying $\alpha[1{\rightarrow}3]$ and $\alpha[1{\rightarrow}6]$ epitopes[2]]. A thymus independent class 2 (TI-2) antigen form of this antigen, alone or linked to lipopolysaccharide (LPS) a thymus independent, class 1 [TI-1] mitogen, or to *Limulus polyphemus* hemocyanin (LPH), a thymus dependent (TD) antigen were studied. The systemic response displays late maturation of the plaque-forming cells (PFC) (FIGURE 1, TABLE 1) and reveals restriction as to: (a) $\alpha[1{\rightarrow}3]$ epitope-specificity (FIGURE 1, TABLE 1); (b) λ_1 L-chain isotype (TABLE 1); (c) V_h-and D_h-related idiotype (Id)-paratopes IdX and IdI (TABLE 1); (d) C_h isotype $\mu > \gamma_3$, a switch to C_α which is T-, and age-dependent (FIGURES 1, 2, TABLE 1); and (e) a significant decline in response post immunization (FIGURE 2, TABLE 1), and with age (TABLE 1), in normal but not in nude mice.

The ontogeny in nonimmune mice of the $\alpha[1{\rightarrow}3]$ epitope-specific B-precursors underlying the systemic response showed early acquisition of λ_1, $\alpha[1{\rightarrow}3]$ epitope immunocompetence, followed by V_h- D_h-related IdX and IdI immunocompetence and the mature frequency precursor repertoire secreting $\alpha[1{\rightarrow}3]$ epitope-specific, monofocal antibody, by day 55, remaining high through maturity in normal mice (TABLE 2). It remained at day <7 level through maturity in germfree mice (TABLE 2). The C_h isotype associated with the $\alpha[1{\rightarrow}3]$-specificity was $\mu > \gamma_3 > \gamma_{2b} > \gamma_{2a}$ and α; the $\gamma_{2b}{\rightarrow}\gamma_{2a}$ expression was T-dependent; and the μ to α was T-and age-dependent. The precursors expressed $\mu > \alpha$ in spleens, $\mu = \alpha$ in mesenteric lymph nodes, and $\mu < \alpha$ in Peyer's patches (TABLE 3). An $\alpha[1{\rightarrow}3]$ epitope-specific, κ potential, minimally expressed in BALB/c, increased exponentially in Ig_h-1^b allogeneic homing (FIGURE 3) without effecting the $\mu{:}\alpha$ ratios. The high level of $\alpha[1{\rightarrow}3]$ epitope-specific precursors expressing α in Peyer's patches, and the low level of $\alpha[1{\rightarrow}3]$ epitope-specific precursors of any isotype or Id in germfree mice, show that the $\alpha[1{\rightarrow}3]$ epitope and reactive Id paratopes are stimulated by environmental antigens. The lag in the BALB/c response to dextran, and the restriction in the expressed L and H isotypes (TABLE 1, FIGURE 1), in the face of an early available repertoire of $\alpha[1{\rightarrow}3]$ committed isotype diverse

*This work was supported in part by a Yamagiwa-Yoshida Memorial International Cancer Study Grant of the International Union Against Cancer.

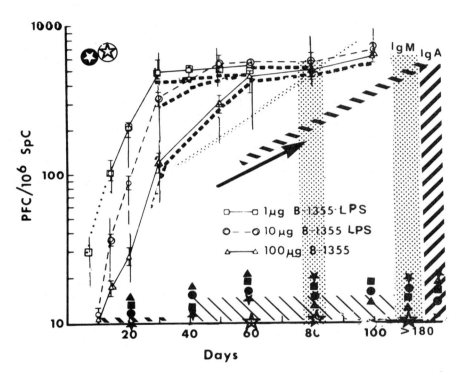

FIGURE 1. Ontogeny of plaque-forming-cell (PFC) responses by BALB/c to a single immunization with dextran B-1355 or B-1355-lipopolysaccharide (LPS).[1,2] Shown are mean and standard deviations, of PFC/10^6 splenocytes taken day 5 post immunization from 8 mice from each age group: $\alpha(1{\rightarrow}3)$ epitope-specific λ_1 ($\square$, O, $\triangle$):κ ($\blacksquare$, $\bullet$, $\blacktriangle$): $\alpha(1{\rightarrow}6)$ epitope-specific λ_1($\bigstar$): κ($\bigstar$); μ ; λ_3\\; α ; IdX---. Note the PFC restriction to the $\alpha(1{\rightarrow}3)$ epitope-specificity, and λ_1 L chain isotype and the age dependent, $C\mu \rightarrow C\alpha$ switch, and the lag in the PFC responses to B-1355 relative to the PFC co-responses or responses by littermates to polyvinylpyrrolidone, a thymus indpendent (TI $\bigstar$) antigen, and to trinitrophenyl coupled sheep erythrocytes (TNP-SRBC), a thymus dependent (TD$\bigotimes$) antigen, shown on the upper left for reference of ontogenic maturation.

TABLE 1

ANTI-$\alpha(1 \to 3)$ EPITOPE-SPECIFIC, ANTIBODY PLAQUE-FORMING CELL RESPONSES
BY BALB/C EUTHYMIC MICE*

Age in Days	L		C_h			IdH		
	$\lambda_1^+ \kappa$	λ_1	μ	α	γ_3	IdX	IdI	Id⁻
7	25	25	25	0	0	0	0	25
28	128	120	110	3	5	117	3	8
55	428	420	306	114	8	402	60	22
180	959	919	504	430	25	889	112	69
(180)	(229)	(201)	(100)	(119)	(10)	(151)	ND	(72)
≥350	1490	1415	780	681	30	1375	189	115
618	615	520	240	360	15	465	ND	149

*Shown are mean plaque-forming cells (PFC) per 10^6 splenocytes, taken from eight mice for each age group. They were assessed by a slide technique using B-1355-sheep erythrocyte and B-512 F-sheep erythrocyte indicators for $\alpha(1 \to 3)$ and $\alpha(1 \to 6)$ epitopes,[1,2] five days after a single i.p. immunization with 1 μg B-1355 per 1 gr body weight (three days after a series of four injections[1,2]). L-chain λ_1 and κ and V_h- and D_h-related IdX and IdI idiotypes evaluated by inhibition of PFC at plateau levels with λ_1-, κ-, IdX- and IdI-specific antibody.[1-3] Alpha and γ_3 PFC developed in presence of 2×10^{-5} M 2-mercaptoethanol inhibitory for the μ PFC, with $C_{h\alpha}$ and $C_{h\gamma_3}$-subclass-specific affinity purified antibody.[1,2] $\alpha(1 \to 6)$ eiptope-specific antibody FPC within background levels 3–15 PFC/10^6 splenocytes. Values differ significantly (p < 0.01).

TABLE 2

FREQUENCY OF $\alpha(1 \to 3)$-RESPONSIVE CLONAL PRECURSORS IN BALB/C Ig_h-1^{al} MICE
CONVENTIONALLY REARED* AND GERMFREE†

Source of BALB/c Donor Cells*†	Day	Number of Clones Producing ng Antibody/Day			$\alpha(1 \to 3)$ dex Specific Clonal Precursor per 10^6 B-cells‡	Percentage Clones Expressing	
		0.5–2	2–5	>5		IdX	IdI 104E + J-558
Spleen*	7	8	2	0	0.9–1.4	<1	0
	28	6	2	2	9.3	68	≃20
	55	9	14	5	15.5	65	≃36
	>300	8	17	15	21.9	60	≃35
Spleen†	<55	6	0	0	0.7	ND	ND
	[<55]	[8]	0	0	[8]	[1.4]	—
	>300	6	2	0	2.1	20§	0
Peyers Patches*	55	8	8	4	14.5	—	—
	>300	22	20	10	25.9	38¶	ND
Mesenteric Lymph nodes*	55	8	2	0	16.1	58	15
	>300	6	7	6	23.2	65	≃33

Frequency of B-precursors responsive to the $\alpha(1 \to 3)$ epitope determined by limiting dilution analysis in a splenic fragment focus assay.[2,3] Quantification of the $\alpha(1 \to 3)$ epitope-specific idiotype IdX and IdI monofocal antibody generated by the B-precursors in the splenic foci was by radioimmunoassay.[2,3]

*Precursors were from conventionally reared BALB/c mice.

†Precursors were from germfree BALB/c mice. [ ] Numbers inside brackets record dinitrophenyl (DNP)-specific Id-460 clonotypes for reference of ontogeny of maturation.

‡Frequency of precursors responding with $\alpha(1 \to 3)$ epitope-specific monofocal antibody per 10^6 Ig^+ B^4 cells after correction for homing and cloning efficiency of the donor B-cells in the recipient spleen.[5]

§IdX/analysis revealed partial identity only.[3]

¶The IdX-IdI profile of Peyer's patches differs significantly from that of the splenic precursors.

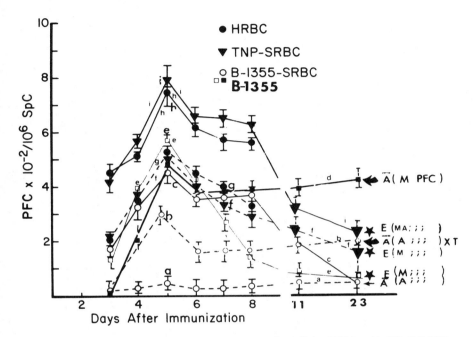

FIGURE 2. Kinetics of systemic *in vivo* responses at the cellular PFC level to (TI-2) B-1355 or (TD) B-1355-sheep erythrocytes (SRBC), B-1355-*Limulus polyphemus* hemocyanin (LPH), TNP-SRBC and/or horse erythrocytes (HRBC). Curves (O---O, O---O, O——O, ■——■, □——□, ▼---▼; ●---●, ●——●, ▼——▼) beginning with the lowest and reading upwards, show: a. O---O α ←PFC to B-1355 by BALB/c athymic mu/nu[←Ā(A-PFC)]. b. O---O α ←PFC to B-1355-LPH by BALB/c athymic nu/nu reconstituted with BALB/c heterozygous athymic nu/+ enriched LPH-T$_H^4$[←Ā(A-PEC)]XT. c. O——O μPFC to B-1355 -SRBC by BALB/c euthymic [*E(M-PFC)]. d. ■——■← μPFC to B-1355 by BALB/c athymic mu/nu [←Ā(M-PFC)]. e. □——□μPFC to B-1355 by BALB/c euthymic [*E(M-PFC)]. f. ▼---▼ μPFC to TNP-SRBC by BALB/c euthymic [*E(M-PFC)]. g. ●---● μPFC to HRBC by BALB/c euthymic. h. ●——● μ+γ$_1$ PFC to HRBC by BALB/c euthymic. i. ▼——▼ μ+α PFC to TNP-SRBC by BALB/c euthymic [*E(MA-PFC)]. *Indicates the significantly reduced levels of PFC (μ = M; α = A; μα-MA) responses/10^6 SpC by the BALB/c euthymic (*E), relative to the athymic (←Ā) at day greater than 23 post immunization.

TABLE 3

C_h ISOTYPES OF $\alpha(1 \to 3)$ RESPONSIVE CLONAL PRECURSORS

Source of BALB/c Donor Cells*†	(day)	BALB/c Recipient Primed With	Stimulating Antigen	No. of Clones Analyzed	Percent of Clones Expressing					
					μ	γ_3	α	$\mu\gamma_3$	$\mu\alpha$	$\mu\gamma_2\alpha$
No. cells		+/+§ LPH	B-1355-LPH	0	0	0	0	0	0	0
		nu/nu	B-1355	5	97	0	0	3	0	0
		nu/nu‡LPH	B-1355-LPH	6	98	0	0	2	0	0
Spleen* +/+	[14]	+/+§ LPH	B-1355-LPH	12	73	4	0	17	3	3
	[55]	+/+§ LPH	B-1355-LPH	28	65	6	5	21	2	1
	[185]	+/+§ LPH	B-1355-LPH	30	32	11	9	32	10	6
	[320]	+/+§ LPH	B-1355-LPH	45	25	8	27	15	18	7
Peyer's patches* +/+	[55]	+/+§ LPH	B-1355-LPH	20	22	6	52	8	10	2
	[185]	+/+§ LPH	B-1355-LPH	41	19	2	59	10	8	2
	[320]	+/+§ LPH	B-1355-LPH	52	12	4	62	7	13	2
Spleen† nu/+	[345]	nu/nu‡	B-1355-LPH	41	25	9	22	17	18	9
Spleen† nu/+	[345]	nu/nu‡	B-1355	15	92	1	0	7	0	0
Spleen(†) nu/+	[345]	nu/nu‡	B-1355-104E	20	30	10	17	12	27	4

*Donors' B-cells were from euthymic (+/+) unprimed mice.

†Donors' cells (selectively enriched for T-, B-depleted by affinity anti-Ig columns[4]) were from Limulus polyphemus hemocyanin (LPH)† or α 104E MP[†]-primed, heterozygous, athymic (nu/+) mice.

‡Recipient athymic (nu/nu) nonirradiated mice, reconstituted with the LPH-or 104E-primed T from the heterozygous, athymic nu/+ mice (lines 11–13), not reconstituted (lines 2–3).

§Recipient euthymic (+/+) mice were primed with LPH[2] six weeks before use and were irradiated (1300 rad) 4 hours before being reconstituted with the donors' cells. Splenic fragments prepared from the recipients each containing a donor clone,[4] were cultured with the dextran. Recorded clonotypes identified by the monofocal antibody generated by the donor precursors in the recipient fragment cultures, having reactivity for dextran B-1355 and lacking reactivity for dextran B-512F.[2] Mesenteric lymph node* B-precursors expressed $\mu(38\%, 36\%) = \alpha(38\%, 40\%)$ at age days 185 and 320.

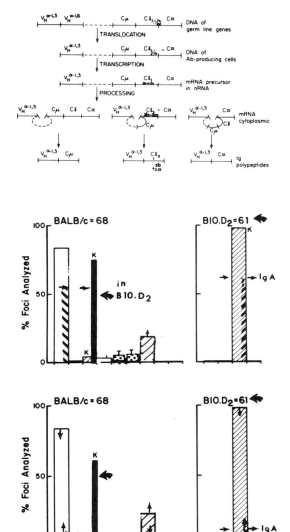

FIGURE 3. Upper schema: C_h isotypes associated with the response to the $\alpha(1{\rightarrow}3)$ epitope and the switch of the C_h gene product, associated with the V_h-D_h from $C_{h\mu} \rightarrow C_{h\alpha}$ and $C_{h\gamma 3} \rightarrow C_{h\gamma 2b} \rightarrow C_{h\gamma 2a}$. (B-1355 does not elicit antibody in the $C_{h\gamma 1}$). Lower schema: The $C_{h\mu}$ to $C_{h\alpha}$ switch is identical in BALB/c precursors during 10 generations of culture-homing in syngeneic BALB/c fragments and in allogeneic B10.D2 fragments. The BALB/c, *al* allogroup secreting principally λ_1, and the B10.D2, Ig_h-1^b allogroup secreting κ. BALB/c precursors homing in the syngeneic fragments secreted principally λ_1, and in the allogeneic fragments κ, indicating that the C_h μ—α switch is independent of the associated L chain isotype.

B-precursors (TABLES 2, 3) do not reflect lack of, and restricted L-,C_h-and V_h-B-precursor commitment, but functional regulatory constraints in the epitope induced B-precursor selective expansion and maturation to response (FIGURES 3 vs. 1) (TABLES 2, 3 vs. 1). The decline in systemic response with age is due not to a decrease in precursor frequency but to deregulation in the Id-B-precursor expansion to systemic response (TABLES 2 vs. 1, FIGURE 2) The relationship noted in this study between the systemic response to polysaccharide and the polysaccharide-specific precursor pool is consistent with: (a) gut-associated microflora playing a critical role in the acquisition of the specific B-precursor repertoire and commitment to α expression; (b) genes linked to Ig_h-1 allotype controlling the λ_1 and κ B-precursor expansion; (c) V_h-and D_h-related Id immunocompetence imposing functional constraints and regulation in the epitope selection process and in the induced precursor maturation to systemic response; and (d) T-dependent deregulation in the precursor expansion to systemic response with age. These interrelated phenomena lead to a lag in systemic response, its restricted expression and its decline with age, despite the high level of immunocompetent precursors available.

REFERENCES

1. BELL, C. 1979. Scand. J. Immunol. **9:** 197 & 209.
2. BELL, C. 1982. Scand. J. Immunol. **15:** 71.
3. BELL, C. 1983. Immunology. In press.
4. BELL, C. & H. WIGZELL. 1977. Eur. J. Immunol. **7:** 726.
5. KLINMAN, N. R., A. R. PICKARD, N. H. SIGAL, P. J. GEARHART, E. S. METCALF & S. K. PIERCE. 1976. Ann. Immunol. (Inst. Pasteur). **127C:** 489.

INDUCTION OF (PARTIAL) SYSTEMIC TOLERANCE IN PRIMED RATS SUBJECTED TO PROLONGED ORAL ADMINISTRATION OF ANTIGEN

Kurt J. Bloch, Robert Perry, Margot Bloch, and W. Allan Walker

Massachusetts General Hospital
Boston, Massachusetts 02114

Although it has been repeatedly shown that enteric administration of antigens to unprimed animals blunts the immune response to parenteral challenge with antigen, limited information is available on the response of primed animals. This preliminary report concerns the effect of repeated enteric administration of protein antigen on serum level of anti-protein antibodies and on the response to a second parenteral injection of antigen and alum.

Sprague-Dawley rats weighing 250–300 g were immunized with 100 μg bovine serum albumin (BSA) and egg albumin (EA) plus 20mg alum injected intraperitoneally. Beginning two weeks later, rats were fed five times each week by gavage for six weeks with either 100 mg EA or 100 mg bovine serum albumin. The anti-BSA antibody response was measured by the Farr assay. The titer of anti-BSA antibody initially increased in rats fed either BSA or EA, but thereafter, the titer declined more in the BSA-fed animals. Upon reimmunization with BSA and alum injected intraperitoneally at week 9, all rats fed with EA showed a rise in anti-BSA antibodies. In rats fed earlier with BSA, the response was blunted or failed to occur. Feeding of antigen had no effect on the primary response to sheep erythrocytes (SRBC) administered at the time of rechallenge with bovine serum albumin.

In another experiment, all rats were initially immunized with an intraperitoneal injection of 100 μg BSA plus 20 mg alum. At 5 weeks, rats received 100 mg BSA by gavage 5 times a week for 11 weeks; control rats were injected with a single 10 μg dose of BSA, and then sham-fed daily. Animals fed BSA, showed an initial increase in serum anti-BSA antibodies that was mimicked by the injected control group. On continued feeding of antigen, there was a fall in titer of anti-BSA antibodies to levels below those of the controls.

Upon parenteral reinjection with antigen and alum after week 16, all of the parenterally boosted rats showed a rise in titer of anti-BSA antibody. This rise in titer either failed to occur or was blunted in rats repeatedly exposed to antigen by feeding.

The fall in titer of serum antibodies in rats fed the corresponding antigen might have been due to systemic uptake of immunologically intact antigen and subsequent neutralization of serum antibody. To test this possibility, rats were immunized with BSA plus alum injected intraperitoneally. Beginning at week 4, rats were injected intravenously five times each week with 100, 10, or 0 μg bovine serum albumin. Rats repeatedly injected with antigen maintained elevated levels of serum antibodies throughout a five-week course. These results suggest that the fall in level of serum antibodies in rats fed antigen is not due to neutralization of antibody by absorbed antigen. The mechanism(s) by which enteric administration of antigen in primed rats induces partial tolerance to the antigen remains to be determined.

In conclusion, in rats primed by intraperitoneal injection of a protein, BSA

787

and alum, subsequent feeding of the protein boosted the serum antibody response. Prolonged feeding of the protein was accompanied by a fall in serum anti-BSA antibodies in most animals. Upon reinjection of BSA and alum administered intraperitoneally, the serum anti-BSA antibody response was blunted in BSA-fed, but not in sham-fed rats. The effect of prolonged feeding of protein antigen on the serum antibody level was unlikely to be due to neutralization of serum antibody by systemically absorbed, immunologically intact antigen. Finally, it should be noted that feeding was conducted according to one dosage schedule; possibly administration of greater quantities of protein antigen might accelerate the fall in serum antibody and the degree of unresponsiveness to reimmunization.

SALIVARY IgA TO CARIOGENIC MICROORGANISMS IN CHILDREN: CORRELATION WITH CARIES ACTIVITY

Ronald W. Bolton and Gwen L. Hlava

College of Dentistry
University of Nebraska Medical Center
Lincoln, Nebraska 68583

Prior research has shown that increased salivary IgA levels result in decreased caries activity in laboratory animals. Salivary IgA is presumed to prevent the adherence of cariogenic microorganisms to hard surfaces. This study investigated the influence, if any, that salivary IgA specific for oral microorganisms might have on caries activity in children. To date, limited published information exists that documents salivary IgA activity to oral microorganisms in caries-active and caries-free children. The questionable role that salivary immunoglobulin may have in the regulation of caries activity in children prompted this study.

Stimulated whole saliva from 89 children, aged 3–14 years, was evaluated for IgA, reactive to antigens from cariogenic microorganisms, by an enzyme-linked immunosorbent assay. Children with one or more active carious lesions in need of restoration were placed in the active caries group (AC). No detectable caries (NDC) patients had no carious involvement of the teeth at the time of saliva collection.

Children aged 3–11 years with NDC had significantly higher levels of salivary IgA to *Streptococcus mutans* serotype *c* than did the AC children ($p < 0.05$). Saliva was also examined for IgA specific for *Lactobacillus casei*, glucan, and glycerol-teichoic acid (TA). Salivary IgA levels to *L. casei* were not significantly different between the NDC and AC groups in the three to five year and six to eight year groups ($p > 0.5$). In the 9–11 year and 12–14 year groups, however, the AC patients had significantly higher IgA levels to *L. casei* ($p < 0.01$ for both groups).

Active caries children in all age groups displayed significantly higher levels of salivary IgA to both glucan and glycerol-teichoic acid ($p < 0.01$ for each group with each antigen).

The higher levels of IgA to *S. mutans* observed in the NDC children does not necessarily indicate increased immunological responses directly to *S. mutans*, but probably reflects the individual's genetic ability to respond to some of the cross-reacting antigens found in the normal oral flora. Two such specificities were examined in this investigation, glucan and glycerol-teichoic acid. Salivary IgA levels to these antigens were positively correlated with caries, thus indicating no protective role. Therefore, some other substance, possibly glucosyltransferase, may have served as a protective antigen in children.

The information presented above suggests that naturally occurring salivary IgA may provide some protection against caries in children; however, the immunological specificity remains undefined. Comparison of the present investigation with previous adult human studies indicates that salivary IgA-response patterns to cariogenic microorganisms may differ during childhood, probably because the immune system is still under development, not reaching maturity until puberty.

IgA IN LIVER DISEASE

K. G. Chandy,* E. Elias,† S. Hubscher,‡ M. Khan,* J. Berg,§
and D. Burnett*

Departments of Immunology,* Medicine,† and Pathology‡
University of Birmingham
Department of Clinical Chemistry,§
East Birmingham Hospital
Birmingham, England

Secretory component (SC) mediated transport of polymeric IgA (pIgA) from blood to bile, through hepatocytes, has been demonstrated in rats.[1] Evidence suggests that a similar, though probably less efficient transport system may exist in man.[2-4] The hypothesis that circulating pIgA is removed by the liver in man was tested by studying the distribution of IgA and SC in eight liver biopsies, and by measuring total IgA, monomeric IgA (mIgA), pIgA, and secretory IgA (sIgA), in the sera of 26 controls and 76 patients with liver disease. Total and pIgA levels were significantly elevated (p < 0.005) in patients with liver disease but mIgA was not raised. Elevated serum pIgA concentrations in liver disease probably reflect failure of normal hepatic clearance of pIgA by either of two routes.

1. Secretory component was localized by immunocytochemical methods in epithelial cells lining bile ductules, but not on hepatocytes, bile canaliculi or sinusoids, in the absence of cholestasis. Bile ductules and blood vessels in the portal tract lie in close apposition with no anatomical barriers separating the two structures.[5,6] pIgA may therefore diffuse through fenestrations in blood vessels in the portal tract[6] and be transported by SC through ductal cells into bile. Serum sIgA concentrations were raised in all patient groups with liver disease, levels being strongly related to markers of cholestasis (serum alkaline phosphatase, bilirubin, bile acids, 2p < 0.001). This elevation of concentration suggests that raised serum pIgA in some patients was due to reflux of sIgA into blood as a result of biliary obstruction. This observation is supported by evidence of similar distribution of bile pigments, IgA, and SC in dilated canaliculi and hepatocytes in the presence of cholestasis.

2. IgA was found lining sinusoids, within hepatocytes and sinusoidal phago-cytes, suggesting that these cells may remove IgA from sinusoidal blood. This evidence is supported by the observation that isolated hepatocytes bind pIgA, but not mIgA, probably by means of a carbohydrate receptor.[7] Hepatocyte IgA, however, is probably not transported into bile because IgA is not apparent in bile canaliculi, in the absence of cholestasis. IgA within hepatocytes or sinusoidal phagocytes is probably catabolized. Patients with hepatocellular disease had significantly elevated serum pIgA, consistent with impairment of its removal by route two. Similarly, patients with porto-systemic shunts had elevated serum pIgA levels, probably due to bypass of the liver.

REFERENCES

1. ORLANS, E., J. PEPPARD, J. REYNOLDS & J. HALL. 1978. J. Exp. Med. 147: 588–592.
2. KUTTEH, H. W., S. J. PRINCE, J. O. PHILLIPS, J. G. SPENNEY & J. MESTECKY. 1982. Gastroenterology 82: 184–193.

3. NAGURA, H., P. D. SMITH, P. K. NAKANE & W. R. BROWN. 1981. J. Immunol. **126:** 587–595.
4. DELACROIX D., C. DIVE, J. P. VAERMAN, A. MACPHERSON & H. J. F. HODGSON. 1981. Clin. Sci. **61:** 23p–24p.
5. STERNLIEB, I. 1972. Gastroenterology **63:** 321–327.
6. TANIKAWA, K. 1979. Ultrastructural Aspects of The Liver and its Disorders, 2nd edit Igaku-Shoin, Tokyo.
7. HOPF, U., P. BRANDTZAEG, T. H. HUTTEROTH, K. H. MEYER-ZUM-BÜSCHENFELDE. 1978. Scand. J. Immunol. **8:** 543–549.

EXPRESSION OF ANTI-PHOSPHOCHOLINE IgA AND IgE ANTIBODIES IN (CBA/N × BALB/c)F$_1$ MICE FOLLOWING SECONDARY STIMULATION WITH *ASCARIS SUUM*

Ellen R. Clough and John J. Cebra

University of Pennsylvania
Philadelphia, Pennsylvania 19104

CBA/N animals have a genetic defect: they do not mount a normal primary response to phosphocholine (PC) even when this determinant is attached to the highly immunogenic carrier, hemocyanin (Hy).[1] Because this defect is x-linked and recessive, (CBA/N × BALB/c)F$_1$ males express the defect, whereas the females are phenotypically normal. Although it had been reported that these animals could not respond at all to PC, Kishimoto et al.[2] found that after priming defective animals with a single low dose of PC-Hy in alum, they could detect a serum anti-PC IgE response in the absence of a response of other isotypes. We confirmed these findings,[3] and in addition, using the Klinman clonal precursor assay,[4] were able to show that male and female mice make comparable secondary responses to two doses of PC-Hy, even though the males never make a normal primary response. Thus initial priming with PC-Hy served to silently expand the pool of PC-reactive cells in the absence of detectable secreted product. The cells could then be detected following secondary stimulation.

In the present studies, defective males and normal female controls were primed with an initial dose of 1 μg PC-Hy in 2 mg alum to silently expand the pool of PC-reactive cells. They were then boosted by stomach intubation with 10^4 embryonated *Ascaris suum* eggs. The Klinman assay was performed at 2–3 weeks and 12 weeks following *Ascaris* infection. *Ascaris*, a gut nematode with PC-determinants on its surface, hatches in the stomach and migrates through the wall of the gut. This intraduodenal priming with a PC-bearing nematode was used to explore pathways of B-lymphocyte differentiation, particularly with regard to IgA and IgE expression.

The isotype profiles of clones derived from male and female mice after a single dose of PC-Hy or after *Ascaris* stimulation alone are very similar. Included in each group is a high proportion of clones that are primary in nature, producing some IgM. Few clones express IgE and few are committed to IgA production. The PC-reactive cells, however, that were first stimulated with PC-Hy and then by *Ascaris*, give rise to clones that express more secondary isotypes (TABLE 1). Between 3 and 12 weeks, as the response to *Ascaris* becomes chronic, there is a trend toward a higher percentage (35%) of clones that express IgE. Of these, 62% also make IgG, 38% make IgA, whereas only 8% make IgM. In addition, there are parallel increases in clones that express some IgE, and those that express IgG ± IgA without IgM. Twelve weeks following *Ascaris* infection there is an increase in the percentage of clones making IgA only, particularly in the Peyer's patches.

These studies indicate that the potential to express IgE is not unique to a small subset of B-lymphocytes, but is probably a normal feature of chronic stimulation. The fact that two doses of 1 μg PC-Hy in alum used in previous experiments were as effective as *Ascaris* infection in stimulating IgE expression indicates that the potential to express IgE may not be unique to nematode infection. Rather these parasites may simply circumvent controls that normally operate against IgE expression *in vivo*. Mucosal delivery of antigen made possible by *Ascaris* infection, however, did increase the frequency of clones committed to exclusive IgA production. These results argue in favor of a linear pathway of B-cell differentiation with respect to isotype potential. Thus a clone derived from a single μ-bearing cell need not be predestined to produce a certain isotype. IgE, for example, can be coexpressed with any isotype. Our data, based on 90 IgE-producing clones, support this conclusion and show that with chronic B-cell stimulation, clones tend toward coexpression of IgE with IgG, IgA, or IgG + IgA.

TABLE 1

CHARACTERISTICS OF α-PC SECRETING CLONES FROM B-CELLS DERIVED FROM F_1 MALE AND FEMALE MICE AT INTERVALS FOLLOWING SECONDARY STIMULATION WITH *ASCARIS SUUM*

	Percent Clones Expressing Particular Isotypes											
	Males						Females					
	PP		MLN		SP		PP		MLN		SP	
Week	2/3	12	2/3	12	2/3	12	2/3	12	2/3	12	2/3	12
Some IgM	91	44	21	—	48	67	36	33	14	0	35	38
IgG + IgA, no IgM	9	22	50	—	48	33	32	44	71	33	46	25
Some IgE	0	11	50	—	65	67	11	44	85	100	38	50
IgA only	0	33	14	—	7	0	25	33	14	0	15	25
Some IgA	36	78	28	—	41	44	75	67	43	100	61	25
Some IgG$_1$	55	44	28	—	65	33	39	33	57	0	42	25
Some IgG$_2$	18	67	43	—	21	67	15	44	14	0	27	50
Some IgG$_3$	0	22	0	—	14	44	4	33	14	33	19	0
Total clones	11	9	14	0	29	9	26	9	7	3	26	8
Frequency/10^5	3	6.1	5.6	<0.3	6	3.5	7.2	6.5	2.7	0.1	6.9	8.5

REFERENCES

1. MOND, J. J., R. LIEBERMAN, J. K. INMAN, D. E. MOSIER & W. PAUL. 1977. J. Exp. Med. **146:** 1138.
2. KISHIMOTO, T., S. SHIGEMOTO, T. WATANABE & Y. YAMAMURA. 1979. J. Immunol. **123:** 1039.
3. CLOUGH, E. R., D. A. LEVY & J. J. CEBRA. J. Immunol. **126:** 387.
4. KLINMAN, N. R. 1969. Immunochemistry **6:** 757–759.

IgA HYBRIDOMAS TO CELL-SURFACE COMPONENTS OF PATHOGENIC BACTERIA*

Dawn E. Colwell, Katherine A. Gollahon, Ichijiro Morisaki,
Jerry R. McGhee, and Suzanne M. Michalek

Department of Microbiology
and
Institute of Dental Research
The University of Alabama in Birmingham
Birmingham, Alabama 35294

Immunoglobulin A (IgA) is the major isotype of antibody found in external secretions of humans and other mammals. It is well known that secretory IgA (sIgA) provides the host with local defense against potentially pathogenic agents including microorganisms (e.g., bacteria and viruses), allergens, and other toxic substances. The precise mechanisms by which IgA effects immunity at mucosal surfaces, however, are largely unknown. Furthermore, progress in this area has been delayed because of the unavailability of sufficient quantities of purified antigen-specific IgA antibodies for studies of functional mechanisms.

Hybridoma technology now offers a means of obtaining an abundant source of highly pure IgA. Previous studies from this laboratory have described a method for generating high numbers of hybridomas producing IgA isotype, antigen-specific antibodies.[1] One method used long-term intravenous (i.v.) administration of increasing doses of either whole killed *Escherichia coli* cells to C3H/HeN mice or whole killed *Salmonella typhimurium* cells to CAF_1 (BALB/c × A/J) mice (10–15 injections per mouse over a 5–10 week period). Another method used gastric intubation of germfree BALB/c mice or germfree Fischer rats with whole killed *Streptococcus mutans* cells. X63-Ag8.653 nonimmunoglobulin-producing murine myeloma cells[2] were fused with spleen cells from immunized animals as outlined in FIGURE 1, resulting in the formation of stable hybridoma cell lines that secrete antibodies with specificity for cell-surface antigens of *E. coli* (IgA, 36; IgG, 18; IgM, 22), *S. typhimurium* (IgA, 180; IgG, 143; IgM, 7), and *S. mutans* (mouse-mouse hybrids: IgA, 52; IgG, 29; IgM, 50, and rat-mouse hybrids: IgA, 163; IgG, 183; IgM, 105), as determined by enzyme-linked immunosorbent assays (ELISA) using microtiter plates coated with whole bacterial cells. Stable cell lines (IgA, 17; IgG, 4; IgM, 28) were also established from hybridomas generated by the fusion of myeloma cells with spleen cells from BALB/c mice given a single i.v. injection of purified *S. mutans* 6715 serotype carbohydrate (serotype g).

Hybridoma antibodies that bound to *S. mutans* whole cells were examined by ELISA for specificity to purified cell-surface components of *S. mutans*, including serotype carbohydrate, dextran, lipoteichoic acid, and cell-surface protein. The IgA antibodies tested were predominantly directed against carbohydrate antigens. The specificity of hybridoma antibodies against gram-negative bacteria for lipopolysaccharide was determined by hemagglutination for antibodies produced by representative hybrids against *E. coli* (IgA, 2; IgG, 7; IgM, 10) and *S.*

*This work was supported by United States Public Health Service Contract DE 02426 and Grants DE 04217, DE 02670, and CA 13148. Suzanne M. Michalek is the recipient of Research Career Development Award DE 00092.

794

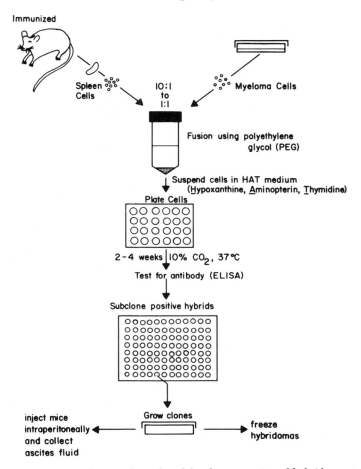

FIGURE 1. Experimental protocol employed for the generation of hybridomas to pathogenic bacteria.

TABLE 1

INDUCTION OF IgA HYBRIDOMAS TO BACTERIAL PATHOGENS

Monoclonal Antibodies To	Species	Percent IgA Hybridomas*	Major Antibody Specificities
Streptococcus mutans	Mouse	40 (52/131)	Serotype carbohydrate, glucan, surface protein and lipoteichoic acid
	Rat	36 (163/448)	
Escherichia coli	Mouse	47 (36/76)	Lipopolysaccharide, protein
Salmonella typhimurium	Mouse	55 (180/330)	Lipopolysaccharide

*Numbers in parentheses represent the number of IgA hybridomas divided by the number of hybrids tested.

typhimurium (IgA, 2; IgG, 6; IgM, 8). The numbers and antigenic specificities of IgA-secreting hybridomas are summarized in TABLE 1. Immunochemical analysis of antibodies produced by various hybridoma lines reveals that the IgA antibodies are primarily polymeric in form.

The finding that a significant proportion of hybridomas generated by the fusion of myeloma cells with spleen cells from mice either gastrically intubated with whole killed *S. mutans* cells or immunized by a single i.v. injection of purified serotype carbohydrate secrete antibody of the IgA isotype may suggest a correlation between the administration of a carbohydrate antigen and the enhanced stimulation of an IgA response.

These antibodies are being used in *in vitro* and *in vivo* studies of infection and immunity at mucosal sites, in diagnostic studies of *S. mutans*, and in studies concerning the anatomical distribution of IgA-secreting cells and the transport of IgA molecules in the mammalian circulatory system.

REFERENCES

1. COLWELL, D. E., K. A. GOLLAHON, J. R. McGHEE & S. M. MICHALEK. 1982. IgA hybridomas: a method for generation in high numbers. J. Immunol. Methods **54:** 259–266.
2. KEARNEY, J. F., A. RADBRUCH, B. LIESGANG & K. RAJEWSKY. 1979. A new mouse myeloma cell line that has lost immunoglobulin expression but permits the construction of antibody-secreting hybrid cell lines. J. Immunol. **123:** 1548–1550.

REGULATION OF IgA SUBCLASSES
IN POKEWEED MITOGEN STIMULATED CULTURES

Mary Ellen Conley

Division of Allergy-Immunology
Department of Pediatrics
Joseph Stokes Jr. Research Institute
Children's Hospital of Philadelphia
Philadelphia, Pennsylvania 19104

William J. Koopman

Division of Rheumatology
Department of Medicine
Veterans Administration Hospital
University of Alabama
Birmingham, Alabama 35294

Studies on the human IgA subclasses, IgA_1 and IgA_2 have provided a new approach for investigation of IgA B-cell differentiation and cell-migration patterns. Although 80% of the IgA B-cells in the peripheral circulation express surface IgA_1 and 20% bear IgA_2, the subclass distribution in pokeweed mitogen (PWM) stimulated cultures is completely different. At day 7, 50% of the IgA-plasma cells in a PWM stimulated culture are positive for cytoplasmic IgA_1 and 50% are positive for IgA_2.

To further investigate regulation of IgA subclasses in PWM cultures, IgA_1 and IgA_2 were measured in culture supernatants by a solid phase radioimmunoassay using subclass specific monoclonal anti-subclass antibodies. At day 7, IgA_2 constituted less than 10% of the IgA in 15 experiments (range 0.2–9.0%).

To determine if this imbalance was due to a delay in IgA_2 release, or failure of the assay to detect IgA_2, culture supernatants and lysates of cell pellets were assayed for IgA_1 and IgA_2 at day 5, day 7, day 9, and day 12 of culture. At all time points the amounts of IgA_1 and IgA_2 in cell-pellet lysates were approximately equal, whereas less than 10% of the IgA in culture supernatants was IgA_2. This proportion did not increase over time. In all experiments there was more IgA_2 in the cell pellets than in the culture supernatants—in some cases as much as 90 times more. By contrast, there was always more IgA_1 in culture supernatants than in cell pellets—sometimes as much as 30 times more.

To determine if IgA_2 were selectively lost or destroyed in culture supernatants, purified IgA_2 myeloma proteins were added at the beginning of the culture period. When 4000 ng/ml of an $IgA_2\kappa$ (Am2+) or an $IgA_2\lambda$ (Am2−) were added at day 0, 3320 ng/ml or 2680 ng/ml respectively were retrieved in the supernatant at day seven.

Because production of J-chain may be required for secretion of polymeric immunoglobulins, plasma cells from seven day cultures were stained by double contrast immunofluorescent techniques with rhodamine-tagged anti-J-chain and fluorescein-tagged anti-IgA_1, anti-IgA_2, or anti-total IgA. On all slides, over 90% of the cells stained for IgA, or either of the IgA subclasses were also stained for J-chain.

These results demonstrate that although 50% of the IgA-plasma cells in a

PWM-stimulated culture express IgA_2, as demonstrated by immunofluorescent staining, less than 10% of the IgA released into the culture supernatants is IgA_2. This discrepancy cannot be explained by selective loss or destruction of IgA_2, failure of the assay system to detect in vitro synthesized IgA_2, delayed maturation of IgA_2-plasma cells, or failure of IgA_2-plasma cells to synthesize J-chain. These results further suggest that maturation of IgA_2-plasma cells into antibody-secreting cells may require additional signals of differentiation and that cells with the phenotypic appearance of plasma cells may not be at the final stages of differentiation.

TRANSFER OF IgA INTO RAT BILE: ULTRASTRUCTURAL DEMONSTRATION

P. J. Courtoy, J. N. Limet, J. Quintart, Y.-J. Schneider, J. P. Vaerman, and P. Baudhuin

International Institute of Cellular and Molecular Pathology and Department of Pathology University of Louvain Brussels, Belgium

Several ligands are internalized in rat hepatocytes by receptor-mediated endocytosis. Whereas most of them (e.g. galactose-exposing proteins) will eventually be digested in lysosomes, polymeric IgA (pIgA) is selectively transferred into bile.[2-4] In order to investigate by electron microscopy the transepithelial transfer of pIgA with a direct probe, we have prepared conjugates of horseradish peroxidase (HRP) with monoclonal human pIgA and examined their fate in rat liver after i.v. injection. The HRP-pIgA conjugate behaved like native pIgA with respect to *in vitro*, binding to cultured rat hepatocytes and *in vivo*, transfer into bile[1] and subcellular distribution in liver upon differential and isopyknic centrifugation.

HRP-pIgA was mostly found in hepatocytes and to a much lesser extent in sinusoidal cells. One minute after injection, numerous small pits and profiles (~100 nm) were labeled along the sinusoidal and lateral plasmalemma of the hepatocytes. These profiles were generally embedded in a dense microfilamentous meshwork. Where this matrix was less prominent, the profiles were covered by a coat suggestive of clathrin, surrounded by a pale halo.

In less than five minutes, HRP-pIgA was, in addition, found in larger irregular vesicles (>200 nm) with no apparent coat. Labeling was seen on the internal aspect of their membrane, and their content was otherwise electron-lucent (FIGURE 1). Hence, these structures resemble the "receptosomes" described by Willingham and Pastan.[6] These findings are similar to those observed with HRP-pIgA in cultured rat hepatocytes.[1] Within 15 minutes, labeled vesicles selectively migrated to the biliary pole, where they clustered around bile canaliculi. Some lysosomes were also labeled, but never Golgi stacks and rims. By 30 minutes, these vesicles could still be observed around bile canaliculi that also became labeled at this time (FIGURE 2).

In conclusion, transepithelial transfer of pIgA into bile includes (1) selective internalization through coated pits, (2) transfer into larger vesicles that may be related to the "receptosomes," (3) migration of the vesicles to the biliary pole, (4) clustering around bile canaliculi, and (5) membrane fusion with the plasmalemma enclosing bile canaliculi and the discharge into bile. Hence, the initial steps of this pathway are identical to those described for ligands that will be digested in lysosomes.[5] Possible involvement of lysosomes in pIgA transfer as well as the sorting mechanism of the two classes of ligands are presently under investigation.

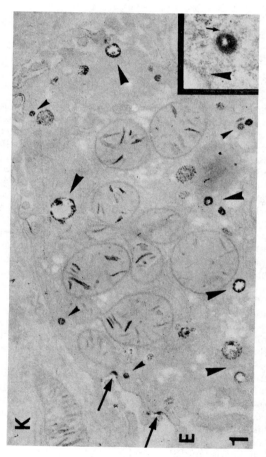

FIGURE 1. Internalization of HRP-pIgA five minutes after i.v. injection: Note the focal labeling of the plasmalemma (arrows), the internalization of HRP-pIgA through small vesicles (small arrowheads) and transfer into larger vesicles with electron-lucent content (large arrowheads). Kupffer's cells (K) and endothelial cells (E) are not labeled (×24,000, unstained). Inset: the peripheral small vesicles are coated. Adjacent plasmalemma (arrow-head) is not labeled (×78,000, stained).

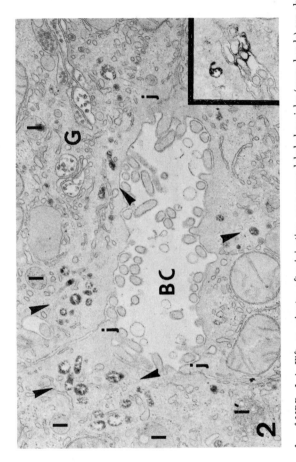

FIGURE 2. Biliary transfer of HRP-pIgA: Fifteen minutes after injection, numerous labeled vesicles (arrowheads) are clustered around a bile canaliculus (BC). Notice their typical electron-lucent content. Golgi apparatus (G) and several lysosomes (L) except one (L') are not labeled. J: tight junctions (×24,000, stained). Inset: thirty minutes after injection, the bile canaliculus is also labeled (×19,000, stained).

REFERENCES

1. Courtoy, P. J., J. Limet, P. Baudhuin, Y.-J. Schneider & J. P. Vaerman. 1981. Cell Biol. Int. Rep. **5:** 57.
2. Renston, R. H., A. L. Jones, W. D. Christiansen, G. T. Hradek & B. J. Underdown. 1980. Science **208:** 1276–1278.
3. Takahashi, I., P. K. Nakane & W. R. Brown. 1982. J. Immunol. **128:** 1181–1187.
4. Vaerman, J. P., I. Lemaître-Coelho, J. N. Limet & D. Delacroix. 1982. *In* Recent Advances in Mucosal Immunity. W. Strober, L. Å. Hanson and K. W. Sell, Eds.: 233–250. Raven Press. New York.
5. Wall, D. A., G. Wilson & A. L. Hubbard. 1980. Cell **21:** 79–93.
6. Willingham, M. C. & I. Pastan. 1980. Cell **21:** 67–77.

DISTRIBUTION OF IgA$_1$ AND IgA$_2$ SUBCLASSES IN HUMAN TISSUE: CORRELATION WITH THE PRESENCE OF J-CHAIN*

S. S. Crago, W. H. Kutteh, S. J. Prince, J. Radl,† J. J. Haaijman,†
and J. Mestecky

*University of Alabama in Birmingham
Birmingham, Alabama 35294*

†*Institute of Experimental Gerontology
TNO, Rijswijk,
The Netherlands*

More than 90% of serum IgA is present in the monomeric form and falls into the IgA$_1$ subclass, whereas external secretions contain predominantly polymeric secretory IgA with an equal distribution of IgA$_1$ and IgA$_2$. Previous studies examined the distribution of IgA$_1$- and IgA$_2$-plasma cells in various human tissues,[1] but made no attempt to correlate these findings with the molecular form of the IgA. This study examines the distribution of IgA$_1$- and IgA$_2$-containing cells in various human tissues, using monoclonal reagents specific for each subclass. We also attempt to correlate the production of IgA$_1$ or IgA$_2$ with the presence of cytoplasmic J-chain.

Cell suspensions were made from tonsils; mediastinal, mesenteric, and axillary lymph nodes; and spleen. Cytocentrifuge preparations were fixed in ethanol:acetic acid. Tissues from small and large intestine and retroperitoneal lymph nodes were frozen in liquid nitrogen, sectioned on a cryotome and fixed in ethanol:acetic acid. To determine the distribution of IgA$_1$- and IgA$_2$-containing cells, slides were incubated with commercially obtained monoclonal reagents specific for IgA$_1$ (BRL) or IgA$_2$ (B-D) followed by tetramethylrhodamine isothiocyanate (TRITC)-labeled anti-mouse IgG or with directly labeled (TRITC) anti-IgA$_1$ or anti-IgA$_2$ (a gift of Dr. J. Radl), followed by fluorescein isothiocyanate (FITC)-labeled polyclonal anti-human IgA (Behring). To correlate the presence of cytoplasmic J-chain with subclass distribution, cells were stained with TRITC-labeled anti-human J-chain followed by FITC-labeled monoclonal anti-IgA$_1$ or monoclonal anti-IgA$_2$ (indirect method).

The majority of IgA-containing cells present in tonsils; spleen; mediastinal, mesenteric, axillary, or retroperitoneal lymph nodes; or bone marrow contained primarily IgA$_1$; whereas relatively more IgA$_2$ was present in small and large intestine (TABLE 1). These findings indicate that tissues not associated with mucosal surfaces are populated primarily by IgA$_1$-containing cells, whereas mucosal surfaces are relatively enriched in IgA$_2$-containing cells, reflecting the distribution of IgA subclasses in serum versus external secretions. There also appears to be relatively more J-chain in IgA$_2$-containing cells from the tissues examined. The presence of J-chain, however, in IgA$_1$-containing cells, particularly in the gut, suggests the production of polymeric IgA by these tissues.

*This work was supported in part by United States Public Health Service Grants AI-10854 and AI-07051.

TABLE 1

DISTRIBUTION OF IGA SUBCLASSES AND J-CHAIN IN HUMAN TISSUES

Tissue	Percent of IgA Cells that are IgA$_1$	Percent of IgA$_1$ Cells Containing J-Chain	Percent of IgA Cells that are IgA$_2$	Percent of IgA$_2$ Cells Containing J-Chain
Tonsil (4)*	90.6% [87.7–94.0]†	43.3% [14.6–72.0]	9.4% [6.0–12.3]	75.8% [63.6–88.8]
Mediastinal lymph node (2)	90.1% [87.1–93.1]	30.6%	9.9% [6.9–12.9]	14.2%
Axillary lymph node (3)	78.1% [76.5–80.0]	ND	21.1% [18.6–23.5]	ND
Mesenteric lymph node (1)	59.5%	22.2%	12.5%	14.5%
Retroperitoneal lymph node (1)	69.2%	ND	30.8%	ND
Spleen (4)	87.5% [85.3–88.2]	23.9% [11.1–32.0]	11.8% [11.1–14.7]	34.2% [20.7–55.6]
Bone Marrow (4)	88.0% [73.5–100.0]	29.0% [19.0–41.7]	13.5% [6.0–20.0]	28.7% [0.0–50.0]
Large intestine (1)	31.8%	ND	77.4%	ND
Small intestine (2)	56.0% [55.1–56.9]	46.9% [31.6–62.2]	44.0% [43.1–44.9]	70.7% [50.0–91.3]

*Number of specimens examined
†Range

REFERENCE

1. ANDRÉ, C., F. ANDRÉ & C. FARGIER. 1978. Distribution of IgA$_1$ and IgA$_2$ plasma cells in various normal tissues and in the jejunum of plasma IgA-deficient patients. Clin. Exp. Immunol. **33:** 327–331.

DIVERGENT SHIFTS IN T-LYMPHOCYTE SUBPOPULATIONS AMONG MUCOSAL LYMPHOID TISSUES OF MICE WITH INCREASING AGE*

Cathy A. Crowley, Andrew W. Wade, and Myron R. Szewczuk†

Department of Microbiology and Immunology
Queen's University
Kingston, Ontario, Canada K7L 3N6

The pattern of shifts in subpopulations of nonimmune T-lymphocytes in various lymphoid tissues with age was studied. Tissues including spleen, thymus, bone marrow, mediastinal (or bronchial) lymph nodes, mesenteric lymph nodes, Peyer's patches, intraepithelial lymphocytes, and lamina propria lymphocytes of the small intestine were obtained from various aged (2–30 months) C57BL/6J male mice. The percentage of cells bearing the Thy-1.2, Lyt-1, Lyt-2 phenotypic cell-surface markers in the various tissues was examined using monoclonal antibodies and epi-immunofluorescent microscopy study. The results are summarized in TABLE 1.

TABLE 1

SHIFTS IN PERCENTAGE OF POSITIVE CELLS WITH AGE

Tissue	THY-1.2	LYT-1	LYT-2	LYT-1/LYT-2
Spleen	↔	↑	↓	↑
Thymus	↔	↑	↓	↑
BM	↔	↑	↔	↑
BLN	↓	↔	↓↑	↑↓
MLN	↔	↔	↑↓	↓↑
PP	↓	↓	↓	↓
IEL	↑	↔	↑↓	↓↑
LPL	↔	↔	↓	↑

A marked increase was found in the ratio of Lyt-1:Lyt-2 positive cells within the spleen, thymus, and bone marrow (BM) with age. This rise in the ratio of Lyt-1:Lyt-2 positive cells is a reflection of a rise in relative numbers of Lyt-1 cells with a corresponding age-related decline in Lyt-2 cells. No change occurred in these tissues with respect to relative numbers of Thy-1.2 cells. By contrast, a more divergent shifting of these subpopulations of lymphocytes occurred in the mucosal-associated lymphoid tissues. The bronchial lymph nodes (BLN) showed with age, a decrease in relative numbers of Thy-1.2 cells, no change in Lyt-1 cells, and an initial increase in Lyt-2 cells up until 12 months of age. At 12 months of age, the Lyt-2 population reached a peak and then declined. This pattern was reflected in an initial increase in the ratio of Lyt-1:Lyt-2 cells followed by a

*This work was supported in part by a grant from the Medical Research Council of Canada, MA-7347, and the Gerontology Research Council of Ontario.
†Gerontology Research Council of Ontario Scholar.

decline in the 20-month and 30-month old animals. The subpopulations within the Peyer's patches (PP) decreased steadily in relative numbers with age. In the lamina propria lymphocyte population (LPL), no change was seen in Thy-1.2 or Lyt-1 populations, yet Lyt-2 subpopulation declined in relative numbers steadily with age. This situation was seen as a steady rise in the ratio of Lyt-1:Lyt-2 cells within the lamina propria. Cells positive for Thy-1.2 in the mesenteric lymph node (MLN) revealed no change with age, whereas in the intraepithial lymphocytes, (IEL) this subpopulation increased in older animals. No change in relative numbers of Lyt-1 cells was seen for both IEL and MLN. The relative numbers, however, of Lyt-2 cells within IEL and MLN showed an initial increase up until 12 months of age and thereafter showed a decline. This response is seen again in the ratio of Lyt-1:Lyt-2 cells as an initial decrease in the ratio and a subsequent increase with age. The results of the present study indicate a difference in relative proportion of subpopulations of T-lymphocytes within the mucosal-associated lymphoid system. These results lend support for the hypothesis that the mucosal-associated lymphoid system differs from the systemic system in its immune competence with age.

SPECIFIC IMMUNE RESPONSE IN HUMAN MILK
TO ORAL IMMUNIZATION WITH FOOD PROTEINS*

José R. Cruz

Institute of Nutrition of Central America and Panama
Guatemala City, Guatemala

Lars Å. Hanson

Department of Clinical Immunology
University of Göteborg
Göteborg, Sweden

Human milk contains antibodies against a wide variety of microorganisms and their products.[3,4] These antibodies are induced by antigenic challenge at the intestinal level, where lymphocytes programmed to secrete IgA are primed, and once committed, migrate to and home in the mammary gland, where they release specific IgA antibodies.[3] Specific antibodies against food components that have also been found in human milk[1] may prevent the development of allergies in the breast-fed infant by inhibiting the absorption of undegraded molecules by the immature intestine.[5] Goldblum[2] has reported that intestinal antigenic challenge with microorganisms results in the appearance of cells in human milk that release specific IgA, in the absence of a rise in the titer of antibodies.

With the purpose of determining if oral immunization with food proteins induces an immune response in human milk in addition to the time and magnitude of such response, six lactating women from Guatemala (mean age 25.5 years) were immunized orally with a protein extract of Vigna sinensis (cowpea). Starting on the fifth day post partum, and for five consecutive days, each mother received 2 g of protein in gelatin capsules. Two unimmunized mothers (29 and 27 years old) were used as controls.

Milk samples were obtained daily from the fifth to the ninth day postpartum and on days 11, 18, 25, and 33. Specific antibodies were determined by means of the enzyme-linked immunosorbent assay (ELISA), using the same protein preparation as antigen to coat the microplates. The samples were tested at dilutions of 1:20, 1:40, 1:80, 1:160, and 1:320, and the bound antibody was detected with alkaline, phosphatase-labeled swine antihuman IgA (Orion Diagnostica, Helsinki, Finland).

Five of the six women, orally immunized, showed no anti-cowpea antibody (<1:20) in their milk at the beginning of the study; four of them produced specific IgA antibodies between the 7th and 21st day; one mother did not have a measurable response. In the only subject with high anti-cowpea IgA antibodies before the immunization, they decreased to undetectable levels for two weeks and then rose again. The two mothers who did not receive cowpea protein remained negative throughout the study. If milk antibodies directed against food components play a role in the prevention of food allergies among children, it is possible to induce the production of such antibodies by immunization of lactating women.

*Kellogg of Central America provided financial support for the presentation of these data.

808

REFERENCES

1. CRUZ, J. R., B. GARCIA, J. J. URRUTIA, B. CARLSSON, & L. Å. HANSON. 1981. J. Pediatr. **99:** 600.
2. GOLDBLUM, R. M., S. AHLSTEDT, B. CARLSSON, L. Å. HANSON, U. JODAL, G. LIDIN-JANSON, & A. SOHL-ÅKERLUND. 1975. Nature (London) **257:** 797.
3. HANSON, L. Å., B. CARLSSON, J. R. CRUZ, B. GARCIA, J. HOLMGREN, S. R. KHAN, B. S. LINDBLAD, A.-M. SVENNERHOLM, B. SVENNERHOLM, & J. URRUTIA. 1979. In Immunology of Breast Milk. p. 145. Raven Press. New York.
4. HOLMGREN, J., L. Å., HANSON, B. CARLSSON, B. S. LINDBLAD & J. RAHIMTOOLA. 1976. Scand J. Immunol. **5:** 867.
5. WALKER, W. A. 1978. Arch. Dis. Child. **53:** 527.

ACKNOWLEDGMENTS

The assistance of Olga Román, Irma Pérez, Emma López, Catalina Monzón, and Roberto Rosales is highly appreciated.

EIMERIA TENELLA: CONTROL OF PARASITIC BEHAVIOR THROUGH MUCOSAL IMMUNITY AND IN-FEED IMMUNIZATION

P. J. Davis and P. Porter

Unilever Research
Bedford MK44 1LQ England

Eimeria tenella presents a complex antigenic challenge within the mucosa and submucosa of the chicken cecum. To effectively counter this type of attack, the whole spectrum of immune defense is marshaled at the gut mucosa, providing a comprehensive model of mucosal immunity in action.[1] There is a major response from the secretory IgA system, during and following infection with *E. tenella*.[1,2] Secretory antibodies can be detected in the bile and gut contents, whereas abundant IgA-secreting plasma cells appear in the lamina propria. Despite the presence of intraluminal secretory antibodies that *in vitro* can recognize and bind the surface membrane antigens of the parasite, the invasive forms, sporozoites, can evade this first line of defence,[3-5] perhaps by shedding their surface antigens—effectively becoming "antigenically modulated" parasites. This effect was also demonstrated *in vitro* with monolayers of chick kidney cells and sporozoites pretreated with various extracts of immune and nonimmune gut contents (TABLE 1). Thus, antigenic modulation was shown, in that immune cecal contents inhibited penetration by only 47% (cf. 98% inhibition with immune serum). Consequent damage to the sporozoite was shown by the inhibition of intracellular development with sporozoites exposed to immune and nonimmune cecal contents. Preexposure to nonimmune cecal contents could create a state of antigenic modulation by means of the intestinal proteases present. This aspect of the host-parasite relationship can illuminate our understanding of the "immune exclusion" role of secretory antibodies, because the sporozoite must imitate, at the cellular level, the events taking place at the molecular level in antigen absorption.

TABLE 1

THE EFFECTS ON SPOROZOITE PENETRATION AND INTRACELLULAR DEVELOPMENT *IN VITRO* OF SERA, EXTRACTS OF CECAL TISSUE AND EXTRACTS OF CECAL CONTENTS

Test Effect	Status of Donor	Test Samples		
		Serum	Cecal Tissue	Cecal Contents
Inhibition of penetration	U.C.*	Nil	Nil	Nil
	I*	98%	47%	47%
Inhibition of intracellular development	U.C.*	Nil	Nil	73%†
	I*	96%†	56%	80%†
Activity ascribed to:		IgG	IgG	IgA and/or intestinal proteases

*U.C. = Uninfected control; I = Immune
†Significant difference from standard, untreated sporozoites (p = <0.05%, Duncan's multiple range test).

Effective mucosal immunity in the chicken can only be achieved with live vaccines. This immunity was best achieved by dispersing the oocysts in a wet premix consisting of starch paste, which assisted their even distribution in the final diet, and offered considerable protection. Other effective oocyst vehicles included solutions of Xanthan Gum and any other polysaccharide formulation with similar qualities. Each bird was thus given a very small trickle dose of live, virulent *E. tenella* oocyst for the first 3–5 weeks of life. The resultant subclinical infections were monitored by means of oocyst output, and where appropriate, by weight gains and histology. Full protective immunity could consistently be produced by the fourth week of life. During immunization, increasing immunological pressure was brought to bear on the parasites, and by the third week, the destructive second generation schizonts became deformed and small, taking up superficial locations instead of migrating deep into the submucosa.

REFERENCES

1. DAVIS, P. J. 1981. Immunity to Coccidia. *In* Avian Immunology. M. E. Rose, L. N. Payne and B. M. Freeman, Eds.: 361–385. British Poultry Science Limited. Edinburgh.
2. WIESNER, J. 1979. Biliary IgA from infected chickens as agglutinating factor for *Eimeria tenella* sporozoites. J. Protozool. **26:** 46–47A.
3. HORTON-SMITH, C., P. L. LONG & A. E. PIERCE. 1963. Behaviour of invasive stages of *Eimeria tenella* in the immune fowl (Gallus domesticus). Exp. Parasitol. **14:** 66–74.
4. LEATHEM, W. D. & W. L. BURNS. 1967. Effects of the immune chicken on the endogenous stages of *Eimeria tenella*. J. Parasit. **53:** 180–185.
5. ROSE, M. E. & P. HESKETH. 1976. Immunity to coccidiosis. Stages of the life cycle of *Eimeria maxima* which induce, and are affected by the response of the host. Parasitology **73:** 25–37.

IgA-SIZE AND IgA-SUBCLASS DISTRIBUTION IN SERUM AND SECRETIONS*

D. L. Delacroix,†‡ K. B. Elkon,§¶ and J. P. Vaerman‡

Gastroenterology Laboratory
University Clinic of St. Luke
‡Experimental Medicine Unit
International Institute of Cellular and Molecular Pathology
Catholic University of Louvain Brussels, Belgium
§Royal Postgraduate Medical School
London, England

The predominance of polymeric IgA (pIgA) in secretions and of monomeric IgA (mIgA) in serum is well known,[1] as is the larger proportion of IgA_2 in colostrum than in serum.[2] Data on IgA subclasses in other secretions are still lacking. A larger proportion of IgA_2- or pIgA-staining plasmacytes is found in mucosae than in bone marrow and peripheral lymphoid organs.[3-6] Hence, pIgA and IgA_2 in serum are regarded by some as the particular contribution of mucosal plasmacytes to blood IgA, whereas serum mIgA would derive mostly from bone marrow.[3,6-8] A link between pIgA and IgA_2 was also suggested when peripheral blood lymphocytes, stimulated in vitro with pokeweed mitogen for seven days, produced predominantly pIgA, with about 40% of IgA cells staining for IgA_2.[9]

We compared the IgA size and IgA-subclass distributions in secretions and sera with normal, low, or high IgA levels. mIgA and pIgA were measured by immunoradiometric assay[10] after sucrose density gradient ultracentrifugation and IgA_1 and IgA_2 by immunoradiometric assay or radial immunodiffusion, using homemade antisera.[11]

In 34 normal adult sera, 5–22% ($\bar{x} = 13\%$) of total IgA was pIgA, compared to 5–36% ($\bar{x} = 21\%$) for IgA_2. In all secretions studied,[11] the IgA_2 percentage was higher ($p < 0.05$) than in the corresponding sera (FIGURE 1); IgA_2 percentage was lower ($p < 0.05$) in bile ($\bar{x} = 26\%$) than in other secretions (>30%), probably because 50% of pIgA in bile (versus 2% in saliva) derives from plasma.[12] IgA_2 was distributed in both pIgA and mIgA in bile and serum after sucrose density gradient ultracentrifugation (FIGURE 2); in serum, IgA_2 percentage was similar in mIgA and pIgA.

Sera from 22 infants[13] (6–240 days old) had a much higher ($p < 0.001$) pIgA percentage (8–72%, $\bar{x} = 36\%$), but not IgA_2 percentage, than sera of adults. Sera from IgA-deficient adults[13] had higher ($p < 0.005$) IgA_2 percentage (16–38%, $\bar{x} = 34\%$), but not pIgA percentage, when compared to normal adults.

In diseases with high serum IgA,[14] a preferential contribution of pIgA was found in all parenchymal liver diseases ($\bar{x} = 19\%$), acute or chronic, but also in systemic sicca syndrome ($\bar{x} = 19\%$), Crohn's disease ($\bar{x} = 20\%$), and ileojejunal bypass ($\bar{x} = 20\%$). Such an increased pIgA percentage was accompanied by an increased IgA_2 percentage only in alcoholic cirrhosis and Crohn's disease. In

*This work was supported by the FRSM and the FNRS, Brussels, Belgium.

†Correspondence to: D. L. Delacroix, UCL-ICP-MEXP, 75, avenue Hippocrate, B-1200 Brussels, Belgium

§Present address: Hospital for Special Surgery, New York, N.Y. 10021.

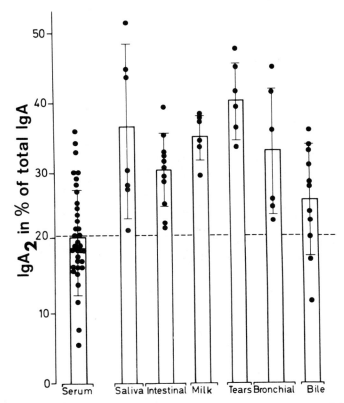

FIGURE 1. Proportions of IgA$_2$ in 34 normal sera and in various secretions. Columns give means ± SD.

autoimmune diseases, a shift to IgA$_1$ occurred. In Berger's disease and biliary obstruction, no change in pIgA percentage was found.

In conclusion, the IgA$_2$ and pIgA characters are not closely linked; other tissues than mucosae probably contribute *in vivo* to pIgA in serum, as suggested *in vitro*.[9]

REFERENCES

1. HEREMANS, J. F. 1974. *In* the Antigens. M. Sela, Ed.: Vol. **2**: 365–522. Academic Press. New York.
2. GREY, H. M., C. A. ABEL, W. J. YOUNT & H. G. KUNKEL. 1968. J. Exp. Med. **128**: 1223–1236.
3. RADL, J., H. R. E. SCHUIT, J. MESTECKY & W. HIJMANS. 1974. Adv. Exp. Med. Biol. **45**: 57–65.
4. BRANDTZAEG, P. 1973. Nature (London) New Biol. **243**: 142–143.
5. ANDRE, C., F. ANDRE & M. C. FARGIER. 1878. Clin. Exp. Immunol. **33**: 327–331.
6. SKVARIL, F. & A. MORELL. 1974. Adv. Exp. Med. Biol. **45**: 433–435.
7. BENNER, R., W. HIJMANS & J. J. HAAIJMAN. 1981. Clin. Exp. Immunol. **46**: 1–8.

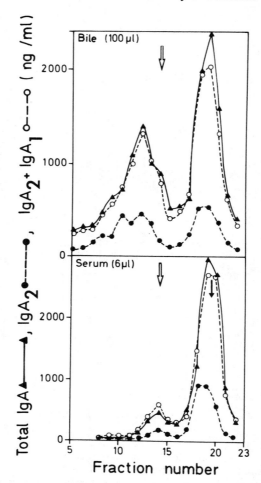

FIGURE 2. Size distribution of IgA$_1$ and IgA$_2$ in serum and bile. Open arrows: position of [^{125}I]dimeric IgA; thin arrow: position of IgG by optical density. Sedimentation from right to left.

8. KUTTEH, W. H., S. J. PRINCE & J. MESTECKY. 1982. J. Immunol. **128:** 990–995.
9. KUTTEH, W. H., W. J. KOOPMAN, M. E. CONLEY, M. L. EGAN & J. MESTECKY. 1980. J. Exp. Med. **152:** 1424–1429.
10. DELACROIX, D. L., J. P. DEHENNIN & J. P. VAERMAN. 1982. J. Immunol. Methods. **48:** 327–337.
11. DELACROIX, D. L., C. DIVE, J. C. RAMBAUD & J. P. VAERMAN. 1982. Immunology. **47:** 383–385.
12. DELACROIX, D. L., H. J. F. HODGSON, A. McPHERSON, C. DIVE & J. P. VAERMAN. 1982. J. Clin. Invest. **70:** 230–241.
13. DELACROIX, D. L., E. LIROUX & J. P. VAERMAN. 1983. J. Clin. Immunol. **3:** In press.
14. DELACROIX, D. L., K. B. ELKON, A. P. GEUBEL, H. J. F. HODGSON, C. DIVE & J. P. VAERMAN. 1983. J. Clin. Invest. In press.

EFFECT OF ADJUVANTS ON LOCAL sIgA RESPONSES*

Jeffrey L. Ebersole, Martin A. Taubman, and Daniel J. Smith

Forsyth Dental Center
Boston, Massachusetts 02115

Secretory IgA (sIgA) antibodies at mucosal surfaces have been shown to provide a protective function against a variety of viral and bacterial diseases. sIgA antibodies in saliva have been shown to inhibit dental caries in various animal model systems. The induction of sIgA antibody in salivary secretions has been accomplished by both parenteral and enteral administration of antigens. To optimize protection by sIgA antibodies, however, methods must be developed to maximize the response. This study investigated the effect of various adjuvants on the induction of salivary IgA-antibody responses to defined antigens in rats.

Adult Sprague-Dawley rats (90–120 days old) were injected in the salivary gland vicinity with either high epitope density ($DNP_{54}BGG$) or low density (DNP_7BGG) conjugates (dinitrophenylated bovine gamma globulin). The antigens were mixed in phosphate-buffered saline (PBS), CFA or with 10^9 heat-killed *Bordetella pertussis* (UBP (unbound *B. pertussis*); Connaught Laboratories Limited, Ontario, Canada). Also, the antigens were bound by adsorption to $Al(OH)_3$ or covalently linked to *B. pertussis* (bound *B. pertussis* or BBP) with carbodiimide. Serum and pilocarpine-stimulated saliva were collected until 67 days postinjection, and the rats were boosted in the salivary gland vicinity on day 87 with homologous antigen/adjuvant combinations. Serum and salivary antibodies to the dinitrophenyl (DNP) hapten were determined in an enzyme-linked immunosorbent assay (ELISA), and levels were expressed as ELISA units based on a reference standard with 100 ELISA units.

After primary and secondary immunization, serum IgG and IgM levels were greatest with complete Freund's adjuvant (CFA). $Al(OH)_3$, BBP, and UBP each elicited significantly increased primary and secondary serum IgG responses; however, the UBP and BBP elicited much greater IgM responses than the $Al(OH)_3$. By contrast, local injection of $Al(OH)_3$ and antigen induced levels of serum IgA that were similar to those with CFA as adjuvant. Minimal levels of salivary IgG were detected after injection of antigens in PBS; however, inclusion of adjuvant with $DNP_{54}BGG$ elicited significantly greater levels of salivary IgG, with CFA providing the greatest enhancement after primary or secondary injection. Only CFA and BBP significantly enhanced the salivary IgG anti-DNP response to the low epitope density antigen (DNP_7BGG). Primary immunization with either antigen in PBS resulted in salivary IgA antibody. All adjuvants tested were equally effective for increasing salivary IgA responses to $DNP_{54}BGG$, whereas $Al(OH)_3$ was superior for inducing local secondary responses of the IgA isotype. Similarly, $Al(OH)_3$ was the most active adjuvant for eliciting primary and secondary IgA responses to DNP_7BGG.

Examination of the kinetics of the salivary IgA response demonstrated that each adjuvant was capable of inducing an earlier onset, higher peak level, and longer duration of IgA antibody after secondary local injection. These findings are characteristic of immunologic memory and suggest that the adjuvant materials

*This work was supported in part by Grant DE-04733 and DE-00075 from the National Institute of Dental Research.

may be useful in enhancing the protective capabilities of the sIgA immune system.

The results suggest that selection of adjuvant materials may have a substantial effect on isotype distribution of antibodies in serum and secretions. Also, the findings indicate that $Al(OH)_3$ may be the adjuvant of choice for elicitation of secretory IgA antibodies through local immunization.

IMMUNOREGULATION ABNORMALITIES IN PATIENTS WITH IgA NEPHROPATHY*

J. Egido, R. Blasco, and J. Sancho

Fundación Jiménez Díaz
Madrid, Spain

IgA nephropathy is characterized by the presence, in the glomerular mesangium, of IgA, and sometimes C3 and other immunoglobulins, in the absence of signs and symptoms of systemic disease. Our aim in this report was to study the cellular bases that could explain the high serum levels of IgA frequently found in these patients. Taking into account the existence of familial IgA nephropathies and the occasional association of this nephritis with some HLA antigens,[1] we also decided to study a group of healthy relatives of these patients.

MATERIALS AND METHODS

Peripheral blood mononuclear cell suspensions (PBM) were obtained from fresh heparinized blood, drawn from 27 patients, 15 normal controls, and 25 healthy relatives, by standard Hypaque-Ficoll density centrifugation. PBM at a concentration of 2×10^6 cells/ml were incubated in the presence or absence of 10 μl/ml of pokeweed mitogen (PWM) in conditions previously published.[2] At the end of day 7, culture tubes were centrifuged and the amounts of IgA, IgG, and IgM secreted into the culture media were detected by a radioimmunoassay, as previously described.[3] T-cell subsets were identified in whole mononuclear cells by using specific monoclonal antibodies (OK series). A suppressor-cell assay generated by concanavalin A was performed by incubating PBM simultaneously with doses of Con A, ranging from 1.25 to 100 μg/ml, and PWM. Both mitogens were added at the beginning of the culture. T-helper cell function was examined in an in vitro assay of immunoglobulin production, by adding PWM to cultures containing allogeneic mixtures of control B-cells with T-cells from either controls or patients with IgA nephropathy.

RESULTS AND COMMENTS

After in vitro PWM-stimulation the amount of IgA produced by PBM from patients was significantly higher (560 ± 97 ng/ml) than in controls (231 ± 57) p < 0.0025. No differences were seen in IgM and IgG synthesis. There were no differences in the percentages of OKT3$^+$ cells between patients and controls. Twenty out of 27 patients had significantly high percentages of OKT4$^+$ helper-cells (greater than 2 SD of mean from controls), with normal or elevated percentages of OKT8$^+$ cells. All patients showed some abnormalities in the generation of specific IgA-suppressor cells at variable doses of Con A. Low doses of Con A (2.5 μg/ml) induced a certain suppression of the IgA synthesis in the

*This work was supported by a grant from the Fondo de Investigacion Sanitaria de la Seguridad Social (FIS).

817

patients that was not observed in the majority of the controls. By contrast, higher doses of Con A (50 μg/ml) produced significantly less IgA suppression than controls. Normal IgA suppression values were found at 10 μg/ml of Con A. Importantly, no significant differences were seen in the percentages of suppression of IgG and IgM synthesis in most of the patients. T-cells obtained from patients were significantly more efficient than T-cells from controls in providing specific IgA-helper activity for normal allogeneic B-cells.

Some of these immunological abnormalities were also seen in the 25 patients' relatives studied (seven families). Thus, PBM from 10 subjects produced, after in vitro polyclonal stimulation, significantly higher amounts of IgA than the controls. Eleven subjects had elevated percentage of OKT4+. Two subjects presented a specific absence in the suppression of IgA with 50 μg/ml of Con A, whereas another 10 relatives showed an increase in the suppression of IgA with 2.5 μg/ml above the values seen in any control of Con A. Most of these alterations were seen in one of the parents, therefore the possible pattern of inheritance, if any, seems vertical.

The observation of an increased production of IgA by PWM-stimulated PBM from patients with IgA nephropathy seems specific for this immunoglobulin, as there were no significant changes in the production of IgG and IgM. Because the in vitro response of human PBM cells to PWM requires the active participation of T-helper lymphocytes, this increased response could represent, a priori, an abnormality in either B-cell or T-helper cell function. Although we cannot discard the existence of a B-cell alteration, the significant increased activity of IgA T-helper cells, together with the subtle abnormalities of IgA-suppressor cells, and results noted in healthy patients' relatives, point to a T-cell anomaly.

Our data also suggest that the immune regulation abnormalities in the IgA synthesis observed in these patients have probably some genetic basis and might be the first step in the pathogenesis of IgA nephropathy.

REFERENCES

1. EGIDO, J., J. SANCHO, R. BLASCO, F. RIVERA & L. HERNANDO. 1983. In Advances in Nephrology. J. Hamburger, J. Crosmer, J.P. Grünfeld, & M.H. Maxwell, Eds.: Vol. 12. Year Book Medical Publishers. Chicago. In press.
2. LÓPEZ TRASCASA, M., J. EGIDO, J. SANCHO & L. HERNANDO. 1980. Clin. Exp. Immunol. 42: 247.
3. EGIDO, J., R. BLASCO & J. SANCHO. 1982. Clin. Exp. Immunol. 47: 309.

PEYER'S PATCH ACCESSORY CELLS BEAR I-A*

John H. Eldridge, Yun Lee, Hiroshi Kiyono, David M. Spalding,
K. A. Gollahon, Gary W. Wood, William J. Koopman,
and Jerry R. McGhee

Departments of Microbiology, Pathology, and Medicine
Institute of Dental Research
and
Comprehensive Cancer Center
The University of Alabama in Birmingham
University Station
Birmingham, Alabama 35294

Peyer's patches (PP) are discrete lymphoreticular follicles located along the gastrointestinal tract of mammals, and represent a first line of defense to environmentally encountered antigens. In addition, the close proximity of this lymphoid population to the endogenous gut microflora exposes them to a variety of biologically active bacterial products such as the lipopolysaccharide of the gram-negative organisms. The PP contain a significant percentage of precursor IgA B-lymphocytes, and following oral administration of antigen, sensitized precursor cells for the IgA response migrate from these sites to populate and secrete in the gut lamina propria and other, more distant, mucosal sites.[1] Complete differentiation of B-cells to plasma cells within the PP is not observed, and this sensitization without terminal differentiation has been attributed to a paucity of accessory cells (MØ) within this tissue. Recent work from our laboratory has shown that enzymatic dissociation of PP with Dispase® releases lymphoreticular cells containing a higher proportion of MØ and that this population will support in vitro immune responses to thymic-dependent antigens.[2]

In order for the MØ to function as an antigen-presenting accessory cell in the induction of T-dependent immune responses, homology at the I-A subregion of H-2 between the MØ and the antigen-specific T-cell is required. Expression of I-A on the MØ has been shown to be under T-cell control. The C3H/HeJ mouse strain is lipopolysaccharide nonresponsive, and exhibits elevated T_h-cells and IgA responses when compared to the normal C3H/HeN strain. We have examined the PP adherent accessory cells from these mouse strains in order to determine whether I-A gene product(s) are expressed and/or required for induction of immune responses by PP MØ and whether PP MØ in C3H/HeJ mice exhibit an altered frequency of I-A expression.

Irradiated splenic or PP adherent cells were able to reconstitute the in vitro direct plaque-forming cell (PFC) response of glass wool passaged splenic cells to sheep red blood cells (SRBC) (TABLE 1). Treatment of the adherent cells with monoclonal anti-I-A^k (hybridoma 11–5.2) plus rabbit C abolished the MØ function of C3H/HeN (H-2^k) but not BALB/c (H-2^d) adherent cells.

The I-A status of normal and adherent cell populations from spleens and PP of C3H/HeN and C3H/HeJ mice were compared using fluorescein conjugated

*This work was supported by United States Public Health Service Grants DE 04217, AI 14807, CA 13148, AM 03555, and DE 02670.

TABLE 1

C3H/HeN ADHERENT ACCESSORY CELLS BEAR I-A^{k}*

Cells added to culture			Direct Anti-SRBC PFC/culture ± S.D.	
Glass wool passaged spleen	Adherent cells from spleen	Adherent cells from PP	BALB/c	C3H/HeN
+	−	−	2 ± 3	3 ± 5
−	+	−	0	2 ± 3
−	−	+	3 ± 3	4 ± 2
+	+	−	935 ± 23	1323 ± 111
+	−	+	1222 ± 48	1463 ± 116
+	+(Anti-IA)†	−	1282 ± 20	1271 ± 32
+	−	+(Anti-IA)	1370 ± 46	1230 ± 52
+	+(C)‡	−	1278 ± 30	1295 ± 43
+	−	+(C)	1285 ± 111	1256 ± 21
+	+(Anti-IA&C)§	−	1217 ± 33	0
+	−	+(Anti-IA&C)	1326 ± 64	9 ± 7

*Two-hour adherent cells (1500 rads)
†Treated with anti-IA only (hybridoma 11–5.2)
‡Treated with complement only
§Treated with anti-IA and complement

anti-I-A^{k} in conjunction with latex phagocytosis and fluorescent labeling of MØ (rabbit anti-murine MØ and rhodamine conjugated goat anti-rabbit IgG).

Within the normal and adherent cell populations of the two strains, equivalent numbers of MØ staining (MØ$^{+}$) cells were identified (TABLE 2). Double labeling with anti-I-A^{k} and anti-MØ demonstrated that both strains possessed similar

TABLE 2

DISTRIBUTION OF I-A^{k} BEARING ACCESSORY CELLS

Strain	Tissue	Population	Percent of Total Cells*	
			MØ$^{+}$	MØ$^{+}$I-A^{k+}
BALB/c	SP	Adherent	27.8	<0.2
BALB/c	PP†	Adherent	45.0	<0.1
C3H/HeN	SP	Normal	8.9 ± 2.2	4.0 ± 1.6 (44)‡
C3H/HeN	SP	Adherent	31.5 ± 3.5	13.7 ± 0.9 (43)
C3H/HeJ	SP	Normal	10.9	4.8 (44)
C3H/HeJ	SP	Adherent	31.9	12.9 (39)
	Mechanical Release			
C3H/HeN	PP	Normal	3.4	2.3 (68)
C3H/HeJ	PP	Normal	3.8	2.8 (73)
	Enzymatic Release†			
C3H/HeN	PP	Normal	10.9 ± 1.2	8.1 ± 0.7 (74)
C3H/HeN	PP	Adherent	44.1 ± 3.9	29.3 ± 3.2 (66)
C3H/HeJ	PP	Normal	9.7	6.3 (65)
C3H/HeJ	PP	Adherent	49.9	34.8 (70)

*MØ staining—Rabbit anti-mouse MØ serum and RBITC-goat anti-rabbit IgG; I-A^{k} staining—FITC anti-I-A^{k} (hybridoma 11-5.2)
†Dispase® prepared
‡Percent of MØ$^{+}$ that also stain for I-A^{k}

percentages of I-A^k bearing (I-A$^+$) MØ$^+$ cells within their normal and adherent spleen populations. The PP adherent population from both strains contained a higher percentage of I-A$^+$ MØ$^+$ cells relative to the splenic adherent cells. Quantitatively similar results were obtained when I-A^k labeling was performed in conjunction with latex ingestion. Comparison of the MØ present in the normal spleen and PP with their respective adherent population indicates that Dispase$^®$ digestion does not selectively release I-A$^+$ MØ and that there is no preferential adherence or phagocytosis by I-A$^+$ as opposed to I-A$^-$ MØ in any population examined.

These results indicate that Dispase$^®$-prepared PP cells contain accessory cells, that a highly enriched population can be obtained by adherence, and that a high percentage of the PP accessory cells bear I-A.

REFERENCES

1. CRAIG, S. W. & J. J. CEBRA. 1971. Peyer's patches: an enriched source of precursors for IgA-producing immunocytes in the rabbit. J. Exp. Med. **134:** 188.
2. KIYONO, H., J. R. McGHEE, M. J. WANNEMUEHLER, M. V. FRANGAKIS, D. M. SPALDING, S. M. MICHALEK & W. J. KOOPMAN. 1982. *In vitro* immune responses to T cell-dependent antigen by cultures of dissociated murine Peyer's patch. Proc. Natl. Acad. Sci. USA **79:** 596–600.

IMMUNOFLUORESCENT AND IMMUNOCYTOCHEMICAL LOCALIZATION OF SECRETORY COMPONENT AND IMMUNOGLOBULINS IN HUMAN LIVER

Cynthia Foss-Bowman, Albert L. Jones, Sussan Dejbakhsh,
and Ira S. Goldman

Cell Biology Laboratory
Veterans Administration Medical Center
San Francisco, California 94121
Department of Laboratory Medicine, Medicine, and Liver Center
University of California at San Francisco
San Francisco, California 94143
Pathology Department
Santa Rosa Community Hospital
Santa Rosa, California 95402

INTRODUCTION

Rodent hepatocytes have a pathway of sIgA transport similar to intestinal epithelium with dimeric IgA binding to the plasma membrane receptor secretory component (SC), endocytosis, intracellular vesicular transport, and sIgA secretion into the bile canaliculus. sIgA and various IgA fragments are present in human bile,[1] but whether the human hepatocyte transports sIgA is debated. One report suggests that biliary epithelium is primarily responsible for sIgA secretion into human bile,[2] whereas another shows SC and immunoglobulins (Igs) in human hepatocytes.[3] Immunofluorescent studies show a variety of hepatocyte IgA patterns.[4-6] Recently our group has shown that perfused human liver wedge biopsies transport IgA, although in amounts less than observed in rats (A.L. Jones, I.S. Goldman, S.J. Burwen, unpublished results).

Because specimen processing so drastically affects the results of immunocytochemical procedures and because no studies have systematically considered these variables, we conducted a comparison study of different conditions in the demonstration of SC and Igs in human liver.

METHODS AND MATERIALS

Nine human liver wedge biopsies from normal patients and those with hepatobiliary diseases, two human colon biopsies, and four adult rat liver biopsies were processed variously (and most often simultaneously) for immunofluorescence with quick freezing and cryostat section fixation with air drying, alcohol or formalin; peroxidase-antiperoxidase cytochemistry with formalin or Bouins fixation or paraformaldehyde, periodate-lysine-paraformaldehyde (PLP), or Karnovsky fixation and using different antibody systems and different substrates; and electron immunocytochemistry (EMIC) with different fixatives and pre- and postembedding techniques. Appropriate blocking and adsorbed antibody controls were used.

RESULTS

Human livers showed positive hepatocyte, sinusoidal, and ductular staining for SC and Igs in varying patterns that depended on technique and hepatobiliary pathology. Bouins fixation showed a rather even diffuse pattern, whereas formalin showed a more patchy variable pattern with negative to intensely positive cells. These patterns were similar with air dried tissue for immunofluorescence and sharper with ethanol-fixed sections. Alcoholic livers showed hepatocytes congested with SC and Igs. Controls were appropriately negative.

Electron immunocytochemistry showed that the liver is unable to withstand caustic etching techniques and is less successfully handled with techniques used for colon. Initial studies at the light level show positive staining with 1% paraformaldehyde, PLP, and weak staining with Karnovsky's fix on frozen sections.

CONCLUSIONS

Secretory component and IgA as well as IgG and IgM are present in human hepatocytes and biliary epithelium. Their presence is not artifactual secondary to uneven fixation, because similar patterns are seen in four micron air-dried or ethanol-fixed tissue. Their demonstration, however, is highly dependent on processing variables and can be modulated by varying fixation, antibody titers and ratios, and substrates. The demonstration of an antigen in a tissue must exhaustively consider these variables. Techniques worked out in one tissue may not be applicable in another (e.g. colon versus liver). These differences may be related to different relative amounts of antigens or their different milieus.

Human hepatocytes may well transport IgA as rodent hepatocytes do or may have different or additional pathways.[1]

REFERENCES

1. KUTTEH, W. H. 1982. Gastroenterology **82:** 184.
2. NAGURA, H. 1982. Immunology **126:** 587.
3. HSU, S. & P. L. HSU. 1980. Gut **21:** 985.
4. KATER, L. 1979. Am. J. Clin. Pathol. **71:** 51.
5. HOPF, U. 1978. Scand. J. Immunol. **8:** 543.
6. HOPF, U. 1976. J. Immunol. **117:** 639.

ROLE OF IgA ANTIBODY IN PHAGOCYTOSIS BY HUMAN POLYMORPHONUCLEAR LEUKOCYTES*

S. N. Goldstine, A. Tsai, and C. J. Kemp

School of Dentistry
Case Western Reserve University
Cleveland, Ohio 44106

M. W. Fanger

Dartmouth Medical School
Hanover, New Hampshire 03755

Previous studies have indicated that human oral and peripheral blood polymorphonuclear leukocytes (PMN) possess separate receptors for IgG and IgA antibody and that a significant proportion of these cells appear to possess both receptors. The purpose of this study was to determine the role of the receptors for IgA in PMN phagocytosis.

Human PMN were prepared from peripheral blood by gradient centrifugation on Ficoll-Hypaque and subsequent dextran sedimentation of the PMN-erythrocyte pellet. Ox red blood cells (ORBC) were sensitized with either rabbit serum IgG or rabbit colostral IgA antibodies or both and washed prior to use as target cells. Polymorphonuclear leukocytes and ORBC target cells were incubated at a 1:10 ratio for 10 minutes at 37° C, centrifuged, and reincubated for an additional 20 minutes.

The supernatant was removed, lysing buffer was added to remove extracellular ORBC, and cytocentrifuge slides were prepared. The percentage of phagocytosis was evaluated by counting the number of positive PMN per 100 PMN on Wright's stained slides.

The results indicated that blood PMN could bind ORBC coated with IgA, but could not phagocytize these target cells. IgA was able, however, to enhance IgG-mediated phagocytosis. The percentage of cells that phagocytized ORBC was increased two to three fold by the addition of IgA antibodies to ORBC sensitized with suboptimal amounts of IgG. The average number of phagocytized ORBC per PMN was also increased using these target cells. Additional studies indicated that both isotypes must be on the same target cell to obtain enhanced phagocytosis, and that IgM antibody was not capable of enhancing IgG-mediated phagocytosis.

The data suggest that during the process of phagocytosis the receptor for IgA on peripheral blood PMN may have functional characteristics similar to those of the PMN receptor for complement; that is, the receptor for IgA plays a role in attachment of IgA-sensitized target cells, but does not trigger ingestion of the target cells. In addition, these receptors also appear to be able to mediate enhancement of IgG-mediated phagocytosis, effectively lowering the IgG dose necessary for optimal phagocytosis. Thus, IgA-mediated enhancement of PMN phagocytosis may play an important role in host defense of oral mucosal surfaces that are bathed with both IgA and IgG antibodies.

*This work was supported in part by United States Public Health Service Grants DE05789 and AI19053.

COMPARATIVE STUDY OF THE SALIVARY AND SERUM ANTIBODY, AND CELL-MEDIATED RESPONSES TO LOCAL INJECTION OF *STREPTOCOCCUS MUTANS* RIBOSOMES AND WHOLE CELLS

R. L. Gregory,*† I. L. Shechmeister,† and S. Rosen‡

†Department of Microbiology
Southern Illinois University
Carbondale, Illinois 62901
and
‡College of Dentistry
Ohio State University
Columbus, Ohio 43210

Streptococcus mutans has been established as the most important causative agent of dental caries in humans by a number of investigators.[1] There are seven distinct cariogenic serotypes (a–g) of this organism. Although immunized animals are protected from caries,[2] recent studies demonstrated that rabbit antisera against antigens of *S. mutans* cell walls cross-reacted with human heart and muscle tissues *in vitro*,[3] mitigating the use of a vaccine from cell walls of this agent.

Ribosomal vaccines have been used successfully to protect experimental animals against many bacterial and fungal pathogens, including *Hemophilus influenzae, Mycobacterium tuberculosis, Salmonella typhimurium, Streptococcus pneumoniae, S. pyogenes, Pseudomonas aeruginosa,* and *Histoplasma capsulatum.* In addition, the *S. typhimurium, P. aeruginosa, S. pyogenes,* and *S. pneumoniae* ribosomal vaccines provided protection against challenge by strains or serotypes different from those used to obtain the ribosomal immunogens.[4]

In order to eliminate cell-wall antigens that may cross-react with human tissues, we prepared a ribosomal preparation from *S. mutans* 6715 (serotype g). This material stimulated a humoral and cell-mediated response in rabbits against 6715 ribosomes and cells, but not against human tissues.[5] We report here the immunogenicity of 6715 ribosomes in conventional and gnotobiotic rats. In addition, it was hoped that such a sample would stimulate antibodies with activities against many of the serotypes of *S. mutans* and therefore would eliminate the need for a polyvalent vaccine against dental caries.

Conventional Wistar and gnotobiotic Sprague-Dawley rats were immunized in the salivary gland region (SGR) with 6715 ribosomes and cells; salivas and sera were collected and the presence of antibodies against the immunogens were determined using either passive hemagglutination (PHA), microbial agglutination (MA) or an enzyme-linked immunosorbent assay (ELISA). Leukocytes were examined for cell-mediated responses using tritiated thymidine uptake in transformed lymphocytes (TL) and inhibition of migration (IM). Serum from rabbits injected intramuscularly in the hind legs with 6715 ribosomes were examined in a MA assay for cross-reactivity against various serotypes of *S. mutans.*

*Present address: Department of Microbiology, University of Alabama in Birmingham, Birmingham, Ala. 35294.

SUMMARY OF IMMUNE RESPONSES FROM CONVENTIONAL WISTAR AND GNOTOBIOTIC SPRAGUE-DAWLEY RATS

Type of Rat	Injected with:	Sample	PHA Titer Against 6715 Ribosomes	MA Titer Against 6715 Cells	Absorbance (405 nm) Values of ELISA Against 6715: Ribosomes	Cells	Transformation Index* of Leukocytes Treated with the Following Agents: 6715 Ribosomes	6715 Cells	Migration Index† of Leukocytes Treated with 6715 Ribosomes
Conventional Wistar	ribosomes and FCA	saliva	64	1	0.390 ($p < 0.01$)‡	0.205 ($p < 0.05$)	NA§	NA	NA
		serum	1,280	16	0.215 ($p < 0.05$)	0.167	NA	NA	NA
		leukocytes	NA	NA	NA	NA	5.9	0.3	0.71
	ribosomes and phosphate-buffered saline	saliva	4	0	0.215 ($p < 0.01$)	0.185 ($p < 0.10$;NS)	NA	NA	NA
		serum	2	1	0.152 ($p < 0.20$;NS)	0.315 ($p < 0.01$)	NA	NA	NA
		leukocytes	NA	NA	NA	NA	1.3	1.4	0.96
	cells and FCA	saliva	64	1	0.125 ($p < 0.01$)	0.383 ($p < 0.01$)	NA	NA	NA
		serum	2,560	32	0.221 ($p < 0.05$)	0.195 ($p < 0.05$)	NA	NA	NA
		leukocytes	NA	NA	NA	NA	0.7	0.6	1.02
Gnotobiotic Sprague-Dawley	ribosomes and FCA	saliva	80	8	ND¶	ND	NA	NA	NA
		serum	5,120	160	ND	ND	NA	NA	NA
	cells and FCA	saliva	32	16	ND	ND	NA	NA	NA
		serum	1,280	512	ND	ND	NA	NA	NA

*Transformation index >3.0 was considered significant.
†Migration index <0.80 was considered significant.
‡Statistical significance between titers of saliva or sera from immunized animals and normal rat saliva or serum using Student's *t*-test; NS = not significant.
§Not applicable.
¶Not determined.

TABLE 2

AGGLUTINATION OF VARIOUS *STREPTOCOCCUS MUTANS*
WITH ANTI- *S. MUTANS* 6715 RIBOSOME SERUM

Serotype	Strain	MA Titer
a	AHT	2,048
a	E-49	2,048
b	BHT	128
b	FA-1	64
c	V318	1,024
c	V310	512
c	GS-5	256
c	Ingbritt	128
c	10449	128
c	KPSK2	64
c	8S1	2,048
d	SL1	512
d	B13	256
d	O1	64
e	LM7	256
f	OMZ-175	2,048
g	KIR	512
g	6715	512

High PHA and MA titers and ELISA values against ribosomes and whole cells were obtained in both salivas and sera of animals immunized in the SGR with ribosomes mixed with Freund's complete adjuvant (FCA) (TABLE 1). Only high ELISA values against both ribosomes and whole cells, however, were found in salivas and sera from rats injected in the SGR with ribosomes alone. Animals vaccinated with 6715 ribosomes and FCA in the SGR developed TL and IM indices against the ribosomes that were significantly higher than control animals, but not against whole cells. Serum of rabbits injected with 6715 ribosomes cross-agglutinated representative strains of all seven serotypes of S. mutans. (TABLE 2). Preliminary data indicate that 6715 ribosomes protected gnotobiotic rats from dental caries, and the results of the present study suggest that such a preparation may also protect animals from lesions caused by any of the seven serotypes of this organism.

ACKNOWLEDGMENTS

We are grateful to Dr. S.M. Michalek, Department of Microbiology, University of Alabama in Birmingham, Birmingham, Ala., for providing the facilities for doing the protection studies.

REFERENCES

1. McGHEE, J. R. & S. M. MICHALEK. 1981. Ann. Rev. Microbiol. 35: 595–638.
2. BOWEN, W. H., B. COHEN, M. F. COLE & G. COLMAN. 1975. Br. Dent. J. 139: 45–58.
3. HUGES, M., S. MACHARDY, A. SHEPPARD & N. WOODS. 1980. Infect. Immun. 27: 576–588.
4. D'HINTERLAND, L. D. 1980. Arzneim. Forsch. 30: 122–125.
5. GREGORY, R. L. 1982. Ph.D. Dissertation. Southern Illinois University, Carbondale, Illinois.

GENERATION AND MIGRATION PATTERNS OF INTESTINAL T- AND B-LYMPHOCYTES IN RESPONSE TO LOCAL ANTIGEN

A. J. Husband, A. W. Cripps, and R. L. Clancy

Faculty of Medicine
The University of Newcastle
Newcastle NSW 2308, Australia

We investigated the way in which IgA B-cells and T-cells respond to mucosally presented antigen.

In our first experiment, rats bearing double Thiry-Vella loops were primed i.p. with ovalbumin and tetanus toxoid in oil adjuvant; 14 days later the thoracic duct was cannulated, the proximal loop immunized with ovalbumin in saline, and the distal loop immunized with tetanus toxoid in saline. IgA-specific antibody-containing cells were enumerated by immunofluorescence at various times after infusion of thoracic duct lymphocytes (TDL). In some rats tritiated thymidine was infused i.v. 18 hours after TDL injection.

Early after injection, equal numbers of anti-ovalbumin-containing cells (AOCC) were detected in both loops and were evenly distributed throughout the lamina propria. In the distal (tetanus toxoid) loop, AOCC retained their even distribution, but decreased in number and were absent by 18 hours. In the proximal (ovalbumin) loop AOCC continued to increase in numbers, and the increase was accounted for by accumulation around and below the crypt region. When sections from rats infused with tritiated thymidine were examined by combined immunofluorescence and autoradiography, at 40 hours after TDL injection, 16.2 ± 3.4% of AOCC were labeled.

These results demonstrated that (1) the initial appearance of IgA cells in the intestinal lamina propria occurs independently of antigen, (2) there is no special-ized site within the intestinal lamina propria for IgA-specific cells to enter the tissue, (3) in the immunized intestine, specific cells progressively accumulate around the crypt regions, and (4) a proportion of this specific accumulation can be accounted for by proliferation within the lamina propria.

In a second experiment, Wistar rats were immunized intraduodenally with DA rat spleen cells. Rats were killed at various times after immunization and T-lymphocytes were assayed for reactivity in mixed lymphocyte culture against mitomycin-treated spleen cells from rats of the DA inbred stain.

Secondary mixed lymphocyte culture reactivity of mesenteric lymph node (MLN) cells reached a peak at day 7 after immunization. At this time the response in peripheral lymph nodes (PLN) and spleen was much less than in MLN, and isolated gut lamina propria lymphocytes showed greater reactivity than PLN or spleen cells, but not as great as MLN.

These results indicate that the intestine is capable of mounting a mucosally generated T-lymphocyte response to mucosally presented alloantigens, and that these activated T-cells migrate to MLN and gut lamina propria to a greater extent than to PLN. In future experiments, we intend to determine whether T-cells follow the same migration pathway described for IgA cells (i.e. PP → MLN → thoracic duct → mucosal lamina propria), and whether the T-cells involved in induction of IgA responses behave in a similar manner to the T-cells responding here to alloantigens.

828

MURINE PEYER'S PATCH T-HELPER CELL CLONES THAT PREFERENTIALLY SUPPORT IgA RESPONSES*

Hiroshi Kiyono, Lisa M. Mosteller, John H. Eldridge, Suzanne M. Michalek, William J. Koopman, and Jerry R. McGhee

Departments of Microbiology, Pathology, and Medicine
Institute of Dental Research and Comprehensive Cancer Center
The University of Alabama in Birmingham
Birmingham, Alabama 35294

A major source of precursor cells for IgA responses are the gut-associated lymphoreticular tissues (GALT), commonly termed Peyer's patches (PP), that contain antigen-sensitive T- and B-cells and accessory cells.[1] Oral immunization with thymic dependent antigen, for example, sheep erythrocytes (SRBC), induces significant T-helper (T_h) cell activity in the Peyer's patches.[2] Furthermore, dissociated PP cell cultures from mice orally primed with SRBC support high IgA responses *in vitro*.[1]

The availability of methods for induction and continuous culture of antigen-specific T_h-cell clones has been a major recent advance and will facilitate our understanding of the cellular and molecular events involved in T-cell help for antibody responses. In the present study, we have adapted the method of Watson to directly isolate and grow T-cells from murine Peyer's patches.[3]

Dissociated and purified PP T-cells from mice primed with SRBC by gastric intubation were cultured in the presence of interleukin 2 or T-cell growth factor (TCGF), irradiated splenic feeder cells, and sheep erythrocytes. Wells exhibiting clone growth were subcloned by limiting dilution and expanded in macroculture plates.

Twenty-one clones have been characterized that exhibit helper activity for IgA responses to SRBC and have been designated PP T_h A clones. Two broad categories of T_h A clones have been maintained in continuous culture in the presence of T-cell growth factor and feeder cells. The first group supports IgM and largely IgA anti-SRBC plaque-forming cell (PFC) responses (e.g. IgM = 755 ± 40, IgG_1 = 0, IgG_2 = 0, IgA = 2263 ± 102), whereas the second group supports low IgM, IgG_1, IgG_2 and high IgA PFC responses (e.g. IgM : 241 ± 18, IgG_1 = 209 ± 11, IgG_2 = 164 ± 17, IgA = 1876 ± 71). Cloned T_h A cells are antigen specific and require full histocompatibility to promote *in vitro* IgA responses. All T_h A clones tested are Thy-1.2$^+$, Lyt-1$^+$, and Lyt-2$^-$, Ig$^-$, and I-A$^-$. Clones of T_h A cells bear Fc receptors for IgA and do not possess receptors for IgM and IgG isotypes.

In summary, T_h A clones have been successfully propagated in continuous culture for over seven months. Twenty-one clones have been characterized that preferentially, but not exclusively, support antigen-specific IgA responses. It should now be possible to determine at both the cellular and molecular level, the precise requirements for differentiation of precursor IgA B-cells into mature cells producing the IgA isotype.

*This work was supported by United States Public Health Service Grants DE 04217, CA 13148, and DE 02670.

REFERENCES

1. KIYONO, H., J. R. McGHEE, M. J. WANNEMUEHLER, M. V. FRANGAKIS, D. M. SPALDING, S. M. MICHALEK & W. J. KOOPMAN. 1982. *In vitro* immune response to a T cell-dependent antigen by cultures of disassociated murine Peyer's patch. Proc. Natl. Acad. Sci. USA. **79:** 596–600.
2. KIYONO, H., J. L. BABB, S. M. MICHALEK & J. R. McGHEE. 1980. Cellular basis for elevated IgA responses in C3H/HeJ mice. J. Immunol. **125:** 732–737.
3. WATSON, J. 1979. Continuous proliferation of murine antigen-specific helper T lymphocytes in culture. J. Exp. Med. **150:** 1510–1519.

THE INFLUENCE OF PREGNANCY AND LACTATION ON TRANSPORT OF POLYMERIC IgA ACROSS EPITHELIAL SURFACES

R. Kleinman, P. Harmatz, D. McClenathan, B. Bunnell,
K. J. Bloch, and W. A. Walker

Pediatric Gastrointestinal and Nutrition Unit
Clinical Immunology and Allergy Unit
Massachusetts General Hospital
Department of Pediatrics and Medicine
Harvard Medical School
Boston, Massachusetts 02114

IgA has been identified as the major immunoglobulin in tears, breast milk, bile, and other external secretions. Although transport of IgA from serum into bile has been confirmed in the experimental animal, the source of IgA in other external secretions remains controversial. The purpose of the present study is to determine whether serum IgA is transported into tears and breast milk, to compare the transport with serum IgA into bile, and to examine the effect of lactation on the transport of IgA into external secretions in the rat. IgA with anti-dinitrophenyl activity was prepared by ammonium sulphate precipitation of the ascites fluid from mice bearing MOPC-315 plasmacytoma. Animals that had been lactating for less than 48 hours or control female Sprague-Dawley rats were injected with two ml of the 50% ammonium sulphate fraction of the ascites fluid. Tears, bile, and breast milk were obtained from separate animals. Two hours after an intravenous injection of the ammonium sulphate fraction of MOPC-315 ascites, tears were collected under light ether anesthesia. Bile was obtained for three hours from a catheter placed in the common bile duct under light ether anesthesia, and breast milk was obtained 24 hours after injection of the MOPC-315 protein into lactating animals from the stomachs of the suckling infant rats. Gastric contents from these infant rats were diluted in phosphate buffered saline, homogenized, and defatted by centrifugation. The IgA in each secretion was identified by immunoprecipitation with rabbit anti-mouse coated polyacrylamide beads and [125I]dinitrophenylated[10] bovine serum albumin. In order to test the effect of the processing of these secretions, equal amounts of MOPC-315 protein were added to bile and breast milk prior to homogenization and defatting. No loss of immunoprecipitable activity occurred as a result of these procedures.

In two separate samples of 20 microliters of tears obtained from six different lactating animals, all of whom had received two ml of the MOPC-315 protein, 6 × 10^2 cpm precipitated from the tears. Nonlactating animals who had also received the MOPC-315 protein had less than 1×10^2 precipitable cpm in their tears. In the three-hour collection of bile from two lactating animals who had received two ml of the MOPC-315 protein, 12.2 × 10^7 cpm precipitated. In two nonlactating animals who had received the same amount of the MOPC-315 protein, less than 4×10^7 counts precipitated in the three-hour bile collection. In lactating animals who had received two ml of the MOPC-315 protein, the mean number of counts precipitated from the gastric contents of each litter of six different lactating animals was approximately 12 × 10^3 counts. Less than 4×10^2 counts were

831

precipitated from the milk of lactating animals who had received no MOPC-315 protein. (FIGURE 1)

In conclusion, these studies have demonstrated that serum-derived IgA can be detected in tears and breast milk, as well as in the biliary secretions of lactating animals. Furthermore, lactation appears to enhance the movement of serum-derived IgA into tears and bile. The rat extraocular lacrimal gland contains very few plasma cells. It would, therefore, appear that such IgA as is present in tears would most likely derive from serum; these studies have confirmed this phenom-

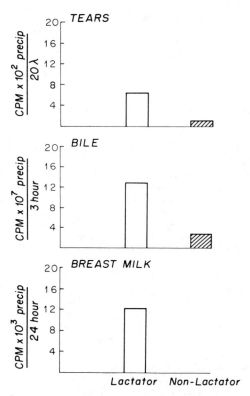

FIGURE 1. Transport of IgA across epithelial surfaces.

enon. The influence of lactation on IgA transport has not been previously reported. The mechanism of enhanced transport during lactation is not known, but may be related to an increase in epithelial-cell receptors for IgA. Secretory component is the putative membrane receptor for IgA. Others have demonstrated an increase in secretory component and IgA concentration in secretions of the rat uterus under estrogen stimulation. This enhanced transport of IgA into external secretions in lactating animals may contribute to the reduced serum levels of IgA seen in lactating animals.

CHARACTERISTICS OF IgA-SECRETING HYBRIDOMAS DERIVED FROM GUT-ASSOCIATED LYMPHOID TISSUE

Jack L. Komisar, Juliet A. Fuhrman, and John J. Cebra

University of Pennsylvania

Philadelphia, Pennsylvania 19104

The frequency of IgA-secreting hybridomas resulting from fusions in which spleen cells are used as a primed plasmablast source is very low. A high frequency of IgA-secreting hybridomas, however, may be obtained by using extensively primed gut-associated lymphoreticular tissues as fusion partners. The hybridomas so derived may secrete both monomeric and polymeric IgA. Some of the hybridoma cells have membrane IgA.

The methods used for producing and screening the monoclonal antibodies have been described.[1] Briefly, cell lines were generated that secreted antibodies that reacted with the phenol/water-extracted lipopolysaccharide (LPS) of *Salmonella typhimurium* and that of a slow lactose-fermenting strain of *Escherichia coli* (serotype 081:H21[2]) isolated from the gastrointestinal tract of a normal mouse.[3] These hybridomas were made by injecting a BALB/c mouse once intravenously with 10^7 heat-killed *E. coli* cells, and five times, over the course of four months, with 50 μg of *E. coli* trichloroacetic acid-extracted LPS intraperitoneally. A pool of Peyer's patch and mesenteric lymph node cells from this mouse was fused with Sp2/0-Ag14 cells. Culture supernatants were screened by radioimmunoassay.

Hybridomas secreting monoclonal antibodies to *Vibrio cholerae* toxoid were made by priming BALB/c mice intraduodenally with five μg of cholera toxin, waiting four months, and transferring Peyer's patch cells intravenously to a sublethally (500 rad) irradiated recipient. The recipient received 125 μg of cholera toxoid intraperitoneally at the time of cell transfer. The spleen was taken nine days later, and the cells were fused with Sp2/0-Ag14 cells. Culture supernatants were screened by antigen-specific radioimmunoassay.[4]

To determine the state of polymerization of the immunoglobulin, hybridoma culture supernatants were chromatographed on Ultrogel AcA 22 (LKB Instruments, Rockville, Md.) by the method of Kutteh et al.[5] Two of the anti-toxoid hybridomas had appreciable monomeric and polymeric IgA, whereas one, AC1.2, had mostly monomeric IgA. The 32G2 anti-LPS hybridoma had almost exclusively dimeric and higher molecular weight polymers of IgA.

IgA hybridomas 32B6 and 32E10 that we prepared, and two anti-phosphoryl-choline-producing hybridomas prepared by Julia Hurwitz, 3F2 (IgA) and 6A6 (IgG$_{2b}$), were tested for the presence of membrane immunoglobulin (mIg) by immunofluorescence. All but 32E10 had demonstrable mIg. Patching of mIg was seen under conditions (0–4° C) that do not allow B-cells to exhibit this phenomenon.

All hybridomas we have tested that are positive for membrane or cytoplasmic immunoglobulin are phenotypically heterogeneous, even shortly after recloning. Cytoplasmically staining cells are not always the same cells that show mIg.

We believe that hybridomas may be useful in studying the role of various cell-surface molecules that occur on subpopulations of normal cells that ordinarily are present in low frequencies, such as the IgA-bearing B-cell or plasmablast.

TABLE 1

IgA-Secreting Hybridomas Mentioned in This Paper

Hybridoma	Antigenic Specificity	Predominant Forms of Immunoglobulin	Membrane Staining
AC1.1	cholera toxoid	monomer	NT*
AC11	cholera toxoid	monomer and dimer	NT
BC10	cholera toxoid	monomer and dimer	NT
32G2	lipopolysaccharide	dimer and polymer	positive
32E10	lipopolysaccharide	NT	negative
32B6	lipopolysaccharide	NT	positive
3F2†	phosphorylcholine	polymer	positive

*NT = Not tested
†Hybridoma made by Julia Hurwitz

REFERENCES

1. KOMISAR, J. L., J. A. FUHRMAN & J. J. CEBRA. 1982. J. Immunol. **128:** 2376–2378.
2. ØRSKOV, I. & F. ØRSKOV. 1981. Personal communication.
3. SCHAEDLER, R. W., R. DUBOS & R. COSTELLO. 1965. J. Exp. Med. **122:** 59–66.
4. FUHRMAN, J. A. & J. J. CEBRA. 1981. J. Exp. Med. **153:** 534–544.
5. KUTTEH, W. H., S. J. PRINCE, J. O. PHILLIPS, J. G. SPENNEY & J. MESTECKY. 1982. Gastroenterology **82:** 184–193.

I-A DISTRIBUTION ON MURINE PEYER'S PATCH AND SPLENIC LYMPHOCYTES*

Yun Lee, John H. Eldridge, Hiroshi Kiyono, and
Jerry R. McGhee

*Departments of Microbiology and Pathology
Institute of Dental Research
Comprehensive Cancer Center
The University of Alabama in Birmingham
Birmingham, Alabama 35294*

Gut-associated lymphoreticular tissue (GALT), for example, Peyer's patches (PP), represents a major inductive site for IgA responses to orally encountered antigens. This tissue contains sufficient numbers of accessory cells and T- and B-lymphocytes for *in vitro* responses to thymic-dependent antigens.[1] It remains unclear at present why local immune responses do not occur in GALT. One suggestion has been that PP cells lack proper expression of Ia antigens. In this regard, Krco et al.[2] have suggested that murine PP B-cells express Ia antigen and that a subpopulation of T-cells also expresses these H-2 I region determinants. Because our laboratory has recently developed an enzyme (Dispase) procedure for the release of the total PP cell population, we have undertaken studies with fluorochrome-conjugated monoclonal anti-I-A^k antibody (hybridoma 10-5.2) to determine the presence of I-A antigen on T- and B-lymphocytes from murine Peyer's patches. Peyer's patches from either C3H/HeN or C3H/HeJ mice were dissociated to single cells with Dispase, and the lymphocyte population was enriched to >96% on Ficoll-Hypaque gradients.

When this PP lymphocyte population was assessed for I-A^k, approximately 53% of cells were I-A$^+$. Spleen lymphocyte populations from C3H/HeN or C3H/HeJ mice prepared on Ficoll-Hypaque exhibited approximately 51% I-A$^+$ cells, whereas control BALB/c (H-2^d) splenic or PP lymphocytes were negative. Double-labeling experiments that used fluorescein isothiocyanate (FITC)anti-I-A^k and tetramethylrhodamine (TRITC)anti-immunoglobulin (Ig; K + λ) reagents identified 99% of PP and 96% of spleen Ig$^+$ cells (B-cells) as positive for surface I-A^k (TABLE 1). Additional double stainings with TRITC-anti-I-A^k and monoclonal FITC-anti-Thy-1.2 indicated that <1% of splenic and PP T-cells bear I-A^k antigen. Fractionation of C3H/HeN PP lymphocytes into enriched T- and B-cell populations using nylon wool columns followed by antibody plus complement-mediated specific cytolysis and examination of I-A^k labeling on the fluorescence-activated cell-sorter (FACS) confirmed the double-labeling results.

In further experiments, both splenic and PP B-cell populations were enriched by passage through glass and nylon wool columns followed by treatment with anti-Thy-1.2 and rabbit C. These B-cells were subsequently stained with anti-I-A^k and subjected to FACS analysis. The intensity of staining for I-A^k on PP B-cells was significantly greater than that seen with splenic B-cells (FIGURE 1). Both mechanically dissociated (nonenzyme treated) PP and enzyme-treated splenic lymphocytes were examined, and no alteration of fluorescence intensity due to

*This work was supported by United States Public Health Service Grants DE 04217, CA 13148, and DE 02670.

TABLE 1

DOUBLE-LABELING OF C3H/HeN LYMPHOCYTES FOR I-A^k IN CONJUNCTION WITH IG($\kappa + \lambda$)
AND Thy-1.2

Cell Source	Percent of Total Cells with the Surface Phenotype*			
	I-A^{k+}Ig$^+$	I-A^{k+}Ig$^-$	I-A^{K-}Ig$^+$	I-A^{k-}Ig$^-$
Spleen†	50 ± 3 (96)‡	1 ± 1	2 ± 1	47 ± 2
Peyer's patches§	52 ± 5 (>99)	1 ± 1	<1	47 ± 6
	I-A^{k+}Thy-1.2$^+$	I-A^{k+}Thy-1.2$^-$	I-A^{k-}Thy-1.2$^+$	I-A^{k+}Thy-1.2$^-$
Spleen	1 ± 1	58 ± 14	23 ± 12	18 ± 3
Peyer's patches	1 ± 1	52 ± 5	34 ± 7	13 ± 3

*Results presented as the mean ± SD of three experiments.
†Ficoll-Hypaque prepared, >98% lymphocytes by Wright-Giemsa Staining.
‡Percent of total Ig$^+$ cells also I-A^{k+}.
§Dispase and Ficoll-Hypaque prepared, >96% lymphocytes by Wright-Giemsa staining.

enzyme exposure was observed with cells from either source. Gaiting the FACS to exclude the small proportion of higher light scattering cells did not significantly alter either the percentage or mean fluorescence intensity of any of the cell populations examined. Together with the fact that the average surface areas of the splenic and PP B-cells are essentially identical, as determined by light scattering, these data indicate that C3H PP B-cells bear a significantly higher density of surface I-A than their splenic B-cells.

In summary, our results clearly demonstrate that PP lymphocytes bear H-2 I-A subregion encoded antigen. The vast majority of I-A bearing lymphocytes are B-cells, and only a small number of I-A$^+$ T-cells are present. Furthermore, the PP

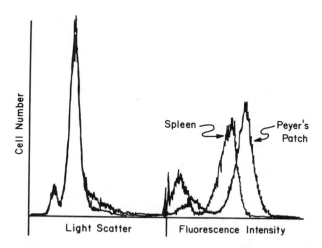

FIGURE 1. Enriched C3H/HeN B-cell populations were prepared from Ficoll-Hypaque passaged spleen and Dispase plus Ficoll-Hypaque passaged Peyer's patch cells by fractionation on nylon wool followed by treatment with anti-Thy-1.2 + C.
Spleen B-cell population: 79% Ig$^+$, 76% I-A^{k+}, and <3% Thy-1.2$^+$
Peyer's Patch B-cell population: 81% Ig$^+$, 82% I-A^{k+}, and <2% Thy-1.2$^+$

B-cell population possesses more detectable cell-surface I-A molecules than are observed on splenic B-cells, and this higher level of I-A expression is neither the result of the enzymatic isolation procedure nor a larger surface area of the PP B-cells.

REFERENCES

1. KIYONO, H., J. R. MCGHEE, M. J. WANNEMUEHLER, M. V. FRANGAKIS, D. M. SPALDING, S. M. MICHALEK & W. J. KOOPMAN. 1982. *In vitro* immune responses to a T cell-dependent antigen by cultures of disassociated murine Peyer's patch. Proc. Natl. Acad. Sci. USA **79:** 596–600.
2. KRCO, C. J., S. J. CHALLACOMBE, P. LAFUSE, C. S. DAVID & T. B. TOMASI, JR. 1981. Expression of Ia antigens by mouse Peyer's patch cells. Cell. Immunol. **57:** 420–426.

HEPATIC UPTAKE AND TRANSFER INTO BILE OF POLYMERIC IgA, ANTI-SECRETORY COMPONENT IgG, HAPTOGLOBIN-HEMOGLOBIN COMPLEX, GALACTOSYLATED SERUM ALBUMIN, AND HORSERADISH PEROXIDASE: A COMPARATIVE BIOCHEMICAL STUDY IN THE RAT

J. N. Limet, J. Quintart, P. J. Courtoy, J. P. Vaerman,
and Y.-J. Schneider

International Institute of Cellular and Molecular Pathology
Brussels, Belgium

The clearance and disposal by rat hepatocytes of polymeric IgA (pIgA), haptoglobin-hemoglobin (HpHb), and galactosylated serum albumin (galSA) were studied. Anti-secretory component (SC) IgG was included because it presumably follows the pIgA pathway.[2] These four ligands were compared to horseradish peroxidase (HRP), a tracer of fluid-phase endocytosis.

Within three hours after i.v. injection, 60% of pIgA and 14% of anti-SC IgG but much smaller amounts of HpHb, galSA, or HRP were transferred into bile (FIGURE 1). Secreted material was analyzed by isokinetic centrifugation. Polymeric IgA was transferred as secretory IgA. Anti-SC IgG was secreted as lower (40%) or higher (60%) molecular weight material, with respect to native IgG. The smaller component is compatible with SC-associated Fab fragments; the larger probably represents immune complexes (FIGURE 2).

At different times after i.v. injection, livers were perfused and homogenized. The particulate fractions contained 45 to 90% of liver-associated label and were further analyzed by isopyknic centrifugation in sucrose gradients. After five minutes, all four ligands were found in structures equilibrating at a density of 1.13 g/ml that were distinct from galactosyltransferase (Golgi), 5'nucleotidase (plasma membrane), and cathepsin B (lysosomes). HRP was associated with 5'nucleotidase (FIGURE 3A). Within 20 minutes, HRP had shifted to a lysosomal distribution; this shift occurred more slowly (within 45 minutes) for galSA and HpHb. By contrast, minor proportions of liver-associated pIgA or anti-SC IgG were found at densities higher than 1.13 g/ml, first at the same density as 5'nucleotidase (20 minutes, FIGURE 3B) and later on, as cathepsin B (45 minutes, FIGURE 3C). At this time, the integrity of anti-SC IgG in the 1.13 g/ml and 1.20 g/ml fractions was checked by isokinetic centrifugation. In the 1.13 g/ml fraction, no degradation product could be detected, even after prolonged incubation at neutral or acidic pH. The 1.20 g/ml fraction contained mostly degradation products.

In conclusion, the pathways of receptor-mediated endocytosis (explored by the four ligands) and fluid-phase endocytosis (traced with HRP) are different. Upon isopyknic centrifugation of liver particulate fractions, receptor-bound ligands initially coequilibrate at a low density in structures that could be specialized in their collection and transport. These structures can be precisely demonstrated by electron microscopy.[1,3] Where and how pIgA, or anti-SC IgG (mostly transferred into bile) are sorted from the other ligands (eventually digested in lysosomes) remains to be elucidated. Our finding of the molecular

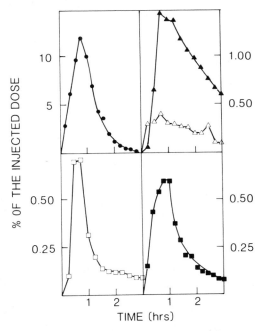

FIGURE 1. Transfer into bile of pIgA (●), anti-SC IgG (▲), rat IgG (Δ), galSA (□) and HpHb (■). Notice the differences in scale. Kinetics are similar.

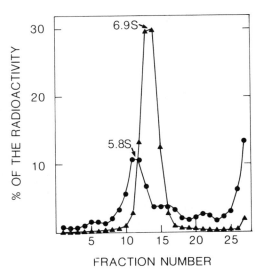

FIGURE 2. Size distribution of native anti-SC IgG (▲) and anti-SC-associated radioactivity after transfer into bile (●).

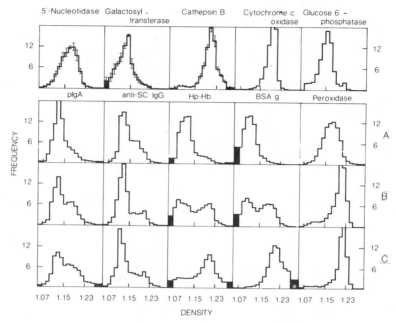

FIGURE 3. Distribution upon isopyknic centrifugation of liver particulate fractions, respectively 5 (A), 20 (B), and 45 minutes (C) after i.v. injection. Top panel: marker enzymes.

trimming of at least some anti-SC antibodies found in bile, which could not occur in the light density structures, points to some involvement of the lysosomes in the SC-mediated pIgA pathway.

REFERENCES

1. Courtoy, P. J., J. N. Limet, J. Quintart, J.-P. Vaerman, Y.-J. Schneider & P. Baudhuin. 1983. Ann. N.Y. Acad. Sci. This issue.
2. Lemaître-Coelho, I., R. Meykens & J.-P. Vaerman. 1982. Protides Biol. Fluids Proc. Colloq. **29:** 419–422.
3. Wall, D. A., G. Wilson & A. L. Hubbard. 1980. Cell **21:** 79–93.

PREVENTION AND TREATMENT OF GASTROINTESTINAL INFECTIONS IN INFANTS BY USING IMMUNOBIOLOGICAL METHODS

R. Lodinová, B. Korych, Z. Bartáková, and H. Braná

Institute for the Care of Mother and Child, Prague

Institute of Medical Microbiology and Immunology
Charles University, Prague

Resident Nursery, Plzeň

Czechoslovakia Academy of Sciences
Prague, Czechoslovakia

Gastrointestinal infections represent a serious problem, especially in mature and premature newborn infants deprived of breast-feeding. Colonization of the intestine using a live nonenteropathogenic *Escherichia coli* strain 083 applied orally, induced a serum and local antibody response in mature as well as premature infants.[1] Strain 083 represents a classical type of *E.coli*; its antigenic and pathogenic properties have been verified in newborn germfree piglets.[2] The strain does not produce enterotoxins and does not possess any K antigens (as determined by the WHO Reference Center in Copenhagen). *E.coli* 083 carries no plasmid, and the frequency of a transferable R plasmid from an effective donor into this strain is 100 times lower using a standard conjugation method, in comparison with strain *E.coli* 600.

The unusual ability of *E.coli* 083 to colonize and predominate in the intestine for several months has been used as a preventive measure against enteric infections. Strain 083 prevented colonization of the gut with microbial pathogens and displaced the ones present (FIGURE 1). Treatment of gastrointestinal infections by oral administration of an inactivated mixture of six selected enteropathogenic *E.coli* strains[3] was highly effective in mature and premature infants during the first three months of life. It significantly reduced the need for treatment with oral antibiotics, decreased the number of carriers, and induced a specific local antibody response in the intestine (TABLE 1).

Oral administration of partly purified colostral antibodies prepared after immunization of cows with six enteropathogenic *E.coli* strains[4] was also very effective for treatment of gastrointestinal infections in mature and premature newborns (TABLE 2).

These immunobiologic methods used for prevention and treatment of gastrointestinal infections in infants are safe and effective, reducing the need for antibiotics. Oral colonization with live *E.coli* strain 083 and administration of an inactivated polyvalent vaccine induces complex immune reactions in the intestine that cannot be completely explained at present.

841

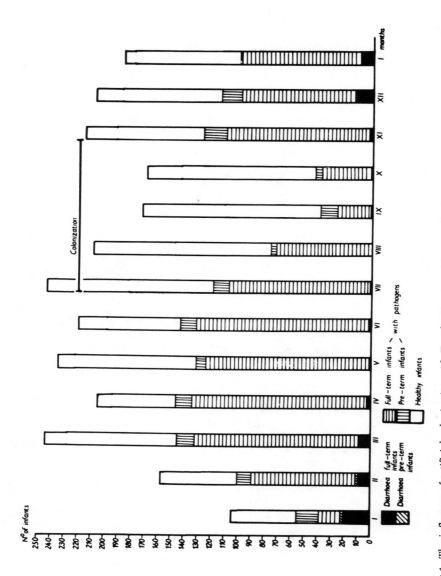

FIGURE 1. The influence of artificial colonization with *E. coli* 083 on gastrointestinal infections and on the presence of bacterial pathogens in stools of newborn infants.

TABLE 1

THE COURSE OF ILLNESS IN INFANTS WITH GASTROINTESTINAL INFECTIONS AFTER ORAL ADMINISTRATION OF AN INACTIVATED MIXTURE OF ENTEROPATHOGENIC *E. COLI* STRAINS, COMPARED WITH INFANTS TREATED WITH ANTIBIOTICS, DURING SIX DAYS OF TREATMENT

Day	Time of Recovery							Total	Total Number of Infants
	1	2	3	4	5	6	Longer		
Premature infants treated with the vaccine	—	4	21	6	11	4	—	46	60
	—	6.6	35	10	18.3	6.6	—	Percent of cured infants	
	—	6.6	41.6	51.6	69.7	76.5	—	Ratio percent/day	
Premature infants treated with antibiotics	—	—	3	7	11	3	7	24	31
	—	—	9.6	22.5	35.5	9.6	22.5	Percent of cured infants	
	—	—	9.6	32.1	67.6	77.2	99.7	Ratio percent/day	
Mature infants treated with the vaccine	—	—	5	5	5	—	1	15	21
	—	—	23.8	23.8	23.8	23.8	4.7	Percent of cured infants	
	—	—	23.8	47.6	71.4	71.4	76.1	Ratio percent/day	
Mature infants treated with antibiotics	—	—	—	1	5	3	1	9	10
	—	—	—	10	50	30	10	Percent of cured infants	
	—	—	—	10	60	90	100	Ratio percent/day	

TABLE 2

THE COURSE OF ILLNESS IN INFANTS WITH GASTROINTESTINAL INFECTIONS AFTER ORAL ADMINISTRATION OF IMMUNE COLOSTRUM AS COMPARED WITH INFANTS TREATED WITH ANTIBIOTICS DURING FIVE DAYS OF TREATMENT

Day	Time of Recovery						Total	Total Number of Infants
	1	2	3	4	5	Longer		
Premature infants treated with colostrum	—	2	13	8	2	1	26	33
	—	6.0	39.3	24.2	6.0	3.0	Percent of cured infants	
	—	6.0	45.3	69.5	75.5	78.5	Ratio percent/day	
Premature infants treated with antibiotics	—	—	3	—	5	6	14	14
	—	—	21.4	—	35.7	42.8	Percent of cured infants	
	—	—	21.4	21.4	57.1	99.9	Ratio percent/day	
Mature infants treated with colostrum	—	2	6	2	10	—	20	24
	—	8.3	25	8.3	41.6	—	Percent of cured infants	
	—	8.3	33.3	41.6	83.2	—	Ratio percent/day	
Mature infants treated with antibiotics	—	—	1	2	5	7	15	15
	—	—	6.6	13.3	33.3	46.6	Percent of cured infants	
	—	—	6.6	19.9	53.2	99.8	Ratio percent/day	

REFERENCES

1. LODINOVÁ, R., V. JOUJA & V. WÁGNER. 1973. Pediatr. Res. **7:** 659–669.
2. TLASKALOVÁ, H., J. ŠTERZL, P. HÁJEK, M. POSPÍŠIL, I. ŘÍHA, H. MARVANOVÁ V. KAMARÝTOVÁ, L. MANDEL, J. KRUML & F. KOVÁŘŮ. 1970. *In* Developmental Aspects of Antibody Formation and Structure. J. Šterzl, I. Říha, Eds.:767. Academia Prague.
3. KORYCH, B., R. LODINOVÁ. 1980. Proc. Symp. Microbiol. Soc. Czech. 29.
4. KORYCH, B., B. PROKEŠOVÁ, R. LODINOVÁ. 1982. Ed. Biol. Soc. Czech. Acad. Sci. Prague. Proc. Third Congress Czech. Immunol. Soc. Czechoslovakia. 156.

EFFECTS OF SEX DIFFERENCES AND GONADAL HORMONE ALTERATIONS ON THE ACCUMULATION OF MESENTERIC LYMPHOBLASTS IN THE SMALL INTESTINE*

S. Mirski, A. D. Befus, and J. Bienenstock

Host Resistance Program
Department of Pathology
McMaster University
Hamilton, Ontario, Canada L8N 3Z5

Local immunity at mucosal surfaces is integrated by cell migration in a common mucosal immune system.[1] A complete understanding of the mechanisms that control this selective mucosal localization would be invaluable when attempting to stimulate local immunity.

The immune system is profoundly influenced by gender differences and gonadal steroids. Sex hormones influence the accumulation of lymphoblasts in sex hormone target tissues[2,3] and the secretion of IgA, IgG, and secretory component in the uterus.[4,5] Gender and gonadal steroids affect the morphology of high endothelial post-capillary venules in lymph nodes.[6] These factors are thus implicated in the modulation of lymphocyte circulation. We have, therefore, examined sex differences in the accumulation of mesenteric lymph node (MLN)-derived lymphoblasts in the small intestine 24 hours after adoptive transfer in CBA/J mice.

We have detected a sex-related difference in the number of MLN lymphoblasts localized in the small intestine after adoptive transfer. Autoradiography revealed a twofold greater accumulation of lymphoblasts from male donors than from female donors (FIGURE 1). The sex of the recipient had no effect on MLN-lymphoblast localization in the small intestine. Because autoradiography is a very laborious method of assessing lymphoblast localization, we attempted to study this phenomenon using [^{125}I]iododeoxyuridine-labeled MLN lymphoblasts and gamma counting. Radiocounting did not reveal any difference in the localization patterns of lymphoblasts from male or female donors. Autoradiography of the same tissues again demonstrated, however, a twofold greater accumulation of male than female lymphoblasts in the small intestine. Because gonadal hormones might cause the gender differences in localization, we performed adoptive transfers using gonadectomized donors. Neither oophorectomy nor orchidectomy of MLN lymphoblast donors had any effect on localization compared to sex-matched sham gonadectomized donors.

The observation that the gender of the lymphoblast donor, but not the recipient, is important in influencing localization to the small intestine is consistent with results from studies of other factors. In transfer experiments using MLN lymphoblasts from vitamin A and protein-calorie deficient rats[7] and different age groups of mice (Mirski, Befus, and Bienenstock, unpublished), the condition of the lymphoblast donor rather than the recipient was of primary importance in modulating lymphoblast localization.

*This work was supported by the Medical Research Council of Canada.

The mechanisms by which the sex difference in the donor lymphoblast population might result in greater accumulation of male cells in the small intestine include differential trapping of cells in other tissues, better selective entry or selective retention of cells in mucosae, and greater proliferation of cells after transfer. Certainly recent work by Husband[8] and ourselves (McDermott and Bienenstock, unpublished) suggests that the number of lymphoblasts with lamina propria of the small intestine is augmented by division after transfer. The observation of a greater localization of male than female MLN lymphoblasts in the small intestine using autoradiography, but not radiocounting of the same

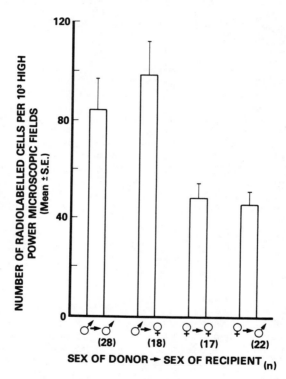

FIGURE 1. The effect of the sex of the donor and the recipient on the number of [³H]thymidine or [¹²⁵I]iododeoxyuridine-labeled mesenteric lymph node-derived lymphoblasts that localize in the small intestine 24 hours after adoptive transfer.

tissues, might be explained if there was more division in the male lymphoblast population after transfer, resulting in more labeled cells in the small intestine without an increase in radioactivity.

Although neither oophorectomy nor orchidectomy of lymphoblast donors had any effect on localization, this situation did not preclude the sex difference in localization being due to hormonal influences; their effect may be more complex than these experiments were designed to reveal. We plan to investigate further the influence of sex steroids on lymphoblast localization by using gonadectomy and treatment with gonadal steroids of the opposite sex, and by altering the hormonal environment before puberty, because there may be permanent changes in the immune system that become manifest upon sexual maturation.

REFERENCES

1. BIENENSTOCK, J. & A. D. BEFUS. 1980. Immunology **41:** 249–270.
2. McDERMOTT, M. R., D. A. CLARK & J. BIENENSTOCK. 1980. J. Immunol. **124:** 2536–2539.
3. WEISZ-CARRINGTON, P., M. E. ROUX, M. McWILLIAMS, J. M. PHILLIPS-QUAGLIATA & M. E. LAMM. 1978. Proc. Natl. Acad. Sci. USA **75:** 2928–2932.
4. SULLIVAN, D. A. & C. R. WIRA. 1981. J. Steroid Biochem. **15:** 439–444.
5. WIRA, C. R. & C. P. SANDOE. 1980. Endocrinology **106:** 1020–1026.
6. KITTAS, C. & L. HENRY. 1980. J. Pathol. **132:** 121–131.
7. McDERMOTT, M. R., D. A. MARK, A. D. BEFUS, B. S. BALIGA, R. M. SUSKIND & J. BIENENSTOCK. 1982. Immunology **45:** 1–5.
8. HUSBAND, A. J. 1982. J. Immunol. **128:** 1355–1359.

ANTIBACTERIAL PROPERTIES OF MILK:
IgA-PEROXIDASE-LACTOFERRIN INTERACTIONS

Zina Moldoveanu, Jorma Tenovuo, Kenneth M. Pruitt,
Britta Mansson-Rahemtulla, and Jiri Mestecky

Department of Microbiology
Department of Biochemistry
University of Alabama in Birmingham
Birmingham, Alabama 35294

Mammalian exocrine secretions contain peroxidase enzymes that catalyze the oxidation of naturally occurring components to generate antibacterial products.[1,2] The oxidizing power is provided by hydrogen peroxide (derived from leukocytes and peroxidogenic, commensal bacteria). Halides and thiocyanate (SCN^-, derived from diet) are utilized as electron donors. In bovine milk and in human saliva, the peroxidase enzymes are similar in structure and catalytic properties and are secreted from acinar cells.[3] The peroxidase in human milk, however, is similar in chromatographic behavior to myeloperoxidase derived from human leukocytes.[4] Human salivary peroxidase reacts with antibodies directed against bovine lactoperoxidase, but these same antibody preparations gave no detectable reaction with the peroxidase in human colostrum.[4]

We found that human colostral peroxidase could use Cl^- as well as SCN^- as electron donors. We conclude that the peroxidase in human milk is derived from milk leukocytes and is similar to myeloperoxidase in structure and catalytic behavior. Because the $Cl^- : SCN^-$ molar ratio in human milk is greater than 100, antibacterial properties of human milk under physiological conditions may be due to, in part, oxidized forms of Cl^-.

Other components of milk and saliva may interact with the peroxidase system and modify its antibacterial effects. Peroxidase was shown by chromatographic and immunodiffusion experiments to bind immunoglobulins and other secretory proteins (FIGURE 1). The binding was nonspecific, but did have a stabilizing effect on the enzyme. Peroxidase system inhibition of glucose-stimulated acid production by *Streptococcus mutans* NCTC 10449 (serotype *c*) was enhanced when the system was combined with sIgA or lactoferrin (FIGURE 2). The enhancement was not dependent on specific antibodies to *S. mutans* in the preparations of IgA or of lactoferrin (tested by agglutination assays), or on the stabilizing effect of binding between peroxidase and these proteins. Lactoferrin did not form complexes with lactoperoxidase. The direct antibacterial effects were due to the oxidation products of the peroxidase system, because these effects could be reversed in every case by addition of excess reducing agent (mercaptoethanol). Our results suggest that various factors in milk may interact synergistically to produce enhanced antibacterial effects.

REFERENCES

1. MORRISON, M. & G. R. SCHONBAUM. 1976. Ann. Rev. Biochem. **45:** 861–888.
2. THOMAS, E. L. 1981. Biochemistry **20:** 3273–3280.

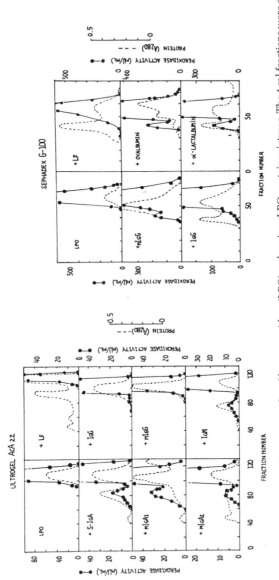

FIGURE 1. Molecular permeation chromatography of lactoperoxidase (LPO) and various LPO-protein mixtures. The 1 ml fractions were assayed for peroxidase activity,[5] protein concentration (A_280), and immunoglobulin or other protein content (single radial immunodiffusion).

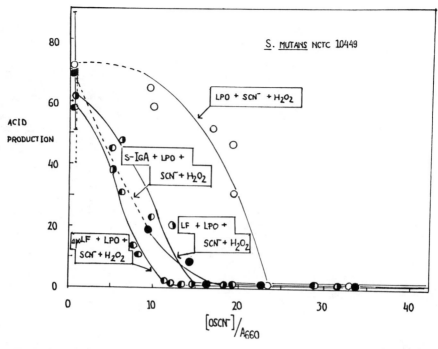

FIGURE 2. Rate of glucose-stimulated acid production by *Streptococcus mutans* NCTC 10449 exposed to various concentrations of hypothiocyanate (OSCN⁻). Quantity of bacteria was estimated by absorbance measurement (A_{660}). Acid production was measured by recording quantity of standard base added by pH *stat.* in order to maintain pH = 6.5. Acid production units are nmoles/*min.* divided by volume (ml) of bacterial suspension and by A_{660}. Units of OSCN⁻/A_{660} are μM.

3. MORRISON, M., P. Z. ALLEN, J. BRIGHT & W. JAYASINGHE. 1965. Arch. Biochem. Biophys. **111:** 126–133.
4. MOLDOVEANU, Z., J. TENOVUO, J. MESTECKY & K. M. PRUITT. 1982. Biochim. Biophys. Acta **718:** 103–108.
5. SHINDLER, J. S., R. E. CHILDS & W. G. BARDSLEY. 1976. Eur. J. Biochem. **65:** 793–800.

AUGMENTATION OF IgA RESPONSES AND CARIES IMMUNITY BY ORAL ADJUVANTS*

Ichijiro Morisaki, Mitsuo Torii, Shigeyuki Hamada,†
Jerry R. McGhee, and Suzanne M. Michalek

Department of Microbiology
Institute of Dental Research
The University of Alabama in Birmingham
Birmingham, Alabama 35294

Previous studies on caries immunity in experimental animals have employed various immunization regimens with either whole bacteria, purified cell walls, or in some cases purified antigen, and major routes have included either local or oral administration of antigen. Studies of local immunization have included use of adjuvant to potentiate immune responses.[1] Local injection of killed *Streptococcus mutans* (the principal etiologic agent of dental caries) whole cells in complete Freund's adjuvant (CFA) into the salivary gland region of rats induces a local salivary antibody response and caries immunity. In these and in similar studies,[1] the presence of secretory IgA (sIgA) antibodies in saliva correlated with caries reductions. Although promising, these studies using local injection of antigen in adjuvant, such as CFA, are not suitable for human use because of the adverse side effects of local inflammation.

Numerous recent studies[1] have indicated that stimulation of gut-associated lymphoreticular tissue (GALT), for example, Peyer's patches (PP), with antigen results in sensitized lymphoid cells capable of populating distant mucosal tissues, including salivary glands. Final differentiation of antigen-sensitized precursor IgA B-cells into plasma cells secreting antibody with specificity to the ingested antigen takes place in mucosal tissues. This method of induction of secretory immune responses offers the most practical approach for eliciting protective salivary IgA antibodies to *S. mutans*.

In the present study, we have evaluated the effectiveness of orally administered particulate and soluble forms of *S. mutans* antigens to induce salivary IgA-immune responses and the ability of oral adjuvants to potentiate this response. Germfree Fischer rats were given *S. mutans* whole cells (WC), purified cell walls (CW), or cell wall lysate (CWL) alone or with the adjuvants muramyl dipeptide (MDP), *S. mutans* peptidoglycan (PG), or liposomes by gastric intubation. Saliva and serum samples were collected from individual rats and assessed for antibody levels, isotype, and specificity by enzyme-linked immunosorbent assay (ELISA). Salivary IgA and IgG antibody responses were assessed, whereas IgM, IgG, and IgA levels were determined in serum. Finally rat molars were scored for levels of caries.

Particulate *S. mutans* antigen forms (WC and CW) were more effective than soluble antigen (CWL) in inducing salivary IgA-antibody responses. The presence of salivary IgA antibodies correlated with protection against *S. mutans*-induced

*This work was supported by United States Public Health Service Contract DE 02426. Suzanne M. Michalek is the recipient of Research Career Development Award DE 00092.

†Present address: Department of Dental Research, National Institute of Health, 2-10-35, Kamiosaki, Shinagawa-ku, Tokyo, 141, Japan.

dental caries. Gastric intubation of the adjuvants MDP, PG, or liposome with
S. mutans WC or CW resulted in a significant potentiation of the salivary IgA
response and greater caries protection than was obtained in animals given
antigen alone.

When individual specificities of sIgA in saliva were determined to individual
CW components, most antibody was directed to serotype carbohydrate and
glucan. Significant sIgA antibody levels to lipoteichoic acid were also seen. Caries
protection correlated directly with sIgA antibody levels to carbohydrate antigens.

In summary, particulate antigens including both WC and purified CW of
S. mutans induce good salivary immune responses, especially sIgA responses,
when given by gastric intubation to gnotobiotic rats. Further, these responses are
potentiated, following gastric intubation of the adjuvants MDP, PG, or liposomes,
with antigen. Finally, the presence of sIgA antibodies to carbohydrate antigens
correlated with caries protection.

REFERENCE

1. McGHEE, J. R. & S. M. MICHALEK. 1981. Immunobiology of dental caries: Microbial
   aspects and local immunity. Annu. Rev. Microbiol. 35: 595–638.

EVIDENCE THAT TOLERANCE OF CELL-MEDIATED IMMUNITY IN MICE FED OVALBUMIN IS DUE TO SUPPRESSOR CELLS ACTIVATED BY INTESTINALLY DERIVED PROTEIN MOIETIES

A. McI. Mowat,* S. Strobel, M. G. Pickering,
H. E. Drummond, and A. Ferguson

Gastrointestinal Unit
Western General Hospital and University of Edinburgh
Edinburgh, Scotland

There is increasing evidence that T-suppressor cells (T_s) are associated with the tolerance of cell-mediated immunity that is found in mice fed ovalbumin (OVA). Cyclophosphamide (CY) inhibits T_s in mice, and in earlier work, we found that CY pretreatment allowed active cell-mediated immunity to develop in the small intestine of mice fed OVA. In the present study, we examined the role of T_s in oral tolerance by investigating whether CY would also inhibit the induction of systemic tolerance after a feed of OVA. We also tested the hypothesis that serum factors are involved in the activation of T_s in OVA-fed mice.

BALB/c mice were fed 2 or 25 mg of OVA and immunized 14 days later with OVA in Freund's complete adjuvant. Systemic delayed-type hypersensitivity (DTH) was assessed 21 days after immunization by intradermal footpad test. One group of mice received 100 mg/kg of CY two days before a feed of OVA. Systemic DTH was significantly reduced in mice fed both 2 and 25 mg of OVA, with 88% and 64% suppression of control values, respectively. In mice fed 25 mg of OVA and pretreated with CY, DTH responses were midway between those of control and tolerant mice and were not significantly different from either group. By contrast, CY pretreatment of mice fed 2 mg of OVA restored their DTH response to control levels. Parallel studies of the hemagglutinating antibody response showed excellent tolerance after a feed of 25 mg of OVA (93% suppression) and partial abrogation by CY. A feed of 2 mg of OVA had no significant effect on systemic antibody responses. These results indicated that systemic DTH was readily suppressed by even low doses of fed OVA and that this state of tolerance was abrogated by CY.

Next, we investigated protein molecules present in the serum after a feed of OVA to determine if they were responsible for the suppressed DTH; we also tried to determine if these factors acted by inducing suppressor cells. Furthermore, these studies were based on the ability of CY to inhibit T_s. Because CY also damages the small intestine, it is possible that its effect on immunity to fed OVA could reflect altered uptake of OVA by the CY-treated intestine. We therefore studied the effect of CY on the presence of immunogenic OVA in the serum of OVA-fed mice.

Mice were fed 25 mg of OVA or H_2O and bled one hour later; 0.8 ml serum was transferred i.p. to syngeneic recipients that were immunized one week later with OVA in Freund's complete adjuvant. Serum from mice fed OVA produced

---

*Address correspondence to: A. McI. Mowat, Department of Bacteriology and Immunology, Western Infirmary, Glasgow G11 6NT, Scotland.

significant suppression (70%) of systemic DTH in recipients but had no effect on their antibody responses. Treatment of donor mice with CY two days before a feed of OVA did not alter the ability of serum from OVA-fed mice to suppress DTH responses of recipients. These results indicated that CY did not influence the nature of immunogenic OVA absorbed from the intestine, and in addition, suggested that antigenic molecules present in serum after a feed of OVA caused the suppressed DTH in OVA-fed mice. When recipient mice were given CY before receiving serum, no reduction of systemic DTH occurred in recipients of OVA-fed serum. Once again, systemic humoral immunity was unaffected. The tolerance we observed in serum recipients could have been due to the quantity of OVA reaching the serum after feeding; however, i.v. or i.p. injection of mice with doses of OVA similar to those found after feeding did not affect subsequent immunity to OVA.

We conclude that systemic DTH is highly susceptible to suppression after a feed of OVA and postulate that this suppression is due to the induction of CY-sensitive T_s by intestinally derived protein moieties.

DIFFERENTIAL IMMUNODEPRESSION OF MONOMERIC IgA BUT NOT POLYMERIC IgA BY PATIENTS WITH IgG MYELOMA

M. M. Newkirk, M. H. Klein, and B. J. Underdown

University of Toronto
Toronto, Ontario, Canada M5S 1A8

The humoral immune deficiency associated with multiple myeloma is characterized by reduced serum levels of polyclonal immunoglobulins. The nature of the deficiency in polyclonal IgA production in patients with IgG myeloma has not been fully characterized. We analyzed the IgA polymeric compartment of the serum in such patients using an ^{125}I-labeled secretory component binding assay.

This assay does not detect the trace amounts of secretory IgA reported to be present in normal human serum. Normal levels of polymeric IgA (0.14 ± 0.01 mg/ml) were found in the serum of the patients tested with IgG myeloma. Because, however, the serum IgA (measured by Nephelometry or Radial Immunodiffusion) was depressed in 40% of the patients, the polymeric IgA represented a significantly elevated percentage of the total IgA. The mean serum IgA level in the IgG myeloma patients was 0.96 mg/ml compared to 1.31 mg/ml for the normal controls. In normal controls, the polymeric IgA represents 11% of the total IgA, whereas in immunodepressed patients, this compartment represents a significantly elevated proportion (35%) of the total serum IgA (p < 0.004). An analysis of the normal controls that had serum IgA levels lower than <0.9 mg/ml showed that there was not a similar significant elevation in the polymeric compartment. Levels of total IgA in saliva collected from such patients were not significantly different from that of normal controls.

Thus, these studies suggest that the immunodepression secondary to IgG myeloma primarily affects monomeric IgA, but not polymeric IgA synthesis, in patients with IgG myeloma. The production of IgA in the human is somewhat compartmentalized with the primary site of monomer synthesis being the bone marrow and spleen, whereas the mucosal plasmacytes produce up to 80% of their IgA as polymers. The mechanism by which the neoplastic plasma cells cause the suppression of the polyclonal immunoglobulins is not clearly understood. Our findings suggest that the suppression of polyclonal immunoglobulins may be a site-specific phenomenon. The fact that the primary site of the neoplasia is the bone marrow may explain why monomeric IgA synthesis is affected, whereas the compartmentalized production of polymeric IgA by mucosal plasmacytes remains normal.

CHARACTERIZATION OF THE ANTIGENIC REGIONS OF AN *E. COLI* PILUS PROTEIN

William Paranchych, Elizabeth Worobec, Laura S. Frost, and
Robert S. Hodges

Department of Biochemistry
University of Alberta
Edmonton, Alberta, Canada, T6G 2H7

The virulence of several enterotoxigenic *E. coli* strains is dependent in part on their ability to colonize the upper intestinal tract. In many cases, this colonizing capacity is promoted by filamentous surface structures known as pili. We are interested in characterizing the antigenic determinants of several types of pili, and asking whether the resulting antigenic peptides could be used as synthetic vaccines.

Using EDP208 conjugative pili as a model system, we have shown that they are composed of a single polypeptide subunit of 11,500 daltons with a blocked N-terminus.[1] The subunits are arranged in a helical array of 3.6 units per turn of 1.28 nm pitch to form hollow cylinders 8.0 nm wide with a central hole of 2.0 nm.[2]

In the present study, the N-terminal region of the pilin subunit is characterized and shown to be the major antigenic determinant. The N-terminal blocking moiety was identified as an *N*-acetyl group by ^{1}H NMR (nuclear magnetic resonance) analysis of an N-terminal tripeptide isolated from pronase digests of EDP208 pilin. Limited acid hydrolysis of the tripeptide allowed its sequence to be determined as Ac-NH-Thr-Asp-Leu. Trypsin digestion of pilin monomers resulted in cleavage at Lys[12] to yield an N-terminal dodecapeptide, ET1 ($M_r \simeq$ 1500) and the remaining C-terminal fragment, ER ($M_r \simeq$ 10,000). The sequence of the dodecapeptide was determined to be: Ac-NH-Thr-Asp-Leu-Leu-Ala-Gly-Gly-Lys-Asp-Val-Asp-Lys.

ET1 was subsequently synthesized by solid phase methodology, coupled to bovine serum albumin (BSA), and subjected to immunological studies. Antisera prepared against intact EDP208 pili as well as the synthetic ET1-BSA conjugate were used in experiments using the enzyme-linked immunosorbent assay (ELISA) and electrophoretic transfer of proteins from SDS (sodium dodecyl sulphate)-polyacrylamide gels to nitrocellulose sheets. Both experimental approaches showed strong reactivity between the synthetic dodecapeptide and antisera raised against whole pili. It was also found that antiserum raised against the synthetic peptide was reactive against intact pilus protein, indicating that the N-terminal dodecapeptide is the major antigenic determinant of the EDP208 pilus protein. Additional studies showed that the C-terminal fragment, ER, may contain a second, weaker antigenic site.

REFERENCES

1. ARMSTRONG, G. D., L. S. FROST, P. A. SASTRY & W. PARANCHYCH. 1980. Comparative studies on F and EDP208 conjugative pili. J. Bacteriol. **141**: 333–341.
2. FOLKHARD, W., K. R. LEONARD, J. DUBOCHET, D. A. MARVIN & W. PARANCHYCH. 1979. Abstr. 03-3-S116, 11th Int. Congr. Biochem. Structure of bacterial pili by X-ray diffraction and electron microscopy. 181.

ELIMINATION OF CIRCULATING ANTIGEN INTO BILE BY ENDOGENOUS IgA ANTIBODY IN RATS

Jane V. Peppard, Eva Orlans,
Andrew W. R. Payne, and Elizabeth M. Andrew*

Chester Beatty Research Institute
Belmont, Surrey, England
*National Institute for Medical Research
London, England

The active transfer of polymeric IgA from blood to bile in several species, by a mechanism that involves secretory component (SC) of rats, is now well documented.[1] That an antigen that is combined with polymeric IgA antibody can also be carried across the liver into bile by this mechanism has been demonstrated using several model systems.[2-4] These models showed that antigen-antibody complexes combining polymeric IgA, but not IgM, IgG, or monomeric IgA, injected intravenously (i.v.) would traverse the liver and appear in bile, using SC as a receptor.

We were interested in determining whether endogenously produced polyclonal IgA antibody would mediate in the same way the transhepatic clearance of i.v. injected antigen *in vivo*. To stimulate an IgA-antibody response to a soluble antigen in rats, insoluble immune complexes of chicken antibody and antigen were injected into Peyer's patches. This injection elicited an antibody response to chicken IgG (CGG) detected by radioimmunoassay in both blood and bile, beginning at about three days after immunization. Serum antibody was predominantly of the IgM and IgG isotypes, whereas bile antibody was all IgA. Rats immunized in this fashion 5 days before were given bile duct cannulae and [^{125}I] CGG was injected i.v.; up to 22% (TCA precipitable) of the injected dose of [^{125}I] CGG was recovered in the bile in 24 hours, whereas in control (unimmunized) rats, a maximum of 0.4% was collected. The [^{125}I] CGG was intact antigenically in that it was precipitated by anti-chicken IgG sera. In contrast, however, to previous experiments of ours using a "model" system,[2] it was difficult to show that the radiolabeled protein was combined with IgA or SC after being transported. Only those samples of bile tested immediately after collection contained small amounts of such complexes.

These experiments, described completely in Reference 5, show that polyclonal polymeric IgA antibodies would perform the function *in vivo* of "mopping up" specific antigen from the systemic circulation by clearance through the liver, and would presumably also function at the gut epithelial surface, should antigen manage to penetrate from the gut. It seems likely, however, from these observations that most of the antigen carried by such IgA, which may be of low affinity, would, at least in bile, be present free, and not in combination with IgA and SC. Whether this dissociation is carried out by the action of bile or within the transporting cell itself remains to be seen.

REFERENCES

1. ORLANS, E., J. PEPPARD, A. W. R. PAYNE, B. M. FITZHARRIS, B. M. MULLOCK, R. H. HINTON & J. G. HALL. 1983. Comparative aspects of the hepato-biliary transport of IgA. Ann. N.Y. Acad. Sci. **409:** This volume.

2. PEPPARD, J. V., E. ORLANS, A. W. R. PAYNE & E. ANDREW. 1981. Elimination of circulating complexes containing polymeric IgA by excretion in the bile. Immunology **42:** 83–89.
3. RUSSELL, M. W., T. A. BROWN and J. MESTECKY. 1981. Role of serum IgA. Hepatobiliary transport of circulating antigen. J. Exp. Med. **153:** 968–976.
4. SOCKEN, D. J., E. R. SIMMS, B. R. NAGY, M. M. FISHER & B. J. UNDERDOWN. 1981. Secretory component-dependent hepatic transport of IgA antibody-antigen complexes. J. Immunol. **127:** 316–319.
5. PEPPARD, J. V., E. ORLANS, E. ANDREW & A. W. R. PAYNE. 1982. Elimination into bile of circulating antigen by endogenous IgA antibody in rats. Immunology **45:** 467–472.

SELECTIVE HEPATOBILIARY TRANSPORT OF MONOCLONAL IgG, BUT NOT IgM ANTI-IDIOTYPIC ANTIBODIES, BY IgA*

John O. Phillips, Michael W. Russell, Thomas A. Brown, and
Jiri Mestecky

University of Alabama in Birmingham
Birmingham, Alabama 35294

Recent investigations with rodent models have demonstrated the selective hepatobiliary transport of polymeric IgA (pIgA) and IgA immune complexes from blood into bile.[1-3] This IgA-mediated clearance has been demonstrated for haptenated protein antigens complexed with hapten-specific mouse IgA in the mouse system and for rabbit anti-idiotypic (anti-Id) IgG complexed to human IgA in the rat system.[4,5] In this study we have examined the ability of the mouse IgA-myeloma protein J558 to mediate the transport of allogeneic or syngeneic monoclonal IgG and syngeneic monoclonal IgM anti-Id antibodies from serum into bile.

Monoclonal IgM and IgG_1 anti-Id antibodies to J558 were iodinated and injected intravenously into mice with or without J558. One hour after injection, bile and corresponding serum samples were analyzed for total radioactivity. Injection of monoclonal $[^{125}I]IgG$ anti-Id antibody with J558 resulted in a dramatic increase in total radioactivity recovered in bile relative to injection of $[^{125}I]IgG$ alone (TABLE 1). Monoclonal anti-Id $[^{125}I]IgM$ with J558 was not preferentially transported into bile relative to injection of $[^{125}I]IgM$ alone (TABLE 1). The radioactivity in bile of mice injected with the $[^{125}I]IgG/J558$ mixture sedimented as high molecular weight forms when analyzed by sucrose density gradient ultracentrifugation, whereas the bile of mice receiving $[^{125}I]IgG$ alone contained only low molecular weight radiolabeled fragments. Radioactivity recovered in the bile

TABLE 1

HEPATOBILIARY TRANSPORT OF ANTI-IDIOTYPIC ANTIBODIES BY J558 IGA

| Anti-idiotype Injected | Radioactivity (mean ± SD)* Recovered in: | | Bile:Serum Ratio | p† |
	Serum cpm/μl	Bile cpm/μl		
IgG_1 alone	8884 ± 2115	476 ± 190	0.054	—
IgG_1 + J558 (50 μg)	3477 ± 155	6263 ± 1921	1.941	<0.001
IgM alone	4054 ± 670	968 ± 206	0.239	—
IgM + J558 (50 μg)	3332 ± 229	1136 ± 143	0.341	>0.2

*Minimum of four mice used per group.
†Student's t-test on log transformed data.

*This work was supported by United States Public Health Service Grants AI-10854 and AM-28537.

859

of mice receiving [^{125}I]IgM with or without J558 sedimented only as low molecular weight fragments.

IgA appears to mediate the hepatobiliary clearance of IgA-IgG idiotype anti-Id immune complexes. Immune complexes of IgA-IgM are not effectively transported, possibly because of their size, as has been suggested by Socken et al.[6] It is conceivable that IgA anti-Id antibodies might regulate the idiotypic network by removing idiotypes from the circulation.

ACKNOWLEDGMENTS

We wish to thank John Kearney and Bob Stohrer for generously providing the anti-Id antibodies.

REFERENCES

1. ORLANS, E., J. PEPPARD, J. REYNOLDS & J. HALL. 1978. J. Exp. Med. 147: 588–592.
2. JACKSON, G. D. F., I. LEMAITRE-COELHO, J.-P. VAERMAN, H. BAZIN & A. BECKERS. 1978. Eur. J. Immunol. 8: 123–126.
3. FISHER, M. M., B. NAGY, H. BAZIN, & B. J. UNDERDOWN. 1979. Proc. Natl. Acad. Sci. USA 76: 2008–2012.
4. PEPPARD, J., E. ORLANS, A. W. R. PAYNE, & E. ANDREW. 1981. Immunology 42: 83–89.
5. RUSSELL, M. W., T. A. BROWN, & J. MESTECKY, 1981. J. Exp. Med. 153: 968–976.
6. SOCKEN, D. J., E. S. SIMMS, B. R. NAGY, M. M. FISHER & B. J. UNDERDOWN. 1981. J. Immunol. 127: 316–319.

THE CLEARANCE KINETICS AND HEPATIC
LOCALIZATION OF IgA-IMMUNE COMPLEXES IN MICE*

Abdalla Rifai† and Mart Mannik

Division of Rheumatology
University of Washington School of Medicine
Seattle, Washington 98195

To characterize the *in vivo* behavior of IgA-immune complexes, covalently cross-linked polymers were prepared with dimeric (dIgA) and monomeric IgA (mIgA). The affinity-labeling antigen, bis-2,4-dinitrophenyl pimelic ester, was used to cross-link specifically purified dIgA and mIgA anti-dinitrophenyl obtained from MOPC-315 plasmacytoma. The cross-linked polymers were separated from the nonpolymerized dIgA and mIgA by gel filtration. Following intravenous injection, heavy polymers ($> 1.2 \times 10^6$ M.W.) of dIgA and mIgA, that were excluded from the gel, were rapidly eliminated from circulation. The disappearance curves consisted of a single exponential component. During the first 2.5 minutes, more than 80% of the polymers were removed with a $t_{1/2}$ of less than one minute.

Clearance of intermediate-latticed complexes, a composite of a relatively heterogeneous population of polymers, was determined by gradient polyacrylamide gel electrophoresis (GPAGE) analysis of sequential plasma specimens obtained from mice at 0.5, 5, 10, 30, and 60 minutes after injection of either pooled dIgA or mIgA complexes. The gradient gel profiles showed a rapid decrease in the concentration of complexes that was directly proportional to the size of the complexes. To determine the minimal size required for rapid elimination from circulation, the area of the curves remaining under each peak in GPAGE was calculated and plotted as the percent of trichloroacetic acid-precipitable radioactivity remaining in circulation against time (FIGURE 1). In this manner the influence of a progressive increase in lattice on the clearance of either dIgA or mIgA complexes was defined. It should be noted that a dimer of mIgA, 45–60% of gel fraction, behaved similarly to unreacted dIgA. Complexes that were composed of three dIgA or six mIgA units, 15–25% of gel fraction, delimited the size above which the complexes were rapidly eliminated. By graphic peeling, curves for the complexes localized in 5–15% of the gel gradient contained a slow component that represented 19% and 27% of the dIgA and mIgA polymers, respectively. The presence of such a slow component could be attributed to the spillover of smaller complexes in the major peak, localized in 15–25% of the gradient gel. Thus, if the initial fast component of the polymers in 5–15% of the gel gradient was corrected for presence of small complexes, IgA-immune complexes with a lattice structure of eight mIgA or four dIgA antibodies were rapidly removed from circulation as a single exponential component similar to the heavy polymers.

The major organ responsible for removal of IgA-immune complexes was the

*This work was supported by grants AM 07108 and AM 26249 from the National Institute of Arthritis, Diabetes, Digestive, and Kidney Diseases.

†Present address: Department of Pathology and Laboratory Medicine, Health Science Center at Houston, The University of Texas, Houston, Texas 77025.

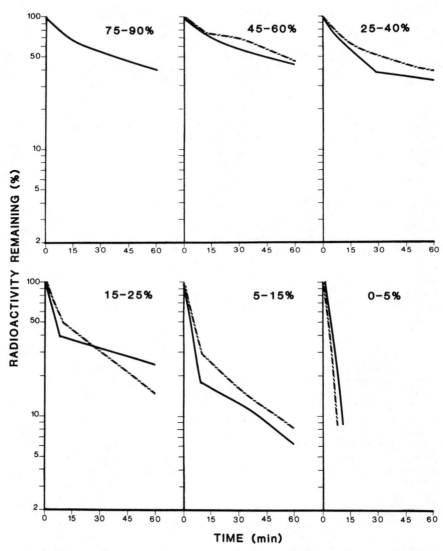

FIGURE 1. Clearance kinetics of dIgA (———) and mIgA (——) immune complexes according to their size after the injection of intermediate-latticed polymers. The numbers, in the upper right-hand corner of each panel, represent percent of the gradient gel length where the polymer's peak localized. The 0.5 minute sample was considered as the 100% value at zero time.

liver. To determine whether the hepatic clearance of circulating IgA-immune complexes could be attributed to preferential uptake by hepatocytes or Kupffer cells, the cellular distribution of bound radiolabeled complexes was examined in separated parenchymal and nonparenchymal cells, 10 minutes after infusion of heavy polymers. The data, expressed as the ratio of nonparenchymal cell to parenchymal cell binding (NPC/PC), indicated that the soluble IgA-immune complexes, both with dIgA or mIgA, were taken up efficiently by the nonparenchymal cells with NPC/PC ratios similar to heavy polymers of IgG-immune complexes.

These results indicate that immune complexes of dIgA and mIgA behave similarly in circulation. The disappearance of these immune complexes from the blood is directly related to the lattice structure; the mononuclear phagocyte system is quantitatively important in the removal of circulating large-latticed IgA-immune complexes.

MONOCLONAL ANTIBODIES IN IDENTIFICATION OF MACROPHAGES/NATURAL KILLER CELLS IN MURINE INTESTINAL MUCOSA*

Michael J. Roy† and William R. Brown

Gastroenterology Division
Veterans Administration Medical Center and
University of Colorado School of Medicine
Denver, Colorado 80220

Macrophages residing in the lamina propria of the small intestine could play important roles in intestinal immune responses. Intestinal macrophages, however, are difficult to identify and isolate, in large part because no specific marker is available to monitor their dissociation and purification. We report here that M1/70, a monoclonal antibody that reacts with a membrane polypeptide, Mac-1, on murine macrophages[1] and natural killer (NK) cells[2] bind Mac-1 antigen-bearing (Mac-1) cells in the intestinal lamina propria and in preparations of intestinal lamina propria cells.

Mac-1 cells were stained by the indirect fluorescent antibody staining technique. Acetone-fixed sections of tissue were stained with M1/70 (Accurate Scientific, Westbury, N.Y.) or nonimmune rat IgG as primary antibody and fluoresceinated Fab'₂ fragments of rabbit anti-rat IgG (Cappel Labs, West Chester, Pa.) as the second antibody. Intestinal leukocytes were isolated following either collagenase[3] or Dispase[4] digestion of lamina propria.

Indirect fluorescence immunocytochemistry demonstrated Mac-1 cells in spleen, mesenteric lymph nodes, and intestinal lamina propria, but not in the liver. Mac-1 cells were sometimes found adjacent to follicles in Peyer's patches, but never in the follicles themselves. Mac-1 cells in lymphoid organs were round, whereas intestinal Mac-1 cells were dendritic and restricted to the lamina propria. Duodenum or jejunum contained four times more Mac-1 cells than ileum.

Leukocytes, removed from the intestinal mucosa by enzymatic digestion or mechanical disruption, were stained for Mac-1 cells. Intestinal epithelial-layer cell populations contained no Mac-1 cells. Collagenase digestion or mechanical disruption of intestinal lamina propria released very few Mac-1 cells, whereas Dispase digestion dissociated Mac-1 cells.

This study demonstrated that the lamina propria contains cells bearing the Mac-1 antigen, with Mac-1 cells more numerous in the middle and upper portions of the small intestine than in the ileum. The finding that Mac-1 appears on cells in some organs but not others may be further evidence that Mac-1 is on macrophage-like cells only at certain stages of differentiation. Alternatively, Mac-1 cells might represent a subpopulation of macrophage-like or NK cells. Mac-1 cells were not released from intestinal mucosa either by mechanical disruption or by collagenase digestion, methods commonly employed[3] in the preparation of intestinal leukocytes. The monoclonal antibody M1/70 that local-

*This work was supported by the National Foundation for Ileitis and Colitis.

†Present address: Department of Experimental Pathology, Division of Pathology, Walter Reed Army Institute of Research, Washington, D.C. 20307.

864

izes intestinal Mac-1 cells might be useful in monitoring the isolation or purification of intestinal macrophages or NK cells.

REFERENCES

1. SPRINGER, T. A. 1980. Cell surface differentiation in the mouse. In Monoclonal antibodies. Hybridomas: A New Dimension in Biological Analyses. R. H. Kennet and T. J. McKearn, Eds.: 185. Plenum Press. New York.
2. HOLMBERG, L. A., T. A. SPRINGER & K. A. AULT. 1981. Natural killer activity in the peritoneal exudates of mice infected with Listeria monocytogenes: Characterization of the natural killer cells by using a monoclonal rat anti-murine macrophage antibody (M1/70). J. Immunol. 127: 1792.
3. DAVIES, M. D. J. & D. M. V. PARROTT. 1981. Preparation and purification of lymphocytes from the epithelium and lamina propria of murine small intestine. Gut 22: 481.
4. KIYONO, H., J. R. MCGHEE, M. J. WANNEMUEHLER, M. V. FRANGAKIS, D. M. SPALDING, S. M. MICHALEK, & W. I. KOOPMAN. 1982. In vitro immune responses to a T-cell-dependent antigen by cultures of disassociated murine Peyer's patch. Proc. Natl. Acad. Sci. USA 79: 596.

POTENTIATION OF THE SECRETORY IgA RESPONSE BY ORAL AND ENTERIC ADMINISTRATION OF CP 20,961*

Donald H. Rubin, Arthur O. Anderson, and Deborah Lucis

University of Pennsylvania
Philadelphia, Pennsylvania 19104

Suzanne M. Michalek

University of Alabama in Birmingham
Birmingham, Alabama 35294

A protective immune response against gastrointestinal pathogens requires that specific secretory IgA antibodies be generated and transported across the appropriate mucosal surfaces.[1] Oral priming has been shown to be superior to parenteral inoculation in generating such a response.[2] With the exception of intraperitoneal priming, immunization by other parenteral routes may cause depression of subsequent IgA responses. In addition, inactivated, attenuated or toxoided antigens often fail to exhibit the essential immunogenic properties needed for protective mucosal immunity. Thus the development of adjuvants to enhance the immunogenicity of enteric vaccines is essential.[3]

We have performed the following studies to determine the effectiveness of the lipoidal amine adjuvant N, N-dioctadecyl-N', N'-bis (2-hydroxyethyl) propane-diamine (CP 20,961) in enhancing mucosal immunity against cholera toxin, reovirus serotype 1/Lang, and S. mutans. Cholera toxin binds to all intestinal epithelial cells; serotype reovirus 1/Lang binds only to the membranous cells overlying Peyer's patches. S. mutans is an oral pathogen responsible for dental caries and binds to teeth and oral mucosal membranes.

Intraduodenal (ID) priming[1] with 10 μg of cholera toxin in a soybean oil lipid emulsion containing 0.3 mg CP 20,961 resulted in fourfold enhancement of toxin-specific IgA in intestinal secretions, as measured by enzyme-linked immunosorbent assay (ELISA). Maximal titer was achieved 14 days following a single ID priming dose of CP 20,961 and toxin (TABLE 1 and FIGURE 1).

Mice were primed ID with live reovirus, 10^8 plaque-forming units (pfu), in the presence or absence of the CP 20,961 adjuvant. The recovery of reovirus in intestinal homogenates from mice receiving virus plus adjuvant or virus alone was similar (1.9 $\times$ 10^6 pfu/ml. and 2.0 $\times$ 10^6 pfu/ml., respectively). Reovirus specific IgA levels present in the intestines were determined by ELISA (TABLE 2). Secretory antibody levels were approximately 2.5 times higher in mice that received reovirus plus adjuvant compared to mice that received reovirus alone. Maximal antibody titers were achieved on day 7 in both groups. The antibody titers decreased by day 14, but this decrease was much less for the adjuvant-treated group than that seen for reovirus alone. It is not known whether the earlier appearance of high antibody titers with reovirus is due to the capacity of reovirus to replicate or its preferential accumulation in Peyer's patches. In both

*This work was supported by Biomedical Research Support Grant 5 507 RR 05415 20, Pfizer Central Research, and National Institutes of Health Grant 1 R22 A1 1855-01 to D.H. Rubin.

TABLE 1

LEVELS OF CHOLERA TOXIN SPECIFIC ANTIBODY IN INTESTINAL SECRETIONS

Experimental Group	Antibody Levels by ELISA Units*					
	IgA			IgG		
	Day 3	Day 7	Day 14	Day 3	Day 7	Day 14
Cholera toxin 10 μg	0	41	187	0	15	0
Cholera toxin + CP 20,961 0.3 mg.	28	165	754	0	9	12
Reovirus 10^{10} particles	0	0	0	0	0	0
CP 20,961 alone	0	0	0	0	0	0

*As determined by ELISA using monospecific antisera to α and γ heavy chains. Values expressed as the mean optical density reading at 405 nm ($\times 10^{-3}$) of duplicate tests per sample (1/20 dilution of original) per group.

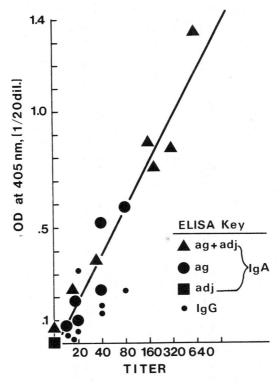

FIGURE 1. There is a direct correlation between the optical density (OD) at 405 nm of ELISA samples diluted 1/20 before incubation with substrate and the antibody titer as measured by dilution to greater than 60% reduction in OD.

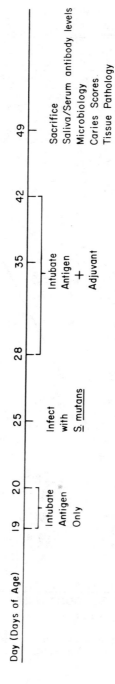

FIGURE 2. Germfree rats were treated as above. Please note that each rat was exposed to *S. mutans* antigens five times in addition to being infected with *S. mutans* six days after initial priming with antigen. CP 20,961 was added to the three booster doses that were given 21, 14, and 7 days before measuring titers in saliva.

TABLE 2

LEVELS OF REOVIRUS SPECIFIC ANTIBODY IN INTESTINAL SECRETIONS AFTER PRIMARY IMMUNIZATION

| | Antibody Levels by ELISA Units* | | | | | |
| | IgA | | | IgG | | |
Experimental Group	Day 3	Day 7	Day 14	Day 3	Day 7	Day 14
Reovirus 10^{10} particles (p) (1/Lang)	529	588	234	60	0	15
Reovirus 10^{10} p + CP 20,961 0.3 mg	63	1352	849	55	78	0
Reovirus 10^{10} p, 10^4 pfu (UV† inac)	0	0	867	0	0	0
Reovirus (as above) + CP 20,961	345	160	220	0	0	100
Cholera toxin 10 µg	0	0	0	0	0	0
CP 20,961 alone	ND	0	0	0	0	0

*As determined by ELISA using monospecific heavy chain antisera. Values expressed as the mean optical density reading at 405nm ($\times 10^{-3}$) of duplicate tests per sample (1/20 dilution of original) per group after two hours of incubation with substrate.

†UV = ultraviolet light at 14 cm for 30 minutes.

TABLE 3

ENHANCEMENT OF *S. MUTANS* SPECIFIC sIGA IN SALIVA BY CP 20,961

| | Level of anti-*S. mutans* Antibodies (EU)* | | | | |
| | Saliva | | Serum | | |
Experimental Group	IgA	IgG	IgM	IgG	IgA
Infected only	6.5	<5	<5	<5	<5
S. mutans 6715 WC	25.2	7.5	6.1	35.2	8.5
S. mutans 6715 WC + CP 20,961	80.0	30.0	5.3	105.0	10.0
S. mutans 6715 WC + Liposomes†	320.0	80.0	7.9	55.0	20.0
CP 20,961 only	<5	<5	<5	<5	<5

*As determined by ELISA using monospecific anti-rat α, γ, and μ. Values expressed as ELISA units (EU), where EU equal the mean reciprocal of the dilution per sample per group giving an optical density reading at 405 nm of 0.1 after 1.5 hours of incubation with substrate.

†The liposomes contained CP 20,961.

TABLE 4

REDUCTION OF DENTAL PLAQUE IN *S. MUTANS* IMMUNE GNOTOBIOTIC RATS

Experimental Group	Plaque Score*	Number of Viable *S. mutans* (CFU $\times 10^6$)†
Infected only	15.3 ± 0.4	6.40 ± 0.35
S. mutans 6715 WC	9.2 ± 0.6	3.96 ± 0.53
S. mutans 6715 WC + CP 20,961	7.3 ± 0.4	2.96 ± 0.21
S. mutans 6715 WC Liposomes‡	6.1 ± 0.3	1.88 ± 0.09
CP 20,961 only	16.0 ± 0.9	6.75 ± 0.48

*Represents mean value of smooth surface plaque on one mandible per rat per group ± SEM.

†Represents mean number of CFU (colony-forming unit approximately equal to number of bacteria recovered) in plaque from one mandible per rat per group as determined on blood and Mitis-Salivarius agar ± SEM.

‡The liposomes contained CP 20,961.

cases the CP 20,961 increased the magnitude but not the kinetics of the antibody and tissue response (TABLE 1 and 2).

In the *S. mutans* and dental caries study, groups of germfree rats were orally immunized with *S. mutans* 6715 WC alone or in combination with CP 20,961, according to the protocol depicted in FIGURE 2. *S. mutans* specific antibodies in serum and saliva samples from the five groups of animals were assessed by ELISA. Approximately threefold higher salivary IgA- and IgG-antibody levels were seen in rats treated with antigen and CP 20,961 compared to rats given *S. mutans* alone (TABLE 3). When liposomes prepared from CP 20,961 were used, the salivary IgG and IgA levels were enhanced tenfold. CP 20,961 did not enhance serum antibody levels when used orally. Plaque scores and microbiology are presented in TABLE 4. It is clear that oral immunization with *S. mutans* 6715 WC results in reduced molar plaque and microbial counts when compared with infected controls. Administration of CP 20,961 with antigen resulted in a further reduction in plaque levels and organisms recoverable.

In summary, the results indicate that the lipoidal amine CP 20,961 elicited an increase in specific IgA in secretions for all three antigens studied.

REFERENCES

1. FUHRMAN, J. A. & J. J. CEBRA. 1981. J. Exp. Med. **153:** 535–544.
2. PIERCE, N. F. & F. T. KOSTER. 1980. J. Immunol. **124:** 307–311.
3. ANDERSON, A. O. & J. A. REYNOLDS. 1979. J. Reticuloendothelial Soc. **26:** 667–680.

IgA-MEDIATED HEPATOBILIARY CLEARANCE
OF BACTERIAL ANTIGENS*

Michael W. Russell, Thomas A. Brown, Rose Kulhavy,
and Jiri Mestecky

Department of Microbiology
Institute of Dental Research
University of Alabama in Birmingham
Birmingham, Alabama 35294

In rodents, serum polymeric IgA, alone or complexed with antigens, is transported through the liver into bile.[1-4] This transport suggests a physiological role for IgA in the elimination of circulating antigens, such as those generated by infecting organisms, that might not otherwise be degradable.

[125]I-labeled pneumococcal type III polysaccharide (SIII) and ^{125}I-labeled C-carbohydrate (PnC) were mixed as appropriate, with murine ascitic fluids containing anti-SIII hybridoma antibodies of IgA, IgG$_3$, and IgM classes (200 μg Ig per ml),[4] or with purified anti-phosphocholine myeloma or hybridoma antibodies of the IgA, IgG$_3$ and IgM classes, all of the T15 idiotype (100 μg Ig per ml).[5] These mixtures (0.1 ml containing 2-5 × 10^6 cpm) were injected intravenously in young BALB/c mice, from which serum and bile samples were collected one hour later.[4]

With both antigens, complexes containing IgA or IgG$_3$ were cleared rapidly from the circulation, but only those containing IgA were effectively transported into bile (FIGURE 1). The clearance of SIII-IgM complexes may have been due to the presence of some contaminating IgG$_{2b}$ antibody. Analysis of the injection mixtures by sucrose density gradient ultracentrifugation showed that all classes of antibodies formed complexes with the appropriate antigens, and in bile, the radiolabeled antigens, when injected with IgA antibodies, were present in peaks corresponding to complexed and intact antigens. By contrast, when the antigens were injected alone or with IgG$_3$ or IgM antibodies, the small amount of radioactivity present in the bile corresponded to free and degraded antigen.

We have previously found, using M315 IgA and dinitrophenyl-human serum albumin, that hepatobiliary transport of antigen depends on polymeric, not monomeric, IgA, and that failure of IgG and IgM to mediate this process is not due to inadequate affinity for the antigen.[4,5] The present experiments used anti-PnC antibodies of different isotype but of the same idiotype, and therefore of similar antigen-binding activity and affinity. Analysis of the anti-SIII and anti-PnC IgAs by ultracentrifugation revealed the presence of both polymeric and monomeric components in all of them, and fractionation studies have suggested that the polymers are the effective forms (unpublished observations).

The IgG$_3$ and IgM, but not IgA, antibodies that were used for these experiments can protect mice against lethal infection with type III pneumococci.[6] The present data suggest instead, however, that serum polymeric IgA can eliminate potentially harmful antigens by a noninflammatory mechanism.

*This work was supported by United States Public Health Service Grants AI-10854, DE-02670, and AM-28537.

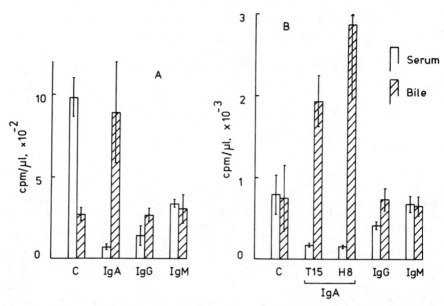

FIGURE 1. Serum and bile levels of ^{125}I-labeled SIII (A) or ^{125}I-labeled PnC (B) in mice one hour after injection together with specific immunoglobulins as shown. Bars represent mean ± S.D. (N = 4). C = control (no specific immunoglobulin).

ACKNOWLEDGMENTS

We are very grateful to K. Schroer and J. L. Claflin for providing the antibodies.

REFERENCES

1. ORLANS, E., J. PEPPARD, J. REYNOLDS, & J. HALL. 1978. J. Exp. Med. **147:** 588–592.
2. JACKSON, G. D. F., I. LEMAITRE-COELHO, J.-P. VAERMAN, H. BAZIN, & A. BECKERS. 1978. Eur. J. Immunol. **8:** 123–126.
3. SOCKEN, D. J., E. S. SIMMS, B. NAGY, M. M. FISHER & B. J. UNDERDOWN. 1981. J. Immunol. **127:** 316–319.
4. RUSSELL, M. W., T. A. BROWN & J. MESTECKY. 1981. J. Exp. Med. **153:** 968–976.
5. BROWN, T. A., M. W. RUSSELL & J. MESTECKY. 1982. J. Immunol. **128:** 2183–2186.
6. BRILES, D. E., J. L. CLAFLIN, K. SCHROER & C. FORMAN. 1981. Nature (London) **294:** 88–90.

INDUCTION OF IgA EXPRESSION BY B-CELLS
RESPONSIVE TO THYMUS-INDEPENDENT ANTIGENS

Roberta D. Shahin, Peter A. Schweitzer, and John J. Cebra

University of Pennsylvania
Philadelphia, Pennsylvania 19104

Thymus-independent antigens have been defined as those that can induce formation of specific antibodies in an athymic animal. This response is predominantly IgM or IgG$_3$ *in vivo*. We present evidence that the B-cell population responding to thymus-independent antigens is multipotential with respect to clonal isotype potential, and that this response may be influenced by external signals from T-cells and accessory cells.

The frequency and isotype potential of antigen-sensitive cells was determined using the Klinman splenic fragment assay. Donor cells were injected intravenously into the tail veins of unprimed or carrier-primed, lethally irradiated recipients at limiting dilution. After 16 hours, recipient spleens were removed and diced; the fragments were distributed into microtiter plates, and challenged with antigen. Supernatants were collected and analyzed for specific antibody by radioimmunoassay.

Thymus-independent antigens elicited predominantly IgM and IgG$_3$ immunoglobulins in the serum of mice when administered parenterally. *In vitro* B-lymphocytes responsive to the thymus-independent antigens trinitrophenylated (TNP)-Ficoll, bacterial levan, or a pneumococcal vaccine, however, were able to stimulate clonal expansion and the heavy chain class switch, as judged by multiple isotype production by B-lymphocytes at a limiting dilution. The isotypes expressed *in vitro* included IgG$_1$, IgG$_2$, and IgA.

In order to determine whether B-lymphocytes responsive to thymus-independent antigens could be affected by "bystander" effects, cultures stimulated with (TNP)-Ficoll or pneumococcal vaccine were costimulated with phosphocholine-hemocyanin or hemocyanin (Hy). The irradiated recipients had been immunized with Hy in complete Freund's adjuvant five to eight weeks previously to generate Hy-specific T-cell help. Also, treatment of the donor-cell inoculum with anti-Thy-1 plus complement followed by stimulation with levan *in vitro* was performed to assess any contribution of T-cells in the donor inoculum.

Our data indicate that when "bystander" Hy-specific cells are stimulated, a decrease in the proportion of clones producing IgM is observed with an increase in the proportion expressing IgG and/or IgA; the greatest increase is seen in IgG$_3$, IgG$_1$, and IgA expression. Elimination of Thy-1 positive cells in the donor inoculum leads to an increase in IgM-producing clones and an accompanying effect of fewer clones expressing IgG$_2$ and clones producing IgA only.

Antigenic determinants frequently associated with common gut flora are often carbohydrate moieties that induce a classic thymus-independent response in the mouse. We classify these as environmental antigens on the basis of the relatively high frequency of antigen-sensitive B-lymphocytes reactive to them in adult mice, and the high proportion of these cells in Peyer's patches committed to generating clones exclusively expressing IgA. BALB/c mice, germfree for up to one year of life, have a low frequency of PC and inulin-reactive cells. Neonatal mice resemble germfree mice in their low numbers of inulin-reactive B-cells; however, there is a naturally occurring rise in frequency of inulin-sensitive cells detectable at five weeks of age. This rise can be prematurely induced by deliberate parenteral priming shortly after birth with either the T-dependent. inulin-hemocyanin or the T-independent bacterial levan that bears the inulin linkage. In addition, immunization of young adults with TNP-Ficoll stimulates an increase of antigen-sensitive cells scored in a thymus-dependent manner, although the isotype potential of these cells is not changed.

Although the frequencies of inulin-reactive cells from mice primed at birth with the T-dependent or T-independent form of the antigen are identical, bacterial levan priming results in the expression of IgM primarily, whereas inulin-Hy results in expression of all isotypes.

T-cells can be isolated from the Peyer's patches of adults primed intraduodenally with cholera toxin. This priming regimen results in the almost exclusive production of IgA. When nylon wool purified T-cells from the Peyer's patches of toxin-primed adults are mixed into the donor inoculum of spleen cells from a levan-primed neonate, the pattern of isotype expression is shifted from predominantly IgM production to production of IgM and IgA.

CONCLUSIONS

Thymus-independent antigens stimulate the expression of multiple immunoglobulin isotypes.

Thymus-independent antigens can prime for a subsequent thymus-dependent response.

T-cells, accessory cells, or factors present in a predominantly IgA response may influence the expression of B-lymphocytes that normally express only IgM. Also, these effects can shift patterns of isotype expression observed in vitro in response to thymus-independent antigens toward the expression of greater IgG and IgA.

AGING AND THE SALIVARY IMMUNE RESPONSE IN HAMSTERS*

Daniel J. Smith, Jeffrey L. Ebersole, and Martin A. Taubman

Forsyth Dental Center
Boston, Massachusetts 02115

Several reports have suggested that the systemic and secretory immune systems may not be affected in an identical fashion by the aging process. The purpose of the present study is to describe in hamsters the effect of aging on the levels of IgA in saliva and serum, and to explore certain aspects of the IgA-immune response to a soluble antigen. The antigen used for subcutaneous injection was glucosyltransferase (GTF), a defined soluble antigen of the oral pathogen, *Streptococcus mutans*. Young (two- to three-month old) and aged (approximately two years old) National Institute of Health white hamsters, raised at Forsyth Dental Center, were used. This colony did not naturally harbor *S. mutans* in its oral flora. IgA concentrations were measured by radial immunodiffusion, and IgA and IgG antibody activity to GTF was measured by a radioisotopic functional inhibition assay and by an enzyme-linked immunosorbent assay (ELISA), using GTF bound to polystyrene microtiter plates. Hamsters were injected in the salivary gland region with 30 μg of GTF in complete Freund's adjuvant. Serum and saliva were sampled prior to immunization, 11, 16, 22, and 28 days after primary immunization, and 8 days after a secondary injection with an equivalent GTF dose.

Salivary volume and mean salivary IgA concentration were slightly higher in the old animals prior to the experiment. Whereas both of these parameters showed appreciable variation, the mean secretion rate of IgA in the aged hamsters was at least 30% higher than in younger animals, and was significantly different (p < 0.02) in one of the two experiments. Serum IgA levels were at least tenfold, and serum IgG levels were approximately twofold higher in aged hamsters. Salivary IgA-antibody responses of aged hamsters were generally lower than those of young hamsters after both primary and secondary immunization. The amount of antibody activity per milligram of immunoglobulin was significantly lower in aged hamsters on all occasions tested during the primary response to injected glucosyltransferase. All hamsters responded to injection of GTF in complete Freund's adjuvant with serum IgG antibody and serum GTF-inhibitory activity (response among all isotypes). Aged hamster serum responses were generally more variable than serum responses of young hamsters. Secondary serum IgG-antibody responses were more elevated in the young animals. The peak primary and peak secondary GTF-inhibitory responses were, with one exception, greater in the younger animals.

The demonstration of elevated IgA levels in the serum of aged hamsters agrees with observations in other rodent systems. In addition, the levels of secretory IgA were also somewhat higher in two-year-old compared with two- to three-month old hamsters. These elevated IgA levels may represent the result of accumulated antigenic exposures in the older animals. The capacity to demon-

*This work was supported by National Institutes of Health Grants DE-04333 and DE-00075.

strate a salivary IgA-antibody response to the soluble GTF antigen was impaired in the older animals. This impairment, however, might have been somewhat offset by the increased secretion rate of salivary IgA. Serum IgG antibody and GTF-inhibitory responses (total isotypes) were generally less vigorous in aged hamsters following a second injection of antigen. Thus, both systemic and secretory immune systems in aged hamsters of this strain gave evidence of reduced ability to respond to soluble antigen administered in complete Freund's adjuvant.

THE NATURE OF IgA IN SECRETIONS FROM CHILDREN

Christian Hjort Sørensen

The Gentofte University Hospital
Hellerup, Denmark

INTRODUCTION

In vivo degradation of IgA in vaginal and intestinal secretions, caused by bacterial IgA proteases, has previously been described.[1,2] As *Hemophilus influenzae* and *Streptococcus pneumoniae*, which both produce IgA proteases, are frequently encountered as members of the nasopharyngeal flora, part of the IgA contained in nasopharyngeal secretions (NPS) may be present in degraded form, that is, as Fab_α and Fc_α fragments. The purposes of this study were (1) to determine the ratio of secretory IgA (sIgA) to IgA in secretions from children; (2) to study the prevalence and clinical distribution of Fc_α fragments in secretions; and (3) to evaluate the stability of secretory component (SC) in sIgA after reaction with bacterial IgA proteases.

MATERIALS

Nasopharyngeal secretions (NPS) were obtained from 100 children consecutively admitted for adenoidectomy because of recurrent upper respiratory tract infections and/or hyperplasia of the adenoids. Fifty of these children, who suffered from recurrent acute otitis and/or secretory otitis, and middle ear effusions (MEE), all of the mucoid type, were aspirated through a tympanocentesis. Detailed anamnestic information was obtained on each child. Atopy was diagnosed in the pediatric and dermatological clinics prior to the operation. None of the children had had acute otitis or received any medical therapy for three weeks prior to the examination. Bacterial IgA proteases isolated from *Hemophilus influenzae* and *Streptococcus pneumoniae* were used in the in vitro experiments to study the degradation of IgA.

METHODS

Quantitation of sIgA and IgA was performed by double-antibody sandwich enzyme-linked immunosorbent assay,[3] (ELISA), using horseradish peroxidase conjugated antisera in the final antibody layer (Dakopatts, Copenhagen). Human colostrum sIgA was used as a standard. Degradation of IgA into Fab_α and Fc_α fragments was studied by rocket immunoelectrophoresis with intermediate gel technique (Tris-barbital buffer, pH 8.6). Presence of Fc_α fragments was determined qualitatively by comparing with the results obtained in samples having IgA cleaved by bacterial IgA proteases during two hours of incubation.

TABLE 1

Secretory IgA (sIgA) and IgA Levels in Nasopharyngeal Secretions (NPS) and
Middle Ear Effusions (MEE) from Children with Secretory Otitis with or
without Previous Episodes of Acute Otitis

		NPS			MEE		
	N‡	sIgA g/l	IgA g/l	sIgA/IgA Percentage	sIgA g/l	IgA g/l	sIgA/IgA Percentage
Secretory otitis	16	1.6*	2.0	73 (53–91)†	1.7	9.3	23 (14–36)
Secretory otitis with Acute otitis	15	1.4	1.8	79 (66–89)	2.0	8.9	28 (17–43)

*Median values.
†Interquartile range.
‡N = number of patients.

RESULTS

The concentrations of sIgA and IgA were equally distributed in the groups of children investigated (TABLE 1). The levels of sIgA and IgA in NPS and MEE varied substantially. In NPS the ratio sIgA:IgA was significantly higher compared with the MEE ratio (Wilcoxon matched pairs signed-ranks test).

IgA cleavage products were demonstrated in 18.6% (11–28%, 95% confidence limits) of NPS and in 4% (0–14%) of middle ear effusions. A significantly high prevalence of Fc_α fragments was found in NPS from allergic children (drug allergy, atopic dermatitis, atopic disposition), compared with the prevalence in nonallergic children (TABLE 2). Nevertheless, recurrent acute otitis was not correlated to the presence of Fc_α fragments in NPS (TABLE 2).

Incubation of NPS and colostrum sIgA with bacterial IgA proteases caused a reduction in the sIgA content as measured by the ELISA. Median recovery of sIgA was 80% (71–86%) in colostrum sIgA and 65% (47–83%) in NPS, respectively.

TABLE 2

In Vivo Prevalence of IgA Cleavage Products in Naso-pharyngeal Secretions
Related to History of Allergy and Episodes of Acute Otitis

			Allergy		Acute Otitis	
	N†	Age Years Median	+ (N = 17)	− (N = 80)	+ (N = 54)	− (N = 43)
			Percentage		Percentage	
+ IgA cleavage	18	3.5 (2.6–5.1)*	64.7	8.8	18.5	18.6
IgA intact	79	4.8 (4.1–5.7)	35.3	91.2	81.5	81.4

*Interquartile range.
†N = number of patients.

DISCUSSION

Evaluation of the local IgA-immune response in secretions from children demands clarification of both the sIgA and IgA levels, owing to the substantial deviation found in the secretions (TABLE 1). Also, possible IgA cleavage products in the individual secretions must be demonstrated.

The high prevalence of IgA cleavage products in secretions from allergic children gives rise to the following hypotheses: (1) high percentages of IgA protease-producing bacteria in the nasopharyngeal flora; (2) the ratio of IgA_1 to IgA_2 is displaced, favoring the presence of IgA_1, the known substrate for IgA proteases; and (3) a decreased production of neutralizing antibodies to bacterial IgA proteases.

In theory, cleavage of $sIgA_1$ by IgA proteases would not influence the results obtained with the ELISA sandwich technique. Nevertheless, incubation of NPS and sIgA with IgA proteases caused a reduction in the sIgA content. Possible explanation would be liberation of SC from part of the dimeric Fc_α fragments.

REFERENCES

1. BLAKE, M., K. K. HOLMES & J. SWANSON. 1979. J. Infect. Dis. **139:** 89.
2. MEHTA, S. K., A. G. PLAUT, N. J. CALVANICO & T. B. TOMASI, JR. 1973. J. Immunol. **111:** 1274.
3. SØRENSEN, C. H. 1982. Scand. J. Clin. Lab. Invest. **42:** 577.

IDENTIFICATION OF A NONADHERENT ACCESSORY
CELL IN MURINE PEYER'S PATCHES

D. M. Spalding, W. J. Koopman, and J. R. McGhee

University of Alabama in Birmingham
Birmingham, Alabama 35294

Peyer's patches (PP) have been considered functionally incompetent because specific antibody-producing plasma cells are not identifiable in PP after oral or parenteral immunization, and *in vitro* models have demonstrated that PP are incapable of mounting specific antibody responses. An explanation forwarded for this functional inadequacy of PP has been a deficiency of functional accessory cells (AC) in Peyer's patches. It has recently been demonstrated, however, that PP cells obtained by enzymatic dissociation (with Dispase) are fully capable of *in vitro* mitogenesis, polyclonally activated immunoglobulin production, and primary *in vitro* antibody responses. These studies have indicated that PP possess functional AC. We have begun to characterize the AC population of PP and contrast it with the AC population of spleen (Sp).

We have used oxidative mitogenesis (using sodium periodate) as an assay for accessory-cell activity. This assay has previously been demonstrated to require accessory cells, and dendritic cells are known to be the most potent stimulating population in the spleen. In our oxidative mitogenesis assay, irradiated (1500 R) stimulator populations to be assessed are cocultured with periodate-modified Sp T-cells (obtained by nylon wool purification), and pulsed with tritiated thymidine (^{3}HTdR) at 24 hours. Cultures are harvested 24 hours later, and ^{3}HTdR incorporation is assessed. Using this assay, enzymatic (Dispase) dissociation of PP releases a cell population with at least 5- to 7-fold more AC activity than obtained with conventional (mechanical) dissociation. By contrast, an insignificant increase in accessory-cell activity is seen when Sp is enzymatically dissociated. Four murine strains (CD1, CBA/J, BALB/c, and C3H/HeN) show comparable results, and in these strains PP AC activity approaches spleen on a per cell basis. Artifactual alterations of PP populations by enzyme treatment have been eliminated as the source of increased accessory-cell activity. Experiments have been performed with total, adherent, and nonadherent populations as stimulators and reveal that AC activity released from PP is attributable to a radioresistant cell that resides predominantly (>75%) in the nonadherent fraction, whereas in Sp >85% of the activity is present in the initially adherent fraction. Persistently adherent Fc receptor-bearing cells (macrophages) have been isolated from Sp and PP and are inactive as stimulator cells in this assay. Accessory-cell activity of PP is enriched in the cell pellicle obtained from flotation on dense bovine serum albumin columns (p = 1.078). The activity, again resides in the nonadherent fraction. Experiments using C3H/HeN (H-2^k) mice have demonstrated that the AC activity of PP is due to an Ia-bearing cell, as cytotoxicity with anti-Ia^k and rabbit complement abolishes AC activity of PP populations. Thus PP contains abundant accessory-cell activity in a cell population that is radioresistant, predominantly nonadherent, low density, Ia bearing, and lacking Fc receptors. These characteristics suggest a relationship with the Sp dendritic cell (described by Steinman and Cohn), but the appearance only after enzymatic dissociation and the lack of adherence are distinctive physical properties that suggest differences in cell lineage or developmental stage. Characterization of the PP AC cell with anti-33D1 (kindly provided by R. Steinman, Rockefeller University) is currently in progress. Differences in the immunologic functions of Sp and PP may be, in part, related to differences in accessory-cell types present in the organs.

ESTRADIOL REGULATION OF SECRETORY
COMPONENT IN THE RAT UTERUS*

David A. Sullivan‡ and Charles R. Wira†

*Department of Physiology
Dartmouth Medical School
Hanover, New Hampshire 03755*

Estradiol increases significantly the levels of IgA in rat uterine secretions.[1,2] Recently, we found that this response involves strictly polymeric IgA, which accumulates against an apparent tissue to lumen concentration gradient.[3] These results suggest that estrogen action may be mediated through effects on secretory component (SC), because at other mucosal sites, SC controls the movement of polymeric IgA into external secretions.[4] The purpose of the present study was to confirm quantitatively, and extend our previous qualitative finding,[5] that hormones regulate SC in the uterus.

Uterine luminal secretions were obtained from either intact Sprague-Dawley rats (150–200 g) during the estrous cycle or hormonally treated, ovariectomized rats, as previously described.[6] Ovariectomies were performed 7–10 days prior to experimentation. Uterine tissue cultures were established after three days of estradiol or saline injections to ovariectomized rats. Free SC and IgA levels in uterine secretions and culture media were measured by radioimmunoassay.[5,7,8]

As shown in FIGURE 1, SC levels in uterine secretions were highest at the proestrous and lowest at the diestrous stages of the estrous cycle. Secretory component content remained partially elevated during estrous. These variations in SC levels were paralleled by those of IgA and were most likely due to estrogen influence, because serum estrogen concentrations are maximal at proestrous.[9] This hypothesis is supported by our finding that estradiol, but not progesterone, treatment significantly increased SC levels in uterine lumina of ovariectomized rats (TABLE 1). In other studies, we have observed that the estradiol effect on uterine SC is both dose- and time-dependent. The time-course experiments, that demonstrated that luminal SC content was highest after three daily injections of estradiol to ovariectomized rats, also showed that increases in IgA levels occurred concomitantly with those of secretory component. Both SC and IgA responses were antagonized when rats received progesterone prior to estradiol.

To determine whether estrogen stimulation of uterine SC content could be observed *in vitro*, individual uterine horns from rats administered estradiol *in vivo* were incubated in culture media. As demonstrated in FIGURE 2, incubation media containing uteri from estradiol-treated rats had significantly greater concentrations of SC than those of control uteri. In addition, the presence of cycloheximide in the culture significantly decreased the effect of estradiol on SC accumulation.

These results indicate that estradiol regulates SC levels in the rat uterus. Moreover, given the close correlation between uterine SC and IgA accumulation

*This work was supported by Research Grant AI 13541 from the National Institutes of Health.

†To whom requests for reprints should be addressed.

‡Present address: Eye Research Institute of Retina Foundation, 20 Staniford Street, Boston, Mass. 02114.

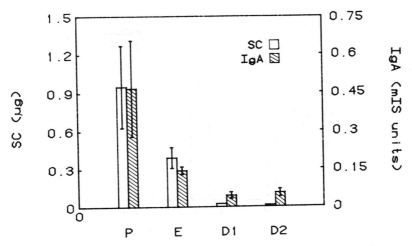

FIGURE 1. Secretory component and IgA levels in uterine secretions during the estrous cycle. Secretions were obtained from intact rats following two consecutive four-day cycles at proestrus (P; 6), estrus (E; 7), diestrus, day one (D1; 6), and diestrus, day two (D2; 6). Both SC and IgA contents at proestrus were significantly (p < 0.05) greater than those at estrus, which, in turn, were significantly (p < 0.001) higher than levels at both stages of diestrus. Measurements of IgA are reported in IS (immunocytoma serum) units, which equal the IgA content in one mg of lyophilized IR 22 immunocytoma serum after reconstitution to one ml.

during the estrous cycle and following hormone treatment, our findings suggest that IgA movement from tissue to lumen is mediated through estrogen control of secretory component. This hypothesis is consistent with our previous observation that IgA in uterine secretions is bound to secretory component.[5] Because cycloheximide decreased the effect of estradiol on uterine SC *in vitro*, these studies further suggest that estrogens may regulate the synthesis of secretory component.

ACKNOWLEDGMENTS

We wish to thank Dr. B. Underdown (University of Toronto, Canada) for his gift of rat SC and rabbit anti-rat SC and Dr. H. Bazin (University of Louvain,

TABLE 1

EFFECT OF STEROID HORMONES ON SECRETORY COMPONENT LEVELS IN UTERINE SECRETIONS OF OVARIECTOMIZED RATS

Treatment	Dose	Secretory Component (μg)
Saline	0.9%	0.042 ± 0.024
Estradiol	2 μg	7.95 ± 2.81*
Progesterone	2 mg	0.004 ± 0.001

*Significantly (p < 0.05) greater than control. Each value represents the mean ± S.E. of five samples.

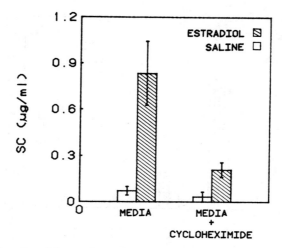

FIGURE 2. Effect of cycloheximide on the accumulation of SC in culture media of uteri incubated *in vitro*. Uterine horns were obtained from rats treated with either estradiol (one μg/day for three days) or saline. Prior to incubation, uterine vasculature was perfused with 0.9% saline to remove residual blood, as previously described.[6] Uteri (three to five per group) were placed in two mls of media (RPMI 1640, 10% fetal calf serum, and gentamycin) and incubated for 20.5 hours at 37° C under an atmosphere of 95% O_2–5% CO_2. Secretory component accumulation in media from uteri of estradiol-treated rats was significantly ($p < 0.05$) greater than in control media. The presence of cycloheximide (100 μg/ml) significantly ($p < 0.01$) reduced the estradiol effect on secretory component.

Belgium) for his contribution of IR 22 immunocytoma serum and goat anti-rat IgA.

REFERENCES

1. WIRA, C. R. & C. P. SANDOE. 1977. Sex steroid hormone regulation of IgA and IgG in rat uterine secretions. Nature (London) **268:** 534–536.
2. WIRA, C. R., D. A. SULLIVAN & C. P. SANDOE. 1983. Estrogen-mediated control of the secretory immune system in the uterus of the rat. Ann. N.Y. Acad. Sci. **409:** This volume.
3. SULLIVAN, D. A. & C. R. WIRA. 1983. Mechanisms involved in the hormonal regulation of immunoglobulins in the rat uterus. Uterine immunoglobulin response to multiple estradiol treatments. Submitted to Endocrinology.
4. BIENENSTOCK, J. & A. D. BEFUS. 1980. Mucosal immunology. Immunology **41:** 249–270.
5. SULLIVAN, D. A. & C. R. WIRA. 1981. Estradiol regulation of secretory component in the female reproductive tract. J. Steroid Biochem. **15:** 439–444.
6. WIRA, C. R. & C. P. SANDOE. 1980. Hormonal regulation of immunoglobulins: Influence of estradiol on immunoglobulins A and G in the rat uterus. Endocrinology **106:** 1020–1026.
7. SULLIVAN, D. A. & C. R. WIRA. 1983. Mechanisms involved in the hormonal regulation of immunoglobulins in the rate uterus: Uterine immunoglobulin response to a single estradiol treatment. Endocrinology **112:** 260–268.
8. SULLIVAN, D. A. & C. R. WIRA. Unpublished information.
9. NEQUIN, L. G., J. ALVAREZ & N. B. SCHWARTZ. 1979. Measurement of serum steroid and gonadotropin levels and uterine and ovarian variables throughout 4 day and 5 day estrous cycles in the rat. Biol. Reprod. **20:** 659–670.

EXPRESSION OF IMMUNOGLOBULIN ISOTYPES BY LYMPHOID CELLS ISOLATED FROM THE LAMINA PROPRIA OF MOUSE SMALL INTESTINE

Jeenan Tseng

Department of Experimental Pathology
Division of Pathology
Walter Reed Army Institute of Research
Washington, D. C. 20307

A striking feature of the gut lamina propria (GLP) is the preponderant presence of plasma cells of the immunoglobulin A (IgA) class. This feature has been known for many years, yet the cellular mechanism is still unknown. A straightforward way of investigation is to isolate lymphoid cells from the GLP and study their characteristics and functions. We isolated GLP lymphoid cells from the small intestine of mice by stripping the epithelium with dithiothreitol and ethylenediamine tetraacetate, dispersing the lymphoid cells by collagenase digestion, and purifying cells by Ficoll-Metrizoate gradient centrifugation. Our lymphoid-cell preparations (viability > 95%) contained approximately 22% Ig-containing (cIg) cells, 18% B-cells, 41% T-cells, 10% myeloid cells, and less than 5% epithelial cells. The cell preparation appears to represent the lymphoid and myeloid constituents residing in the gut lamina propria.

The cIg cells were mainly (96%) cells containing IgA (cIgA cells), with most (3.7%) of the remaining being IgM- and IgG_2-containing cells (cIgM and $cIgG_2$ cells, respectively). Most (80%) cIgA cells possessed only IgA on the membrane; IgM-, IgD-, or IgG_2-bearing cIgA cells were not seen. The $cIgG_2$ cells did not bear any membrane Ig, whereas most (80%) cIgM possessed only IgM on the surface. The cIgA cells had different nuclear to cytoplasmic ratios, suggesting that they are at different stages of differentiation.

The GLP B-cells were characterized by a predominant presence of IgM-bearing cells that included cells bearing only IgM (mIgM cells) and cells bearing IgM and IgD (mIgM-mIgD cells); cells bearing only IgA (mIgA cells) were present in large numbers. Essentially, B-cells bearing only IgD, IgG_2, or two isotypes of IgA and IgD, and IgM and IgA were not present, although these cells were minorities in mesenteric lymph nodes. In mesenteric lymph nodes, mIgM-mIgD cells were the majority (74%); in GLP, however, these cells were less common (40%). Strikingly, cells bearing C3 receptors were scarce in the gut lamina propria. The GLP B-cells lost their membrane Igs rapidly when cultured. This loss was apparently not due to the isolation procedure, cell death, the effect of contaminated epithelial cells, or the presence of a certain cell type in the GLP, because splenic cells isolated by the same procedure did not show any correlation with the disappearance of membrane Ig. Viability of the GLP cell cultures, and mixed cultures of epithelial (or GLP) cells and splenic cells did not show any similar correlation. Because GLP B-cells were mainly mIgM cells, easily made tolerable, it appears that a tolerance induction against environmental antigens may be actively occurring in the gut lamina propria. In culture, GLP B-cells were best stimulated by concanavalin A (Con A), and Con A plus lipopolysaccharide to further divide and generate cIgA and cIgM, but not $cIgG_2$, cells. Interestingly, all the cIgA cells induced were nondividing cells, whereas some of the cIgM cells induced were dividing cells.

A large portion of GLP T-cells, although detectable by the cytotoxicity test, seems to possess very small amounts of Thy-1 antigen on the membrane, as a relatively small portion of the T-cells could be stained with fluorescent anti-Thy-1 reagent. Gut lamina propria T-cells, however, consisted of both helper and suppressor cells, as was revealed by the generation of cIgM and cIgA cells in lymphoid-cell cultures stimulated with Con A plus lipopolysaccharide. Under mitogen stimulations in culture, when GLP T-cells were titrated against B-cells of spleen and Peyer's patches, no profound expression of IgA nor suppression of IgM and IgG_2 was seen. Taken together, all these results suggest that GLP B-cells have several distinct characteristics and T-cells specific for IgA expression may not preferentially reside in the gut lamina propria.

IMPAIRMENT OF SECONDARY
MEMORY B-LYMPHOCYTES
BY ORAL IMMUNIZATION OF AGING MICE*

Andrew W. Wade and Myron R. Szewczuk†

Department of Microbiology and Immunology
Queen's University
Kingston, Ontario, Canada K7L 3N6

It has been previously shown that mucosal lymphoid tissue differs from that of the systemic immune system in its lack of an age-associated decline in primary immune responsiveness. It was of interest to determine whether this effect could be observed in various lymphoid tissues of aged mice upon secondary antigenic stimulation.

Male C57BL/6J mice were immunized with trinitrophenylated (TNP) bovine gamma globulin either in soluble form or in complete Freund's adjuvant, presented either intraperitoneally (i.p.) or intragastrically (i.g.). Three weeks later the mice were boosted either i.p. or i.g., and the anti-TNP plaque-forming cells were assayed seven days later. Kinetic studies revealed peak secondary responses seven days after boosting in the spleen, mediastinal (BLN) and mesenteric lymph nodes (MLN).

When mice were initially presented with antigen i.p., no age-related decline in secondary immune responsiveness was observed in the three tissues, whether the animals were challenged i.p. or i.g. A consistent fourfold reduction in anti-TNP plaque-forming cells was seen when the animals were boosted i.g. as opposed to those boosted i.p. In both cases, peak splenic secondary responses were observed at eight months of age, whereas the mucosal-associated response (MLN and BLN) peaked at 20 months.

By contrast, when mice were initially primed with antigen i.g., there was both an age-related decline in immune responsiveness in all three tissues and a reduction of anti-TNP plaque numbers below that seen following primary stimulation. This effect was observed in these animals regardless of whether they were boosted i.p. or i.g.

The data lend further support for the hypothesis that the mucosal immune system is distinct from that of the systemic system. The findings in the present study suggest that there is an impairment of secondary memory B-lymphocytes following oral immunization.

*This work was supported in part by Medical Research Council of Canada Grant Ma-7347, and the Gerontology Research Council of Ontario.
†Gerontology Research Council of Ontario Scholar.

IMMUNE REGULATION OF SUPPRESSION IN OFFSPRING OF ORALLY TOLERIZED MICE*

Michael J. Wannemuehler, Suzanne M. Michalek, and
Jerry R. McGhee

Department of Microbiology
The University of Alabama in Birmingham
Birmingham, Alabama 35294

The ability to induce oral tolerance in sheep erythrocytes (SRBC) by gastric intubation (GI) of mice has been extensively studied in this laboratory.[1] Mice given SRBC for prolonged periods (14–60 days) by GI were shown to develop systemic unresponsiveness to the antigen. This effect was demonstrated in the spleen and Peyer's patches of GI mice. The mechanism entailed in the development of suppression was shown to be a T-suppressor cell that originated in the Peyer's patches. This proposal would be consistent with the current theory of the secretory immune system and the ability of cells to migrate to distant lymphoid tissue.[2] To investigate this hypothesis further, we gave female C3H/HeN mice SRBC by GI, and we examined the splenic plaque-forming cell (PFC) response in the offspring (four to six weeks old).

Previous studies by Auerbach and Clark[3] demonstrated that the parenteral injection of a soluble antigen into female mice could result in tolerance in offspring. This phenomenon was attributed to the transfer of antigen-antibody complexes or a tolerogenic form of the antigen alone. More recently, Peri and Rothberg[4] have demonstrated transfer of suppression from rabbit dams to their kits by feeding bovine serum albumin. Their results, however, indicated that parenteral administration of the antigen did not induce the tolerant state in the young rabbits. To extend these findings and incorporate the model of oral tolerance developed in this laboratory,[1] we fed female mice a 50% SRBC suspension and determined the anti-SRBC response in resultant litters.

Offspring from mice given SRBC for 14 or more consecutive days demonstrated a suppressed splenic response to intraperitoneally administered SRBC (TABLE 1). Furthermore, it was shown that mice borne by untreated females but nursed on orally tolerized females were also suppressed (TABLE 1). Subsequent experiments demonstrated that newborn pups allowed to nurse on a tolerized female for only 48 hours showed splenic suppression ranging from 20–70 percent. In vitro data also demonstrated that splenic cultures from offspring of GI females were also suppressed in their anti-SRBC response. The anti-SRBC PFC response of tolerant pups began to reappear at about eight to nine weeks of age. The tolerance appeared to be passively transferred by way of the milk (TABLE 1) as demonstrated by the suppression of mice borne by an untreated female and subsequently nursed by a SRBC-tolerant female. Currently, experiments are underway to determine whether the suppression is the result of antibody, antibody-antigen complex, T-suppressor cells, or suppressor factors.

*This work was supported by United States Public Health Service Grants AI 07051, DE 04217, CA 13148, and DE 02670.

TABLE 1

ANTI-SRBC RESPONSE IN OFFSPRING NURSED BY C3H/HEN MICE GIVEN SRBC BY
GASTRIC INTUBATION

Group*	Number of Mice	Anti-SRBC PFC/10^7 Spleen Cells
Born and nursed by GI female	16	150 ± 40
Born by GI female and nursed by an untreated female	15	730 ± 150
Born by an untreated female and nursed by a GI female	9	210 ± 40
Control	9	1,660 ± 290

*Mice were four to six weeks of age at the time of the assay.

REFERENCES

1. MICHALEK, S. M., H. KIYONO, M. J. WANNEMUEHLER, L. M. MOSTELLER & J. R. MCGHEE. 1982. J. Immunol. **128:** 1992.
2. MCDERMOTT, M. R. & J. BIENENSTOCK. 1979. J. Immunol. **122:** 1892.
3. AUERBACH, R. & S. CLARK. 1975. Science **189:** 811.
4. PERI, B. & R. M. ROTHBERG. 1981. J. Immunol. **127:** 2520.

IgA-ANTIBODY RESPONSE TO VASECTOMY*

Steven S. Witkin, Jon M. Richards, J. Michael Bedford, and
Gerald Zelikovsky†

Department of Obstetrics and Gynecology
Cornell University Medical College
New York, New York 10021
†Department of Urology
New York University Medical Center
New York, New York 10016

The findings of sperm antibodies in fluids collected from the epididymis during vasovasotomy[1] suggest that a local-antibody response may occur within the male reproductive tract. To examine the IgA response to vasectomy, we analyzed sera from 35 men obtained prior to vasectomy and at timed intervals after vasectomy. Using each man's prevasectomy serum as a control, 15%, 18%, and 28% of the men exhibited at least a 50% increase in IgA that was reactive with human spermatozoa by two weeks, two months, or four months postvasectomy, respectively. Detection was by an enzyme-linked immunosorbent assay (ELISA).[2] Comparable results were obtained when measuring IgA reactivity to seminal fluid. During this same time interval, 7% of the men developed an IgG-antibody response to spermatozoa. Of the 11 sera positive for IgA-sperm antibody during the four months following vasectomy, only one was also positive for IgG-sperm antibody; none of the 14 samples positive for IgA-seminal fluid antibody were positive for sperm antibody. It appeared that men with an IgA response to vasectomy did not have an IgG response; the converse was also true. Using an ELISA for sperm-related antigen in serum,[3] it was also determined that of the 15 men who were sera positive in this assay, 14 were negative for IgA antibody to seminal fluid. Similarly, only 2 of the 15 sera with IgA antibody to seminal fluid had circulating immune complexes as detected by a Raji cell ELISA;[3] 11 sera without IgA-seminal fluid antibody were positive for circulating immune complexes. The IgA antibody to seminal fluid in sera of vasectomized men was shown to be 11S by sucrose gradient centrifugation and to be unreactive with seminal fluids from vasectomized men. This finding is consistent with the possibility that the IgA antibody is secretory IgA and is reactive with an antigen produced proximally to the point of ligation in vasectomy. To determine whether the epididymis might be a site of male genital-tract IgA production, the relative amounts of IgG and IgA in epididymal fluids obtained from five rabbits were determined by ELISA. The ratio of IgG:IgA was 0.84 ± 0.12. In marked contrast the IgG:IgA ratio in rabbit serum was 12.2. This fact is consistent with our hypothesis that IgA was being produced within the epididymis.

These data lead us to propose that the stimulation of a vigorous local IgA response to intraepididymal antigens following vasectomy in some men limits the release of these antigens into the circulation and consequently greatly lowers the incidence of IgG-sperm antibodies and sperm-related circulating immune complexes[3] in these individuals.

*This work was supported by National Institutes of Health Grants HD-16587 and HD-16586.

890

REFERENCES

1. LINNET, L. & P. FOGH-ANDERSON. 1979. J. Clin. Lab. Immunol. **2:** 245–248.
2. WITKIN, S. S., G. ZELIKOVSKY, R. A. GOOD & N. K. DAY. 1981. Clin. Exp. Immunol. **44:** 368–374.
3. WITKIN, S. S., G. ZELIKOVSKY, A. M. BONGIOVANNI, N. GELLER, R. A. GOOD & N. K. DAY. 1982. J. Clin. Invest. **70:** 33–40.

Index of Contributors

(Italic page numbers refer to comments made in discussion.)